Health Opportunities Through Physical Education

Health Opportunities Through Physical Education

Charles B. Corbin
Arizona State University

Karen E. McConnell
Pacific Lutheran University

Guy C. Le Masurier
Vancouver Island University

David E. Corbin
University of Nebraska Omaha

Terri D. Farrar
Pacific Lutheran University

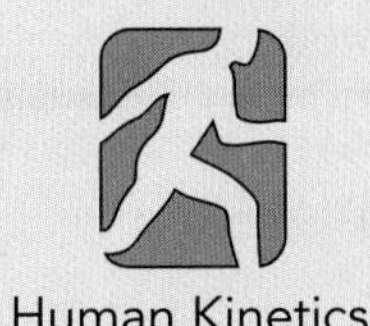

Human Kinetics

Library of Congress Cataloging-in-Publication Data has been applied for.

ISBN: 978-1-4504-9741-1 (print)

The web addresses cited in this text were current as of October 28, 2013, unless otherwise noted.

Acquisitions Editors: Ray Vallese and Scott Wikgren; **Developmental Editors:** Melissa Feld and Ray Vallese; **Managing Editors:** Derek Campbell and Rachel Fowler; **Copyeditor:** Tom Tiller; **Indexer:** Nancy Ball; **Permissions Manager:** Dalene Reeder; **Graphic Designer:** Nancy Rasmus; **Graphic Artists:** Denise Lowry and Nancy Rasmus; **Cover Designer:** Keith Blomberg; **Photographs (front and back covers and part openers):** PhotoDisc, © Human Kinetics, Stephen Coburn, Monkey Business, Michael Svoboda; **Photographs (interior):** © Human Kinetics, unless otherwise noted; **Photographs in Illustrations:** Upper left photo in figure 24.2 and photo on right in figure 30.2: PhotoDisc/Barbara Penoyar; lower right photo in figure 24.2 and photo on left in figure 30.2: PhotoDisc/Kevin Peterson; first and second photos in figure 29.1: Photodisc; third photo in figure 29.1: © Shannon Fagan | Dreamstime.com; fourth photo in figure 29.1: Photodisc/Getty Images; photo in figure 30.3: Suprijono Suharjoto/fotolia.com; photo on right in figure 30.4: iStockphoto/Eduardo Jose Bernardino; photo on right in figure 30.5: Monkey Business/fotolia.com; photo on right in figure 36.2: PhotoDisc; **Photo Asset Manager:** Laura Fitch; **Visual Production Assistant:** Joyce Brumfield; **Photo Production Manager:** Jason Allen; **Art Manager:** Kelly Hendren; **Associate Art Manager:** Alan L. Wilborn; **Art Style Development:** Joanne Brummett; **Illustrations:** © Human Kinetics, unless otherwise noted; **Printer:** Courier Companies, Inc.

We thank Truly Fit in Urbana, Illinois, for assistance in providing the location for the photo shoot for this book.

Printed in the United States of America 10 9 8 7 6 5 4 3 2 1

The paper in this book was manufactured using responsible forestry methods.

Human Kinetics
Website: www.HumanKinetics.com

United States: Human Kinetics
P.O. Box 5076
Champaign, IL 61825-5076
800-747-4457
e-mail: humank@hkusa.com

Canada: Human Kinetics
475 Devonshire Road Unit 100
Windsor, ON N8Y 2L5
800-465-7301 (in Canada only)
e-mail: info@hkcanada.com

Europe: Human Kinetics
107 Bradford Road
Stanningley
Leeds LS28 6AT, United Kingdom
+44 (0) 113 255 5665
e-mail: hk@hkeurope.com

Australia: Human Kinetics
57A Price Avenue
Lower Mitcham, South Australia 5062
08 8372 0999
e-mail: info@hkaustralia.com

New Zealand: Human Kinetics
P.O. Box 80
Torrens Park, South Australia 5062
0800 222 062
e-mail: info@hknewzealand.com

E6320

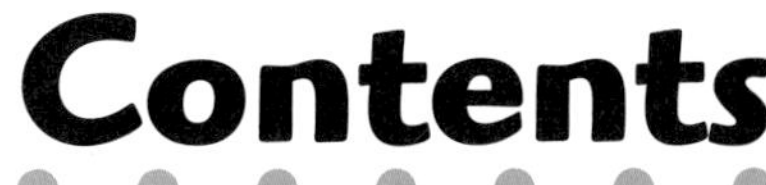

Contents

Introduction

Do you want to be fit, healthy, and well? Do you want to look your best and feel good? *Health Opportunities Through Physical Education* (*HOPE*) is based on the proven HELP philosophy: **h**ealth for **e**veryone for a **l**ifetime in a **p**ersonal way.

H = health

E = everyone

L = lifetime

P = personal

The HELP philosophy allows you to take control of your future fitness, health, and wellness.

HOPE helps you understand and apply concepts and principles of fitness, health, and wellness; understand and use self-management skills (also called skills for healthy living) that promote healthy lifestyles for a lifetime; be an informed consumer and critical user of fitness, health, and wellness information; and adopt a healthy lifestyle now and later in life.

HOPE was created by a team of established authors who are winners of numerous awards for textbook excellence, including several Texty Awards from the Text and Academic Authors Association.

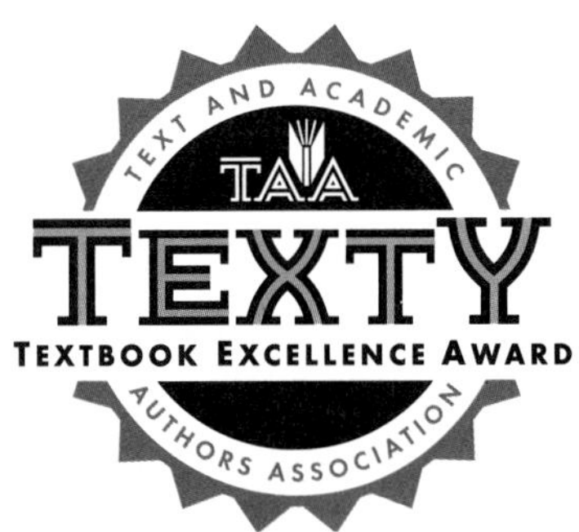

HOPE is divided into two parts. **Part 1, Fitness for Life,** focuses on physical activity, which contributes to lifelong fitness, health, and wellness. Other factors (determinants) that influence fitness, health, and wellness are also highlighted. **Part 2, Health for Life,** focuses more on health and wellness. Each chapter includes two lessons to help you learn key concepts relating to fitness, health, and wellness. As you read through the first several chapters of each part, you will notice that some key concepts presented in part 1 are also covered in part 2. There are several reasons for this repetition. First, the information is presented as a review in part 2 to help you remember important ideas presented early in part 1. Second, the information provides you with a foundation for learning concepts presented in the later chapters of part 2. In some schools, material from this book is presented in reverse order—that is, part 2 is taught before part 1. Presenting key concepts in the early chapters of both parts of this book ensures that you have the basic information for learning key concepts, regardless of the order in which the material is presented.

Take the guided tour on page 3 to learn about all of the features of part 1 of this textbook. You will take a similar tour at the beginning of part 2 (page 423). As mentioned previously, there are many similar features in part 1 and part 2. However, some features that focus on fitness and physical activity (part 1) have slightly different names than those that focus on health and wellness (part 2). The table at the end of this introduction provides you with information about the differing features in both parts of the book.

In addition to the textbook features, *HOPE* includes several other components:

- **Student web resource:** You have access to a variety of resources at www.HOPEtextbook.org/student. These resources aid your understanding of the textbook content. You'll find worksheets, interactive review questions, vocabulary pop-ups, and expanded discussions of topics that are marked by web icons throughout this book. Video clips also demonstrate how to do self-assessments and other exercises in part 1.
- **Teacher web resource:** Your teacher has access to a special web resource with lessons and activities that you can do to enhance your understanding of the information in this textbook.

Now read on, and enjoy *HOPE*!

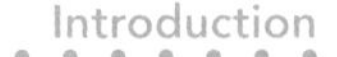

FEATURES IN *Health Opportunities Through Physical Education*

Part 1	Part 2	Description
2020 Health Goals	2020 Health Goals	Health goals for the nation for the year 2020 are described in both parts of the book.
Self-Assessment	Self-Assessment	This feature includes tools to help you evaluate your own fitness, health, and wellness. It is included in both parts of the book.
Taking Charge	Making Healthy Decisions	Both features help you take charge of fitness, health, and wellness decisions.
Self-Management	Skills for Healthy Living	Self-management skills and healthy living skills are similar skills that help you adopt healthy lifestyles and make good decisions.
Taking Action	Living Well News	Taking Action gets you active, and Living Well News (part 2) provides current health information.
Fit Fact	No equivalent in part 2	This feature communicates important facts. There is no equivalent in part 2.
No equivalent in part 1	Healthy Communication	This feature encourages you to use and expand interpersonal communication skills while sharing your views about various health topics.
Fitness Technology	Health Technology	Both features emphasize technology; fitness is emphasized in part 1 and health in part 2.
Science in Action	Health Science	These features provide scientific information relevant to the two parts of the book.
Consumer Corner	Consumer Corner	Both features help you become an informed consumer.
Lesson Review	Comprehension Check	Both features help you review information in the lessons.
Chapter Review	Chapter Review	This feature helps you review your knowledge and understanding of chapter content.
Academic Connection	Academic Connection	Both features relate concepts from other academic subject areas to fitness, health, and wellness.
No equivalent in part 1	Diverse Perspectives	This feature helps you understand another's point of view. This feature is not in part 1.
No equivalent in part 1	Advocacy in Action	This feature presents personal, school, and community advocacy challenges. This feature is not in part 1.
No equivalent in part 1	Connect	Reflect on family, peer, media, or technology influences related to a specific topic in a chapter. This feature is not in part 1.

PART 1

Fitness for Life

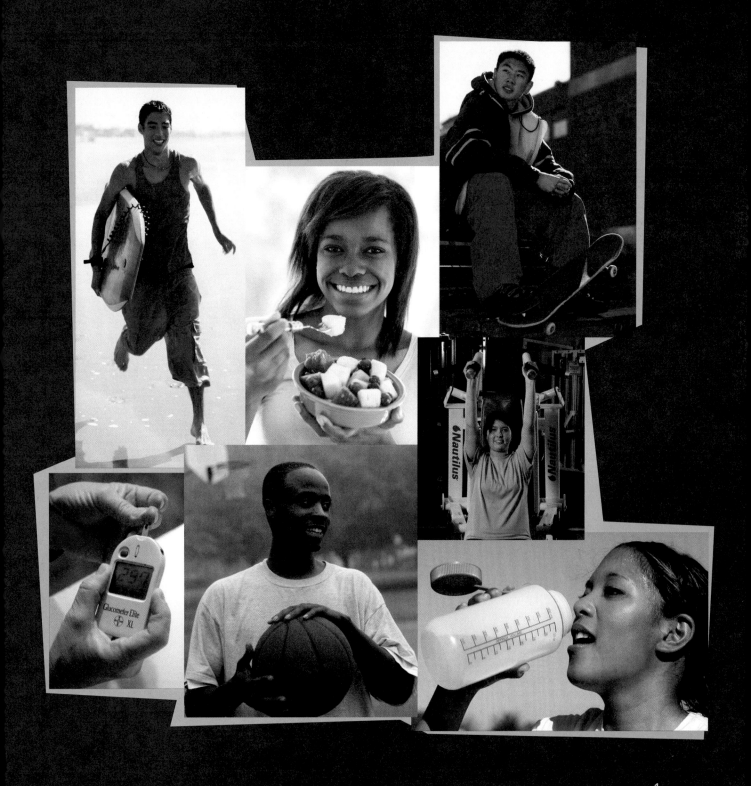

Touring Part 1

Do you want to be healthy and fit? Do you want to look your best and feel good?

Health Opportunities Through Physical Education helps you become a physically literate person so that you can

- understand and apply important concepts and principles of fitness, health, and wellness;
- understand and use self-management skills that promote healthy lifestyles for a lifetime;
- be an informed consumer and critical user of fitness, health, and wellness information; and
- adopt healthy lifestyles now and later in life.

Health Opportunities Through Physical Education will help you meet your fitness and physical activity goals. Take this guided tour to learn about all of the features of part 1. Two lessons are included in each chapter to help you learn key concepts relating to fitness, health, and wellness.

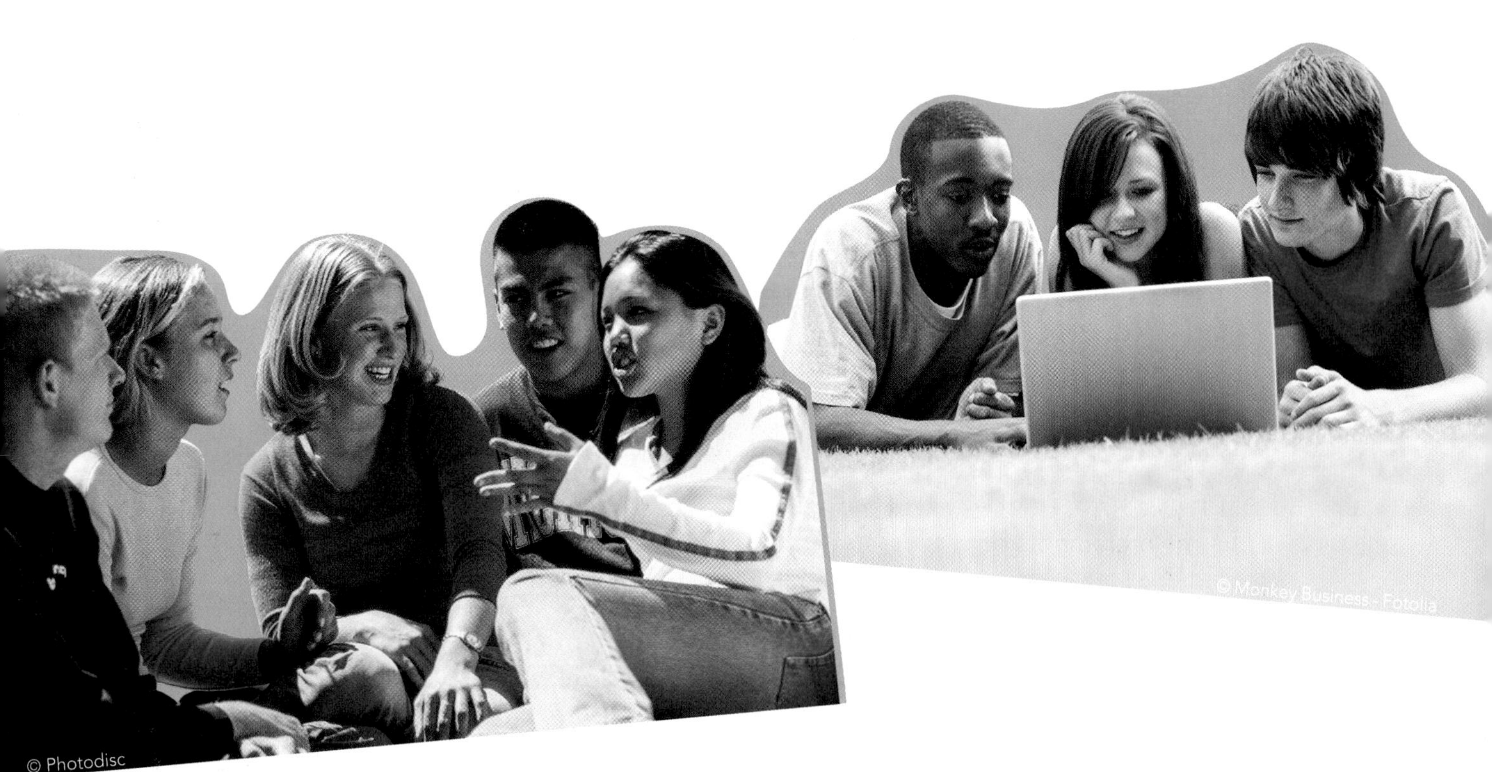
© Photodisc
© Monkey Business - Fotolia

UNIT OPENER: Provides a brief overview of the content in each unit.

HEALTHY PEOPLE 2020 GOALS: Lists national health goals covered in each unit.

FEATURES: Lists the Self-Assessment, Taking Charge, Self-Management, and Taking Action features in each unit.

STUDENT WEB RESOURCES: Provides the web address for finding additional information in each lesson.

UNIT III

Moderate and Vigorous Physical Activity

Healthy People 2020 Goals

- Increase the percentage of teens who meet aerobic activity guidelines.
- Increase overall cardiovascular health.
- Reduce the risk of heart disease and other chronic diseases.
- Increase education to promote health-enhancing behaviors and reduce health risks.
- Reduce the percentage of teens with high blood pressure and other health risks.
- Improve teens' understanding of health promotion and disease prevention.
- Reduce overweight and obesity among teens.
- Reduce sport and recreation injuries.
- Improve community facilities (s… environment (such as sidewalks).
- Increase physical education in
- Increase the percentage of tee
- Improve health literacy and in

Self-Assessment Features in This

- Walking Test
- Step Test and One-Mile Run
- Assessing Jogging Techniqu

Taking Charge Features in This

- Learning to Manage Time
- Self-Confidence
- Activity Participation

Self-Management Features in

- Skills for Managing Time
- Skills for Building Self-Con
- Skills for Choosing Good A

Taking Action Features in Thi

- Your Moderate Physical A
- Target Heart Rate Worko
- Your Vigorous Physical Ac

2

Adopting a Healthy Lifestyle and Self-Management Skills

In This Chapter

LESSON 2.1
Adopting Healthy Lifestyles

SELF-ASSESSMENT
Practicing Physical Fitness Tests

LESSON 2.2
Learning Self-Management Skills

TAKING CHARGE
Building Knowledge and Understanding

SELF-MANAGEMENT
Skills for Building Knowledge and Understanding

TAKING ACTION
Fitness Trails

Student Web Resources
www.HOPEtextbook.org/student

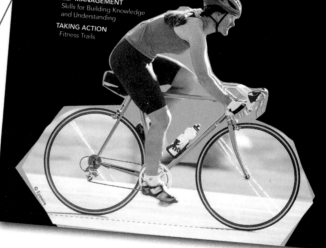

© Eyewire

CHAPTER OPENER: Provides a brief overview of the content of the chapter.

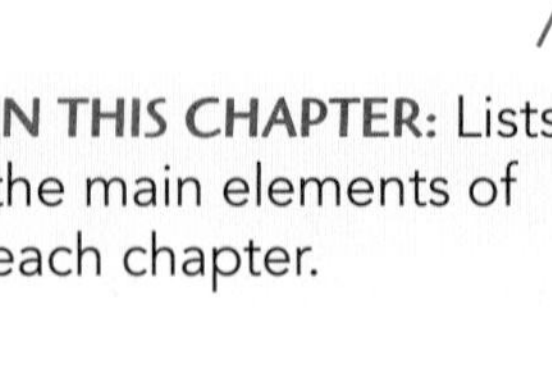

IN THIS CHAPTER: Lists the main elements of each chapter.

LESSON OBJECTIVES: Describes what you will learn in each lesson.

LESSON VOCABULARY: Lists key terms in each lesson, which are defined in the glossary and on the student website.

CONSUMER CORNER: Provides information to help you become a good consumer and avoid quackery.

WEB ICONS: Indicate that additional information is available on the student website.

FIT FACT: Offers interesting information about key topics.

FITNESS TECHNOLOGY: Helps you become aware of new technological information related to fitness, health, and wellness and helps you try out and use new technology.

Lesson 13.2

Energy Balance

Lesson Objectives

After reading this lesson, you should be able to

1. explain how to use the FIT formula for fat control,
2. describe how many calories are expended in doing various physical activities,
3. explain how physical activity helps a person maintain a healthy body fat level, and
4. describe some common myths about fat control.

Lesson Vocabulary

calorie, calorie expenditure, calorie intake, energy ba

Do you know how many **calories** you expend in a typical day? Do you know how many calories you consume in a typical day? One major health goal is to achieve and maintain an acceptable level of body fat throughout your life. To do this, you must balance the calories you consume and the calories you expend. In this lesson, you'll learn the FIT formula for fat control and appropriate activities for gaining weight and losing body fat.

Balancing Calories

The term *calorie* is commonly used to describe the amount of energy in a food. The true term is *kilocalorie* (a unit of energy or heat), but when talking about diet and nutrition, *calorie* is typically use... Energy balance refers to balan... and calorie expen...

FIT FACT

One pound of f... Therefore, you c... kilogram) of fat... fewer than you no... or by burning 3,... normal in physical... provides more calo... will cause you to g... you can gain a poun... calories more than y... given time or by exp... fewer than usual in p... a given time.

CONSUMER CORNER: TV Tactics—Creating Needs

You've now learned about developing a strategy and using tactics to achieve a goal. Companies also develop strategies and tactics. Sometimes their strategies help them but are not good for you. For example, a company's strategy may be to get you to buy something you don't really want or need. To help them carry out their str... companies buy advertising in ... such as television, the ... zines, radio, ... com...

every day. Of course, not all advertisements are deceptive, but many are. It takes a very critical eye to detect the mess... ...ng conveyed in ads and to di... ...good and bad infor...

Lesson 16.2

FITNESS TECHNOLOGY: Motion Analysis Systems

Many technological advances have helped people become more skilled at a variety of sport activities. One of the most noteworthy is the use of motion analysis systems, which can be as simple as a basic video camera and playback system or as complicated as a high-speed video camera and software that helps analyze whether a performer's movements (biomechanics) are efficient and effective. Whether simple or complex, a motion analysis system video-records a person performing a sport or activity. Next, a skill-learning expert, such as a sport pedagogist or coach, views the video and analyzes the performer's movements. For example, football players and coaches routinely review game footage together to look at defensive and offensive formations, as well as opponents' tactics. High-powered systems allow users to analyze the action in very slow motion and generate computer analysis to provide information that helps the performer make corrections. Motion analysis systems can be used for many kinds of activity (such as softball pitching and tennis) but are especially popular among golfers, who use the biomechanical feedback to improve their swings.

Using Technology

Make a video of your performance of a motor skill. Analyze the performance using information you've learned from an instructor or from information gained in the Science in Action student activity.

Movement sequences can be studied to provide feedback for improved performance.

Lesson 6.1

ability that includes both eye–hand coordination (the ability to use your hands and eyes together, as in hitting a ball) and eye–foot coordination (the ability to use your eyes and feet together, as in kicking a ball). You may be good in one area but not as good in another. In addition to working on the areas that need improvement, you should consider selecting activities for your program that match your strengths.

Once you've assessed your skill-related fitness abilities, you can develop a profile of your results to help you select lifetime sports and other activities.

In this lesson, you'll learn both how to do that and how to make plans for becoming proficient in your chosen activities.

Building a Skill-Related Fitness Profile

One student, Sue, did all of the skill-related physical fitness assessments presented in this chapter, then developed a profile for her skill-related fitness

Skill Learning and Injury Prevention 121

EXERCISES: Provide instructions and pictures to teach you correct technique for exercises.

SELF-ASSESSMENT: Helps you learn more about your fitness and behaviors that affect your health and wellness and helps you prepare a personal plan for improvement.

HEEL RAISE

1. Place a board that is 2 inches (5 centimeters) thick on the floor. Stand with the balls of your feet on the board and the handles even with your shoulders.
2. Grasp the handles with your palms facing away from your body. Keep your hands and arms stationary during the lift.
3. Rise onto the balls of your feet, then lower to the starting position.

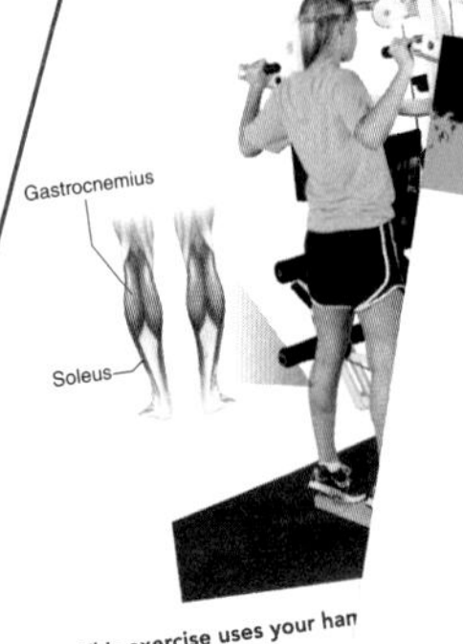

This exercise uses your han

LAT PULL-DOWN

1. Sit on the bench (or floor, depending on the machine). Adjust the seat height so that your arms are fully extended when you grab the bar.
2. Grab the bar with your palms facing away from you. Your arms should be at least shoulder-wid
3. Pull the bar down
4. Return to the star

SELF-ASSESSMENT: Walking Test

Many of the self-assessments you perform in this course require very intense physical activity. If you're a very active person and are quite fit, the mile run or PACER may be the best way to estimate your cardiorespiratory endurance, but the walking test is also a good one. The test is especially good for people who are beginners, who haven't done a lot of recent activity, or who are regular walkers but do not regularly get more vigorous activity. The walk test is also good for older people and for those who cannot do running tests due to joint or muscle problems. As directed by your teacher, record your scores and fitness ratings for the walking test. You can then use the information in preparing your personal physical activity plan. If you're working with a partner, remember that self-assessment information is personal and considered confidential. It shouldn't be shared with others without the permission of the person being tested.

1. Walk a mile at a fast pace

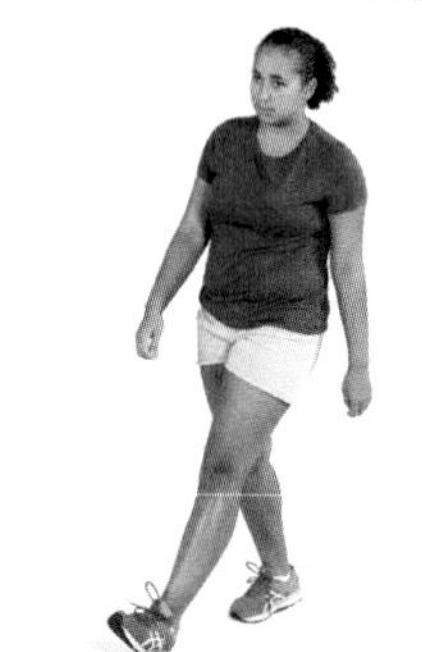

The walking test is a good assessment for beginners ... a lot of vigorous activity.

...priate chart to determine ...ating. Locate your heart ...column of the chart and ...e along the bottom row. ...ere the row and column ...rmine your rating.

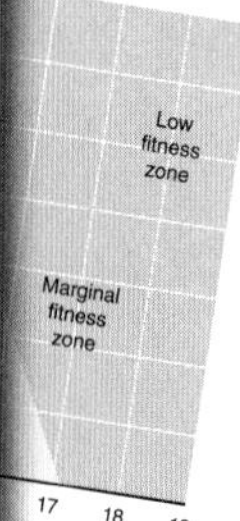

...r males).

...al Activity 151

Lesson 3.1

SCIENCE IN ACTION: Optimal Challenge

Scientists in many fields have collaborated to find ways to help people stay active, eat well, and stick with other healthy lifestyle behaviors. They have discovered that in order to be successful, you must set goals that provide "optimal challenge." The key is giving effort (trying hard). If a challenge is too easy, there's no need to try hard—it's not really a challenge. On the other hand, if a goal is too hard, we fail, which may lead us to give up or quit because our effort seems hopeless (see figure 3.2).

An optimal challenge requires *reasonable* effort. Meeting an optimal challenge provides us with success and makes us want to try again. In fact, providing optimal challenge is one reason that video games are so popular. They challenge you by making the task more difficult as you improve, and this optimal challenge makes you want to play again and again. You can use optimal challenge when setting your own goals to help yourself succeed.

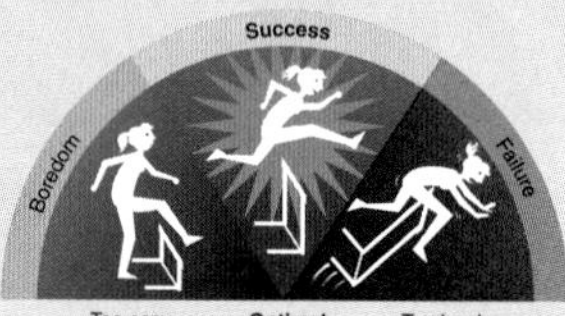

Figure 3.2 Some challenges can lead to boredom or failure, but optimal challenges can lead to success.

Student Activity

Imagine that you want to help a friend learn a skill—for example, hitting a tennis ball or a golf ball. How could you use optimal challenge to help your friend learn the skill?

day (figure 3.1*b*). Process goals make good short-term goals because you can easily monitor your progress and, with effort, succeed. In contrast, *product* goals do not make especially good short-term goals, because they can be discouraging, especially for a person who is just beginning to change. For example, if you chose a product goal of performing, say, 25 push-ups, it might (depending on your current fitness level) take you so long to meet the goal that you would give up. But a short-term process goal—such as performing 5 to 10 push-ups each day for two weeks—would be possible for you to achieve with effort. Thus, as you meet a series of short-term process goals, you work toward meeting long-term product goals.

The Taking Charge and Self-Management features in this chapter focus on setting goals for physical activity and building physical fitness. Elsewhere in the book, you'll get the chance to set long-term goals for fitness, health, and wellness (product goals) and for making healthy lifestyle changes (process goals) that lead to good fitness, health, and wellness. You'll also get the chance to set short-term goals that help you move toward achieving your long-term goals.

> "If you want to live a happy life, tie it to a goal, not to people or things."
>
> —Albert Einstein, Nobel Prize–winning physicist

Lesson Review

1. How does the SMART formula help you set goals?
2. How can you use long-term and short-term goals to plan your program? In your answer, use fitness and physical activity examples.
3. What is the difference between a process goal and a product goal? In your answer, use fitness and physical activity examples.

64

SCIENCE IN ACTION: Helps you understand how new information is generated using the scientific method.

FITNESS QUOTES: Provide quotes from famous people about fitness, health, and wellness.

LESSON REVIEW: Helps you review and remember the information you learned in the lesson.

TAKING CHARGE AND SELF-MANAGEMENT: Provide guidelines for learning self-management skills that help you adopt healthy behaviors.

TAKING CHARGE: Improving Physical Self-Perception

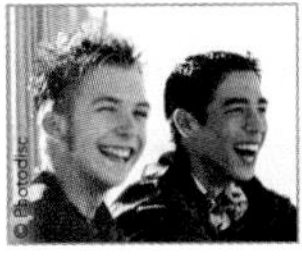

Each person has a mental picture of himself or herself. If you think you do well in a certain activity, you'll probably take part in that type of activity. If you feel embarrassed about your appearance or ability level while doing an activity, you'll probably avoid that activity. Here are two very different examples of physical self-perception.

Michael was not sure that he wanted to go back to school after the summer break. It seemed as if all of his friends had grown taller in the last few months, but he had stayed the same height. Michael felt embarrassed and a little jealous, even though none of his friends seemed to notice. His height certainly did not alter his ability to play tennis. In fact, his friends still called him "King of the Court" because he usually won.

Raul was one of the shortest people in his class, but his height did not stop him from being involved in activities. He realized that he had never been a great basketball player, but he still liked to play with his friends from school. He also discovered that height had nothing to do with his ability to go hiking, nor did it prevent him from being a good wrestler.

For Discussion

Michael had a negative self-perception because of his height. What can he do to change his negative perception? How does Raul keep a positive self-perception? What else can a person do to develop a positive self-perception? Consider the guidelines presented in the Self-Management feature as you answer the discussion questions.

FOR DISCUSSION: Helps you take charge by making good decisions.

SELF-MANAGEMENT: Skills for Self-Perception

A self-perception is an idea you have about your own thoughts, actions, or appearance. It is influenced by how you think other people view you. Some of the many kinds of self-perception are academic, social, and artistic. In part 1 of this book, the focus is on physical self-perceptions—the way you view your physical self.

Four aspects of physical self-perception are strength, fitness, skill, and physical attractiveness. People with good physical self-perceptions are happy with their current strength and fitness levels; they also feel that their skills are adequate to meet their needs, and they like the way they look. We know that people who have positive physical self-perceptions are more likely to be physically active than those who do not. The following list provides guidelines you can use to maintain or improve your physical self-perceptions.

- **Assess your physical self-perceptions.** You may use the worksheet provided by your teacher.
- **Consider your self-assessment results.** Use the self-assessment worksheet to determine whether you have any areas in which your physical self-perceptions are especial[ly lo]w (strength, fitness, skill, or physical
- **Perform r... improve y... tice regul... skills.** Re... you look... can help
- **Consid... yourse...** standa... ing lik... or in t... life th... they... app... cial... You

star has an eating disorder or practices healthy habits. Consider your heredity and set realistic standards for yourself.

- **Think positively.** Almost all people have a physical characteristic that they would like to change. But studies show that the things people don't like about themselves are rarely seen as problems by other people. You're often your own worst critic, and thinking positively can help you present yourself in a positive way.
- **Do not let the actions of a few insensitive people cause you to feel negatively about yourself.** There will always be some people who are insensitive to others' feelings. These people often have low self-perceptions and try to build themselves up by tearing other people down. Recognize that criticism from these people is their problem, not yours.
- **Consider how your behavior and actions influence the way other people view you.** Acting cheerful and friendly has as much to do with how others perceive you as your physical characteristics.
- **Realize that all people have some imperfections.** Try to build on your strengths and improve your areas of weakness.
- **Find a realistic role model and be a role model for others.** Instead of trying to be like someone who is totally unlike you, find someone you admire who has characteristics you can realistically achieve. And, just as you look to others for models, remember that others may look to you as a model. Providing a positive model for others can help you think positively about yourself.

Academic Connection: Quartiles

Various statistics can be used to describe scores for a group of people. The term *quartile* is used to describe the scores for each quarter of a distribution. In the following example, each number represents a score (in inches) on the waist girth test for 36 15-year-old females. The distribution is divided into quartiles (25 percent of scores per quartile, listed in different colors).

A good fitness rating for waist girth for 15-year-old females is 32 inches or less. Which color of quartile includes scores for the good fitness range? What percentage of girls were in the good fitness zone for waist girth? What percentage of girls had scores that did not qualify them to be in the good fitness zone?

Distribution of Waist Girth Scores (Inches) for 15-Year-Old Females

						34									
					33	34	35								
				32	33	34	35	36							
	28		30	32	33	34	35	36	37	38	39	40			
27	28	29	30	32	33	34	35	36	37	38	39	40	41	42	43

Check Your Answers

The red quartile includes scores in the good fitness range, so 25 percent of the girls were in the good fitness zone. That also means that 75 percent, or three quartiles, of the girls were not in the good fitness zone.

ACADEMIC CONNECTION: Relates concepts from other academic subject areas to fitness, health, and wellness.

TAKING ACTION: Lets you try out teacher-directed activities that can help you become fit and active for a lifetime.

CHAPTER REVIEW: Helps you reinforce what you've learned in the chapter's two lessons.

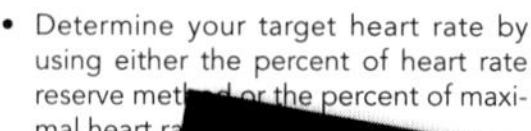

TAKING ACTION: Target Heart Rate Workouts

Cardiorespiratory endurance is important for living a long and healthy life. It's also essential for competing, participating in your favorite physical activities, and maintaining a healthy body weight. As you've learned in this chapter, you must do vigorous physical activity above your threshold of training and in your target zone to build cardiorespiratory endurance. **Take action** by doing vigorous activity that fulfills the FIT formula: at least three days each week (addressing F for frequency in the FIT formula), in your target heart rate zone (addressing I for intensity), and for at least 20 minutes each session (addressing T for time). Consider the following tips as you take action by performing a target heart rate workout.

- Determine your target heart rate by using either the percent of heart rate reserve met[...] or the percent of maximal heart ra[...]
- Before ch[...] consider y[...]
- Before do[...] a 5-minu[...] warm-up.
- Check y[...] ceived e[...] you're r[...] workou[...]
- After y[...] cool-d[...]

Take action by doing a workout that elevates your heart r[...]

[...]ties Through Physical Education

CHAPTER REVIEW

Reviewing Concepts and Vocabulary

As directed by your teacher, answer items 1 through 5 by correctly completing each sentence with a word or phrase.

1. Factors that affect your fitness, health, and wellness are called ________.
2. Factors influencing fitness, health, and wellness over which you have little control are called ________.
3. Factors influencing fitness, health, and wellness over which you have the most control are called ________.
4. The steps that lead you from dependence to independence are referred to together as the ________.
5. The fitness test used to assess cardiorespiratory endurance by running when signaled by a beep is called the ________.

For items 6 through 10, as directed by your teacher, match each term in column 1 with the appropriate phrase in column 2.

6. sedentary person	a. just bought exercise equipment
7. inactive thinker	b. is active most days of the week
8. planner	c. is sometimes active
9. activator	d. is considering becoming active
10. active exerciser	e. is inactive

For items 11 through 15, as directed by your teacher, respond to each statement or question.

11. Explain what a self-management skill is and why it can be useful.
12. What are some of the fitness test items used in major fitness test batteries such as Fitnessgram, and what do they measure?
13. Describe the five stages of change.
14. What are fitness trails, and how can they be useful in staying active?
15. What are some guidelines for building knowledge and understanding?

Thinking Critically

Write a paragraph to answer the following question.

Of all the self-management skills described in lesson 2, which one would most help you be more active or eat better? Give the reasons for your answer.

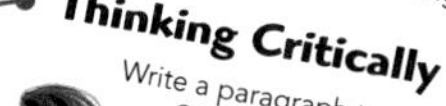

Project

Assume that you are the head of a marketing company assigned to create an ad campaign promoting healthier eating and more active living. Prepare a script for a television commercial for the promotion. If resources are available, create a video of the commercial.

59

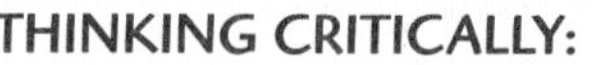

THINKING CRITICALLY: Requires the use of critical-thinking skills to apply chapter information.

PROJECT: Provides an enrichment activity for use outside the classroom.

UNIT I

Building a Foundation

Healthy People 2020 Goals

- Live high-quality, longer lives.
- Reduce preventable disease, injury, and early death.
- Increase awareness and understanding of what determines good health.
- Encourage all people to adopt healthy lifestyles that promote lifetime health, fitness, and wellness.
- Create environments that promote health, fitness, and wellness for all.

Self-Assessment Features in This Unit

- Physical Fitness Challenges
- Practicing Physical Fitness Tests
- Assessing Muscle Fitness

Taking Charge Features in This Unit

- Learning to Self-Assess
- Building Knowledge and Understanding
- Setting Goals

Self-Management Features in This Unit

- Skills for Learning to Self-Assess
- Skills for Building Knowledge and Understanding
- Skills for Setting Goals

Taking Action Features in This Unit

- The Warm-Up
- Fitness Trails
- Exercise Circuits

1

Fitness, Health, and Wellness for All

In This Chapter

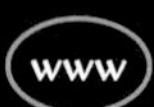

Student Web Resources

www.HOPEtextbook.org/student

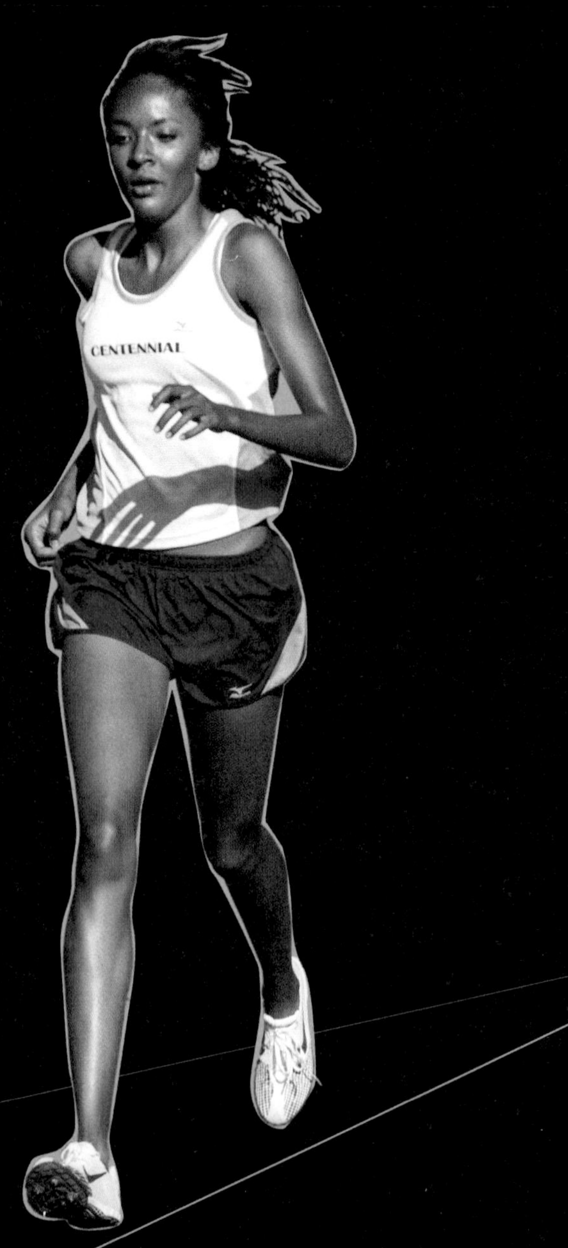

Lesson 1.1

Scientific Foundations

Lesson Objectives

After reading this lesson, you should be able to

1. describe the scientific method;
2. define *health and medical science* and *nutrition science*;
3. define *kinesiology* and list the seven types of science it encompasses; and
4. describe and differentiate the warm-up, the workout, and the cool-down.

Lesson Vocabulary

biomechanics, calisthenics, cool-down, dietitian, dynamic warm-up, exercise anatomy, exercise physiology, exercise psychology, exercise sociology, health and medical science, kinesiology, motor learning, motor skill, nutrition science, sport pedagogy, stretching warm-up, warm-up, workout

Science is the study of knowledge based on observation and experimentation. In school, you study various sciences, such as natural science (focused on nature), social science (focused on individual and social behavior), and mathematics (focused on numbers and their operations). Examples of natural science include biology, chemistry, and physics; examples of social science include psychology, sociology, and geography; and examples of mathematics include algebra, geometry, and calculus.

FIT FACT

Many of the names of sciences end with "-ology," which means "the study of."

The Scientific Method

Scientists of all types use the scientific method to discover new knowledge and establish principles that help us make good decisions and solve problems. A simplified form of the scientific method is presented here. The steps—identifying a problem, establishing a hypothesis, collecting information, and interpreting information—are shown in figure 1.1.

The information presented in part 1 of this book is based on studies that use the scientific method as described in figure 1.1, and each chapter in part 1 includes a special feature called Science in Action. This feature helps you see how research in **health and medical science, kinesiology** (exercise science), and **nutrition science** can help us make good decisions about fitness, health, and wellness.

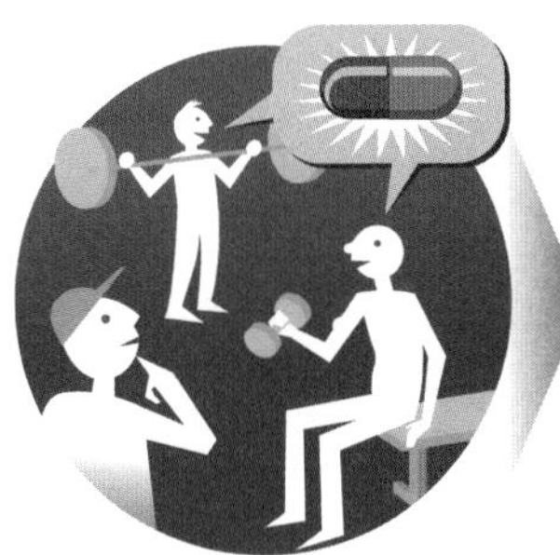

Problem
Friends are considering taking a dietary supplement. Should I take one?

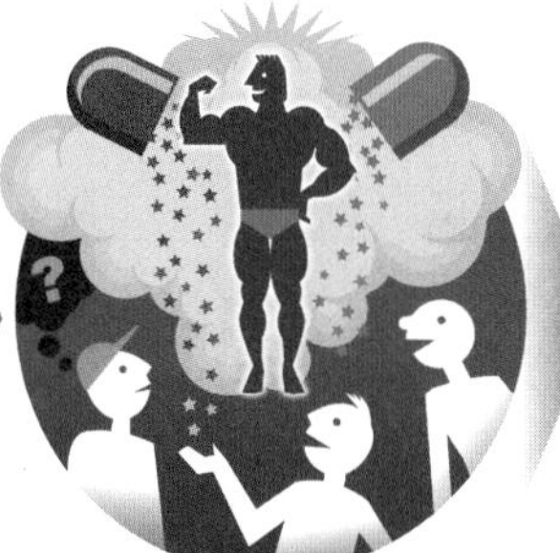

Hypothesis
They think a supplement might help them get fit faster.

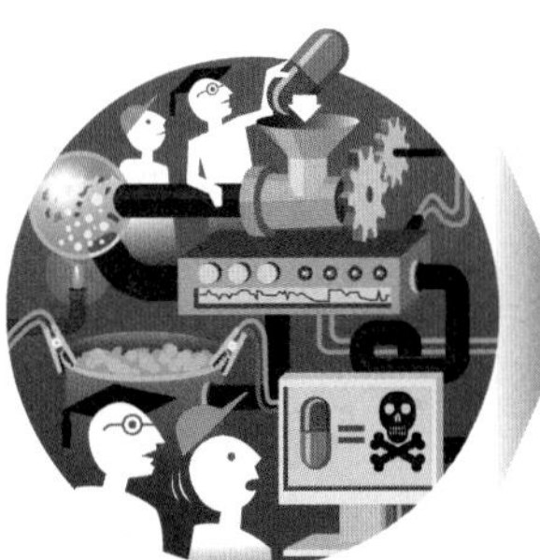

Collect information
Conduct a search for information about benefits and risks associated with the supplement.

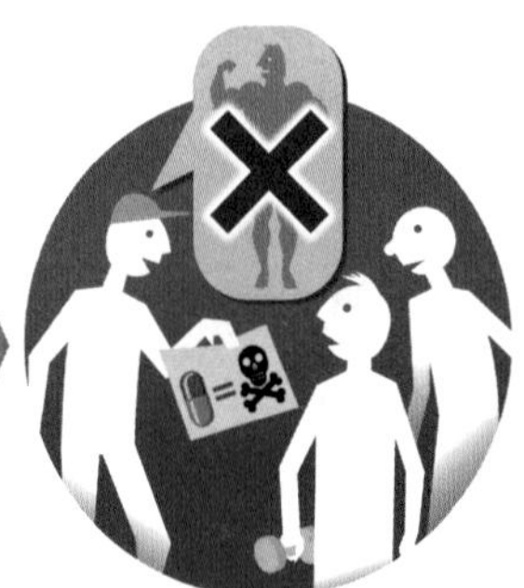

Interpret information
Analysis and conclusion: the risks are greater than the benefits. Don't take the supplement.

FIGURE 1.1 A simplified form of the scientific method.

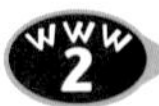

You've probably used the scientific method yourself when conducting experiments in science classes. You've also read studies that used the scientific method. But you may not have thought about using the scientific method in your personal life. As you work your way through part 1 of the book, you'll learn to use the scientific method to help you solve problems and make healthy lifestyle decisions. You'll also use the scientific method to plan programs for building your fitness, health, and wellness.

Health and Medical Science

Medicine is the art and science of healing. Historically, the practice of medicine has been focused on diagnosing and treating disease. In prehistoric times, people often associated illness with demons and evil influences. But as early as 2000 BC, Egyptians performed surgery and began to build a more scientific base for medicine. Modern medical practitioners use evidence-based approaches, and research studies are required before medical procedures and medicines are approved.

Because of advances in health and medical science, life expectancy in the United States has increased dramatically over the last century. In 1900, the life expectancy for Americans was 47 years. Over the next century, it almost doubled, reaching nearly 80 years. Health and medical scientists have developed medicines that treat bacterial infections, and as a result infectious diseases such as typhoid fever and smallpox, which used to be among the leading causes of death, have been conquered. Before 1900, fewer than 100 medicines were available to doctors. Now there are more than 10,000, and in the United States they must be tested before the government's Food and Drug Administration (FDA) approves them. With infectious illness reduced, the main causes of early death in developed countries today are heart disease, cancer, diabetes, and other chronic diseases related to unhealthy lifestyles.

Health science focuses on preventing disease and promoting wellness and high quality of life. Some health scientists study personal health issues in order to help individuals prevent disease and promote wellness. Public health scientists, on the other hand, study patterns of health and illness among populations in order to help prevent epidemics of illness; thus they are sometimes called epidemiologists.

> "Physical fitness is not only one of the most important keys to a healthy body; it is the basis of dynamic and creative intellectual activity."
>
> —John F. Kennedy, U.S. president

Kinesiology (Exercise Science)

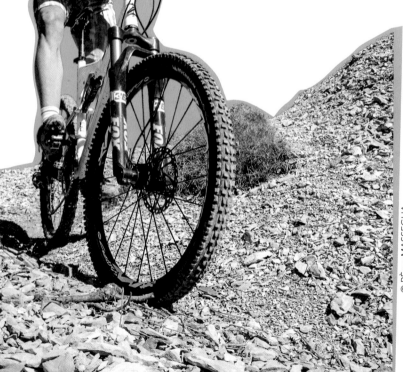

The past two centuries have sometimes been called the golden age of medicine because they have seen many of the most significant advances in health and medical science. Toward the end of the 20th century, a relatively new science called kinesiology emerged as more and more evidence accumulated showing the health and wellness benefits of physical activity and exercise. The U.S. National Research Council now recognizes kinesiology as a major area of science along with other major branches such as those listed at the beginning of this chapter.

Put simply, kinesiology is the study of human movement. There are, of course, many types of human movement. Some involve small muscle movements, such as the movement of your eyes when reading, the movement of your fingers when typing, and the movement of your hands when playing a musical instrument. Kinesiology is the study of all human movement, but it focuses on large-muscle physical activity; in fact, the phrase "physical activity" is a very general term for large muscle movement. There are many types of physical activity, including moderate activities such as walking, vigorous activities such as aerobics, sport and recreational activities, and exercise for muscle fitness and flexibility. These activity types are included in the Physical Activity Pyramid, which is described in more detail throughout part 1 of this book.

FIT FACT

One national health goal established by the U.S. Department of Health and Human Services (USDHHS) is to eliminate disparities in fitness, health, and wellness. People who study kinesiology look for ways of helping *all* people be active, fit, healthy, and well—regardless of race, ethnicity, social or economic class, disability, age, sex, or gender identity.

The general category of kinesiology includes seven sciences. The most prominent are featured in this chapter and in special features that appear throughout this book. They include **exercise physiology, exercise anatomy, biomechanics, exercise psychology, exercise sociology, motor learning,** and **sport pedagogy**. These sciences provide the foundation for our current understanding of the health benefits of physical activity and exercise. Exercise professionals, including physical education teachers, study all of the sciences in kinesiology as part of their training. You don't need to know as much about kinesiology as your teachers, but an understanding of the sciences of kinesiology will help you to understand the information in part 1 of this book.

Exercise Physiology

Physiology is a branch of biology focused on the study of body systems. More specifically, exercise physiology is a branch of kinesiology that explores how physical activity affects body systems. For example, exercise physiologists study the cardiovascular, respiratory, skeletal, muscular, and other body systems to see how they are affected by exercise. Understanding the basic principles of exercise physiology is essential for planning physical activity programs for promoting lifelong fitness, health, and wellness.

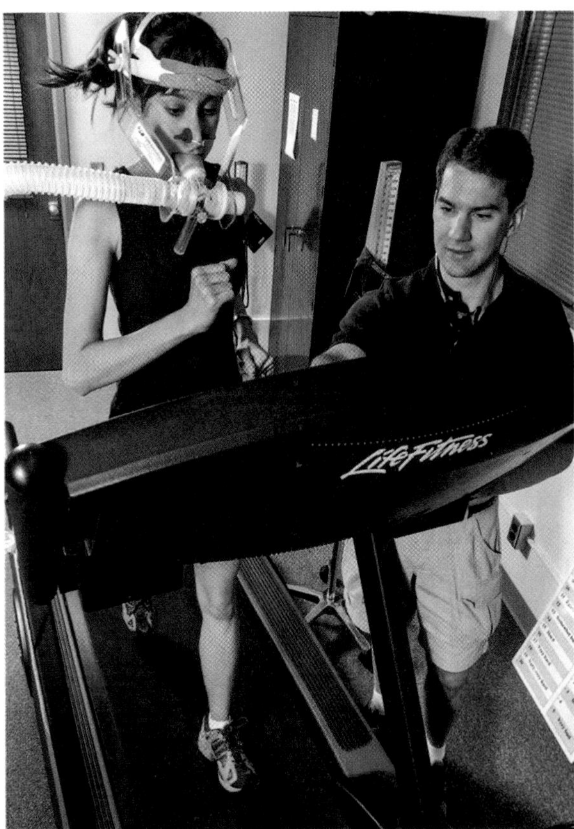

Exercise physiology is the branch of kinesiology that explores how physical activity affects body systems.

Exercise Anatomy

Human anatomy is a branch of biology focused on studying the structure of the human organism. Scientists who study human anatomy focus on the tissues that make up the body (muscle, bone, tendon, ligament, skin, organ). Scientists who study exercise anatomy are especially interested in understanding how we use our muscles—and how our muscles work together with our bones, ligaments, and tendons—to produce movement. Understanding exercise anatomy can help you choose good exercises for building your personal fitness program.

Biomechanics

The human body is much like a machine. It uses a complex system of levers (bones) that are moved by the force produced when you contract your muscles. Biomechanics is the branch of kinesiology that seeks to understand the human machine in motion through the principles of physics. Knowing the basic principles of biomechanics can help you move efficiently and avoid injury.

Exercise Psychology

Psychology is commonly referred to as the science of mind and behavior. More specifically, exercise psychology focuses on the study of human behavior in all types of physical activity, including sport and exercise for fitness. Exercise psychology, including sport psychology, can help motivate people to be active, set realistic goals, and perform better in sports.

Exercise Sociology

Sociology is the study of society and social relationships. Within this broad field, exercise sociology focuses on social relationships and interactions in physical activity, including sports. Exercise sociology has helped people understand teamwork and cooperation; social responsibility; and cultural and ethnic differences in physical activity. Understanding key principles of exercise and sport sociology will help you experience positive social interactions in your physical activity.

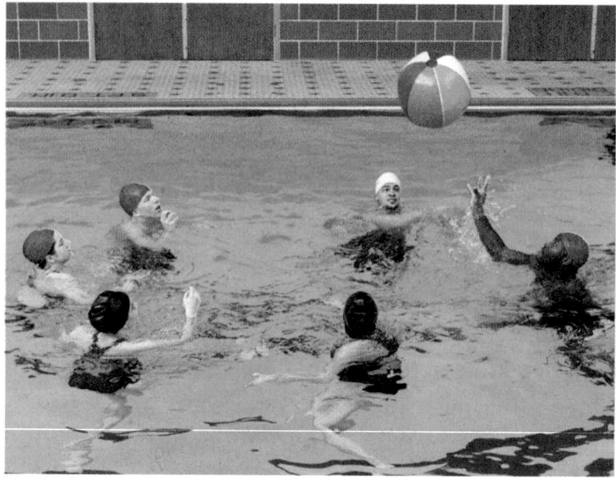

Exercise sociology is the branch of kinesiology that focuses on social relationships and interactions in physical activity, including sports.

Motor Learning

When you see the word *motor*, you may think of an automobile engine, but the term *motor learning* in part 1 of this book refers to skill learning. When you perform a movement skill (also called a **motor skill**), your brain sends a signal through a nerve that tells the relevant muscles to contract. Nerves and muscle fibers that work together to produce

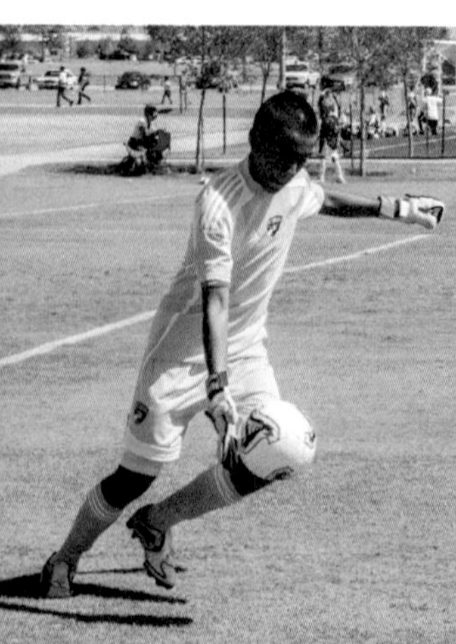

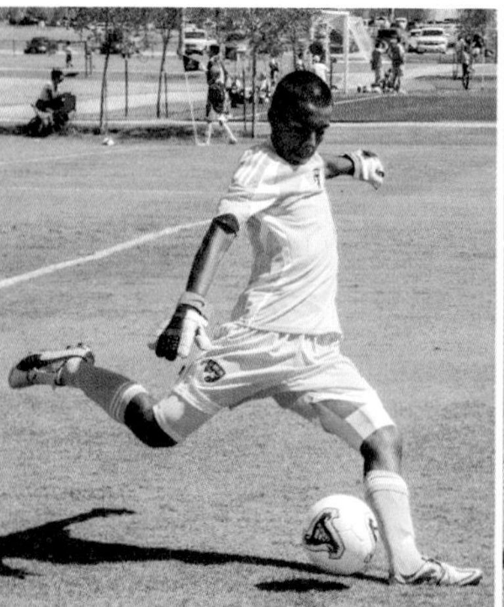

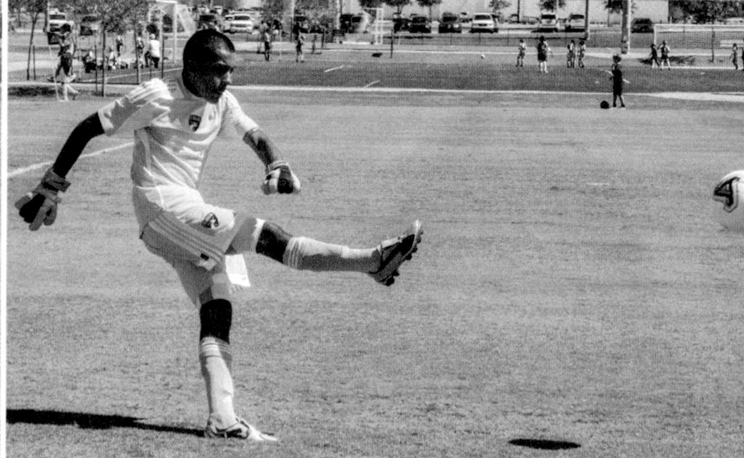

Biomechanics is the branch of kinesiology that seeks to understand the human body in motion through the principles of physics.

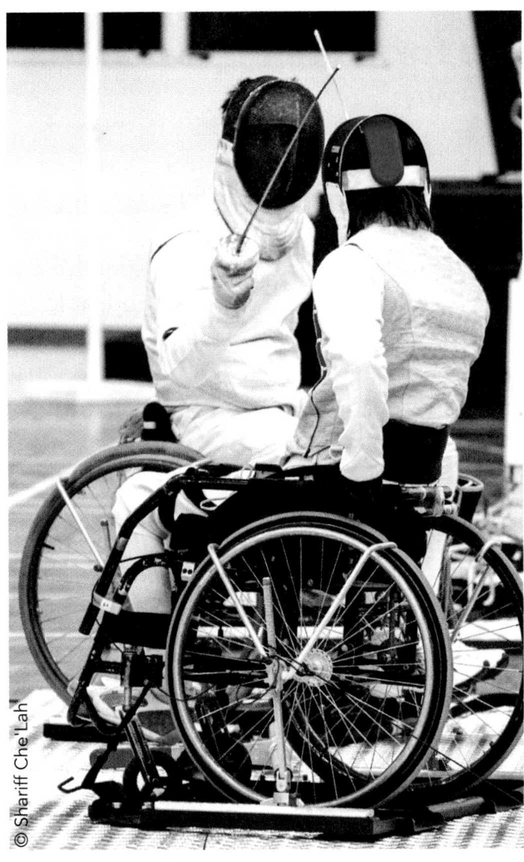

Motor learning is the branch of kinesiology that involves the study of nerves and muscles to see how they work together to perform motor skills.

movement are called a motor unit. Performing a motor skill, such as throwing a ball, requires action by many motor units (nerves and muscles). People who study motor learning have developed rules and principles that help us learn motor skills and control movements. In this book, you'll learn the best ways to develop and practice the skills used in all of the activities presented in the Physical Activity Pyramid.

Physical Education and Sport Pedagogy

Pedagogy is the art and science of teaching. People who study pedagogy as a science focus on discovering the best ways to teach. Sport pedagogy is the study of teaching and learning in many different physical activity settings, including school physical education, on sports teams, and in fitness clubs. The word *sport* is used broadly to include more than just traditional American sports. In other regions of the world, *sport* is used similarly to the term *physical activity*. So sports, or sporting activities, include activities such as riding a bike, taking a hike, performing muscle fitness exercises, and performing traditional sports such as basketball, volleyball, or tennis. People who study pedagogy as a science focus on developing a better understanding of the most appropriate approaches to teaching and the many factors that influence learning. They apply learning principles to help students meet important educational objectives. Examples include applying motor learning principles to help students improve their skills, applying management principles to increase physical activity during classes, and using motivational principles to encourage full participation and optimal learning.

FITNESS TECHNOLOGY: World Wide Web

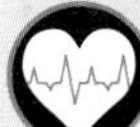

The World Wide Web has given many people immediate access to all kinds of health and fitness information. As you'll learn elsewhere in part 1, some of the information available on the web is good. However, much of it is inaccurate, especially health information. In each chapter of part 1, you'll find a web address that leads you to sound information about fitness, health, and wellness. Look for special web symbols included throughout the book; just type in the address from the first page of the chapter, and you'll find good, reliable information. These web pages will also give you links to other good sources of fitness and health information.

Using Technology

Access the web address provided at the beginning of each chapter in part 1. You will find additional information related to topics in each lesson. Explore the topics to learn more. Explore some of the websites provided to find good fitness and health information.

SCIENCE IN ACTION: Guidelines for Warming Up and Cooling Down

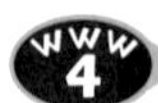

The time you spend doing physical activity each day is your physical activity session. The activity session has three phases: warm-up, workout, and cool-down. The **warm-up** is the activity you perform before your workout in order to get ready for it. The **workout** is the main part of your activity session. It can involve exercise to build fitness, participation in a competitive event, or activity done just for fun. The **cool-down** is the activity you perform after your workout to help you recover. You can use the information presented here about warming up and cooling down to prepare yourself for the various workouts described in part 1 of this book.

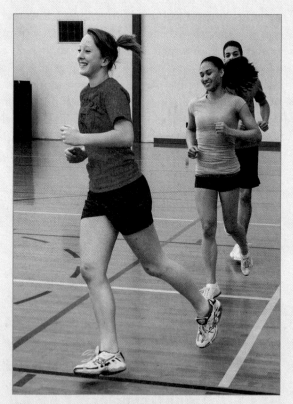

The general warm-up helps your heart and other body systems get ready for more vigorous physical activity.

The Warm-Up

Experts have studied the warm-up for nearly 100 years. For many years, exercise physiologists thought that a **stretching warm-up** was the preferred method of getting ready for a workout. For this reason, the most common type of warm-up includes static stretching (slowly stretching a muscle beyond its normal length and holding the stretch for several seconds). The American College of Sports Medicine (ACSM) notes that a warm-up improves range of motion and may reduce the risk of injury. But some recent research has raised questions about whether the traditional stretching warm-up really prevents injury. Additionally, questions have been raised about the effects of a stretching warm-up on certain types of performance. The best evidence now suggests that your warm-up can vary depending on the workout you plan to perform. Here are some warm-up guidelines:

You don't need to perform a warm-up prior to a workout of low to moderate intensity (such as walking or slow jogging). Low to moderate physical activity is used as a general warm-up as recommended by ACSM, so a workout consisting of low- to moderate-intensity exercise doesn't require a special warm-up.

ACSM recommends 5 to 10 minutes of general warm-up involving low- to moderate-intensity physical activity prior to a vigorous workout or competition. The goal is to increase your body and muscle temperature. This general warm-up helps your heart and other body systems get ready for more vigorous exercise. The general warm-up can include walking, jogging, and **calisthenics**, such as those included in a **dynamic warm-up** (see the Taking Action feature near the end of the chapter).

The National Strength and Conditioning Association (NSCA) recommends a series of dynamic exercises prior to a workout or competition that requires strength, speed, and power. Examples of dynamic exercises include jogging, skipping, hopping, jumping, and calisthenics using your arms, legs, shoulders, and hips (see this chapter's Taking Action feature). You can also perform sport-related movements that use your body parts similarly to how you'll use them in sport competition. Examples include jumping and shooting drills for basketball and swinging a club or bat with gradually increasing intensity. Dynamic warm-up exercises are good for increasing your body temperature and for getting your muscles ready for more vigorous exercise. They can serve as all or part of the general warm-up recommended by ACSM.

A stretching warm-up may be performed prior to a workout or competition, including activities that require strength, speed, and power, if the stretch is not held too long. The NSCA recommends dynamic movement exercises as the preferred warm-up before activities requiring strength, speed, and power. For this reason, some may choose not to perform a stretching warm-up before these activities. However, for those who enjoy a stretching warm-up, stretching exercises can be included as long as each stretch is not held for more than 60 seconds, even prior to a strength, speed, and power workout. Recent research indicates that as long as the stretches don't exceed 60 seconds, they don't inhibit performance. Research also indicates that abruptly stopping a stretching warm-up after regularly performing one increases risk of injury. If you choose a stretching warm-up you should use a variety of stretching exercises to address all of your major muscle groups and joints (see this chapter's Taking Action feature). Stretches should be held for 15 to 30 seconds. Stretching is more effective when your muscles are warm, so you should stretch only after performing a general warm-up.

Stretching exercises used to build flexibility, rather than for warming up, are best performed as a separate part of your workout. The stretching warm-up and the stretching workout are not the same thing. A stretching warm-up is used to prepare you for physical activity. The stretching workout includes exercises to build flexibility, a health-related component of physical fitness. ACSM recommends that stretching for flexibility be done after the general warm-up as part of the workout or as a separate workout session after the cool-down. The flexibility workout is typically much more comprehensive than a warm-up. You will have the opportunity to study flexibility and the flexibility workout later in part 1 of this book.

The Cool-Down

After a workout, your body needs to recover from the demands of physical activity; to aid this process, ACSM recommends a cool-down of 5 to 10 minutes after a vigorous workout. The cool-down usually consists of slow to moderate activity, such as walking or slow jogging, that allows your heart and muscles to gradually recover. The cool-down helps prevent dizziness and fainting. Hard exercise increases the flow of blood to your muscles; for example, running causes more blood to be pumped to your arms and legs than to your head. If you suddenly stop running, the blood can pool in your legs. This leaves your heart with less blood to pump to your brain, which may cause you to feel dizzy or faint. But if you continue moving after a hard run, your muscles will squeeze the veins of your legs. This helps return the blood to your heart, which can then pump more blood to your brain, making you less likely to feel dizzy or faint. The following list provides some more cool-down guidelines.

- Do not lie down or sit down immediately after vigorous activity.
- Gradually reduce the intensity of activity during the cool-down (for example, if you were running, slow to a jog, then a walk, and then consider gentle stretching).
- Walk or do other moderate total body movements.
- You may choose to do some of the stretching exercises presented in the chapter titled Flexibility after your general cool-down while your muscles are still warm.

Student Activity

How does the information in this feature change the way you would warm up before, and cool down after, a workout?

Nutrition Science

Nutrition science is the study of how plants and animals use food to grow and sustain life. This book, of course, focuses on human nutrition. Nutrition scientists study nutrients (carbohydrate, protein, fat, vitamin, and mineral) to better understand which ones contribute to healthy growth and development. One type of nutrition science—food science—is the study of the chemical makeup of food. Another type—food technology—focuses on food processing, packaging, preservation, and safety. **Dietitians** are experts who help people apply principles of nutrition in daily life.

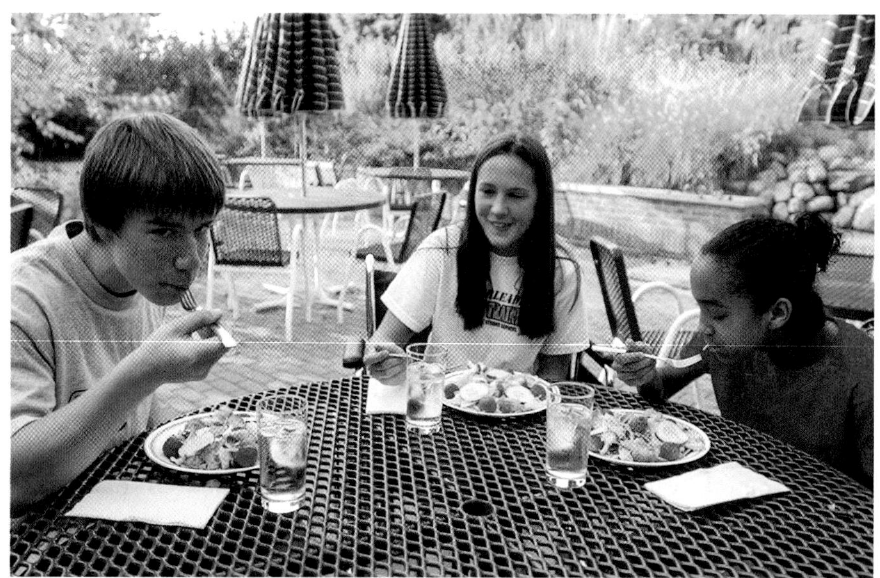

For healthy growth and development, apply the principles of nutrition in daily life.

Lesson Review

1. What is the scientific method and what are its four steps?
2. What are the *health and medical* and *nutrition sciences*, and how do they relate to fitness, health, and wellness?
3. What is *kinesiology*, and what are the seven types of science it encompasses?
4. What are the warm-up and the cool-down, and how are they best performed?

SELF-ASSESSMENT: Physical Fitness Challenges

Each chapter of this book includes a feature titled Self-Assessment. In most chapters, the self-assessment is designed to help you determine your personal fitness level. You'll record and analyze your assessment results. In this self-assessment, you'll try 11 challenges. They're called challenges rather than tests because *they are not meant to be tests of fitness; nor are they meant to be exercises that you do to get fit.* Instead, trying these challenges is a fun way to better understand the differences between the various parts of physical fitness. Please do not draw conclusions about your fitness based on your performance in these challenges. As you work your way through this book, you'll learn many self-assessments to help you determine your true fitness level.

The cardiorespiratory endurance and flexibility challenges will help you warm up before performing the other challenges. You may also want to consider additional warm-up exercises recommended by your teacher.

PART 1: Health-Related Physical Fitness Challenges

Running in Place (cardiorespiratory endurance)

1. Determine your resting heart rate for one minute. To do this, use your fingers to feel your pulse at your wrist or neck, then count your pulse (heartbeats) for one minute.
2. Run 120 steps in place for one minute. Count one step every time a foot hits the floor.
3. Rest for 30 seconds, then count your pulse (heart rate) for one minute. People with good cardiorespiratory endurance recover quickly after exercise. Is your heart rate after this exercise within 15 beats per minute of your resting heart rate before running in place?

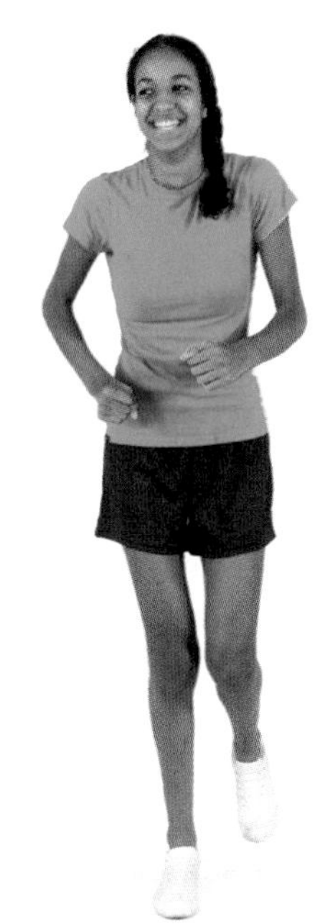

This challenge focuses on cardiorespiratory endurance.

Two-Hand Ankle Grip (flexibility)

1. Squat with your heels together. Lean the upper body forward and reach with your hands between your legs and behind your ankles.
2. Clasp your hands in front of your ankles.
3. Interlock your hands for the full length of your fingers. Keep your feet still.
4. Hold the position for five seconds.

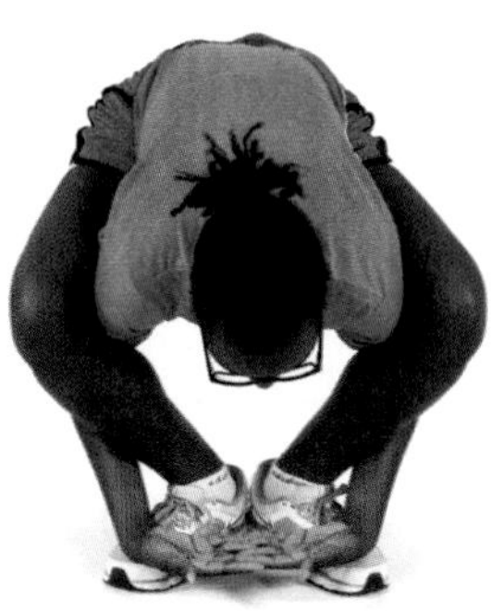

This challenge focuses on flexibility.

Single-Leg Raise (muscular endurance)

1. Bend forward at your waist so that your upper body rests on a table and your feet are on the floor.
2. Raise one leg so that it is extended straight out behind you. Complete several such raises with each leg. Performing multiple repetitions (8 or more) requires muscular endurance. Stop if you reach 25 with each leg.

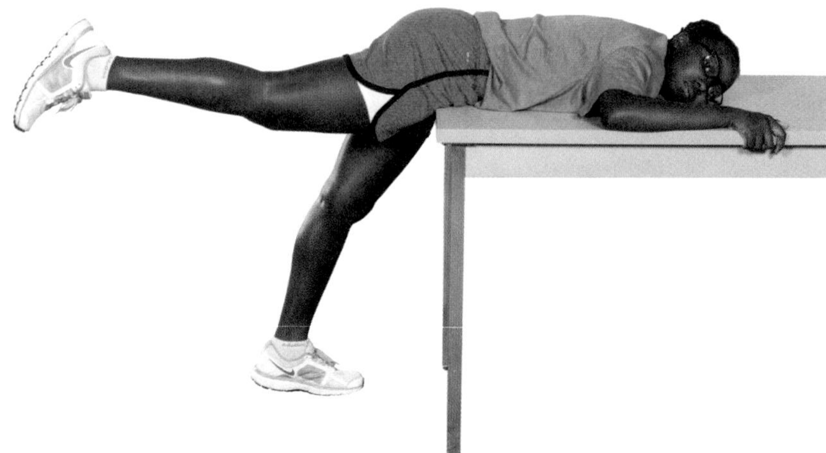

This challenge focuses on muscular endurance.

Arm Skinfold (body fat level)

1. Let your right arm hang relaxed at your side. Have a partner gently pinch the skin and the fat under the skin on the back of your arm halfway between your elbow and shoulder. Together the skin and fat under the skin is called a skinfold.
2. Several skinfolds in different body locations can be used to determine the total amount of fat in the body. At this point there is no need to measure the skinfold. The skinfold on the arm is used only to illustrate the concept of body composition.

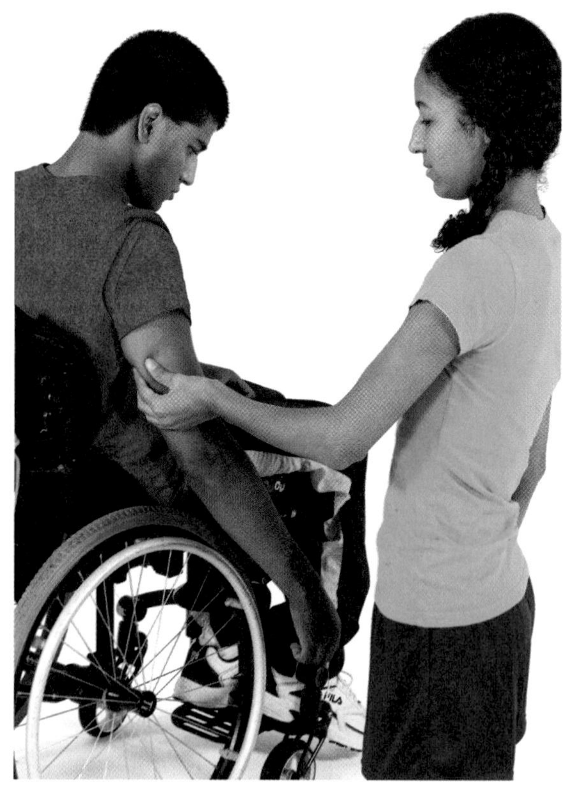

This challenge focuses on body composition.

90-Degree Push-Up (strength)

1. Lie facedown on a mat or carpet with your hands under your shoulders, your fingers spread, and your legs straight. Your legs should be slightly apart and your toes should be tucked under.
2. Push up until your arms are straight. Keep your legs and back straight—your body should form a straight line.
3. Lower your body by bending your elbows until your upper arms are parallel to the floor (elbows at a 90-degree angle), then push up until your arms are fully extended. Do one push-up every three seconds. You may want to have a partner say "up-down" every three seconds to help you. Performing up to 5 push-ups requires muscular strength.

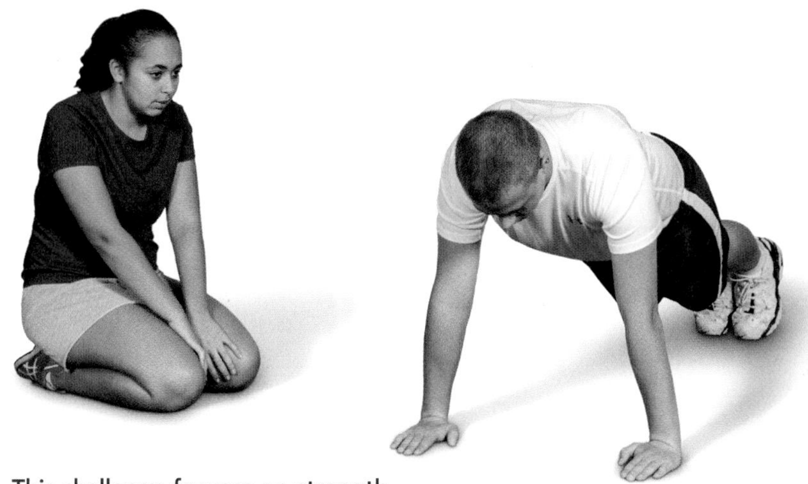

This challenge focuses on strength.

Knees-to-Feet (power)

1. Kneel so that your shins and knees are on a mat. Hold your arms back. Point your toes straight backward.
2. Without curling your toes under you or rocking your body backward, swing your arms upward and spring to your feet.
3. Hold your position for three seconds after you land.

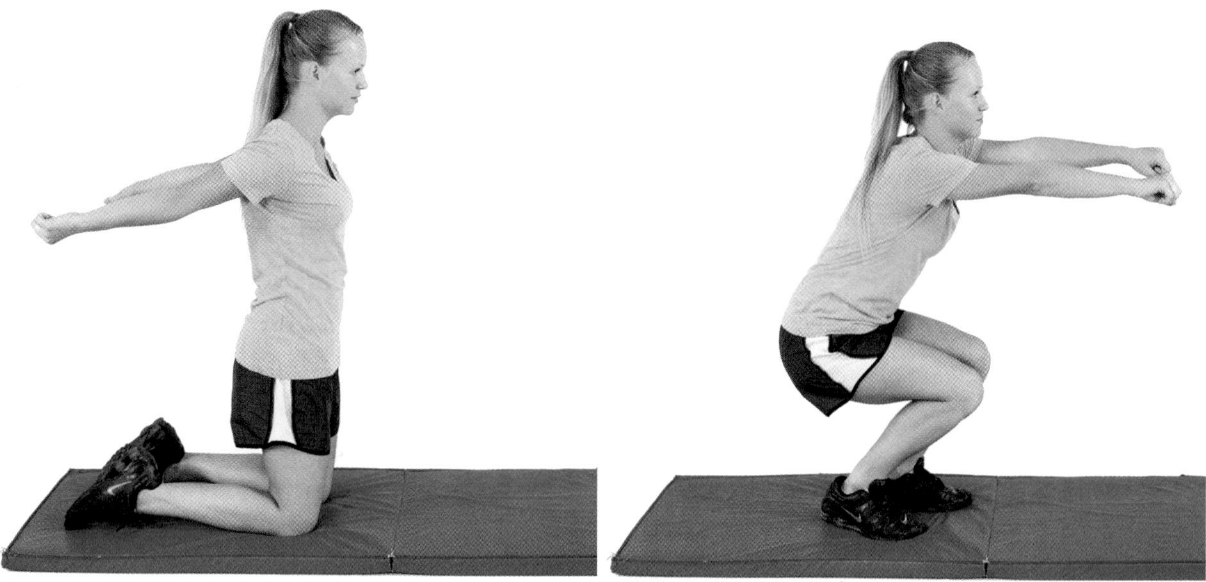

This challenge focuses on power.

PART 2: Skill-Related Physical Fitness Challenges

Line Jump (agility)

1. Balance on your right foot on a line on the floor.
2. Leap onto your left foot so that it lands to the right of the line.
3. Leap across the line onto your right foot; land to the left of the line.
4. Leap onto your left foot, landing on the line.

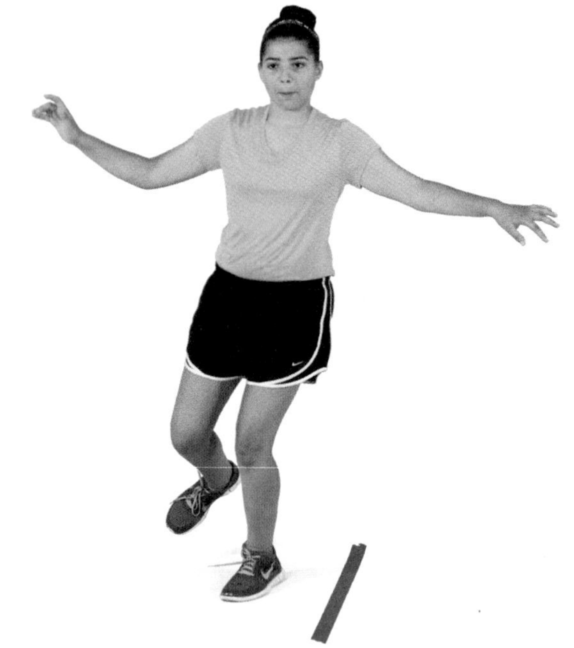

This challenge focuses on agility.

Double Heel Click (speed)

1. Jump into the air and click your heels together twice before you land.
2. Your feet should be at least three inches (eight centimeters) apart when you land.

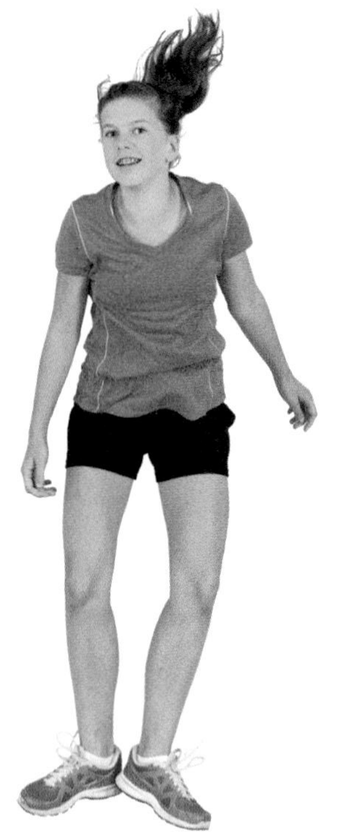

This challenge focuses on speed.

Backward Hop (balance)

1. With your eyes closed, hop backward on one foot five times.
2. After the last hop, hold your balance for three seconds.

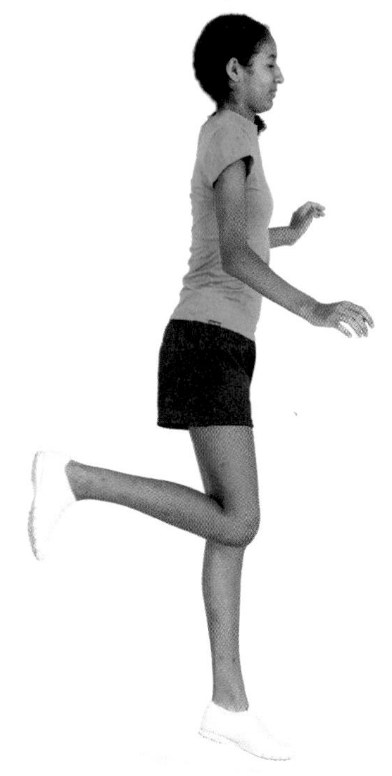

This challenge focuses on balance.

Double-Ball Bounce (coordination)

1. Hold a volleyball in each hand. Beginning at the same time with each hand, bounce both balls at the same time, at least knee high.
2. Bounce both balls three times in a row without losing control of them.

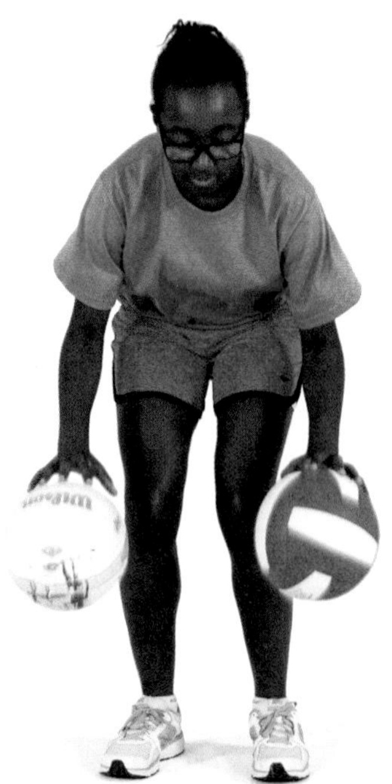

This challenge focuses on coordination.

Coin Catch (reaction time)

1. Point your right elbow outward in front of you. Your right hand, palm up, should be beside your right ear. If you're left-handed, do this activity with your left hand.
2. Place a coin as close to the end of your elbow as possible.
3. Quickly lower your elbow and grab the coin in the air with the hand of the same arm.

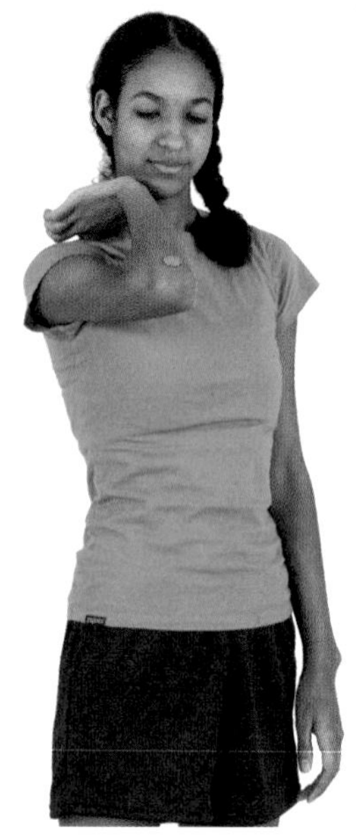

This challenge focuses on reaction time.

Lesson 1.2

Lifelong Fitness, Health, and Wellness

Lesson Objectives

After reading this lesson, you should be able to

1. define *physical fitness*, *health*, and *wellness* and describe how they are interrelated;
2. describe the five components of health and wellness;
3. describe the six parts of health-related physical fitness and the five parts of skill-related physical fitness; and
4. define *self-assessment* and explain how it is important to good fitness, health, and wellness.

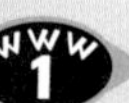

Lesson Vocabulary

agility, balance, body composition, body fat level, cardiorespiratory endurance, coordination, flexibility, functional fitness, health, health-related physical fitness, hypokinetic condition, muscular endurance, physical fitness, power, public health scientist, reaction time, skill-related physical fitness, speed, strength, wellness

If you could have one wish come true, what would it be? Some people would wish for material things, such as money, a new car, or a new house. But after thinking about it, most people indicate that they would wish for good fitness, health, and wellness for themselves and their family. If you possess health, fitness, and wellness, you can enjoy life to its fullest. Without them, no amount of money will allow you to do all of the things you would like to do. More than 90 percent of all people, including teens, agree that good health is important because it helps you feel good, look good, and enjoy life with the people you care about most.

As you read this book, you'll learn more about healthy lifestyle choices that can help you be fit, healthy, and well. You'll learn how to prepare a healthy personal lifestyle plan and how to use self-management skills to stick with your plan. The goal of this book is to help you become an informed consumer who makes effective decisions about your lifelong fitness, health, and wellness.

> The first wealth is health.
>
> —Ralph Waldo Emerson, poet

Before you can start developing a plan, you need some basic information. In this lesson, you'll learn definitions for some key words used throughout this course. You'll better understand the meaning of the words *fitness*, *health*, and *wellness*, and you'll learn about their components.

What Is Health? What Is Wellness?

Early definitions of **health** focused on illness. The first medical doctors concentrated on helping sick people overcome their health problems; in other words, their main job was treating people who were ill.

But in 1947, the World Health Organization (WHO), which now includes representatives from 194 countries, issued a statement indicating that health meant more than freedom from disease or illness. This recognition led people to develop a more comprehensive definition of health, which now includes **wellness**. According to the WHO statement, the sheer fact of not being sick doesn't mean you are well. Wellness is the positive component of health that includes having a good quality of life and a good sense of well-being exhibited by a positive outlook on life.

Figure 1.2 shows that a healthy person both is not ill (the blue circle) and has a strong wellness component (the green circle). Illness is the negative component of health that we want to treat or prevent, whereas wellness is the positive component of health that we want to promote.

Total health

Freedom from illness and debilitating conditions

Wellness (quality of life)

FIGURE 1.2 Being healthy means having wellness in addition to not being ill.

Health and wellness have many components, and a chain is often used to show how the components are linked (figure 1.3). For a chain to be strong, each link must be strong. Likewise, to have good health and wellness, you must have all of the health and wellness components, not just one or two. The goal is to promote the positive while avoiding the negative in each component, as shown in figure 1.3. If you're happy, informed, involved, fit, and fulfilled, then you have incorporated the positive aspects of the health components into your life. You possess wellness, and your risk of illness is reduced. The bottom line is this: Health is freedom from disease and debilitating conditions as well as optimal wellness in all five components (physical, emotional-mental, social, intellectual, and spiritual).

Personal Health and Community Health

One major goal of this book is to help each reader achieve good personal health, including wellness. Another important goal is to promote community health, which refers to the health of a group rather than an individual—from small groups such as families and networks of friends, to larger groups such as towns and cities, and on to very large groups such as states and countries. Just as each person sets health goals, communities do so as well. Your school is a community, and many schools have a coordinated school health program (CSHP). A CSHP program has many components including physical education, health education, wellness programs, and other programs designed to improve the personal health of students and the health of the school community.

One example of a large-scale program designed to promote health in a large community is the Healthy People 2020 project, in which the U.S. Department of Health and Human Services has set national health goals to be accomplished by

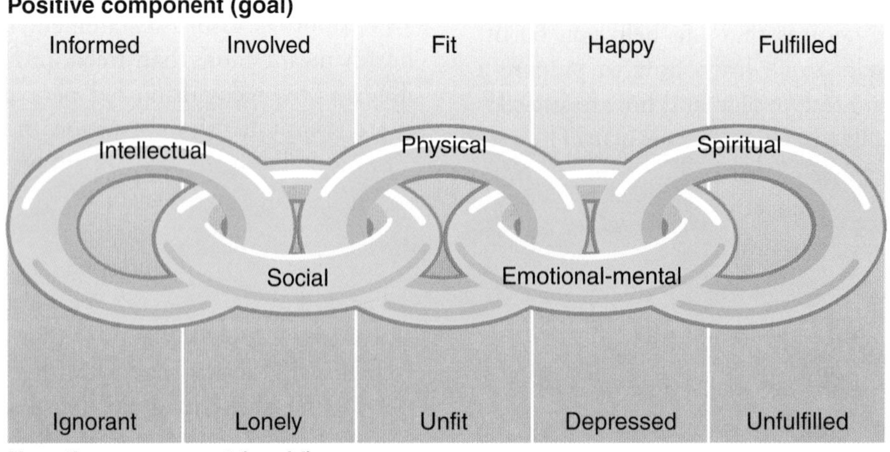

FIGURE 1.3 The total health and wellness chain.
Based on Corbin et al. 2011.

the year 2020. The project is part of an ongoing program. Every 10 years, experts from more than 400 groups nationwide work together to develop health goals for the nation. **Public health scientists** and other experts from every state and many federal and private agencies develop the goals. Many of the Healthy People 2020 objectives are described on the unit opening pages of this book.

What Is Physical Fitness?

Physical fitness refers to the ability of your body systems to work together efficiently to allow you to be healthy and perform activities of daily living. Being efficient means doing daily activities with the least effort possible. A fit person is able to perform schoolwork, meet home responsibilities, and still have enough energy to enjoy sport and other leisure activities. A fit person can respond effectively to normal life situations, such as raking leaves at home, stocking shelves at a part-time job, and marching in the band at school. A fit person can also respond to emergency situations—for example, by running to get help or aiding a friend in distress.

FIT FACT

Studies indicate that fitness scores in the United States have declined in recent years for recruits in physically demanding lines of work, such as policing, fire fighting, and the military.

WWW 3

The Parts of Physical Fitness

Physical fitness is made up of 11 parts—6 of them health related and 5 skill related. All of the parts are important to good performance in physical activity, including sports. But the 6 are referred to as contributing to **health-related physical fitness** because scientists in kinesiology have shown that they can reduce your risk of chronic disease and promote good health and wellness. These parts of fitness are **body composition**, **cardiorespiratory endurance**, **flexibility**, **muscular endurance**, **power**, and **strength**. They also help you function effectively in daily activities.

As the name implies, **skill-related physical fitness** components help you perform well in sports and other activities that require motor skills. For example, **speed** helps you in sports such as track and field. These 5 parts of physical fitness are also linked to health but less so than the health-related components. For example, among older adults, **balance**, **agility**, and **coordination** are very important for preventing falls (a major health concern), and **reaction time** relates to risk for automobile accidents. Each part of physical fitness is described in more detail in the two following features: The Six Parts of Health-Related Fitness and The Five Parts of Skill-Related Fitness.

FIT FACT

Cardiorespiratory endurance is also referred to as cardiovascular fitness and aerobic fitness. The Institute of Medicine, an independent U.S. nonprofit organization, reviewed names for this fitness component and chose cardiorespiratory endurance, especially for use with youth. They chose the name because this type of fitness requires the cardiovascular and respiratory systems to work well together (cardiorespiratory) to allow your entire body to function for a long time without fatigue (endurance).

Health-Related Physical Fitness

Think about a runner. She can probably run a long distance without tiring; thus she has good fitness in at least one area of health-related physical fitness. But does she have good fitness in all six parts? Running is an excellent form of physical activity, but being a runner doesn't guarantee fitness in all parts of health-related physical fitness. Like the runner, you may be more fit in some parts of fitness than in others. The feature named The Six Parts of Health-Related Fitness describes each part and shows an example. As you read about each part, ask yourself how fit you think you are in that area.

The Six Parts of Health-Related Fitness

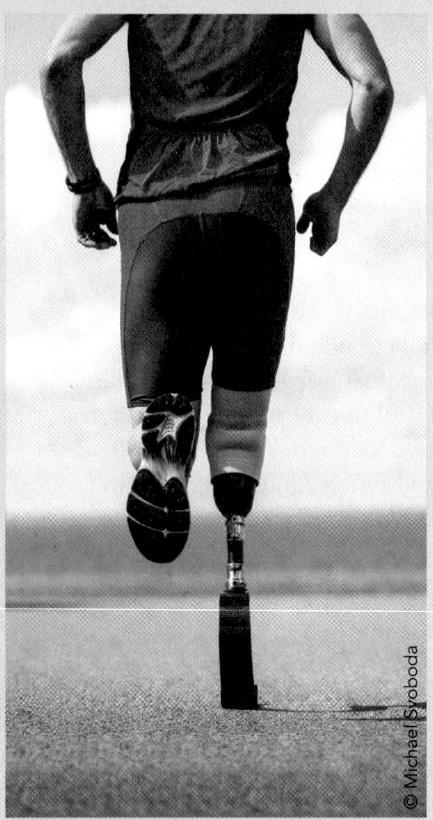

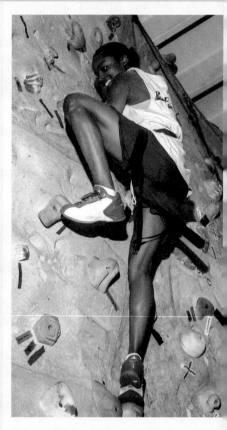

Cardiorespiratory endurance is the ability to exercise your entire body for a long time without stopping. It requires a strong heart, healthy lungs, and clear blood vessels to supply your large muscles with oxygen. Examples of activities that require good cardiorespiratory endurance are distance running, swimming, and cross-country skiing.

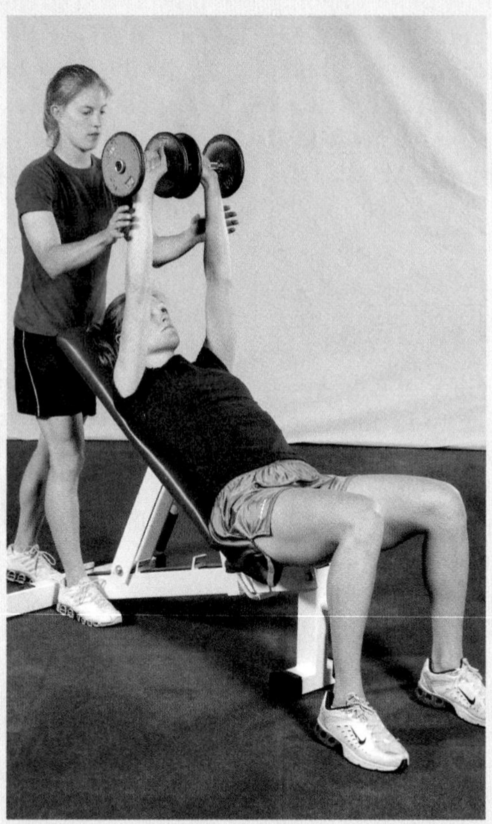

Strength is the amount of force your muscles can produce. It is often measured by how much weight you can lift or how much resistance you can overcome. Examples of activities that require good strength are lifting a heavy weight and pushing a heavy box.

Muscular endurance is the ability to use your muscles many times without tiring—for example, doing many push-ups or curl-ups (crunches) or climbing a rock wall.

How do you think you rate in each of the six health-related parts of fitness? To be healthy, you should be fit for each of the six parts. Totally fit people are less likely to develop a **hypokinetic condition**—a health problem caused partly by lack of physical activity—such as heart disease, high blood pressure, diabetes, osteoporosis, colon cancer, or a high **body fat level**. You'll learn more about hypokinetic conditions in other chapters of part 1. People who are physically fit also enjoy better wellness. They feel better, look better, and have more energy. You don't have to be a great athlete in order to enjoy good health and wellness and be physically fit. Regular physical activity can improve anyone's health-related physical fitness.

Skill-Related Physical Fitness

Just as the runner in our example may not achieve a high rating in all parts of health-related physical fitness, she also may not rate the same in all parts of skill-related physical fitness. Though most sports

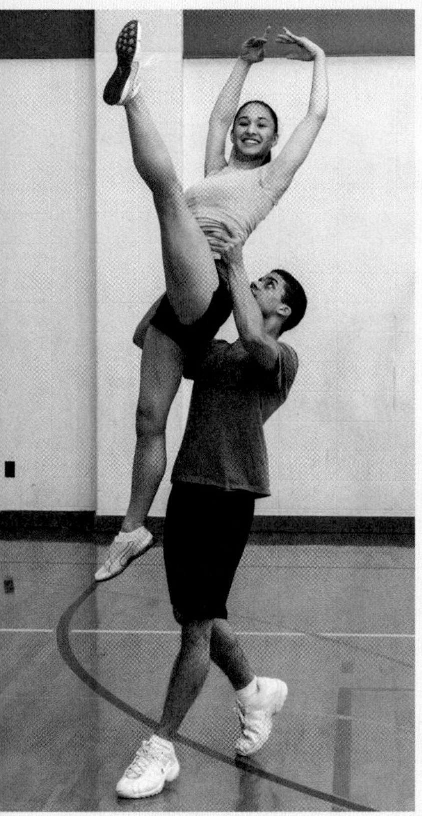

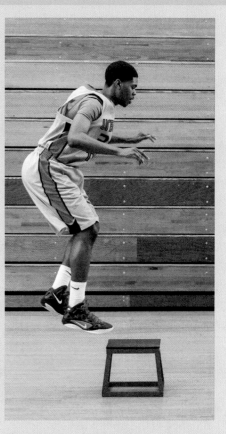

Flexibility is the ability to use your joints fully through a wide range of motion without injury. You are flexible when your muscles are long enough and your joints are free enough to allow adequate movement. Examples of people with good flexibility include dancers and gymnasts.

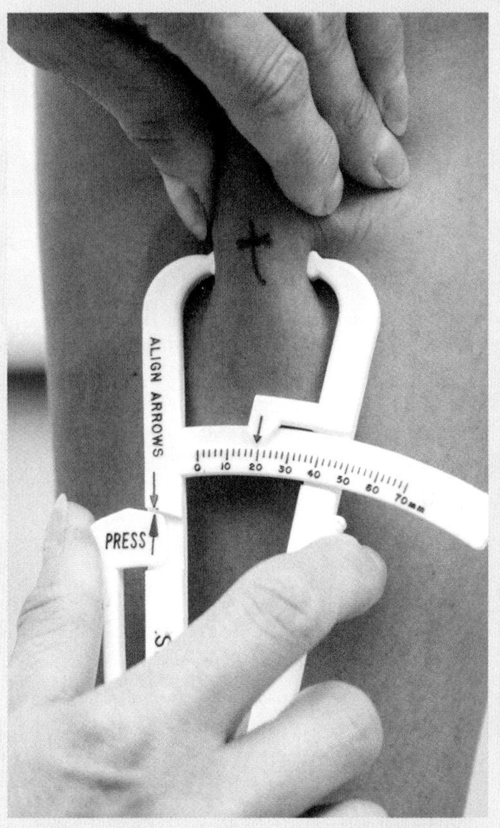

Body composition refers to the different types of tissues that make up your body, including fat, muscle, bone, and organ. Your level of body fat is often used to assess the component of body composition related to health. Body composition measures commonly used in schools include body mass index (based on height and weight), skinfold measures (which estimate body fatness), and body measurements such as waist and hip circumferences.

Power is the ability to use strength quickly; thus it involves both strength and speed. It is sometimes referred to as explosive strength. People with good power can, for example, jump far or high, put the shot, and speed-swim.

require several parts of skill-related fitness, different sports can require different parts. For example, a skater might have good agility but lack good reaction time. Some people have more natural ability in some areas than in others. No matter how you score on the skill-related parts of physical fitness, you can enjoy some type of physical activity.

Remember, too, that good health doesn't come from being good in skill-related physical fitness. It comes from doing activities designed to improve your health-related physical fitness, and it can be enjoyed both by great athletes and by people who consider themselves poor athletes.

As noted earlier, health-related fitness offers a double benefit. It not only helps you stay healthy but also helps you perform well in sport and other activities. For example, cardiorespiratory endurance helps you resist heart disease and helps you perform well in sports such as swimming and cross-country running. Similarly, strength helps you perform well in sports such as football and wrestling, muscular endurance is important in soccer and tennis,

The Five Parts of Skill-Related Fitness

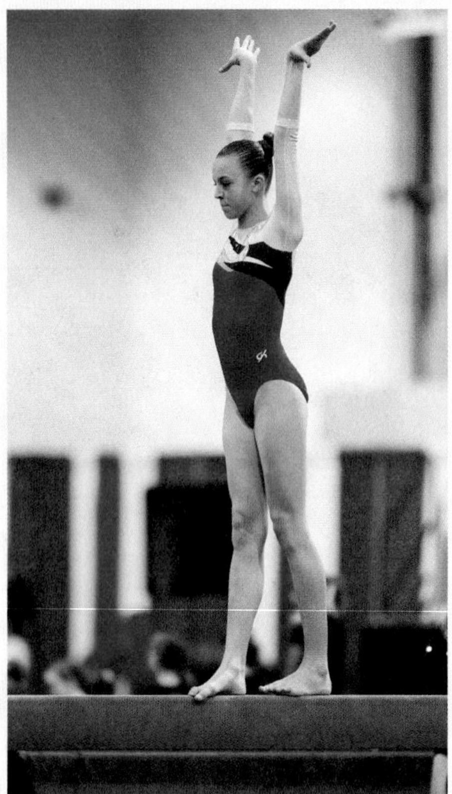

Balance is the ability to keep an upright posture while standing still or moving. People with good balance are likely to be good, for example, at gymnastics and ice skating.

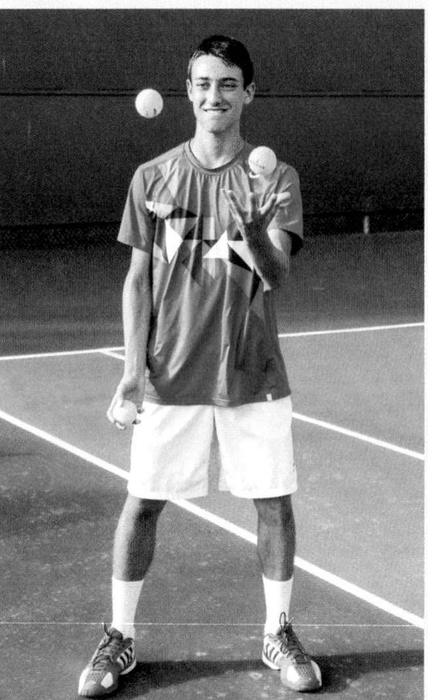

Coordination is the ability to use your senses together with your body parts or to use two or more body parts together. People with good eye–hand or eye–foot coordination are good at juggling and at hitting and kicking games, such as soccer, baseball, volleyball, tennis, and golf.

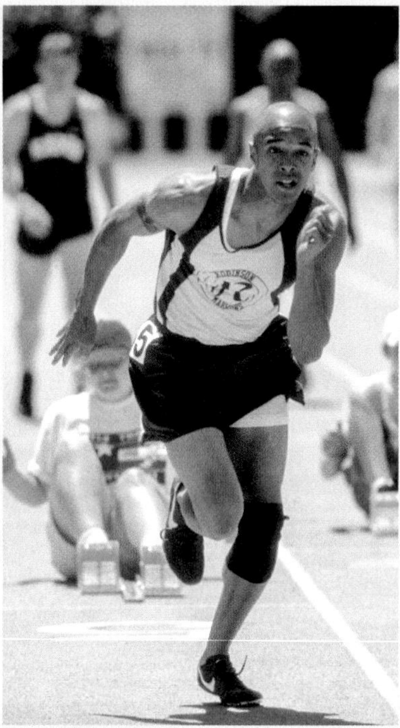

Speed is the ability to perform a movement or cover a distance in a short time. For example, people with good leg speed can run fast, and people with good arm speed can throw fast or hit a ball that is thrown fast.

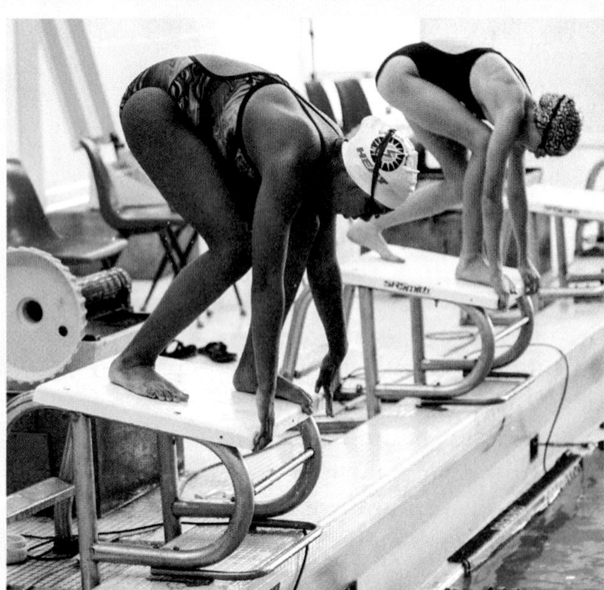

Reaction time is the amount of time it takes you to move once you recognize the need to act. People with good reaction time can make fast starts in track and swimming and can dodge fast attacks in fencing and karate.

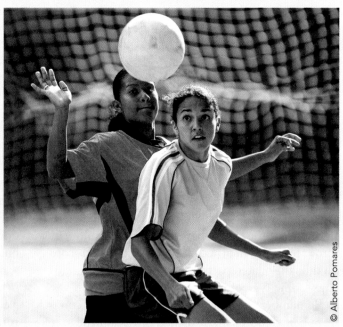

Agility is the ability to change the position of your body quickly and control your body's movements. People with good agility are likely to be good, for example, at wrestling, diving, soccer, and ice skating.

FIT FACT

Power, formerly classified as a skill-related part of fitness, is now classified as a health-related part of fitness. A report by the independent Institute of Medicine provides evidence of the link between physical power and health. The report indicates that power is associated with wellness, higher quality of life, reduced risk of chronic disease and early death, and better bone health. Power, and activities that improve power, have also been found to be important for healthy bones in children and teens.

flexibility helps in sports such as gymnastics and diving, power helps in track activities such as the discus throw and the long jump, and having a healthy amount of body fat makes your body more efficient in many activities.

Functional Fitness

Functional fitness refers to the ability to function effectively when performing normal daily tasks. You have functional fitness if you can do your schoolwork, get to and from school, participate in leisure activities without fatigue, respond to emergency situations, and perform other daily tasks safely and without fatigue (for example, driving a car or doing housework and yardwork). From this point of view, health-related fitness not only helps you stay healthy but also helps you function; for example, it helps you avoid fatigue when working or playing. Similarly, skill-related fitness not only helps you perform well in sports but also can help you function in life, such as when you need to stop quickly while driving a car. As you work your way through this book, you'll learn how each part of health- and skill-related fitness contributes to your functional fitness.

Fitness, Health, and Wellness Are Interrelated

Fitness, health, and wellness are all states of being, and you can maximize all three by living a healthy lifestyle. The interrelationship of fitness, health, and wellness is shown in figure 1.4 by the overlapping circles. For example, if you're active on a regular basis, your fitness improves. That reduces your risk of disease, which improves your health. Your wellness and quality of life are also improved because you feel better and can better enjoy the activities of daily life.

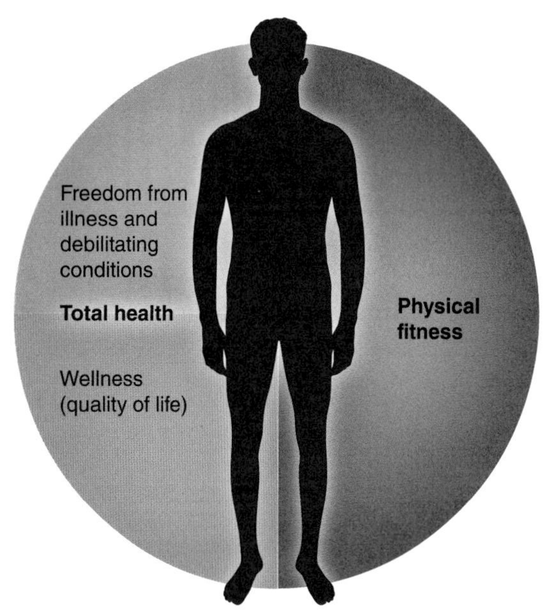

FIGURE 1.4 Interrelationship of fitness, health, and wellness.

Lesson Review

1. What is meant by the terms *physical fitness*, *health*, and *wellness*, and how they are interrelated?
2. What are the five components of health and wellness, and how are they defined?
3. What are the six parts of health-related physical fitness and the five parts of skill-related physical fitness, and how are they defined?
4. What is self-assessment, and how it is important to good fitness, health, and wellness?

TAKING CHARGE: Learning to Self-Assess

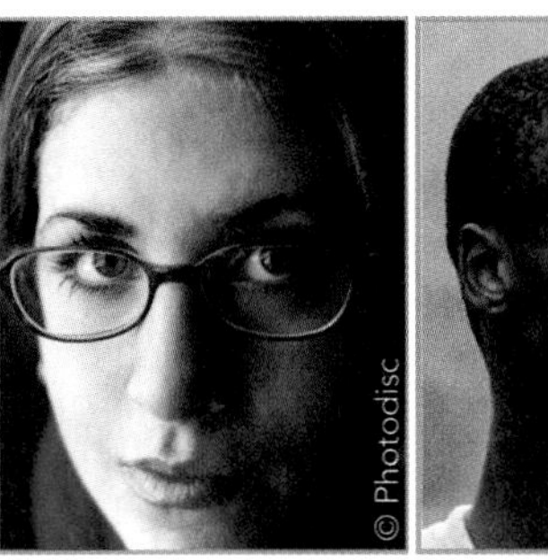
© Photodisc

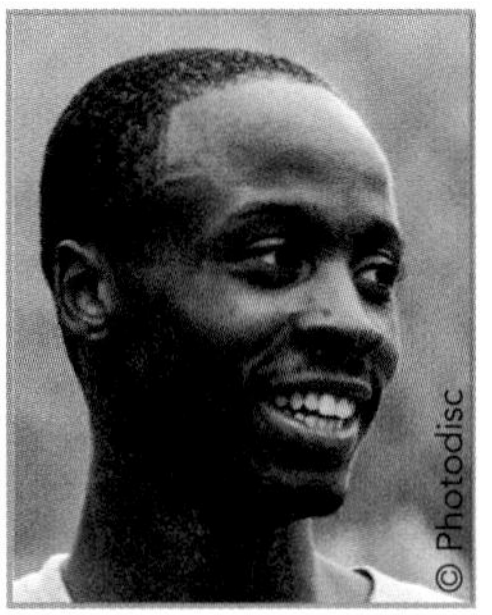
© Photodisc

Self-management skills help you adopt a healthy lifestyle both now and throughout life. Self-assessment is a type of self-management skill that enables you to test yourself to see what you can do. You can perform many kinds of self-assessment. For example, you can assess your physical fitness, eating patterns, stress level, health risks, knowledge, and ability to perform in a sport. This book includes many self-assessments focused on physical fitness, as well as some that address health, wellness, and healthy lifestyle choices. The following example focuses on health-related physical fitness.

Julia and Troy were friends who wanted to know more about their health-related physical fitness. They had taken fitness tests in school but had learned little about why they were doing the tests or how to test themselves. They wanted to learn how to assess their own fitness.

Julia remembered some of the tests she had taken in elementary school, such as running a 50-yard (about 46-meter) dash and performing something called a "shuttle run." Troy had not taken a fitness test in physical education, but he had been tested for his baseball team to see how far he could throw a ball and how fast he could run to first base.

Julia and Troy thought about doing a self-assessment that included all of the tests Julia had been given in school and all of the tests Troy had done for his baseball team. But they weren't sure how to do the tests in the correct way, and they weren't sure that these were the best tests. What they really wanted to learn was how to do a self-assessment for health-related physical fitness.

For Discussion

Discuss a plan of self-assessment that Julia and Troy could follow to determine their health-related physical fitness. Did the tests Julia performed in elementary school assess health-related physical fitness? Did the tests Troy performed for his baseball team measure health-related physical fitness? What do you think the tests they performed really measured?

The guidelines in the following Self-Management feature will help you as you answer the discussion questions above and will be useful as you try the various self-assessments included in part 1 of this book.

SELF-MANAGEMENT: Skills for Learning to Self-Assess

Before you go on a trip, you use a map to make plans. The map helps you decide where you want to go. Assessing your own fitness is much like using a map. You can assess your current fitness and physical activity in order to help you learn where you need to improve and make your plans for doing so. You can also use the assessment information to develop strategies and tactics to commit to your plan. Use the following guidelines as you learn to do personal fitness and activity self-assessments.

- **Try a wide variety of tests.** Fitness and physical activity include many parts, and performing a variety of self-assessments enables you to get a total picture of your fitness and activity needs. You will learn various self-assessment techniques in this class.
- **Choose self-assessments that work best for you.** You'll try all the self-assessments you learn in this book, but ultimately you won't need to use them all. You should choose at least one assessment for each type of health-related physical fitness and one assessment to determine your current activity level. After you've tried many self-assessments, you'll be prepared to select the ones that work best for you.

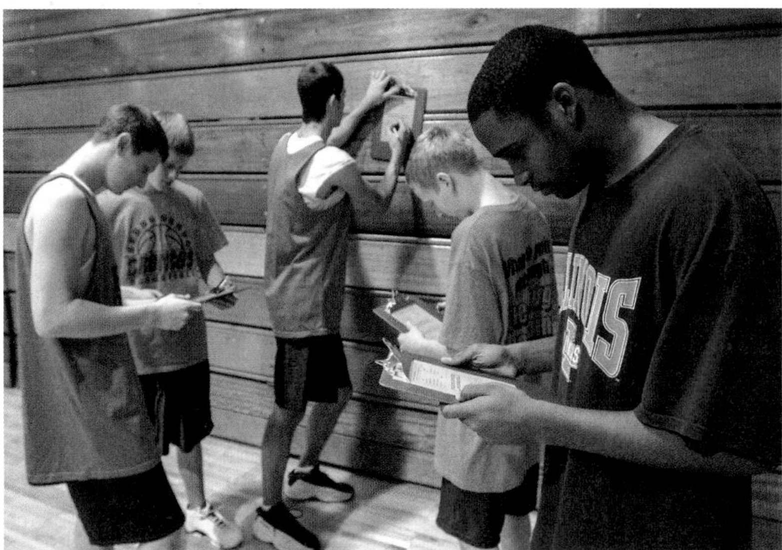

Learning to assess your own fitness is an important life skill.

- **Practice.** When you first drive a car, it's not easy, but your skill improves with practice. Similarly, the first time you do self-assessments, you'll make mistakes, but the more you practice, the better you'll get. So, once you decide which assessments to use on a regular basis, practice using them!
- **Use self-assessments for personal improvement.** Once you've learned to use self-assessments, repeat them from time to time to monitor your progress. Avoid making assessments too often, but check yourself periodically to see how you're doing. It takes several weeks to see improvement in health-related physical fitness after starting a new activity program. Avoid daily or even weekly self-assessments in favor of self-assessing after several weeks when improvement is more likely.
- **Use health standards rather than comparing yourself with others.** Sometimes people are discouraged when they get test results, often because they had unrealistic expectations. Rather than comparing yourself with others, evaluate yourself in relation to health standards and to your own previous performances. This type of comparison helps you stay realistic. *The standards used in part 1 of this book are based on the level of fitness needed for good health and wellness—not on comparisons of one person with another.*
- **Information from self-assessments is personal.** Self-assessments are done to gain information that will help you build an accurate personal profile and plan for healthy active living. In many assessments you will work with a partner. Partners must agree to keep test results private. Information may be submitted to an instructor, parent, or guardian—again with the expectation that information is kept private. Information should not be shared with others without the permission of the person being tested. Think of doing a self-assessment like hiring a personal trainer. A personal trainer would have you do a series of tests to determine your strengths and weaknesses and then work with you to come up with a plan to meet your goals. The personal trainer would keep your information totally confidential.

TAKING ACTION: The Warm-Up

As noted in the Science in Action feature in lesson 1, your warm-up should vary depending on the workout you plan to perform. Because *Health Opportunities Through Physical Education* includes many types of activity, the type of warm-up you perform will vary from day to day. Before engaging in low- to moderate-intensity activity, no warm-up is typically necessary, though you may choose to do one if you wish. The activities in the warm-up you use prior to vigorous activity will vary depending on the nature of your workout activity. For vigorous activities that involve strength, speed, and power, you may choose a dynamic warm-up. If you prefer a stretching warm-up prior to vigorous activities, the stretches should last 15 to 30 seconds. Be sure not to stretch longer than 60 seconds, because that can result in reduced performance in some activities. You will **take action** here by trying both a stretching warm-up and a dynamic warm-up. After you've tried them, you can work with your teacher and use the guidelines in the Science in Action feature to create warm-up activities for each type of workout you're planning to do. WWW 4

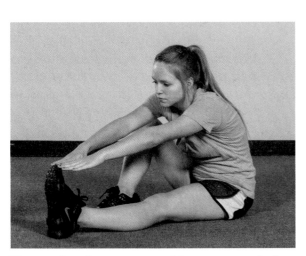

Those who choose a stretching warm-up before vigorous exercise should hold stretches for 15 to 30 seconds.

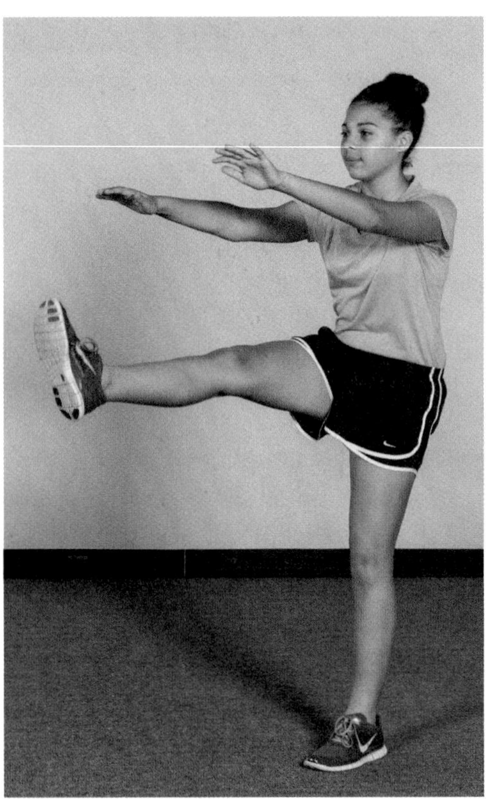

For vigorous activities that do involve strength, speed, and power, you can use a dynamic warm-up.

CHAPTER REVIEW

Reviewing Concepts and Vocabulary

As directed by your teacher, answer items 1 through 5 by correctly completing each sentence with a word or phrase.

1. The study of human movement is called ______________.
2. The ______________ is a series of steps that can help you make good decisions and solve problems.
3. The science that uses principles of physics to understand the human machine is called ______________.
4. A hypokinetic condition is a health problem caused by ______________.
5. The part of fitness that refers to the types of body tissue is called ______________.

For items 6 through 10, as directed by your teacher, match each term in column 1 with the appropriate phrase in column 2.

6. muscular endurance	a. movement of the body using larger muscles
7. agility	b. positive component of health
8. pedagogy	c. ability to change body position quickly
9. physical activity	d. art and science of teaching
10. wellness	e. ability to use muscles continuously without tiring

For items 11 through 15, as directed by your teacher, respond to each statement or question.

11. What is physical fitness?
12. How do health-related physical fitness and skill-related physical fitness differ?
13. Explain how the understanding of health has changed over time.
14. What are some important factors to consider when choosing a warm-up before your workout?
15. What are some guidelines for using self-assessments?

Thinking Critically

Write a paragraph to answer the following question.

You are asked to make an important decision about your fitness, health, or wellness. How would you use the scientific method to make that decision?

Project

Interview several healthy older adults about their fitness, health, and wellness. Ask questions such as these: How would you rate your health? How would you rate your wellness? How would you rate your health-related physical fitness? (Ask the person to use ratings such as good fitness, marginal fitness, and poor fitness.) How do you think teens rate their fitness, health, and wellness compared to people your age? Present the information to a group such as your class or family members.

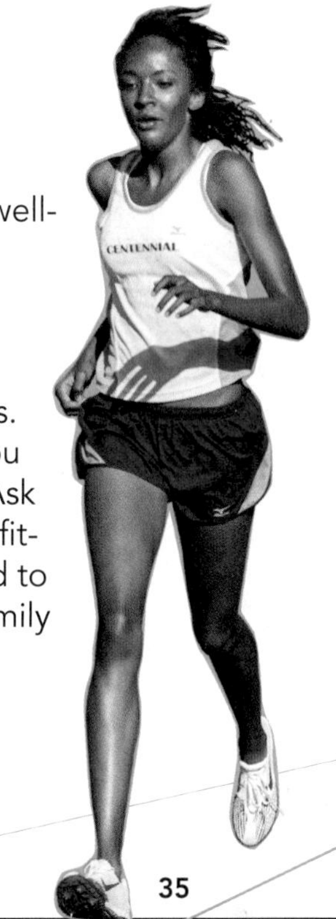

2

Adopting a Healthy Lifestyle and Self-Management Skills

In This Chapter

Student Web Resources

www.HOPEtextbook.org/student

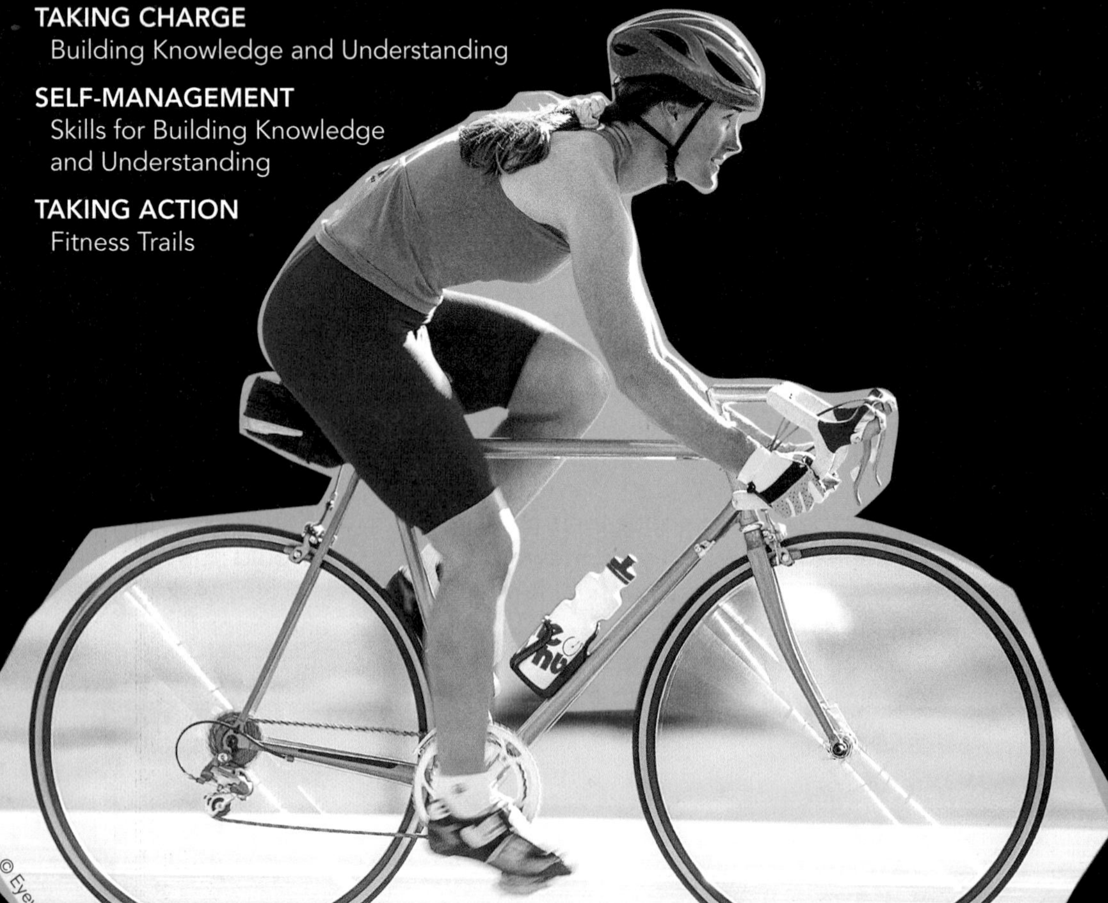

Lesson 2.1

Adopting Healthy Lifestyles

Lesson Objectives

After reading this lesson, you should be able to

1. name and describe the five types of determinants of fitness, health, and wellness;
2. name and describe the five benefits of a healthy lifestyle; and
3. explain the Stairway to Lifetime Fitness, Health, and Wellness and how it can be used.

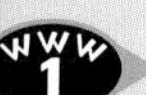

Lesson Vocabulary

determinant, priority healthy lifestyle choice, self-management skill, state of being

Let's take a moment to consider the nature of fitness, health, and wellness. Each is a **state of being** that an individual person can possess to his or her benefit. If you possess fitness, you can work and play efficiently. If you possess health and wellness, you are free from disease and can enjoy a good quality of life. These states are interrelated, so if you do something to change one, you affect the others. Your fitness, health, and wellness are also affected by many other factors. Medical and scientific experts refer to these factors as **determinants**, and the U.S. government's Healthy People 2020 project suggests that all people learn about them in order to stay fit, healthy, and well.

> "One who has health has hope; and one who has hope has everything."
>
> —Ancient proverb

Determinants of Fitness, Health, and Wellness

As shown in figure 2.1, your fitness, health, and wellness are affected by five types of determinants: personal, environmental, health care, social and individual, and healthy lifestyle choices. Some are more within your control than others. The figure shows the determinant types in varying shades of orange—the lighter the color, the less control you have; the darker the color, the more control.

Personal Determinants

You have relatively little control, or none at all, over personal determinants, such as heredity, age, sex, and disability; thus they are shaded in light orange in the figure. Nonetheless, these factors can greatly affect your fitness, health, and wellness. For example, a person might inherit genes that put him or her at risk for certain diseases, and disease risk also increases with age. Sex is also a factor. For example, males, especially after the teen years, tend to have more muscle than females do. As for age, up to a certain point in life, muscles grow, and some parts of fitness improve just because of normal changes in the body. We also know that women have a longer life expectancy than men. Another potential factor is disability, which can affect a person's capacity to perform certain tasks but does not necessarily affect his or her health or quality of life.

You'll learn more about personal determinants and their effects on fitness, health, and wellness in other chapters of this book. Although you cannot control personal determinants, you can be aware of them. Being aware can help you decide to alter other determinants over which you do have control.

FIT FACT

A disability is an objective condition (impairment), while a handicap is the inability to do something you would like to do. A disabled person is not necessarily handicapped. We are all physically different, and various personal determinants affect what you can and cannot do. Understanding your own strengths and limitations helps you be the best you can be and allows you to help others be the best they can be.

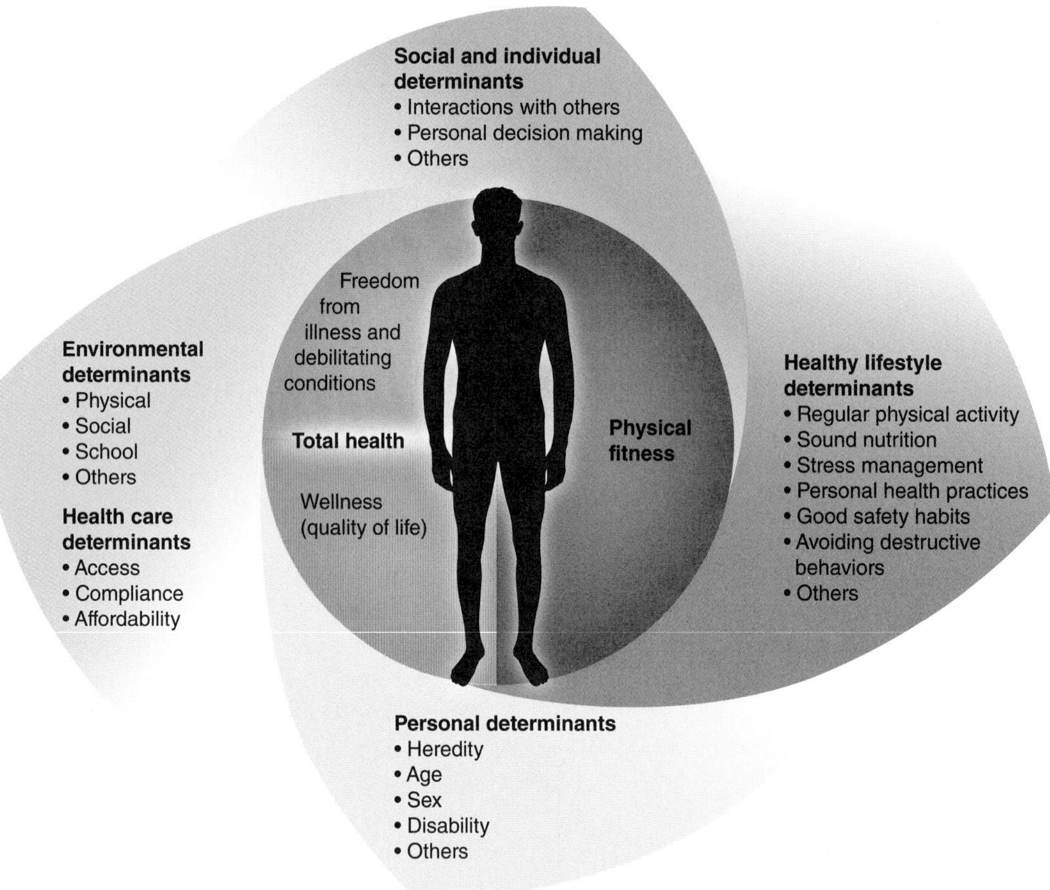

FIGURE 2.1 The five determinants of fitness, health, and wellness.

Adapted, by permission, from C. Corbin et al., 2013, *Concepts of fitness and wellness: A comprehensive lifestyle approach*, 10th ed. (St. Louis, MO: McGraw-Hill). © The McGraw-Hill Companies.

Environmental and Health Care Determinants

Fitness, health, and wellness are also affected by environmental and health care determinants. In figure 2.1, they are colored in a darker shade of orange than the personal determinants because you have more control over them. For example, as an adult, you can choose to live or work in a healthy environment; you can also recycle in order to help protect the environment. There are other ways you can take action to improve the environment but, of course, there are limits on your control. For example, you cannot directly control the quality of the air in your neighborhood. Environmental determinants are discussed throughout this book.

Health care refers to being able to see a doctor or other health-care professional as needed and having access to health-care facilities and medicine. Health care also includes opportunities to learn about prevention of illness and promotion of wellness. People who receive good health care live longer and have higher-quality lives compared to those who don't. This factor is shown in a darker shade of orange because you have some control over it. Having access to good health care, seeking it when needed, and complying with health care recommendations are all important to your health and wellness.

Social and Individual Determinants

As an individual in a free society, you have the freedom to make choices and decisions that affect your fitness, health, and wellness. For example, you choose your friends and make decisions about how you interact with them, and these social choices make a difference. Teens who choose friends who avoid destructive habits and practice healthy ones are

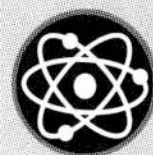 SCIENCE IN ACTION: Heredity and Fitness, Health, and Wellness

Exercise physiologists have studied human genes to determine whether heredity plays a role in fitness, health, and wellness. Their studies show that the genes we inherit from our parents do make a difference. For example, some people inherit genes that make them more likely to have a specific disease; other genes make it more likely that a person will be able to build muscle mass. And of course genes make a difference in how tall you are and how much you weigh. Recently, scientists have also discovered that, because of genetics, people respond differently to exercise. They learned this by studying groups of people who all did the same exercise. People who got big benefits are called responders, and those who benefited less are called nonresponders.

Even though heredity surely makes a difference in your fitness, health, and wellness, scientists also emphasize that making healthy lifestyle choices can help counteract heredity. Early in life, heredity plays a major role in your health, fitness, and wellness. However, people who practice a healthy lifestyle throughout life are among the healthiest people regardless of their heredity. What you inherit matters, but over the long haul what you do can be even more important.

Student Activity

Choose one part of health-related fitness and describe how your own heredity influences it.

more likely to be fit, healthy, and well themselves. Individual determinants are also important. Being a good consumer—for example, by using good information to choose healthy foods—is a way each individual can contribute to good fitness, health, and wellness. In figure 2.1, social and individual determinants are colored in a relatively dark shade of orange because you can exercise a lot of control over the choices you make, both as an individual and with your friends and other people. Personal decision making and peer interaction are discussed in special features throughout part 1 of this book.

Healthy Lifestyle Choices

By far the most important determinants of your fitness, health, and wellness are your lifestyle choices. A healthy lifestyle is made up of behaviors that you adopt to improve your fitness, health, and wellness. Because you generally have a lot of control over these determinants, they are colored in dark orange in figure 2.1. With good information and good **self-management skills**, you can adopt each of the healthy lifestyle behaviors illustrated in the figure. Self-management skills help you become more active and eat better; they also help you adapt well in stressful situations. You'll learn more about self-management skills in lesson 2.

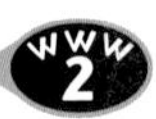

Adopting a healthy lifestyle gives you many benefits. First, it reduces your risk of disease and early death. In fact, nearly 60 percent of early deaths result from unhealthy lifestyle choices. Healthy choices, on the other hand, can help you prevent and treat various illnesses. For example, eating well and being active can help prevent heart disease and manage diabetes. You might assume that because illness and disease are more common in later life, you don't have to worry about them now. You might even share an attitude that is common among teenagers: "I'm young and healthy; it can't happen to me." But evidence indicates that the disease process begins early in life. Therefore, choosing and adopting a healthy lifestyle early in your life can do a lot to prevent disease and illness later on.

FIT FACT

Healthy living pays off. For example, Oakland County, Michigan, cut health insurance costs by 15 percent after starting a program to promote healthy lifestyle choices.

Benefits of a Healthy Lifestyle for Teens

Living a healthy lifestyle helps you not only later in life—you can also enjoy many benefits now. Examples include looking and feeling good, learning better, enjoying daily life, and effectively handling emergencies.

Looking Good

Do you care about how you look? Experts agree that regular physical activity is one healthy lifestyle choice that can help you look your best. Others are proper nutrition, good posture, and good body mechanics.

Feeling Good

People who do regular physical activity also feel better. If you're active and therefore physically fit, you can resist fatigue, you're less likely to be injured, and you're capable of working more efficiently. National surveys indicate that active people sleep better, do better in school, and experience less depression than people who are less active. Research indicates that regular activity can increase brain chemicals called endorphins that give you a sensation of feeling great after exercise such as a run. You can also help yourself feel your best by eating well and managing stress wisely (for diet and stress management strategies, see the separate chapters on nutrition and stress).

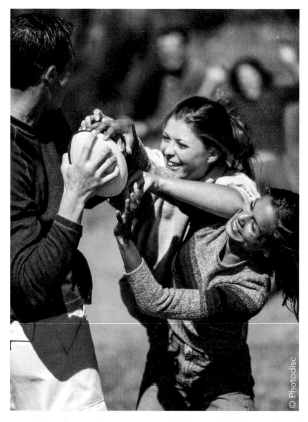

© Photodisc

Regular physical activity can help you feel good and look your best.

Learning Better

In recent years, scientists have found that you learn better if you are active, eat well, get enough sleep, and manage stress effectively. More specifically, studies show that teens who are active and fit score

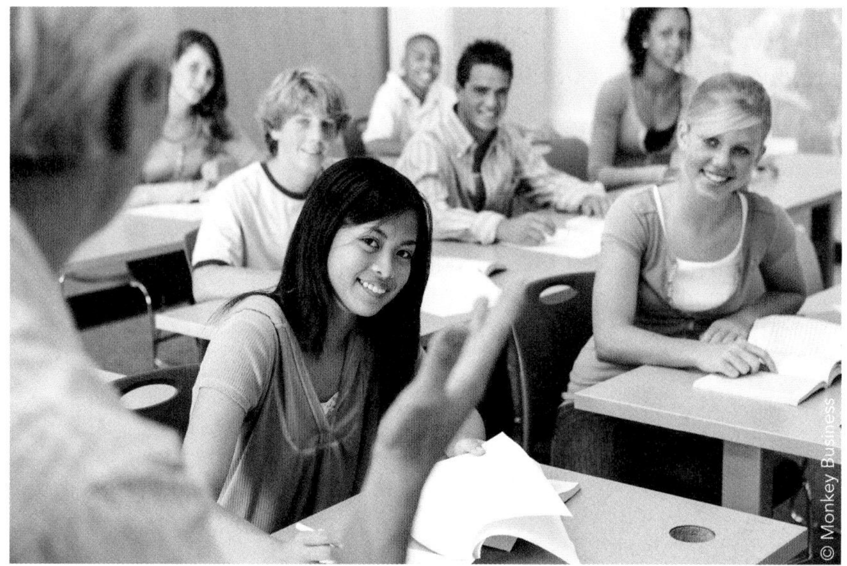

© Monkey Business

Physical activity and other healthy lifestyle choices can help you learn better.

better on tests and are less likely to be absent from school. In addition, teens who are active and eat regular healthy meals, especially breakfast, are more alert at school and less likely to be tired in the classroom. And recent studies show that regular exercise and good fitness are associated with high function in the parts of the brain that promote learning.

Enjoying Life

Everyone wants to enjoy life. But what if you're too tired on most days to participate in the activities you really like? Regular physical activity increases your physical fitness, which is the key to being able to do more of the things you want to do. People who are fit, healthy, and well are able to enjoy life to the fullest.

Meeting Emergencies

Sometimes challenging situations arise suddenly in life. You can prepare yourself to meet emergencies, as well as day-to-day demanding situations, by engaging in regular physical activity and making other healthy lifestyle choices. For example, if you're physically fit and active, you'll be able to run for help, change a flat tire, and offer various kinds of assistance to others as needed.

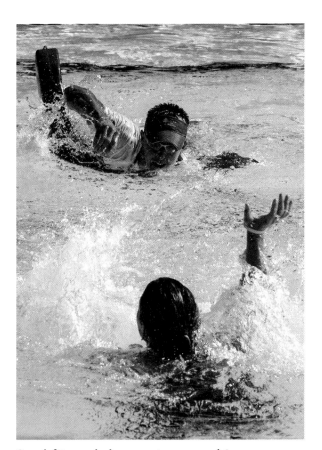

Good fitness helps you to respond in emergency situations.

Program Overview

Throughout this book, you'll learn how determinants influence your fitness, health, and wellness. We focus especially on three **priority healthy lifestyle choices** that are very important in helping you prevent disease, get and remain fit, and enjoy a good quality of life. These three choices are regular physical activity, sound nutrition, and effective stress management. The fact that these are choices means, of course, that they are largely in *your* control.

Stairway to Lifetime Fitness, Health, and Wellness

Do you live a healthy lifestyle? Do you eat well? If you eat meals at home, then you probably do eat well, but will you continue doing so when you're on your own? Are you physically active? Many teens are. But will you remain active as you grow older? Will you do the same kinds of activity you do now? If you answered no to any of these questions, you need to begin developing a lifetime plan for practicing a healthy lifestyle. One way to accomplish this goal is to climb what is called the Stairway to Lifetime Fitness, Health, and Wellness. As you can see in figure 2.2, when you climb this stairway, you move from a level of dependence to a level of independence. You move from having others make decisions for you to making good decisions on your own.

Step 1: Making Healthy Lifestyle Choices—Directed by Others

Think about the way you eat, the various physical activities you're involved in, and your other lifestyle practices—even simple things such as brushing your teeth. When you were a kid, other people made most decisions about your lifestyle at home, at school, and in the community. As you've grown older, you've started making more decisions for yourself. As an adult, you'll be almost totally responsible for making your own decisions. School programs will no longer serve as your incentive to

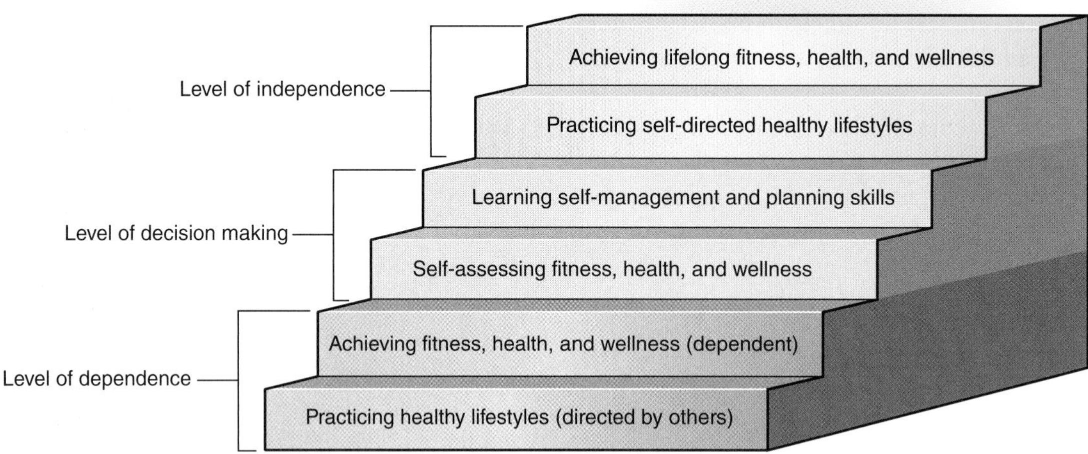

FIGURE 2.2 The Stairway to Lifetime Fitness, Health, and Wellness.

exercise, and other opportunities for physical activity will probably decrease. You'll also choose your own food. Living out the healthy lifestyle choices made for you (or facilitated) by other people is a good first step, but it's up to you to keep climbing the stairway.

Step 2: Achieving Fitness, Health, and Wellness—Dependent

The first step is about taking action based on what others expect. If you stick with the healthy living practices described in step 1, you will improve your fitness, health, and wellness (step 2). The resulting fitness, health, and wellness that you enjoy are dependent on others. In other words, you are not primarily responsible; others are. For example, if you get fit because of exercise prescribed by coaches and physical education teachers, you are dependent on them for the benefit you gain from the exercise. You may also eat well because of choices made by a parent who buys the food and prepares most or all of your meals. It's good that others help you to be active and adopt healthy lifestyles (step 1). It's also good when these lifestyles lead to fitness, health, and wellness (step 2). But it's not until you move to the third step in the stairway that you begin to make your own decisions.

Step 3: Self-Assessment

Self-assessments help you set appropriate goals, make good decisions, and become more independent. A self-assessment is an evaluation that you make of yourself. You can evaluate (self-assess) your fitness, health, and wellness, as well as the lifestyle choices that produce them. In this book, you'll try self-assessments of many kinds (one in each chapter). Once you learn to self-assess, you'll have reached the third step on the stairway. You can use the skill of self-assessment throughout your life to help you develop and implement your lifetime plan.

Step 4: Self-Management Skills and Self-Planning

Self-management skills help you implement healthy lifestyle choices that lead to good fitness, health, and wellness. One self-management skill was discussed in the previous step—self-assessment—and many others are discussed throughout part 1 of this book (one per chapter). A brief introduction to these self-management skills is provided in the next lesson of this chapter. After you've learned a variety of self-management skills, you'll be equipped to move on to the next step of the stairway.

Step 5: Practicing a Self-Directed Healthy Lifestyle

With this step, you will move to the level of decision making and problem solving. You'll have learned *why* fitness, health, and wellness are important; *what* your personal needs are; and *how* to plan for a lifetime. Because no two people have identical needs, no two people will have exactly the same program. But you will now have the necessary tools (self-management skills) to succeed in independent planning. You'll be able to develop your own personal fitness, health, and wellness programs by implementing the healthy choices discussed in part 1 of this book. In a way, then, this step is much like

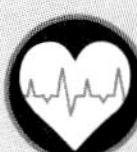

FITNESS TECHNOLOGY: Fitnessgram

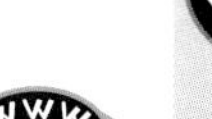

Fitnessgram is a fitness self-assessment program developed by a group of science advisors at the Cooper Institute in Dallas, Texas. The program provides instructions for assessing your fitness by using a variety of health-related test items. It also includes software that allows you to build a personal fitness report by entering your data into a computer. Fitnessgram has been adopted as the national assessment program for both the President's Council on Fitness, Sports, and Nutrition (PCFSN) and the Society of Health and Physical Educators (SHAPE America). You'll learn how to perform and practice the items in the Fitnessgram test battery in this chapter's Self-Assessment feature. Other chapters in part 1 of this book provide more information about each test item and how to determine fitness ratings using Fitnessgram.

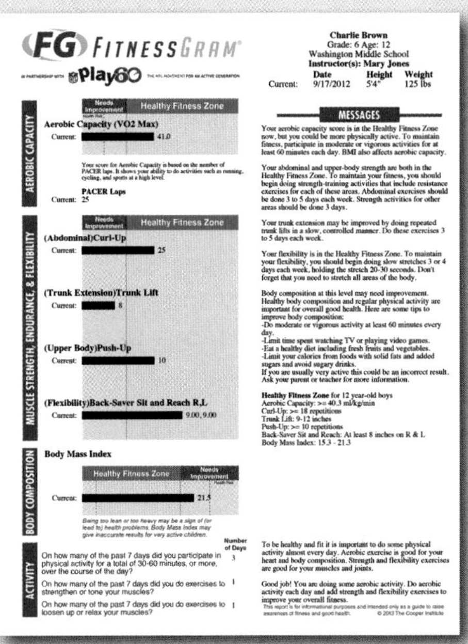

FG FITNESSGRAM®
In partnership with Play60 The NFL movement for an active generation

Charlie Brown
Grade: 6 Age: 12
Washington Middle School
Instructor(s): Mary Jones

	Date	Height	Weight
Current:	9/17/2012	5'4"	125 lbs

AEROBIC CAPACITY

Needs Improvement | Healthy Fitness Zone

Aerobic Capacity (VO2 Max)
Current: 41.0

Your score for Aerobic Capacity is based on the number of PACER laps. It shows your ability to do activities such as running, cycling, and sports at a high level.

PACER Laps
Current: 25

MUSCLE STRENGTH, ENDURANCE, & FLEXIBILITY

Needs Improvement | Healthy Fitness Zone

(Abdominal)Curl-Up
Current: 25

(Trunk Extension)Trunk Lift
Current: 8

(Upper Body)Push-Up
Current: 10

(Flexibility)Back-Saver Sit and Reach R,L
Current: 9.00, 9.00

BODY COMPOSITION

Body Mass Index

Healthy Fitness Zone | Needs Improvement

Current: 21.5

Being too lean or too heavy may be a sign of (or lead to) health problems. Body Mass Index may give inaccurate results for very active children.

ACTIVITY

	Number of Days
On how many of the past 7 days did you participate in physical activity for a total of 30-60 minutes, or more, over the course of the day?	3
On how many of the past 7 days did you do exercises to strengthen or tone your muscles?	1
On how many of the past 7 days did you do exercises to loosen up or relax your muscles?	1

MESSAGES

Your aerobic capacity score is in the Healthy Fitness Zone now, but you could be more physically active. To maintain fitness, participate in moderate or vigorous activities for at least 60 minutes each day. BMI also affects aerobic capacity.

Your abdominal and upper-body strength are both in the Healthy Fitness Zone. To maintain your fitness, you should begin doing strength-training activities that include resistance exercises for each of these areas. Abdominal exercises should be done 3 to 5 days each week. Strength activities for other areas should be done 3 days.

Your trunk extension may be improved by doing repeated trunk lifts in a slow, controlled manner. Do these exercises 3 to 5 days each week.

Your flexibility is in the Healthy Fitness Zone. To maintain your flexibility, you should begin doing slow stretches 3 or 4 days each week, holding the stretch 20-30 seconds. Don't forget that you need to stretch all areas of the body.

Body composition at this level may need improvement. Healthy body composition and regular physical activity are important for overall good health. Here are some tips to improve body composition:
-Do moderate or vigorous activity at least 60 minutes every day.
-Limit time spent watching TV or playing video games.
-Eat a healthy diet including fresh fruits and vegetables.
-Limit your calories from foods with solid fats and added sugars and avoid sugary drinks.
If you are usually very active this could be an incorrect result. Ask your parent or teacher for more information.

Healthy Fitness Zone for 12 year-old boys
Aerobic Capacity: >= 40.3 ml/kg/min
Curl-Up: >= 18 repetitions
Trunk Lift: 9-12 inches
Push-Up: >= 10 repetitions
Back-Saver Sit and Reach: At least 8 inches on R & L
Body Mass Index: 15.3 - 21.3

To be healthy and fit it is important to do some physical activity almost every day. Aerobic exercise is good for your heart and body composition. Strength and flexibility exercises are good for your muscles and joints.

Good job! You are doing some aerobic activity. Do aerobic activity each day and add strength and flexibility exercises to improve your overall fitness.

This report is for informational purposes and intended only as a guide to raise awareness of fitness and good health. © 2013 The Cooper Institute

Reprinted by permission from Fitnessgram.

Using Technology

From time to time, the Fitnessgram science advisors make changes based on new research related to the fitness test items or the method of rating fitness for each test. You can stay up to date with changes in Fitnessgram by accessing the student section of the Health Opportunities Through Physical Education website.

the first step in the stairway, but now you're making your own decisions instead of having other people make decisions for you.

Step 6: Achieving Lifelong Fitness, Health, and Wellness

When you reach the top step of the stairway, you will have taken responsibility for your own lifetime fitness, health, and wellness. You'll have moved from depending on others to making independent decisions, and you'll now implement the programs you developed in the previous step. You'll continue to use self-assessment and other self-management skills (such as self-monitoring) to modify your plans as your needs and interests change. You'll also use other self-management skills to overcome barriers that might prevent you from sticking to your plan.

Making Healthy Lifestyle Choices

This book and this class are designed to help you make healthy lifestyle choices that enable you to achieve lifetime fitness, health, and wellness. In the remaining chapters of part 1, you'll learn how to climb the stairway and reach the highest step.

Lesson Review

1. What are the five types of determinants, and which are most in your personal control?
2. What are the major benefits of healthy lifestyle choices such as regular physical activity and good nutrition?
3. What is the Stairway to Lifetime Fitness, Health, and Wellness, and how can it be used?

SELF-ASSESSMENT: Practicing Physical Fitness Tests

In part 1 of this book, you'll read about many physical fitness tests. The overall goal is to be able to select appropriate tests (self-assessments) to use both now and throughout your life. Several groups have developed physical fitness assessments specifically for young people. One of these, called Fitnessgram (see the Fitness Technology feature), is the most widely used test battery in the United States and is also used in many other countries. A test battery is a group of items designed to test several parts of fitness, and the Fitnessgram test battery assesses various parts of health-related physical fitness.

There are other test batteries in addition to Fitnessgram. The ALPHA-FIT test battery includes multiple test items that assess health-related physical fitness. It was developed in Europe and, like Fitnessgram, is used throughout the world. ALPHA-FIT contains some of the same items as Fitnessgram but also some different ones. For example, ALPHA-FIT includes the long jump and grip strength tests. These same two test items are included in the Institute of Medicine (IOM) Fitness Test Battery developed for youth fitness surveys in the United States. Recent research has shown a relationship between grip strength and long jump tests and good health.

Before using a physical fitness test, learn about the test and what it measures, then practice each test item that you plan to use. Practice helps you get better at taking the test properly, so that you're truly measuring fitness rather than just learning test-taking skills. For best results, give your best effort when doing the self-assessment. For now, the goal is not to determine a score or rating on the test items but to practice the tests so that you know how to perform them properly. Since body composition assessments are not performance tests, they don't require practice and thus are not described here, but you'll learn more about them later.

Remember that self-assessment information is personal and is considered confidential. It should not be shared with others without the permission of the person being tested. Record your results as directed by your teacher.

Test of Cardiorespiratory Endurance

PACER
(Progressive Aerobic Cardiovascular Endurance Run, or 20-meter shuttle run)

This test is included in Fitnessgram, ALPHA-FIT, and the IOM Fitness Test Battery.

1. The test objective is to run back and forth across a 20-meter (almost 22-yard) distance as many times as you can at a predetermined pace (pacing is based on signals from a special audio recording provided by your instructor).
2. Start at a line located 20 meters from a second line. When you hear the beep from the audio track, run across the 20-meter area to the second line, arriving just before the audio track beeps again, and touch the line with your foot. Turn around and get ready to run back.
3. At the sound of the next beep, run back to the line where you began. Touch the line with your foot. Make sure to wait for the beep before running back.
4. Continue to run back and forth from one line to the other, touching the line each time. The beeps will come faster and faster, causing you to run faster and faster. The test is finished when you twice fail to reach the opposite side before the beep.

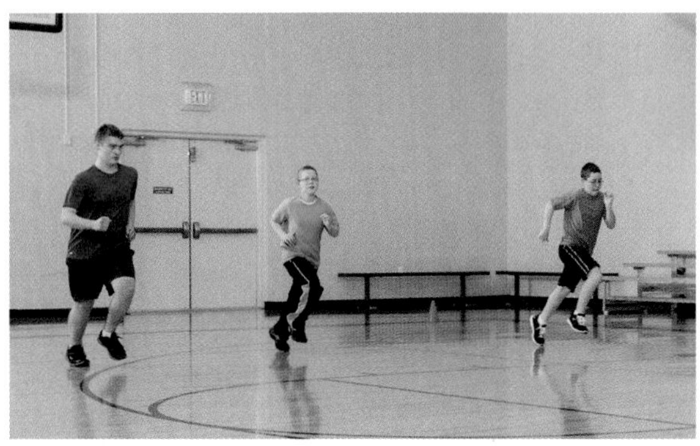

The PACER is a good test of cardiorespiratory endurance.

Practice Tips

- Practice running at the correct pace so that you arrive just before the beep that signals you to change directions.
- Practice adjusting your pace as the beeps come faster and faster.

Tests of Muscle Fitness

Curl-Up (abdominal muscle strength and muscular endurance)

This test is included in Fitnessgram.

1. Lie on your back on a mat or carpet. Bend your knees approximately 140 degrees. Your feet should be slightly apart and as far as possible from your buttocks while still allowing your feet to be flat on the floor. (The closer your feet are to your buttocks, the more difficult the movement is.) Your arms should be straight and parallel to your trunk with your palms resting on the mat.
2. Place your head on a piece of paper. The paper will help your partner judge whether your head touches down on each repetition. Place a strip of cardboard (or rubber, plastic, or tape) 4.5 inches (about 11.5 centimeters) wide and 3 feet (about 1 meter) long under your knees so that the fingers of both hands just touch the near edge of the strip. You can tape the strip down or have a partner stand on it to keep it stationary.
3. Keeping your heels on the floor, curl your shoulders up slowly and slide your arms forward so that your fingers move across the cardboard strip. Curl up until your fingertips reach the far side of the strip.
4. Slowly lower your back until your head rests on the piece of paper.
5. Repeat this procedure so that you do one curl-up every three seconds. A partner can help you by saying "up, down" every three seconds.

Practice Tips

- Practice keeping your buttocks and heels in the same location (that is, not moving them) as you do repetitions.
- Practice doing one repetition (up, down) every three seconds.
- Practice reaching to the end of the strip for each repetition.
- Practice lowering your head to the mat on each repetition.
- Next, practice as many repetitions as you can (up to 15). Have a partner check your form to make sure you are performing each curl-up correctly.

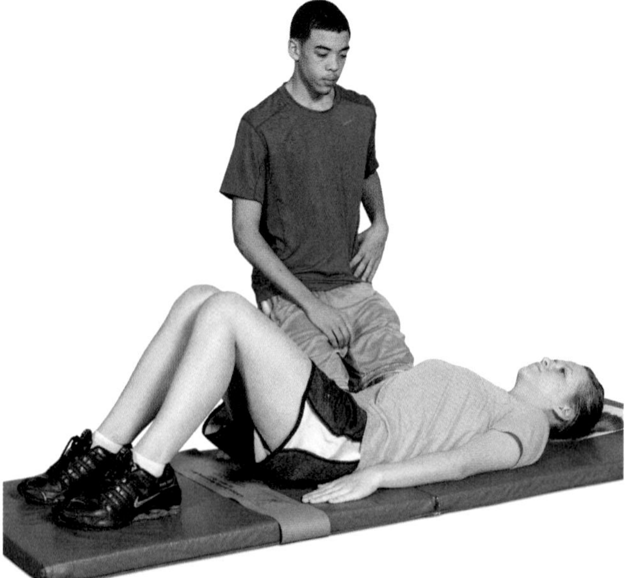

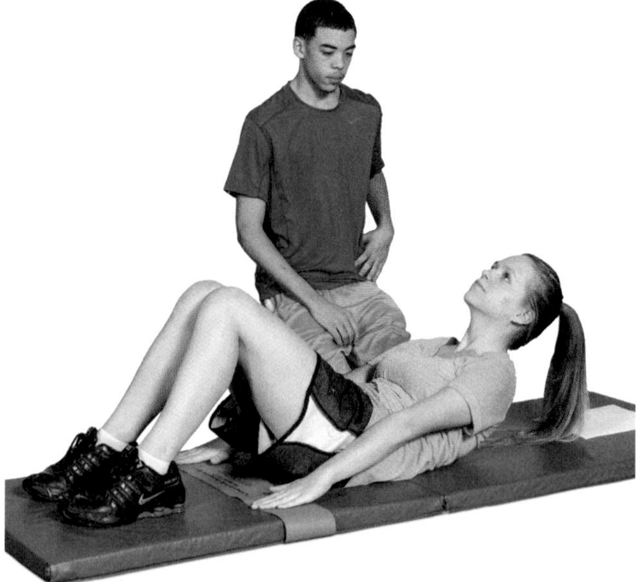

When properly performed, the curl-up is a good measure of muscle fitness of the abdominal muscles.

Push-Up (upper body strength and muscular endurance)

This test is included in Fitnessgram.

1. Lie facedown on a mat or carpet with your hands (palm down) under your shoulders, your fingers spread, and your legs straight. Your legs should be slightly apart and your toes tucked under.
2. Push up until your arms are straight. Keep your legs and back straight. Your body should form a straight line from your head to your heels.
3. Lower your body by bending your elbows until your upper arms are parallel to the floor (elbows at a 90-degree angle), then push up until your arms are fully extended. Do one push-up every three seconds. You may want to have a partner say "up, down" every three seconds to help you.

Practice Tips

- Practice lowering until your elbows are bent at 90 degrees. You may want to have a partner hold a yardstick parallel to the floor (at the elbow) to help you determine when your elbows are properly bent.
- Practice pushing up all the way so that your arms are at full extension at the top of each push-up.
- Practice doing one repetition (up, down) every three seconds.
- Next, practice as many repetitions as you can (up to 15). Have a partner check your form to make sure you are performing each push-up correctly.

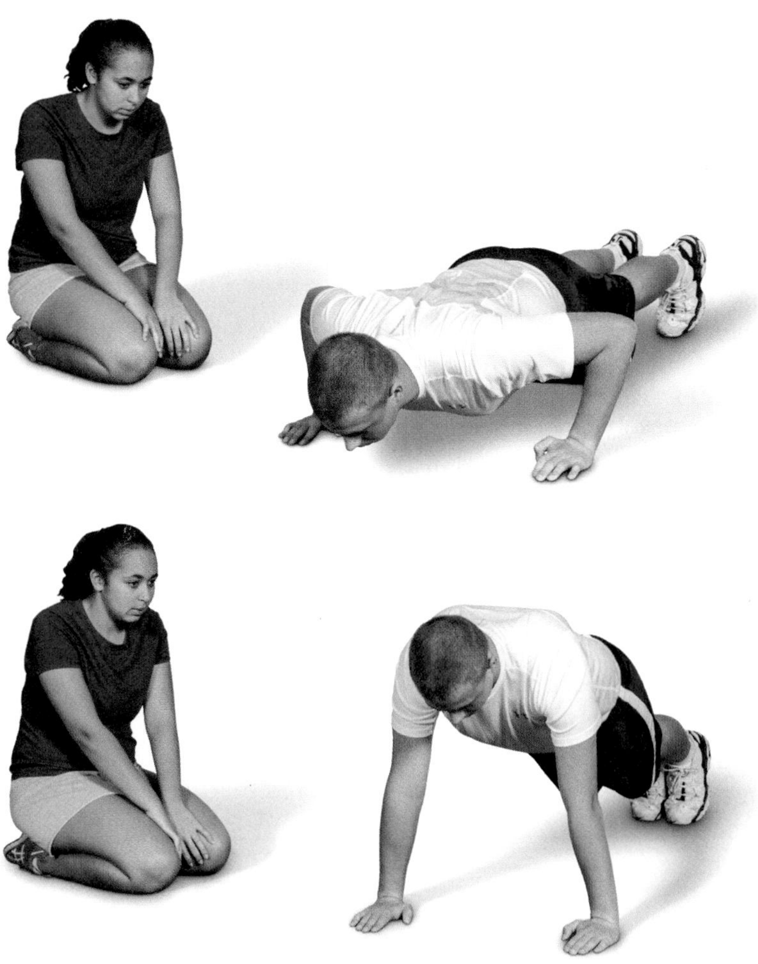

The 90-degree push-up is a measure of muscle fitness of the upper body.

Handgrip Strength (isometric hand and arm strength)

This test is included in ALPHA-FIT and the IOM Fitness Test Battery.

1. Use a dynamometer to measure isometric strength. Adjust the dynamometer to fit your hand size.
2. Squeeze as hard as possible for two to five seconds. Your arm should be extended with your elbow nearly straight. Do not touch your body with your arm or hand.
3. Repeat with each hand. Alternate hands to allow a rest between each attempt.
4. Results are most often reported in kilograms (a kilogram equals about 2.2 pounds). To get your score in pounds, multiply your score in kilograms by 2.2.

Practice Tips

- Try the grip at different settings to see which enables you to perform the best.
- Try bending your knees a bit as you squeeze to help maintain good balance, which may help your score.

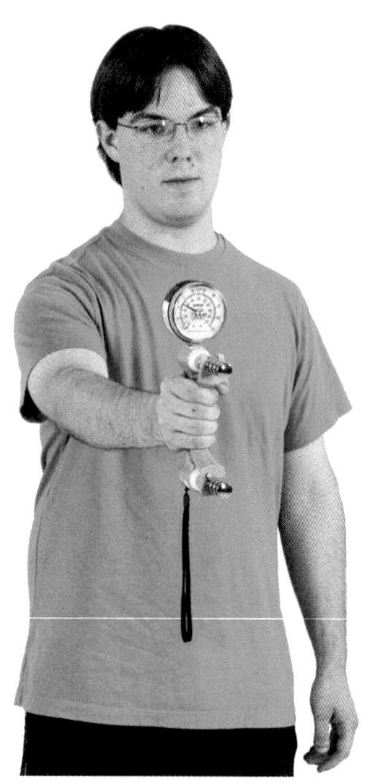

The handgrip strength test measures muscle fitness, and scores are related to total body strength.

Standing Long Jump (leg power, or explosive strength)

This test is included in ALPHA-FIT and the IOM Fitness Test Battery.

1. Use masking tape or another material to make the necessary line on the floor.
2. Stand with your feet shoulder-width apart behind the line on the floor. Bend your knees and hold your arms straight in front of your body at shoulder height.
3. Swing your arms downward and backward, then vigorously forward as you jump forward as far as possible, extending your legs.
4. Land on both feet and try to maintain your balance on landing. Do not run or hop before jumping.

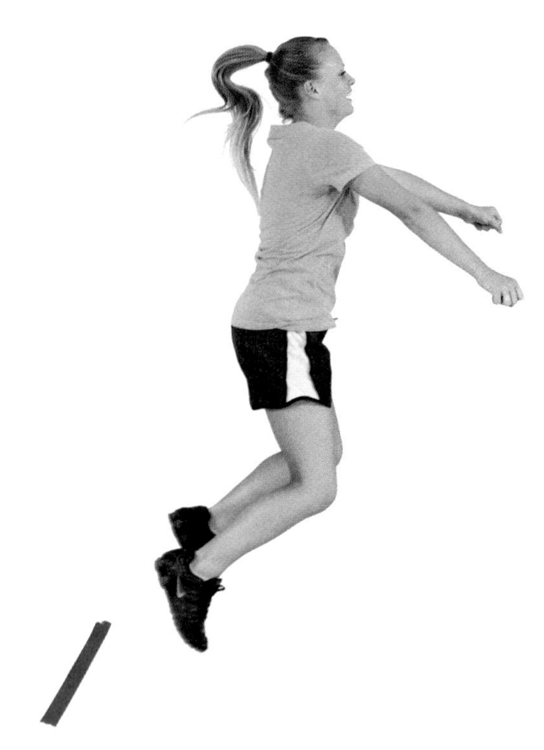

The standing long jump is a test of power (explosive strength).

Practice Tips

- For best performance, lean forward just before you jump. Practice to get the best timing of the lean followed by the forward arm swing just before you jump.
- Try the test several times so that you can land without losing your balance. To help you avoid falling when you land, keep your arms extended in front of you. Also bend your knees when you land to help you absorb the shock of landing and to help you maintain your balance.
- Try bending your knees more or less before different jumps to see which amount of knee bend gives you the best jump.

Test of Muscle Fitness and Flexibility

Trunk Lift (back muscle fitness and back and trunk muscle flexibility)

This test is included in Fitnessgram.

1. Lie facedown with your arms at your sides and your hands under or just beside your thighs.
2. Lift the upper part of your body very slowly so that your chin, chest, and shoulders come off the floor. Lift your trunk as high as possible, to a maximum of 12 inches (30 centimeters). Hold this position for three seconds while a partner measures how far your chin is from the floor. Your partner should hold the ruler at least 1 inch (2.5 centimeters) in front of your chin. Look straight ahead so that your chin is not tipped abnormally upward.

Caution: The ruler should not be placed directly under your chin, in case you have to lower your trunk unexpectedly.

Practice Tips

- Practice lifting your trunk 12 inches (30 centimeters) off the floor. Hold the trunk off the floor at 12 inches (do not lift higher) for three seconds.
- Practice three to five times to see if you are able to hold the lift for the required three seconds.
- Practice looking straight ahead so that your chin is not tipped up.

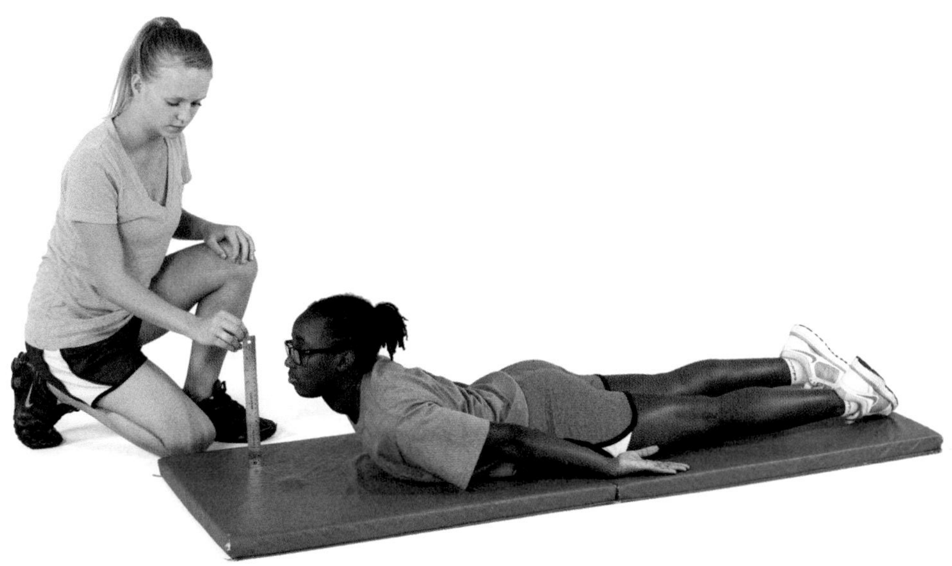

The trunk lift measures muscle fitness of the back and trunk muscles as well as flexibility.

Test of Flexibility

Back-Saver Sit-and-Reach (range of motion, or flexibility, of the hip)

This test is included in Fitnessgram.

1. Place a measuring stick, such as a yardstick or meter stick, on top of a box that is 12 inches (30 centimeters) high with the stick extending 9 inches (23 centimeters) over the box and the lower numbers toward you. You may use a flexibility testing box if one is available.
2. To measure the flexibility of your right leg, fully extend it and place your right foot flat against the box. Bend your left leg, with the knee turned out and your left foot 2 to 3 inches (5 to 8 centimeters) to the side of your straight right leg.
3. Extend your arms forward over the measuring stick. Place your hands on the stick, one on top of the other, with your palms facing down. Your middle fingers should be together with the tip of one finger exactly on top of the other.
4. Lean forward slowly; do not bounce. Reach forward with your arms and fingers, then slowly return to the starting position. Repeat four times. On the fourth reach, hold the position for three seconds and observe the measurement on the stick below your fingertips.
5. Repeat with your left leg.

Practice Tips

- Do the PACER practice or another general warm-up before practicing this test.
- Practice keeping your extended leg straight (a very slight bend is okay).
- Practice keeping your other leg bent and the foot of that leg about 2 to 3 inches (5 to 8 centimeters) from your straight leg.
- Practice keeping one middle finger on top of the other.
- Practice holding your stretch for three seconds.
- Practice three to five times with each leg.

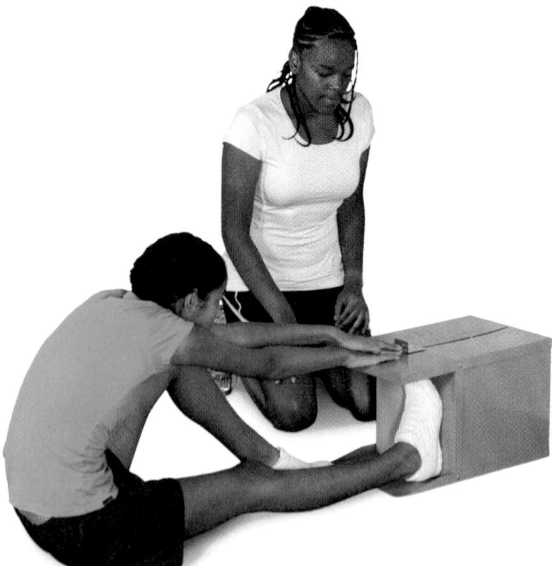

The back-saver sit-and-reach measures flexibility (range of motion) of the hip.

Lesson 2.2

Learning Self-Management Skills

Lesson Objectives

After reading this lesson, you should be able to

1. describe the stages of change in adopting a healthy lifestyle,
2. describe several self-management skills, and
3. explain how to use self-management skills for living a healthy life.

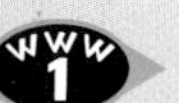

Lesson Vocabulary

exercise, motor skill, physical activity, sedentary, skill

In the first lesson of this chapter, you learned about what it means to live a healthy lifestyle. You also learned about many determinants of health, fitness, and wellness. In this lesson, you'll learn about making lifestyle changes to enhance your fitness, health, and wellness. First, you'll learn about the stages of change. People do not change overnight; change takes time, and people who are making a change typically progress through five stages. These stages were identified by psychologists working to help people stop smoking. They found that most smokers do not quit all at once but go through stages instead. Later, exercise psychologists and nutrition scientists found that these five stages of change apply to other lifestyle choices, such as physical activity and nutrition. Understanding these stages can help you make positive changes in your lifestyle.

FIT FACT

Physical activity refers to movement that uses your large muscles. Thus it includes a wide range of pursuits, such as sport, dance, recreational activities, and activities of daily living. Exercise is a form of physical activity specifically designed to improve your fitness.

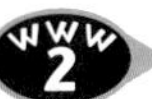

Stages of Change for a Healthy Lifestyle

Healthy lifestyle behaviors—such as being active, eating well, and managing stress—are within your control. With effort, most anyone can make healthy lifestyle changes in these areas. There are five stages of change for modifying behaviors to improve fitness, health, and wellness: precontemplation (not thinking of change), contemplation, planning for change, taking action to change, and maintenance. Figure 2.3 shows the five stages of change for physical activity.

- **Precontemplation:** A person at stage 1 chooses not to be active. Another word for being inactive is **sedentary**, and more than one-third of all adults are sedentary and thus are included in this stage. You might think there are no sedentary teens, but there are. It's true that this category includes fewer teens than adults, but nearly one in four teens can also be included here. In an ideal world, all people would be active exercisers, but sometimes people move slowly from one stage to the next.
- **Contemplation:** A sedentary person might read about the importance of physical activity and even start to think about being active—but take no action. This person has moved from being sedentary to being an inactive thinker (stage 2). An inactive thinker does little physical activity but is thinking about becoming active.
- **Planning:** At stage 3, a person starts planning to be active. For example, he or she might visit an exercise facility or buy a new tennis racket. The person has now become a planner, even though he or she is not yet active.

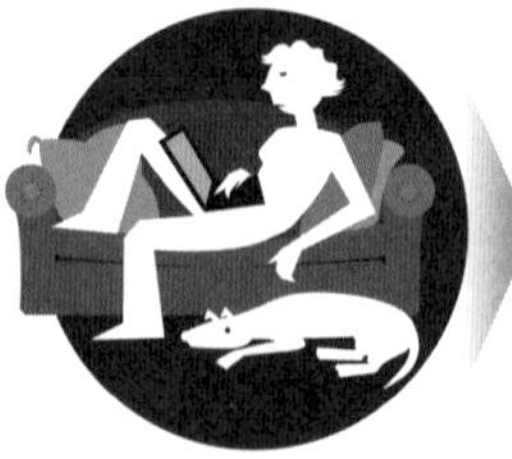
Sedentary
I'm inactive, and I plan to stay that way.

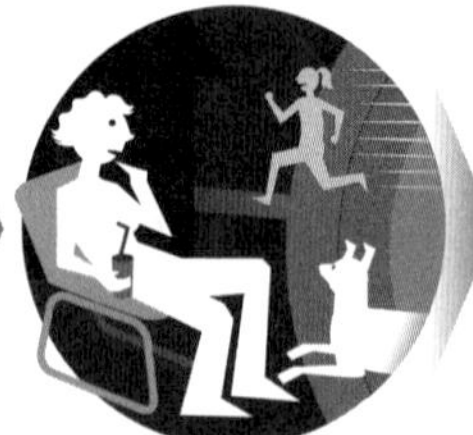
Inactive thinker
I'm inactive, but I'm thinking about becoming active.

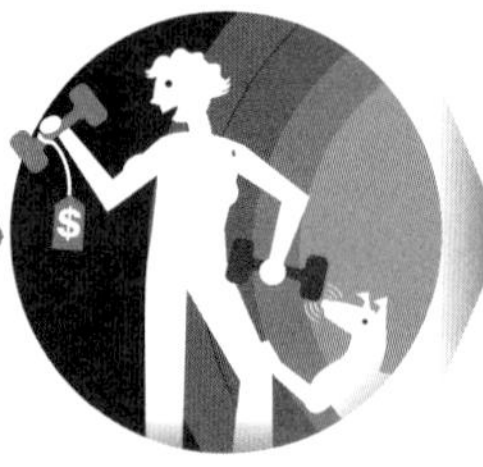
$
Planner
I'm taking steps to start to be active.

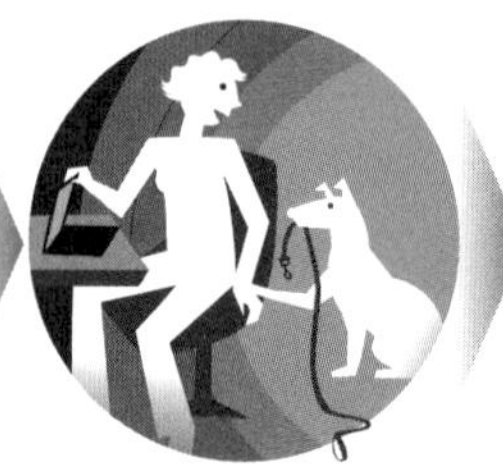
Activator
I'm active, but not yet as active as I should be.

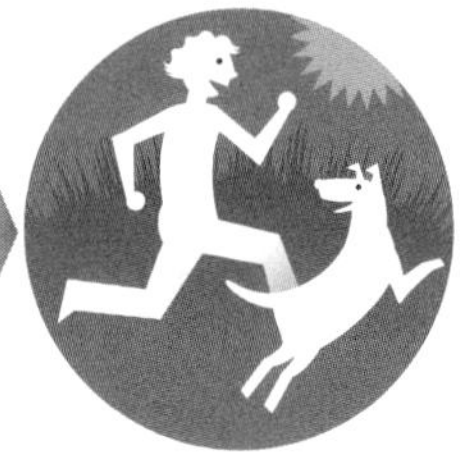
Active exerciser
I'm regularly active and have been for some time!

FIGURE 2.3 The five stages of change for physical activity.

- **Taking action:** Stage 4 involves actually becoming active. The person, now an activator, goes to the exercise facility to work out, for example, or plays tennis with a friend.
- **Maintenance:** Stage 5 involves maintaining regular activity. The ultimate goal is to help all people progress to the stage of the active exerciser (stage 5). When this stage is reached, a person is active on a regular basis for a long time (at least several months).

The same five stages of change apply to other healthy lifestyle choices. For example, figure 2.4 shows the stages as they might relate to eating well. Only about 1 in every 4 teens eats the recommended number of fruits and vegetables each day, and about 1 in 10 have avoided eating meals for as long as 24 hours. Teens who do not eat well are at stage 1, whereas those who do eat well on a regular basis are at stage 5. For any healthy lifestyle choice, the goal is to move to stage 5.

Living a healthy lifestyle means making good choices in various areas of your life. You can be at one level of change in one area and at another level in a different area. For example, perhaps you're not active on a regular basis but are thinking about becoming more active; therefore, you're at stage 2 for physical activity. At the same time, you might regularly eat well and therefore be at stage 5 for healthy eating.

FIT FACT

Changes in behavior don't always occur from stage 1 to 5 without interruption. Sometimes people move forward a few stages, then fall back a stage, and then move forward again. With effort, progress is made gradually from one stage to another.

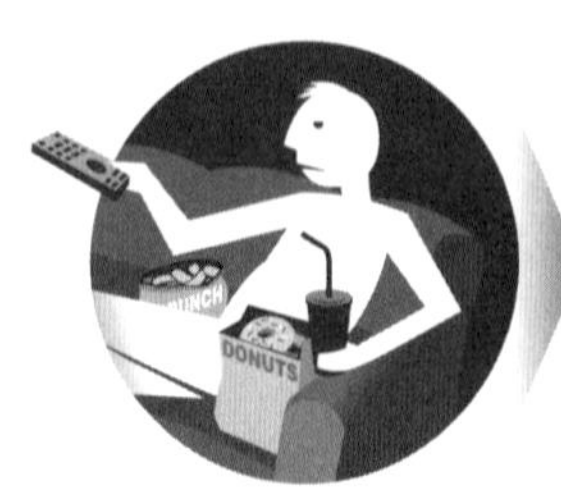
DONUTS
Unhealthy eater
I don't eat well, and I don't plan to.

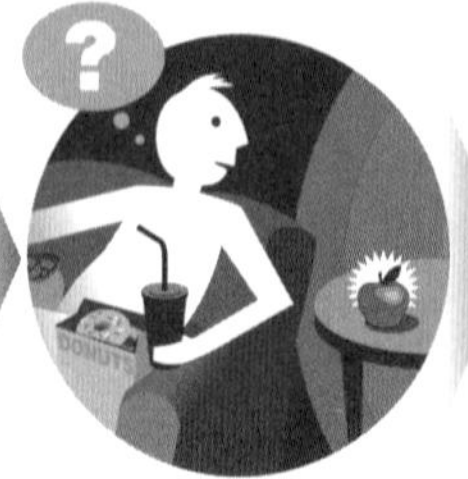
?
DONUTS
Thinker
I don't eat well, but I'm thinking about eating better.

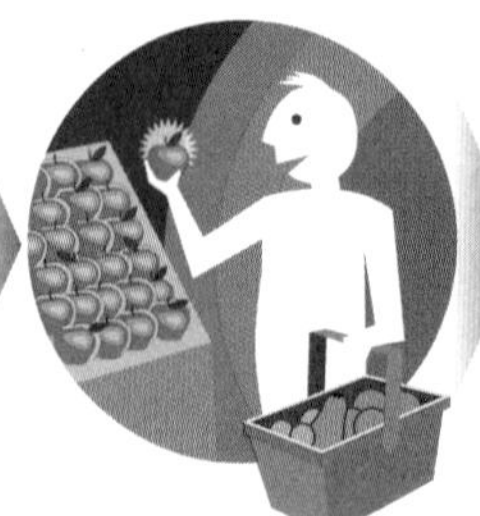
Planner
I'm taking steps to eat better.

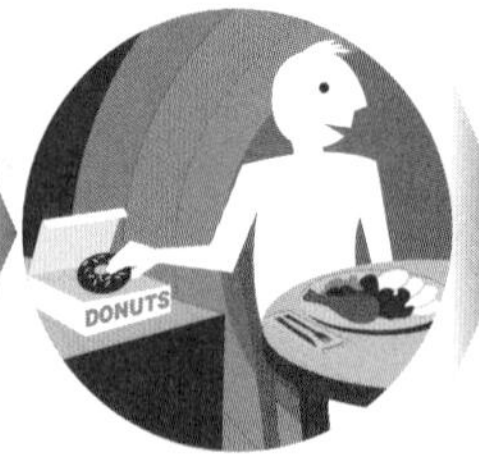
DONUTS
Improved eater
I eat well some of the time, but I need to do better.

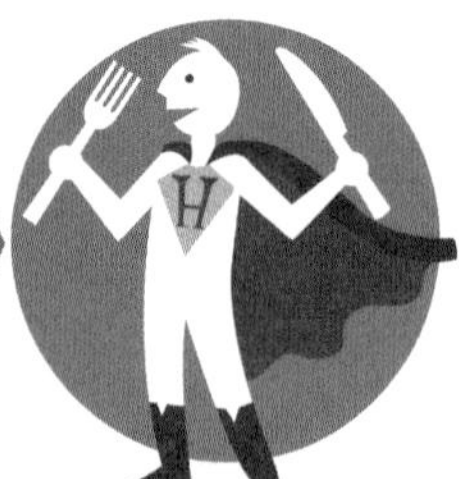
H
Healthy eater
I regularly eat healthy meals and avoid empty calories.

FIGURE 2.4 The five stages of change for eating well.

Self-Management Skills: Adopting a Healthy Lifestyle

How do you change your lifestyle? How do you move from stage 1 to stage 5 for being active or eating well?

The best way is to learn self-management skills for change. A **skill** is an ability that allows you to perform a specific task effectively. You improve your skills through practice. For example, writing and typing are skills that help you communicate; if you practice them, you get better at doing them. Similarly, **motor skills**—such as throwing, kicking, and catching—help you perform better in sports and games. They also improve with practice.

Self-management skills are abilities that help you change your lifestyles. There are three kinds: those that help you begin to change, those that help you make change, and those that help you maintain change (see figure 2.5).

> "Happiness lies, first of all, in health."
>
> —George William Curtis, author and social reformer

Skills That Help You Think About Change

Table 2.1 lists the names and descriptions of 21 self-management skills. Some of these are especially helpful to people who need to make changes but have not begun a plan of action (people in stages 1 and 2). *Self-assessment* skills, for example, help you see that you need to make changes and determine what changes to make. *Building knowledge and understanding* helps you see why it is important to change. Knowing the benefits of healthy lifestyle choices—such as being active and eating right—can also motivate you to make positive changes. More specifically, *identifying risk factors* for disease helps you see the need to adopt a healthy lifestyle not only for now but also for your future.

Two other self-management skills that help you begin to change are *positive attitude* and *self-confidence*. If you think you can make a change and you feel good about the change, then you're more likely to be motivated to actually do it! You'll learn more about the self-management skills that help you start making changes as you progress through part 1 of this book.

Skills That Help You Make Changes

Once you have reached stage 3 of the change process, you're ready to take action, but you must

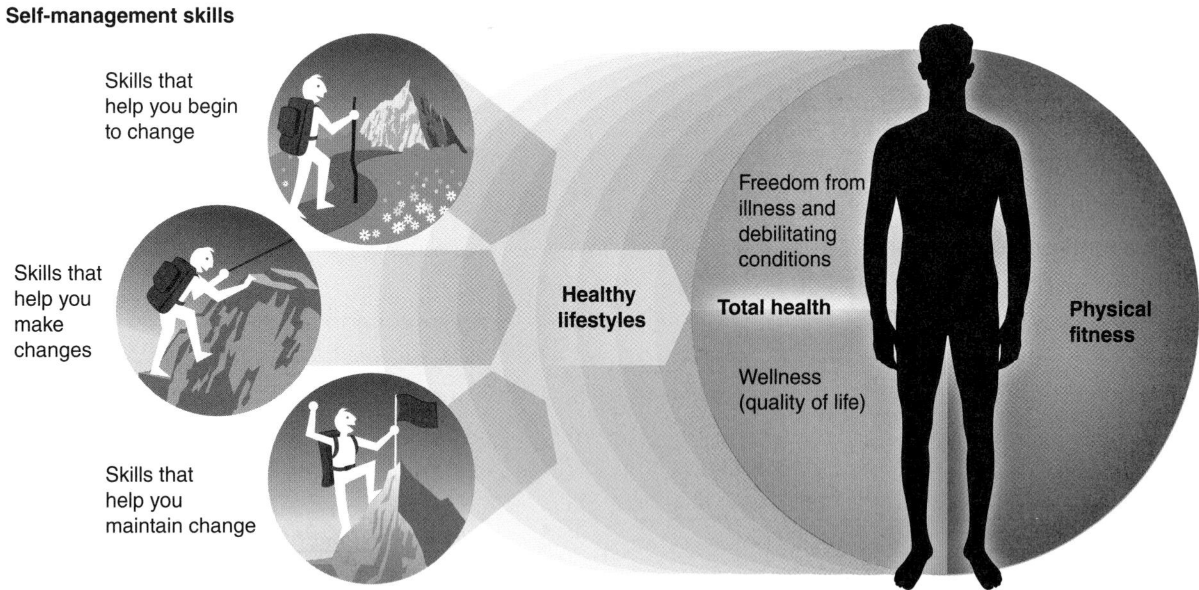

FIGURE 2.5 Self-management skills help you change your lifestyles to improve your fitness, health, and wellness.

TABLE 2.1 Self-Management Skills for Fitness, Health, and Wellness

	Skill	Description
		Skills that help you think about change
1	Self-assessment	This skill helps you see where you are and what to change in order to get where you want to be.
2	Building knowledge and understanding	You can use a modified form of the scientific method to solve problems—such as how to make healthy changes in your life.
3	Identifying risk factors	Identifying your health risks enables you to assess and then reduce them.
4	Positive attitude	This skill helps position you to succeed in adopting healthy lifestyles.
5	Self-confidence	This skill helps you build the feeling that you're capable of making healthy changes in your lifestyles.
		Skills that help you make changes
1	Goal setting and self-planning	These skills create a foundation for developing your personal plan by setting goals that are SMART (specific, measurable, attainable, realistic, and timely) and preparing a written schedule.
2	Time management	This skill helps you be efficient so that you have time for the important things in your life.
3	Choosing good activities	This skill involves selecting the activities that are best for you personally so that you will enjoy and benefit from doing them.
4	Learning performance skills	This skill helps you to perform well and with confidence. For example, learning motor skills helps you become active, learning stress management skills helps you avoid or reduce stress, and learning nutrition skills helps you eat well.
5	Improving self-perception	This skill helps you think positively about yourself so that you're more likely to make healthy lifestyle choices and feel that they will make a difference in your life.
6	Stress management	This skill involves preventing or coping with the stresses of daily life.
		Skills that help you maintain changes
1	Self-monitoring	This skill involves keeping records (logs) to see whether you are in fact doing what you think you're doing.
2	Overcoming barriers	This skill helps you find ways to stay active despite barriers, such as lack of time, temporary injury, lack of safe places to be active, inclement weather, and difficulty in selecting healthy foods.
3	Finding social support	This skill enables you to get help and support from others (such as your friends and family) as you adopt healthy behaviors and work to stick with them.
4	Saying no	This skill helps keep you from doing things you don't want to do, especially when you're under pressure from friends or other people.
5	Preventing relapse	This skill helps you stick with healthy behaviors even when you have problems getting motivated.
6	Thinking critically	This skill enables you to find and interpret information that helps you make good decisions and solve problems in living a healthy lifestyle.
7	Resolving conflicts	This skill helps you solve problems and avoid stress.
8	Positive self-talk	This skill helps you perform your best and make healthy lifestyle choices such as being active by thinking positive thoughts rather than negative ones that detract from success.
9	Developing good strategy and tactics	This skill helps you focus on a specific plan of action and successfully execute the plan.
10	Finding success	Finding success is not technically a skill, but it comes from using a variety of self-management skills to change behavior. If you use the self-management skills described here and believe that they will help you succeed, you are much more likely to achieve success.

know how to take the *right* action. Six of the self-management skills help you begin to actually make the lifestyle changes that are right for you (see table 2.1). *Goal setting and self-planning* skills help you design a plan for change. *Time management* skills help you make time for carrying out your personal plan. Goal setting, self-planning, and time management skills apply to all types of lifestyle change.

Other self-management skills that help you become more active are *choosing good activities* and *learning performance skills*. As you do so, the skill of *improving self-perception* helps you think positively about yourself. Also, people who think positively and know how to *manage stress* are more likely to make changes because they believe that change is possible and aren't worried about confronting change.

Skills That Help You Maintain Changes

The remaining self-management skills presented in table 2.1 help you stick with your healthy lifestyle changes. Once you've made a lifestyle change (that is, achieved stage 4 or 5 in that area of your life), these skills help you stay there. *Self-monitoring* helps you track your progress. You can also learn to *overcome barriers*, *find support from others*, and *say no* to those who might deter you. And you can learn specific skills that help keep you from quitting your healthy lifestyle (*preventing relapse*).

Several other skills can also help you stay on the right track. Learning to *think critically* helps you make good decisions and avoid mistakes that can hurt your health. Learning to *resolve conflicts* helps you avoid stress. Using *positive self-talk* and *good strategy and tactics* helps you *find success* so that you are much more likely to stick with your lifestyle plan.

This book is intended to help you live an active, healthy life. To accomplish this goal, you must learn about and practice each of the self-management skills listed in table 2.1.

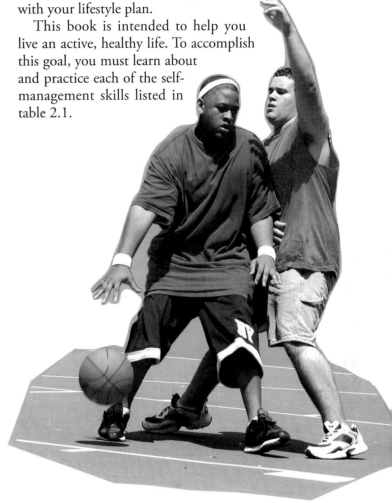

Lesson Review

1. What are the five stages of change, and how are they useful to you?
2. What are some examples of self-management skills for each of the different stages of change?
3. How can you use self-management skills for living a healthy life?

TAKING CHARGE: Building Knowledge and Understanding

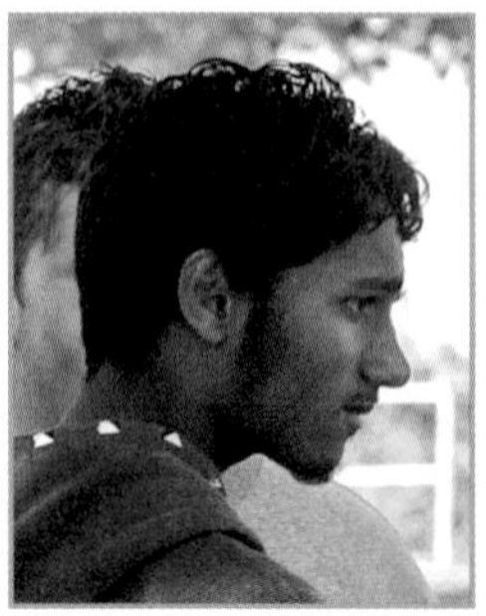

Anish's mother, Mrs. Bhalla, made a New Year's resolution to be more active. She did not know a lot about how to exercise, so she searched the web for information about fitness programs. She found a website with the following claim: "Get fit in five minutes a day without getting sweaty!" Anish was concerned because he had learned in class that it takes weeks of regular exercise to improve fitness.

Anish told his mom, "I think you need to get more knowledge and understanding about fitness and physical activity before you get started." But his mother decided to try the plan. Several months later, her fitness had not improved, and she felt discouraged.

At this point, she talked with Anish about the fitness and activity strategies he was learning at school. They both decided that it was important for her to gain good knowledge about fitness before trying a new program. Anish had also learned the value of understanding the "why" of exercise if a person wants to get best results: Why should I exercise (what are the benefits)? Why is this plan best for me (what are my personal needs)?

Anish and his mother agreed that she would learn along with him as he studied fitness and physical activity at school so that she could do things right the next time she tried.

For Discussion

Mrs. Bhalla made one good decision and one bad decision. How can someone who wants to make a healthy New Year's resolution avoid making a bad decision about fitness and physical activity? Why do you think people choose programs such as the one Mrs. Bhalla tried? Is it possible to get fit in five minutes a day? How might Anish help his mother in the future? Consider the guidelines presented in the following Self-Management feature as you answer these discussion questions.

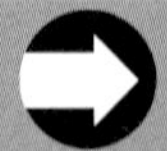

SELF-MANAGEMENT: Skills for Building Knowledge and Understanding

Knowledge based on sound information can help you make good decisions. But knowledge alone does not always lead to good decisions. You must understand the information you take in. A person with knowledge knows facts, but a person with understanding comprehends the significance of the facts and can use that understanding to make good decisions.

In this book, you learn knowledge about fitness, health, and wellness. You also build higher-level understanding that helps you apply the information you've learned. The following guidelines will help you use this book to build both your knowledge and your understanding.

- **Learn the facts first.** Learning the facts is a necessary first step toward building higher-level understanding.
- **Use the scientific method.** Investigate (collect information) to gain as many facts as possible. The facts help you analyze and test hypotheses. For example, you might have a hypothesis that you can get fit in five minutes a day. After gaining the facts and analyzing them, you would learn that the hypothesis is false. The scientific method helps you understand the information you learn and make sound decisions.
- **Ask why.** When studying healthy lifestyle choices, ask yourself "why" questions: Why do I need this? Why should I believe this information? Why will this information be beneficial?
- **Consult reliable sources.** Whether you're consulting a website, magazine

article, or book, check with trusted people to help you find good sources. Your knowledge and understanding are only as good as the sources you use. The chapter titled Making Good Consumer Choices provides more information about how to find reliable source material.

- **Try to apply.** When learning new information, ask, "How can I apply this?" Applying new information to real situations helps you understand it, which in turn helps you apply it more effectively. For example, regarding the dangers of fat in your diet, ask yourself questions like these: What else do I need to know? How much fat is too much? What changes can I make in my diet to reduce my fat intake?
- **Put it all together.** When you learn about something new, you often find many pieces of information. Taking time to fit the pieces together will help you make sense of what you've learned. Another word for "putting all the facts together" is *synthesizing*. For example, if you know you feel stressed out, and you know that there are several reasons for the stress, how do you use all of the information together—synthesize it—to make a good decision?

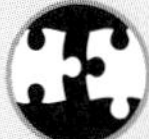

ACADEMIC CONNECTION: Accurate Use of Words

English language arts is an area of academic study that focuses on preparing students who are college and career ready in reading, writing, speaking, listening, and language. Learning to use words accurately and knowing how similar words differ are important in the study of the English language and in achieving literacy (being educated).

In this chapter, and in other parts of this book, factors influencing fitness, health, and wellness are discussed. Health experts typically refer to the factors as determinants. The word *sex* is used throughout the book to describe whether you are biologically male or female. Your sex is one determinant that influences your fitness, health, and wellness. The word *gender* has a similar but slightly different meaning. It refers to social or cultural roles of people (masculine or feminine). For example, in the past some activities were identified as gender appropriate for males only (masculine) or females only (feminine). Over time, stereotypes have diminished, opening up more activity opportunities for both males and females. In this book, activities are not identified as masculine or feminine. Activities are considered appropriate for both sexes (male and female). *Gender* is also a word used in grammar to categorize pronouns (such as *he* or *she*) and other parts of speech.

The use of words sometimes changes over time. In recent years the word *gender* has been used more frequently to indicate a person's sex (male or female). In the sciences, the preferred term is *sex* rather than *gender* when indicating whether a person is male or female, and for this reason *sex* is the term used in this book (in this context).

TAKING ACTION: Fitness Trails

Fresh air, nature, and fitness? Yes, please! Most communities have natural spaces where you can walk, jog, run, or bike. Some communities have also created fitness trails—pathways through parks or woodlands designed especially for walking, jogging, and running. Some fitness trails include human-made or natural structures intended for particular exercises. These structures allow walkers, joggers, and runners to mix their movement activity with muscle fitness and flexibility exercises. Fitness trails are sometimes considered "outdoor gyms," and there's probably one near you!

Take action by learning about, visiting, or even helping create a fitness trail near you. Many fitness trails are already well established by city or county park and recreation departments or federal agencies such as the U.S. National Park Service. Although they may differ from remote trails, urban areas can have fitness trails.

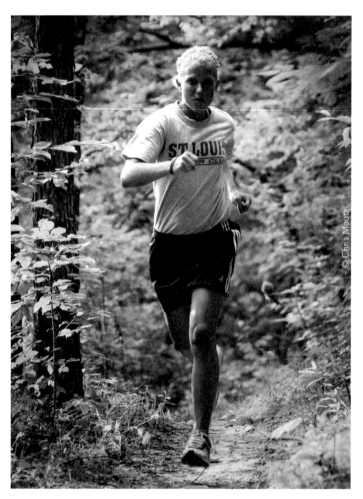

Being outdoors dramatically increases the amount of activity that people perform.

Reviewing Concepts and Vocabulary

As directed by your teacher, answer items 1 through 5 by correctly completing each sentence with a word or phrase.

1. Factors that affect your fitness, health, and wellness are called ______________.
2. Factors influencing fitness, health, and wellness over which you have little control are called ______________.
3. Factors influencing fitness, health, and wellness over which you have the most control are called ______________.
4. The steps that lead you from dependence to independence are referred to together as the ______________.
5. The fitness test used to assess cardiorespiratory endurance by running when signaled by a beep is called the ______________.

For items 6 through 10, as directed by your teacher, match each term in column 1 with the appropriate phrase in column 2.

6. sedentary person	a. just bought exercise equipment
7. inactive thinker	b. is active most days of the week
8. planner	c. is sometimes active
9. activator	d. is considering becoming active
10. active exerciser	e. is inactive

For items 11 through 15, as directed by your teacher, respond to each statement or question.

11. Explain what a self-management skill is and why it can be useful.
12. What are some of the fitness test items used in major fitness test batteries such as Fitnessgram, and what do they measure?
13. Describe the five stages of change.
14. What are fitness trails, and how can they be useful in staying active?
15. What are some guidelines for building knowledge and understanding?

Thinking Critically

Write a paragraph to answer the following question.

Of all the self-management skills described in lesson 2, which one would most help *you* be more active or eat better? Give the reasons for your answer.

Project

Assume that you are the head of a marketing company assigned to create an ad campaign promoting healthier eating and more active living. Prepare a script for a television commercial for the promotion. If resources are available, create a video of the commercial.

3

Goal Setting and Program Planning

In This Chapter

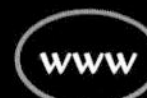

Student Web Resources

www.HOPEtextbook.org/student

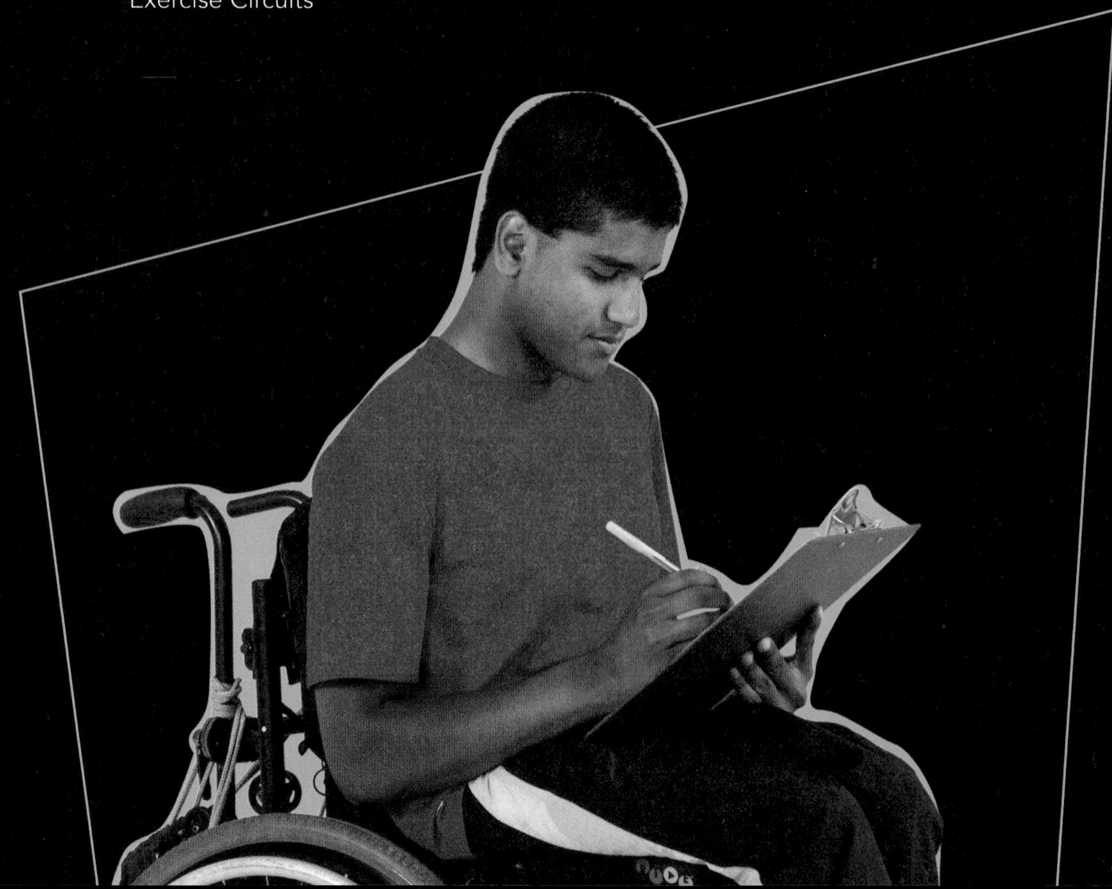

Lesson 3.1

Goal Setting

Lesson Objectives

After reading this lesson, you should be able to

1. explain the SMART formula for setting goals,
2. explain how long-term and short-term goals differ, and
3. describe process and product goals and explain how they differ.

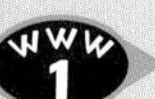

Lesson Vocabulary

acronym, goal setting, long-term goal, mnemonic, process goal, product goal, short-term goal, SMART goal

How do you turn your dreams into realities? Successful people use **goal setting** as part of their overall planning to achieve success; they decide ahead of time what they plan to accomplish, then go about doing it. You can use goals to plan a personal fitness program, a program of good eating, or any other type of program. In this lesson, you'll learn to use long-term and short-term goals. You'll also learn about other goals that can help you make good lifestyle choices, such as being physically active and eating well.

SMART Goals

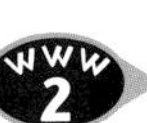

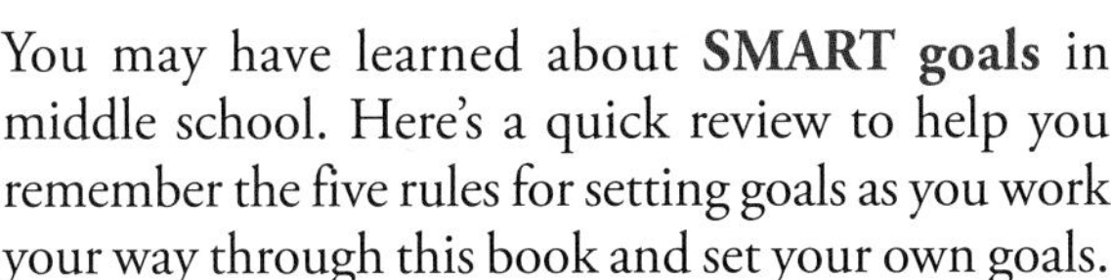

You may have learned about **SMART goals** in middle school. Here's a quick review to help you remember the five rules for setting goals as you work your way through this book and set your own goals.

S = specific. Your goal should include details of what you want to accomplish.

M = measurable. You should be able to measure your progress and accurately determine whether you've accomplished your goal.

A = attainable. Your goals should challenge you. They should not be too easy or too hard.

R = realistic. You should be able to reach your goal if you put in the time and effort and have the necessary resources.

T = timely. Your goal should be useful to you at this time in your life and can be met in the time allotted.

FIT FACT

A **mnemonic** (pronounced ni-mon'-ik) is a trick for remembering something. The mnemonic SMART helps us remember five guidelines for creating goals. Specifically, SMART is an **acronym**, which means that each letter in the word is the first letter of a key word related to goal setting.

SMART Long-Term Goals

Long-term goals take you months or even years to accomplish, whereas you can reach **short-term goals** in a short time, such as a few days or weeks. One example of a long-term goal is saving money to help pay for college expenses. If you plan to save $2,400, you could make your long-term goal earning that amount.

In order to earn that much, you might have to work on weekends and during summers throughout high school. Saving money takes time. If your job allowed you to save $100 a month, it would take you two years to save the $2,400. Now let's see whether this would be a SMART goal.

Specific. $2,400 is a very specific long-term goal. You know the amount of money you need.

Measurable. The $2,400 goal is measurable. You can count your money to see how close you are to reaching your goal.

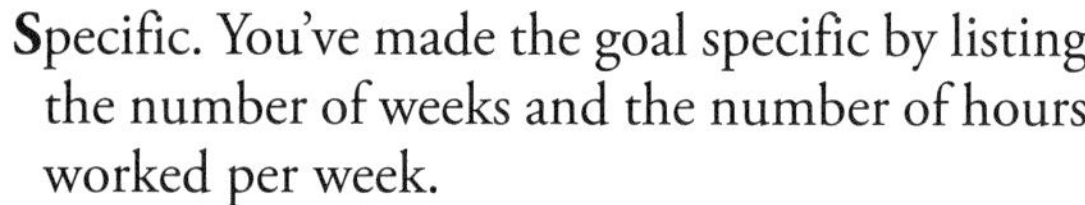

Attainable. The goal might be too hard for a person without a job, but you have one. It won't be easy, but you make enough money each hour to make your goal possible.

Realistic. For someone else, the $2,400 goal might not be realistic. But if you put in the time and stick with your job, saving $100 a month for two years is possible. You must also consider other commitments, such as homework, activities, and family responsibilities.

Timely. The goal of saving $2,400 in two years has a specific and workable time line that fits your planned entrance into college.

SMART Short-Term Goals

Short-term goals can usually be reached in a few days or weeks. Thus you might set a series of short-term goals to help you accomplish a long-term goal. For example, to meet your long-term goal of saving $2,400, you might set a short-term goal of working five hours a week at $8 an hour for two weeks. Doing so would be a manageable way to start working toward meeting your long-term goal. After completing this short-term goal, you could establish a new one.

Let's now consider whether this short-term goal would be a SMART one.

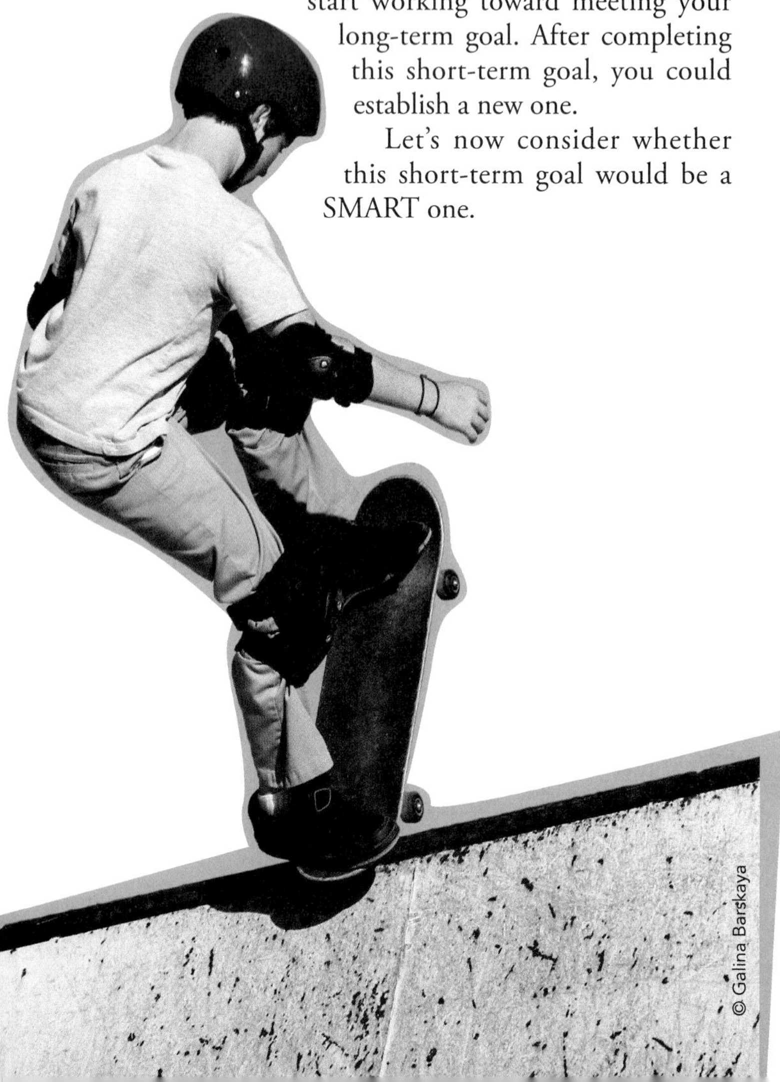
© Galina Barskaya

Specific. You've made the goal specific by listing the number of weeks and the number of hours worked per week.

Measurable. You can measure your progress toward the goal by tracking your work hours each week.

Attainable. Your short-term goal is attainable because it depends only on your making the effort to fulfill your work schedule. You could have set a goal of working more hours per week, but that might not be attainable.

Realistic. Setting a realistic number of work hours depends on other factors, such as homework, activities, and family responsibilities. However, you have the time to work five hours a week and still meet other responsibilities, so this is a realistic goal.

Timely. Working five hours a week for two weeks is a timely goal because you've specified the time frame for completing the goal and it fits your current schedule.

Product and Process Goals

The long-term goal of earning $2,400 is a **product goal**. A product is something tangible that results from work or effort. It's not what you do, but what you get as a result of what you do. Examples of product goals for fitness, health, and wellness include being able to perform 25 push-ups, being able to run a mile in six minutes, and losing five pounds (figure 3.1*a*). In each case, the goal is a product or outcome of work and effort. Product goals make

FIT FACT

Each year, millions of Americans make New Year's resolutions to eat better and exercise more. And each year, many of them fail to stick with their resolutions. Scientists have discovered that one of the main reasons for this failure is that people choose long-term goals that cannot be accomplished in the time allotted. In other words, they fail to set SMART goals. This pattern illustrates why scientists urge people to focus short-term goals on lifestyle change rather than on results such as fitness or weight loss.

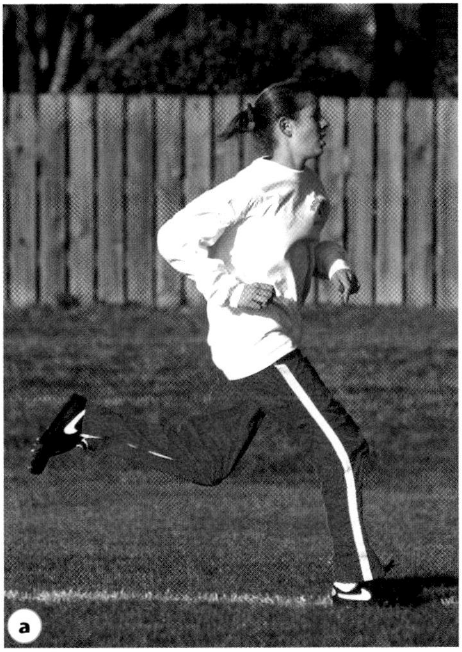

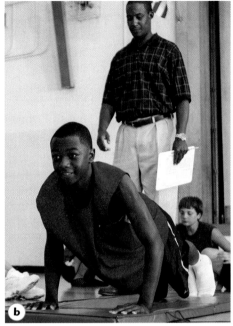

FIGURE 3.1 Product and process goals: *(a)* Running a mile in eight minutes is a product goal, and *(b)* doing five push-ups a day for three weeks is a process goal.

appropriate long-term goals because it may take you a fair amount of work and time to reach them.

Process goals involve performing a behavior, such as working a certain number of hours to earn money. Process refers to what you do rather than to the product resulting from what you do. Examples for fitness, health, and wellness include exercising 60 minutes and eating five fruits and vegetables every

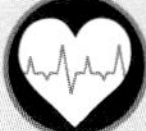

FITNESS TECHNOLOGY: Smartphones and Tablet Computers

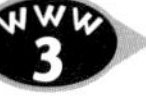

The first computers were so large that they filled entire rooms. Over time, computers got smaller and smaller. Today's smartphones are very small computers that can do many tasks that formerly required desktop or laptop computers. Smartphones use software, or applications (also known as apps), to perform a wide variety of functions. Some companies have developed smartphone apps that can help you plan and monitor your physical activity and nutrition. For example, you can record your self-assessment results and your program schedule and track your exercise and food intake. These apps can also be used on tablet computers, which are larger than smartphones but still very portable.

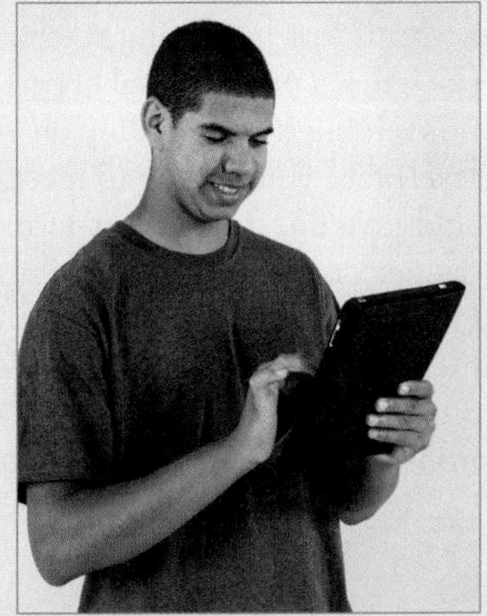

Smartphone and computer tablets have apps that help you meet healthy lifestyle goals.

Using Technology

Create an idea for a fitness or health app. Describe the app and how it would be used.

SCIENCE IN ACTION: Optimal Challenge

Scientists in many fields have collaborated to find ways to help people stay active, eat well, and stick with other healthy lifestyle behaviors. They have discovered that in order to be successful, you must set goals that provide "optimal challenge." The key is giving effort (trying hard). If a challenge is too easy, there's no need to try hard—it's not really a challenge. On the other hand, if a goal is too hard, we fail, which may lead us to give up or quit because our effort seems hopeless (see figure 3.2).

An optimal challenge requires *reasonable* effort. Meeting an optimal challenge provides us with success and makes us want to try again. In fact, providing optimal challenge is one reason that video games are so popular. They challenge you by making the task more difficult as you improve, and this optimal challenge makes you want to play again and again. You can use optimal challenge when setting your own goals to help yourself succeed.

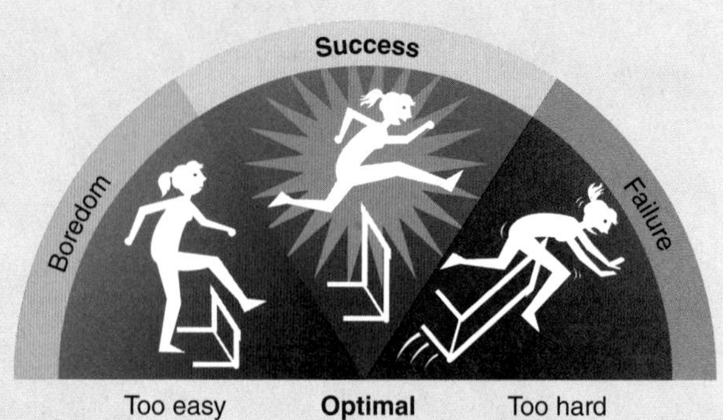

Figure 3.2 Some challenges can lead to boredom or failure, but optimal challenges can lead to success.

Student Activity

Imagine that you want to help a friend learn a skill—for example, hitting a tennis ball or a golf ball. How could you use optimal challenge to help your friend learn the skill?

day (figure 3.1*b*). Process goals make good short-term goals because you can easily monitor your progress and, with effort, succeed. In contrast, *product* goals do not make especially good short-term goals, because they can be discouraging, especially for a person who is just beginning to change. For example, if you chose a product goal of performing, say, 25 push-ups, it might (depending on your current fitness level) take you so long to meet the goal that you would give up. But a short-term process goal—such as performing 5 to 10 push-ups each day for two weeks—would be possible for you to achieve with effort. Thus, as you meet a series of short-term process goals, you work toward meeting long-term product goals.

The Taking Charge and Self-Management features in this chapter focus on setting goals for physical activity and building physical fitness. Elsewhere in the book, you'll get the chance to set long-term goals for fitness, health, and wellness (product goals) and for making healthy lifestyle changes (process goals) that lead to good fitness, health, and wellness. You'll also get the chance to set short-term goals that help you move toward achieving your long-term goals.

> "If you want to live a happy life, tie it to a goal, not to people or things."
>
> —Albert Einstein, Nobel Prize–winning physicist

Lesson Review

1. How does the SMART formula help you set goals?
2. How can you use long-term and short-term goals to plan your program? In your answer, use fitness and physical activity examples.
3. What is the difference between a process goal and a product goal? In your answer, use fitness and physical activity examples.

SELF-ASSESSMENT: Assessing Muscle Fitness

This book's chapters on fitness, health, wellness, and self-management skills introduce you to national and international fitness test batteries and give you a chance to practice test items to make sure that you know how to do them properly. In this self-assessment, you'll perform four of the tests that measure your muscle fitness: curl-up, push-up, handgrip strength, and long jump. For each item, you'll learn how to rate your performance. Later, when you've taken all of the tests included in Fitnessgram, you can use your scores and ratings to prepare a Fitnessgram report. For the tests included in this chapter, you'll record your scores and ratings as directed by your teacher so that you can use the information when you plan your personal fitness program. If you're working with a partner, remember that self-assessment information is personal and considered confidential. It shouldn't be shared with others without the permission of the person being tested.

Curl-Up (abdominal muscle strength and muscular endurance)

1. Lie on your back on a mat or carpet. Bend your knees approximately 140 degrees. Your feet should be slightly apart and as far as possible from your buttocks while still allowing your feet to be flat on the floor. Your arms should be straight and parallel to your trunk with your palms resting on the mat.
2. Place your head on a piece of paper. Place a strip of cardboard (or rubber, plastic, or tape) 4.5 inches (about 11.5 centimeters) wide and 3 feet (about 1 meter) long under your knees so that the fingers of both hands just touch the near edge of the strip.
3. Keeping your heels on the floor, curl your shoulders up slowly and slide your arms forward so that your fingers move across the cardboard strip. Curl up until your fingertips reach the far side of the strip.
4. Slowly lower your back until your head rests on the piece of paper.
5. Repeat the curl-up procedure so that you do one curl-up every three seconds. A partner could help you by saying "up, down" every three seconds. You are finished when you can't do another curl-up or when you fail to keep up with the three-second count.
6. Record the number of curl-ups you completed, then find your rating in table 3.1 and record it.

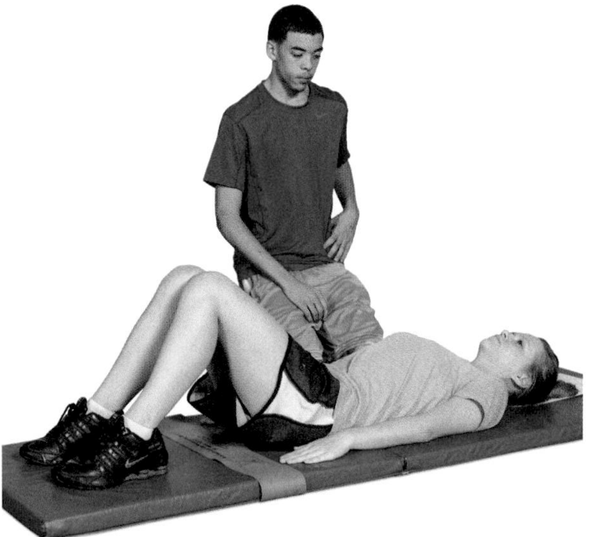

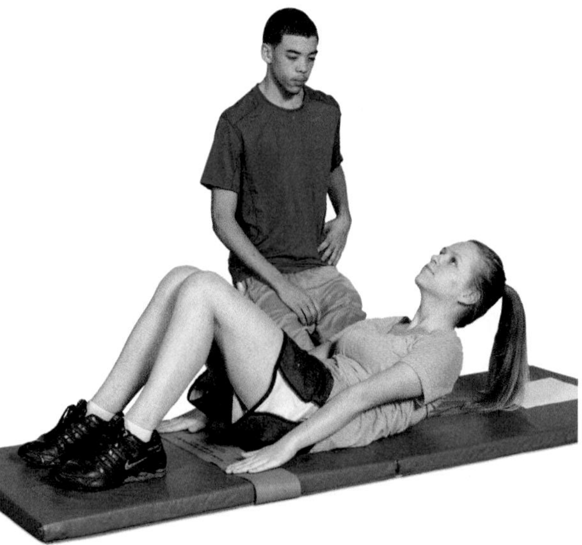

The curl-up assesses muscle fitness of the abdominal muscles.

TABLE 3.1 Rating Chart: Curl-Up (Number of Repetitions)

	13 years old		14 years old		15 years or older	
	Male	Female	Male	Female	Male	Female
High performance	≥41	≥33	≥46	≥33	≥48	≥36
Good fitness	21–40	18–32	24–45	18–32	24–47	18–35
Marginal fitness	18–20	15–17	20–23	15–17	20–23	15–17
Low fitness	≤17	≤14	≤19	≤14	≤19	≤14

Data based on *Fitnessgram*.

Push-Up (upper body strength and muscular endurance)

1. Lie facedown on a mat or carpet with your hands (palm down) under your shoulders, your fingers spread, and your legs straight. Your legs should be slightly apart and your toes tucked under.
2. Push up until your arms are straight. Keep your legs and back straight. Your body should form a straight line from your head to your heels.
3. Lower your body by bending your elbows until your upper arms are parallel to the floor (elbows at a 90-degree angle), then push up until your arms are fully extended.
4. Do one push-up every three seconds. You may want to have a partner say "up, down" every three seconds to help you. You are finished when you are unable to complete a push-up with proper form for the second time or are unable to keep the pace for a second time.
5. Record the number of push-ups you performed, then find your rating in table 3.2 and record it.

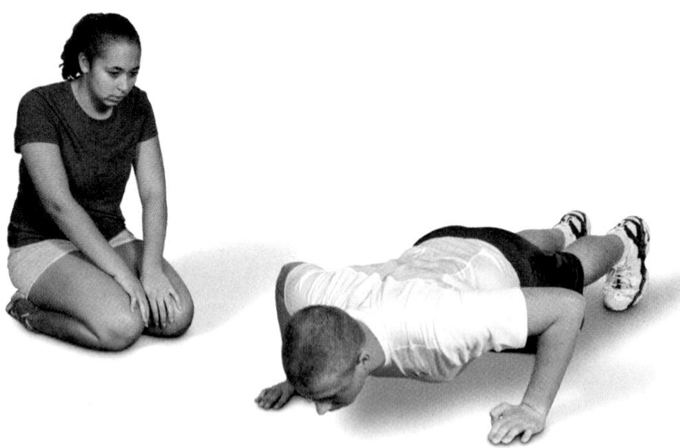
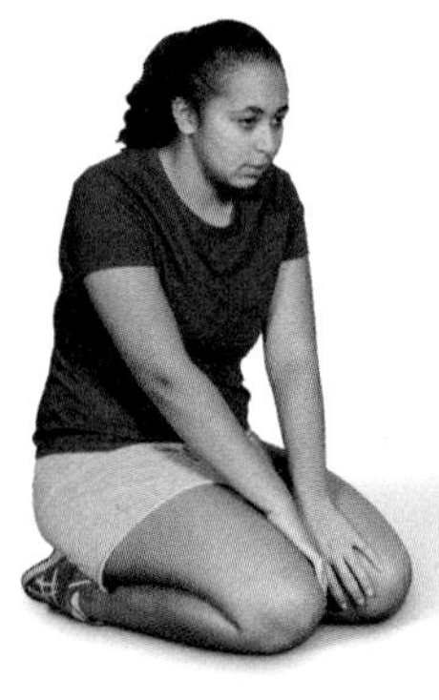
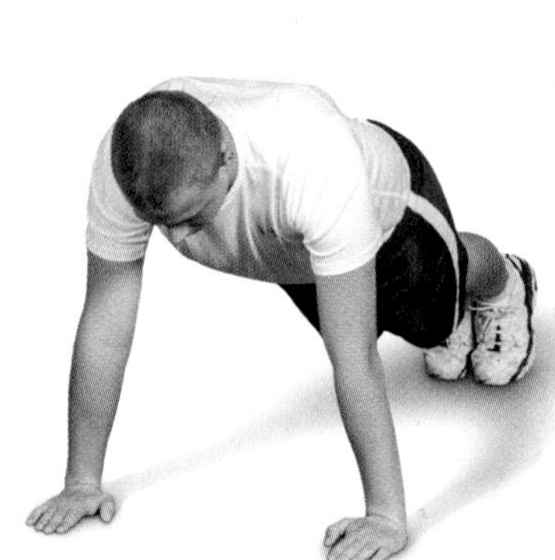
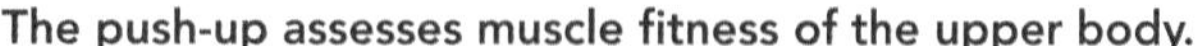

The push-up assesses muscle fitness of the upper body.

TABLE 3.2 Rating Chart: Push-Up (Number of Repetitions)

	13 years old		14 years old		15 years old		16 years or older	
	Male	Female	Male	Female	Male	Female	Male	Female
High performance	≥26	≥16	≥31	≥16	≥36	≥16	≥36	≥16
Good fitness	12–25	7–15	14–30	7–15	16–35	7–15	18–35	7–15
Marginal fitness	10–11	6	12–13	6	14–15	6	16–17	6
Low fitness	≤9	≤5	≤11	≤5	≤13	≤5	≤15	≤5

Data based on *Fitnessgram*.

Handgrip Strength (isometric hand and arm strength)

1. Use a dynamometer to measure isometric strength. Adjust the dynamometer to fit your hand size.
2. Squeeze as hard as possible for two to five seconds. Your arm should be extended with your elbow nearly straight. Do not touch your body with your arm or hand.
3. Results are most often reported in kilograms (a kilogram equals about 2.2 pounds). To get your score in pounds, multiply your score in kilograms by 2.2.
4. Do two tests with each hand. Record your best score for each hand. Add your best right-hand score to your best left-hand score, then divide the total by two to get your average score.
5. Record your average score, then find your rating in table 3.3 and record it.

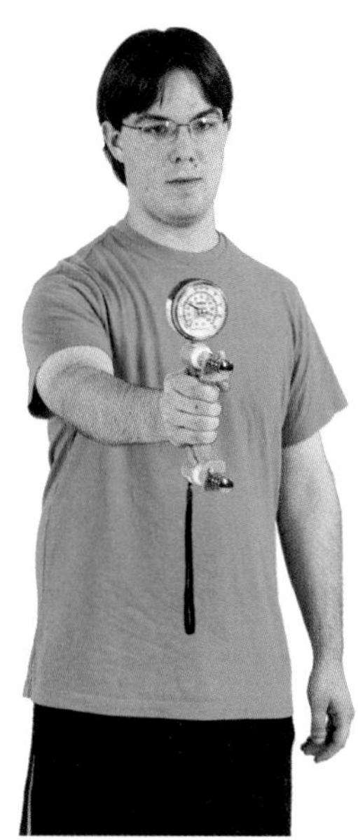

The handgrip strength test assesses isometric hand and arm strength.

TABLE 3.3 Rating Chart: Handgrip Strength in Pounds

	13 years old		14 years old		15 years old		16 years old		17 years or older	
	Male	Female	Male	Female	Male	Female	Male	Female	Male	Female
High performance	≥65	≥57	≥80	≥60	≥91	≥61	≥107	≥62	≥112	≥71
Good fitness	58–64	54–56	71–79	58–59	82–90	59–60	100–106	60–61	104–111	65–70
Marginal fitness	52–57	50–53	63–70	55–57	74–81	56–58	93–99	57–59	97–103	59–64
Low fitness	≤51	≤49	≤62	≤54	≤73	≤55	≤92	≤56	≤96	≤58

Ratings are based on the average of the best right-hand and left-hand scores.

Standing Long Jump (leg power, or explosive strength)

1. Use masking tape or another material to make the necessary line on the floor.
2. Stand with your feet shoulder-width apart behind the line on the floor. Bend your knees and hold your arms straight in front of your body at shoulder height.
3. Swing your arms downward and backward, then vigorously forward as you jump forward as far as possible, extending your legs.
4. Land on both feet and try to maintain your balance on landing. Do not run or hop before jumping.
5. Perform the test two times. Record the better of your two scores in inches (1 inch equals 2.54 centimeters), then find your rating in table 3.4 and record it.

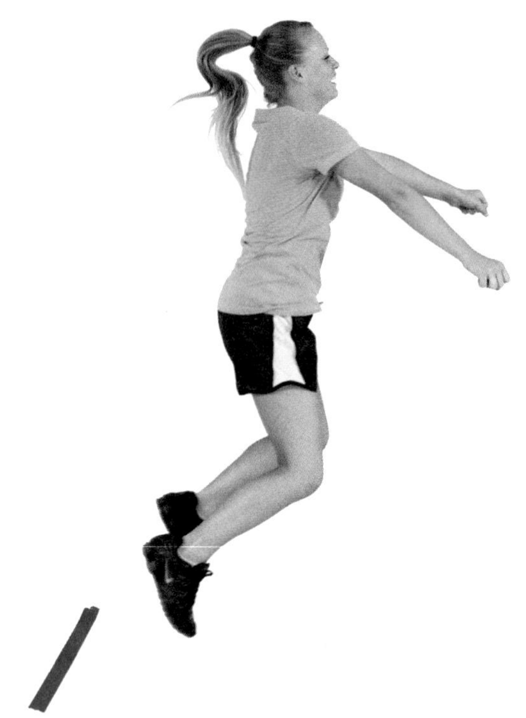

The standing long jump assesses leg power.

TABLE 3.4 Rating Chart: Standing Long Jump in Inches

	13 years old		14 years old		15 years old		16 years old		17 years or older	
	Male	Female	Male	Female	Male	Female	Male	Female	Male	Female
High performance	≥73	≥59	≥80	≥60	≥85	≥61	≥88	≥62	≥91	≥68
Good fitness	67–72	57–58	73–79	58–59	78–84	59–60	82–87	60–61	86–90	63–67
Marginal fitness	61–66	54–56	67–72	55–57	73–77	56–58	77–81	57–59	80–85	58–62
Low fitness	≤60	≤53	≤66	≤54	≤72	≤55	≤76	≤56	≤79	≤57

Lesson 3.2

Program Planning

Lesson Objectives

After reading this lesson, you should be able to

1. describe the five steps in program planning,
2. describe and explain the purpose of a personal needs profile, and
3. describe what you would include in a written program plan.

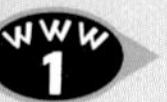

Lesson Vocabulary

personal lifestyle plan, personal needs profile, personal program

Have you ever prepared a written plan to change a healthy lifestyle? If not, would you know how to prepare a good plan? You can use self-management skills to help you adopt healthy lifestyles. You've already learned about the self-management skill of goal setting. In this lesson, you'll learn about another self-management skill—self-planning—in which you prepare personal plans for various aspects of a healthy lifestyle, such as being active, eating well, and managing stress. Eventually, you'll put all of these plans together to prepare a comprehensive **personal lifestyle plan**.

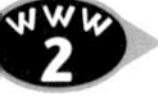

The Five Steps of Program Planning

The steps used in program planning are similar to the steps used in the simplified scientific method. They are described in detail in the sections that follow.

Step 1: Determine Your Personal Needs

The first step toward preparing a good **personal program** plan is to collect information about your personal needs. Throughout this book, you'll do many self-assessments of personal fitness, physical activity patterns, foods you eat, and other health-related areas. You'll use the information you gather to build a personal fitness, physical activity, or nutrition profile. This personal profile will help you focus on your own personal needs as you plan your program. If you don't know your needs, it will be difficult to perform the next steps in personal program planning such as considering program options (step 2) or setting goals (step 3). For example, before planning a fitness and activity program, you assess your fitness level and physical activity patterns. Before planning a nutrition program, you assess your eating habits. In fact, before you plan to change *any* aspect of your lifestyle, you should perform a self-assessment in that particular area.

FIT FACT

Nearly three in four Americans say they eat a balanced diet, but the typical teen eats less than a third of the recommended fruits and vegetables.

Once you complete your self-assessment in a specific lifestyle area, you summarize your scores and ratings in a chart called a **personal needs profile**. You'll build a personal needs profile for each healthy lifestyle plan you develop as you work your way through part 1 of this book. The following example addresses muscle fitness and muscle fitness exercises. It will help you see what a profile looks like.

Jordan is a freshman in high school. She had always wanted to play on the lacrosse team and felt that improving her muscle fitness would help her be a better player. She also felt that building muscle fitness would help her look better. To evaluate her current muscle fitness, Jordan performed three self-assessments: the curl-up, the push-up, and the long jump. She also answered some questions about her current muscle fitness activities. She summarized her results in a personal needs profile (see figure 3.3).

Activity self-assessment	Yes	No	Comment
Do you do muscle fitness exercises 2 or 3 days per week?		✔	Stretch every day for 10 min.
Fitness self-assessments	**Score**	**Rating**	
Push-up	6	Marginal	
Curl-up	19	Good fitness	
Standing long jump	57 in. (145 cm)	Marginal	

FIGURE 3.3 Jordan's personal needs profile.

Step 2: Consider Your Program Options

After determining your personal needs, the next step is to consider your program options. For physical activity, you determine what types of activity are available to you. Since Jordan was interested in muscle fitness, she used a checklist of the muscle fitness activities available to her. As you can see from the chart (figure 3.4), there are many types of muscle fitness exercise. Jordan checked elastic band exercises, calisthenics, and isometric exercises because she could do them at home and had the necessary equipment. She decided to hold off on considering other types of exercise until she learned more about them.

	Elastic band exercises		Calisthenics		Free weights		Resistance machine exercises		Isometric exercises
✔	Arm curl	✔	Prone arm lift		Bench press		Bench press	✔	Biceps curl
✔	Arm press	✔	Push-up		Biceps curl		Biceps curl	✔	Bow exercise
✔	Upright row	✔	Bridging		Dumbbell row		Lat pull-down	✔	Hand push
✔	Leg curl	✔	Curl-up		Seated French curl		Seated row	✔	Back flattener
✔	Two-leg press	✔	Trunk lift		Seated press		Triceps press	✔	Knee extender
✔	Toe push	✔	High-knee jog		Half squat		Hamstring curl	✔	Leg curl
		✔	Side leg raise		Hamstring curl		Heel raise	✔	Toe push
		✔	Stride jump		Heel raise		Knee extension	✔	Wall push
					Knee extension				

FIGURE 3.4 Jordan's exercise options for muscle fitness.

Step 3: Set Goals

The next step in self-planning is to set SMART goals. Jordan reviewed the example of writing SMART goals to save money for college, then used the SMART formula to write down her own long-term and short-term goals (see figure 3.5). She chose exercise (process) goals for her short-term goals. For her long-term goals, she listed fitness (product) goals.

You are never too old to set another goal or to dream a new dream. ”

—C.S. Lewis, author

Short-term goals	Long-term goals
1. Perform the push-up and elastic band biceps curl exercises 3 days a week.	1. Perform 10 push-ups.
2. Perform the long jump, the elastic band leg curl, and the elastic band toe push exercises 3 days a week.	2. Long-jump 59 in. (about 1.5 m).
3. Perform the curl-up exercise for the abdominal muscles 3 days a week.	3. Perform 25 curl-ups.

FIGURE 3.5 Jordan's goals for fitness and physical activity included both short-term and long-term goals.

S = specific. Jordan set her goals for muscle fitness and physical activity by choosing specific exercises and a specific number of exercise days per week. She grounded these decisions in the information recorded in her personal needs profile.

M = measurable. Jordan made her goals measurable by deciding the number of weeks, the number of exercise days per week, and, for her long-term fitness goals, the number of repetitions or distance for each outcome.

A = attainable. To keep her goals attainable, Jordan's short-term goals addressed only activity (not fitness). She chose fitness goals for her long-term goals. She took this approach because muscle fitness takes time to build, which means that short-term fitness goals are often not attainable. In addition, for her long-term fitness goals, she chose scores that are higher than she can currently perform—but not too high. For her activity goals, Jordan chose two weeks of exercise as her short-term goal. In this way, she will first focus on her short-term goal as a step toward achieving her long-term goal. Jordan also sought out help from her physical education teacher in selecting her exercises and setting attainable goals.

R = realistic. Because Jordan has various commitments—such as homework, family activities, and school activities—she limited the number of her goals (both short- and long-term) so that she has a realistic chance to meet them all.

T = timely. Jordan also set a specific amount of time for reaching both her long-term and her short-term goals. Since she needs more muscle fitness to make the lacrosse team, she needs to improve her fitness in time for tryouts.

Step 4: Structure Your Program and Write It Down

In the fourth step, you use information gained during steps 1, 2, and 3 to structure your program. Once you establish your goals, you prepare a detailed written plan. As you work through part 1 of this book, you'll create written plans for several programs; they will all be similar to Jordan's planning.

Jordan used a chart to prepare her exercise plan for muscle fitness. Since muscle fitness exercises should not be done every day, Jordan's teacher helped her decide which days to do each exercise and how many to do. Her teacher also helped her select the right elastic band to use in her exercises. Jordan decided on the best time of day based on her free time and the times when she most enjoyed exercising. She also considered times when she was

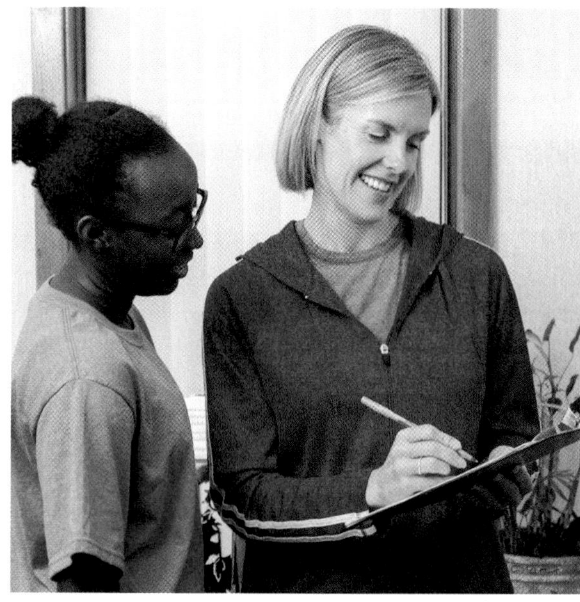

Experts can provide assistance in choosing exercises and determining how often to perform them.

Day	Activity (exercise)	Time	Repetitions	Completed Week 1	Completed Week 2
Mon.	Warm-up (jog)	4 p.m.	5 min	✔	✔
	Biceps curl (exercise band)		3 sets of 10	✔	✔
	Toe push (exercise band)		3 sets of 10	✔	✔
	Curl-up		2 sets of 15	✔	✔
	Long jump		3 sets of 10	✔	✔
Tues.	Warm-up (walk)	4 p.m.	5 min	✔	✔
	Push-up		2 sets of 5	✔	✔
	Leg curl		3 sets of 10	✔	✔
Wed.	Warm-up (jog)	4 p.m.	5 min	✔	✔
	Biceps curl (exercise band)		3 sets of 10	✔	✔
	Toe push (exercise band)		3 sets of 10	✔	✔
	Curl-up		2 sets of 15	✔	✔
	Long jump		3 sets of 10	✔	✔
Thurs.	Warm-up (walk)	4 p.m.	5 min	✔	
	Push-up		2 sets of 5	✔	
	Leg curl		3 sets of 10	✔	
Fri.	Warm-up (jog)	4 p.m.	5 min	✔	✔
	Biceps curl (exercise band)		3 sets of 10	✔	✔
	Toe push (exercise band)		3 sets of 10	✔	✔
	Curl-up		2 sets of 15	✔	✔
	Long jump		3 sets of 10	✔	✔
Sat.	Warm-up (walk)	4 p.m.	5 min	✔	✔
	Push-up		2 sets of 5	✔	✔
	Leg curl		3 sets of 10	✔	✔
Sun.	No exercise				

FIGURE 3.6 Jordan's two-week written program plan.

not likely to be interrupted. A sample of Jordan's written plan is shown in figure 3.6. The last column allowed Jordan to checkmark each day on which she did her exercises.

Step 5: Keep a Log and Evaluate Your Program

After you've tried your program for some time (the exact amount of time depends on your goals), evaluate it. Did you meet your goals? Was your program plan a good one? After your evaluation, make a new plan using the program planning steps.

Jordan tried her plan for two weeks. She placed checkmarks beside the days on which she completed the exercises in her plan. As you can see in figure 3.6, she missed her planned exercises on only one day during the two-week period. Given this success, she decided to keep doing the same plan for another two weeks on her way to meeting her long-term goals. She hoped to reach her long-term goal in eight weeks.

 CONSUMER CORNER: Too Good to Be True

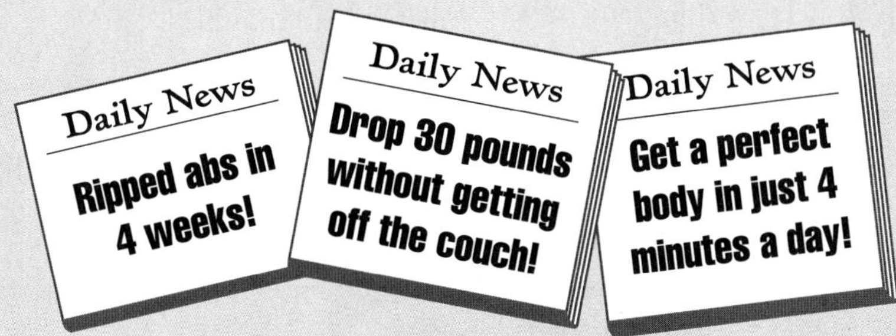
Daily News
Ripped abs in 4 weeks!
Daily News
Drop 30 pounds without getting off the couch!
Daily News
Get a perfect body in just 4 minutes a day!

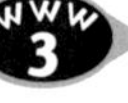

These are just a few examples of headlines you'll see in magazines, newspapers, and TV and web ads. The fitness and health industry is big business. Unfortunately, many companies try to make money by promising big results with little effort. They use marketing campaigns that prey on people who want quick results. You're becoming a critical consumer of fitness, health, and wellness information. Use the tips presented here to make good decisions and avoid falling victim to false claims.

Consumer guideline	Consumer action
Evaluate the source of the information.	Avoid testimonials by famous people (such as athletes and movie stars) who are not experts. Use information from experts in health, medicine, nutrition, and kinesiology who use the scientific method. Use information from government sources (such as the U.S. Food and Drug Administration) and reliable professional organizations (such as the American Heart Association). Use the scientific method to evaluate the information.
Be suspicious of claims that promise quick results and are inconsistent with information presented in this book.	Compare claims with facts you've learned from this book and other reliable sources. Beware: If a claim seems too good to be true, it probably isn't true.
Be suspicious of "special offers" that say you must take advantage immediately or they will no longer be available.	Avoid quick action. "Special offers" that quickly expire are designed to get you to act fast without taking the time to make a good decision.
Check the credentials of the person or company doing the promotion.	Check to see if people who claim to be experts really are. Do they have a college degree or advanced degree? Are they certified by a well-known, legitimate organization? People with university degrees in kinesiology, physical education, and physical therapy are generally well equipped to give you sound advice about exercise. The same is true for a certified strength and conditioning specialist (CSCS), American College of Sports Medicine certified personal trainer (CPT), certified health fitness specialist (CHFS), certified group exercise instructor (CGEI), or registered clinical exercise physiologist (RCEP). For nutrition needs, a registered dietitian (RD) is well qualified to give you information.

Using Self-Planning Skills

You can use the five steps of program planning presented in this lesson to help you do your self-planning—that is, to plan your own program. Once you've developed a personal program plan, you're on your way to becoming independent rather than dependent on others.

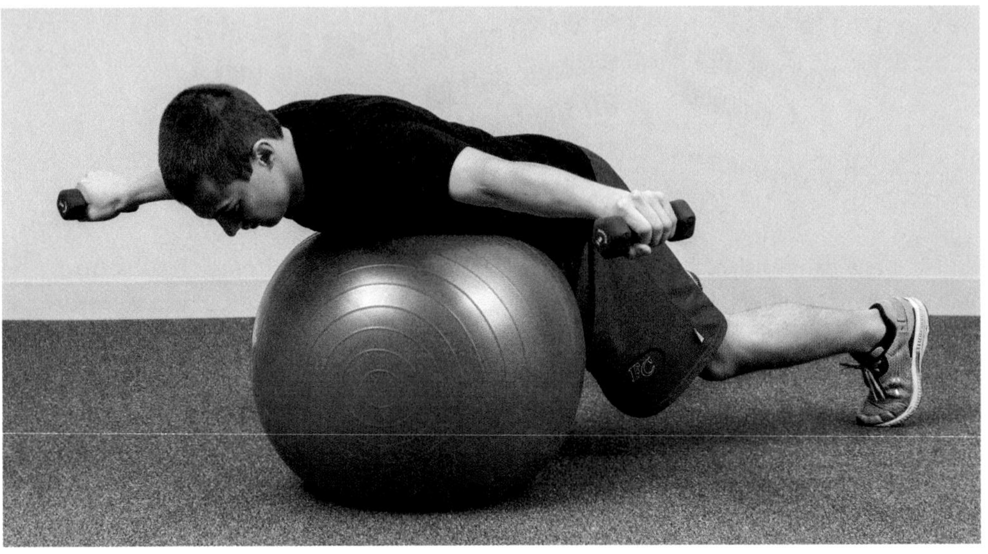

Keeping a log or journal of the activities you perform can help you determine if you have met your goals.

Lesson Review

1. What are the five steps in program planning? Describe each step.
2. What information do you need when preparing your personal needs profile?
3. What are some things you should write down when doing your personal program plan?

TAKING CHARGE: Setting Goals

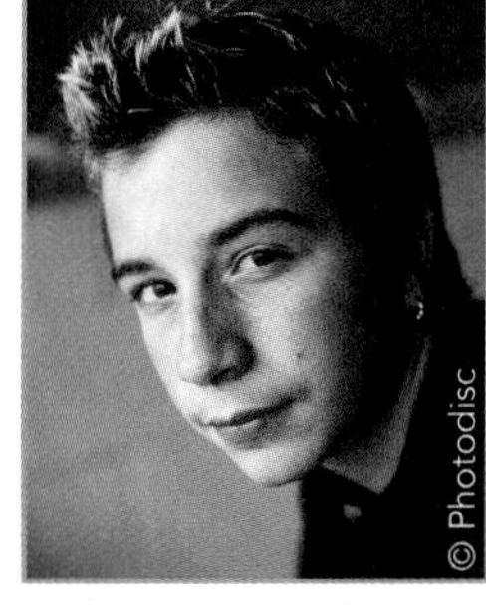
© Photodisc

You probably know people who are sedentary or who eat a lot of unhealthy food. They may be in stage 1 of the process of change for physical activity or nutrition. They may have tried to make lifestyle changes but been ineffective because they failed to set good goals. This feature highlights SMART goals for physical activity.

Ms. Booker, a physical education teacher, noticed that Kevin seemed a bit listless in class. She stopped by his desk and asked, "Are you all right, Kevin? You seem a bit tired."

Kevin said, "I'm okay. I was in a hurry this morning so I missed breakfast."

Later, as she passed through the cafeteria, Ms. Booker couldn't help noticing that Kevin was eating food from a vending machine for lunch. He was sitting by himself at an isolated table.

Ms. Booker walked over, sat down, and asked, "Are you feeling better now?"

Kevin replied, "Yes, but I know I need to eat better."

Ms. Booker said, "Maybe you need to make a plan to eat better. Do you remember the SMART formula we learned in class? Maybe you could use the formula to set some goals." Kevin agreed that this was a good idea.

For Discussion

How could Kevin use the SMART formula to set good nutrition goals? What might be some good long-term goals for him? What might be some good short-term goals? What kinds of advice do you think Ms. Booker gave Kevin about goal setting? What advice would you have for Kevin? Consider the guidelines presented in the following Self-Management feature as you answer these discussion questions.

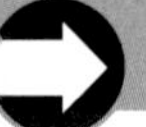

SELF-MANAGEMENT: Skills for Setting Goals

Now that you know more about different types of goal setting, you can begin developing some goals of your own. Use the following guidelines to help you as you identify and develop your personal goals.

- **Know your reasons for setting your goals.** People who set goals for reasons other than their own personal improvement often fail. Ask yourself, *Why is this goal important for me?* Make sure you're setting goals for yourself based on your own needs and interests.
- **Choose a few goals at a time.** As you work your way through this book, you'll establish goals for fitness, physical activity, food choices, weight management, stress management, and other healthy lifestyle behaviors. But rather than focusing on all of these goals at once, you'll choose a few goals at a time. Trying to do too much often leads to failure. Choosing a few goals at a time can help you be successful.
- **Use the SMART formula.** The SMART formula helps you set goals that are specific, measurable, attainable, realistic, and timely.
- **Set long-term and short-term goals.** The SMART formula helps you establish both long-term and short-term goals. When setting short-term goals, focus not on results but on making good lifestyle changes (that is, focus on process goals).
- **Put your goals in writing.** Writing down a goal represents a personal commitment and increases your chances of meeting that goal. You'll get the opportunity to write down your goals as you do the activities in this book.
- **Self-assess periodically and keep logs.** Doing self-assessments helps you set your goals and determine whether

you've met them. Focus on improvement by working toward goals that are slightly higher than your current self-assessment results.

- **Reward yourself.** Achieving a personal goal is rewarding. Allow yourself to feel good. Congratulate yourself for your accomplishment.
- **Revise if necessary.** If you find that a goal is too difficult to accomplish, don't be afraid to revise it. It's better to revise your goal than to quit because you didn't reach an unrealistic goal.
- **Consider maintenance goals.** Improvement is not always necessary. Once you reach the highest level of change, setting a goal of maintenance can be a good idea. For example, an active, fit person cannot continue to improve in fitness forever. At some point, enough is enough, and following a regular workout schedule to maintain good fitness is a reasonable goal. Likewise, once you achieve the goal of eating well, maintaining your healthy eating pattern is a worthwhile goal.

ACADEMIC CONNECTION: Mnemonics and Acronyms

Earlier in this chapter, you learned the meaning of the words *mnemonic* and *acronym*. SMART is a mnemonic device, or memory aid, that helps you remember the five guidelines for creating goals. SMART is also an acronym because each letter in SMART is the first letter of a guideline for setting goals. FIT is another useful mnemonic and acronym that can be used to remember the frequency, intensity, and time of physical activity when the type of activity is already established.

Health organizations are often referred to using an acronym. For example, most people recognize that the acronym AMA refers to the American Medical Association. The AMA does not promote the use of the acronym, but people frequently use it. Since AMA does not have a separate meaning, as is the case for SMART and FIT, it is not considered a mnemonic.

Not all mnemonics are acronyms. In addition to acronyms, poems or rhymes, songs, lists, and other devices can be used as mnemonics. For example, a rhyme is commonly used as a mnemonic to remember how many days there are in each month ("Thirty days have September, April, June, and November"), and the alphabet song is a mnemonic that helps children learn the alphabet. As you continue your study of fitness, health, and wellness, you may want to make up your own mnemonics and acronyms to help you remember important information.

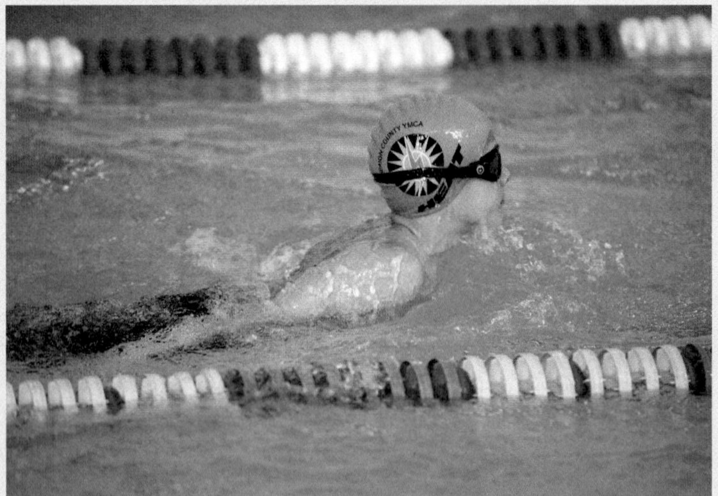

Swimmers on this team used the acronym TEAM (Together Everyone Achieves More) to help them achieve their goals.

TAKING ACTION: Exercise Circuits

An exercise circuit consists of several stations, each of which features a different exercise. Typically, you move from one station to the next without resting between them. Exercise circuits are popular because they include a variety of exercises, which helps make the workout interesting. Circuits can be designed to focus on either health-related or skill-related fitness components, and they can be performed in a variety of places—indoors or outdoors, at home or elsewhere. They also have the advantage of not requiring a lot of equipment, though you might enjoy bringing some favorite music to listen to while performing the circuit. **Take action** to create and use an exercise circuit. Try the following tips.

- Before starting the circuit, perform a dynamic warm-up.
- Plan stations that address all parts of your body: lower, middle, upper.
- Avoid having two stations in a row that challenge the same body part.
- Pace yourself so that you can be active for the whole time at each station and keep moving between stations.
- Use correct technique at each station; if your technique fails due to fatigue, take a break.
- After doing the circuit, perform a cool-down.

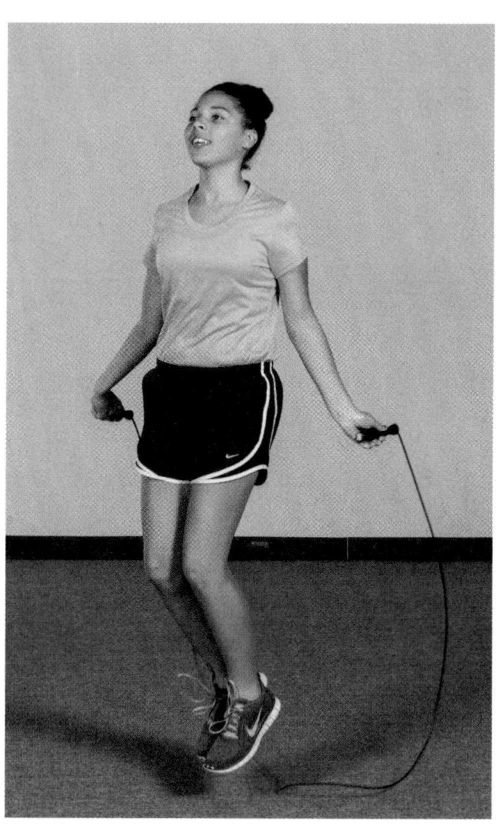

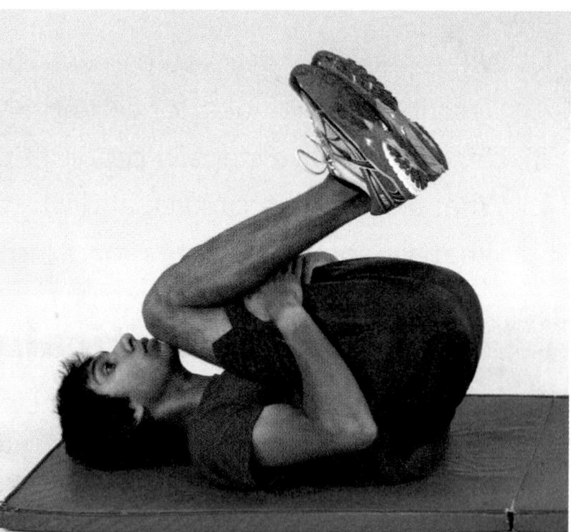

Exercise circuits use a variety of exercises at several stations.

Reviewing Concepts and Vocabulary

As directed by your teacher, answer items 1 through 5 by correctly completing each sentence with a word or phrase.

1. The acronym used to remember the characteristics of effective goals is ______________.
2. Performing several exercises three days a week for two weeks is an example of a ______________-term goal.
3. Deciding to walk 30 minutes a day for the next two months is an example of a ______________-term goal.
4. Being able to run a mile in six minutes (a kilometer in four) is an example of a ______________ goal.
5. Deciding to do flexibility exercises three days a week is an example of a ______________ goal.

For items 6 through 10, as directed by your teacher, match each term in column 1 with the appropriate phrase in column 2.

6. step 1	a. setting goals
7. step 2	b. considering program options
8. step 3	c. structuring your program
9. step 4	d. determining your personal needs
10. step 5	e. evaluating your program

For items 11 through 15, as directed by your teacher, respond to each statement or question.

11. What are some tests you can use to assess and rate your muscle fitness?
12. Describe the five rules for setting SMART goals.
13. Describe the five steps in program planning.
14. What are exercise circuits, and why are they useful in staying active?
15. What are some guidelines for using the self-management skill of goal setting?

Thinking Critically

Write a paragraph to answer the following question.

Why is it important to understand the concept of optimal challenge when setting goals? Provide an example to help you make your point.

Project

Imagine that you are hired as a health consultant in December to help clients make New Year's resolutions for eating better and being more active. Prepare a brief booklet that contains advice for making *effective* New Year's resolutions.

UNIT II

Becoming and Staying Physically Active

Healthy People 2020 Goals

- Increase the percentage of teens who meet national physical activity guidelines.
- Increase aerobic activity among teens.
- Reduce the percentage of people who do no leisure-time physical activity.
- Increase daily physical education and out-of-school physical activity among teens.
- Reduce computer use to less than two hours a day for teens.
- Increase trips taken by walking and biking.
- Help people live high-quality, longer lives free from preventable disease, injury, and early death.
- Reduce heart disease, stroke, cancer, diabetes, high blood pressure, osteoporosis, and back problems.
- Increase the percentage of people who receive information about risk factors.

Self-Assessment Features in This Unit

- Body Composition and Flexibility
- PACER and Trunk Lift
- Assessing Skill-Related Physical Fitness

Taking Charge Features in This Unit

- Reducing Risk Factors
- Learning to Self-Monitor
- Improving Performance Skills

Self-Management Features in This Unit

- Skills for Reducing Risk Factors
- Skills for Learning to Self-Monitor
- Skills for Improving Performance

Taking Action Features in This Unit

- Walking for Health
- Physical Activity Pyramid Circuit
- Safe Exercise Circuit

4

Getting Started in Physical Activity

In This Chapter

www **Student Web Resources**
www.HOPEtextbook.org/student

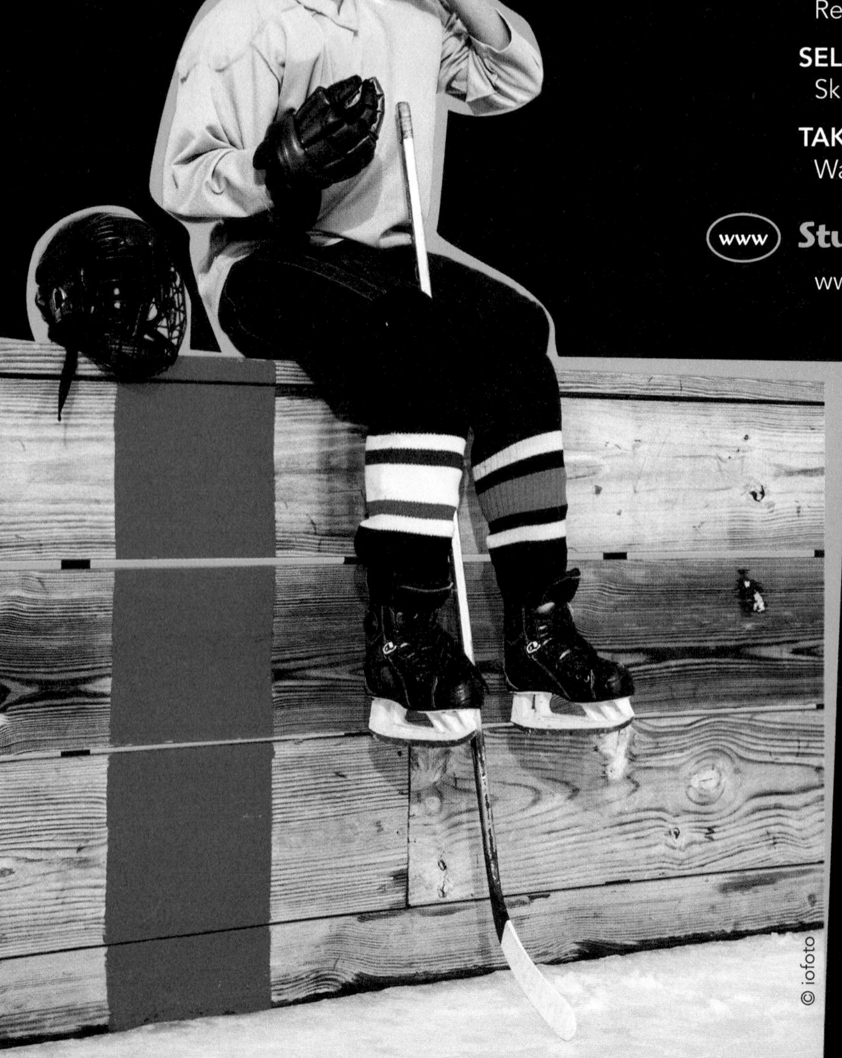

Lesson 4.1

Safe and Smart Physical Activity

Lesson Objectives

After reading this lesson, you should be able to

1. describe medical readiness and explain how to assess it,
2. explain how the environment affects physical activity, and
3. describe some steps in dressing appropriately for physical activity in normal environments.

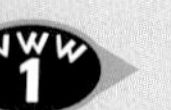

Lesson Vocabulary

air quality index, graded exercise test, heat index, humidity, hyperthermia, hypothermia, Physical Activity Readiness Questionnaire (PAR-Q), wind-chill factor

Are you prepared to be active? Whether you're a beginner or you've been physically active for some time, you need to know how to exercise safely in all conditions. If you're a beginner, the first step is to be physically and medically ready. As a young person, you probably won't have a problem with physical and medical readiness, but you should answer some simple questions about yourself just to be sure. You should also be ready for a variety of environmental conditions—such as heat, cold, pollution, and high altitude—that could necessitate a change in your exercise habits. In this lesson, you'll learn how to prepare yourself for physical activity.

> "An ounce of prevention is worth a pound of cure."
>
> —Benjamin Franklin, statesman and scientist

Medical Readiness

Have you ever been injured during physical activity? Do you know how to prepare yourself for exercise so as to avoid injury and participate safely? Before you begin a regular physical activity program for health and wellness, you should assess your medical and physical readiness. For this purpose, experts have developed a seven-item questionnaire called the **Physical Activity Readiness Questionnaire (PAR-Q)**. If you answer yes to any of the seven questions, you are advised to seek medical consultation before beginning or continuing an exercise program. You can get a copy of the questionnaire from your teacher. You may also want to show the PAR-Q to your parents or other adults who are important to you. Of course you should consider any current health problems as you prepare for exercise. For example, some people have short-term illnesses such as a cold or the flu that will alter their plans for exercise. Others, with chronic conditions such as asthma, will have to alter their exercise according to their doctor's instructions. Older people are more likely to be at risk when doing exercise. You may want to encourage older adults who are important to you to answer the PAR-Q questions before they begin an exercise program.

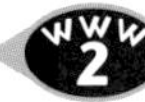

As for yourself, you may even be *required* to have a medical examination if you're going to participate in an interscholastic sport or other program of similar intensity, such as a community sport or other rigorous physical challenge. Medical exams help ensure that you are free from disease and can also help you prevent health problems in the future. You should also answer the questions included in the sport readiness questionnaire available from your teacher.

Later in life, you may need to do a **graded exercise test**, which is administered by a health professional and is sometimes called an exercise stress test. The test is done on a treadmill and can help identify people at high risk for health problems such as heart attacks (figure 4.1). It is an expensive test and is not necessary for everyone, and a health professional can use screening to determine whether it is appropriate for you. Even seemingly fit athletes can be at risk, although risk is low among

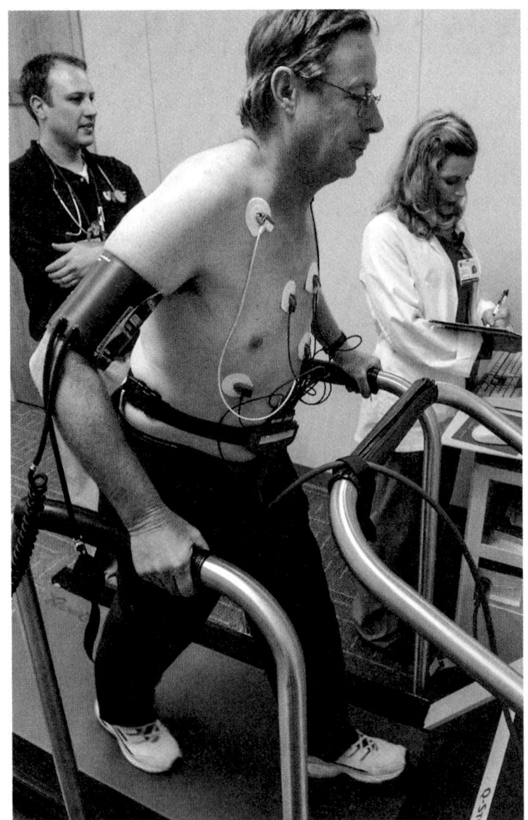

FIGURE 4.1 The graded exercise test can be using to screen adults with risk factors.

young athletes. Nevertheless, outstanding runners and baseball and football players thought to be in good health have died from heart attacks, especially among older athletes. For example, Gaines Adams, a professional football player, died unexpectedly from an undetected heart condition in 2010. Jim Fixx, a famous runner and author, died of heart problems that could probably have been addressed if he had performed a graded exercise test. Most young people will not perform this test unless it is recommended by a doctor after medical screening.

Readiness for Extreme Environmental Conditions

Environmental conditions play an important role in determining when and how strenuously you should exercise. Whether you are just beginning a physical activity program or have been exercising for a while, you must understand how environmental conditions can affect your body during exercise. Your body can adapt to environmental factors such as heat, cold, altitude, and air quality. That adaptability is why people who have been exposed to an environment for a long time can function better in it than those who have just become exposed. This lesson presents guidelines to help you adapt to weather and other environmental factors in order to prevent injury and health problems. All people should follow these guidelines, but they are especially important for people who are new to exercise or new to a particular environment.

Hot, Humid Weather

Be careful when performing physical activity in high heat and **humidity**, which can cause your body temperature to rise too high—a situation referred to as **hyperthermia** or overheating. When exercise causes your body temperature to rise, you start to perspire (sweat). As your sweat evaporates, your body is cooled. But when the humidity is high, evaporation is less effective in cooling your body, and hyperthermia is more likely to occur. Hyperthermia causes three main conditions, which are described in table 4.1.

TABLE 4.1 Heat-Related Conditions

Condition	Definition
Heat cramps	Muscle cramps caused by excessive heat exposure and low water consumption.
Heat exhaustion	Condition caused by excessive heat exposure and characterized by paleness, clammy skin, profuse sweating, weakness, tiredness, nausea, dizziness, muscle cramps, and possibly vomiting or fainting. Body temperature may be normal or slightly above normal.
Heatstroke	Condition caused by excessive heat exposure and characterized by high body temperature up to 106°F (41°C); hot, dry, flushed skin; rapid pulse; lack of sweating; dizziness; and possibly unconsciousness. This serious condition can result in death and requires prompt medical attention.

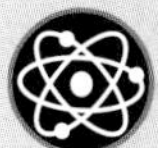

SCIENCE IN ACTION: Science Prepares Us for Safe Exercise

In the 1950s, people who had heart attacks were advised to stay in bed for months and avoid being active. Such myths about physical activity were common. For example, some athletes were told not to drink water during practice because it could make them "water-logged" and impair their performance. We have come a long way since then. Scientists who study medicine, nutrition, and kinesiology have made discoveries that make exercise safer and more effective. Here are two examples of science in action.

- **Exercise physiologists working with medical doctors developed cardiac rehabilitation programs.** They found that well-planned exercise after a heart attack is better than bed rest. In cardiac rehabilitation programs, people who have had a heart attack enroll in an exercise program under the care of a registered clinical exercise physiologist approved by the American College of Sports Medicine (ACSM). The physiologist works with a physician to plan an effective program of recovery for the patient. Exercise physiologists were also responsible for developing many of the tests now used in screening for heart disease, such as the graded exercise test described earlier in this chapter.
- **Nutrition scientists working with exercise physiologists have developed sport drinks that help people resist heat-related conditions.** The drinks contain electrolytes, which help the body retain fluid. They also contain a limited amount of sugar, which can be helpful for people performing long bouts of exercise. Scientists conducted many research studies to find the right combination of ingredients.

Student Activity

Identify a product or program related to fitness or health that has been developed recently based on new scientific discoveries.

FIT FACT

Hyper means too much or excessive, and *thermia* refers to heat, so *hyperthermia* means too much heat. *Hypo* means too little or less than normal, so *hypothermia* means too little heat.

Use the following guidelines to prevent and cope with heat-related conditions.

- **Begin gradually.** As your body becomes accustomed to physical activity in hot weather, it becomes more resistant to heat-related injury. Start with short periods of activity and gradually increase the duration.
- **Drink water.** In hot weather, your body perspires more than usual to cool itself. In order to replace the water your body loses through perspiration, you need to drink plenty of water before and after activity.
- **Wear proper clothing.** Wear porous clothing that allows air to pass through to cool your body. Also wear light-colored clothing—lighter colors reflect the sun's heat, whereas darker colors absorb it. Clothing made of fibers that wick away moisture and keep you cool (for example, Coolmax) are now available.
- **Rest frequently.** Physical activity creates body heat. Periodically stop to rest in a shady area to help your body lower its temperature.
- **Avoid extreme heat and humidity.** You can use the heat index chart shown in figure 4.2 to determine whether the environment is too hot and humid for activity. If the **heat index** is too high, you should postpone or cancel your activity. You should do physical activity in the caution zones only if you are well adapted to hot environments and follow all of the basic guidelines. The amount of time

it takes to adapt to these conditions varies from person to person.

- **If heat-related injury occurs, get out of the heat and cool your body.** Find shade; apply cool, wet towels to your body; spray your body with water; drink water; and seek medical help if heatstroke occurs.

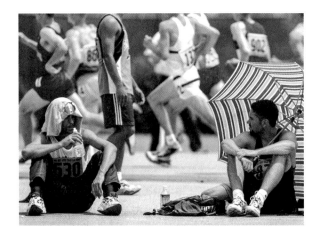

When you exercise in hot weather, wear light-colored clothing and drink plenty of water to help cool your body.

Cold, Windy, and Wet Weather

It can also be dangerous to exercise in cold, windy, and wet weather. Extreme cold can result in **hypothermia**, or excessively low body temperature. Hypothermia is accompanied by shivering, numbness, drowsiness, muscular weakness, and confusion or disorientation. Extreme cold can also cause a condition called frostbite, in which a body part becomes frozen. A person with frostbite often feels no pain, thus making the condition even more dangerous. Use the following guidelines when exercising in cold, windy, and wet weather.

- **Avoid extreme cold and wind.** Before dressing for physical activity, use the chart in figure 4.3 to determine the **wind-chill factor**. Exercising when the temperature is cold and the wind is blowing is especially dangerous because the air feels colder. The wind-chill chart shows how long it takes to get frostbite when your skin is exposed to various wind-chill levels. Experts agree that if the time to frostbite is 30 minutes or less, you should postpone activity. If you're active when the wind-chill factor is excessive, be sure to dress properly and be aware of the symptoms of frostbite:
    - Skin becomes white or grayish yellow and looks glossy.
    - Pain may be felt early and then subside, though often feeling is lost and no pain is felt.
    - Blisters may appear later.
    - The affected area feels intensely cold and numb.
- **Dress properly.** Wear several layers of lightweight clothing rather than a heavy jacket or coat. The clothing closest to your body (base layer) helps wick away body moisture to keep

Heat index

As humidity increases, air can feel hotter than it actually is. This chart shows how hot it feels as humidity rises.

Relative humidity (%) \ Air temperature (°F)	70	75	80	85	90	95	100	105	110	115	120
100	72	80	91	108	132						
90	71	79	88	102	122						
80	71	78	86	97	113	136					
70	70	77	85	93	106	124	144				
60	70	76	82	90	100	114	132	149			
50	69	75	81	88	96	107	120	135	150		
40	68	74	79	86	93	101	110	123	137	151	
30	67	73	78	84	90	96	104	113	123	135	148
20	66	72	77	82	87	93	99	105	112	120	130
10	65	70	75	80	85	90	95	100	105	111	116
0	64	69	73	78	83	87	91	95	99	103	107

Caution zone

Danger zone

FIGURE 4.2 Heat index chart.

Wind (mph) \ Temperature (°F)	30	25	20	15	10	5	0	−5	−10	−15	−20	−25
5	25	19	13	7	1	−5	−11	−16	−22	−28	−34	−40
10	21	15	9	3	−4	−10	−16	−22	−28	−35	−41	−47
15	19	13	6	0	−7	−13	−19	−26	−32	−39	−45	−51
20	17	11	4	−2	−9	−15	−22	−29	−35	−42	−48	−55
25	16	9	3	−4	−11	−17	−24	−31	−37	−44	−51	−58
30	15	8	1	−5	−12	−19	−26	−33	−39	−46	−53	−60
35	14	7	0	−7	−14	−21	−27	−34	−41	−48	−55	−62
40	13	6	−1	−8	−15	−22	−29	−36	−43	−50	−57	−64
45	12	5	−2	−9	−16	−23	−30	−37	−44	−51	−58	−65
50	12	4	−3	−10	−17	−24	−31	−38	−45	−52	−60	−67
55	11	4	−3	−11	−18	−25	−32	−39	−46	−54	−61	−68
60	10	3	−4	−11	−19	−26	−33	−40	−48	−55	−62	−69

Frostbite occurs in 30 minutes or less

FIGURE 4.3 Wind-chill chart.

you warm and dry. Silk and special wicking materials made of synthetic fibers such as Polartec are good for this layer. Cotton is not recommended for the base layer because it tends to get wet and stay wet. The second layer is often called the insulating layer. This layer helps retain body heat but should also wick away moisture. Polyester fleece and wool are good for this layer. The outer layer is designed to protect you against wind and moisture (rain, snow) but should also allow heat and moisture to be released. For this reason jackets made of plastic, rubber, or other materials that do not "breathe" are not recommended. Jackets made of synthetic fibers (for example, Gore-Tex) that breathe are recommended. Wearing a jacket with a zipper allows you to regulate heat retained and released by the body. Wear a high collar on one of the inner layers. If needed, wear a knit cap, ski mask, or mittens (which keep hands warmer than gloves do).

- **Avoid exercising in weather that is icy or cold and wet.** These conditions can cause special problems. Your shoes, socks, and pant legs can get wet, which increases your risk of foot injuries and falls.

Pollution and Altitude

The effectiveness and safety of your exercise can also be affected by conditions other than weather, such as air pollution and altitude. Air pollution can affect your ability to breathe, and experts have identified levels of pollution (ozone and particulate matter) that are unhealthful. Pollution levels are rated by means of an **air quality index** that ranges from good to very unhealthful. When the air pollution level is high, you can find warnings on radio, television, and reliable

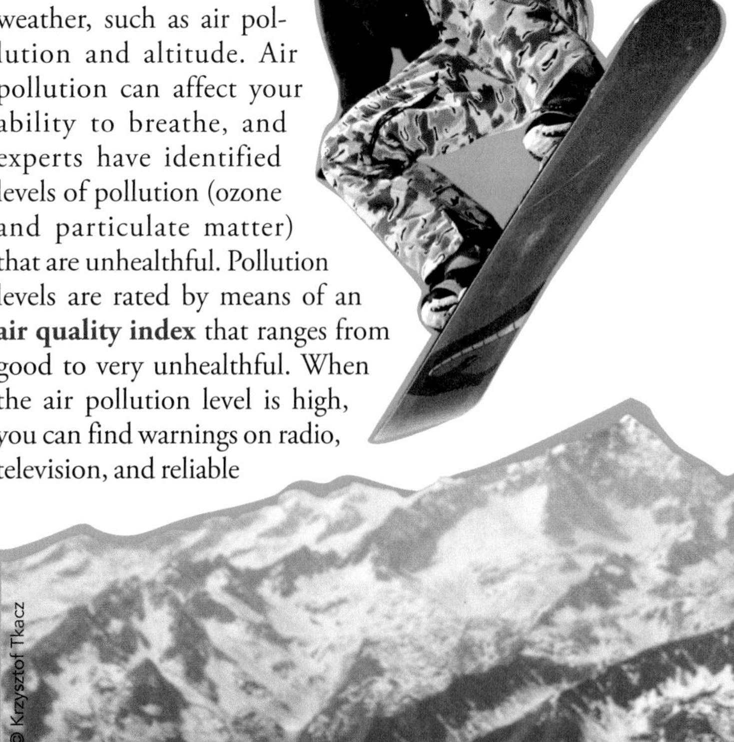

FIT FACT

Health scientists recently discovered an inaccuracy in the wind-chill factor system that had been used for years. Specifically, the importance of wind had been overemphasized. Now, Canadian experts aided by U.S. scientists have developed a new formula, which is used in the wind-chill chart shown in figure 4.3.

websites. During such times, avoid exercising outdoors. A table showing air quality levels is available in the student section of the Health Opportunities Through Physical Education website.

People who live at high altitude are able to exercise there with little trouble, but people who live at lower altitude may have trouble adjusting to being active at higher altitude. It takes time for the body to adjust, even for very fit people. For this reason, if you exercise at a higher altitude than you are used to (for example, if you go skiing), adjust the intensity of your physical activity until your body adapts.

General Readiness: Dressing for Physical Activity

As you've seen, special environmental circumstances—such as intense heat and cold—require special dress for physical activity. But even under normal circumstances, the way you dress has a lot to do with your comfort and enjoyment. Consider the following guidelines when dressing for physical activity.

- **Wear comfortable and appropriate clothing for the environmental conditions.** Guidelines for dressing for cold and hot weather were presented earlier. In addition to following these guidelines, wearing comfortable clothing will make your workout more enjoyable.
- **Use sun screen or wear clothing that protects you from the sun.** These will help protect your skin from harmful ultraviolet rays.
- **Wash exercise clothing regularly.** Clean clothing is more comfortable than soiled clothing, and it reduces the chance of fungal growth and infection.
- **Dress in layers when exercising outdoors.** You can remove layers of clothing as you become warmer while exercising and put them back on when you cool down.
- **Wear proper socks.** Moisture-wicking fabrics are now used in making socks and other apparel (see the Fitness Technology feature). Socks made with these fabrics reduce foot moisture and can help prevent blisters. Thick socks made of cotton or another traditional fabric can help cushion your feet but are not as effective at keeping them dry.
- **Wear proper shoes.** Most people can use a good pair of multipurpose exercise or sport shoes. However, if you plan to do special activities, you might prefer shoes designed just for them. Try shoes on before buying them. When you try them on, wear the kind of socks you normally wear and walk around to see how the shoes feel. They should not feel too heavy, because extra weight makes exercise more tiring. Avoid vinyl or plastic shoes that do not let air pass through to help cool your feet. As an alternative to cloth and leather shoes (which do allow some air passage), new shoes made from fabrics that wick away excess moisture have proven effective in keeping feet dry. Before buying shoes, consider the features shown in figure 4.4.
- **Consider lace-up ankle braces.** Ankle braces can help prevent ankle injuries, especially for activities that involve quick changes in direction, such as basketball and racquetball. Studies show that lace-up ankle braces reduce the number of ankle injuries among those who have a history of them. Some people prefer high-top shoes for sports with high rates of ankle injury.

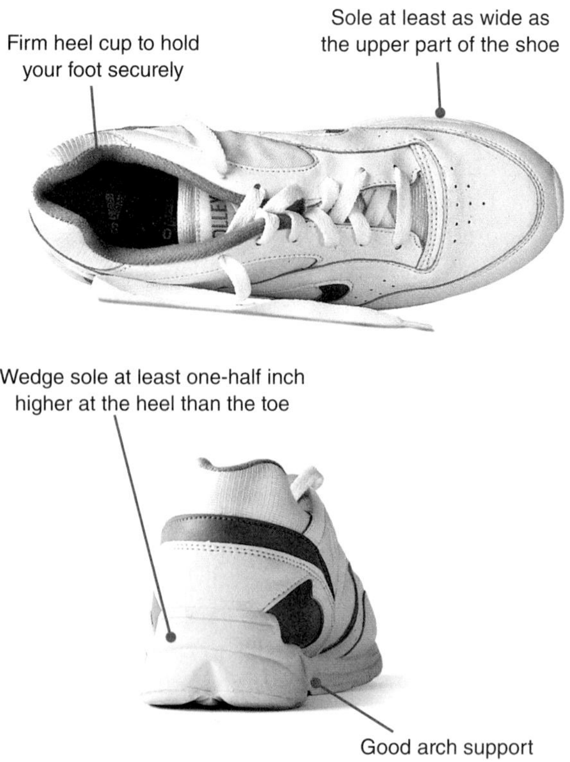

FIGURE 4.4 Characteristics of proper shoes.

FITNESS TECHNOLOGY: High-Tech Exercise Clothing

Modern technology has produced clothing that is especially good for exercising in both hot and cold weather. As noted in the guidelines for exercising in hot or cold environments, clothing made of special synthetic fibers are available that wick moisture away from the body to help it stay cool (for example, Coolmax) or warm (for example, Polartec). Clothing made of wicking fibers can aid your performance in the heat and cold. Jackets made of a synthetic material such as Gore-Tex block the wind but allow your body heat to be released. This type of garment also works well as an outer layer in cold weather. These synthetic fibers are engineered to function in different ways.

Using Technology

Research one type of synthetic fiber used in making exercise clothing in hot or cold environments. What are the special characteristics of the fiber you selected?

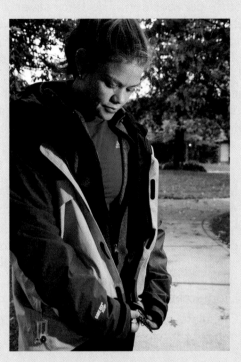

Wearing specially engineered clothing can help you when you exercise in the heat or cold.

Other General Preparation Guidelines

In this chapter, you've learned about medical readiness, environmental factors that affect your activity, and dressing appropriately for activity. Here are some additional steps you can take to make your activity sessions safe and effective.

- **Get fit for your workout.** We all know that you do your workout to get fit. But you also need to be fit enough to do your workout without getting hurt. When you begin a new program, start gradually. As your fitness improves, you can do more. Safe exercise depends on good health-related fitness of all kinds.
- **Warm up before your workout.** Scientists have recently discovered that different types of warm-up are necessary for different kinds of activity. As you continue to work through part 1 of *HOPE*, you'll try a variety of warm-up activities depending on the workout you plan to do.
- **Cool down after your workout.** The cool-down helps you recover after your workout.

Lesson Review

1. What are some steps you can take to make sure you're medically ready to participate in physical activity and sports?
2. What are some environmental factors that can make activity unhealthy or unsafe?
3. What are some guidelines for dressing properly for physical activity in normal environments?

SELF-ASSESSMENT: Body Composition and Flexibility

In this self-assessment, you'll perform two tests: the body mass index (BMI) test and the back-saver sit-and-reach. The BMI is an indicator of your body composition. The back-saver sit-and-reach measures the flexibility of your lower back and your hamstrings (the muscles on the back of your thighs). If you have not done so already, practice this test before performing it for a score. You will have an opportunity later to do other self-assessments of body composition and flexibility. For these two tests, record your scores and fitness ratings as directed by your teacher. These tests give you information that you can use in preparing a Fitnessgram or other fitness report and your personal physical activity plan. If you're working with a partner, remember that self-assessment information is personal and considered confidential. It shouldn't be shared with others without the permission of the person being tested.

Body Mass Index

1. Measure your height in inches (or meters) without shoes.
2. Measure your weight in pounds (or kilograms) without shoes. If you're wearing street clothes (as opposed to lightweight gym clothing), subtract 2 pounds (0.9 kilogram) from your weight.
3. Calculate your BMI using the chart or either of the following formulas.

$$\frac{\text{weight (lb)}}{\text{height (in.)} \times \text{height (in.)}} \times 703 = \text{BMI}$$

$$\frac{\text{weight (kg)}}{\text{height (m)} \times \text{height (m)}} = \text{BMI}$$

4. Use table 4.2 to find your BMI rating, and record your BMI score and rating.

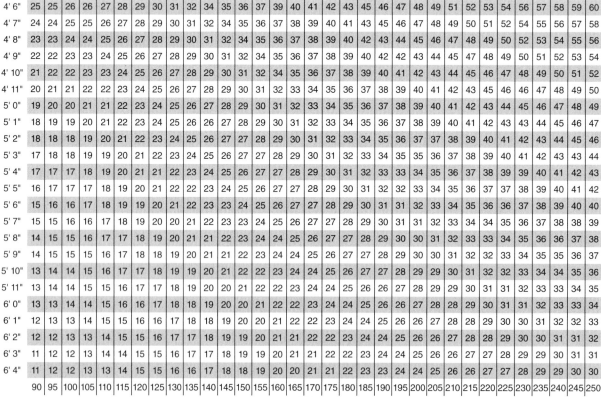

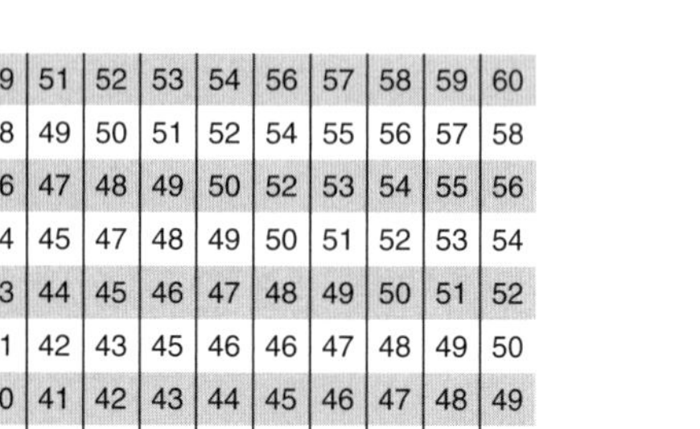

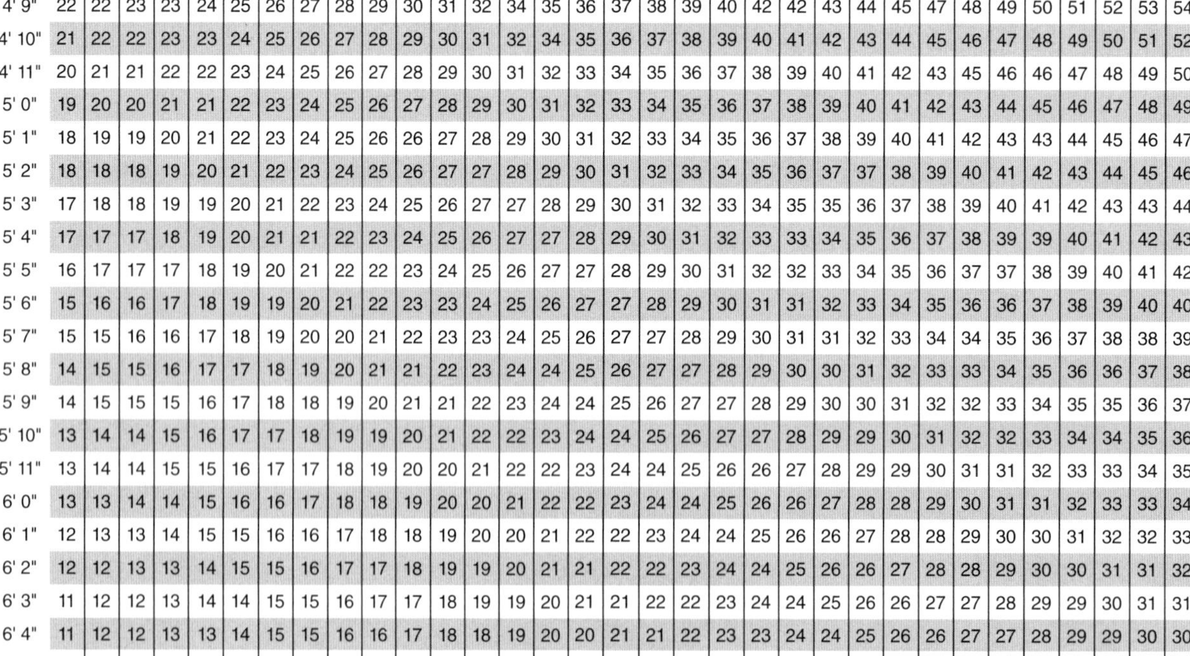

Height	90	95	100	105	110	115	120	125	130	135	140	145	150	155	160	165	170	175	180	185	190	195	200	205	210	215	220	225	230	235	240	245	250
4' 6"	25	25	26	26	27	28	29	30	31	32	34	35	36	37	39	40	41	42	43	45	46	47	48	49	51	52	53	54	56	57	58	59	60
4' 7"	24	24	25	25	26	27	28	29	30	31	32	34	35	36	37	38	39	40	41	43	45	46	47	48	49	50	51	52	54	55	56	57	58
4' 8"	23	23	24	24	25	26	27	28	29	30	31	32	34	35	36	37	38	39	40	42	43	44	45	46	47	48	49	50	52	53	54	55	56
4' 9"	22	22	23	23	24	25	26	27	28	29	30	31	32	34	35	36	37	38	39	40	42	42	43	44	45	47	48	49	50	51	52	53	54
4' 10"	21	22	22	23	23	24	25	26	27	28	29	30	31	32	34	35	36	37	38	39	40	41	42	43	44	45	46	47	48	49	50	51	52
4' 11"	20	21	21	22	22	23	24	25	26	27	28	29	30	31	32	33	34	35	36	37	38	39	40	41	42	43	45	46	46	47	48	49	50
5' 0"	19	20	20	21	21	22	23	24	25	26	27	28	29	30	31	32	33	34	35	36	37	38	39	40	41	42	43	44	45	46	47	48	49
5' 1"	18	19	19	20	21	22	23	24	25	26	26	27	28	29	30	31	32	33	34	35	36	37	38	39	40	41	42	43	43	44	45	46	47
5' 2"	18	18	18	19	20	21	22	23	24	25	26	27	27	28	29	30	31	32	33	34	35	36	37	37	38	39	40	41	42	43	44	45	46
5' 3"	17	18	18	19	19	20	21	22	23	24	25	26	27	27	28	29	30	31	32	33	34	35	35	36	37	38	39	40	41	42	43	43	44
5' 4"	17	17	17	18	19	20	21	21	22	23	24	25	26	27	27	28	29	30	31	32	33	33	34	35	36	37	38	39	39	40	41	42	43
5' 5"	16	17	17	17	18	19	20	21	22	22	23	24	25	26	27	27	28	29	30	31	32	32	33	34	35	36	37	37	38	39	40	41	42
5' 6"	15	16	16	17	18	19	19	20	21	22	23	23	24	25	26	27	27	28	29	30	31	31	32	33	34	35	36	36	37	38	39	40	40
5' 7"	15	15	16	16	17	18	19	20	20	21	22	23	23	24	25	26	27	27	28	29	30	31	31	32	33	34	34	35	36	37	38	38	39
5' 8"	14	15	15	16	17	17	18	19	20	21	21	22	23	24	24	25	26	27	27	28	29	30	30	31	32	33	33	34	35	36	36	37	38
5' 9"	14	15	15	15	16	17	18	18	19	20	21	21	22	23	24	24	25	26	27	27	28	29	30	30	31	32	32	33	34	35	35	36	37
5' 10"	13	14	14	15	16	17	17	18	19	19	20	21	22	22	23	24	24	25	26	27	27	28	29	29	30	31	32	32	33	34	34	35	36
5' 11"	13	14	14	15	15	16	17	17	18	19	20	20	21	22	22	23	24	24	25	26	26	27	28	29	29	30	31	31	32	33	33	34	35
6' 0"	13	13	14	14	15	16	16	17	18	18	19	20	20	21	22	22	23	24	24	25	26	26	27	28	28	29	30	31	31	32	33	33	34
6' 1"	12	13	13	14	15	15	16	16	17	18	18	19	20	20	21	22	22	23	24	24	25	26	26	27	28	28	29	30	30	31	32	32	33
6' 2"	12	12	13	13	14	15	15	16	17	17	18	19	19	20	21	21	22	22	23	24	24	25	26	26	27	28	28	29	30	30	31	31	32
6' 3"	11	12	12	13	14	14	15	15	16	17	17	18	19	19	20	21	21	22	22	23	24	24	25	26	26	27	27	28	29	29	30	31	31
6' 4"	11	12	12	13	13	14	15	15	16	16	17	18	18	19	20	20	21	21	22	23	23	24	24	25	26	26	27	27	28	29	29	30	30

Weight

BMI calculation chart. Locate your height in the left column and your weight in pounds in the bottom row. The box where the selected row and column intersect is your BMI score.

TABLE 4.2 Rating Chart: Body Mass Index

	13 years old		14 years old		15 years old		16 years old		17 years old		18 years old	
	Male	Female	Male	Female	Male	Female	Male	Female	Male	Female	Male	Female
Very lean	≤15.4	≤15.3	≤16.0	≤15.8	≤16.5	≤16.3	≤17.1	≤16.8	≤17.7	≤17.2	≤18.2	≤17.5
Good fitness	15.5–21.3	15.4–22.0	16.1–22.1	15.9–22.8	16.6–22.9	16.4–23.5	17.2–23.7	16.9–24.1	17.8–24.4	17.3–24.6	18.3–25.1	17.6–25.1
Marginal fitness	21.4–23.5	22.1–23.7	22.2–24.4	22.9–24.5	23.0–25.2	23.6–25.3	23.8–25.9	24.2–26.0	24.5–26.6	24.7–27.6	25.2–27.4	25.2–27.1
Low fitness	≥23.6	≥23.8	≥24.5	≥24.6	≥25.3	≥25.4	≥26.0	≥26.1	≥26.7	≥27.7	≥27.5	≥27.2

Data based on *Fitnessgram*.

Back-Saver Sit-and-Reach

1. Place a measuring stick, such as a yardstick or meter stick, on top of a box that is 12 inches (30 centimeters) high with the stick extending 9 inches (23 centimeters) over the box and the lower numbers toward you. You may use a flexibility testing box if one is available.
2. To measure the flexibility of your right leg, fully extend it and place your right foot flat against the box. Bend your left leg, with the knee turned out and your left foot 2 to 3 inches (5 to 8 centimeters) to the side of your straight right leg.
3. Extend your arms forward over the measuring stick. Place your hands on the stick, one on top of the other, with your palms facing down. Your middle fingers should be together with the tip of one finger exactly on top of the other.
4. Lean forward slowly; do not bounce. Reach forward with your arms and fingers, then slowly return to the starting position. Repeat four times. On the fourth reach, hold the position for three seconds and observe the measurement on the stick below your fingertips.
5. Repeat the test with your left leg straight.
6. Record your score to the nearest inch (1 inch equals 2.54 centimeters). Consult table 4.3 to determine your fitness rating for each side of your body.

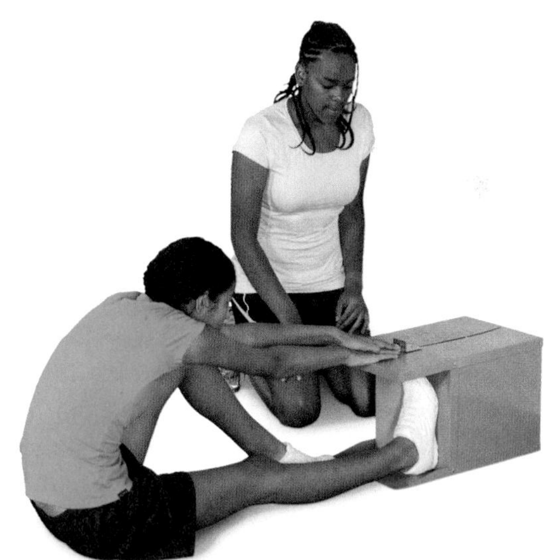
The back-saver sit-and-reach assesses flexibility.

TABLE 4.3 Rating Chart: Back-Saver Sit-and-Reach (Inches)

	13 or 14 years old		15 years or older	
	Male	Female	Male	Female
High performance	≥10	≥12	≥10	≥14
Good fitness	8–9	10–11	8–9	12–13
Marginal fitness	6–7	8–9	6–7	10–11
Low fitness	≤5	≤7	≤5	≤9

Data based on *Fitnessgram*.

Lesson 4.2

Health and Wellness Benefits

Lesson Objectives

After reading this lesson, you should be able to

1. explain, using examples, how physical activity is related to hypokinetic conditions;
2. list some benefits of physical activity that contribute to health and wellness; and
3. explain, using examples, how physical activity is related to hyperkinetic conditions.

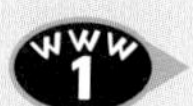

Lesson Vocabulary

activity neurosis, atherosclerosis, blood pressure, cardiovascular disease (CVD), coronary artery disease (CAD), diabetes, diastolic blood pressure, eating disorder, heart attack, hyperkinetic condition, hypertension, metabolic syndrome, osteoporosis, peak bone mass, risk factor, stroke, systolic blood pressure

Have you ever wondered why many people now live twice as long as most people did a few hundred years ago? Do you know the leading causes of death today? Do you understand the roles played by physical activity and nutrition in living a long, high-quality life?

Prior to 1900, the leading cause of death in the United States and other developed countries was pneumonia, and infections from other bacteria and viruses accounted for many of the other common causes of death. Science has found cures or vaccinations for many of these conditions, and today they are no longer the leading health problems for people with access to modern health care. Instead, the leading health threats today are conditions that are hypokinetic—caused in part by sedentary living—such as heart disease, cancer, and stroke (in that order). In this lesson, you'll learn more about how physical activity reduces your risk of hypokinetic conditions and increases your personal wellness; similar benefits are provided by good nutrition.

Hypokinetic Diseases and Conditions

Sedentary living costs the United States billions of dollars each year in health care expenses and loss of productivity. Even more alarming, thousands of people die prematurely every year because they are inactive. Reports issued by major health organizations, including the U.S. Office of the Surgeon General and the American Heart Association, indicate that regular physical activity is one of the best ways to reduce illness and increase wellness in American society. The American College of Sports Medicine (ACSM) lists 27 different health benefits of regular exercise. Sometimes teenagers feel that these statistics are not relevant to them; they think illness happens only to old people. As you'll see next, however, many hypokinetic diseases are now prevalent among teens, and many teens are not active enough to resist these conditions.

> In the United States, physical inactivity is the biggest health problem of the 21st century.
>
> —Dr. Steven Blair, past president of the American College of Sports Medicine

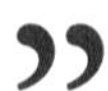

Cardiovascular Disease

Did you know that **cardiovascular disease (CVD)** has been the leading cause of death in the United States each year since 1920? In fact, CVD is a primary or contributing cause of more than half of all deaths in the United States. Currently, about one in every four Americans has at least one form of CVD.

CVD encompasses various conditions, such as **coronary artery disease (CAD)**. *Coronary* means related to the heart, and an *artery* is a kind of blood vessel. Your heart is a muscle that acts as a pump to push blood, and your arteries are the pipelines that carry your blood from your heart to various parts of your body. CAD exists when the arteries become clogged—a condition called **atherosclerosis**, which occurs when substances including fats, such as cholesterol, build up on the inside walls of the arteries. This build-up narrows the openings through the arteries. As a result, the heart must work harder to pump blood. See figure 4.5 for the difference between a clear artery and one that is partially blocked. Atherosclerosis typically develops with age but can begin early in life.

A **heart attack** occurs when the blood supply within the heart is severely reduced or cut off; as a result, an area of the heart muscle can die. The main reasons for heart attacks are arteries blocked by atherosclerosis, blood clots in narrowed arteries, spasms in the muscle of the artery, or a combination of these causes. During a heart attack, the heart may beat abnormally or even stop beating. Treatments often include medicines that stabilize the heartbeat and cardiopulmonary resuscitation (CPR) to restore circulation of oxygen.

Another form of cardiovascular disease is **stroke**, which is the third leading cause of early death in the United States and other developed countries. It occurs when the oxygen supply to the brain is severely reduced or cut off. A stroke can be caused when an artery that supplies blood to the brain bursts or is blocked by a blood clot or atherosclerosis. Because a stroke damages the brain, it can affect a person's ability to move, think, and speak. Some strokes are severe enough to cause death.

A primary risk factor for CVD is **hypertension**, or, as it is commonly called, high blood pressure.

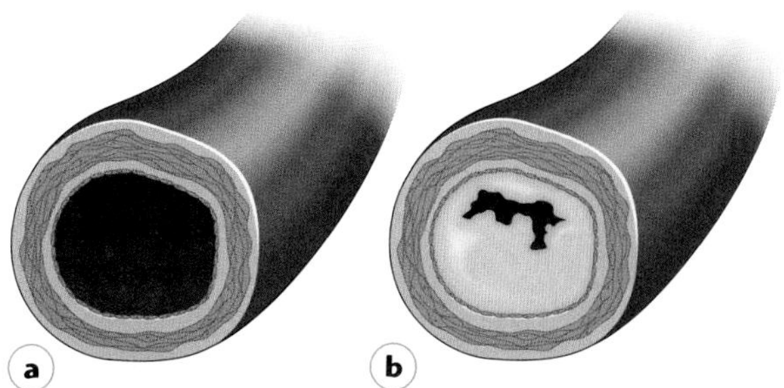

FIGURE 4.5 *(a)* A healthy heart has open arteries. *(b)* An unhealthy heart has clogged arteries that can cause a heart attack.

FIT FACT

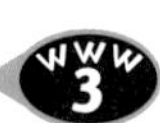

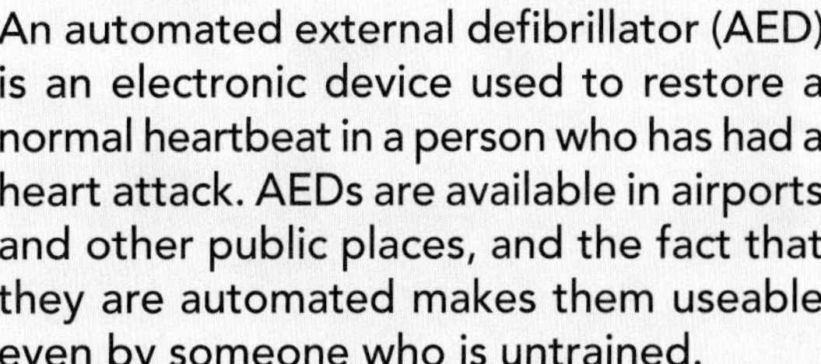

An automated external defibrillator (AED) is an electronic device used to restore a normal heartbeat in a person who has had a heart attack. AEDs are available in airports and other public places, and the fact that they are automated makes them useable even by someone who is untrained.

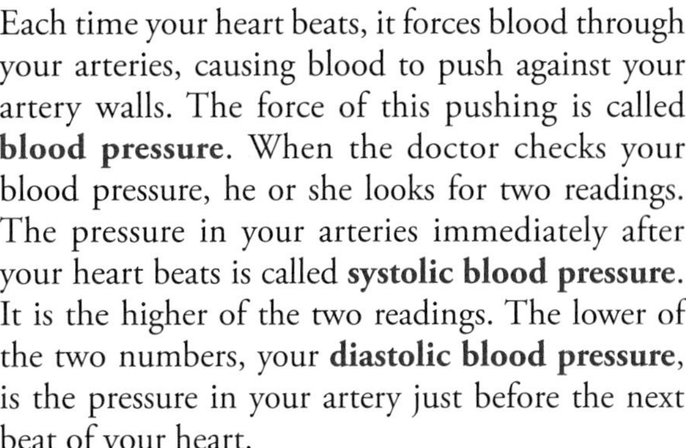

Each time your heart beats, it forces blood through your arteries, causing blood to push against your artery walls. The force of this pushing is called **blood pressure**. When the doctor checks your blood pressure, he or she looks for two readings. The pressure in your arteries immediately after your heart beats is called **systolic blood pressure**. It is the higher of the two readings. The lower of the two numbers, your **diastolic blood pressure**, is the pressure in your artery just before the next beat of your heart.

You can see what counts as normal blood pressure in table 4.4. The table also shows the range for prehypertension, a new category indicating blood pressure that is higher than normal but not high enough to be considered hypertension. People with prehypertension should take precautions to prevent developing even higher blood pressure. There are three stages of high blood pressure. Stage 1 is the least severe and stage 3 the most. When you have your blood pressure checked, you should be rested and relaxed. Blood pressure will be higher if you exercise immediately before taking a reading. Also, your blood pressure is often elevated when you're excited or anxious. The incidence of high blood pressure has decreased in recent years because of improved medicines and early screening. Because high blood pressure is a hypokinetic condition, regular physical activity can help decrease it. A healthy low-sodium diet is also helpful in reducing high blood pressure.

An active person's coronary arteries are more likely to be free from atherosclerosis and generally

TABLE 4.4 Blood Pressure Readings

	Normal	Prehypertension	Stage 1	Stage 2	Stage 3
Systolic	≤119	120–139	140–159	160–179	≥180
Diastolic	≤79	80–89	90–99	100–109	≥110

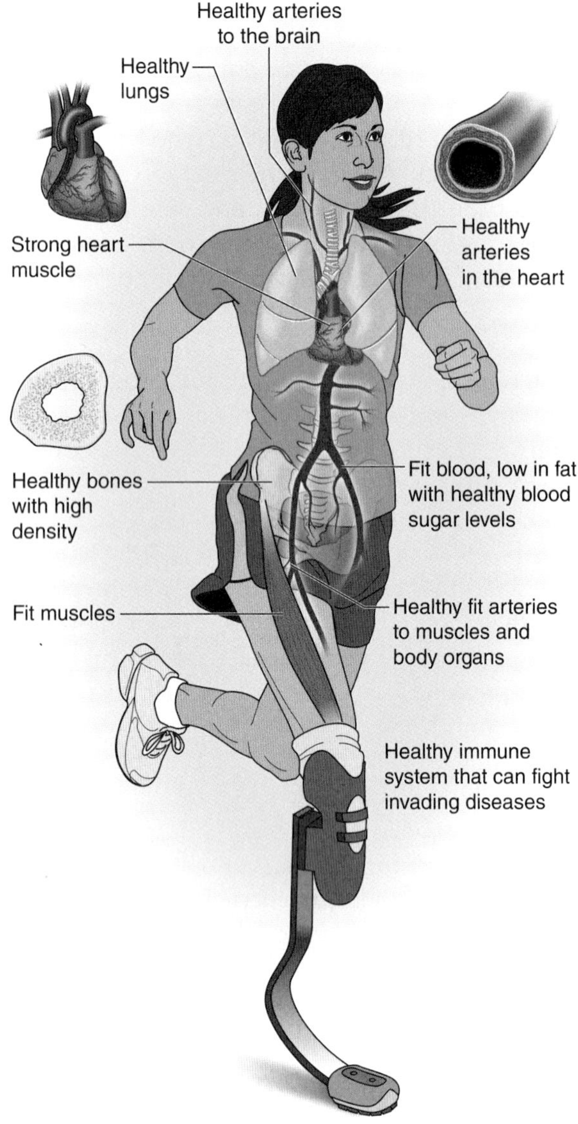

FIGURE 4.6 Physical activity benefits associated with reduced risk of hypokinetic conditions and CVD.

healthy. An active person also has healthy arteries in his or her brain, muscles, and organs; has a strong heart muscle capable of pumping adequate blood to the body; has fit blood that is low in fat, such as cholesterol; and has blood pressure in the healthy range. Regular physical activity not only reduces your risk of heart attack and stroke but also is often prescribed by doctors to help people recovering from these conditions. Figure 4.6 illustrates some ways in which regular physical activity reduces the risk of hypokinetic conditions, including CVD.

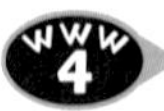

People get CVD for many reasons, each of which is called a **risk factor**. The more risk factors you have, the more chance you have of getting a disease. Two kinds of risk factor exist: primary (more important) and secondary (less important). Because one primary risk factor is sedentary (inactive) living, cardiovascular disease is considered a hypokinetic condition. Other primary risk factors for heart disease include smoking, high blood pressure, high fat levels in the blood, too much body fat, and diabetes. Secondary risk factors include stressful living and excessive alcohol use. More information is available in the Taking Charge feature near the end of this chapter.

As you get older, your doctor will likely test your cholesterol, blood pressure, blood sugar, and other potential CVD risk factors. Your doctor will also provide you a rating or standard for each of these tests that indicates how those levels might affect your health. Research shows that your activity and nutrition influence conditions like high cholesterol, high blood pressure, and other risk factors.

Cancer

According to the American Cancer Society, cancer includes more than one hundred types, all characterized by the uncontrollable growth of abnormal cells. Cancer's uncontrolled cells invade normal cells, steal their nutrition, and interfere with the cells' normal functioning.

Cancer is the second leading cause of death in the United States. When diagnosed early, many forms of cancer can be treated and even cured through surgery, chemical or radiation therapy, or medication. Many of the risk factors for cancer are the same as those for heart disease. We know that the death rate from all forms of cancer is lower in active people than in inactive people. Certain forms of cancer (breast, colon, prostate, and rectal) are considered hypokinetic conditions because people who are physically active are less likely to get them than people who are inactive. It is not clear why physical activity helps reduce the risk of cancer, but, as shown in figure 4.6, one of the health benefits of physical activity is an immune system that is more capable of fighting diseases that invade the body. Another good way to help prevent or minimize cancer is to get regular physical exams.

Diabetes

When a person's body cannot regulate its sugar level, the person has a disease called **diabetes**. A person with diabetes has excessively high blood sugar unless he or she gets medical assistance. Diabetics may also have trouble using insulin effectively because the cells may become resistant to it. Insulin is a hormone made in the pancreas that helps control blood sugar level. Over time, diabetes can damage the blood vessels, heart, kidneys, and eyes. A very high level of sugar in the blood can cause coma and death. Fortunately, several effective medical treatments can help diabetic people regulate their blood sugar and lead a normal life.

There are two types of diabetes. Type 1, which accounts for about 10 percent of cases, is not a hypokinetic condition and is often hereditary. People with type 1 diabetes take insulin. In people without diabetes, the body automatically produce insulin to keep blood sugar in a normal range. At one time, it was thought that people with type 1 diabetes should avoid physical activity. Now we know that physical activity can help people manage diabetes. Most people with type 1 diabetes take a blood sample one or more times a day in order to test their blood sugar. If the level is high, they take insulin to lower their blood sugar. In the past, it was necessary to puncture the skin to take a blood sample, but new technology allows some people with diabetes to wear a computerized watch that automatically tests blood sugar without having to draw blood.

The most common kind of diabetes—type 2—is a hypokinetic condition because people who are physically active are less likely to have it. As shown in figure 4.6, active people are more likely to have a healthy level of blood sugar. Diabetes has many of the same risk factors as heart disease, including sedentary living. Exercise helps reduce your risk of type 2 diabetes by lowering your blood sugar level, helping your body tissues use insulin more efficiently, and helping control body fat. Having too much body fat is a major risk factor for type 2 diabetes. In fact, so many obese people have diabetes that one expert coined the term *diabesity*—a combination of the words *diabetes* and *obesity*.

FIT FACT

Type 2 diabetes used to be called adult-onset diabetes because adults got it, not teens and children. This name is no longer used because in recent years the disease has become common among youth.

Obesity

Obesity, in which a person has a high percentage of body fat, often results from inactivity, though many other factors can contribute. The American Medical Association now classifies obesity as a disease. Having too much body fat contributes to conditions such as heart disease and diabetes. Since 1980, the incidence of obesity among teens in the United States has almost quadrupled, rising from 5 percent to more than 18 percent, and a similar upward trend is found in other developed nations.

Osteoporosis

Osteoporosis exists when bone structure deteriorates (see figure 4.7) and bones become weak. It is most common among older people but has its beginnings in youth. You develop your greatest bone mass—also called your **peak bone mass**—when you're young. People who exercise regularly develop stronger bones than those who are sedentary. Choose physical activities that cause you to bear weight and thus stress your bones in a healthy way. Examples of weight-bearing activities are walking, running, jumping, and resistance training. If you do the right kind of activity when you're young, you'll build a higher peak bone mass. As a result, even if you lose bone mass as you get older, you'll have stronger bones than if you hadn't exercised while young.

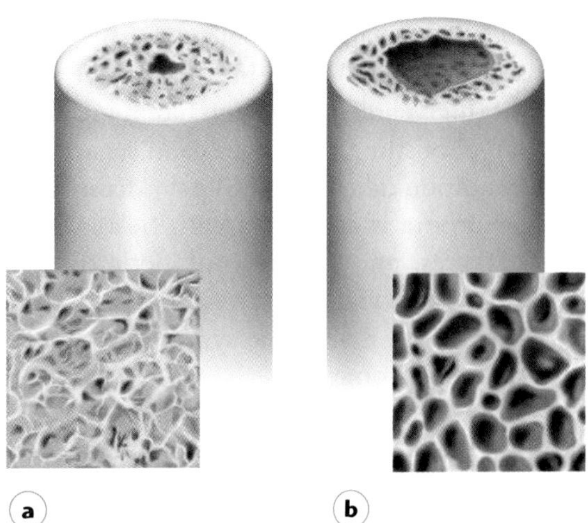

FIGURE 4.7 Osteoporosis involves a decrease in bone density: *(a)* healthy bone in an active person; *(b)* unhealthy bone (osteoporosis) more common among sedentary people.

One contributor to osteoporosis is a lack of sufficient calcium in the diet, especially when a person is young. Women are more likely to have osteoporosis than men because the hormonal changes they experience later in life cause their body to absorb calcium less efficiently. Whether you are female or male, you can maximize your bone health throughout life by getting good nutrition, regular activity, and proper medical attention.

Other Hypokinetic Conditions

Evidence suggests that regular physical activity can also reduce the risk or relieve the symptoms of the following diseases and conditions.

- **Mental health conditions.** One-third of all adults report that they often feel depressed, but people who do regular physical activity are less likely to be depressed. Being active can also help reduce feelings of anxiety and improve brain function in older people.
- **Back problems.** More than 80 percent of all adults experience back pain at some point, but exercise can help reduce the incidence of back problems.
- **Metabolic health conditions.** *Metabolism* is a word that refers to the many chemical reactions that allow the body, and the cells of the body, to live and function effectively. You are metabolically healthy when the chemical reactions work normally, allowing the cells to function well. When this does not happen metabolic problems occur. People with metabolic problems such as high blood fat (high cholesterol), high blood pressure, a large waistline, and high blood sugar have a condition called **metabolic syndrome.** This syndrome is associated with heart disease, diabetes, and other hypokinetic diseases. Regular exercise can improve metabolic health and reduce the symptoms of metabolic syndrome.
- **Immune system conditions.** Regular physical activity has been shown to enhance the function of the immune system, thus helping the body resist infections such as the common cold and the flu.
- **Arthritis.** Moderate activity has been shown to help reduce symptoms of some forms of arthritis.
- **Alzheimer's disease and dementia.** Research shows that doing regular exercise and challenging mental tasks can improve brain health and reduce the risk of memory loss disorders.

Physical Activity and Wellness

As you can see, physical activity plays an important role in preventing hypokinetic diseases and conditions and thus is a key to good health. But remember—health is more than freedom from disease; it also includes positive health, or wellness. As a result, the U.S. government's Healthy People 2020 report incorporates wellness in two of its major goals: high quality of life and sense of well-being. Some of the benefits of physical activity that contribute to wellness are illustrated in figure 4.8.

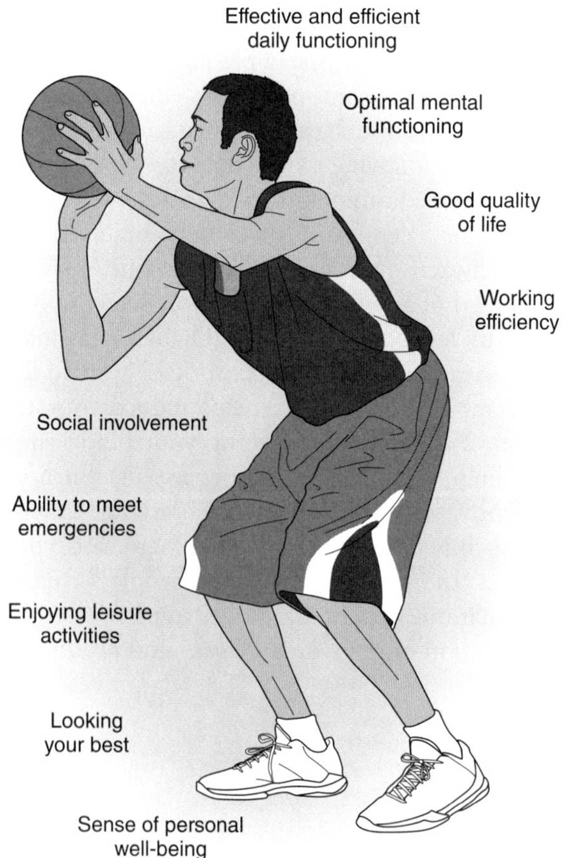

FIGURE 4.8 The wellness benefits of regular physical activity.

FIT FACT

Studies conducted by experts in exercise physiology, exercise psychology, and physical activity show that teens who are fit and active enjoy multiple benefits. For example, they perform better in school and are less likely to be absent or cause discipline problems than unfit, inactive teens.

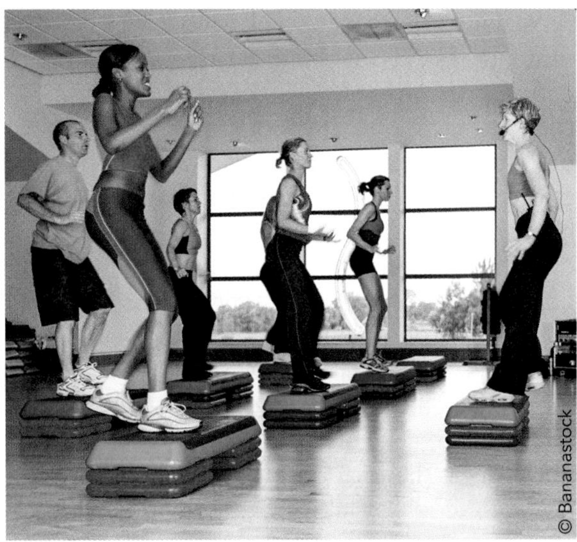
© Bananastock

People who are overly concerned about getting enough exercise may have a condition called activity neurosis.

Hyperkinetic Conditions

You've probably heard the saying "too much of a good thing can be bad." This saying can even be true of physical activity. The fact that some physical activity is good does not mean that more activity is always better. In some cases, people experience **hyperkinetic conditions**—health problems caused by doing too *much* physical activity.

Overuse Injuries

Overuse injuries occur when you do so much physical activity that you suffer damage to a bone, muscle, or other tissue. Examples include stress fractures, shin splints, and blisters.

Activity Neurosis

Neurosis is a condition in which a person is overly concerned or fearful about something. People with an **activity neurosis** are overly concerned about getting enough exercise. They feel upset if they miss a regular workout and often continue physical activity when they are sick or injured. Activity neurosis is more common among aerobic dance instructors, bodybuilders, and runners than other active groups. Aerobic dance instructors often teach many classes and also take classes to improve their dance skills. Some experts believe this can lead to a compulsive need to exercise. Some bodybuilders seek perfection and continue to do more exercise in pursuit of this ideal. Reasons for activity neurosis among runners may be the desire to improve running times or distance.

Body Image and Eating Disorders

People with body image disorders try to achieve their idea of an ideal body by doing excessive exercise. This idealized body is unrealistic and distorted. People with this disorder often perform excessive resistance training and sometimes use dangerous supplements or substances such as steroids. Use of steroids and dangerous supplements or substances is most common among teenage boys and young adult men but can occur in both men and women of all ages. Teenage girls and young women, and to a lesser extent young men, often strive for extreme thinness, which is both unhealthy and unrealistic. An extreme desire to be abnormally thin is associated with several kinds of **eating disorders**. People with these conditions have dangerous eating habits and often resort to excessive activity to expend calories for fat loss. Eating disorders that include abuse of exercise are considered to be hyperkinetic conditions. People with body image disorders and eating disorders often need the help of an expert to overcome their problem.

Lesson Review

1. Name and describe at least four hypokinetic conditions. How can physical activity reduce your risk of getting these conditions?
2. What are some health and wellness benefits of physical activity?
3. How is physical activity related to hyperkinetic conditions? Give examples.

TAKING CHARGE: Reducing Risk Factors

A risk factor is any action or condition that increases your chances of developing a disease. Some risk factors, such as your age and your genetic makeup, are beyond your ability to control or change. But there are also risk factors that you can control—for example, your diet and physical activity. Therefore, your actions can affect the probability that you will get a disease.

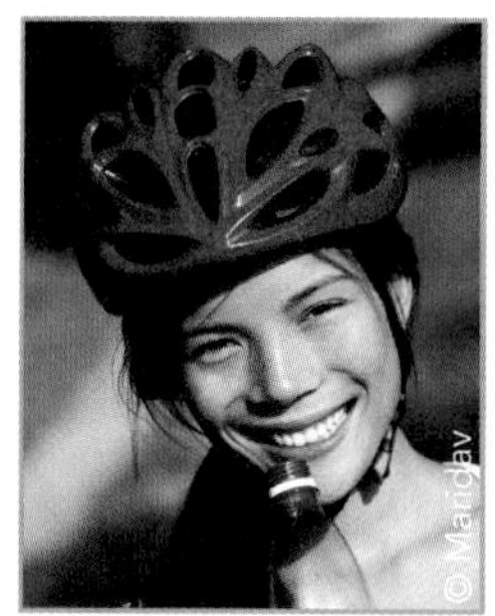

Here's an example. Last summer, Brenda's family took a trip to the mountains, where they planned to hike, raft the rivers, and ride bikes and horses. Unfortunately, Brenda's father did not get to enjoy all of the activities. Brenda was surprised: "I never thought my father had any health problems because he was always busy with work and taking care of the house. He never went to the doctor."

But Brenda's father was a smoker. And though he was busy, he didn't actually do much physical activity because he easily became short of breath. On the trip, Brenda's father found that he couldn't keep up with the rest of the family. While hiking, he became so short of breath that he almost fainted. While riding a bike, he fell far behind the others. And in the evening, while the rest of the family did other things, Brenda's father went to bed.

When they returned home, Brenda's father visited his doctor, who recommended that he change his lifestyle. Specifically, his doctor advised him to stop smoking and get more exercise. He also was warned that if he continued his present lifestyle, he was at risk for heart disease and other health problems.

For Discussion

What controllable risk factors for heart disease did Brenda's father have? What can Brenda's father do to reduce his risk? Is there anything that Brenda can do to help her father reduce his risk? What can Brenda do now to minimize her own disease risk later in life? Consider the guidelines presented in the following Self-Management feature as you answer these discussion questions.

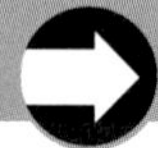

SELF-MANAGEMENT: Skills for Reducing Risk Factors

Of the 10 leading causes of death, 6 can be considered hypokinetic conditions. Many of these conditions can be prevented if you adopt a healthy lifestyle early in life. You can take the following steps, even in your teen years, to reduce your risk of hypokinetic conditions.

- **Know how to identify important risk factors.** In order to lower your disease risks, you must first identify them. Risk factors for hypokinetic disease that are *not* in your control include heredity, sex, age, and diseases such as type 1 diabetes (which increases the risk of heart disease). You do have some control over risk factors such as your body fat, blood pressure, and blood fat, but they are also influenced by heredity. Risk factors over which you have more control are diet, physical activity, tobacco and alcohol use, and exposure to stress.
- **Periodically self-assess your risk factors.** You can't change risk factors if you don't know you have them. Doing a self-assessment helps you plan for reducing your risks and lets you know when you need to seek medical help. Because risk increases with age, it becomes even more important to check your risk factors as you grow older.
- **Learn about your family history.** Heredity is a factor over which you have no control. You can, however, check to see what diseases or conditions your parents or grandparents have had—and thus which ones you may inherit a tendency to develop (for example, heart disease, diabetes, and some forms of cancer). You can then pay special attention to controllable risk factors for those diseases.

- **Take steps to change risk factors that are partially in your control.** Some risk factors are influenced by heredity but can also be modified through healthy lifestyle choices. These risk factors include your blood pressure, your blood fat, your body's ability to regulate sugar, and your body fatness. You can influence these factors through choices such as getting regular physical activity, eating properly, and seeking proper medical care. If you have a family history of any of these risk factors, seek medical help and professional advice about how to make lifestyle changes to reduce your risk.
- **Take steps to change risk factors that are fully in your control.** Some risk factors are well within your control—for example, physical activity, what you eat, tobacco and alcohol use, and your stress level.
- **Use the self-management skills you learn in part 1 of this book to make lifelong changes.** You'll learn many self-management skills throughout part 1 of this book. Use them to change the risk factors that you identify.

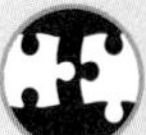

ACADEMIC CONNECTION: Statistics

Statistics is a branch of mathematics dealing with the collection, analysis, and interpretation of data (numerical information). Mathematic literacy is important for meeting college and career readiness standards. Understanding and using some basic statistical concepts can help you not only as you prepare for a career or college and university studies but also in understanding health risks.

The average person is said to be typical. In math, *average* refers to measures of central tendency such as

- the mean, or the sum of all scores divided by the number of scores (11 scores in the following example);
- the median, or the middle score in a number of scores (in the following example, the sixth score from the lowest or sixth score from the highest); and
- the mode, or the most common score in a number of scores (in the following example, the only score that was common to two people).

Calculate the mean, median, and mode for a group of 11 people with the following systolic blood pressure readings in mmHg: 120, 125, 130, 130, 135, 140, 145, 150, 155, 160, 165.Remember that systolic blood pressure is the higher of the two blood pressure numbers and reflects the pressure in your arteries just after the heart beats.

A systolic blood pressure of 120 mmHg is considered to be healthy. Knowing this, would you want to have your blood pressure equal to the average for this group (using any of the three measures of central tendency)?

Check Your Answers

Mean = 141.36; median = 140; mode = 130

TAKING ACTION: Walking for Health

Walking can be done by most people, in most places, and with little or no equipment. Research shows that 30 minutes or more of daily walking can

- help you maintain a healthy weight,
- reduce your risk of hypokinetic disease,
- improve your wellness and mental health,
- strengthen your bones and muscles, and
- increase your chances of living longer.

Because walking is a moderate-intensity activity, it can typically be done while talking with others. As a result, you can use it as a way of not only relaxing and helping your body but also building healthy relationships as you walk and talk with friends and family members. If you have not been active up until now, walking is also a great way to slowly build your fitness before you start an exercise program. In fact, some people have begun with a walking program and ended up running a marathon. If you want to start looking and feeling your best but don't know where to start, **take action** and try walking!

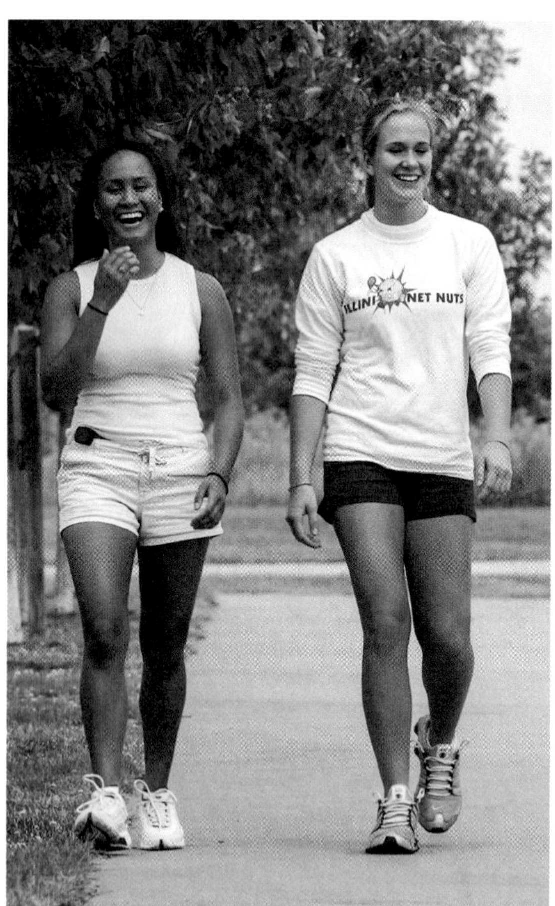

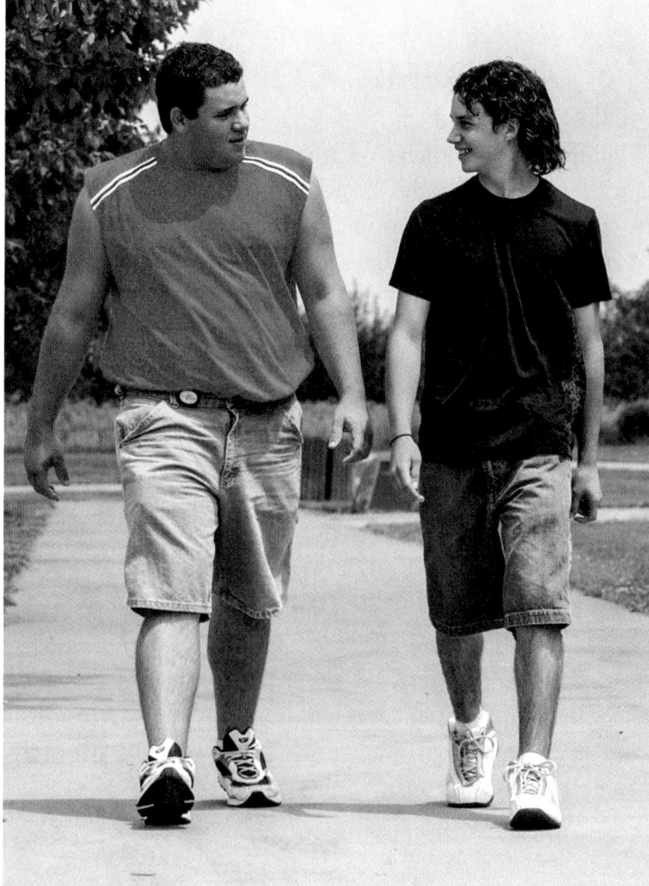

Taking action by walking can improve health and promote social relationships.

CHAPTER REVIEW

Reviewing Concepts and Vocabulary

As directed by your teacher, answer items 1 through 5 by correctly completing each sentence with a word or phrase.

1. The seven questions used to determine readiness for physical activity are called the ______________.
2. The two factors used to determine the heat index are ______________.
3. The measure used to determine whether it is too cold to exercise is called the ______________.
4. Symptoms of frostbite include ______________.
5. Hot, dry, flushed skin; rapid pulse; and lack of sweating are symptoms of ______________.

For items 6 through 10, as directed by your teacher, match each term in column 1 with the appropriate phrase in column 2.

6. electrolytes	a. inability to regulate blood sugar
7. diabetes	b. body composition measure
8. air quality index	c. minerals that help prevent heat injuries
9. hypothermia	d. extremely low body temperature
10. BMI	e. indicator that helps determine whether it is safe to exercise

For items 11 through 15, as directed by your teacher, respond to each statement or question.

11. Describe the three types of heat-related conditions.
12. What are the benefits of physical activity in preventing heart disease?
13. Describe two hyperkinetic conditions.
14. Describe two wellness benefits of physical activity.
15. What are some benefits of walking 30 minutes or more each day?

Thinking Critically

Write a paragraph to answer the following question.

Why is inactivity a primary risk factor for many diseases?

Project

You have been asked to give a speech to a local civic club on the health benefits of physical activity. Prepare a presentation using 10 or more slides.

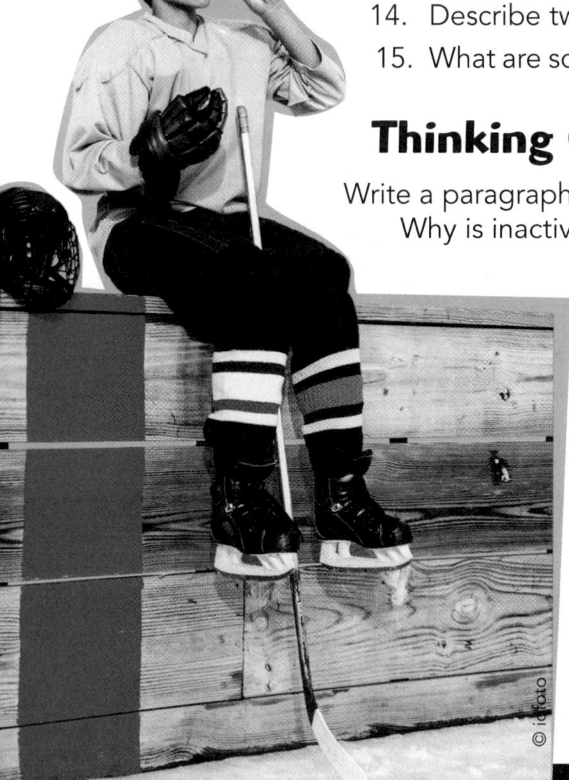

5

How Much Is Enough?

In This Chapter

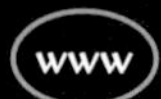

Student Web Resources

www.HOPEtextbook.org/student

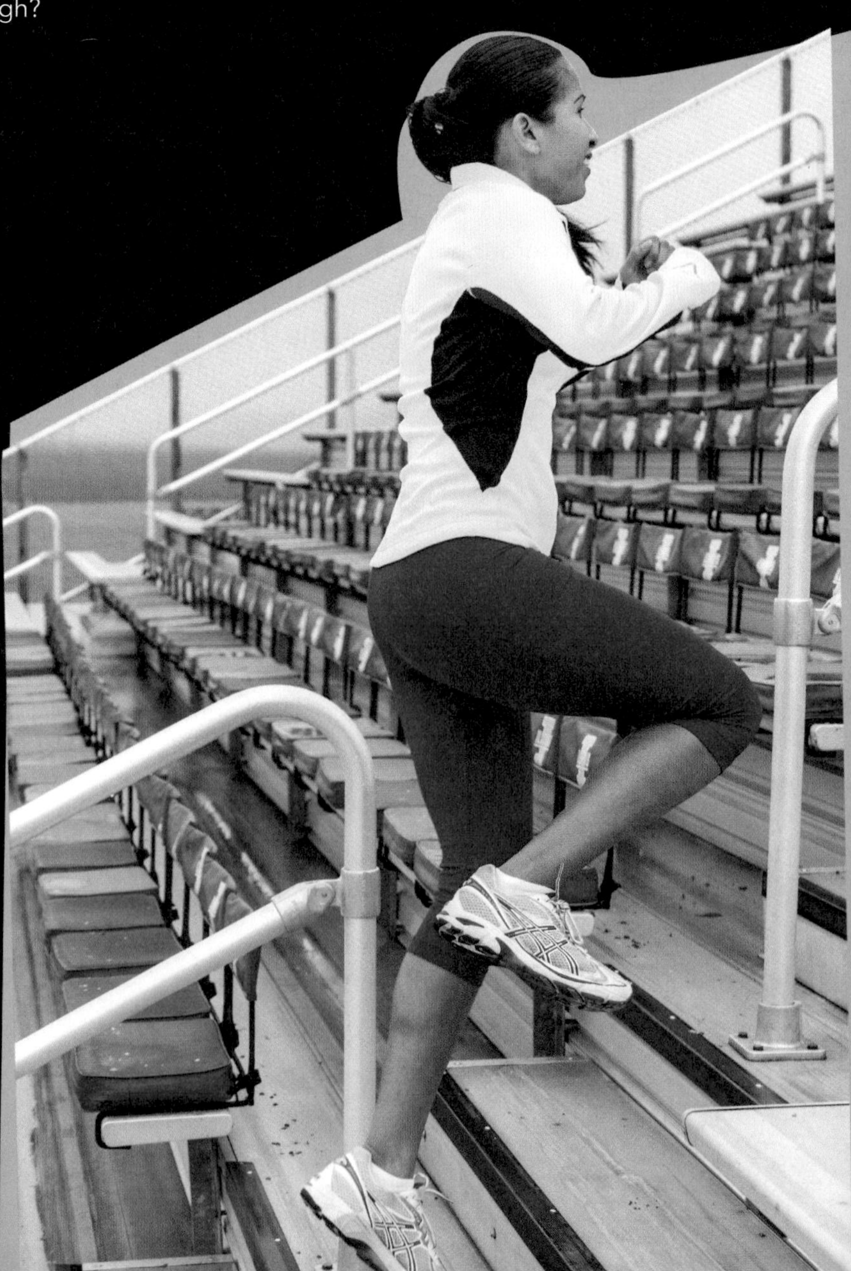

Lesson 5.1

How Much Physical Activity Is Enough?

Lesson Objectives

After reading this lesson, you should be able to

1. name and describe the three principles of exercise;
2. describe the four parts of the FITT formula and discuss how they relate to threshold of training, target ceiling, and fitness target zone; and
3. describe the five types of physical activity included in the Physical Activity Pyramid.

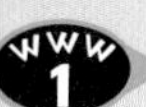

Lesson Vocabulary

fitness target zone, FITT formula, frequency, intensity, Physical Activity Pyramid, principle of overload, principle of progression, principle of specificity, target ceiling, threshold of training, time, type

How much physical activity is enough? This question might seem very simple, but the answer can be complicated, especially if you're just beginning an activity program. In this lesson, you'll develop an understanding of three basic exercise principles as a good first step in answering the question of how much is enough.

Principles of Physical Activity

Consider this example. Mia has been exercising for several months. Every day, she does the same physical activities for about 15 minutes. Her activity program has not changed since she started. Initially, Mia saw some positive results from her program: She was no longer tired at the end of her exercise, and a self-assessment showed that her cardiorespiratory endurance had improved. Lately, however, Mia has felt disappointed because her strength and flexibility haven't been improving as much as they did at first. Mia wants to know what she's doing wrong. For some clues to the answer, let's look at the three principles of exercise: overload, progression, and specificity.

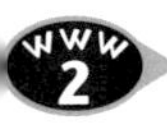

Principle of Overload

The most basic law of physical activity is the **principle of overload**, which states that the only way to produce fitness and health benefits through physical activity is to require your body to do more than it normally does. Increased demand on your body—overload—forces it to adapt. Your body was designed to be active, so if you do nothing (underload), your fitness will decrease, and you will increase your risk of hypokinetic disease.

Since Mia is no longer overloading when she exercises, she is maintaining but no longer gaining increased fitness and health benefits. If she wants to continue improving her strength and flexibility, she'll have to increase the amount of her physical activity.

Principle of Progression

The **principle of progression** states that the amount and intensity of your exercise should be increased gradually. After a while, your body adapts to an increase in physical activity (load), and the activity gets easier for you to perform. When this happens, you can gradually increase your activity.

Figure 5.1 shows the minimum overload you need in order to build physical fitness. This amount is called your **threshold of training**. Performing activity above your threshold builds your fitness and promotes your health and wellness. Since Mia has exercised for several months at the same level, she may now be exercising below her threshold of training for at least some parts of fitness.

This correct range of physical activity is called your **fitness target zone**, typically shortened to just *target zone*. It begins with the threshold of training and has an upper limit called the **target ceiling**. Exercise below the threshold is not enough to produce benefits. Activities above the target ceiling (excessive exercise) can increase risk of injury and

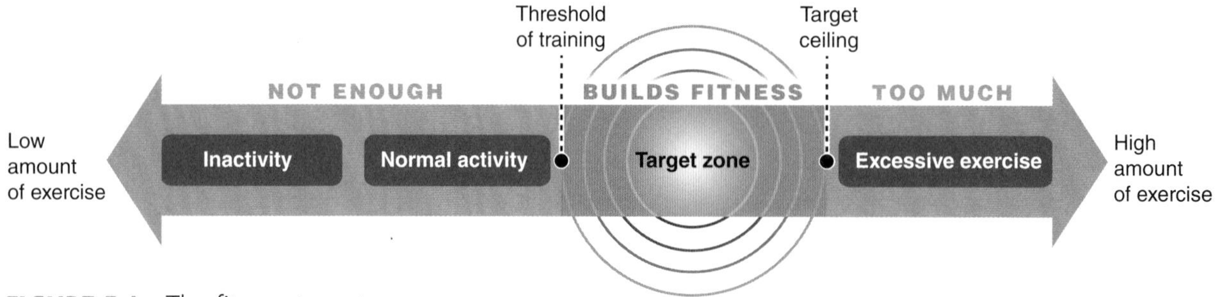

FIGURE 5.1 The fitness target zone.

soreness and may produce less than optimal benefits. Some people think you have to experience pain in order to gain fitness, but the principle of progression provides the basis for rejecting the theory of "no pain, no gain." If you experience pain when you exercise, you're probably overloading too much or too quickly for your body to adjust.

Principle of Specificity

The **principle of specificity** states that the particular type of exercise you perform determines the particular benefit you receive. Different kinds and amounts of activity produce very specific and different benefits. An activity that promotes health benefits in one part of health-related fitness may not be equally good in promoting high levels of fitness in another part of fitness. For example, Mia jogs on a track several days a week, but she does not do stretching exercises as often as she should. She may also need to use more resistance in her muscle fitness exercises.

In addition, exercises performed for specific body parts, such as the calf muscles, may provide benefits only for those parts. For example, if Mia does exercises only for her calf muscles, she will not build the muscles in her back, shoulders, arms, or other parts of her legs.

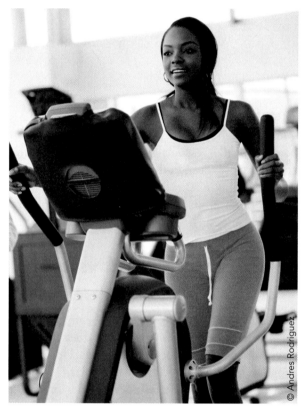

© Andres Rodriguez

Applying the principle of specificity is important for getting optimal benefits.

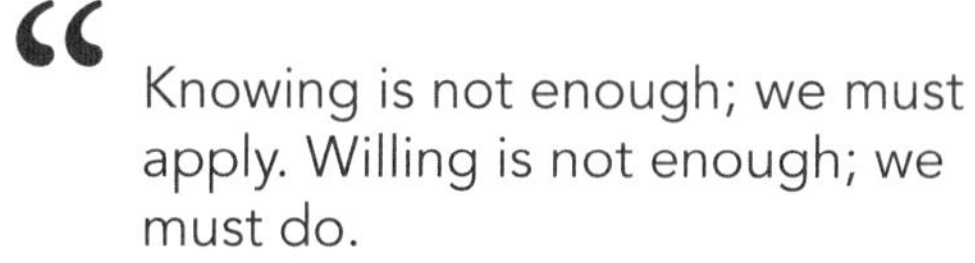

> Knowing is not enough; we must apply. Willing is not enough; we must do.
>
> —Johann Wolfgang von Goethe, writer and artist

FITT Formula

You know that you must do more physical activity than normal to build fitness. You also know that you should gradually increase your physical activity in order to stay within your fitness target zone. But how much physical activity do you need?

To help you apply the principles of exercise, you can use the **FITT formula**. Some people refer to it as the FITT *principle*, but we use the term *formula* in this book because a formula refers to a prescription or recipe. In this case, the prescription is for determining the right amount of physical activity for applying the three exercise principles. In fact, each letter in the acronym FITT represents a key factor in determining how much physical activity is enough: frequency, intensity, time, and type.

- **Frequency refers to how often you do physical activity.** For physical activity to be beneficial, you must do it several days a week. Optimal **frequency** depends on the type of activity you're doing and the part of fitness you want to develop. To develop strength, for example, you might need to exercise two days a week. To lose fat, you should exercise daily.
- **Intensity refers to how hard you perform physical activity.** If the activity you do is too easy, you will not build fitness or gain other benefits. But remember—extremely vigorous activity can be harmful if you don't work up to it gradually. **Intensity** is determined differently depending on the type of activity you do and the type of fitness you want to build. For example, you can use your heart rate to determine your intensity of activity for building cardiorespiratory endurance, whereas you would use the amount of weight you lift to determine the intensity for building strength.
- **Time refers to how long you do physical activity.** As with frequency and intensity, the length of **time** for which you should do physical activity depends on the type of activity you're doing and the part of fitness you want to develop. For example, to build flexibility you should exercise for 15 seconds or more for each muscle group, whereas to build cardiorespiratory endurance you need to be vigorously active for a minimum of 20 minutes.

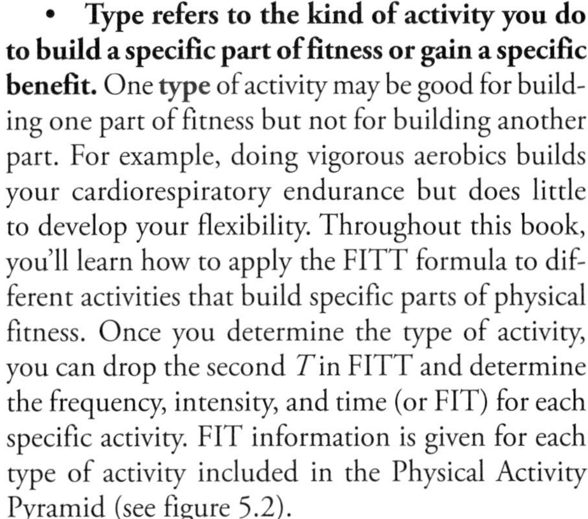

- **Type refers to the kind of activity you do to build a specific part of fitness or gain a specific benefit.** One **type** of activity may be good for building one part of fitness but not for building another part. For example, doing vigorous aerobics builds your cardiorespiratory endurance but does little to develop your flexibility. Throughout this book, you'll learn how to apply the FITT formula to different activities that build specific parts of physical fitness. Once you determine the type of activity, you can drop the second *T* in FITT and determine the frequency, intensity, and time (or FIT) for each specific activity. FIT information is given for each type of activity included in the Physical Activity Pyramid (see figure 5.2).

FIT FACT

FITT is a mnemonic acronym or formula used to remember four key factors in applying the overload principle and related principles: frequency, intensity, time, and type.

Volume and Progression

The American College of Sports Medicine (ACSM) uses the FITT formula for prescribing how much physical activity is enough. It's also important to consider the total amount of physical activity you perform (volume) and the need for progression (principle of progression) in your program, so ACSM sometimes includes the letters VP after FITT, thus making it FITT-VP. In this version, V stands for the volume (amount) of exercise, which is a function of intensity and time. Consider your total volume of activity when developing a personal activity plan. For example, you can do moderate activity for a longer time and do the same volume of activity as for vigorous activity done for a shorter time. As you learn more about the FITT formula you will learn how volume of exercise can be adjusted by altering the intensity and time of the workout. Over a longer time, such as a week, the frequency of exercise also contributes to volume. Doing the same workout four days a week will have twice the volume as doing the workout two days a week.

The P in FITT-VP is to remind people of the importance of progression—that is, applying the FITT formula gradually. As you work through this book, you'll see only the acronyms FIT and FITT, but you should also keep volume and progression (VP) in mind as you develop your personal activity plan.

The Physical Activity Pyramid

National physical activity guidelines for youth developed by the U.S. Department of Health and Human Services (USDHHS) recommend at least 60 minutes of physical activity each day. The five steps of the **Physical Activity Pyramid** (figure 5.2) help you understand the five kinds of physical activity, which build different parts of fitness and produce different health and wellness benefits (recall the principle of specificity). To meet the recommended 60 minutes of daily activity, you can choose from the different types of activity. For optimal benefits, you should perform activities from all parts of the pyramid each week. As you can see, activities at or near the bottom of the pyramid may need to be done more frequently or for a longer time than those near the top of the pyramid to get the same volume of activity.

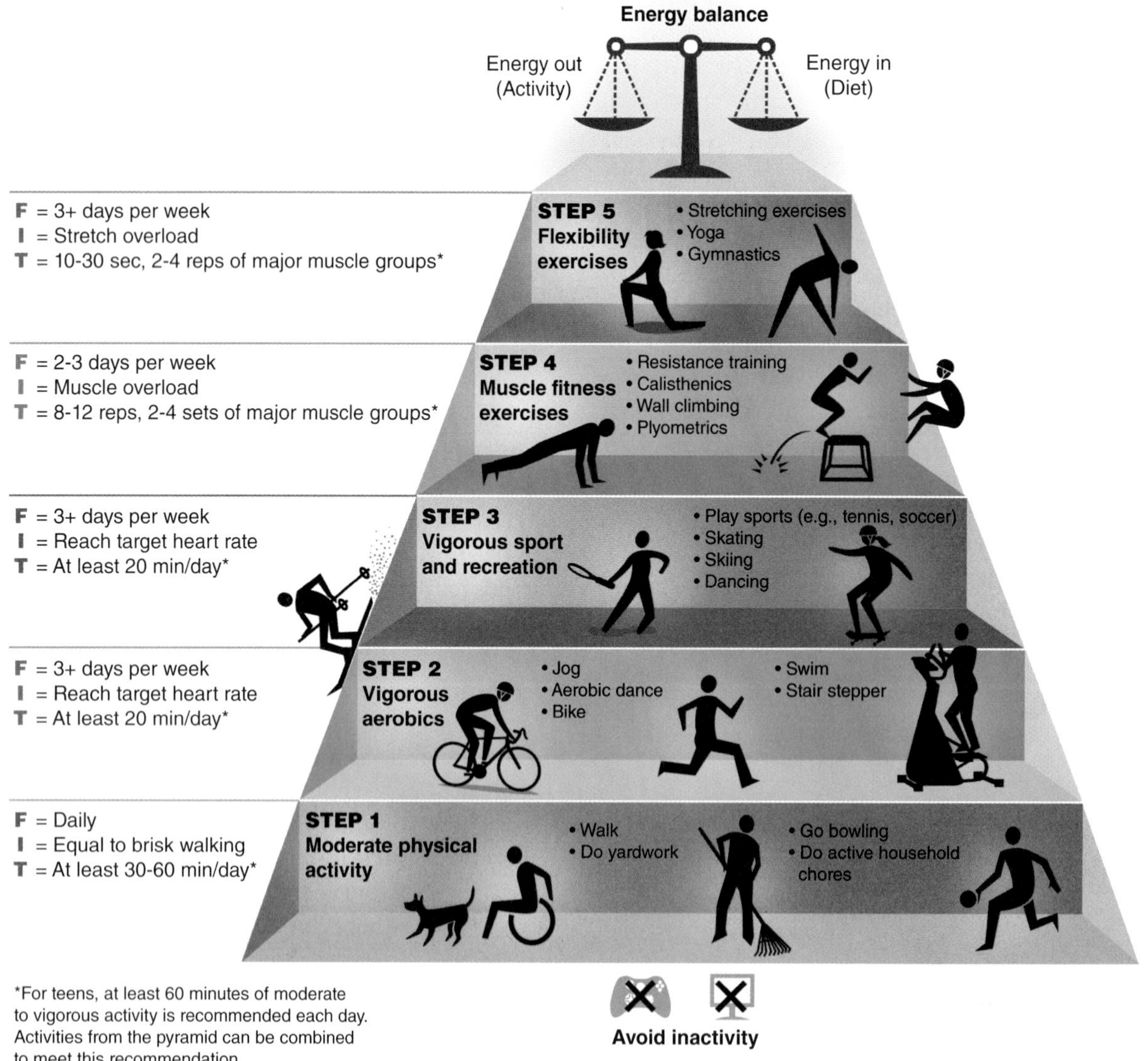

FIGURE 5.2 The new Physical Activity Pyramid for Teens.
Source: C.B. Corbin.

Moderate Physical Activity

Moderate physical activity is the first step in the Physical Activity Pyramid, and it should be performed daily or nearly every day. Moderate activity involves exercise equal in intensity to brisk walking. It includes some activities of normal daily living (also called lifestyle activities), such as yardwork (for example, raking leaves or mowing the lawn) and housework (for example, mopping the floor). It also includes sports that are not vigorous, such as bowling and golf. Some other sports can be either moderate or vigorous; for example, shooting basketballs is typically a moderate activity, whereas playing a full-court game is vigorous. National guidelines recommend 60 minutes of moderate to vigorous activity each day for teens. Moderate activity should account for some of this time each day (30 minutes a day is recommended for adults). It is also associated with many of the health benefits of activity described in part 1 of this book, such as controlling your level of body fat, and is well suited for people of varying abilities.

Vigorous Aerobics

Step 2 of the Physical Activity Pyramid represents vigorous aerobics, which includes any exercise that you can do for a long time without stopping and that is vigorous enough to increase your heart rate, make you breathe faster, and make you sweat. Thus these activities are more intense than moderate activities such as brisk walking. Vigorous aerobics, such as jogging and aerobic dance, are typically continuous in nature. Like moderate activity, they provide many health and wellness benefits, and they're especially helpful for building a high level of cardiorespiratory endurance. You should perform vigorous aerobics (or vigorous sport or recreation) at least three days a week for at least 20 minutes each day in order to meet national activity guidelines.

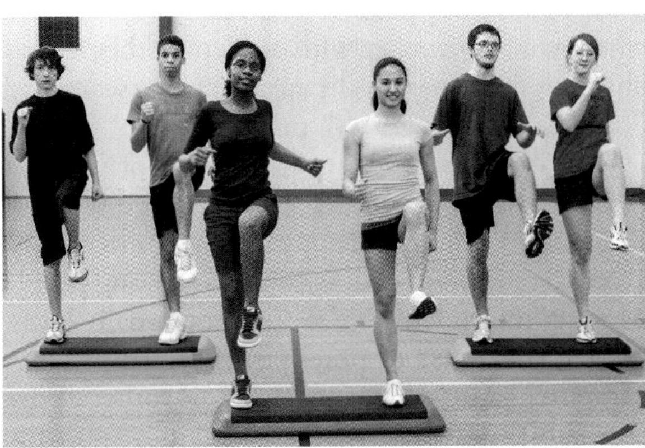

Vigorous aerobic activity helps you build cardiorespiratory endurance.

FIT FACT

The word *aerobic*, meaning "with oxygen," is a scientific term that has been used for decades. It was popularized in the 1968 book *Aerobics*, written by Dr. Ken Cooper, whose work over the years has helped everyday people around the world understand how much activity is needed for fitness and health benefits. In fact, in Portuguese, the English word *jogging* is translated as "coopering"! Dr. Cooper also founded the Cooper Institute, a world-famous health and fitness research organization based in Dallas, Texas.

Vigorous Sport and Recreation

Like vigorous aerobics, vigorous sport and recreation (represented in step 3 of the Physical Activity Pyramid) require your heart to beat faster than normal and cause you to breathe faster and sweat more. As your muscles use more oxygen, your heart beats faster, and you breathe faster and more deeply to meet the oxygen demand. Unlike vigorous aerobics, however, vigorous sport and recreation often involve short bursts of activity followed by short bursts of rest (as in basketball, football, soccer, and tennis). When done for at least 20 minutes a day in bouts of 10 minutes or more at a time, these activities provide similar fitness, health, and wellness benefits to those of vigorous aerobics. They also help you build motor skills and contribute to healthy weight management. As with vigorous aerobics, you can use vigorous sport and recreation to meet national activity recommendation when you do them for at least 20 minutes a day on three days a week.

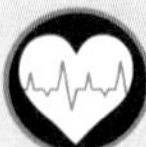

FITNESS TECHNOLOGY: Activitygram

You can use computer technology to keep track of your daily physical activity. Activitygram is a computer program that helps you track your physical activity over a three-day period. You enter any activity you perform for every 30-minute block of time during your waking hours. You also record the type of activity you do and whether its intensity level is resting, light, moderate, or vigorous. The program generates a report showing your total number of activity minutes each day, the amount of activity you did at each step of the Physical Activity Pyramid, and the amounts of moderate activity and vigorous activity you performed.

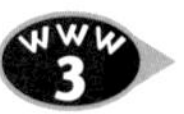

Using Technology

Locate the Activitygram portion of the student section of the Health Opportunities Through Physical Education website. Open the document that explains Activitygram and use the information you find there to estimate the amount of activity you get from each of the different types shown in the pyramid. Ask your instructor for more information about Activitygram.

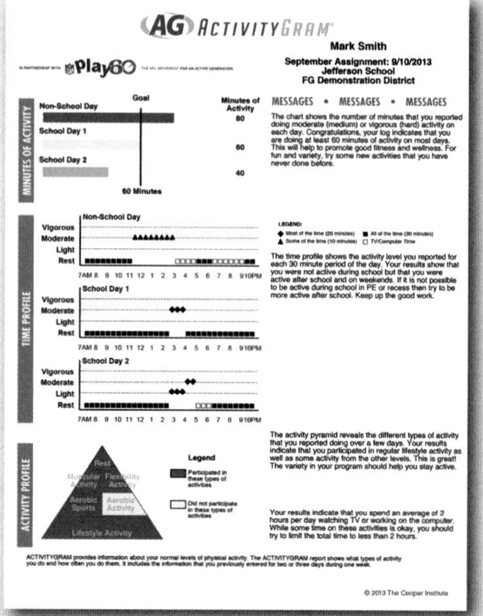

Reprinted by permission from Cooper Institute, 2003, *Activitygram* (Champaign, IL: Human Kinetics).

Muscle Fitness Exercises

Step 4 in the Physical Activity Pyramid represents muscle fitness exercises, which build your strength, muscular endurance, and power. Muscle fitness exercises include both resistance training (with weights or machines) and moving your own body weight (as in rock climbing, calisthenics, and jumping). This type of exercise produces general health and wellness benefits, as well as better performance, improved body appearance, a healthier back, better posture, and stronger bones. These exercises can be used to meet national activity guidelines and should be performed on two or three days a week.

Flexibility Exercises

Step 5 of the Physical Activity Pyramid represents flexibility exercises. According to ACSM, flexibility exercises improve postural stability and balance. There is also some evidence that flexibility exercises may reduce soreness, prevent injuries, and reduce risk of back pain. Flexibility exercises also improve your performance in activities such as gymnastics and dance. They also are used in therapy to help people who have been injured. Two examples of flexibility exercise are stretching and yoga (figure 5.3). To build and maintain flexibility, you should perform flexibility exercise at least three days a week.

Avoiding Inactivity

Just below the Physical Activity Pyramid (see figure 5.2) you'll notice pictures of a television set and a video game controller with an X over them. This illustration emphasizes the fact that being sedentary, or inactive, poses a health risk.

Just as you should do 60 minutes of physical activity each day, drawing from the five types of activity presented in the pyramid, you should also avoid the inactivity that is common among people who log too much "screen time" on a daily basis. Screen time refers to time spent in front of a TV, computer game, phone screen, or any other device that substitutes inactivity for activities from the pyramid. A recent survey of children and teens in the United States found that they watch TV for an average of nearly four hours a day! Sixty-eight

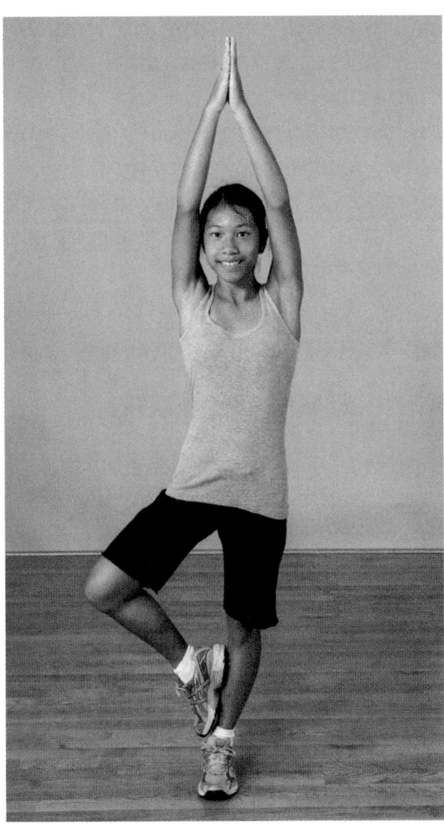

FIGURE 5.3 Yoga is one type of physical activity for improving flexibility.

percent of teens have a TV in their room, and of course many also spend screen time on computers, video games, movies, and cell phones, more than doubling the amount of time they spend watching a screen. Research shows that screen time results in inactivity and increases health risk.

We all need to take time to recover from daily stresses and prepare for new challenges, so periods of rest and sleep are important for good health. Some activities of daily living—such as studying, reading, and even a moderate amount of screen time—are appropriate. But general inactivity or sedentary living is harmful to your health. Your choices from active areas of the pyramid should exceed your choices from the inactivity area.

Balancing Energy

The top of the pyramid presents a balance scale illustrating the need to balance the energy you take in (food) with the energy you put out (activity). Energy balance means that the calories in the food you eat each day are equal to the calories you expend in exercise each day. Balancing your energy in this way is essential to maintaining a healthy body composition.

Patterns of Moderate and Vigorous Activity

A pattern is a schedule you use to accumulate minutes of activity from the pyramid each day and each week. One pattern is continuous activity, in which you do all of your physical activity for the day in one continuous session (for example, 30 minutes of continuous moderate activity).

The second pattern is accumulated activity, in which you do sessions of 10 minutes or more in order to accumulate your targeted daily total (for example, 10 + 10 + 10 = 30). Bouts of less than 10 minutes may provide some health benefits but are not recommended for use in accumulating your recommended daily activity time, because bouts of less than 10 minutes are considered below the threshold of training for getting benefits.

The ACSM refers to a third pattern as that of the "weekend warrior." This pattern is marked by inactivity during most of the week punctuated by relatively long sessions of activity—sometimes for several hours at a time and often all in one day. Adults often do this extended activity on weekends because of their work commitments during the week—thus the name "weekend warrior." This pattern is not recommended and can even be dangerous for people with risk factors because it violates the principle of progression and can lead to soreness and injury. Thus you should do your activity on most days of the week using a continuous or accumulated pattern.

Lesson Review

1. What are the three principles of exercise, and why are they important?
2. What are the four parts of the FITT formula as represented by the letters in the acronym FITT? How are they related to the following concepts: threshold of training, target ceiling, and fitness target zone?
3. What are some characteristics and examples of the five types of activity included in the Physical Activity Pyramid?

SELF-ASSESSMENT: PACER and Trunk Lift

In this assessment, you'll perform two tests: one to assess your cardiorespiratory endurance and another to measure the flexibility and fitness of your back and trunk muscles. If you have not done so already, practice each test before performing them for a score. Record your scores and fitness ratings for the two tests as directed by your teacher. Performing these tests will provide information that you can use in preparing a Fitnessgram report and in preparing your personal physical activity plan. If you're working with a partner, remember that self-assessment information is personal and considered confidential. It shouldn't be shared with others without the permission of the person being tested.

PACER (Progressive Aerobic Cardiovascular Endurance Run, or 20-meter shuttle run)

This test of cardiorespiratory endurance was originally called the 20-meter shuttle run, and that name is still used in many countries. The name PACER, as it is called in Fitnessgram, was the winning entry, submitted by Dr. Jack Rutherford, in a contest designed to create a new name for the test that would be easy to remember.

The test is scored differently by different test batteries. In part 1 of this book, you'll use the number of laps you perform as the score on which your fitness rating is based; laps are also used for scoring by the ALPHA-FIT test. Using laps makes it easy for you to see if you improve after performing your personal activity plan. If you want to do a Fitnessgram report, you'll need to convert your laps score to an aerobic capacity score as described in the student section of the Health Opportunities Through Physical Education website.

Directions

1. The test objective is to run back and forth across a 20-meter (almost 22-yard) distance as many times as you can at a predetermined pace (pacing is based on signals from a special audio recording provided by your instructor).
2. Start at a line located 20 meters from a second line. When you hear the beep from the audio track, run across the 20-meter area to the second line, arriving just before the tape beeps again, and touch the line with your foot. Turn around and get ready to run back.
3. At the sound of the next beep, run back to the line where you began. Touch the line with your foot. Make sure to wait for the beep before running back.
4. Continue to run back and forth from one line to the other, touching the line each time. The beeps will come faster and faster, causing you to run faster and faster. The test is finished when you twice fail to reach the opposite side before the beep.
5. Your score is the number of laps you ran (the number of times you ran the 20-meter distance from one line to the other) before your test was finished. Using laps as your score allows you to easily test yourself to see how you improve over time. This method of scoring provides you with a good indicator of your cardiorespiratory endurance, which is a measure of functional fitness—your ability to function effectively in daily living.

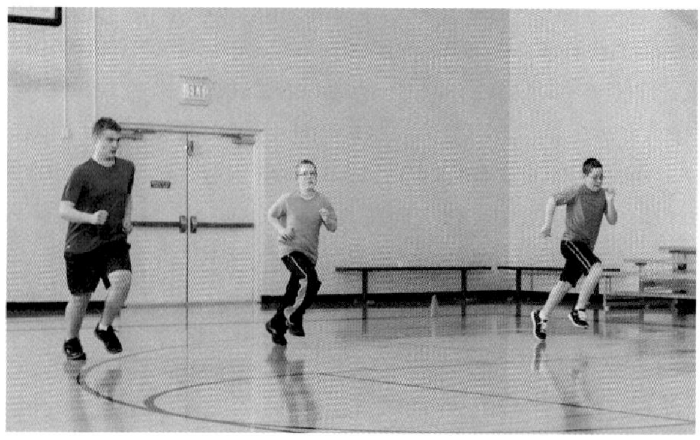

The PACER test assesses cardiorespiratory endurance and can be used to estimate aerobic capacity.

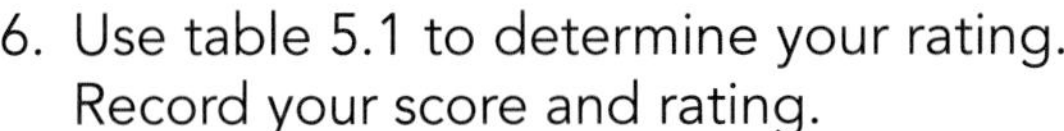

6. Use table 5.1 to determine your rating. Record your score and rating.
7. If you or your teacher would like to prepare a Fitnessgram report card, aerobic capacity score will be used. Aerobic capacity refers to your body's ability to supply oxygen during sustained aerobic activity and is best determined using a treadmill test. Your lap score can be used to estimate your aerobic capacity score. You can use Fitnessgram software with the help of your teacher; alternatively, you can use the charts presented in the student section of the Health Opportunities Through Physical Education website to determine your aerobic capacity score and fitness rating. Aerobic capacity is discussed further in the Cardiorespiratory Endurance chapter.

TABLE 5.1 Rating Chart for PACER

	13 years old		14 years old		15 years old		16 years old		17 years or older	
	Male	Female	Male	Female	Male	Female	Male	Female	Male	Female
High performance	≥36	≥31	≥45	≥34	≥54	≥38	≥60	≥40	≥67	≥50
Good fitness	29–35	25–30	36–44	27–33	42–53	30–37	47–59	32–39	54–66	38–49
Marginal fitness	23–28	19–24	28–35	21–26	32–41	23–29	36–46	25–31	42–53	30–37
Low fitness	≤22	≤18	≤27	≤20	≤31	≤22	≤35	≤24	≤41	≤29

Scores in this table refer to the number of completed laps.

Based on data provided by G. Welk.

Trunk Lift (upper back)

1. Lie facedown with your arms to your sides and your hands under your thighs.
2. Lift the upper part of your body very slowly so that your chin, chest, and shoulders come off the floor. Lift your trunk as high as possible, to a maximum of 12 inches (30 centimeters). Hold this position for three seconds while a partner measures how far your chin is from the floor. Your partner should hold the ruler at least 1 inch (2.5 centimeters) in front of your chin. Look straight ahead so that your chin is not tipped abnormally upward.
3. Do the trunk lift two times (lifting slowly) and record how far from the floor you can lift and hold your chin (for three seconds). Do not record scores above 12 inches (30 centimeters).

   Caution: The ruler should not be placed directly under your chin, in case you have to lower your trunk unexpectedly.
4. Use table 5.2 to determine your fitness rating. Record your score and rating.

TABLE 5.2 Rating Chart for Trunk Lift

Rating	Inches
High performance	11–12
Good fitness	9–10
Marginal fitness	7–8
Low fitness	≤6

To convert inches to centimeters, multiply by 2.54.

Data based on *Fitnessgram*.

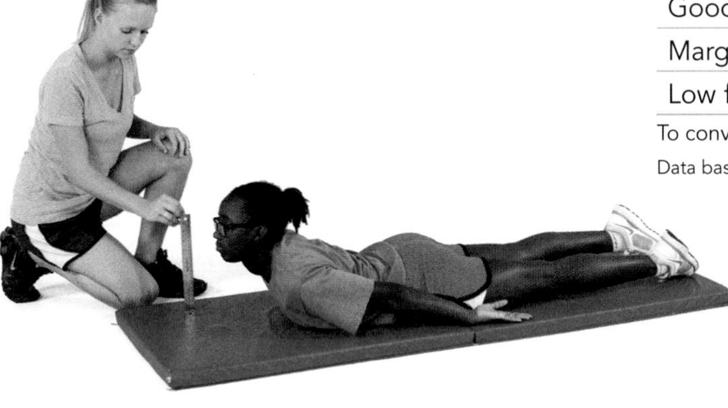

This test measures the flexibility of your back and trunk muscles, as well as the muscle fitness of your back muscles.

Lesson 5.2

How Much Fitness Is Enough?

Lesson Objectives

After reading this lesson, you should be able to

1. describe the four fitness rating categories and how they apply to your physical activity program,
2. identify factors that contribute to fitness, and
3. explain how a person can attain good health and fitness even if some factors make it difficult to succeed.

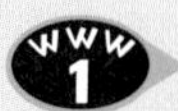

Lesson Vocabulary

criterion-referenced health standard, maturation

You now know that physical activity is necessary to build each part of physical fitness. But exactly how much fitness do you need? In this lesson, you'll learn some ways to decide how much fitness is enough for you.

Fitness Standards and Rating Categories

Sometimes people judge their fitness by comparing themselves with others. If they score higher on a fitness test than most other people, they consider themselves fit. This type of comparison creates several problems. First, it suggests that only a few people can be fit. Second, it suggests that only high test scores are adequate for fitness. In this lesson, you'll learn why neither of these suggestions is true.

Most experts agree that you should judge fitness using **criterion-referenced health standards**. The word *standard* refers to an established amount or quantity. The word *criterion* is a marker used to establish the standard (as it relates to health). So a criterion-referenced standard for health-related fitness refers to the amount of fitness you need in order to achieve good health. This type of standard does not require you to compare yourself with others. It does require you to have enough fitness to

- reduce your risk of health problems,
- achieve wellness benefits,
- function effectively in your daily life,
- meet emergencies, and
- enjoy your free time.

As noted in this chapter's Science in Action feature, you'll learn to do many self-assessments for each of the health-related parts of physical fitness. In part 1 of this book, we use a rating system based on criterion-referenced health standards. It is similar to the rating systems used in test batteries such as Fitnessgram, and we use it here so that you can rate your fitness in all of the tests included in part 1 of this book by means of the same system.

To rate yourself in each of the six parts of health-related physical fitness, you'll use one of the following four categories. If you attain a rating of "good fitness" for all six fitness areas, you'll achieve the basic health and wellness standards of physical fitness.

- **Low fitness.** If you have a low fitness rating, you have an above average risk of developing health problems. You also might not look your best, feel your best, or work and play as efficiently as you could. If you have a low fitness rating, you should work to achieve a marginal fitness rating.
- **Marginal fitness.** Moving from the low to the marginal rating shows important progress in fitness. However, if you have a marginal rating, you should try to get a good fitness rating.
- **Good fitness.** This rating indicates that you have the fitness needed to live a full, healthy life. In fact, achieving a good fitness rating is the goal of most people. To maintain this level of fitness, you'll need to continue being physically active.

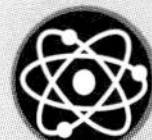

SCIENCE IN ACTION: Personal Fitness Assessment

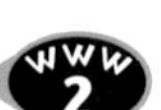

Experts in physical education and exercise physiology have worked together to develop various physical fitness test batteries. A battery is a group of tests designed to assess all parts of physical fitness. As you've learned, Fitnessgram is one fitness test battery used in many schools in the United States and throughout the world. Fitnessgram has been adopted as the national assessment program for both the President's Council on Fitness, Sports, and Nutrition (PCFSN) and the Society of Health and Physical Educators (SHAPE America). ALPHA-FIT is a fitness test battery widely used in Europe. The two batteries contain some similar tests and some that differ from each other.

In part 1 of this book, you'll try many fitness tests. The goal is to help you select test items for your own personal fitness test battery that you can use throughout your life to self-assess your fitness. You will perform all of the test items in the Fitnessgram and ALPHA-FIT batteries, as well as several other tests. For all tests in part 1, you'll use the Fitness for Life rating system, but you can also learn how to use standards and ratings from other test batteries. What's most important is that you learn to test your own fitness and use your personal self-assessment results to plan your own fitness and physical activity.

Student Activity

On the Health Opportunities Through Physical Education website, find the information about the Fitnessgram and ALPHA-FIT test batteries. Specifically, read the information about the two batteries' standards. Compare the standards to see how they differ. Prepare a report in writing or present your report to the class.

- **High performance.** Most experts agree that many health benefits can be achieved without reaching a high performance rating. However, performing the amount of physical activity necessary to reach this rating has additional health benefits because you get more benefits with a greater volume of activity (when not overdone). It should be noted that the fitter you get, the harder it is to improve. Achieving a high performance rating is necessary if you want to be an athlete or perform a physically demanding job, such as firefighter, soldier, or police officer.

Factors Influencing Physical Fitness

Physical activity is the most important thing you can do to improve or maintain your health-related physical fitness. Fortunately, it is also something that you can control. You can choose the kinds of activity you want to do and schedule a regular time to do them. But as figure 5.4 shows, physical activity is not the only factor that contributes to your physical fitness. Other important factors are **maturation**, age, heredity, environment, and lifestyle choices such as nutrition and stress management.

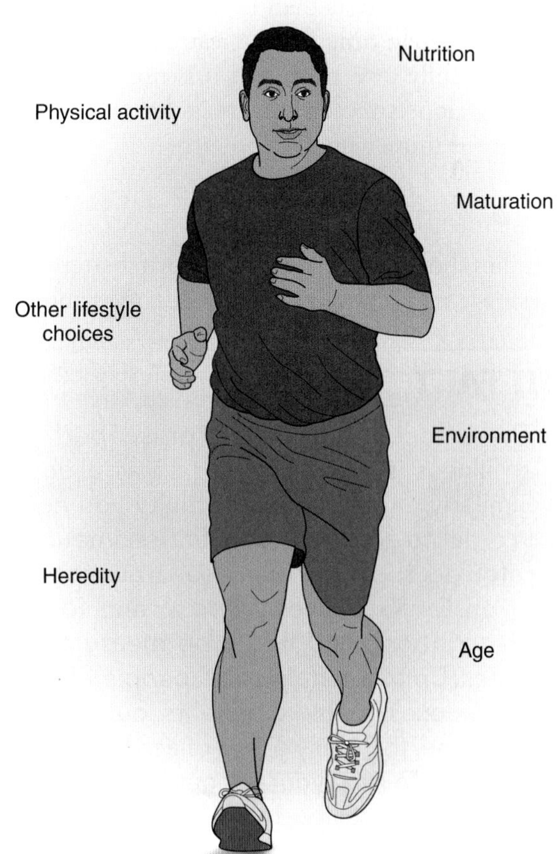

FIGURE 5.4 Various factors influence your physical fitness.

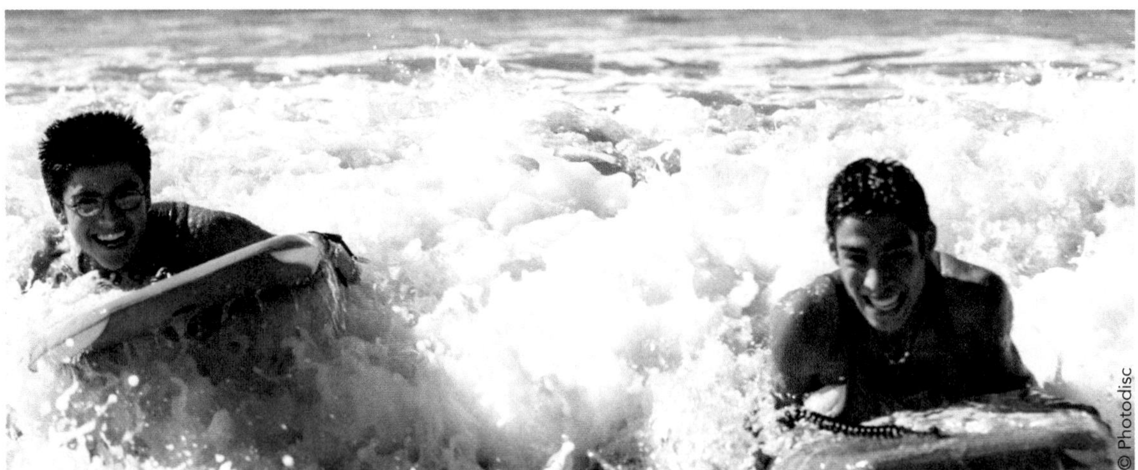

Compare your fitness with criterion-referenced health standards rather than with your friends' fitness levels.

Maturation

Physical maturation means becoming physically full grown and developed. It begins in earnest in your early teen years because of hormones that promote the growth and development of tissues such as muscle and bone. Some people mature earlier than others, and early developers often do better on physical fitness tests than those who mature later. But ultimately time is the great equalizer. We all develop fully over time, and it is not unusual for late developers to achieve fitness levels that equal or exceed those who develop early.

Age

Studies show that older teens perform better on fitness tests than younger teens. Even in the same class, those who are older typically do better than those who are younger. This difference results mostly from the fact that the older you are, the more you've grown and the more physically mature you're likely to be. As you learned earlier, age and maturation do not always parallel each other. However, sometimes one person matures earlier than another, and in such cases a younger but more physically mature person could have an advantage in performing physical fitness tests.

FIT FACT

The amount of medicine prescribed for an illness is often referred to as a dose. Similarly, the amount of activity you need in order to get health benefits is sometimes referred to as an exercise prescription, or an Ex Rx (Ex for exercise and Rx for prescription), and it can be measured in doses. Up to a certain point, people who do more doses get more benefits, but, as with medicine, too many doses of activity can be harmful. To help yourself get just the right number of activity doses for good health and fitness, follow the FIT formula for each type (the last *T* in FITT) of physical activity.

> Do not let what you cannot do interfere with what you can do.
>
> —John Wooden, basketball coach

Heredity

Heredity involves the characteristics we inherit from our parents, including the physical characteristics that influence how we perform on physical fitness tests. For example, some people have more fat cells than others because of heredity. Similarly, some people have more of the muscle fibers that help them run fast, whereas others have more of the muscle fibers that help them run a long time without fatigue. Each person's heredity enables better performance in some areas and makes it harder to perform well in others. Fortunately, fitness is composed of many different parts. Your heredity helps determine the parts of fitness in which you do well and the parts in which you may not do as well.

Environment

Your fitness is also affected by environmental factors, such as where you live (city, suburbs, country), your school environment, and the (un)availability of places to play and do other types of physical activity. Even your social environment can affect your fitness, including the friends you choose. For example, people who live near parks and those who have active friends are typically more active than those who don't.

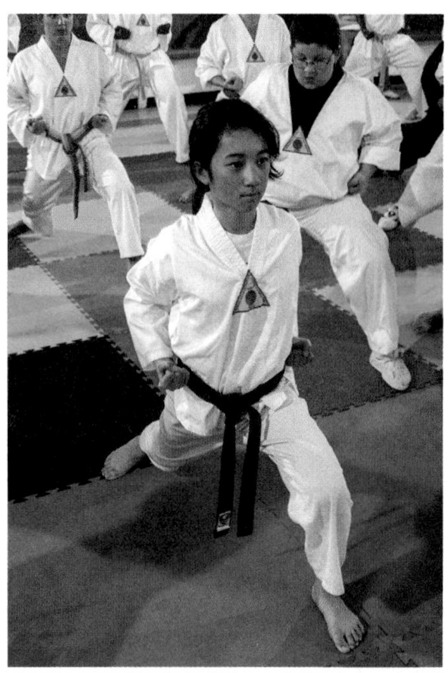

Find an activity that you enjoy and will be able to do later in life.

FIT FACT

Teens who walk or ride a bicycle to school are more active overall than those who do not. Specifically, they get an average of 16 minutes more activity each day, and that difference in itself is more than 25 percent of the recommended amount of daily activity.

Anyone Can Succeed

Because many factors contribute to physical fitness, it is possible for some people who do relatively little physical activity to achieve relatively good fitness scores while they are in their teens. These people probably matured early and inherited physical characteristics that help them do well on physical fitness tests. However, they may also be in danger of concluding that they don't need to do physical activity. This may be true enough if they care only about doing well on fitness tests while they're young, but it will not be true for a lifetime. As people get older, they can no longer gain a fitness advantage from early physical maturation or the energy of youth. Sooner or later, physical inactivity will catch up with even those who enjoy a hereditary advantage. Therefore, if you want lifetime fitness, health, and wellness, you need to perform regular physical activity and make healthy lifestyle choices.

Just as some people enjoy fitness advantages because of age, maturation, and heredity, others face disadvantages. For some people, even if they do physical activity, they still find it hard to get high fitness scores, and they may become discouraged. If you're one of these people, avoid comparing yourself with others. Try to achieve a good fitness rating rather than worrying about getting a high performance rating. Good fitness may be harder to achieve for some people than others, but all people can do it. In fact, studies show that people who are good at sports in school but do not remain active later in life are less healthy and die earlier than those who do regular activity throughout their lives—even if they were not especially good performers when they were young.

Anyone can do physical activity. And no matter who you are, physical activity is crucial to your fitness, health, and wellness. With regular physical activity, you can achieve a good fitness rating in all parts of fitness.

Lesson Review

1. What are the four fitness ratings? How do they apply to your physical activity program?
2. What factors contribute to fitness?
3. How can a person attain good health and fitness even if he or she has factors that make it difficult to build a high level of fitness?

TAKING CHARGE: Learning to Self-Monitor

An activity log is a written account of your physical activities during a specified time. It's a way to keep track of what you do so that you can tell whether you're meeting your activity goals. Self-monitoring refers to any of a variety of techniques for keeping track of your behavior (for example, a log, diary, or step counter).

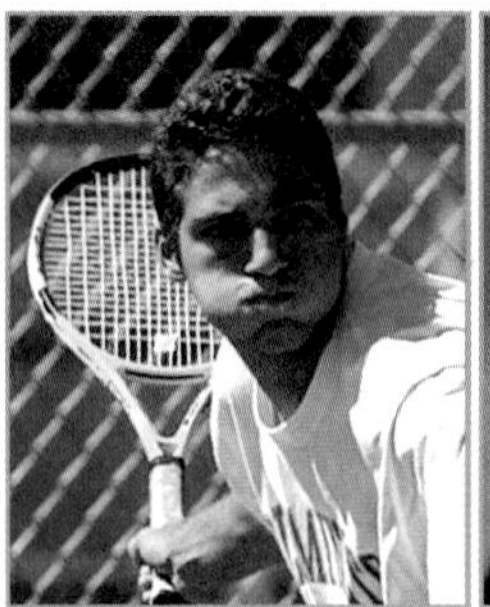

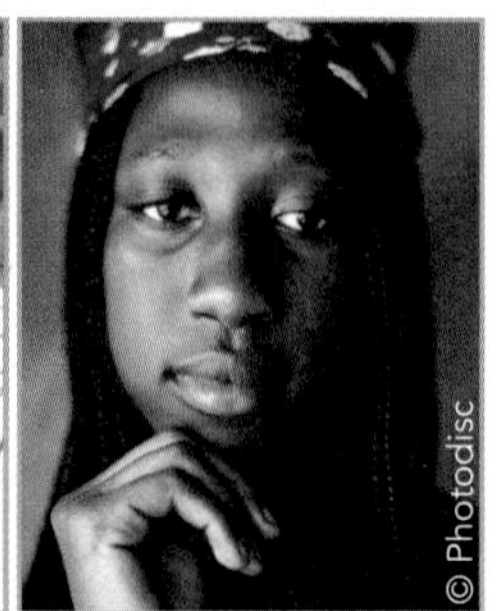

© Photodisc

Mark enjoyed playing tennis on the weekends. He would start out full of energy, but he lacked the endurance to play well for a complete match. His instructor suggested that he do some daily activities to improve his endurance. For several weeks, Mark reported that he faithfully engaged in the activities. But Mark's instructor was a little skeptical based on his level of improvement. Finally, she suggested that Mark keep a log of all the times that he did the activities, and the results were eye opening: "Boy, was I surprised," said Mark. "I usually didn't spend as much time as I thought on each activity. I really thought I was doing well until I saw the results written down."

Erica's situation was different. She had knee surgery and was ordered to limit both the kinds and the amount of her activity and to follow a schedule of rehabilitation exercises. She was also supposed to elevate her leg whenever possible. Erica's leg was often swollen and sore at the end of the day, so her physical therapist suggested that she keep a daily log. Erica discovered that she was spending much more time on her feet than she had intended. As a result, she realized that she had to continue doing her rehabilitation exercises but curtail her other activities so that her knee could heal.

For Discussion

How did keeping a log help Mark and Erica? What are some other ways in which a log might help someone? What other ways might Mark and Erica self-monitor their physical activity levels? Consider the guidelines presented in the following Self-Management feature as you answer these discussion questions.

SELF-MANAGEMENT: Skills for Learning to Self-Monitor

One of the truths of human nature is that adults tend to underestimate how much they eat and overestimate how much physical activity they get. People also make other errors in estimating what they do. For example, we often underestimate how much television we watch and how much money we spend on nonessential items. One name for keeping track of what we do is "self-monitoring." We all self-monitor our behavior in informal ways, but sometimes it's necessary to make formal assessments if we want accuracy. You can self-monitor your behaviors to help you set goals and make plans—and to evaluate whether you're meeting your goals and fulfilling your plans. Self-monitoring of physical activity is sometimes referred to as "record keeping" or "keeping an activity log." Use the following guidelines to effectively monitor your physical activity.

- **Keep a written log.** Make a formal record of your physical activities by using an activity log or a computer program such as Activitygram.
- **Consider using an activity monitor.** Two examples are pedometers and heart rate watches. A pedometer counts the number of steps you take; it is typically worn on your belt or arm. A heart rate monitor uses a strap around your chest and a watchlike device on your wrist. Either of these devices gives you objective information that you can record in your activity log.
- **Record information as frequently as possible.** The longer you wait before you write down what you do, the more likely you are to make an error. Write

things down as soon as possible after you do them.

- **Start by self-monitoring your current activity pattern.** To get an accurate picture of your activity level, monitor yourself for at least three days. At least one of the days should be a weekend day, since most people's activity pattern is different on weekends than on weekdays.
- **Use your current activity pattern to help you determine your goals and plans.** People who are already active can set higher goals than those who are less active (or just beginning).
- **Determine how much activity you do in each area of the Physical Activity Pyramid.** For each type of activity included in the pyramid, determine your frequency, intensity, and time (FIT).
- **Write down your goals and plans and keep records to see whether you fulfill them.** Putting your goals and plans in writing can help you self-monitor. Keep records to see whether you did what you planned to do. Keep a diary or an activity chart.

You can also use these guidelines to self-monitor other behaviors, such as your eating patterns.

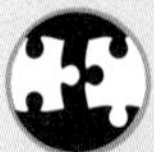

ACADEMIC CONNECTION: Percentages

The term *percentage* is used to express a portion or part of a whole. The whole is 100 percent. In a group of 100 people, one person represents 1 percent of the whole group. As an example, we often describe the activity levels of teens and adults in terms of percentages. Among adults in the United States, 20 percent meet national activity guidelines (150 minutes a week) and 80 percent do not. The percentage of teens meeting national activity guidelines (60 minutes a day) is 29 percent; 71 percent of teens do not meet the goal. You can calculate the percentage of a group that meets a health standard by dividing the number of people in the group who meet the standard by the total number of people in the group.

Scores for the trunk lift test for one group of teens are presented in the following table. A score of nine or higher (shown in boldfaced type) is required to meet the good fitness standard for this test. To determine the percentage of teens meeting the good fitness standard for the trunk lift, count the number who met the standard and divide it by the total number of teens in the group. What percentage of teens in the group meet the good fitness standard?

Distribution of Trunk Lift Test Scores for One Group

					8				
				7	8				
				7	8	**9**	**10**		
			6	7	8	**9**	**10**	**11**	
		5	6	7	8	**9**	**10**	**11**	
3	4	5	6	7	8	**9**	**10**	**11**	**12**
3	4	5	6	7	8	**9**	**10**	**11**	**12**

Check Your Answers

40 percent (16 students met the standard, and there are 40 total students; 16 ÷ 40 = 0.40)

TAKING ACTION: Physical Activity Pyramid Circuit

The Physical Activity Pyramid illustrates how much physical activity you need of different types in order to build fitness, health, and wellness. For example, you need to perform moderate physical activity (the first step of the pyramid) almost every day to get health benefits, whereas you need to perform muscle fitness activities only two or three times per week. The area *below* the pyramid represents inactivity or sedentary living. Aside from sleeping, you should minimize your daily sedentary time. A Physical Activity Pyramid circuit is an exercise circuit with stations that provide opportunities for you to **take action** by performing activities from each step of the Physical Activity Pyramid.

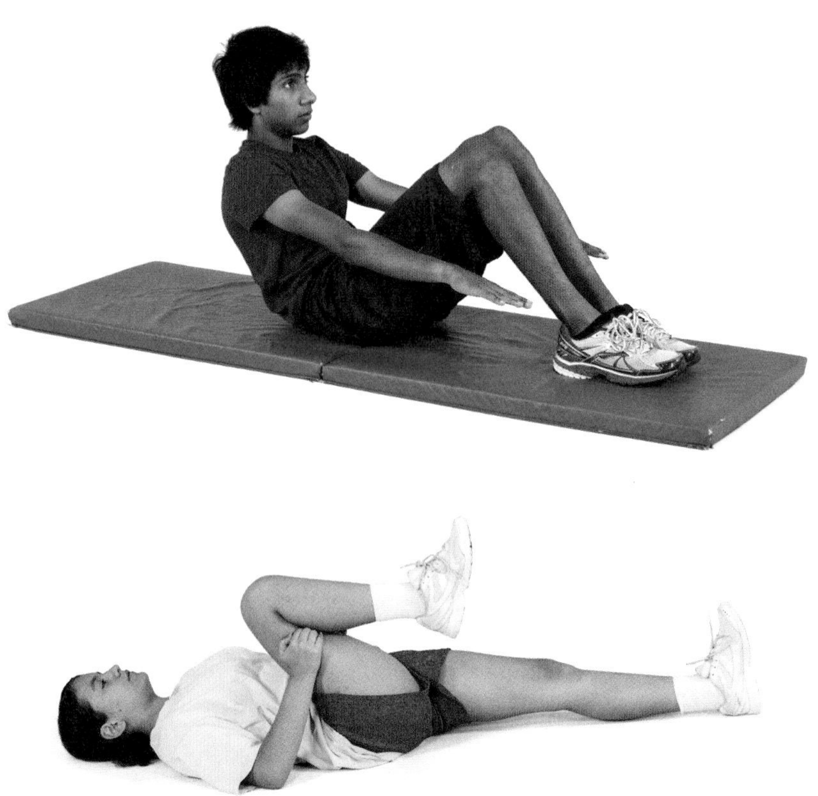

The Physical Activity Pyramid circuit includes activities from each step of the pyramid, including step 4 (muscle fitness) and step 5 (flexibility).

CHAPTER REVIEW

Reviewing Concepts and Vocabulary

As directed by your teacher, answer items 1 through 5 by correctly completing each sentence with a word or phrase.

1. The diagram with five steps that helps you understand the types of physical activity is called the _____________.
2. The minimum amount of overload needed to achieve physical fitness is called the _____________.
3. Age, maturation, _____________, and the environment are factors that affect your physical fitness.
4. If you achieve a _____________ fitness rating, you're probably at the level of fitness you need in order to live a full, healthy life.
5. The preferred standard used to rate fitness based on health is called a _____________.

For items 6 through 10, as directed by your teacher, match each term in column 1 with the appropriate phrase in column 2.

6. target ceiling	a. how hard you perform physical activity
7. intensity	b. gradual increase of exercise
8. progression	c. upper limit of your physical activity
9. specificity	d. performing more exercise than you normally do
10. overload	e. exercising for one fitness part

For items 11 through 15, as directed by your teacher, respond to each statement or question.

11. What is the FITT formula, and what does each of the four letters mean?
12. Why should you develop a lifetime physical activity plan even if you're in the good fitness zone now?
13. Explain why your physical activity program should include activities from all steps of the Physical Activity Pyramid.
14. What are some guidelines for self-monitoring physical activity?
15. Explain why you shouldn't compare yourself with others when assessing fitness.

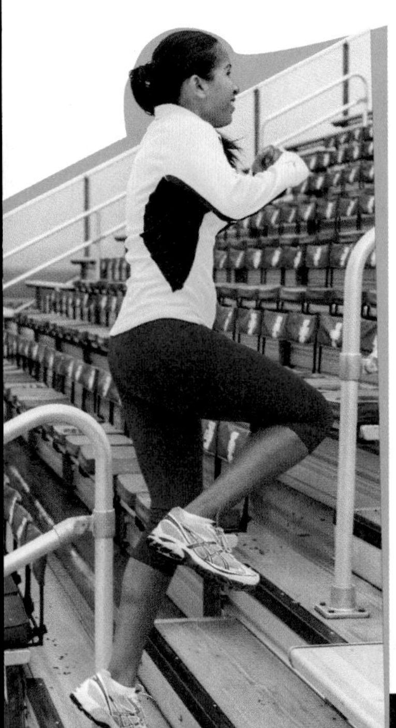

Thinking Critically

A friend tells you that it's important for everyone to attain a high performance fitness rating. Your friend says that if a good rating is the goal, then a high performance rating must be even better. How would you respond? Write a paragraph to explain your answer.

Project

Investigate places in your school and community that offer facilities and equipment for performing activities in the Physical Activity Pyramid. Compile a directory of places, their addresses and phone numbers, their websites, and their facilities and equipment. Distribute the directory to class members or post it on a website that other students can access.

6

Skill Learning and Injury Prevention

In This Chapter

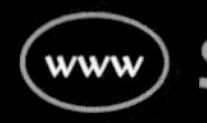

Student Web Resources

www.HOPEtextbook.org/student

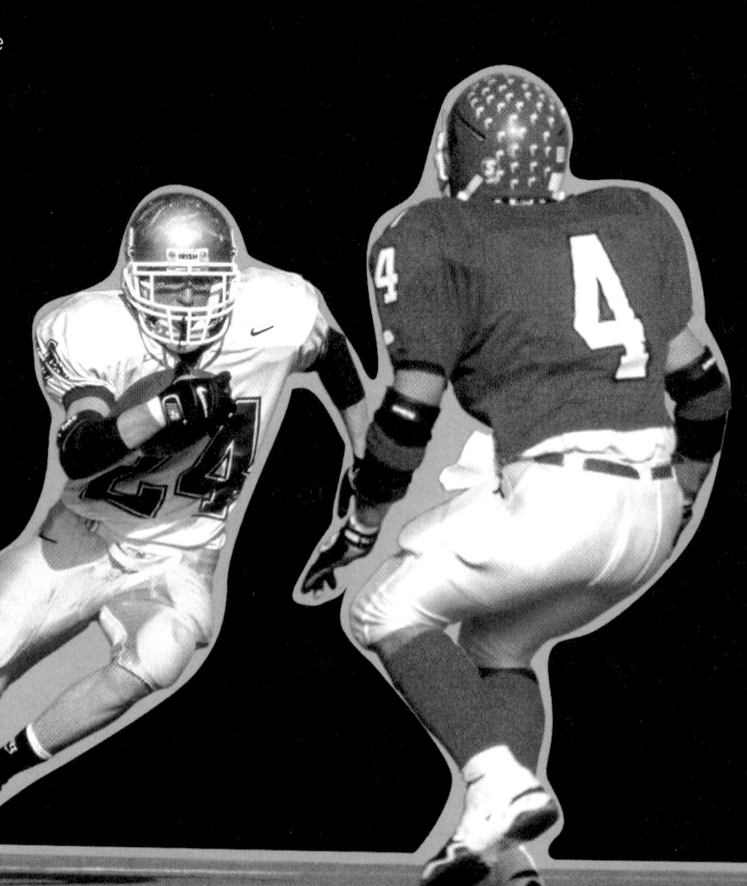

Lesson 6.1

Skills and Skill-Related Physical Fitness

Lesson Objectives

After reading this lesson, you should be able to

1. describe the five parts of skill-related fitness and give examples of each,
2. describe the factors that influence skill-related fitness and explain how to build a skill-related fitness profile,
3. define *motor skill* and describe the factors that influence it, and
4. define *teamwork* and *leadership* and describe some guidelines for building these skills.

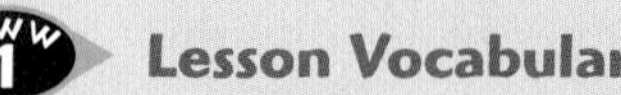

Lesson Vocabulary

agility, balance, coordination, feedback, leadership, motor unit, reaction time, skill, skill-related physical fitness, speed, teamwork

Do you have good skill-related physical fitness? Do you have good skills? Do you know the difference between skill-related fitness and skills? In this lesson, you will learn more about skill-related fitness and skills.

Skill-Related Fitness

You already know that physical fitness is divided into two categories: health-related physical fitness and **skill-related physical fitness**. Health-related fitness is considered the most important because it helps you maintain good health and wellness and perform well in physical activities. Skill-related fitness refers to a group of basic abilities that helps you perform well in sports and activities requiring certain physical skills. These are the five parts of skill-related fitness:

- **Agility:** The ability to change the position of the body quickly and control your body's movements
- **Balance:** The ability to keep an upright posture while standing still or moving
- **Coordination:** The ability to use your senses together with your body parts or to use two or more body parts together
- **Reaction time:** The amount of time it takes you to move once you recognize the need to act
- **Speed:** The ability to perform a movement or cover a distance in a short time

A **skill** is a capability for doing a task that is acquired through knowledge and practice. Skills are specific tasks that people perform. Skills such as those in sports and games are sometimes referred to as physical or motor skills (motor refers to muscles and nerves working together). Physical (or motor) skills include sport and recreational skills such as catching, throwing, swimming, and batting, as well as certain other skills (such as dancing). As you can see, skill-related fitness abilities and physical skills are not the same thing. The various parts of skill-related fitness help you learn particular skills, but they are not skills. If you have good skill-related fitness abilities—such as speed and agility—you'll be able to learn running skills used in football more

FIT FACT

Power was formerly considered to be a part of skill-related fitness because it is important in sport and other physical activities. However, the U.S.-based Institute of Medicine now classifies power as a health-related part of fitness. Ultimately, all parts of fitness are important for both health and skill performance, but the link to health for teens is more established for the health-related parts of fitness than it is for the skill-related parts.

easily. Similarly, if you have good balance, you'll be able to learn gymnastics skills more easily. You'll learn more about skills later in this lesson.

Learning about your own skill-related fitness will help you determine which sports and lifetime activities will be easiest for you to learn and enjoy. Because people differ in their levels of each part of skill-related fitness, different people find success in different activities. In this lesson, you'll learn how to assess your skill-related fitness so that you can choose activities that match your abilities, work to improve your abilities, and find activities that you can enjoy for a lifetime. You'll also learn about skills and how to acquire them.

Factors affecting skill-related fitness include heredity, age, maturation, sex, and training. Figure 6.1 shows how these factors are related.

Heredity

Skill-related fitness abilities are influenced by heredity. For example, some people are able to run fast or react quickly because they inherited these traits from their parents. A person who did not inherit these tendencies may have more difficulty performing well on skill-related fitness tests. However, it is still possible for such a person to improve his or her skill-related fitness by using special training techniques (discussed a bit later). In addition, lack of inherited ability can sometimes be made up for by desire and motivation.

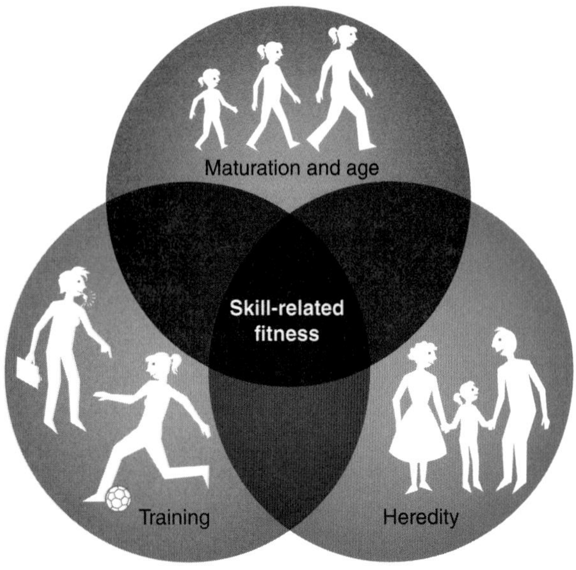

FIGURE 6.1 Various factors influence skill-related fitness.

Maturation and Age

In general, teens who mature early perform better on skill-related fitness tests than those who mature later. Because older teens in the same grade or on the same team are typically more mature, they also often have an advantage in skill-related fitness. Late-maturing teens typically catch up as they grow older.

Training

WWW 2

It has long been thought that changing one's skill-related fitness is hard to do. Because of heredity, this is somewhat true. But recent research has shown that with the right kind of training, you can improve your skill-related fitness, though it takes considerable effort and strong motivation to do so.

The Principle of Specificity

Skill-related fitness is also subject to the principle of specificity. Excelling in one part of skill-related fitness does not mean that you will excel in another. This is often true even when abilities seem closely related, such as reaction time and speed. For example, you might have great speed, meaning you can run fast, but lack good reaction time and thus be unable to get a good start. Apply the principle of specificity to choose a sport or activity that requires the specific skill-related fitness abilities you perform best.

The principle of specificity also tells you that you get what you train for. So if you want to build a specific part of skill-related fitness, train specifically for it.

Assessing Skill-Related Fitness

If you want to learn a lifetime sport or physical activity, a good first step is to assess your skill-related fitness abilities. Doing so helps you to determine your strengths and weaknesses. Self-assessments have two other benefits. They help you choose activities that can improve your skill-related fitness and they help you match your abilities to activities in which you have the greatest chance of success. As you perform the skill-related fitness assessments presented in this chapter, remember that skill-related fitness has many subparts. For example, coordination is a skill-related

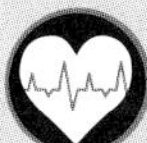

FITNESS TECHNOLOGY: Motion Analysis Systems

Many technological advances have helped people become more skilled at a variety of sport activities. One of the most noteworthy is the use of motion analysis systems, which can be as simple as a basic video camera and playback system or as complicated as a high-speed video camera and software that helps analyze whether a performer's movements (biomechanics) are efficient and effective. Whether simple or complex, a motion analysis system video-records a person performing a sport or activity. Next, a skill-learning expert, such as a sport pedagogist or coach, views the video and analyzes the performer's movements. For example, football players and coaches routinely review game footage together to look at defensive and offensive formations, as well as opponents' tactics. High-powered systems allow users to analyze the action in very slow motion and generate computer analysis to provide information that helps the performer make corrections. Motion analysis systems can be used for many kinds of activity (such as softball pitching and tennis) but are especially popular among golfers, who use the biomechanical feedback to improve their swings.

Using Technology

Make a video of your performance of a motor skill. Analyze the performance using information you've learned from an instructor or from information gained in the Science in Action student activity.

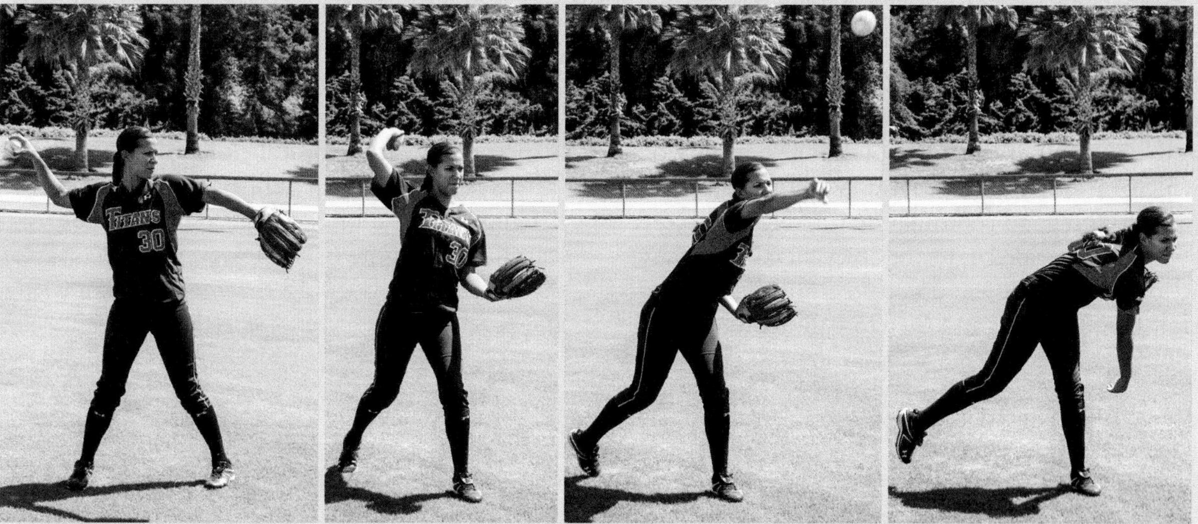

Movement sequences can be studied to provide feedback for improved performance.

ability that includes both eye–hand coordination (the ability to use your hands and eyes together, as in hitting a ball) and eye–foot coordination (the ability to use your eyes and feet together, as in kicking a ball). You may be good in one area but not as good in another. In addition to working on the areas that need improvement, you should consider selecting activities for your program that match your strengths.

Once you've assessed your skill-related fitness abilities, you can develop a profile of your results to help you select lifetime sports and other activities. In this lesson, you'll learn both how to do that and how to make plans for becoming proficient in your chosen activities.

Building a Skill-Related Fitness Profile

One student, Sue, did all of the skill-related physical fitness assessments presented in this chapter, then developed a profile for her skill-related fitness (see table 6.1). Sue's profile helped her identify her strengths and weaknesses, and she used her profile to develop her fitness program.

You can see that Sue has better ability in some parts of fitness than in others. One way she used her profile was to identify areas where she needed to improve her skill-related fitness. She used table 6.2 to choose activities that provided the most benefit for the parts of skill-related fitness that she wanted to improve. For example, Sue didn't do well in agility and balance, so she decided to take tai chi lessons to help her improve. She also didn't do well in reaction time and speed, but she realized that because of her heredity she probably would never be a really fast person with good reaction time. Still, she thought that tai chi might help her improve these abilities to some degree. She also decided not to worry if she wasn't as able as some other people in these parts of fitness.

The second way in which Sue can use her profile is to point her toward physical activities that are well suited to her abilities. Activities that provide the most benefit in a specific part of skill-related fitness also *require* the most fitness in that specific part. For example, Sue scored well in coordination, and bowling is excellent for building coordination, which means that it's also an activity in which a person with good coordination is likely to succeed.

Sue also decided to include bicycling in her activity program because it doesn't require high levels of skill-related fitness and therefore didn't require her to learn new skills. At the same time, bicycling does offer good health benefits.

You can develop your own skill-related fitness profile similar to the one Sue developed (refer back to table 6.1). Use your profile to determine which activities can help you improve where you need to and which activities you can most easily learn and enjoy.

Physical or Motor Skills

To review, a skill is a capability for doing a task that is acquired through knowledge and practice. Physical skills are also referred to as motor skills because learning a skill requires you to use "motor units" in your body. A **motor unit** is made up of nerves that cause muscles to contract and the muscle fibers that do the contracting and thus cause movement. If motor units are used over and over again (as when you practice a skill), you learn to use the nerves and muscles to move efficiently and thus improve your skills.

Skill Learning

The five parts of skill-related fitness are abilities that help you to learn physical skills. For this reason, factors that affect your skill-related fitness such as heredity, maturation, and age also affect your skill learning (see figure 6.1). However, the two factors that affect skill learning the most are knowledge and practice.

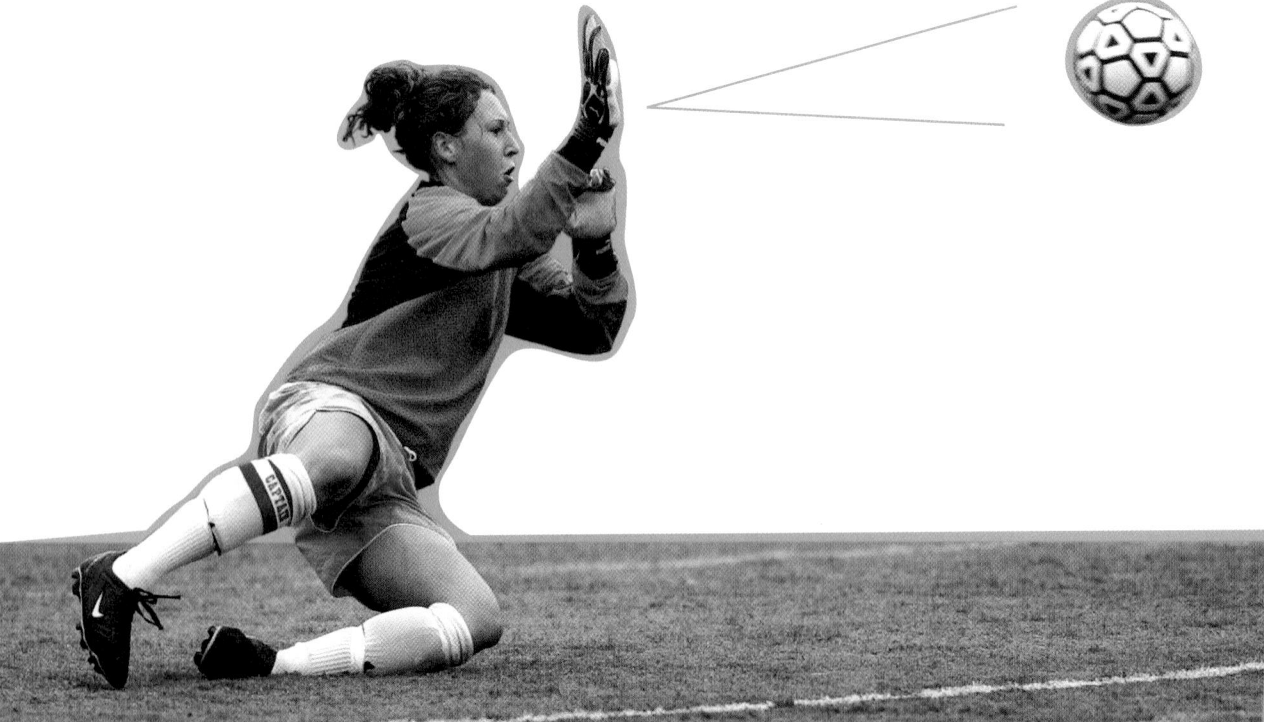

TABLE 6.1 Sue's Skill-Related Fitness Profile

	Skill-related performance rating			
Part of fitness	Low	Marginal	Good	High
Agility	✔			
Balance		✔		
Coordination				✔
Speed		✔		
Reaction time		✔		

TABLE 6.2 Skill-Related Benefits of Sports and Other Activities

Activity	Balance	Coordination	Reaction time	Agility	Speed
Badminton	Fair	Excellent	Good	Good	Good
Baseball	Good	Excellent	Excellent	Good	Good
Basketball	Good	Excellent	Excellent	Excellent	Good
Bicycling	Excellent	Fair	Fair	Fair	Fair
Bowling	Good	Excellent	Poor	Fair	Fair
Circuit training	Fair	Fair	Poor	Fair	Fair
Dance (aerobic or social)	Fair	Good	Fair	Good	Poor
Dance (ballet or modern)	Excellent	Excellent	Fair	Excellent	Poor
Fitness calisthenics	Fair	Fair	Poor	Good	Poor
Extreme sports	Good	Good	Excellent	Excellent	Good
Football	Good	Good	Excellent	Excellent	Excellent
Golf (walking)	Fair	Excellent	Poor	Fair	Poor
Gymnastics	Excellent	Excellent	Good	Excellent	Fair
Interval training	Fair	Fair	Poor	Poor	Fair
Jogging or walking	Poor	Poor	Poor	Poor	Poor
Martial arts	Good	Excellent	Excellent	Excellent	Excellent
Racquetball or handball	Fair	Excellent	Good	Excellent	Good
Rope jumping	Fair	Good	Fair	Good	Poor
Skating (ice or roller)	Excellent	Good	Fair	Good	Good
Skiing (cross-country)	Fair	Excellent	Poor	Good	Fair
Skiing (downhill)	Excellent	Excellent	Good	Excellent	Poor
Soccer	Fair	Excellent	Good	Excellent	Good
Softball (fastpitch)	Fair	Excellent	Excellent	Good	Good
Swimming (laps)	Poor	Good	Poor	Good	Poor
Tai chi	Excellent	Good	Fair	Excellent	Good
Tennis	Fair	Excellent	Good	Good	Good
Volleyball	Fair	Excellent	Good	Good	Fair
Weight training	Fair	Fair	Poor	Poor	Poor

Knowledge

Practice helps you to learn skills. But first you have to have basic information (knowledge) about how to perform skills and how best to practice. Throughout part 1 of this book you will gain information about biomechanical principles that are important for skill learning. You will also learn how to practice properly. For example, the Science in Action feature in this lesson provides information about feedback, or information used to help you perform and practice properly.

Practice

All people, regardless of their skill-related fitness, can learn skills with practice. However, it takes some people longer than others to learn skills, and some people will be better at performing skills than others. Not everyone can become an Olympic athlete, but with practice everyone can learn the basic skills necessary to enjoy some sports and to perform physical tasks efficiently. Considerable evidence shows that people who are dedicated and willing to work hard can even overcome hereditary disadvantages and outperform people who have a hereditary advantage. The key is practice.

Practice involves repeating a skill over and over again. If you repeat a skill, such as a tennis serve, and do it correctly, you will become better at that skill. You'll learn more about skill development in this chapter's Taking Charge and Self-Management features.

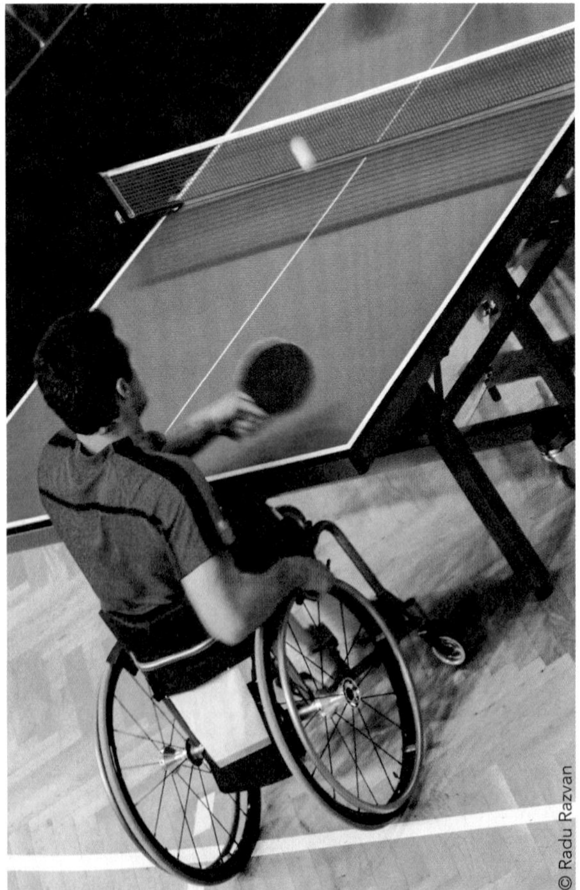

Practice is the key to learning new motor skills.

Three Stages of Skill Learning

When learning to perform a motor skill, you typically move through three stages. The first stage is called the *cognitive stage* because you have to think about what you're doing and apply knowledge to help you perform the skill. During this stage, movements are inefficient and typically slower than at later stages. Verbal feedback helps you to perform the skill properly. The second stage is called the *associative stage* because you begin to associate the knowledge of the skill with the actual movements. You still have to think about what you're doing, but skills start to become more automatic and your performance becomes more efficient and consistent. The final stage of skill learning is called the *autonomous stage* because you perform independent of cognitive control. (*Autonomous* is a word that refers to performing independently without outside control.) You do the movements automatically, and they are much more accurate and efficient.

Practice is the most important factor in skill learning, but practicing a skill *incorrectly* can be

FIT FACT

Having too much feedback can cause "paralysis by analysis," a state of mind in which you can't focus on the few things that are really important. For example, if a softball batter is given too much information—keep your eyes level, keep your elbows up, stride straight forward, lead with your hips, keep your eye on the ball—she may swing and miss the ball entirely. Too much feedback all at once can be more harmful than helpful.

SCIENCE IN ACTION: Feedback

Motor learning is an area of study in the field of kinesiology. Experts in motor learning study the best ways to learn skills. One key to motor or skill learning is **feedback**. Feedback refers to information you receive about your performance that includes suggestions for making changes in order to perform better. Feedback helps you use practice effectively. One of the best forms of feedback is from experts such as teachers and coaches. After watching your performance, they can give you specific comments about how to improve. Another way to receive feedback is to watch a video recording of your performance. Motor learning experts suggest that when you practice, you use one piece of feedback at a time.

Student Activity

Choose a skill used in one of the activities included in the Physical Activity Pyramid. Ask an expert to watch you perform the skill and give you feedback. Write down key points to remember when practicing the skill.

harmful to your skill learning because it may cause you to perform the skill incorrectly. Practice doesn't make perfect—*perfect practice* makes perfect. So it is crucial that you know both what to practice and how to practice it correctly. When first learning a skill (stage 1), you gain knowledge about the skill so that you know what to practice. You rely on cognitive information, including feedback from instructors (see the Science in Action feature). As you improve, you continue to refine your skills but focus more on repeating the skill rather than thinking about it. Even highly skilled athletes, who typically perform at the autonomous stage, practice regularly to keep their skills sharp and to make their performances more consistent and reliable.

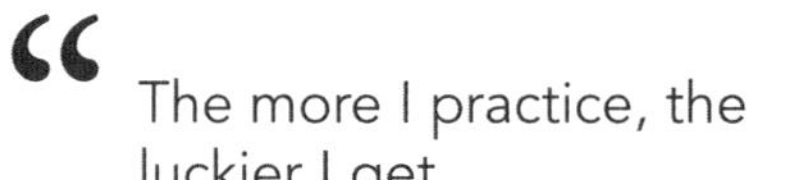

"The more I practice, the luckier I get."

—Gary Player, Hall of Fame golfer (and others)

Teamwork and Leadership Skills

Performance in sport and other activities depends, of course, on motor skills. But teamwork and leadership skills are also important for success, especially in team sports. Team sports require team members to work together, follow the team leader, and play their designated roles so that the team can enjoy success. No team can succeed without good leaders, but even the best leader is ineffective without teammates who play other important roles.

Leadership involves motivating people in a group to work toward a common goal. **Teamwork** involves all team members striving to achieve that common goal through cooperative effort. Team members can play different roles in different situations, perhaps leading in one instance and following in another. This pattern is good because it allows all people to play a variety of roles and helps them enjoy their involvement. Here are some ways to learn and develop your leadership and teamwork skills.

- **Learning and accepting your role.** Listening to coaches and more experienced players can help you define the role that is best for you. Carrying out that role is the best way for you to help your team.
- **Sacrifice.** Success often depends on a team member's willingness to sacrifice personal gain for the benefit of the team.
- **Communication.** Part of being a good leader is being able to convey your ideas clearly—for example, communicating specific feedback to your teammates in a respectful manner. Being a good communicator also involves positive nonverbal communication, such as appearing upbeat instead of dejected after something bad happens. Another important part of communication is good listening, which can help you understand team goals and personal roles and thus exercise effective leadership.

- **Sensitivity.** Teams work best when all members are sensitive to each other's feelings and concerns. Ways to build sensitivity include listening (for example, hearing what others have to say rather than only telling others what to do) and communicating in nonthreatening language (for example, giving positive comments rather than harsh criticism).
- **Trust and respect.** Good leaders are respected because they can be trusted. They keep their promises and are sensitive to fellow team members' feelings. Good leaders communicate and interact effectively with all team members. Trust is built when everyone feels a part of the team.
- **Decision making.** Teams perform best when team members, especially leaders, use critical thinking skills to make good decisions. This can be demonstrated by explaining why decisions are made and how they will help the team.
- **Observation.** Good leaders learn by observing effective leaders and teams that use good teamwork. By observing, you can learn to identify the specific behaviors of good leaders.
- **Practice.** Leadership and teamwork skills are learned in the same way that motor skills are learned—with practice. The reason that team leaders are often older and more experienced is that their experiences have allowed them to practice and develop their leadership skills.

Lesson Review

1. What are the five parts of skill-related fitness, and what are some examples of each part?
2. What factors influence skill-related fitness? How do you build a skill-related fitness profile?
3. What is a motor skill, and what factors influence motor skill?
4. What is involved in teamwork and leadership? What are some guidelines for building these skills?

SELF-ASSESSMENT: Assessing Skill-Related Physical Fitness

You can assess your skill-related fitness abilities by using the following tests. Use tables 6.3 and 6.4 to get your ratings. Record your scores and ratings as directed by your teacher. Keep the following points in mind, especially if you score low.

- You can improve all parts of your skill-related fitness, but it is often harder to improve skill-related fitness abilities than health-related fitness abilities.
- Due to the principle of specificity, you may excel in some and do less well in others.
- Some activities, such as jogging, do not require a high level of skill-related fitness.
- You do not need to excel in skill-related fitness in order to enjoy physical activity.

If you're working with a partner, remember that self-assessment information is personal and considered confidential. It shouldn't be shared with others without the permission of the person being tested.

Part 1: Side Shuttle (agility)

Use masking tape or another material to make five parallel lines 2 to 3 feet (61 to 91 centimeters) long on the floor; space the lines 3 feet apart. Have a partner count while you do the side shuttle. Then count while your partner does it.

1. Stand with the first line to your right. When your partner says "go," step to the right with the right foot, and then slide the left foot over to the right foot. Continue to step-slide until your right foot steps over the last line. Then reverse direction, stepping with the left foot and sliding with the right until your left foot steps over the first line.
   Caution: Do not cross your feet.
2. Repeat the exercise, moving from side to side as many times as possible in 10 seconds. Only one foot must cross the last line.
3. When your partner says "stop," freeze in place until he or she counts your score. Score 1 point for each line you crossed in 10 seconds. Subtract 1 point for each time you crossed your feet.
4. Do the side shuttle twice and record the better of your two scores. Use table 6.3 to determine your rating. Record your rating.

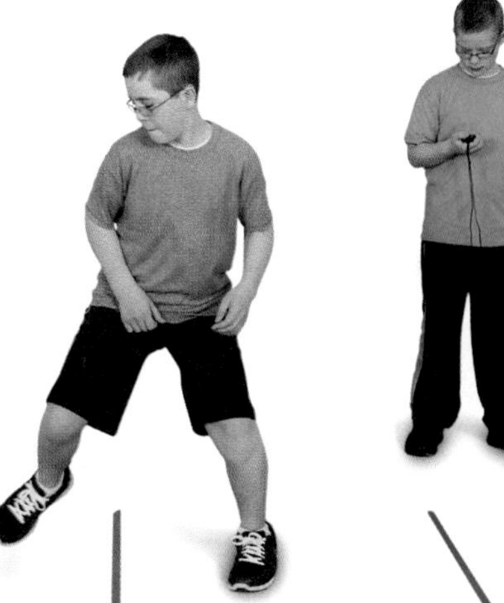

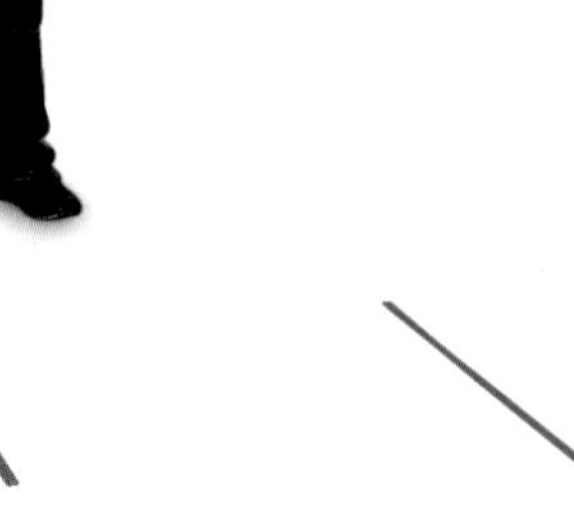

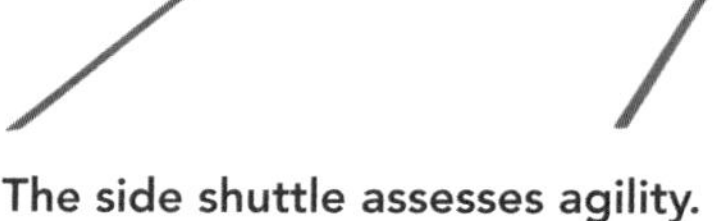

The side shuttle assesses agility.

Part 2: Stick Balance (balance)

You may take one practice try before doing each test for a score.

Test 1

1. Use a square stick (1.5 inches, or about 4 centimeters) that is 1 foot long (30 centimeters). Place the balls of both feet across a stick so that your heels are on the floor.
2. Lift your heels off the floor and maintain your balance on the stick for 15 seconds. Hold your arms out in front of you for balance. Once you begin, do not allow your heels to touch the floor (off of the stick) or your feet to move on the stick.

   Hint: Focus your eyes on a stationary object in front of you.
3. Try the test twice. Give yourself 2 points if you succeed on the first try but fail on the second, 1 point if you fail on the first try but succeed on the second, and 3 points if you succeed on both tries.
4. Record your scores.

Test 2

1. Stand on the stick with either foot. Your foot should run the length of the stick.
2. Lift your other foot off the floor. First, balance for 10 seconds with your base foot flat. Then rise onto the ball of your base foot (with your heel off the stick) and continue balancing for 10 seconds.

   Hint: Balance on your dominant leg—the one you use to kick a ball.
3. Try the test twice. Give yourself 1 point if you balance flat-footed for 10 seconds, 1 point if you balance on the ball of your foot for 10 seconds, and another point if you successfully performed both trials. Your maximum score is 3 points.
4. Add the scores from both stick tests. Use table 6.3 to determine your rating.
5. Record your scores and rating.

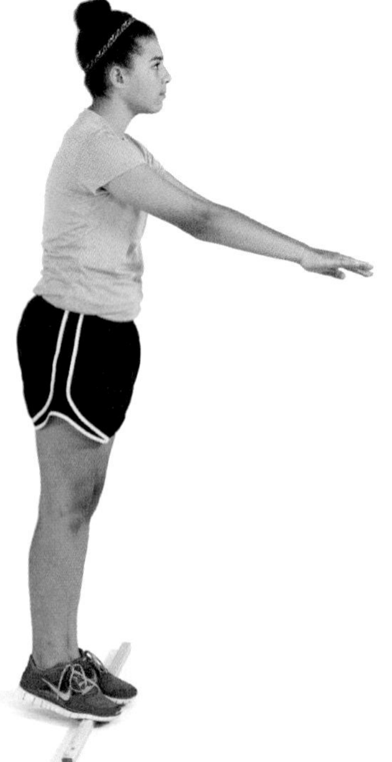

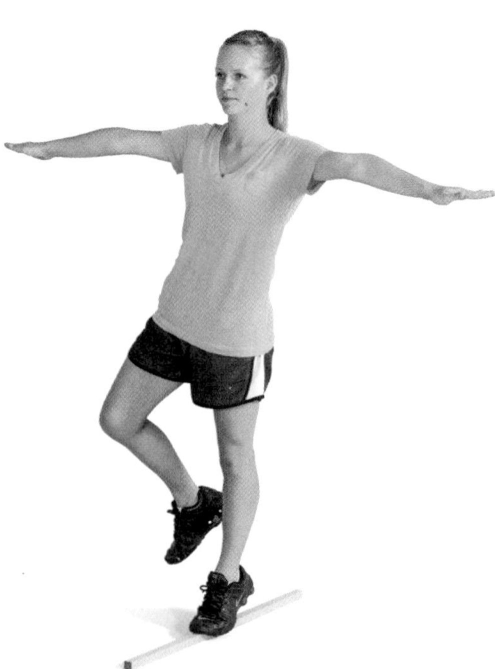

The two stick balance tests assess balance.

Part 3: Wand Juggling (coordination)

1. Take three practice tries before doing this test for a score. Hold a stick in each hand. Have a partner place a third stick across the sticks held in your hands.
2. Using the two sticks you're holding, toss the third stick into the air so that it makes a half turn. Catch it with the sticks you're holding. The tossed stick should not hit your hands.
3. Do this test five times by tossing the stick to the right, then five times by tossing the stick to the left. Score 1 point for each successful catch.

   Hint: Absorb the shock of the catch by giving with the held sticks, as you might do when catching an egg or something breakable.
4. Record your results and use table 6.3 to determine your rating. Record your rating.

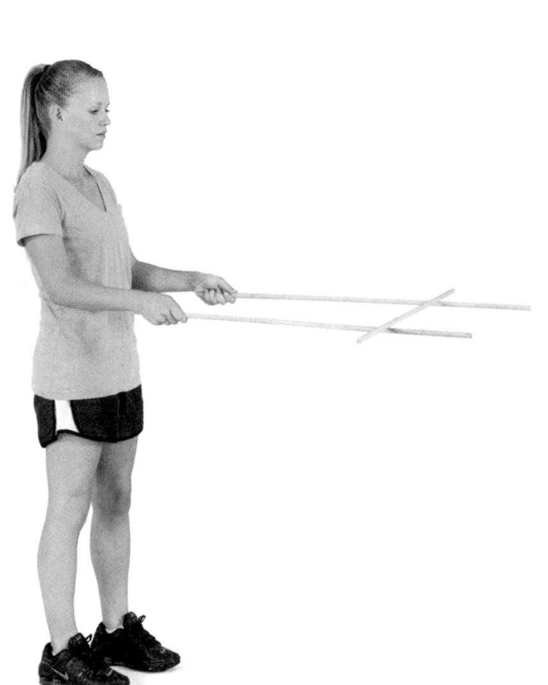

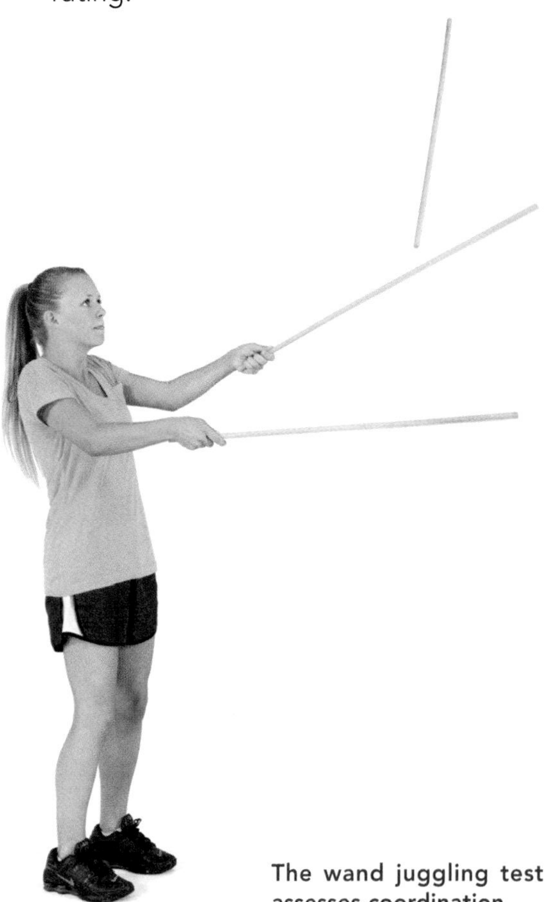

The wand juggling test assesses coordination.

TABLE 6.3 Rating Chart: Agility, Balance, and Coordination

	Side shuttle		Stick balance	Wand juggling
	Male	Female	Male or female	Male or female
Excellent	≥31	≥28	6	9 or 10
Good	26–30	24–27	5	7 or 8
Fair	19–25	15–23	3 or 4	4–6
Poor	≤18	≤14	≤2	≤3

Part 4: Stick Drop (reaction time)

1. Have a partner hold the top of a yardstick (or meter stick) with his or her thumb and index finger between the 1-inch (2.5-centimeter) mark and the end of the stick.
2. Position the 24-inch (61-centimeter) mark on the stick between your thumb and fingers. Do not touch or grip the stick. Your arm should rest on the edge of a table with only your fingers over the edge.
3. When your partner drops the stick without warning, catch it as quickly as possible between your thumb and fingers.
   Hint: Focus on the stick, not your partner, and be very alert.
4. Try this test three times. Your score for each try is the number on the stick at the place where you catch it. Record your scores. Your partner should be careful not to drop the stick after the same waiting period each time. In other words, you should not be able to guess when the stick will drop.
5. Use table 6.4 to determine your rating based on your middle score (the one between your lowest and highest scores). Record your rating.

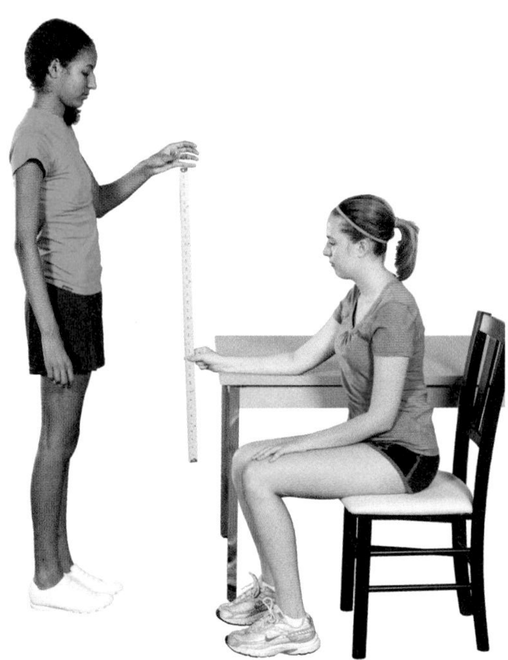

The stick drop test assesses reaction time.

Part 5: Short Sprint (speed)

Use masking tape or other materials to make 10 lines on the floor that are 2 to 3 feet long (61 to 91 centimeters). The first line is a starting line; the second is 10 yards (9.1 meters) from the starting line. The remaining lines are 2 yards (1.8 meters) apart beginning after the 10-yard (9.1-meter) line for a total distance of 26 yards (23.8 meters). Work with a partner who will time you and blow a whistle to signal you to stop.

Try the test once for practice without being timed, then do it for a score.

1. Stand two or three steps behind the starting line.
2. When your partner says "go," run as far and as fast as you can. Your partner will start a stopwatch when you cross the starting line. Three seconds later, your partner will blow the whistle. When the whistle sounds, do not try to stop immediately, but do begin to slow down.
3. Your partner should mark where you were when the three-second whistle blew. Measure the distance to the nearest line. If you were more than halfway to a line, count that line when scoring. Your score is the distance you covered in the three seconds after crossing the starting

line. For example, if you cross five lines after the starting line plus 1 foot, your score is 18 yards because 1 foot is less than half the distance to the next line.

4. Record your score and use table 6.4 to determine your rating. Record your rating.

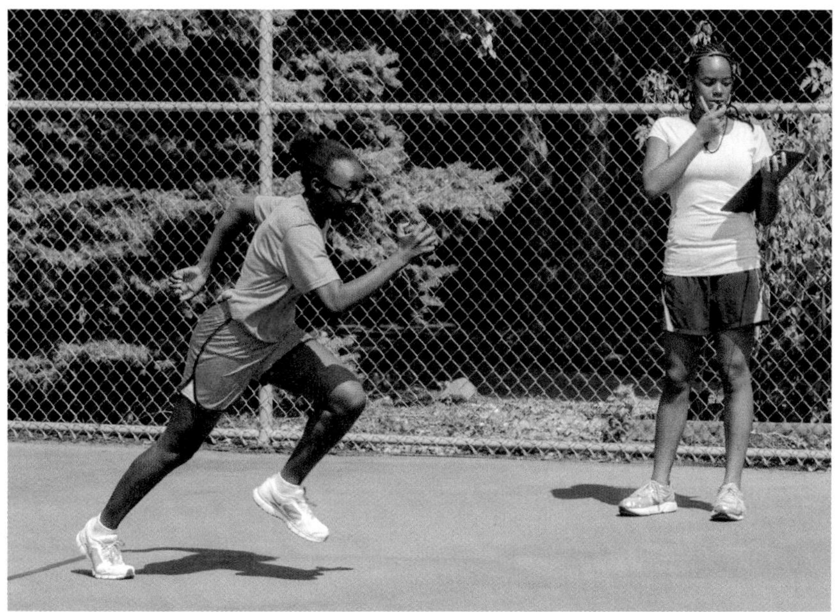

The short sprint test assesses speed.

TABLE 6.4 Rating Chart: Reaction Time and Speed

	Stick drop (inches)	Short sprint (yards run)	
	Male or female	Male	Female
Excellent	≥22	≥24	≥22
Good	19–21	21–23	19–21
Fair	14–18	16–20	15–18
Poor	≤13	≤15	≤14

To convert inches to centimeters, multiply by 2.54. To convert yards to meters, multiply by 0.91.

The rating categories for skill-related physical fitness describe levels of performance ability, not health or wellness.

Lesson 6.2

Physical Activity and Injury

Lesson Objectives

After reading this lesson, you should be able to

1. list and describe some activity-related physical injuries,
2. list some guidelines for preventing injury during physical activity,
3. explain how to apply the RICE formula for treating physical injuries, and
4. identify types of risky exercise.

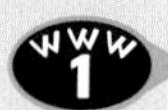

Lesson Vocabulary

biomechanical principles, extension, flexion, ligament, microtrauma, overuse injury, RICE, side stitch, sprain, strain, tendon

Would you know what to do if you sprained your ankle? If you were performing a yoga pose that is risky, would you know it? At this point, you certainly know that physical activity provides many benefits for your health and wellness. But if you don't do it properly, you can injure yourself; fortunately, most injuries are minor and can be prevented by being careful.

Before you start a physical activity program, be sure you're prepared for exercise and know how to exercise safely. In this lesson, you'll learn about some common minor injuries, as well as some basic precautions you can take to avoid them. You'll also learn about some exercises that are considered too risky and about safer alternatives that you can use.

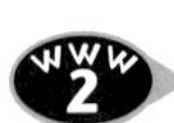

Common Injuries

If you've ever suffered a sport- or exercise-related injury, you may already know that an injury can be quite painful even if it's not serious. Some of the more common minor injuries related to sport and exercise are sprains, strains, blisters, bruises, cuts, and scrapes. More serious but less common injuries include joint dislocation and bone fracture. The body parts injured most commonly in physical activity are the skin, feet, ankles, knees, and leg muscles (see figure 6.2). Parts less likely to be injured are the head, arms, trunk, and internal organs, such as the liver and kidneys.

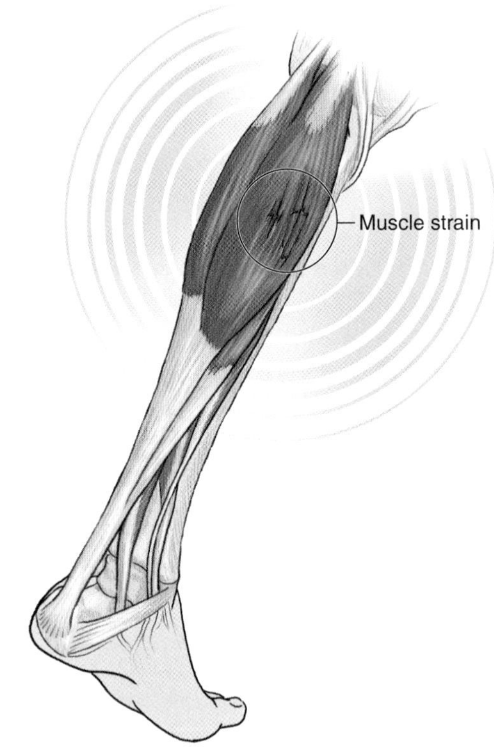

FIGURE 6.2 Muscle strains are a common injury in sport and physical activity.

One type of injury, called an **overuse injury**, occurs when you repeat a movement so much that your body suffers wear and tear. You're most likely familiar with one very common overuse injury—a blister. Another example is shin splints, which involves soreness in the front of the lower leg. Small muscle tears or muscle spasms resulting from overuse are probably the cause. A third example, runner's heel, also involves soreness, in this case usually caused by running or jumping activities that require the heel to repeatedly hit the ground. These injuries are especially common among long-distance runners and other people whose activities involve repeated foot impact.

A **side stitch** is a pain in the side of the lower abdomen that people often experience when participating in a sport (especially running activities). No one is exactly sure what causes the side stitch, but one theory is a spasm in the diaphragm, the muscle tissue involved in breathing. Side stitches are most common among people who are not accustomed to vigorous activity. A side stitch is not really an injury, because the pain goes away if you stop the activity or continue at a more moderate pace. To help relieve a side stitch, press firmly at the point of the pain with your hand while bending forward or backward.

Another type of injury is called **microtrauma.** *Micro* means small—so small it may not show up on an X ray or exam—and *trauma* is another word for injury. So a microtrauma is an invisible injury. This injury often causes no immediate pain, but, with repeated use, symptoms of the damage eventually appear. Many adults today experience back problems, neck aches, and stiff or painful joints caused by microtrauma suffered when they were younger. Some risky exercises that can cause microtrauma are discussed later in this chapter.

FIT FACT

Anabolic steroids are illegal supplements taken by some athletes, including some teens. People who take steroids are trying to enhance their performance but often end up experiencing the opposite effect. Steroids have been identified as a significant cause of injury to tendons and ligaments. Leading sports medicine doctors indicate that steroid use causes athletes to miss many games and can result in career-ending injury or serious health problems.

Preventing Injury

Your body is made up of more than two hundred bones that connect at joints. Different kinds of joints allow different types of movement. For example, synovial joints allow free movement; they include hinge joints (such as your knees and elbows) that allow only **flexion** and **extension**, as well as ball and socket joints (such as your hips and shoulders) that allow additional movements such as rotation. Cartilaginous joints (such as the vertebrae in your back) allow only limited movement. Fibrous joints are referred to as immoveable or fixed; examples are the joints where the bones of your skull connect.

When your muscles contract, they pull your tendons and make your bones move. Your bones act as levers to allow body movement. For example, contracting the muscles at the top of your upper arms (your biceps muscles) provides force that pulls on the tendons connecting to the bones (levers) of your lower arms, thus causing your elbows (hinge joints) to bend as shown in figure 6.3. When used properly, the levers of your body help you move efficiently, but when used incorrectly they can produce forces that cause injury to a joint or other body part.

Different types of injury can affect different types of tissue. A **sprain** is an injury to a ligament that typically results in swelling and pain around the joint. As illustrated in figure 6.4, **ligaments** are

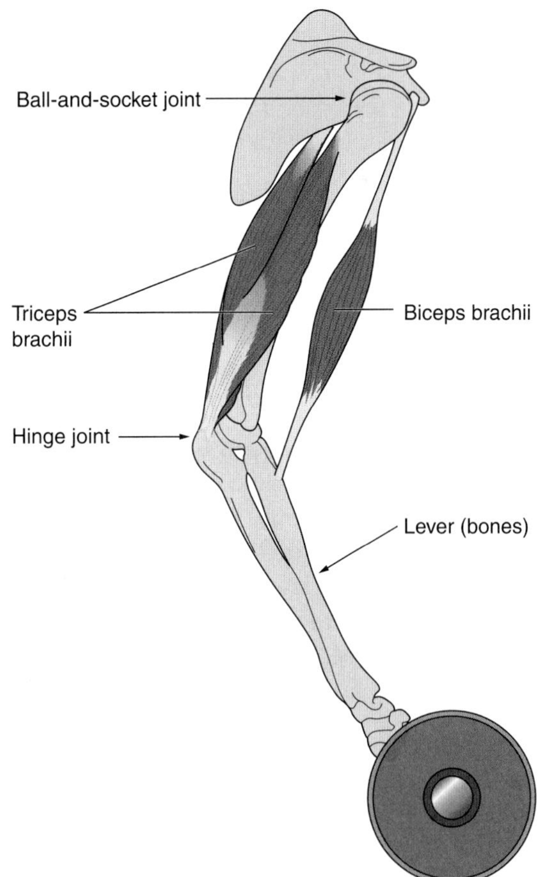

FIGURE 6.3 Your bones act as levers to allow body movement.

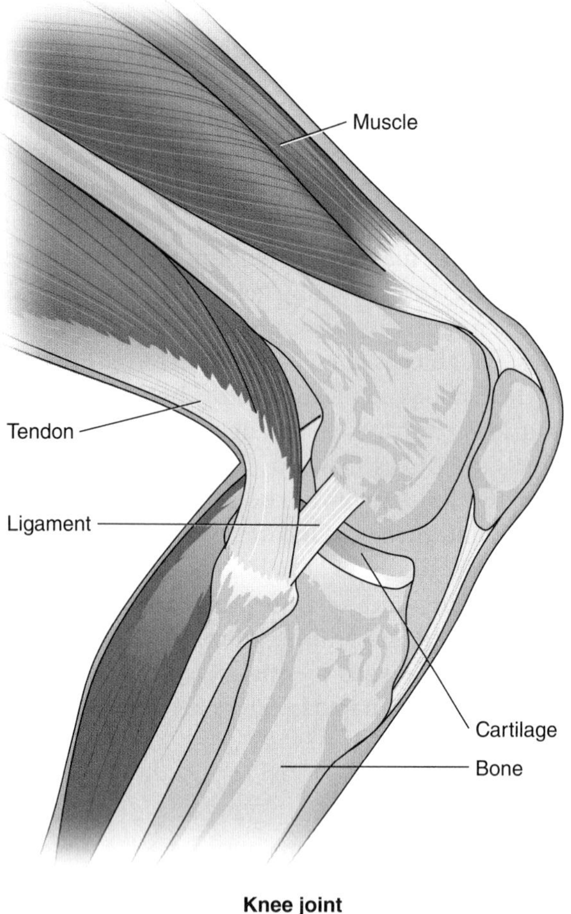

FIGURE 6.4 These tissues are commonly injured.

tough tissues that hold your bones together. The other types of tissue you see in the figure are tendons, muscles, and bones; **tendons** connect muscles to bones. A **strain**, sometimes called a pulled muscle, is an injury to tendon or muscle resulting from tears in the tissues. Like sprains, strains often result in pain and swelling.

Experts in sports medicine have studied injuries that occur in a wide variety of activities, including all of those included in the Physical Activity Pyramid. They have developed the following guidelines to help you prevent injury.

- **Start slowly.** Injuries are more common among beginners. If you haven't been exercising regularly, follow the principle of progression: start slowly, then gradually build up to more vigorous activity.
- **Listen to your body.** Injury can occur when you ignore signs and symptoms that your body is giving you. If you experience pain, pay attention to it. Until you know what is causing the pain, slow your exercise or stop altogether. Most blisters and shin splints can be avoided if you listen to your body.
- **Be fit!** One of the best ways to avoid injury is to be physically fit. A person with a fit heart and lungs and long, strong muscles is less likely to be injured than one who is unfit. Proper physical activity builds total physical fitness, which helps you prevent injury.
- **Use moderation.** Overuse causes many minor injuries in physical activity. For example, about 40 percent of regular runners and 50 percent of aerobic dancers experience injury at some point, usually due to using a body part too intensely or for too long a time.
- **Dress properly.** Some injuries are caused by improper dress; for example, wearing poor shoes and socks can cause blisters or runner's heel. Make sure you dress properly, wear proper shoes, and replace them when they begin to wear down.
- **Avoid risky exercises.** Injury can be caused by certain exercises that violate the rules of biomechanics (see risky exercise descriptions later in this lesson).

FIT FACT

People who are just beginning a physical activity program sometimes get a type of soreness called delayed onset muscle soreness (DOMS). This soreness occurs 24 to 48 hours after a vigorous workout, such as a sport practice. DOMS is caused by microscopic muscle tears. Unlike microtrauma, these tears do not cause permanent damage. To avoid DOMS, progress gradually when you begin an exercise program. It is okay to continue to exercise when you're sore, but if pain persists or is sharp rather than general in nature, stop exercising and seek medical advice.

Simple Treatment of Minor Injuries

When injury occurs, it is often necessary to seek medical help. However, you can take immediate steps to reduce pain and prevent complications—if you know basic first aid and thus can take the right steps. For muscle strains, sprains, and bruises, which are common in sport and other activities, you can follow the **RICE** formula. Each letter in the formula represents a step taken to treat a minor injury:

- **R is for rest.** After first aid has been given, the injured body part should be immobilized for two or three days to prevent further injury. The length of rest depends on the severity of the injury and the response to treatment.
- **I is for ice.** A body part that has been sprained or strained should be immersed in cold water or covered with ice that is wrapped in a towel or placed in a plastic bag. Icing for 20 minutes immediately after injury helps reduce swelling and pain. Apply ice or cold several times a day for one to three days. To relieve the pain of shin splints, apply the ice bag and towel to the front of your leg until the pain subsides (no longer than 20 minutes at a time).
- **C is for compression.** Use an elastic bandage to wrap the injured area in order to help limit swelling. For a sprained ankle, keep the shoe laced and the sock on the foot until compression can be applied with a bandage (the shoe and sock compress the injury). To avoid restricting blood flow, remove the bandage for a few minutes or loosen it if you feel throbbing or it feels too tight.
- **E is for elevation.** Raise the injured body part above the level of your heart to help reduce swelling.

“The more injuries you get, the smarter you get.” 

—Mikhail Baryshnikov, professional dancer

Risky Exercises

Biomechanics experts who study the body's levers and tissues have developed several rules to help you avoid improper movement and therefore prevent injury.

1. Avoid movements that stretch your ligaments.
2. Avoid movements that twist your joints or force them to move in other ways for which they were not designed.
3. Avoid movements that use your body's levers improperly.
4. Balance your muscle development on both sides of your joints so that all of your muscles develop properly. For example, look back at figure 6.3, which shows the muscles of the upper arm. If you overdevelop your biceps muscle with no attention to your triceps, you may eventually become unable to fully extend your arm (your triceps may not be strong enough). You also increase your risk of straining your triceps muscle because this weak muscle will be overstressed by the pull of the stronger biceps.

Some exercises are considered risky because they cause your body to move in ways that violate these rules and basic **biomechanical principles**. Doing these exercises may not cause immediate injury and pain, but if you do them repeatedly they put you at risk for microtrauma. They can result in pain, joint problems, wear-and-tear injuries such as inflammation of tendons and bursas (cushioning tissues in your joints), and wearing away of joint cartilage. Over time, microtrauma caused by risky exercise can result in crippling arthritis or back and neck pain—a leading medical complaint in the United States.

Generally speaking, you should avoid the following exercises (you'll perform some safe substitutes in the Taking Action section). Of course, some athletes may find it impossible to avoid all potentially harmful exercises. For example, gymnasts must perform stunts that require back arching, and softball and baseball catchers must do full squats. These athletes do extra flexibility and strength exercises to prepare their bodies for these activities; in addition, if pain occurs when exercising, they should get medical help immediately.

Hyperflexion Exercises to Avoid

Hyper means too much, and *flexion* means bending at the joint. Hyperflexion exercises cause you to use joints in ways that they are not intended to be used; specifically, they violate rules 1 and 2 because they bend your joints too far and overstretch your ligaments. For example, deep knee bends involve hyperflexion of the knee (figure 6.5). Other hyperflexing exercises to avoid include duckwalks, bicycles (also called shoulder stands), yoga ploughs, sit-ups with the hands behind the neck, and knee pull-downs. Some safer alternatives include the curl-up with the hands across the chest, the half squat, and the hip and thigh stretch.

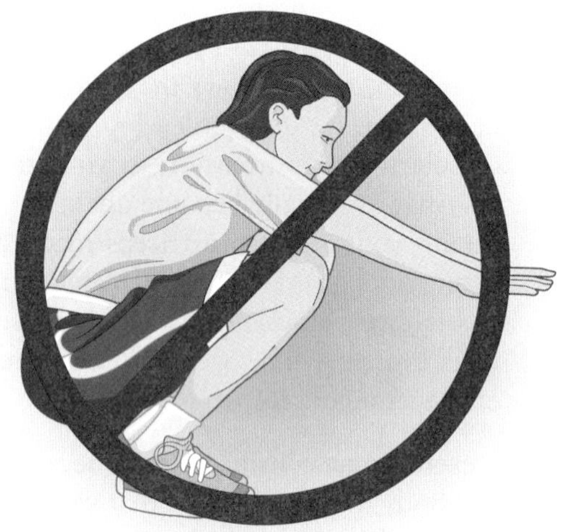

FIGURE 6.5 Avoid hyperflexion exercises, such as deep knee bends.

Hyperextension Exercises to Avoid

Hyperextension is the opposite of hyperflexion. As mentioned earlier, *hyper* means too much. *Extension* means increasing the angle of the bones at a joint. So *hyperextension* means increasing the angle of the joint too much. For example, having some curve in the back is normal, but arching the lower back more than normal involves hyperextension. Exercises that create hyperextension violate rules 2 and 3 because they cause joints such as the vertebrae to move in ways for which they are not intended and because they cause the levers of the body to apply force inappropriately.

Some back arching exercises tend to stretch your abdominal muscles and can injure your spinal discs and joints. These exercises also violate rule 4 because they may shorten your back muscles, which are already too short in most people. Particular caution should be used by people with swayback, weak abdominal muscles, a protruding abdomen, or back problems. (You can learn more about swayback and other back problems in the chapter titled Muscle Fitness Applications.) Risky hyperextension exercises include straight-leg sit-ups, back bends (figure 6.6), rocking horses, cobras, prone swan positions, excessive upper back lifts, and incorrect weightlifting positions in which the back is arched. Safe alternatives include the curl-up, knee-to-nose touch, and the hip and thigh stretch. Some other exercises that hyperextend the spine are neck hyperextensions, neck circling to the rear (figure 6.7),

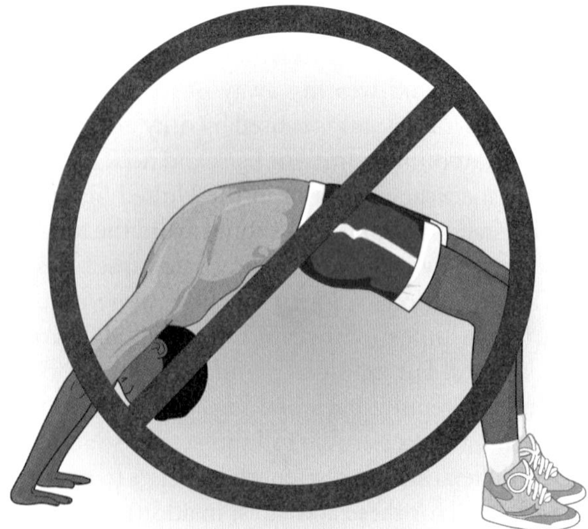

FIGURE 6.6 Avoid hyperextension exercises, such as back bends.

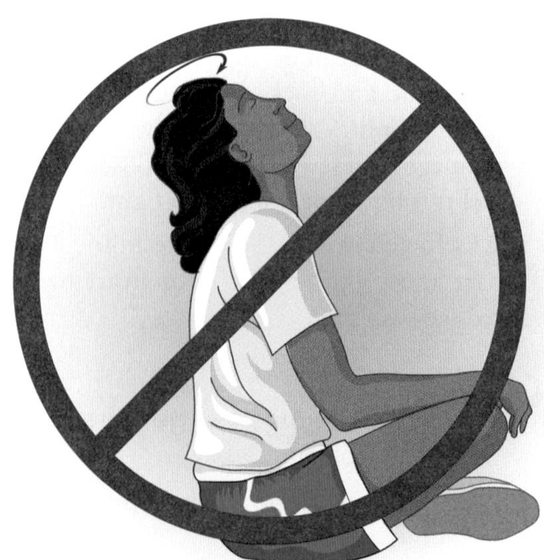

FIGURE 6.7 Avoid hyperextension and exercises that cause friction, such as neck circling to the rear.

rear double-leg lifts, donkey kicks, landing from a jump with the back arched, wrestler's bridges, and backward trunk circling.

Joint-Twisting, Compression, and Friction Exercises to Avoid

Some exercises cause the joints to twist excessively (such as standing windmill toe touches and heroes). Others cause compression at the joints or cause certain structures to rub against each other, creating friction that results in wear and tear. Examples of exercises in this category are hurdle sits, heroes (figure 6.8), double-leg lifts, sit-ups with the hands behind the head, standing straight-leg toe touches, and arm circling with the palms down. Safe alternatives include the back-saver hamstring stretch, the reverse curl, the curl-up, knee-to-nose touch, and the hip and thigh stretch.

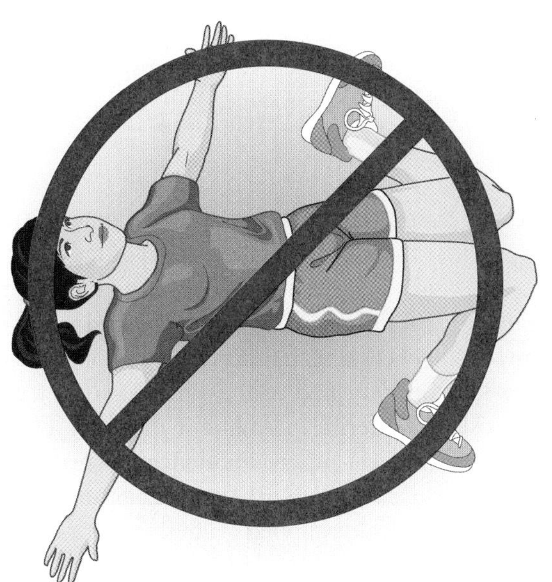

FIGURE 6.8 Avoid exercises that twist or compress your joints, such as heroes.

Improper Strengthening or Stretching Exercises

Some exercises can result in muscle imbalance (thus violating rule 4) because they build muscles that are not especially in need of development rather than muscles that are needed for good health and wellness. These exercises are not risky but are still poor choices. For example, forward arm circling develops already-strong pectorals, but backward arm circling with your palms up is a better choice because it works on the weaker back muscles. Other improper exercises strengthen the already-too-strong muscles that go across the front of your hip joints. These exercises can cause disc injury, abdominal tears, tendon tears, and loose ligaments. Examples of this type of risky exercise include straight-leg sit-ups and double-leg lifts (figure 6.9). Safe alternatives include the curl-up and the reverse curl.

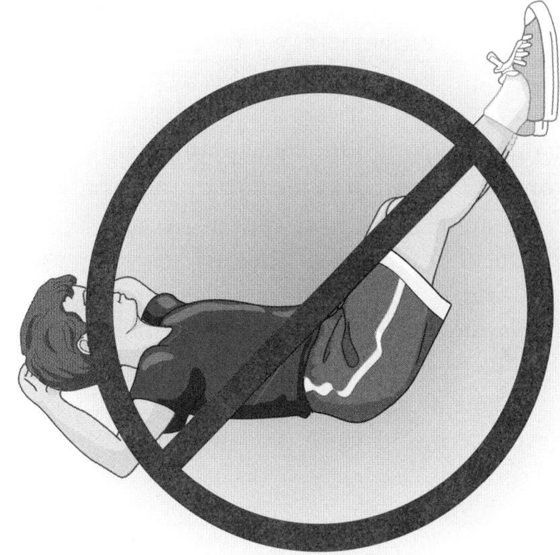

FIGURE 6.9 Avoid exercises that strengthen muscles that may already be too strong, such as the double-leg lift.

Concussions and Other Sport Injuries

Sports medicine is a branch of medical science. Sports medicine experts study injuries in sport to help people take steps to prevent them. One serious sport injury is concussion, a brain injury that occurs when a blow to the head causes the brain to crash into the bones of the skull. Concussions range in severity from mild to severe. A mild concussion may result in dizziness and confusion. A more severe concussion can cause you to pass out; it can also result in temporary or long-term loss of functions such as speaking and moving your muscles and cause other severe symptoms. Fortunately, most sport-related concussions are not severe, and symptoms usually disappear within hours or days. However, having one concussion increases the risk of having another. Repeated blows or jolts to the head can cause cumulative damage even when a concussion is not present.

CONSUMER CORNER: Putting Technology Into Action

Advances in technology have limited the amount of physical activity that many people get each day. Often, they get screen time instead. At the same time, however, technological advances have produced wonderful tools for use in almost every part of our lives, and some of these tools can help you achieve your health and fitness goals.

You can use software (sometimes called applications or "apps") for smartphones, tablets, and computers to help you achieve your health and fitness objectives. You can also access exercise video clips to see how to perform exercises properly. And you can use devices such as pedometers, accelerometers, and heart rate monitors to help with your self-assessment and self-monitoring.

If you decide to use one or more of these devices, consider the following consumer guidelines.

- **Apps.** Check the app to determine if it adheres to the exercise principles described in part 1 of this book.
- **Exercise videos.** View the video. Check to see if it includes any risky exercises. Check to see if the video follows exercise principles described in part 1 of this book.
- **Pedometers.** Check the accuracy of a pedometer with a simple walk test. Set the pedometer to zero, then walk and count exactly 100 steps. Check the pedometer to see if it counted 100 steps; an error of up to 3 steps in 100 is considered acceptable. You may also find that a pedometer counts more accurately in one location on your body than in another. Test the accuracy in different positions on your belt. If the unit does not count accurately in any position, try a different pedometer.

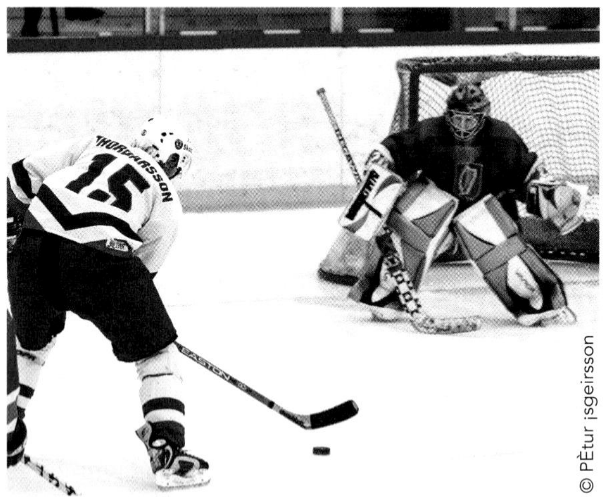

© PÉtur ¡sgeirsson

Wearing helmets can reduce risk of concussion but doesn't eliminate it.

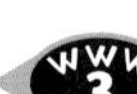

Concussions are more prevalent in collision sports such as hockey and football, but they also occur in other sports, such as soccer and basketball. Examples include head-to-head or head-to-ball contact in soccer and falls and blows to the head in basketball. Repeated concussions increase a person's risk of suffering permanent damage. This is why boxers have a higher incidence of permanent damage than athletes in other sports. Sports medicine experts have developed guidelines for preventing concussions and for allowing athletes to return to action after a concussion.

Lesson Review

1. What are some activity-related physical injuries, and what are the characteristics of the injuries?
2. What steps can you take to prevent injury during physical activity?
3. How can the RICE formula be used to treat physical injuries?
4. What are some types of risky exercise, and why are they considered risky?

TAKING CHARGE: Improving Performance Skills

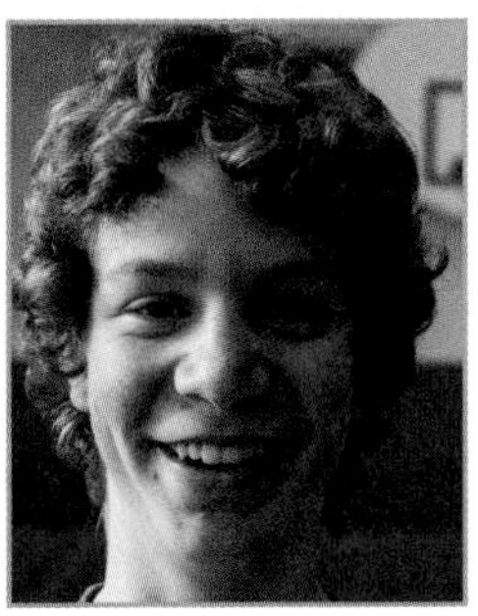

To enjoy a physical activity, you must possess the specific skills needed for that particular sport or game. Performance skills such as kicking, throwing, hitting, and swimming can be learned by most people with practice. It does, however, take some people longer than others to learn skills. Here's an example.

Zack felt that he was never really good at sports. He tried several activities and found that he was not as good at them as other people he knew. He even tried out for sport teams at school—first soccer, then swimming—but didn't make either one. His biggest problem was that he had not learned to play sports when he was young, and now he was behind others who had learned.

Zack wanted to learn a sport but was afraid that he'd be unsuccessful again and that his friends would laugh at him. He performed a self-assessment of his skill-related abilities and was surprised to find that he did pretty well on most of the assessments. He did especially well in coordination and agility, though his speed was not very high.

Before trying out for another team, Zack thought it would be best to try to learn the skills needed for a sport that matched his abilities. His size seemed to be an advantage—he was over 6 feet (1.8 meters) tall and weighed 180 pounds (82 kilograms)—but he wanted to get stronger, and he was not sure which sport would be best for him. He wanted to be on a team but also wanted to learn something that would be fun and interesting.

For Discussion

What advice would you give Zack for choosing a sport? Once he makes his choices, what steps could he take to improve his performance skills? Who could he talk to for help? Zack knew that he needed to practice but wasn't sure exactly *what* to practice. What practice advice would you give him? Consider the guidelines presented in the Self-Management feature as you answer the discussion questions.

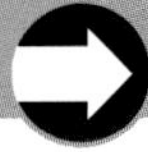

SELF-MANAGEMENT: Skills for Improving Performance

Experts in sport pedagogy and motor learning have studied the best ways to learn sport skills. They have developed guidelines that can help you as you work to improve your skills.

- **Get good instruction.** If you learn a skill incorrectly, it will be hard to improve, even with practice. Good instructors provide feedback that you can use to correct errors and improve your performance.
- **Practice.** Good practice is the key to improving your skills. It involves repeated performance focused on correct technique. Good instruction helps you perform good practice. Many people do not like to practice skills—they just want to play the game. But just playing the game doesn't provide practice in a particular skill, and if you play a game without the proper skills you often develop bad habits that hinder your success.
- **Practice all skills, not just those that you already do well.** Sport requires more than a few skills to become proficient. For example, basketball requires shooting, dribbling, passing, catching, and defensive skills. In order to succeed, you must practice all necessary skills.
- **At first, don't worry about details.** When you first learn a skill, concentrate on the skill as a whole. You can deal with the details after you learn the main skill. As you improve, concentrate on one detail at a time. If you try to concentrate on too many details at once, you may develop what is called "paralysis by analysis," a condition in which you

analyze an activity and try to correct several problems all at once. For example, if you're learning the tennis serve, don't try to work on your ball toss, grip, backswing, and follow-through at the same time. Instead, practice the parts of the skill one at a time.

- **Avoid competing while learning a skill.** Although competition can be fun, competing while you're learning a skill is stressful and does not promote optimal learning. When you compete you only try skills that you are already good at, so you often don't make improvements in areas of need.
- **Think positively.** Experts have shown that if you think negatively, you're likely to perform poorly. But if you think positively while you practice, you'll learn faster and become more confident in your abilities.
- **Choose an activity that matches your skill-related fitness.** As you may recall, heredity can play a role in your sport success. Use the information in your self-assessment of skill-related fitness to help you select a sport in which you're most likely to succeed.
- **Consider mental practice.** Doing mental practice involves imagining that you're performing a skill. Research shows that practicing a skill mentally can improve your performance. You can do mental practice even when you can't do regular practice due to factors such as bad weather or lack of a suitable location or facility.

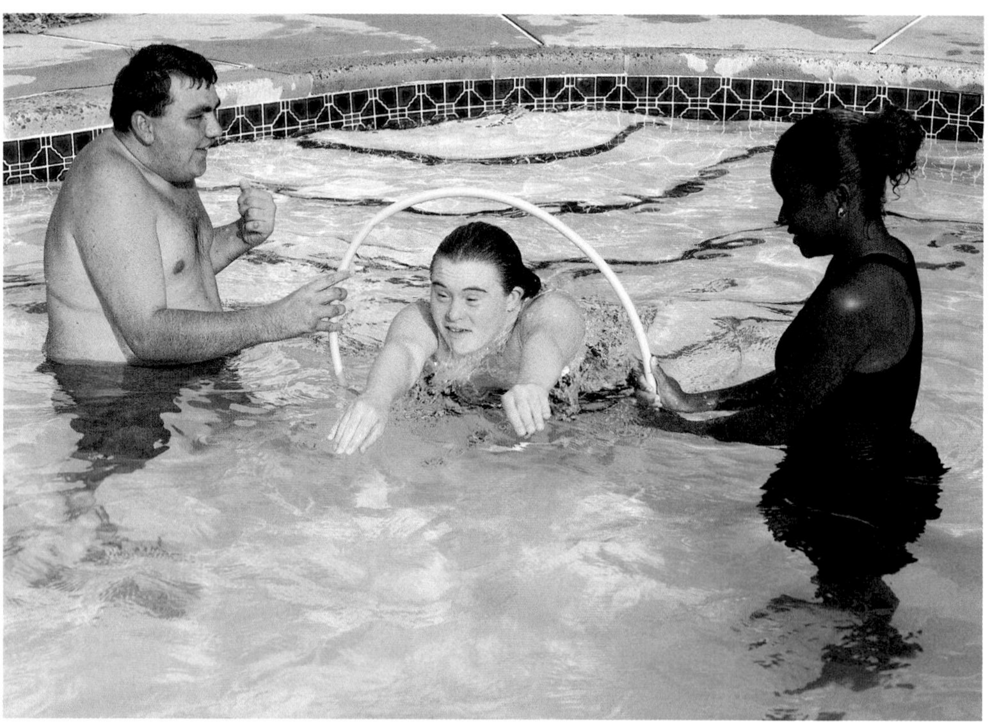

Good instruction and good practice can help you learn new skills.

TAKING ACTION: Safe Exercise Circuit

You now know about risky exercises. Some safe substitutes were listed but not described in detail. You can **take action** by trying some of the safe exercises using a safe exercise circuit. The exercises in the circuit are safe to perform and give you the benefits of risky exercises without the risk. Additional safe exercises are described throughout part 1 of this book.

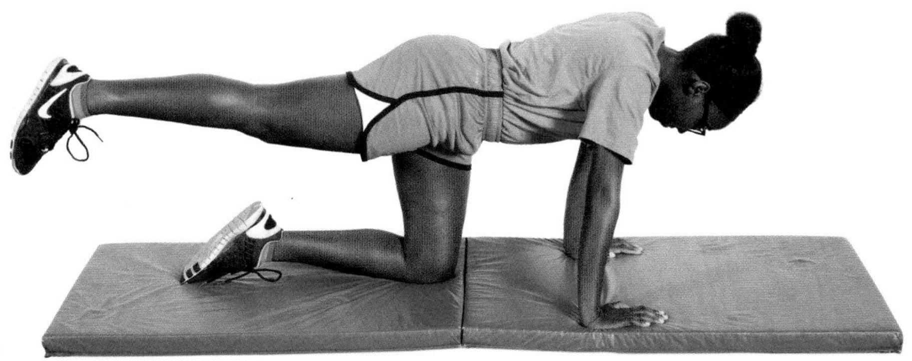

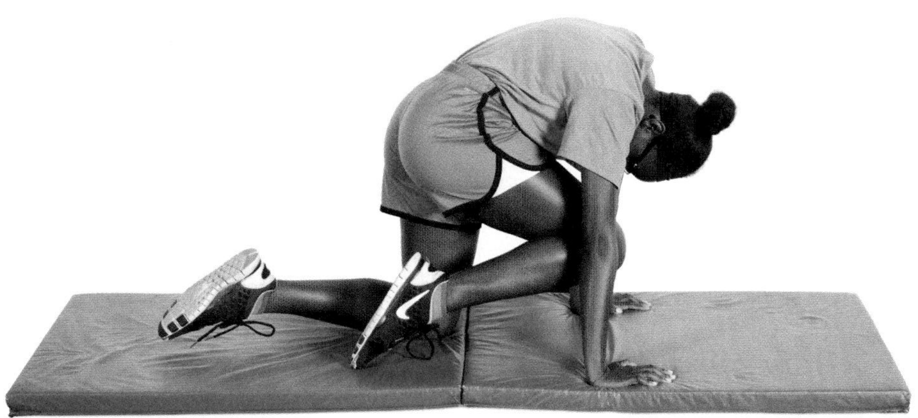

Take action by doing a safe exercise circuit that includes only safe alternatives to risky exercises.

Reviewing Concepts and Vocabulary

As directed by your teacher, answer items 1 through 5 by correctly completing each sentence with a word or phrase.

1. Fitness that improves your ability to learn skills is called ______________.
2. Software programs used on smartphones to help with fitness are called ______________.
3. Information you receive about your performance that helps you improve is called ______________.
4. Invisible body damage caused by heavy repetition of a movement is called a ______________.
5. Soreness that occurs 24 to 48 hours after a workout is called ______________.

For items 6 through 10, as directed by your teacher, match each term in column 1 with the appropriate phrase in column 2.

6. joint	a. connects muscle to bone
7. ligament	b. repetition of a skill to aid improvement
8. tendon	c. holds bones together at a joint
9. skills	d. catching, throwing
10. practice	e. place where bones connect

For items 11 through 15, as directed by your teacher, respond to each statement or question.

11. What are some ways to self-assess your skill-related physical fitness?
12. What is the difference between skill and skill-related physical fitness?
13. Explain how to follow the RICE formula when treating a minor injury.
14. Describe two risky exercises and explain why they are risky.
15. Describe several guidelines for effective skill learning.

Thinking Critically

Write a paragraph to answer the following question.

You're about to begin an exercise program with a group of friends. The leader of your group has selected the exercises. How can you determine whether the exercises are safe?

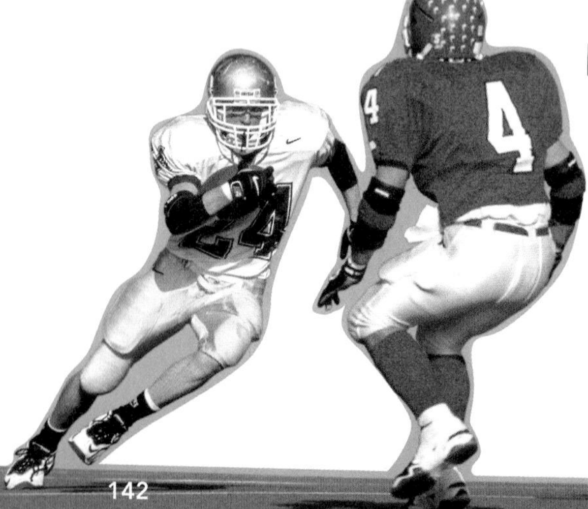

Project

Look through some magazines for articles that feature exercises. Evaluate two exercises to determine whether you think they are safe. Report your findings to your class and discuss the criteria you used to make each evaluation.

UNIT III

Moderate and Vigorous Physical Activity

Healthy People 2020 Goals

- Increase the percentage of teens who meet aerobic activity guidelines.
- Increase overall cardiovascular health.
- Reduce the risk of heart disease and other chronic diseases.
- Increase education to promote health-enhancing behaviors and reduce health risks.
- Reduce the percentage of teens with high blood pressure and other health risks.
- Improve teens' understanding of health promotion and disease prevention.
- Reduce overweight and obesity among teens.
- Reduce sport and recreation injuries.
- Improve community facilities (such as parks) and environment (such as sidewalks).
- Increase physical education in schools.
- Increase the percentage of teens who do in-school and out-of-school activity.
- Improve health literacy and increase the number of high-quality health-related websites.

Self-Assessment Features in This Unit

- Walking Test
- Step Test and One-Mile Run Test
- Assessing Jogging Techniques

Taking Charge Features in This Unit

- Learning to Manage Time
- Self-Confidence
- Activity Participation

Self-Management Features in This Unit

- Skills for Managing Time
- Skills for Building Self-Confidence
- Skills for Choosing Good Activities

Taking Action Features in This Unit

- Your Moderate Physical Activity Plan
- Target Heart Rate Workouts
- Your Vigorous Physical Activity Plan

7

Moderate Physical Activity

In This Chapter

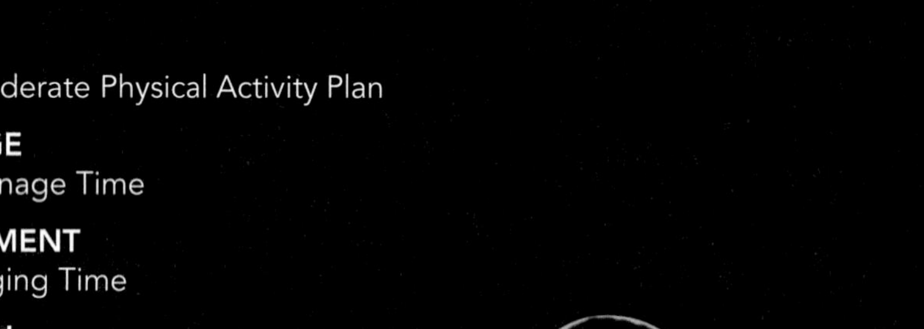

Student Web Resources

www.HOPEtextbook.org/student

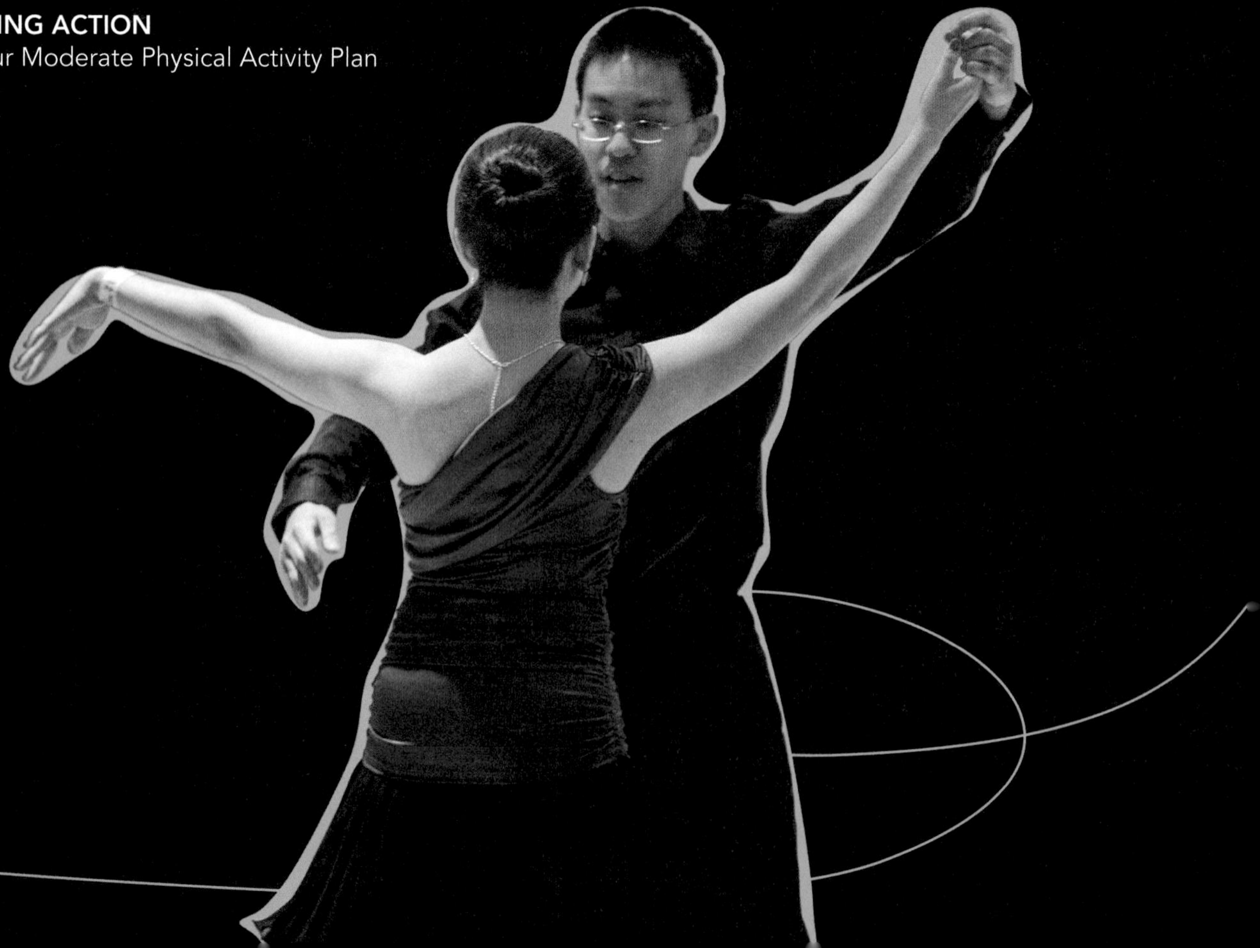

Lesson 7.1

Moderate Physical Activity Facts

Lesson Objectives

After reading this lesson, you should be able to

1. describe the meaning of the term *MET* and why it is important,
2. describe various types of moderate physical activity,
3. describe the FIT formula for moderate physical activity, and
4. describe several methods of self-monitoring moderate activity.

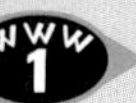

Lesson Vocabulary

accelerometer, lifestyle physical activity, metabolic equivalent (MET), moderate physical activity, pedometer

Have you ever wondered if you can be healthy without feeling pain and getting sweaty during exercise? Do you know the minimum amount of weekly physical activity you need for good health? While it's good to choose activities from each of the five steps of the Physical Activity Pyramid, public health scientists place a high priority on the first step—moderate physical activity. The reason is that moderate physical activities provide many of the health benefits described in this book. These activities are easy to do and can be performed by people of all ages and ability levels. They are sometimes referred to as the foundation of health-enhancing physical activity and thus are appropriately placed at the base of the Physical Activity Pyramid.

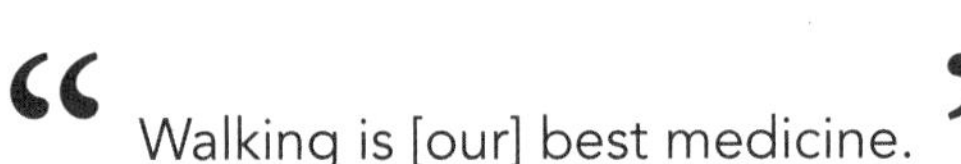

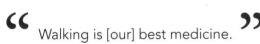

"Walking is [our] best medicine."

—Hippocrates, Greek physician and originator of modern medicine

What Are Moderate Physical Activities?

The term **metabolic equivalent (MET)** comes from the word *metabolism*, which refers to the amount of energy (oxygen) necessary to sustain life. You can use the abbreviated term *MET* to help you determine the intensity of any type of exercise. One MET represents the energy expended while sitting at rest. Physical activities are rated according to their MET value from very light to maximal. The harder the body works, the higher the MET level. For teens, activities requiring less than 2 METs are considered to be very light—for example, eating, reading, and using a computer. Activities that require 2 to 3.9 METs are considered to be light activities; examples include making a bed, washing dishes while standing, preparing food, and walking slowly. These activities are not intense enough to be considered as health-enhancing as those presented in the Physical Activity Pyramid (figure 7.1). However, as you've learned, research has shown that some activity is better than none, and performing light or very light activity does expend energy and thus helps you maintain a healthy weight.

FIT FACT

The amount of energy (the number of METs) used in an activity depends in part on your fitness level. Fit people use fewer METs than unfit people use for the same activity.

Moderate physical activity requires you to use four to seven times as much energy as being sedentary (thus 4 to 7 METs). For most teens, a good example of moderate physical activity is brisk walking. Moderate physical activities are often divided into the following categories: **lifestyle physical activities** done as part of daily life (such as walking to school and doing yardwork or housework), moderate sports (such as bowling and golf), moderate

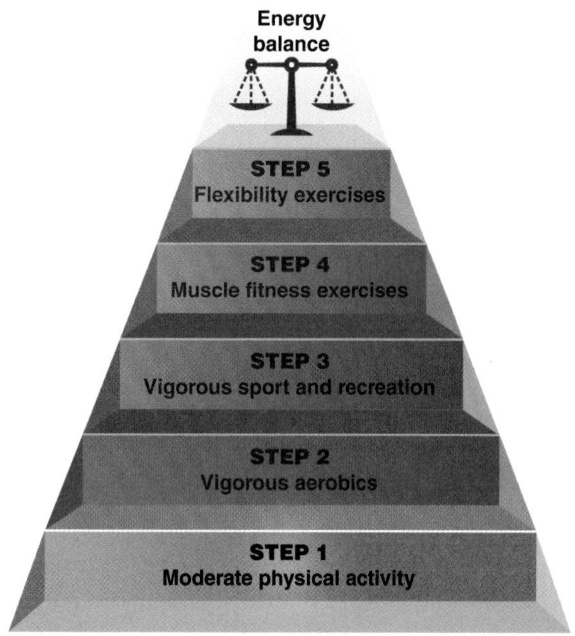

FIGURE 7.1 Step 1 of the Physical Activity Pyramid, moderate physical activity, provides a foundation for all other activities.

recreational activities (such as social dancing and biking slowly), and occupational activities (such as carpentry or landscaping). Table 7.1 presents examples in each of these categories along with the METs for each activity. Some of the activities can require more than 7 METs, and when they are performed at that level they are considered vigorous activities.

Where Do You Get Energy for Moderate Physical Activities?

The human body uses three systems to provide energy for physical activity. For short bursts of very vigorous activity, such as sprinting (for 10 seconds or less), the body uses a high-energy fuel (ATP-PC) stored in the muscles to provide energy. This system is called the ATP-PC system. When the high-energy fuel is used up, a second system takes over. For vigorous activities that last between 11 seconds and about 90 seconds, such as running up and down a soccer field several times or lifting a heavy weight many times, the body uses the glycolytic system to provide energy. A carbohydrate called glucose is stored in the muscles and liver as glycogen, which provides energy to perform vigorous activity in this second system.

TABLE 7.1 Moderate Physical Activities for Teens

Activity type	Description	METs
Lifestyle activities	Walking (brisk)	4.0–5.5
	Yardwork	
	Wood chopping	6.0–7.0
	Push mower (hand)	6.0–7.0
	Push mower (power)	4.0–5.0
	Leaf raking	3.0–4.0
	Shoveling	5.0–7.0
	Housework	
	Floor mopping	3.0–4.0
	Cleaning (heavy)	3.0–4.0
Moderate sports	Bowling	3.0–4.0
	Golf (walking)	3.5–4.5
	Basketball (shooting only)	4.0–5.0
Moderate recreation	Bicycling (slow)	3.0–5.0
	Bicycling (brisk)	5.0–7.0
	Fishing (standing in water)	3.5–4.5
	Social dance	3.0–6.0
Occupational activities	Bricklaying	3.5–4.5
	Carpentry	3.5–5.5
	Heavy assembly work	5.0–6.0

METs for people with low fitness will be higher than those shown in the table; likewise, they will be lower for people with high fitness.

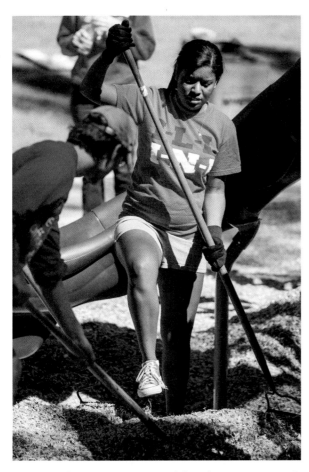

Many moderate activities are lifestyle activities, such as yardwork and housework.

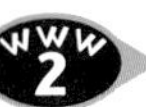

For sustained activity of moderate intensity, such as brisk walking, the body uses the oxidative system (also called the aerobic system) to provide energy. This system allows you to perform activity for many minutes or even hours. Like the glycolytic system, this system uses glucose to provide energy. But since adequate oxygen is available to convert carbohydrate and fat in the body into glucose during moderate activity, the body does not have to rely primarily on glycogen (glucose) stored in the muscles and liver. More information about energy systems is available on the student section of the Health Opportunities Through Physical Education website.

Why Should I Do Moderate Physical Activities?

Experts used to think that in order to gain health benefits you had to do vigorous physical activity (using more than 7 METs). We now know that many health benefits can be achieved by doing moderate physical activity. Here's a summary of the benefits of moderate physical activity.

- Reduced risk of hypokinetic disease, such as heart disease, cancer, diabetes, and other chronic diseases
- Improved bone health
- Fitness benefits for people in the low and moderate fitness zones (whereas vigorous activity is required for fitness improvement in people in the good fitness and high performance zones)
- Healthy weight maintenance as a result of adequate energy expenditure
- Improved wellness and functional fitness, including feeling good, enjoying free time, and doing the things you want to do without undue fatigue
- Improved academic performance (such as improved mental performance resulting from physical activity done before taking a test)

How Much Moderate Physical Activity Is Enough?

National physical activity guidelines in the United States recommend 60 minutes of daily activity for teens. Some of the recommended activity should be vigorous activity performed on at least three days a week, and some should be activity that promotes muscle fitness and bone building performed on at least two days a week. Moderate activity is recommended every day, and for most teens it will be the easiest way to meet the 60-minute recommendation. For adults, the recommendation is 150 minutes of moderate activity per week, which translates to 30 minutes per day on five days a week. For this reason, many experts recommend that teens get at least 30 minutes of moderate activity each day so that they develop the habit of meeting the adult activity guideline.

You need to be familiar with the FIT formulas for moderate physical activity for both teens and adults (see table 7.2). The teen guidelines apply, of course, while you're in school, and the adult guidelines will apply for the rest of your life after school.

 SCIENCE IN ACTION: Sedentary Living

Exercise physiologists have recently learned that extended periods of inactivity can be harmful to your health—the more time people spend sitting, the higher their rate of chronic disease. For this reason, scientists now refer to excessive sedentary living as the "sitting disease." One major reason for sitting among teens today is screen time (whether it be with a television, computer, smartphone, or other device). In fact, teens spend more time sitting now than in the past, and from age 12 to age 16 the amount of sitting and inactivity increases by more than 100 percent.

The danger posed by the sitting disease is the reason that the words "Avoid inactivity" are included under the first step of the Physical Activity Pyramid. Physical activity guidelines published by the Society of Health and Physical Educators (SHAPE America) indicate that youth should not go more than two hours without an activity break. Among adults, many companies now offer activity breaks to reduce sitting time, and some companies provide treadmills beside computers to encourage employees to move while working.

Student Activity

Keep track of the daily time you spend in front of a screen. Do you need to reduce your screen time? If so, how could this be done?

For teens, the goal is to accumulate at least 60 minutes each day, but more is better. Moderate activities can be combined with other activities from the pyramid to meet the goal. Experts now agree that it is best to get your 60 minutes in bouts or activity sessions lasting at least 10 minutes each. In other words, you could do six 10-minute bouts, three 20-minute bouts, two 30-minute bouts, or other combinations that total 60 minutes a day. Accumulating 60 minutes in bouts shorter than 10 minutes each is better than doing nothing, but it does not give you optimal benefits.

TABLE 7.2 FIT Formulas for Health and Wellness Benefits From Moderate Physical Activity

FIT formula	Threshold of training	Target zone
	Teens	
Frequency	Most days of the week	Daily
Intensity	4 METs Moderate activity equal in intensity to brisk walking	4–7 METs At least as intense as brisk walking but less intense than normal jogging
Time	60 min of total activity, some of which should be moderate activity in bouts of ≥10 min*	60 min to several hr of total activity, some of which should be in bouts of ≥10 min*
	Adults	
Frequency	Most days of the week	Daily or most days of the week
Intensity	4 METs** Moderate activity equal in intensity to brisk walking	4–7 METs At least as intense as brisk walking but less intense than normal jogging
Time	30 min in bouts of ≥10 min***	30–60 min in bouts of ≥10 min***

*Using 30 of the 60 minutes on moderate activity would meet the teen and adult guidelines.

**Less fit adults may use activities of 3 to 4 METs.

***At least 150 minutes per week, spread over multiple days.

For adults, the recommendation is for 150 minutes per week because this amount provides many health benefits with a minimum of effort. As with teens, moderate exercise is best done on several days a week (see table 7.2) and in bouts of at least 10 minutes each. Doing more than 30 minutes at a time gives additional benefits and is recommended for maintaining a healthy weight and for achieving good fitness, health, and wellness. Adults can substitute 75 minutes per week of vigorous exercise for the 150 minutes of moderate activity; they can also meet the guidelines by combining moderate and vigorous activity.

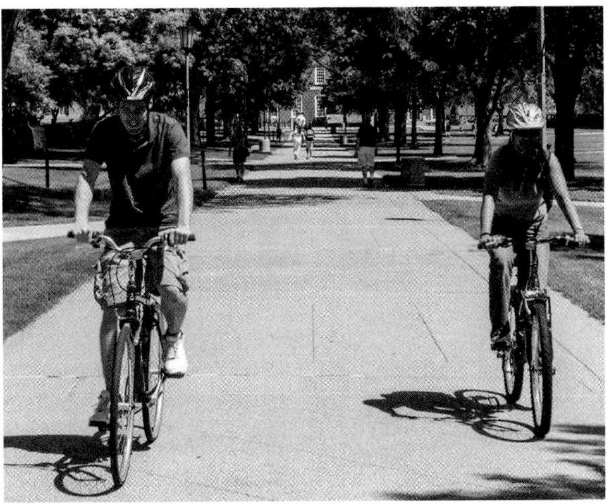

Recreational biking is an example of a moderate physical activity. It's one of many activities you can choose to accumulate your 60 minutes of daily physical activity.

Counting Steps and Movement

Another way to determine how much moderate physical activity you perform is to count the steps you take each day. You can do so by using a pedometer (see the Fitness Technology feature), which automatically tracks your step count; the disadvantage is that a pedometer counts *all* steps that you take, regardless of whether they come in very light, light, or even vigorous activity. Still, wearing a pedometer can help you see how active you really are; you may have the opportunity to wear one in school. The American College of Sports Medicine states that moderate physical activity requires a step rate of 100 steps per minute.

For adults, some experts believe that taking 10,000 steps each day is necessary to be in the target zone for moderate physical activity. Other experts are concerned about this advice because you can reach 10,000 steps without doing any sustained activity (bouts of 10 minutes or more). On the other hand, some people can do 60 minutes of moderate activity each day and still not reach a 10,000-step count. Rather than setting an absolute daily step count, most experts recommend monitoring your activity for a full week and then determining your average daily step count. People who want to increase their activity level can then establish a realistic step goal that is 500 to 1,000 steps per day higher than their average step count. Once they reach this goal, they can, if desired, gradually increase their step count to higher levels.

Studies show that children average 12,500 steps a day (13,000 for boys and 12,000 for girls), whereas teens average 10,000 steps a day (11,000 for boys and 9,000 for girls). To meet the national physical activity guidelines of 60 minutes a day, most teens would require 12,000 steps. However, if you're just beginning, remember the principle of progression. Instead of starting with a high goal such as 12,000 steps per day, work gradually toward a realistic step goal.

FIT FACT

On average, Americans of all ages take about 5,000 steps per day. This is considerably less than the averages in some other countries—for example, 9,000 or more in Australia and Switzerland and 7,000 or more in Japan—where obesity rates are much lower.

The President's Council on Fitness, Sports, and Nutrition offers the Presidential Active Lifestyle Award for people who do regular physical activity. Many types of physical activity can be used to earn the award, including moderate physical activity in which steps are counted with a pedometer.

You can also monitor moderate physical activity by means of other devices, such as an accelerometer (see the Fitness Technology feature) and a heart rate monitor. An accelerometer both counts your steps and gives you a better idea of your exercise intensity than a pedometer can. You can determine the distance you've walked by determining the length of your step (your stride length), then multiplying it by the number of steps you take.

FITNESS TECHNOLOGY: Pedometers and Accelerometers

A **pedometer** is a small, battery-powered device that can be worn on your belt. It counts each step you take and displays the running count on a meter. You simply open the face of the pedometer or push a button to see how many steps you've taken. Some pedometers also contain a small computer that allows you to enter the length of your step (your stride length) and your body weight so that the computer can estimate the distance you walk and the number of calories you expend. More expensive pedometers can also track the total time you spend in activity during the day and the number of bouts of activity that you perform lasting 10 minutes or longer. Less expensive pedometers must be reset at the end of the day, but some more expensive ones can store steps for several days.

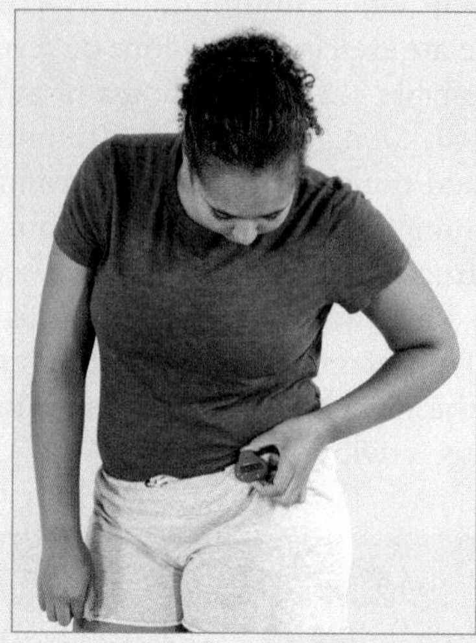

A pedometer counts steps and is a good way to self-monitor moderate activity.

Accelerometers are similar to pedometers but measure physical activity in more detail. Specifically, accelerometers can record the *intensity* of your movements (for more about intensity, see the discussion of METs and recall the I in the FITT formula), as well as the amount of *time* (the first T in the FITT formula) you spend at different intensities. Like a pedometer, an accelerometer is worn on your belt and contains a small computer and a device (the accelerometer itself) that measures the intensity of your movements. Most accelerometers can count your steps taken per day and estimate the calories you expend in activity.

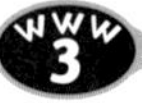

Using Technology

Estimate the number of steps you take on a typical weekday and a typical weekend day. Then wear a pedometer to see how many steps you actually take (weekday and weekend day). See if you're as active as you think you are!

Counting Physical Activity Calories

We know that moderate activity should be done according to the FIT formula summarized in table 7.2. Another way to determine whether you perform enough moderate activity is to count the calories you expend in activity. For example, a teen who weighs 150 pounds (68 kilograms) would expend 300 to 400 calories during 60 minutes of moderate activity, such as brisk walking. Therefore, this number of calories expended per day would be a good goal for moderate activity.

Lesson Review

1. What does the term *MET* mean, and how is it useful?
2. What are some types of moderate physical activity, and what benefits do they provide?
3. What is the FIT formula (in terms of the threshold of training and target zone) for gaining health and wellness benefits from moderate physical activity?
4. What are some methods of self-monitoring moderate activity?

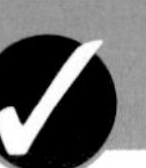

SELF-ASSESSMENT: Walking Test

Many of the self-assessments you perform in this course require very intense physical activity. If you're a very active person and are quite fit, the mile run or PACER may be the best way to estimate your cardiorespiratory endurance, but the walking test is also a good one. The test is especially good for people who are beginners, who haven't done a lot of recent activity, or who are regular walkers but do not regularly get more vigorous activity. The walk test is also good for older people and for those who cannot do running tests due to joint or muscle problems. As directed by your teacher, record your scores and fitness ratings for the walking test. You can then use the information in preparing your personal physical activity plan. If you're working with a partner, remember that self-assessment information is personal and considered confidential. It shouldn't be shared with others without the permission of the person being tested.

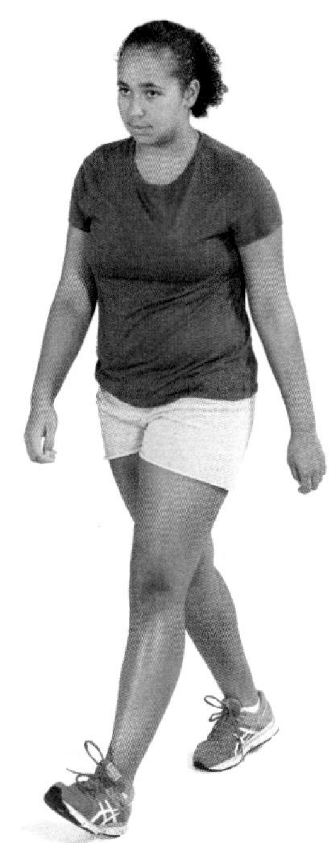

The walking test is a good assessment for beginners or people who don't do a lot of vigorous activity.

1. Walk a mile at a fast pace (as fast as you can go while keeping approximately the same pace for the entire walk).
2. Immediately after the walk, count your heartbeats for 15 seconds. Multiply the result by four to calculate your one-minute heart rate.
3. Use the appropriate chart to determine your walking rating. Locate your heart rate in the left column of the chart and your walking time along the bottom row. Find the point where the row and column intersect to determine your rating.

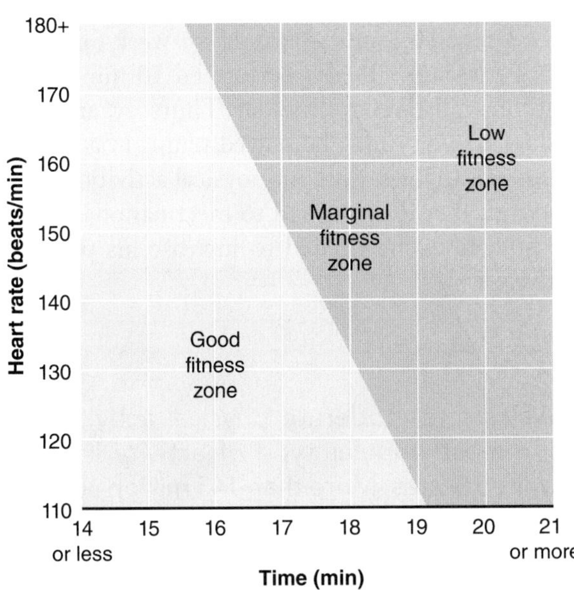

Rating chart for the walking test (for females).

Adapted from the *One Mile Walk Test* with permission of author James M. Rippe, M.D.

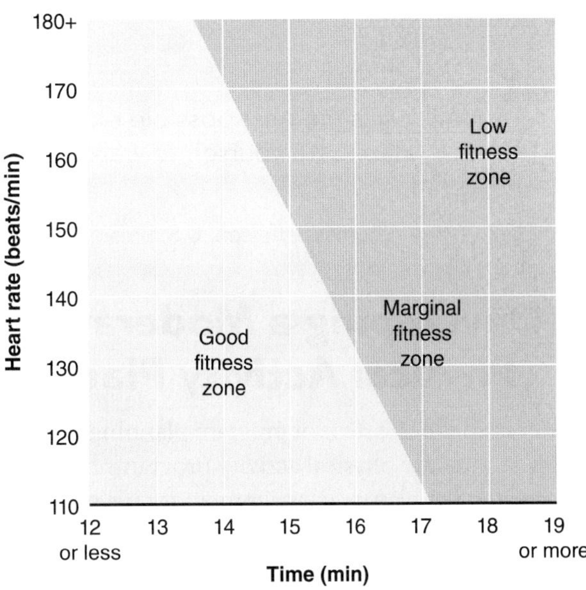

Rating chart for the walking test (for males).

Adapted from the *One Mile Walk Test* with permission of author James M. Rippe, M.D.

Lesson 7.2

Preparing a Moderate Physical Activity Plan

Lesson Objectives

After reading this lesson, you should be able to

1. prepare a moderate physical activity plan using the five planning steps, and
2. carry out your moderate activity plan for several days.

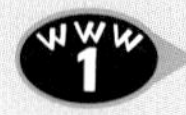

Lesson Vocabulary

calisthenics, habituate

Have you ever created your own fitness plan? Have you ever tracked your daily activities? In this lesson, you'll use the five steps of program planning to develop a moderate physical activity plan for yourself. You'll then carry out that plan. Implementing a good plan will help you meet national physical activity guidelines—both now and later in your life. The most popular physical activities among adults are moderate ones, including walking, biking, yardwork, and home **calisthenics**. If you establish the habit of doing moderate physical activity early in your life, you're more likely to be active as you grow older. And people who **habituate** to activity get multiple health benefits over the course of a lifetime.

> "Walking is the best possible exercise. Habituate yourself to walk very fast."
>
> —Thomas Jefferson, U.S. president

Developing a Moderate Physical Activity Plan

Javier used the five steps of program planning to prepare a moderate physical activity program. Because he created the plan as an assignment for his physical education class, it covered only two weeks. Later, he would get the opportunity to prepare a longer plan. Notice that in doing his planning, Javier used steps similar to those of the scientific method. You can prepare a similar plan.

Step 1: Determine Your Personal Needs

To get started, Javier collected some basic information. First, he answered questions about his moderate physical activity levels in the past week. He also wrote down his fitness test results that related to moderate physical activity. He recorded his results in figure 7.2.

Javier had a good fitness rating for both the PACER and the walking test (see figure 7.2). He also met the national activity guideline of 60 minutes a day on three days of the previous week. His moderate activity included mostly walking to and from school (20 minutes each weekday) and riding his bike for 10 minutes two days a week (Tuesday and Thursday). He also performed 10 minutes of vigorous calisthenics (Tuesday, Thursday, and Saturday). On Saturday he played tennis in addition to his calisthenics. Still, his physical activity profile told him that if he wanted to meet national activity guidelines, he needed to increase his physical activity.

FIT FACT

Walking, a moderate physical activity, is the most popular type of activity in the United States. More than 145 million adults report walking at least 10 minutes a day, most commonly for transportation, for fun, for exercise, or for walking the dog. People with a dog walk more frequently than people who don't have a dog.

Physical fitness profile			
Fitness self-assessments	**Score**	**Rating**	
Walking test	Time: 15:00 Heart rate: 140	Good fitness	
PACER	41 laps	Good fitness	
Physical activity profile			
Day	**Moderate activity (min)**	**All activity (min)**	**Met guideline**
Mon.	30	30	
Tues.	30	60	✔
Wed.	30	30	
Thurs.	30	60	✔
Fri.	30	60	✔
Sat.	30	30	
Sun.	0	0	

FIGURE 7.2 Javier's physical activity and fitness profiles.

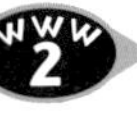

Step 2: Consider Your Program Options

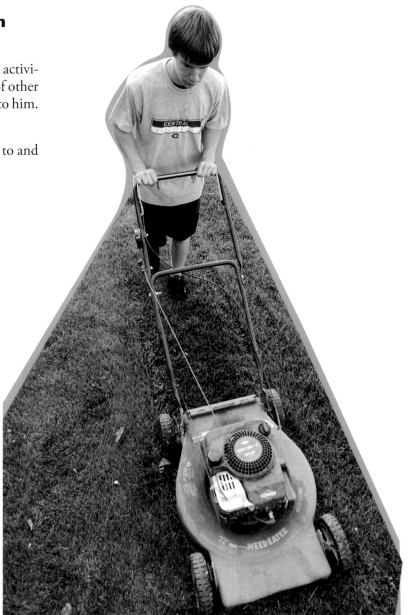

Javier looked at the list of moderate physical activities presented in table 7.1 and created a list of other moderate activities that were easily available to him.

Lifestyle Activities

- More walking in addition to walking to and from school
- Yardwork at home

Moderate Sports

- Bowling
- Shooting baskets

Moderate Recreation

- Fishing
- More bike riding

Occupational or School Activity

- Physical education class activities

Step 3: Set Goals

Since two weeks was too short a time for setting long-term goals, Javier developed only short-term goals for his moderate physical activity plan; as a result, all of his goals were physical activity goals. He did this because he knew that activity goals (process goals) work best as short-term goals. He also knew that if he met his activity goals he would be making progress toward his fitness (product goals). Later, when he prepares a longer plan, he will develop long-term goals, including physical fitness goals. For these first two weeks, Javier decided to focus on moderate activity through the following goals.

1. Continue to perform the same activities that he has regularly been doing.
2. Walk to school and back three days a week (30 minutes each day).
3. Perform 30 minutes of moderate activity on three days each week in physical education class.
4. Rake the yard for 30 minutes on one day every two weeks.
5. Shoot baskets for 30 minutes two days a week.
6. Bike with friends for 30 minutes on two days a week.
7. Mow the neighbor's yard once every two weeks (60 minutes).
8. Go fishing one day a week (includes walking for 60 minutes).
9. Walk with family for 15 minutes on two days a week.

Javier remembered to use SMART goals. His goals listed *specific* activities and amounts of time because he wanted to be able to *measure* his progress. He also tried to make his goals challenging but *attainable* and *realistic*. Finally, he wanted his goals to be *timely*—just right for his life at this time and able to be achieved in the time allotted.

Step 4: Structure Your Program and Write It Down

Javier's plan included at least the recommended 60 minutes of moderate physical activity on each day during the two-week period. On several days, he planned to do more than 60 minutes. As shown in figure 7.3, he wrote down the activities and the times when he planned to perform them.

Week 1				Week 2			
Day	**Activity**	**Time**	**✔**	**Day**	**Activity**	**Time**	**✔**
Mon.	Walk to school* Walk home* Shoot baskets	7:45–7:55 a.m. 3:30–3:40 p.m. 3:45–4:15 p.m.		Mon	Walk to school* Walk home* Shoot baskets	7:45–7:55 a.m. 3:30–3:40 p.m. 3:45–4:15 p.m.	
Tues.	Walk to school* PE class activity* Walk home*	7:45–7:55 a.m. 10:00–10:30 a.m. 3:30–3:40 p.m.		Tues.	Walk to school* PE class activity* Walk home*	7:45–7:55 a.m. 10:00–10:30 a.m. 3:30–3:40 p.m.	
Wed.	Walk to school* Walk home* Ride bike	7:45–7:55 a.m. 3:30–3:45 p.m. 3:45–4:00 p.m.		Wed.	Walk to school* Walk home* Ride bike	7:45–7:55 a.m. 3:30–3:45 p.m. 3:45–4:00 p.m.	
Thurs.	Walk to school* PE class activity* Walk home*	7:45–7:55 a.m. 10:00–10:30 a.m. 3:30–3:40 p.m.		Thurs.	Walk to school PE class activity* Walk home*	7:45–7:55 a.m. 10:00–10:30 a.m. 3:30–3:40 p.m.	
Fri.	Walk to school* PE class activity* Walk home*	7:45–7:55 a.m. 10:00–10:30 a.m. 3:30–3:45 p.m.		Fri.	Walk to school PE class activity* Walk home*	7:45–7:55 a.m. 10:00–10:30 a.m. 3:30–3:40 p.m.	
Sat.	Mow the grass* Ride bike	9:00–9:30 a.m. 1:00–1:30 p.m.		Sat.	Rake the yard* Ride bike	9:30–10:30 a.m. 1:00–1:30 p.m.	
Sun.	Bowling Family walk	2:30–3:30 p.m. 6:30–6:45 p.m.		Sun.	Bowling Family walk	2:30–3:30 p.m. 6:30–6:45 p.m.	

*Activities that Javier was already doing.

FIGURE 7.3 Javier's two-week written program plan.

FIT FACT

Canadian laws provide tax incentives for increasing regular physical activity. Families that enroll children and teens in youth activity programs get an income tax break, and people who buy bicycles get a reduction in sales tax.

Step 5: Keep a Log and Evaluate Your Program

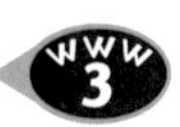

Over the next two weeks, Javier will self-monitor his activities and place a checkmark beside each activity he performs. At the end of two-week period, he'll evaluate his performance to see whether he met his goals. He can then use that evaluation to help him make another activity plan.

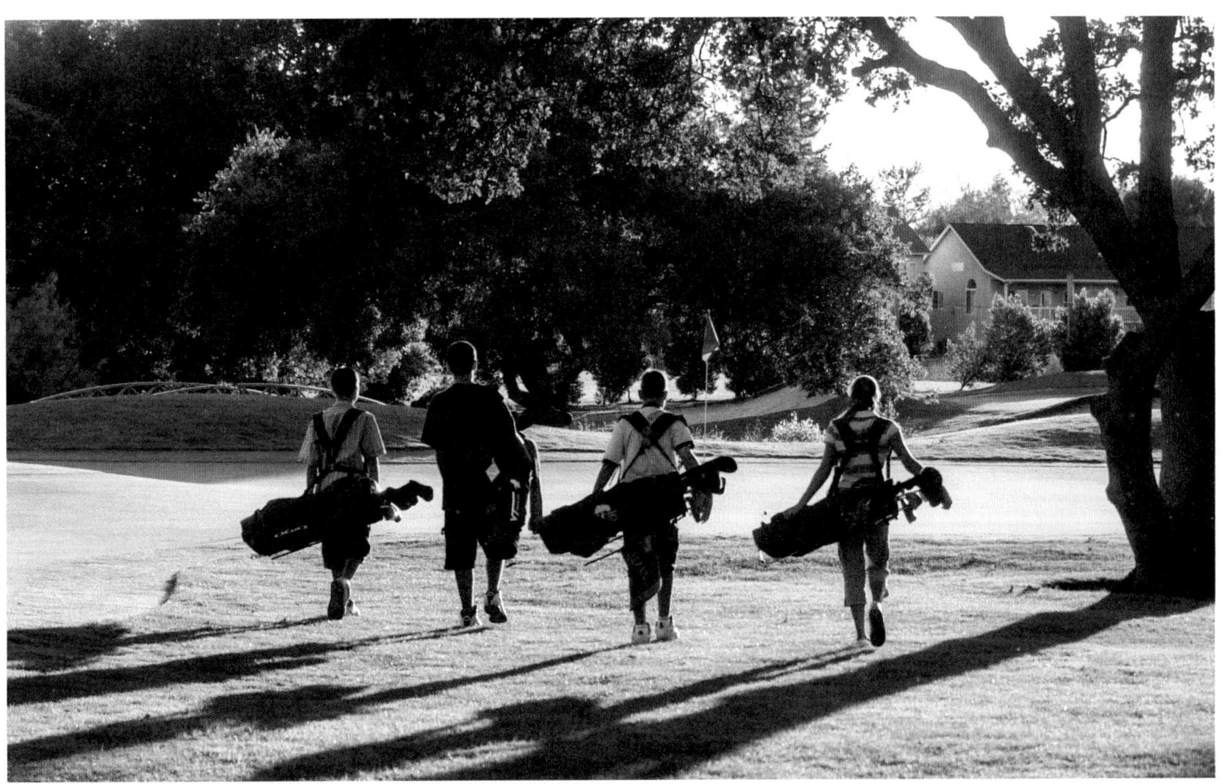

Golfing is a good form of moderate physical activity.

Lesson Review

1. How do you use the five steps in planning to prepare a personal moderate physical activity plan?
2. How can you best implement your personal plan over a span of several days?

TAKING CHARGE: Learning to Manage Time

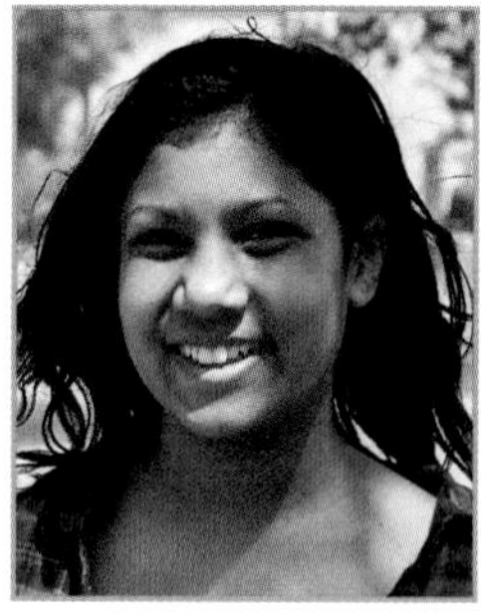

Why can some people always find time for an added activity while others barely have time to do their regularly scheduled activities? For a lot of people, the answer is time management. Good time managers know how to make the best use of their time. They efficiently control their daily schedule in order to complete their activities without wasting time. These people are more likely to find time for regular physical activity.

Here's an example of poor time management. Jennifer lives near some good cross-country ski trails. In the winter, her friends spend a few hours skiing every Monday and Wednesday after school; they also go skiing on weekends. Although they always ask her to join their fun, Jennifer usually refuses. Her common excuse is, "I just don't have the time. I really love skiing, but with three honors classes, homework, and my job at the mall, I barely have time to eat, let alone ski. I wish I could go with you, but I can't. It's impossible! I'll ski next year when my schedule is easier. Then I'll have more spare time."

Jennifer's friends are used to her excuses. In fact, she used many of the same ones last year. Her friends have the same classes and work hours that Jennifer has, but they complete their homework assignments and handle their jobs with time to spare. They do not understand why Jennifer can't manage to find the time to go skiing with them.

For Discussion

What can Jennifer do to manage her time better so that she can do things with her friends? What can her friends do to help? What suggestions can you make to help anyone who would like to manage time better? Consider the time management strategies presented in this chapter's Self-Management feature when answering the discussion questions.

SELF-MANAGEMENT: Skills for Managing Time

How many times do you hear yourself and others say, "I don't have the time"? It seems to be a common complaint. If you're one of those who seems to have too little time, how can you remedy the problem? Many experts believe that learning to manage time is a good solution. In this lesson, you'll learn how to manage your time so that you can be more active.

In 1900, the average person worked more than 60 hours a week. Now the average workweek is less than 40 hours. Similarly, in 1900, many young people were not enrolled in school and were already working long hours in factories and on farms. Now most teens are in school, and those who work limit their work hours.

Fewer working hours has made free time much more abundant now than it was years ago. But work and school aren't the only things that take time. Most of us make other time commitments when we aren't working or going to school. For example, you might have to care for a brother or sister, or you might have committed to a school or community activity such as a club, band, chorus, or sport team. And of course you also spend time on necessary activities such as eating, sleeping, dressing, and getting to and from school or work. The time you spend in all of these activities is called committed time.

Free time, on the other hand, is the time left over after accounting for your school and work time and your other committed time. Some people make so many commitments that they have very little free time. Often, people who say they don't have time for physical activity have not planned their time carefully. Active people manage their time effectively so that they can commit regularly to being active. If you're in the group of people who often say, "I don't have time," the following guidelines can help you.

- **Keep track of your time.** The best way to start managing your time more efficiently is to see what you're doing with it now. You can do this by keeping records (self-monitoring your use of time). Write down what you do during the course of each day. Record when you sleep, when you eat, when you're in school, when you're at work, and when you do all of the other things you do. You might use three categories: school and work, other committed time, and free time. Most people who keep records of their time use are surprised by the results. For example, some people who say they don't have time to exercise spend several hours a day watching television. Others find that they spend a lot of time doing nothing.
- **Analyze your use of time.** Once you've tracked your time for several days, review your records to see how many hours you spend in each of the three categories. You can also identify exactly how you spend your committed time and your free time. Doing so will help you decide whether you're using your time in the way you really want to use it.
- **Decide purposefully what to do with your time.** After you determine how much time you spend doing various activities, decide whether you're managing your time efficiently. Efficient time management enables you to do the things you think are most important. To decide what's most important to you, answer the following questions.
    - What activities did you spend more time on than you wanted to?
    - How much less time could you spend on each?
    - Are the activities you would like to change under your control?
    - What activities do you want to spend more time on?
    - How much more time would you like to spend on these activities?
- **Schedule your time.** After you decide how you would like to spend your time, create a schedule to ensure that you make time for the things you identified as most important. If you feel that regular physical activity is important, you will commit time to doing it. Plan a schedule for one day, making sure you have time to do the most important things.

Sometimes good scheduling allows you to do two things at once. For example, since you have to get to school somehow, what if you did so by walking or riding a bicycle? Thus you would be effectively committing that time to two different purposes. Similarly, if you join a sport team or activity club, the time you commit to that group is also committed to doing physical activity.

TAKING ACTION: Your Moderate Physical Activity Plan

Prepare a two-week moderate physical activity plan using the five steps described in this chapter. Like Javier, consider moderate activities from each activity category: lifestyle activity, moderate sports, moderate recreation, and occupational or school activity. The goal is to accumulate at least 60 minutes of activity each day, including a considerable portion that involves moderate activity. Prepare a written plan and carry out it over a two-week period. Your teacher may give you time in class to do some of the activities in your plan. Consider the following suggestions for **taking action** and building moderate activity into your plan.

- **Lifestyle activity.** Walk or bike to school. If driving, park away from your destination and walk the rest of the way. When you have a choice, take the stairs. Walk while talking on the phone. Work in the yard.
- **Moderate sports.** Consider bowling or shooting baskets with friends.
- **Moderate recreation.** Walk with friends at lunch or go for a walk in the park.
- **Occupational or school activity.** Do yardwork for pay, take an optional physical education class, participate in intramural activities, or start a walking club.

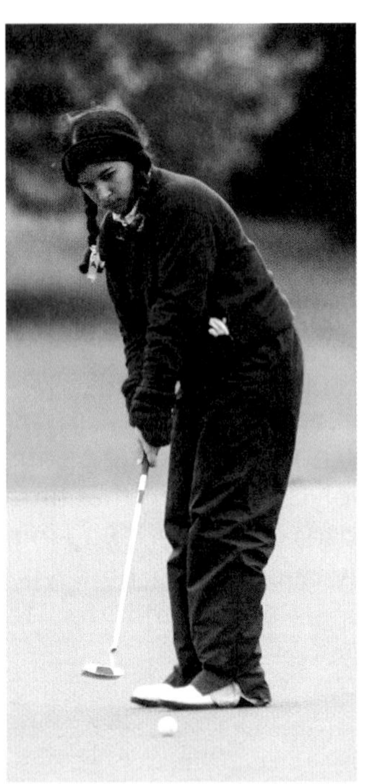

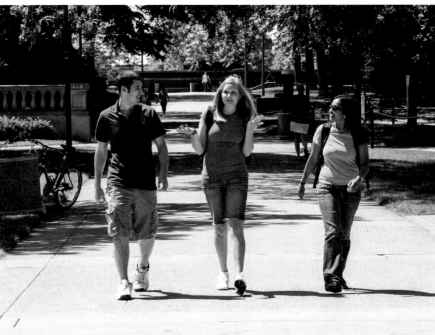

Lifestyle activities can be part of your plan for taking action.

CHAPTER REVIEW

Reviewing Concepts and Vocabulary

As directed by your teacher, answer items 1 through 5 by correctly completing each sentence with a word or phrase.

1. Activity that is equivalent to brisk walking in intensity is considered to be ______________ physical activity.
2. An activity done as part of daily life is called a/an ______________ activity.
3. A device worn on your belt that counts steps is called a/an ______________.
4. Intensity of activity can be expressed in units called ______________.
5. Considering your program options is step ______________ of the planning process.

For items 6 through 10, as directed by your teacher, match each term in column 1 with the appropriate word or phrase in column 2.

6. excessive inactivity	a. mopping
7. yardwork	b. carpentry
8. recreational activity	c. sitting disease
9. occupational work	d. bowling
10. housework	e. mowing

For items 11 through 15, as directed by your teacher, respond to each statement or question.

11. What does *sedentary* mean, and what can be done to reduce sedentary living among teens?
12. Describe several devices that can be used to self-monitor physical activity.
13. How much moderate physical activity is enough?
14. List and describe the five steps for planning a moderate physical activity program.
15. Describe several guidelines for managing time effectively.

Thinking Critically

Write a paragraph to answer the following question.

Teens are often more vigorously active than adults. For this reason, some people say that teens should begin to do more moderate activity to increase their chance of staying active later in life. Do you think you will become more or less active as you grow older? What types of activity do you think you'll do as you grow older?

Project

National polling groups regularly conduct surveys to learn people's opinions about various issues, including health and fitness. Assume that you work for a polling company. Develop a list of questions about moderate activity and ask at least six people to answer them. Try to interview people from different age groups. Analyze your results and prepare a brief news article reporting the results.

8

Cardiorespiratory Endurance

In This Chapter

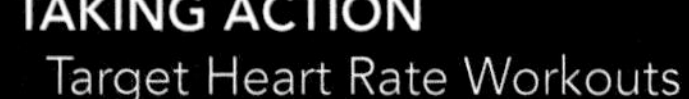

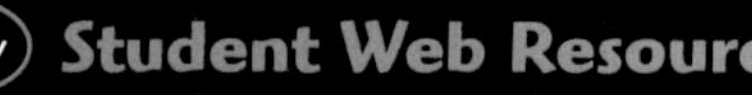

Student Web Resources

www.HOPEtextbook.org/student

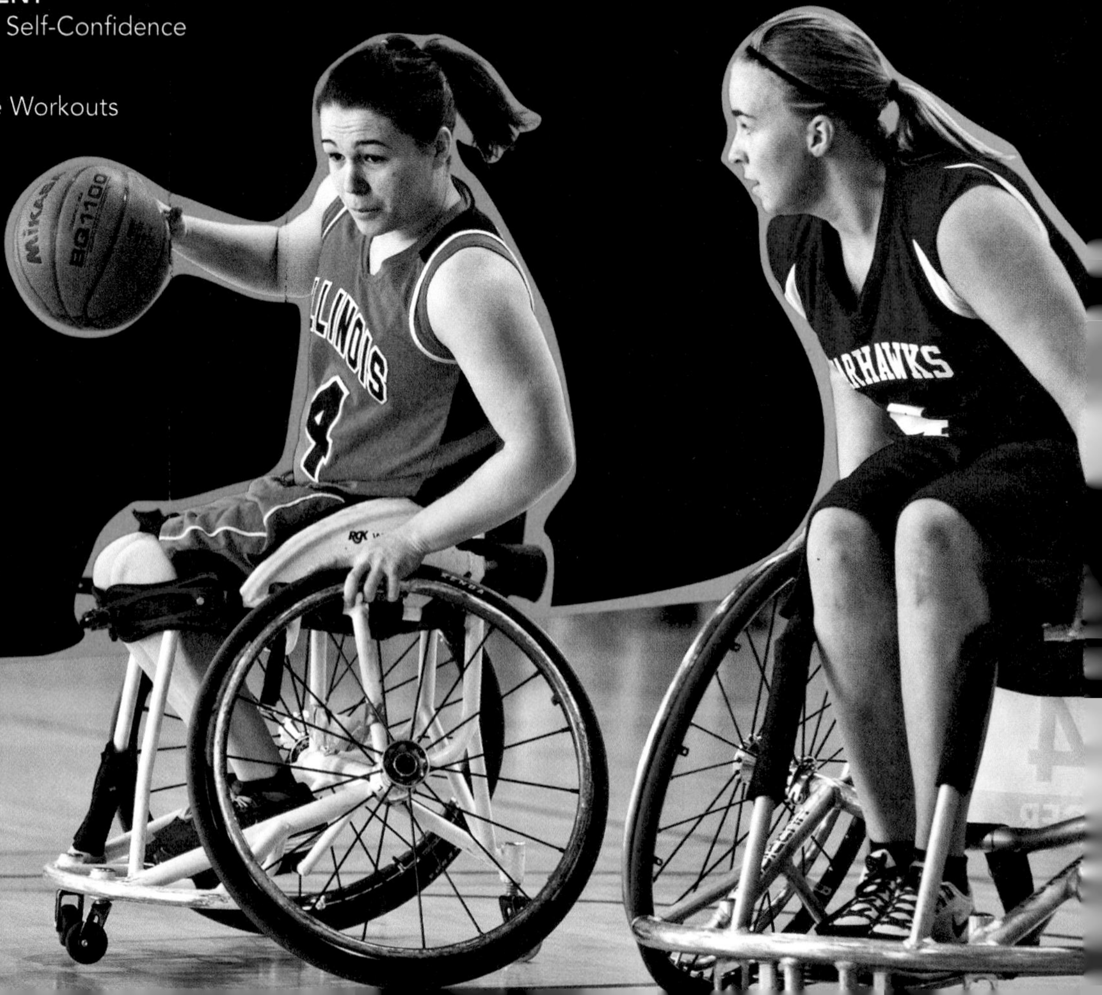

Lesson 8.1

Cardiorespiratory Endurance Facts

Lesson Objectives

After reading this lesson, you should be able to

1. describe the health and wellness benefits of cardiorespiratory endurance;
2. explain how physical activity benefits the cardiovascular, respiratory, and muscle systems;
3. describe some methods for assessing your cardiorespiratory endurance; and
4. determine how much cardiorespiratory endurance is enough.

WWW 1

Lesson Vocabulary

aerobic capacity, artery, cardiorespiratory endurance, cardiovascular system, cholesterol, fibrin, graded exercise test, high-density lipoprotein (HDL), lipoprotein, low-density lipoprotein (LDL), maximal oxygen uptake, respiratory system, vein

Do you have good cardiorespiratory endurance? Do you do enough regular vigorous physical activity to build good cardiorespiratory endurance? Of the 11 parts of fitness, cardiorespiratory endurance is the most important because it gives you many health and wellness benefits, including a chance for a longer life. In addition, the activity that you do to improve your cardiorespiratory endurance helps you look your best. As shown in figure 8.1, cardiorespiratory endurance requires fitness of your heart, lungs, blood, blood vessels, and muscles. In this lesson, you'll learn how proper physical activity improves your cardiorespiratory endurance. You'll also learn how to assess your cardiorespiratory endurance.

Cardiorespiratory endurance is the ability to exercise your entire body for a long time without stopping. It requires a strong heart, healthy lungs, and clear blood vessels to supply your large muscles with oxygen. Examples of activities that require good cardiorespiratory endurance are distance running, swimming, and cross-country skiing. Cardiorespiratory endurance is sometimes referred to by other names, including cardiovascular fitness, cardiovascular endurance, and cardiorespiratory fitness. The term *aerobic capacity* is also used to describe good cardiorespiratory function, but it is not exactly the same as cardiorespiratory endurance (see this chapter's Science in Action feature).

This book uses the term *cardiorespiratory endurance*. The first word in the term is *cardiorespiratory* because two vital systems are involved. Your **cardiovascular system** is made up of your heart, blood vessels, and blood. Your **respiratory system** is made up of your lungs and the air passages that

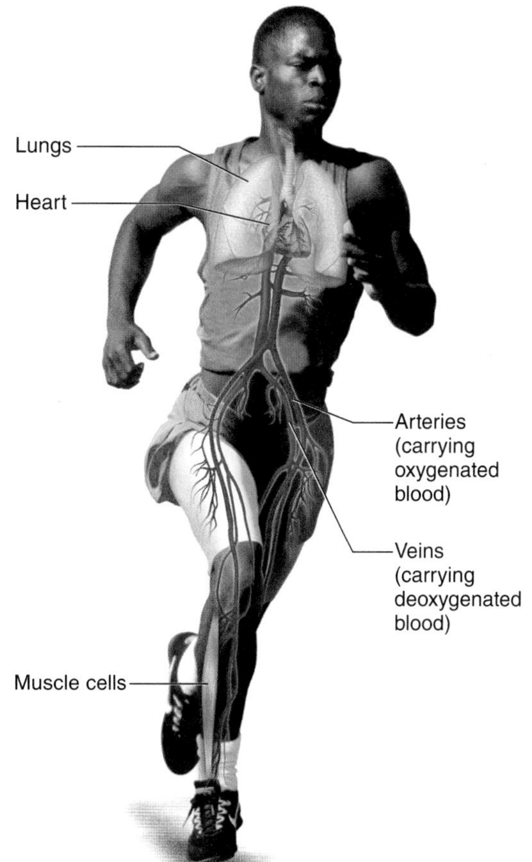

FIGURE 8.1 Cardiorespiratory endurance requires fitness of many parts of the body, including heart, lungs, muscles, and blood vessels.

bring air, including oxygen, to your lungs from outside of your body. In your lungs, oxygen enters your blood, and carbon dioxide is eliminated. Your cardiovascular and respiratory systems work together to bring your muscle cells and other body cells the materials they need and to rid the cells of waste. Together, the two systems help you function both effectively (with the most benefits possible) and efficiently (with the least effort).

The second word in the term *cardiorespiratory endurance* refers to the ability to sustain effort. Together, then, these two words—*cardiorespiratory* and *endurance*—refer to the ability to sustain effort, which hinges on fitness of the cardiovascular (cardio) and respiratory systems.

Benefits of Physical Activity and Cardiorespiratory Endurance

Doing regular physical activity can help you look better by controlling your weight, building your muscles, and helping you develop good posture. Regular physical activity also produces changes in your body's organs, such as making your heart muscle stronger and your blood vessels healthier. These changes improve your cardiorespiratory endurance and wellness and reduce your risk of hypokinetic diseases, especially heart disease and diabetes.

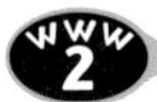

Physical activity provides benefits for both your cardiovascular and respiratory systems. In this lesson, you'll learn how each part of these systems benefits and how all the parts work together to promote optimal functioning and good health.

FIT FACT

In the early 1900s, medical doctors referred to an enlarged heart as the "athlete's heart" because athletes' hearts tend to be large, and enlarged hearts were associated with disease. By midcentury, research showed that the large heart muscle of a trained athlete was a sign of health, not disease.

Heart

Because your heart is a muscle, it benefits from exercise and activities, such as jogging, swimming, and long-distance hiking. Your heart acts as a pump to deliver blood to cells throughout your body. When you do vigorous physical activity, your muscle cells need more oxygen and produce more waste products. Therefore, your heart must pump more blood to supply the additional oxygen and remove the additional waste. If your heart is unable to pump enough blood, your muscles will be less able to contract and will fatigue more quickly.

Your heart's capacity to pump blood is crucial when you're doing physical activity, especially for an extended length of time. Your heart has two ways to get more blood to your muscles—by beating faster and by sending more blood with each beat (this is called stroke volume).

Your resting heart rate is determined by counting the number of heartbeats per minute when you're relatively inactive. A person who does regular physical activity might have a resting heart rate of 55 to 60 beats per minute, whereas a person who does not exercise regularly might have a resting heart rate of 70 or more beats per minute. As a result, a very fit person's heart beats approximately 9.5 million fewer times each year than that of the average person. As you can see in figure 8.2, a fit person's heart works more efficiently by pumping more blood with fewer beats.

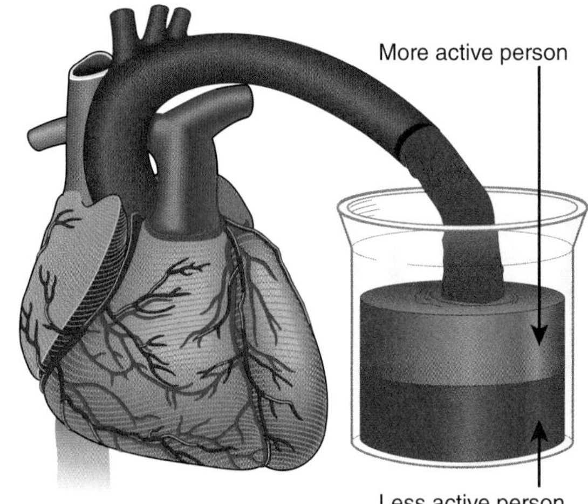

FIGURE 8.2 The heart muscle of a fit, active person pumps more blood per heartbeat than that of a less active person.

Lungs

When you inhale, air enters the lungs, causing them to expand. In the lungs, oxygen is transferred from the air to the blood for transport to the tissues of the body. When you exhale, air leaves the lungs. The diaphragm (a band of muscular tissue located at the base of your lungs) and abdominal muscles (which help move the diaphragm) work to allow you to breathe in and out (figure 8.3*a*). Fit people can take in more air with each breath than unfit people because they have more efficient respiratory muscles. As shown in figure 8.3*b*, a fit person gets more air in the lungs with each breath and therefore can transport the same amount of air to the lungs in fewer breaths. Healthy lungs also have the capacity to easily transfer oxygen to the blood. Together healthy lungs and fit respiratory muscles contribute to good cardiorespiratory endurance.

Blood

Although your body needs a certain amount of fat, excessive amounts trigger formation of fatty deposits along your artery walls. **Cholesterol**—a waxy, fatlike substance found in meat, dairy products, and egg yolk—can be dangerous because high levels can build up in your body without your noticing it.

Cholesterol is carried through your bloodstream by particles called **lipoproteins**. One kind, **low-density lipoprotein (LDL)**, is often referred to as "bad cholesterol" because it carries cholesterol that is more likely to stay in your body and contribute to atherosclerosis. An LDL count below 100 is considered optimal for good health. Another kind, **high-density lipoprotein (HDL)**, is often referred to as "good cholesterol" because it carries excess cholesterol out of your bloodstream and into your liver for elimination from your body. Therefore, HDLs appear to help prevent atherosclerosis. An HDL count above 60 is considered optimal for good health.

In addition to being free of fatty deposits, healthy arteries are free from inflammation, which contributes to arterial clogging. Blood tests can pick up markers of inflammation.

Regular physical activity helps you improve your health and resist disease by reducing your LDL (bad cholesterol) and increasing your HDL (good cholesterol). It also helps reduce inflammation in your arteries and can help prevent the formation of blood clots by reducing the amount of **fibrin** in your blood. Fibrin is a substance involved in making your blood clot, and high amounts of fibrin can contribute to the development of atherosclerosis.

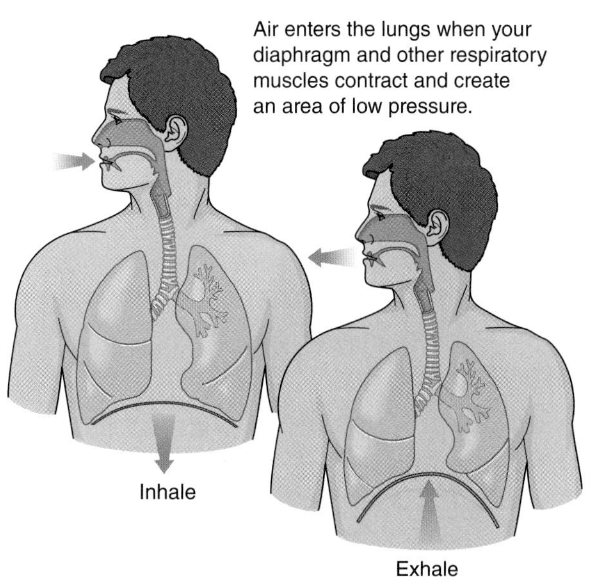
Air enters the lungs when your diaphragm and other respiratory muscles contract and create an area of low pressure.
Inhale
Exhale
a

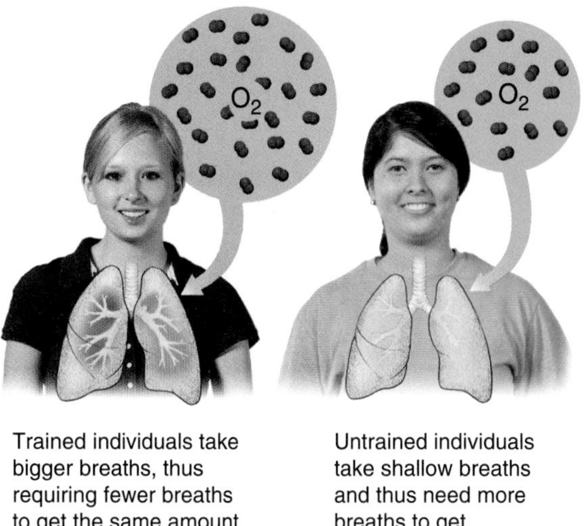
The average lung holds 3 to 5 liters of air.
O2
O2
Trained individuals take bigger breaths, thus requiring fewer breaths to get the same amount of oxygen.
Untrained individuals take shallow breaths and thus need more breaths to get sufficient oxygen.
b

FIGURE 8.3 *(a)* The lungs and diaphragm during inhalation and exhalation; *(b)* fit people can breathe more efficiently than unfit people.

Arteries

Each **artery** carries blood from your heart to another part of your body. The beating of your heart forces blood through your arteries. Therefore, a strong heart and healthy lungs are not very helpful if your arteries are not clear and open. As you now know, fatty deposits on the inner walls of an artery lead to atherosclerosis. An extreme case of atherosclerosis can totally block the blood flow in an artery. The hardened deposits can also allow the formation of blood clots, severely blocking your blood flow. In either case, your heart muscle does not get enough oxygen, and a heart attack occurs.

Regular physical activity also provides other cardiovascular benefits. Scientists have found that people who exercise regularly develop more branching of the arteries in the heart. Figure 8.4 shows that the heart muscle has its own arteries (coronary arteries), which supply it with blood and oxygen. People who exercise regularly develop extra coronary arteries. The importance of this richer network of blood vessels can be shown in two examples.

- After astronaut Ed White died in a fire while training for a mission, an autopsy was performed. Doctors found that one of the major arteries in his heart was completely blocked due to atherosclerosis. However, because of all the physical training that astronauts perform, scientists think White's body had developed an extra branching of arteries in his heart muscle. Therefore, he didn't die of a heart attack when a main artery was blocked. Instead, he had been able to continue a high level of physical fitness training without signs of heart trouble.
- Like White, professional hockey player Richard Zednik had very good cardiorespiratory endurance. This fact became crucial to his survival during a hockey game when his carotid artery was cut by an opponent's skate. For most people, this would be a deadly injury. However, the doctor who performed the rescue surgery reported that because of Zednik's fitness level, he had very healthy and elastic arteries that were large and easy to repair. Zednik made a full recovery.

Veins

Each **vein** carries blood filled with waste products from the muscle cells and other body tissues back to the heart. One-way valves in your veins keep the blood from flowing backward. Your muscles squeeze the veins to pump the blood back to your heart. Regular exercise helps your muscles squeeze your veins efficiently. Lack of physical activity can cause the valves, especially those in your legs, to stop working efficiently, thereby reducing circulation in your legs.

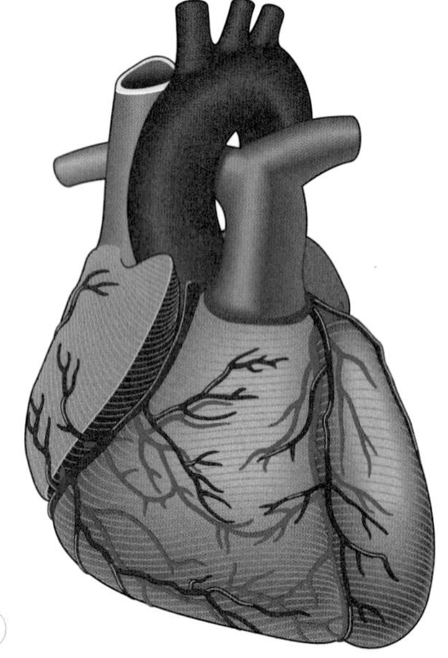

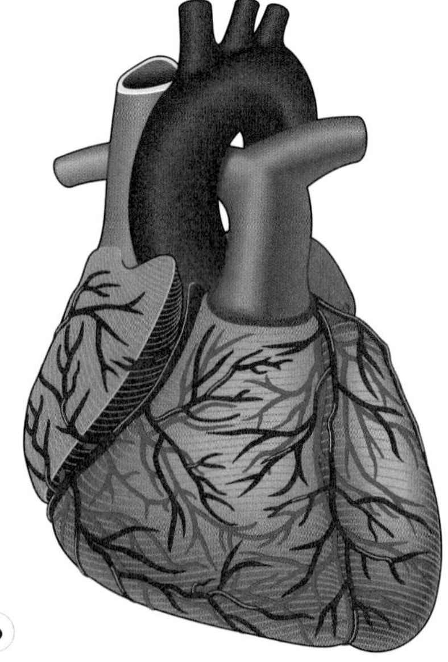

FIGURE 8.4 Blood vessels on the heart: *(a)* the heart of a typical person; *(b)* the heart of a person who exercises regularly.

> “If you don't do what's best for your body, you're the one who comes up on the short end.”
>
> —Julius Erving (Doctor J), Hall of Fame basketball player

Nerves of Your Heart

Your heart muscle is not like your arm and leg muscles. When your arm and leg muscles contract, nerves in them are responding to a message sent by the conscious part of your brain. In contrast, your heart is not controlled voluntarily; it beats regularly without your consciously telling it to do so. Instead, your heart rate is controlled by a part of it called a pacemaker, which sends out an electrical current telling it to beat regularly. People who do regular vigorous aerobic exercise often develop a slower heart rate because the heart pumps more blood with each beat—meaning it has greater stroke volume—and therefore can beat less often. Thus, if you exercise properly, your heart works more efficiently because each heartbeat supplies more blood and oxygen to your body than if you did not exercise. You can also function more effectively during an emergency or during vigorous physical activity.

Muscle Cells

In order to do physical activity for a long time without getting tired, your muscle cells must also function efficiently and effectively. Regular physical activity helps your cells be effective in their use of oxygen and in getting rid of waste materials. Physical activity also helps your muscle cells use blood sugar, with the aid of the hormone called insulin, to produce energy. This function is important for good health.

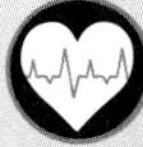

FITNESS TECHNOLOGY: Heart Rate Monitors

One way to count your heart rate is to use your wrist or neck pulse. But it's difficult to do so while you're exercising, so pulse is typically counted after exercise.

To count your pulse during activity, you can use a high-tech device called a heart rate monitor. One type requires you to wear a band around your chest. The band contains sensors that detect electrical stimulation from your heart's nervous system (similar to how an electrocardiogram works). A transmitter in the chest band sends a signal to a receiver located in a special watch worn on your wrist. The receiver picks up the signal and displays your heart rate on the watch. Another type of monitor counts your pulse and displays your heart rate on a watch located on your arm. It does not require the band around your chest.

You can set a heart rate watch to tell you whether you're exercising in your heart rate target zone. You can also set it to keep track of how many minutes you stay in your target zone. Heart rate monitors vary in cost, and some are better than others, so consult with your teacher or another reliable source before buying one. If your school has heart rate watches, you might want to use one to monitor your heart rate during vigorous activity.

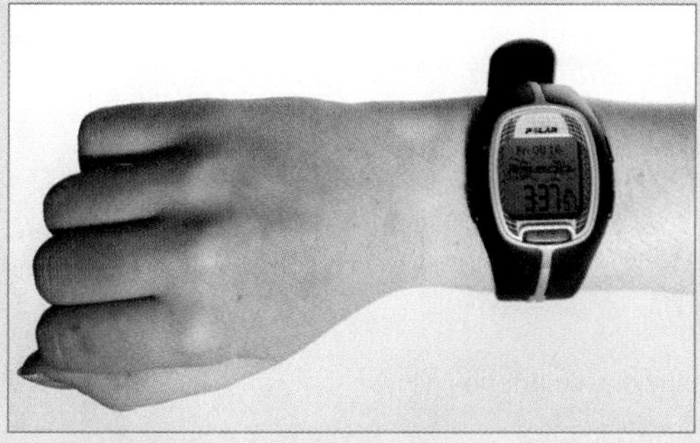

A heart rate watch is helpful for counting your pulse during activity.

Using Technology

Use a variety of sources to evaluate several heart rate monitors. Consider cost, reliability, and ease of use, then decide which monitor would be the best buy.

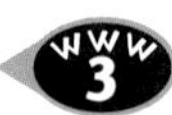

Summary of Benefits

As noted in the previous sections, regular physical activity benefits many different body systems. A summary of these benefits is presented in figure 8.5.

Cardiorespiratory Assessment

You might be curious about your own cardiorespiratory endurance. How good is it? Several tests can help you find the answer.

You can assess the fitness of your cardiorespiratory systems in two settings: in the laboratory and in the field (such as in a gym and or on an athletic field). Two types of laboratory test are the **maximal oxygen uptake** test (also referred to as the $\dot{V}O_2$max test) and the **graded exercise test**.

The maximal oxygen uptake test is considered the best for assessing fitness of the cardiovascular and respiratory systems. It measures how much oxygen you can use when you're exercising very vigorously. To take the test, you run on a treadmill while connected to a special gas meter (figure 8.6). The difficulty increases as the treadmill goes faster

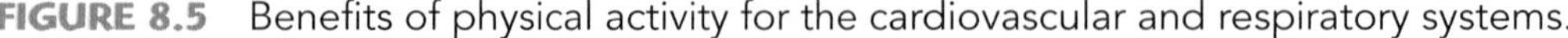

O_2
• Lungs work more efficiently
• Deliver more oxygen to blood
• Healthy lungs allow deeper and less frequent breathing
Lungs
• Heart muscle gets stronger
• Pumps more blood with each beat (stroke volume)
• Beats slower
• Gets more rest
• Works more efficiently
• Helps the nerves slow your heart rate at rest
• Builds muscles and helps them work more efficiently
• Healthy elastic arteries allow more blood flow
• Less risk of atherosclerosis
• Lower blood pressure
• Less risk of a blood clot leading to heart attack
• Development of extra blood vessels
• Healthy veins with healthy valves
• Less bad cholesterol (LDL) and other fats in the blood
• More good cholesterol (HDL) in the blood
• Reduces inflammatory markers in the blood
• Fewer substances in the blood that cause clots
• Use oxygen efficiently
• Get rid of more wastes
• Use blood sugars and insulin more effectively to produce energy

FIGURE 8.5 Benefits of physical activity for the cardiovascular and respiratory systems.

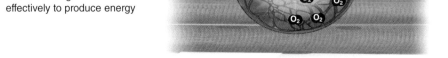

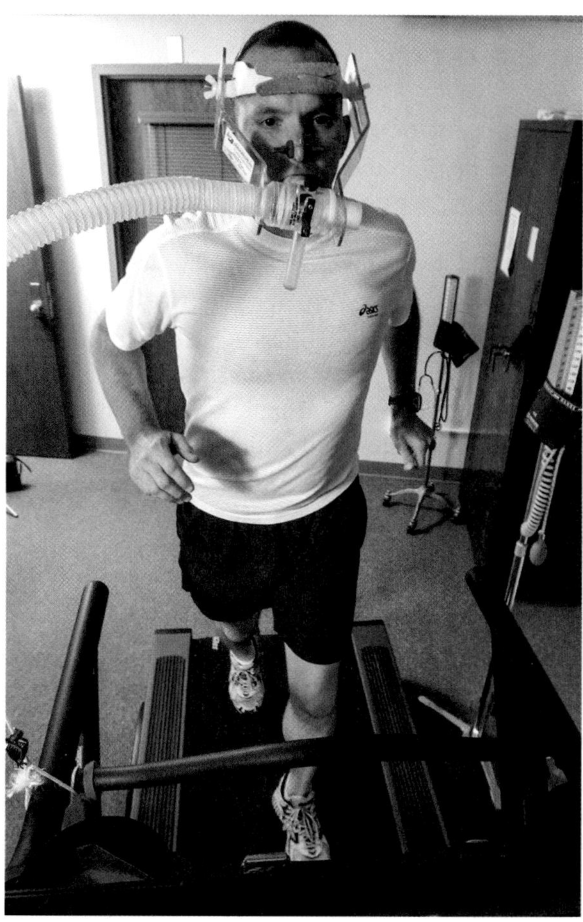

FIGURE 8.6 The maximal oxygen uptake test measures the amount of oxygen you use while running on a treadmill.

and you begin to run uphill. As you exercise, the gas meter measures the amount of oxygen you use each minute. The amount (volume) of oxygen you can use during the hardest minute of exercise is considered your $\dot{V}O_2$max score (see Science in Action).

Medical doctors and exercise physiologists sometimes use another laboratory test called a graded exercise test (or an exercise stress test). This test is used to detect potential heart problems. During the test, your heart is monitored by means of an electrocardiogram while you run on a treadmill.

Both the graded exercise test and the maximal oxygen uptake test are done in a laboratory and require special equipment and people who are trained to administer them. Most people, however, assess their cardiorespiratory endurance using practical nonlaboratory tests called field tests. These tests require little equipment and can be done at home or at school. Scores are determined based on your ability to function (your functional fitness) rather than on the amount of oxygen you can use. Examples include the PACER, the walking test, the step test, and the one-mile run test.

FIT FACT

Studies show that endurance athletes—such as cross-country skiers, cyclists, and distance runners—typically have very high aerobic capacity and score well on field tests of cardiorespiratory endurance.

Interpreting Self-Assessment Results

Self-assessments are not as accurate as laboratory tests of fitness; therefore, you should perform more than one self-assessment for cardiorespiratory endurance. However, self-assessments do give a good estimate of your fitness level, and each assessment has its own strengths and weaknesses. For example, the results of the PACER and the one-mile run (included in this chapter) are influenced by your motivation; if you don't try very hard, you won't get an accurate score. Because these tests require a high level of exertion, they may not be the best tests for people who have not been exercising regularly or who have low fitness.

The walking test, on the other hand, is a good indicator of fitness for most people but is not best for assessing very fit people. It would be a good test for a beginner. The step test (included in this chapter) uses heart rate; therefore, motivation does not influence its results as much as it does some other assessments. But step test results can be distorted if you've done other exercise that might elevate your heart rate before doing the assessment. Your heart rate can also be influenced by emotional factors (stress) and nutritional factors (caffeine) that cause it to be higher than normal. Finally, your results may vary depending on the time of day the assessment is done. For example, fatigue associated with daily activities may result in poorer scores late in the day.

Regardless of which tests you do, practice them before using them to assess your fitness. Practice allows you to pace yourself properly during the test and enables you to perform the tests properly so that you get accurate assessments. Because you may get different ratings on different tests of cardiorespiratory endurance, consider the strengths and weaknesses of each test when making decisions

SCIENCE IN ACTION: Aerobic Capacity

After extensive research, the Institute of Medicine recommended the use of the term *cardiorespiratory endurance* for performance on field tests such as the PACER. Because of this recommendation, we use the term *cardiorespiratory endurance* in this book rather than some of the other commonly used terms (such as *cardiovascular fitness* or *aerobic fitness*). Cardiorespiratory endurance reflects a person's functional fitness—the ability to perform tasks of daily life such as enjoying leisure-time activities and the ability to meet emergencies without undue fatigue.

As noted earlier, the term **aerobic capacity** is similar to, but not exactly the same as, cardiorespiratory endurance. The only true measure of aerobic capacity is your score on a laboratory based maximal oxygen uptake test. Your score on the maximal oxygen uptake test ($\dot{V}O_2$max test) is recorded in liters of oxygen per minute. You may want to adjust your aerobic capacity score (in liters) to account for body size because big people use more liters of oxygen simply because of their size. So aerobic capacity scores are commonly reported as milliliters of oxygen per kilogram of body weight per minute (mL/kg/min).

You can also get an idea of your aerobic capacity in other ways. For example, when used with the Fitnessgram report card, your cardiorespiratory endurance score is converted to an estimated aerobic capacity score. You can find more information and tables for estimating aerobic capacity from PACER scores at the student section of the Health Opportunities Through Physical Education website.

Student Activity

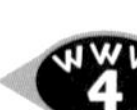

Estimate your aerobic capacity score in milliliters of oxygen per kilogram of body weight per minute (mL/kg/min) using your PACER score. Tables for converting PACER scores to aerobic capacity scores are available in the student section of the Health Opportunities Through Physical Education website.

about which score best represents your fitness. After you've done regular exercise over time, test yourself again to see how much you've improved.

How Much Cardiorespiratory Endurance Is Enough?

To get the health and wellness benefits associated with cardiorespiratory endurance, you should achieve the good fitness zone in the rating charts that accompany each self-assessment in part 1 of this book. Health benefits are associated with moving out of the low and marginal zones and into the good fitness zone. The risk of hypokinetic diseases is greatest for people in the low fitness zone.

Some people aim for especially high cardiorespiratory endurance because they want to perform at a high level in a sport or a physically demanding job, such as being a Marine or a police officer. To be properly fit for such challenges, you must train harder than most people. Achieving the high performance zone will be difficult for some people, and doing so is not necessary in order to get many of the health benefits of fitness. Nevertheless, the higher your cardiorespiratory endurance score, the lower your risk of hypokinetic disease.

Lesson Review

1. What are some health and wellness benefits of cardiorespiratory endurance?
2. How does physical activity affect the various parts of your cardiovascular and respiratory systems?
3. What are some methods for assessing cardiorespiratory endurance and aerobic capacity, and how are they done?
4. How much cardiorespiratory endurance is enough?

SELF-ASSESSMENT: Step Test and One-Mile Run Test

As you've learned, the maximal oxygen uptake test is the best test of fitness of the cardiovascular and respiratory systems. But if you want a quicker, easier, and less expensive test, try the step test or the one-mile run test. Then, after you've done regular exercise over time, test yourself again to see how much you've improved. As directed by your teacher, record your scores and fitness ratings for either test (or both). You can then use the information in preparing your personal physical activity plan. If you're working with a partner, remember that self-assessment information is personal and considered confidential. It shouldn't be shared with others without the permission of the person being tested.

Step Test

1. Use a bench that is 12 inches (30 centimeters) high. Step up with your right foot. Step up with your left foot.
2. Step down with your right foot. Step down with your left foot.
3. Repeat this four-count pattern (up, up, down, down). Step 24 times each minute for three minutes.
4. Immediately after stepping for three minutes, sit and count your pulse. Begin counting within five seconds. Count for one minute.
5. Use table 8.1 to determine your cardiorespiratory endurance rating. Record your heart rate, minutes of stepping, and rating.

Note: The height of the bench and the rate of stepping are both crucial to getting an accurate test result. Sit calmly for several minutes before the test to assure that your resting heart rate is normal.

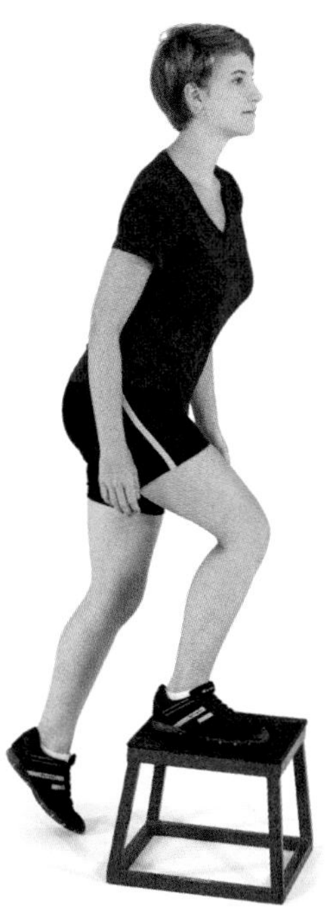

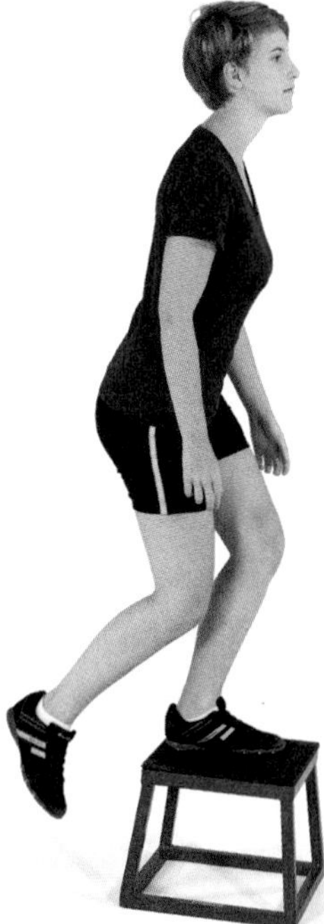

The step test assesses cardiorespiratory endurance.

TABLE 8.1 Rating Chart: Step Test (Heartbeats per Minute)

	13 years old		14–16 years old		17 years or older	
	Male	Female	Male	Female	Male	Female
High performance	≤90	≤100	≤85	≤95	≤80	≤90
Good fitness	91–98	101–110	86–95	96–105	81–90	91–100
Marginal fitness	99–120	111–130	96–115	106–125	91–110	101–120
Low fitness	≥121	≥131	≥116	≥126	≥111	≥121

Those who cannot step for 3 minutes receive a low fitness rating.

One-Mile Run

An alternative test of cardiorespiratory endurance is the one-mile (1.6-kilometer) run. Remember that this test is for your own information; it's not a race. Your goal is a good fitness rating, which indicates reduced risk of hypokinetic disease and enough fitness to function effectively. Some people may strive to achieve the high performance zone, which provides additional health benefits and allows you to perform sports and jobs requiring strong cardiorespiratory endurance.

1. Run or jog for one mile (1.6 kilometers) in the shortest possible time. A steady pace is best. Try to set a pace that you can keep up for the full run. If you start too fast and then have to slow down at the end, you will probably not be able to run for the entire distance. You can use target heart rate or ratings of perceived exertion (RPE) to help you set a good pace. Another indicator is the talk test. If you are unable to talk comfortably while running (for example, talking with a friend), then you are probably running too fast.
2. Your score is the amount of time it takes you to run the full distance. Record your time in minutes and seconds.
3. Find your rating in table 8.2 and record it.

TABLE 8.2 Rating Chart: One-Mile (1.6-Kilometer) Run (Minutes:Seconds)

	13 years old		14 years old		15 years old		16 years old		17 years or older	
	Male	Female	Male	Female	Male	Female	Male	Female	Male	Female
High performance	≤7:45	≤8:40	≤7:30	≤8:25	≤7:15	≤8:10	≤7:00	≤7:45	≤6:50	≤7:35
Good fitness	7:46–10:09	8:41–10:27	7:31–9:27	8:26–10:15	7:16–9:00	8:11–9:58	7:01–8:39	7:46–9:46	6:51–8:26	7:36–9:31
Marginal fitness	10:10–12:29	10:28–13:03	9:28–11:51	10:16–12:48	9:01–11:14	9:59–12:27	8:40–10:46	9:47–12:11	8:27–10:37	9:32–11:54
Low fitness	≥12:30	≥13:04	≥11:52	≥12:49	≥11:15	≥12:28	≥10:47	≥12:12	≥10:38	≥11:55

Based on data provided by G. Welk.

Lesson 8.2

Building Cardiorespiratory Endurance

Lesson Objectives

After reading this lesson, you should be able to

1. define *vigorous aerobic activity* and give several examples,
2. describe the FIT formula for developing cardiorespiratory endurance,
3. describe how to count your resting heart rate and determine your maximal heart rate, and
4. explain how to use two methods for determining your threshold of training and your target zone for building cardiorespiratory endurance.

Lesson Vocabulary

aerobic activity, heart rate reserve (HRR), maximal heart rate, vigorous aerobics

You now know that physical activity is important to your cardiorespiratory endurance. But how much physical activity do you have to do to improve your cardiorespiratory endurance? In this lesson, you'll learn about the best types of activity for building cardiorespiratory endurance. You'll also learn to determine how much physical activity you need in order to build your own cardiorespiratory endurance.

> "To keep the body in good health is a duty; otherwise, we shall not be able to keep our mind strong and clear.

>
> —The Buddha

Physical Activity and Cardiorespiratory Endurance

The term *aerobic* means "with oxygen," and **aerobic activity** is activity that is steady enough to allow your heart to supply all the oxygen your muscles need. Moderate physical activities are considered to be aerobic because you can do them for a long time without stopping. Moderate activities provide many health benefits and can build cardiorespiratory endurance in low-fit people, but they are not intense enough to build cardiorespiratory endurance for most people.

Vigorous aerobics, represented on the second step of the Physical Activity Pyramid for Teens, is the most effective way to build cardiorespiratory endurance. Vigorous aerobic activities are intense enough to elevate your heart rate above your threshold of training and into your target zone for cardiorespiratory endurance. National physical activity guidelines for teens recommend doing vigorous activity on at least three days a week because they promote benefits beyond those provided by moderate activity.

Vigorous sport and recreation activities, represented on the third step of the Physical Activity Pyramid for Teens (figure 8.7), also build cardiorespiratory endurance. Vigorous sports often involve quick bursts of vigorous activity followed by rest, and for this reason they are not totally aerobic. However, they offer the same benefits as vigorous aerobic activity. To be considered vigorous, sports and recreation activities must be intense enough to elevate your heart rate above your threshold of training and into your target zone for cardiorespiratory endurance.

How Much Vigorous Activity Is Enough?

As you're already aware, teens should accumulate 60 minutes of physical activity each day of the week. Some of that recommended activity should be of

Energy balance

STEP 5
Flexibility exercises

STEP 4
Muscle fitness exercises

STEP 3
Vigorous sport and recreation

STEP 2
Vigorous aerobics

STEP 1
Moderate physical activity

FIGURE 8.7 Vigorous activities from steps 2 and 3 are best for building cardiorespiratory endurance.

a vigorous nature. Specifically, you should perform vigorous activity at least three days a week in exercise sessions totaling at least 20 minutes per day. Vigorous activity should be of a high enough intensity that it increases your heart rate above your threshold level and into your target zone.

The FIT formula for building cardiorespiratory endurance is shown in table 8.3. As you can see, both the threshold of training and the target zone are different for people who are sedentary than for people who are regularly active. Sedentary people exercise at a lower intensity and use a different target heart rate zone than more active people.

When using table 8.3, first find your current physical activity level among the options listed in the table's second row. Rows below indicate frequency and length of exercise in days and minutes. The intensity of your exercise is determined by one of two methods of counting heart rate; these two methods are described in the next section of this chapter. Once you learn how to count your heart rate using one of the two methods, you can use table 8.3 to determine your exercise intensity.

FIT FACT

Another way (besides heart rate) to determine intensity is to use rating of perceived exertion (RPE). In this method, you estimate the intensity of your exertion during exercise using numbers from 6 (no exertion) to 20 (maximal exertion). An RPE of 12 to 14 is typically equal to the target zone for cardiorespiratory endurance (see table 8.3). RPE can be used to help you determine your pace during vigorous aerobic activity.

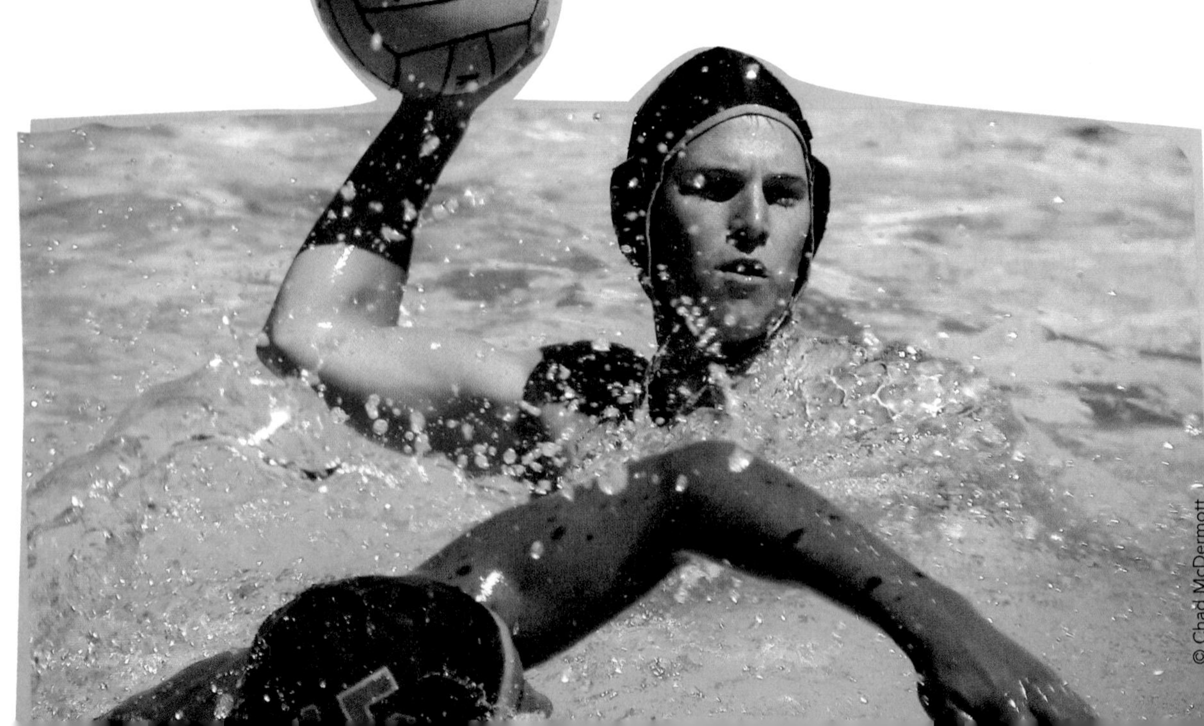

© Chad McDermott

TABLE 8.3 Threshold of Training and Target Heart Rate Zones (FIT Formula) for People With Different Activity Levels

	Threshold of training			Target heart rate zone		
Current activity level	No regular vigorous activity	Some vigorous activity	Regular vigorous activity	No regular vigorous activity	Some vigorous activity	Regular vigorous activity
Frequency	3 days a week for all fitness levels			3–6 days a week for all fitness levels		
Intensity	Percentage			Percentage		
HRR* % max HR**	50 70	60 80	70 84	50–70 70–85	60–80 80–91	70–89 84–95
Time	20 min for all activity levels***			20–90 min for all activity levels***		

*HRR indicates heart rate reserve.

**% max HR indicates percent of maximal heart rate.

***Sessions of at least 10 minutes can be combined to meet time recommendations.

Based on ACSM exercise prescription guidelines.

Heart Rate and Intensity of Physical Activity

Monitoring heart rate is a common technique for determining exercise intensity. This is because taking a pulse count to determine your heart rate is relatively easy to do. But what exactly are we looking for when we take a pulse count? In order to build cardiorespiratory endurance, you need to overload the cardiovascular and respiratory systems. Calculating a target heart rate zone, including your threshold of training and target ceiling, is the scientific approach to providing optimal overload. Once you know your target heart rate zone, you know how high you need to elevate your heart rate to pace your exercise for building cardiorespiratory endurance. The American College of Sports Medicine (ACSM) recommends two methods for determining your target heart rate zone. The first is the percent of heart rate reserve (% HRR) method and the second is the percent of maximal heart rate (% max HR) method.

In this lesson, you'll learn how to use both of these methods to calculate your threshold target heart rate zone. After learning both methods, you'll choose one to use. You can then count your heart rate during or right after exercise to determine whether you're exercising at the right intensity for your target zone.

Counting Resting Heart Rate

To determine your target heart rate zone, you first need to determine your resting heart rate, which is the number of times your heart beats when you're relatively inactive. Use the following instructions.

1. Sit and take your heart rate by using the first and second fingers of your hand to find a pulse at your opposite wrist (your radial pulse) (figure 8.8*a*). Do not use your thumb. Practice so that you can locate your pulse quickly.
2. Count the number of pulses for one minute. Record your one-minute heart rate.
3. Take your resting (seated) heart rate again, this time counting the pulse at your neck (figure 8.8*b*). This is your carotid pulse. Use two fingers (index and middle) of either hand. Place the fingers on the side of your neck. Move until you locate the pulse. Press only as hard as necessary to feel the pulse; be careful not to press too hard.
4. Now take both your wrist and your neck pulse while you are standing. Repeat the pulse count (both wrist and neck) while sitting. Compare your results. Usually, your standing pulse is faster than your sitting pulse.

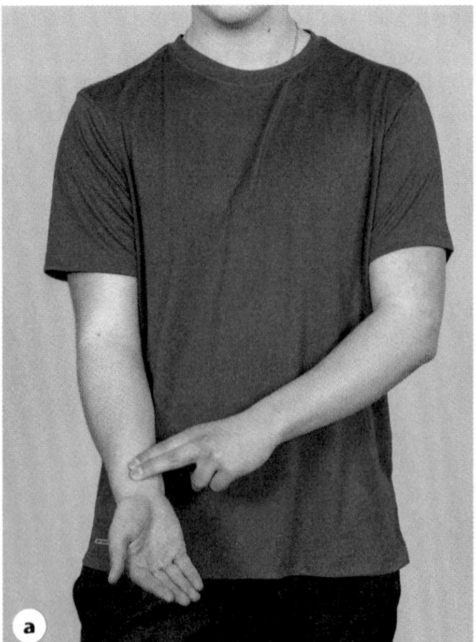

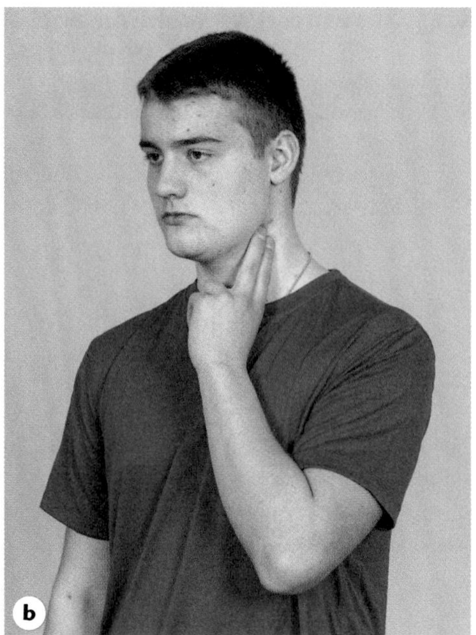

FIGURE 8.8 Use your first and second finger to find a pulse *(a)* at your wrist and *(b)* at your neck.

5. Take a partner's pulse while your partner takes your pulse (both standing). Compare your self-counted heart rate with your heart rate as determined by your partner. You may use different methods of counting, but use the same one as your partner when making comparisons.
6. As directed by your teacher, record your resting heart rate using the methods just described.

Determining Maximal Heart Rate (Max HR)

Maximal heart rate (max HR) is the highest heart rate that a person can reach during the most vigorous exercise. To estimate your max HR, you can count your heart rate after a very vigorous exercise session; or, to determine a more accurate max HR, you can wear a heart rate monitor to see how high your heart rate gets during very vigorous exercise. Be aware, however, that people who are unfit or are not regularly active should *not* do an exercise session vigorous enough to determine max HR.

Because determining a true max HR requires very vigorous activity that isn't appropriate for some people, exercise physiologists have developed several formulas for estimating max HR without doing exercise. Five different formulas are listed by the ACSM for estimating max HR. Each has advantages and disadvantages. Here we use the formula that is most commonly used by exercise experts. It's simple to use, and the estimated max HRs from the formula are very similar to those calculated using a more complex formula for young people including teens. You can use the formula below or estimate your max HR by using table 8.4.

220 – age in years = maximal heart rate

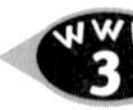

Example for 16-year-old: 220 – 16 = 204

As directed by your teacher, record your estimated max HR. You'll use it when determining your heart rate target zone.

Counting Exercise Heart Rate

It can be difficult to count your pulse during activities such as jogging, but you can get a good estimate of your heart rate during a physical activity by determining your heart rate immediately after exercising. To estimate your heart rate during exercise based on your after-exercise pulse count, use the following instructions.

1. Immediately after exercise, locate your pulse (within 5 seconds).
2. Use either your wrist or neck pulse to count your heart rate for 15 seconds. Multiply your

15-second count by 4 to get your 1-minute heart rate. This method is useful because you can do it quickly and because your heart rate slows down quickly when you stop exercising, which means the longer counts may underestimate what your heart rate was during the exercise. On the other hand, counting for a shorter time can result in error because a single counting mistake is multiplied. You can use table 8.5 to help you determine your 1-minute heart rate from your 15-second count.

3. While you count your heart rate, you may want to continue to walk slowly because slow walking can help you recover faster. If you have trouble counting your heart rate while walking, stand still when you count, then begin moving.

Percent of Heart Rate Reserve Method for Determining Target Heart Rate

To build cardiorespiratory endurance, you must elevate your heart rate above your threshold of training and into your target zone (see table 8.3). The percent of heart rate reserve (% HRR) is one of two methods for determining target heart rate. This method is considered the most accurate, but it is a bit more difficult to calculate than the other method. To use this method, you must know your resting and maximal heart rates and your **heart rate reserve (HRR)**. Table 8.6 provides an example of the calculations for a 16-year-old who has a resting heart rate of 67 and is in the good fitness zone for cardiorespiratory endurance.

1. Begin by determining your resting and max HR as described earlier in this chapter. In the example, the resting HR is 67 and the max HR is 204.
2. Next, determine your heart rate reserve by subtracting your resting heart rate from your maximal heart rate (max HR). In the example, the resting heart rate is 67, so the heart rate reserve is 137.
3. To calculate the threshold heart rate, multiply the heart rate reserve (HRR) by a percentage of the max HR—60 percent (0.6) in the example. As shown in table 8.3, different percentages are used for people of different activity levels; use the percentage that fits your current activity level. This number is

TABLE 8.4 Estimated Maximal Heart Rates

Your age (years)	12	13	14	15	16	17	18	19
Max HR	208	207	206	205	204	203	202	201

Find your age in the top row, then find your estimated max HR immediately below your age.

TABLE 8.5 Heart Rate in 15-Second and 1-Minute Intervals

15-sec rate	1-min rate	15-sec rate	1-min rate	15-sec rate	1-min rate
15	60	27	108	39	156
16	64	28	112	40	160
17	68	29	116	41	164
18	72	30	120	42	168
19	76	31	124	43	172
20	80	32	128	44	176
21	84	33	132	45	180
22	88	34	136	46	184
23	92	35	140	47	188
24	96	36	144	48	192
25	100	37	148	49	196
26	104	38	152	50	200

Find your 15-second heart rate in a shaded column; your 1-minute heart rate is in the white column to the immediate right of it.

then added to the resting heart rate. In the example, the threshold is 149.

4. The target ceiling heart rate is calculated by repeating steps 1 through 3, but in step 3 multiply by a higher percentage—80 percent (0.8) in the example. Refer to table 8.3 to find the percentage you should use for your target zone based on your currently activity level. Then add your resting heart rate. In the example, the target ceiling heart rate is 177.
5. Thus the target heart zone is 149 to 177 (60 to 80 percent of HRR) in the example of the 16-year-old who is in the good fitness zone.

Percent of Maximal Heart Rate Method for Determining Target Heart Rate

The second method, percent of maximal heart rate (% max HR), is not quite as accurate as the HRR method but is easier to calculate. In this method, you do not use your resting heart rate. Table 8.7 provides an example using the % max HR method for a 16-year-old in the good fitness zone for cardiorespiratory endurance.

1. Estimate your maximal heart rate. In the example, the maximal heart rate is 204.
2. In this example, the max HR (204) was multiplied by 80 percent (0.8) to find the threshold heart rate. As noted in table 8.3, different percentages are used for people of different activity levels; use the percentage that fits your current activity level. In the example, the threshold is 163.
3. To calculate the target ceiling rate, repeat steps 1 and 2, but in step 2 multiply by 91 percent (0.91). This number will vary based on your activity level (see table 8.3). In the example, the ceiling rate is 186.

TABLE 8.6 Calculating Heart Rate Target Zone (% HRR Method)

Threshold HR	Step 1: Step 2: Step 3:	204 (max HR)* – 67 (resting HR) 137 (HRR) × 0.6 (threshold %) 82 + 67 (resting HR) 149 (threshold HR)
Target ceiling	Step 1: Step 2: Step 3:	204 (max HR)* – 67 (resting HR) 137 (HRR) × 0.8 (ceiling %) 110 + 67 (resting HR) 177 (target ceiling HR)
Target HR zone	149–177 beats per min	

*The example is for a 16-year-old with a resting HR of 67 with cardiorespiratory endurance in the good fitness zone.

TABLE 8.7 Calculating Heart Rate Target Zone (% max HR Method)

Threshold HR	Step 1: Step 2:	204 (max HR)* × 0.8 (threshold %) 163 (threshold HR)
Target ceiling rate	Step 1: Step 2:	204 (max HR)* × 0.91 (ceiling %) 186 (target ceiling rate)
Target HR zone	163–186 beats per min	

*The example is for a 16-year-old with a resting HR of 67 and cardiorespiratory endurance in the good fitness zone.

4. Thus the target heart rate zone is 163 to 186 (80 to 91 percent of max HR) in the example of the 16-year-old in the good fitness zone for cardiorespiratory endurance. Note that these numbers are slightly higher than those generated with the % HRR method.

Exercise for Ellen

Ellen is a high school sophomore. She took the PACER and the walking test and got a marginal fitness rating in both. She was not surprised, because she rarely did vigorous exercise, but she did want to improve her cardiorespiratory endurance. To do so, she knew that she had to start doing more vigorous activity each week.

Specifically, based on information presented in table 8.3, Ellen learned that she needed to do vigorous exercise at least three (and up to six) days a week. She decided to begin with three, and she chose to jog for 20 minutes on each of the three days because table 8.3 recommended sessions of 20 minutes.

In class, Ellen learned how to use the % HRR and % max HR methods for determining her target heart rate zone. She decided to use the % HRR method. She first determined her maximal heart rate (204 beats per minute) and resting heart rate (67 beats per minute). She then determined that her heart rate reserve (HRR) was 137 by subtracting her resting heart rate from her maximum heart rate (204 – 67 = 137).

Next, she calculated her target heart rate zone, and she did so with the 50 percent to 70 percent range shown in table 8.3 for someone who does no regular vigorous activity. Specifically, she did the following calculations: 50 percent of 137 (her heart rate reserve) is 69, and 70 percent of 137 is 96. Ellen then added 67 (her resting heart rate) to each of these figures to get her threshold heart rate (69 + 67 = 136) and her upper heart rate (96 + 67 = 163). Thus she determined that her target heart rate zone was 139 to 163 beats per minute.

Immediately after each jogging session, Ellen counted her heart rate to see if it was in her target heart rate zone. On a few days, it was below the zone, so she ran a bit faster the next time. Over time, Ellen expects to improve her cardiorespiratory endurance so that she will be in the good fitness zone.

Lesson Review

1. What is vigorous aerobic activity? Give several examples.
2. What is the FIT formula for developing cardiorespiratory endurance?
3. How can you determine your resting heart rate and estimate your max HR?
4. How can you determine your threshold of training and your target heart rate zone for building cardiorespiratory endurance? Describe two methods.

TAKING CHARGE: Self-Confidence

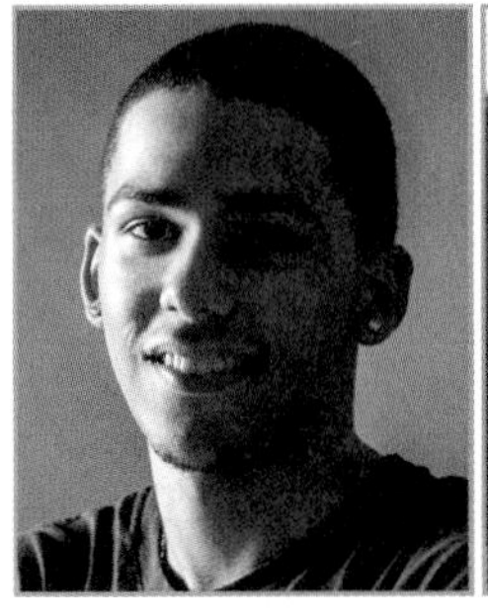

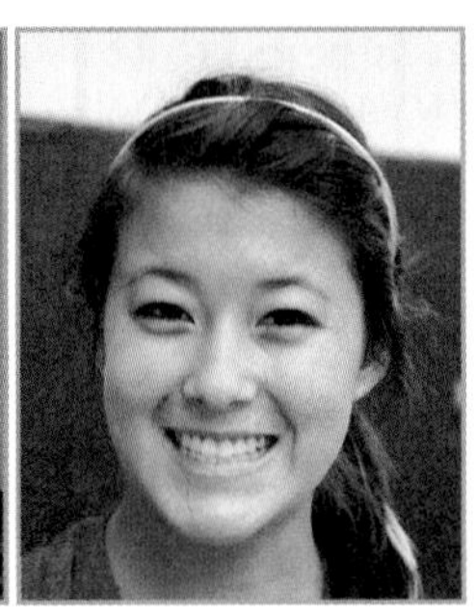

Self-confidence involves believing that you can be successful in an activity. If you think you'll succeed, you have more confidence than if you're unsure about how well you'll do. You're more likely to participate in an activity if your self-confidence is high.

Tony rarely takes part in any physical activity. He went through an awkward stage in his preteen years and thinks that people laugh at the way he runs: "My arms and legs don't seem to work together when I run. I think I look foolish."

Mei, on the other hand, loves any kind of physical activity. Every day, she shoots baskets or rides her bike, and she is a member of multiple teams. Even though she excels in sport, however, she would like to socialize more, but she feels shy around strangers: "I can't think of anything witty or even halfway intelligent to say. When I try to talk, I get tongue tied. It's easier for me to just avoid talking."

Tony and Mei both lack self-confidence but in two different situations. Tony wants to participate in physical activity, and Mei wants to socialize, but they both avoid situations where they might get involved because they feel uncomfortable. Both need to find a way to build their self-confidence so they can succeed in these situations.

For Discussion

For different reasons, people like Tony may avoid trying new activities or may quit an activity prematurely. People like Mei who lack confidence in social situations may avoid them. What are some reasons that people lack self-confidence? How can they increase their self-confidence? What advice can you give Tony to get him to try new activities and stick with them? What advice can you give Mei to help her be more comfortable in social situations? Also consider the guidelines presented in the Self-Management feature when answering the discussion questions.

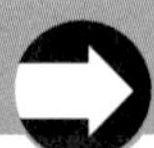

SELF-MANAGEMENT: Skills for Building Self-Confidence

A recent study of teenagers found that one of the best indicators of who will be physically active is self-confidence. A person is self-confident if he or she thinks *I can do that* rather than *I don't think I can*. Some people are not very confident when it comes to physical activity because they think they are not very good at it or that others are better than they are. Does it surprise you to learn that self-confident people are not always the best performers and that some good performers lack self-confidence? In fact, research done with teenagers in schools shows that all students can find some type of activity in which they can be successful, regardless of physical ability. In addition, people who think they can succeed in activity are nearly twice as likely to be active as people who don't think they can succeed.

Building self-confidence is a self-management skill that you can learn. You may want to assess your self-confidence using the worksheet supplied by your teacher. Then, if necessary, you can use the following guidelines to improve your self-confidence.

- **Learn a new way of thinking.** One major reason some people lack self-confidence is that they think their own success depends on how they compare with others. Practicing a new way of thinking means setting your own standards of success rather than comparing yourself with others. These guidelines are designed to help you build self-confidence by developing a new way of thinking.
- **Set your own personal standards for success.** Assess yourself and set standards for success related to your own improvement. Comparing yourself with

others is not necessary for your success, and it can contribute to low self-confidence.

- **Avoid competition if it causes you a problem.** Some people like to compete, but others don't. If competition makes you feel less confident in a physical activity, try to find noncompetitive activities (such as walking, jogging, and swimming) that allow you to feel good about yourself.
- **Set small goals that you're sure to reach.** Setting goals that are a bit higher than your current level is a good idea, but don't set them too high. As you reach one small goal, you can set another. Reaching several small goals builds your self-confidence, whereas not reaching one unrealistic goal can make you less confident.
- **Think and act on positive—not negative—ideas.** When you're involved in a physical activity, think of how you can improve. Talk to yourself about what you did well and what you can practice to improve in the future. Avoid negative self-talk, such as berating yourself for what you didn't do well or referring to yourself in negative terms.

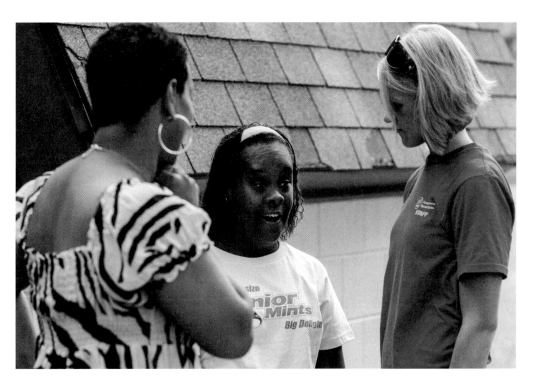

Setting a personal standard of success and getting reinforcement from others can help a person build self-confidence.

TAKING ACTION: Target Heart Rate Workouts

Cardiorespiratory endurance is important for living a long and healthy life. It's also essential for competing, participating in your favorite physical activities, and maintaining a healthy body weight. As you've learned in this chapter, you must do vigorous physical activity above your threshold of training and in your target zone to build cardiorespiratory endurance. **Take action** by doing vigorous activity that fulfills the FIT formula: at least three days each week (addressing F for frequency in the FIT formula), in your target heart rate zone (addressing I for intensity), and for at least 20 minutes each session (addressing T for time). Consider the following tips as you take action by performing a target heart rate workout.

- Determine your target heart rate by using either the percent of heart rate reserve method or the percent of maximal heart rate method.
- Before choosing vigorous activities, consider your level of fitness.
- Before doing vigorous activity, perform a 5-minute cardiorespiratory general warm-up.
- Check your pulse rate or rating of perceived exertion periodically to make sure you're maintaining the intensity of your workout in your target heart rate zone.
- After your vigorous workout, perform a cool-down.

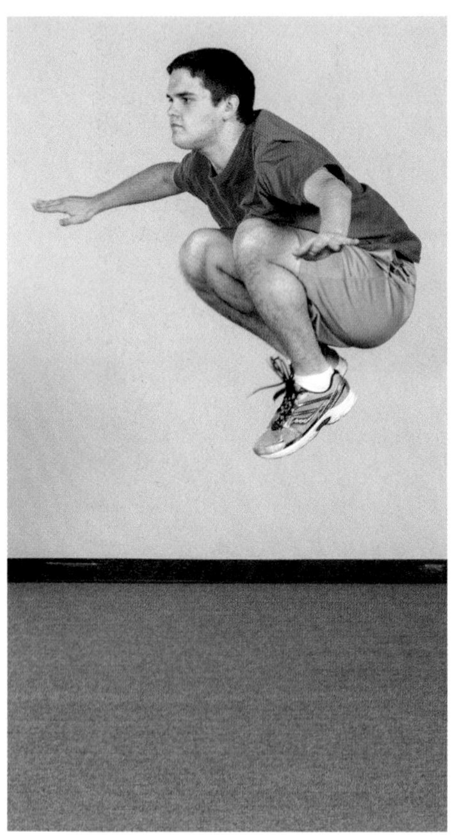

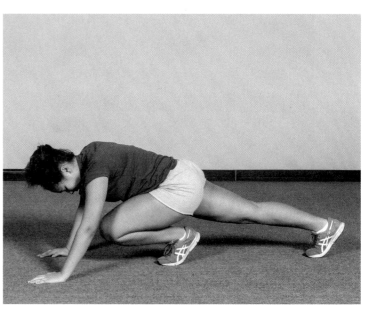

Take action by doing a workout that elevates your heart rate into the target zone.

CHAPTER REVIEW

Reviewing Concepts and Vocabulary

As directed by your teacher, answer items 1 through 5 by correctly completing each sentence with a word or phrase.

1. Vessels that carry blood from the muscles back to the heart are called ______________.
2. The body system that includes your heart, blood vessels, and blood is the ______________ system.
3. The substance in your blood that helps it clot is called ______________.
4. The method for determining exercise intensity by estimating it without measuring it is called rating of ______________.
5. The highest your heart rate ever gets is called your ______________.

For items 6 through 10, as directed by your teacher, match each term in column 1 with the appropriate phrase in column 2.

Column 1	Column 2
6. carotid	a. waxy, fatlike substance in blood
7. cholesterol	b. neck pulse
8. high-density lipoprotein	c. bad cholesterol
9. low-density lipoprotein	d. aerobic capacity
10. maximal oxygen uptake	e. carries bad cholesterol out of the bloodstream

For items 11 through 15, as directed by your teacher, respond to each statement or question.

11. Explain how cardiorespiratory endurance helps your cardiovascular and respiratory systems work more efficiently and thus helps to prevent cardiovascular disease.
12. Define *aerobic capacity*. How does it relate to cardiorespiratory endurance?
13. Describe the two field tests of cardiorespiratory endurance discussed in this chapter.
14. Describe two methods for determining your target heart rate zone.
15. Describe several guidelines for building self-confidence.

Thinking Critically

Write a paragraph to answer the following question.

Sue has a resting heart rate of 76 beats per minute. Bill has a resting heart rate of 54. Assuming that neither has a disease or illness, what are some possible reasons that their resting heart rates differ so much?

Project

Create a poster, slide presentation, or video describing the benefits of physical activity for the cardiovascular and respiratory systems.

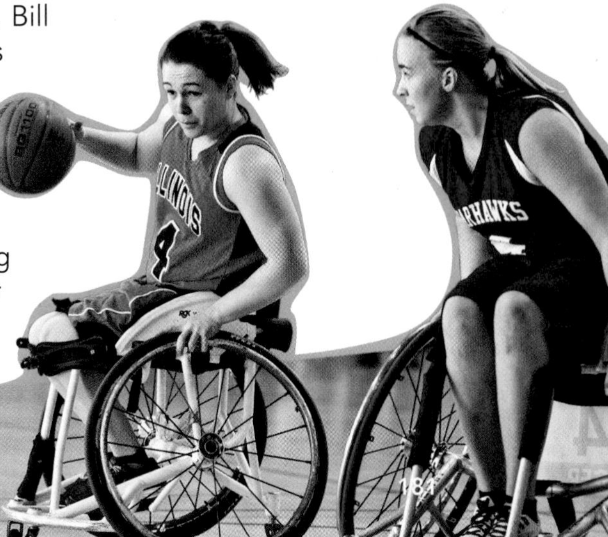

9

Vigorous Physical Activity

In This Chapter

Student Web Resources
www.HOPEtextbook.org/student

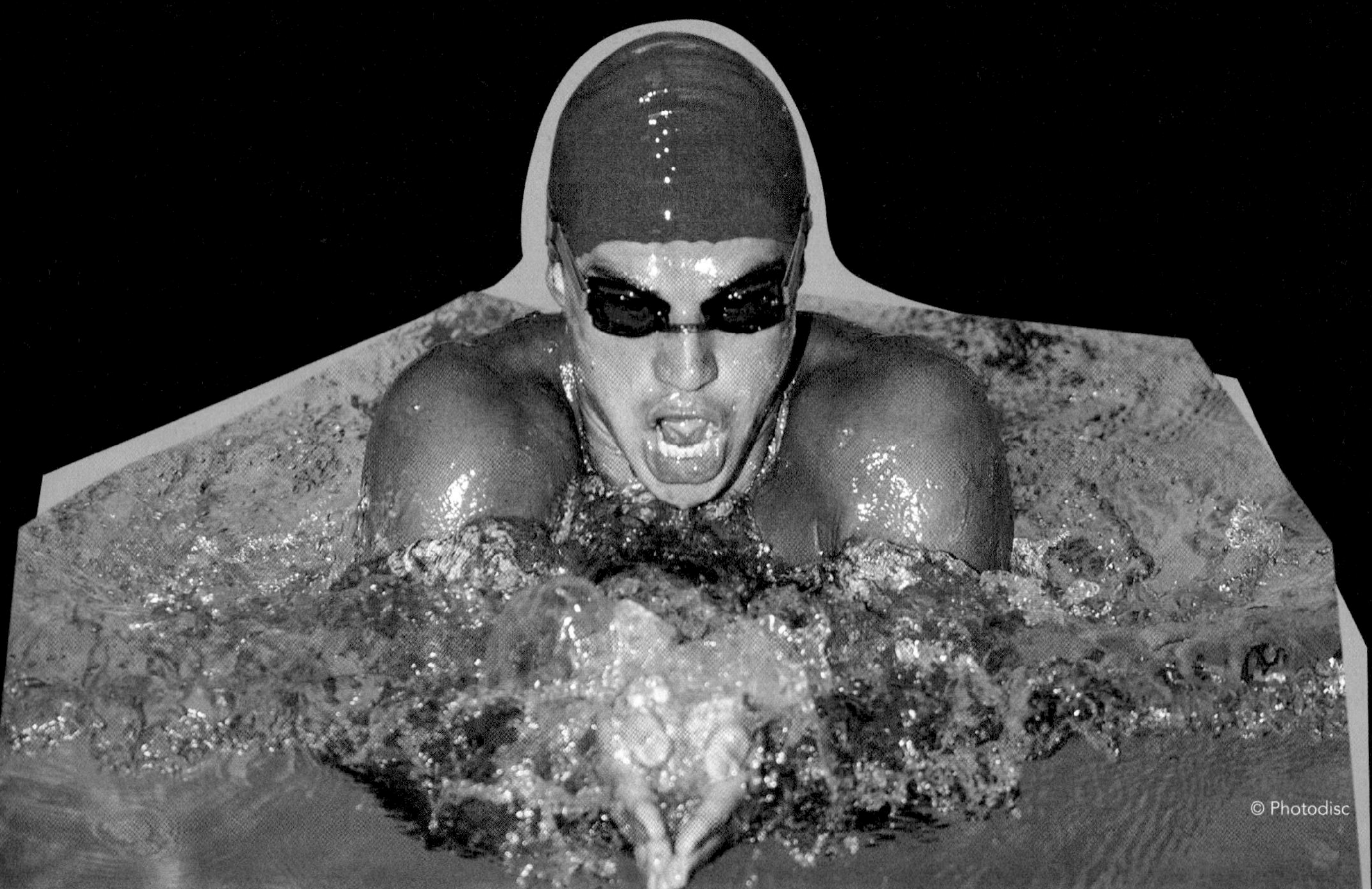

Lesson 9.1

Vigorous Aerobics, Sport, and Recreation

Lesson Objectives

After reading this lesson, you should be able to

1. describe the three types of vigorous activity (one from step 2 and two from step 3 of the Physical Activity Pyramid),
2. describe several types of vigorous aerobic activity (pyramid step 2),
3. define *sport* and describe the four categories of vigorous sport (pyramid step 3), and
4. define *recreation* and *leisure* and describe several types of vigorous recreation (pyramid step 3).

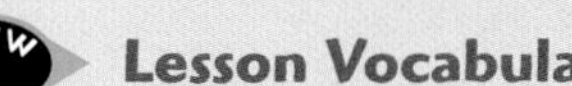

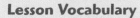

Lesson Vocabulary

aerobic, anaerobic activity, anaerobic capacity, circuit training, leisure time, lifetime sport, recreation, sport, vigorous aerobics, vigorous recreation, vigorous sport

How often do you engage in activities that make you breathe hard and sweat? Did you know that building fitness increases your chances of living longer? The Physical Activity Pyramid shows two types of vigorous physical activity: vigorous aerobics (step 2) and vigorous sport and recreation (step 3) (figure 9.1). Activities included in these steps are more vigorous (requiring 7 METs or more) than the moderate activities included in step 1 (which require 4 to 7 METs) and are especially good for building cardiorespiratory endurance. (As discussed in the Moderate Physical Activity chapter, 1 MET represents the energy you expend when at rest.) The MET count increases as activity becomes more vigorous. Research shows that vigorous physical activity (7+ METs) provides the health benefits of moderate activity—and more. In this lesson, you'll learn more about the many types of vigorous activity.

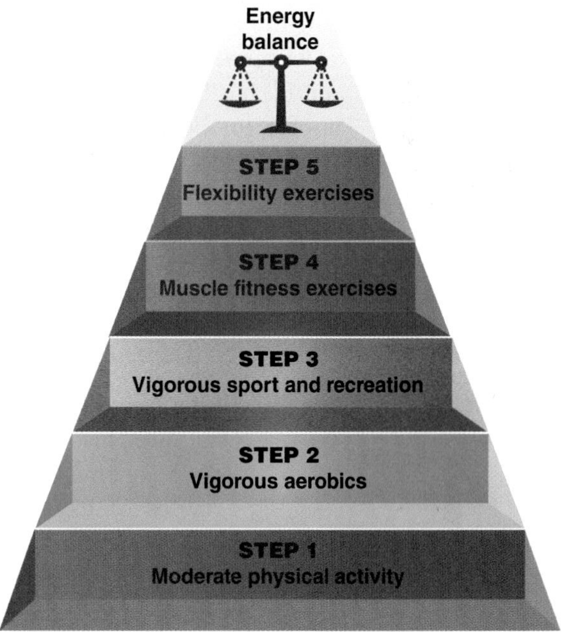

FIGURE 9.1 Vigorous aerobics, sport, and recreation (steps 2 and 3) build cardiorespiratory fitness and have many other health benefits.

Vigorous Aerobic Activity

Most activities included in the Physical Activity Pyramid (including moderate activities) can be considered **aerobic**. But only activities that are intense enough to elevate your heart rate above your threshold of training and into your target zone are considered **vigorous aerobics**. Aerobic activities—such as jogging, aerobic dancing, cycling, and swimming—are among the most popular and most beneficial of all the activities included in the Physical Activity Pyramid. Their popularity results from the following reasons.

- They often do not require high levels of skill.
- They frequently are not competitive.
- They often can be done at or near home.
- They often do not require a partner or group.

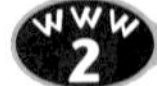

There are many types of vigorous aerobic activity. Some of the most popular are described in the following sections. Some activities could be classified in more than one section of the Physical Activity Pyramid. For example, swimming is a sport, a type of vigorous aerobic activity, and a type of vigorous recreation; in this book, it is classified as a vigorous aerobic activity. Each activity is described only once in this chapter, even if it could fit in multiple places.

Aerobic Dance

Aerobic dance involves continuously performing various dance steps to music. Unlike social dancers, aerobic dancers typically dance by themselves, often following a leader or a video. This activity first became popular in the 1970s and remains one of the most popular forms of aerobic exercise. Forms of aerobic dance include low-impact, high-impact, and step aerobics. Low-impact aerobics is typically done with one foot staying on the ground at all times. This form is best for beginners because it leads to fewer injuries than other forms. High-impact aerobics is typically more vigorous and involves jumping. Step aerobics involves dance steps done on a step or box. Some types of aerobic dance use light weights, rubber bands, and other types of exercise equipment, as well as movements from other activities such as martial arts.

Aerobic Exercise Machines

Types of aerobic exercise machines include treadmills, stair steppers, exercise bicycles, rowing machines, and ski machines. You can purchase these machines for use in your own home or use them in health clubs and schools. They can be effective if used properly, but some people do not find exercise on machines to be as enjoyable as activities that allow them to move more freely. For example, skiing may be more enjoyable than using a ski machine. On the other hand, exercise machines are often convenient and efficient.

Bicycling

Bicycling could be classified as a sport because some people compete in it and as a recreational activity because some do it for fun. If done slowly, it can also be considered a form of moderate physical activity. It is included here because it is often done continuously at a consistent speed that elevates the heart rate. Some forms of cycling, such as BMX and downhill mountain biking, are considered extreme sports.

Cooper's Aerobics

Dr. Ken Cooper, founder of the Cooper Institute in Dallas, Texas, created the term *aerobics*. He has been so successful in promoting physical activity that in Brazil and some other South American countries, some forms of aerobic activity (aerobics), such as jogging, are referred to as "coopering" or "doing the cooper." He also developed a system in which points can be earned for doing vigorous aerobic activities each week.

Circuit Training

Circuit training involves performing several different exercises one after another. The performer does one exercise for a period of time, then moves to the next with only a brief time between exercises. The goal is to keep the heart rate in the target zone. Circuit training can use exercise machines, small equipment such as jump ropes or rubber bands, free weights, or no equipment at all (for example, calisthenics). Doing different activities helps build muscle fitness as well as cardiorespiratory endurance and can increase your enjoyment because of the variety. Sometimes people use music to determine how much time is spent on each exercise. A break in the music signals that it's time to move to the next exercise.

Dance

Dance is one of the oldest art forms and has been a means of expression in many cultures. Some dance forms are not only enjoyable but also excellent forms of vigorous aerobic exercise. More traditional dance activities include modern, ballet, folk, and square dance. Another category of dance is social dance, which includes both more traditional types (such as the waltz, country dancing, and Latin dancing) and newer forms (such as hip-hop and line dancing). Some dance activities have been altered so that traditional steps are used in ways that are similar to aerobic dance. For example, Zumba uses Latin music and Latin dance steps in ways that resemble aerobic dance. All can be good forms of vigorous aerobics if you do them vigorously enough to elevate your heart rate.

Jogging and Running

Jogging and running consistently rank among the most popular forms of vigorous aerobic activity. Jogging is generally considered to be noncompetitive, whereas running is considered to be jogging that is done more seriously. Runners often participate in competitive events such as 5K and 10K races. Jogging and running are combined into one category here because they are very similar. You'll learn more about them in the self-assessment that follows this lesson.

Martial Arts Exercise

Judo and karate are just two of the several hundred martial arts practiced around the world. Different countries throughout the world have different forms. Martial arts can build various parts of fitness, but they are not always good at building cardiorespiratory endurance because they may not involve enough continuous activity to keep the heart rate elevated. Some forms of martial arts, however, have been combined with aerobic dance to create martial arts exercises; examples include Tae Bo and cardio karate. These forms of exercise can build cardiorespiratory endurance but may not be as effective for learning self-defense as more traditional techniques.

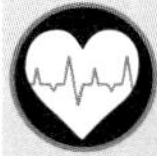

FITNESS TECHNOLOGY: Global Positioning System

The global positioning system (GPS) is a satellite-based system that communicates precise location information to places around the world. Satellites send signals to a receiver, which sends the signal to a computer that analyzes the information. The GPS was developed by the U.S. government to aid in national defense, but the technology is now available for consumer use. GPS technology is quite accurate and has been used in automobiles to help drivers find their way. It is now being used to help bikers, joggers, hikers, and others who perform outdoor physical activities. The GPS can also provide information about how fast you're moving, the distance you've traveled, the altitude you've gained or lost, and the average pace for your total workout. The first GPS systems for use in physical activity were complicated and required arm or leg straps with a receiver as well as a watchlike device worn on the arm. Others required a computer chip built into shoes to pick up the satellite signal. Technology changes rapidly, however, and now GPS devices for use in physical activity are more advanced.

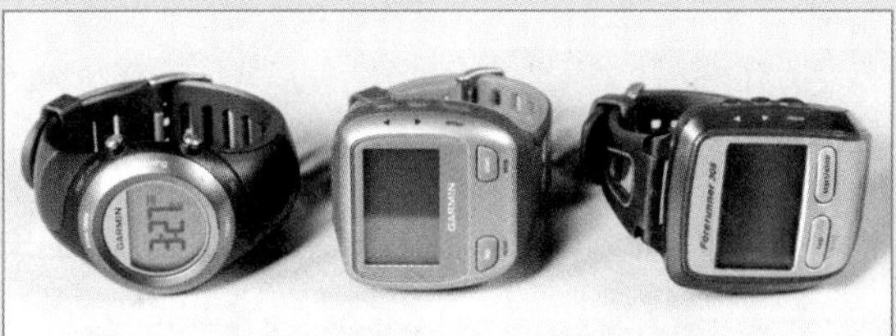

GPS technology can help track your physical activity—for example, these watches can track how far a jogger has run.

Using Technology

Research GPS technology for use in physical activity. Identify the device that you think would be the best buy and give reasons for your choice.

Rope Jumping

Rope jumping has long been used by boxers and other athletes as a method of training. Because it requires moving the arms and legs, as well as the entire body, it can be quite vigorous. For this reason, people sometimes alternate rope jumping with other forms of exercise, such as calisthenics. Practitioners have developed many rope-jumping moves. Rope jumping is inexpensive and can easily be done at home or in your neighborhood. You can also easily transport the needed equipment when traveling.

Swimming

Swimming is both a sport and a form of recreation. It is included here because it is one of the most popular fitness activities among adults and can serve as a good way to improve cardiorespiratory endurance for almost all people. Like water aerobics, it is a good choice for people who are overweight, elderly, or suffering from joint problems. For swimming to be an effective aerobic exercise, however, your heart rate must be elevated, which means that you must swim continuously for many minutes. Many people who swim do not meet either of these standards.

Water Aerobics

Water aerobics, sometimes called aqua dynamics, involves doing calisthenics or dance steps in a swimming pool. This form of aerobic exercise is especially good for people who are overweight, elderly, or suffering from arthritis or other joint problems because the water reduces stress on the joints. For stronger exercisers, water can also be used to provide resistance and thus increase the intensity of exercise.

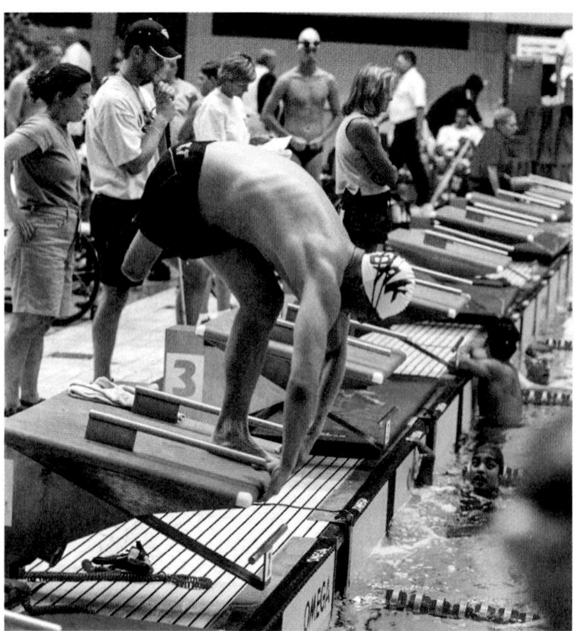

Swimming can be a good form of vigorous aerobics.

Vigorous Sport

Sport involves physical activity that is competitive (has a winner and loser) and follows well-established rules. Some sports, such as golf and bowling, are classified as moderate physical activity (step 1 of the Physical Activity Pyramid). **Vigorous sports** (step 3 of the pyramid) elevate the heart rate above the threshold level and into the target zone for cardiorespiratory endurance.

There are so many vigorous sports that it is impossible to mention them all here. We can, however, mention general categories: team sports; dual sports; individual sports; and outdoor, challenge, or extreme sports. Certain other sports are not considered here either because they are not among the most popular or because they have little relevance to a personal physical activity program (for example, auto racing and horse racing).

Team Sports

Team sports such as football, hockey, soccer, volleyball, and basketball are among the most popular for high school students and for adult spectators. These activities can be very good for helping participants build fitness (though of course they do little for the fitness of spectators!). Team sports can be harder to do after your school years are completed because they require other participants (teammates), as well as special equipment and facilities. Even though baseball and softball involve some vigorous activity and training for these sports is often vigorous, they are usually considered to be moderate activities.

No team sport is among the 10 most popular types of physical activity performed by adults in the United States, but basketball is one of the few listed among the top 20. The 10 most popular activities are mostly either moderate physical activities or vigorous aerobics. Because relatively few people who play team sports when they are young continue to pursue them for a lifetime, it will be important for you to actively seek opportunities to continue

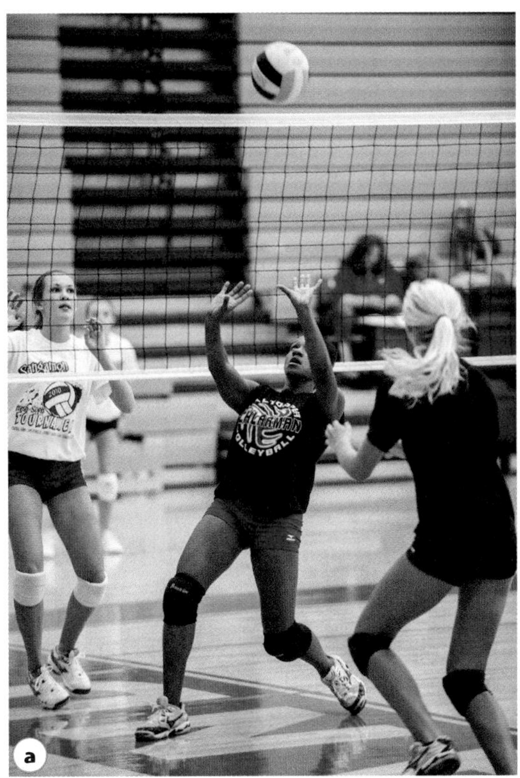

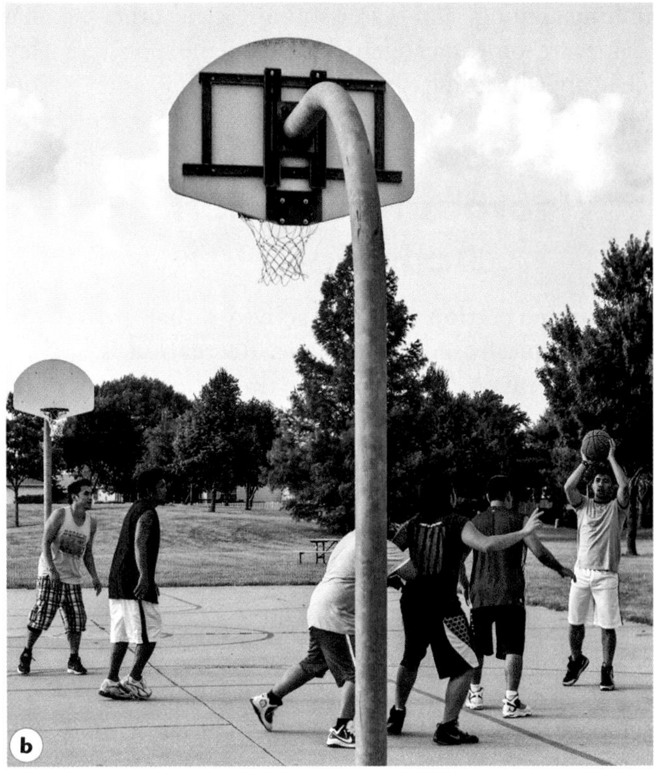

Team sports: *(a)* Volleyball is among the most popular team sports for high school students in the United States; *(b)* basketball is one of the few team sports listed among the top 20 physical activities performed by adults in the United States.

if you want to play team sports as you grow older. Another way to stay active is to begin learning an individual sport, a dual sport, or an aerobic activity that you can enjoy later in life.

Dual or Partner Sports

Dual sports are those you can do with just one other person (the person you are playing against) or with a partner against another set of partners (for example, tennis doubles). Examples include tennis, badminton, fencing, and judo. Because they require fewer people than team sports, dual sports are often referred to as **lifetime sports** because they are easier to continue throughout your life. Tennis is often included in the top 10 participation activities in the United States, partly because it can be done with just one other person and because tennis courts are now available to most people.

Some dual sports are not activities that many people do as adults. For example, wrestling is considered a dual sport but is not often done as a lifetime sport, even though it does develop many important parts of health-related fitness. Dual sports that are not done by many adults are not considered lifetime sports.

Individual Sports

Individual sports are those that you can do by yourself. Golf, gymnastics, and bowling are truly individual sports because you do not have to have a partner or a team to perform them. Many of these sports are also lifetime sports because they are more likely to be done throughout life, although some, such as gymnastics, are not done by many people later in life (and gymnastics often requires a spotter). Skiing and skating are two forms of vigorous recreation that are also sometimes classified as individual sports.

Outdoor, Challenge, or Extreme Sports

Many of the types of vigorous recreation can also be classified as sports. Some vigorous recreation activities are sometimes referred to as outdoor or challenge sports, such as mountain biking, rock climbing, sailing, and water skiing. Some other activities are sometimes referred to as extreme sports, such as snowboarding, skateboarding, surfing, and BMX cycling.

Vigorous Recreation Activities

Vigorous recreation includes activities that are fun and, typically, noncompetitive. **Recreation** is something you do during your free time; therefore, recreational activities are sometimes called leisure activities. Recreation includes both physical activity and other pursuits, such as art and music. Here, of course, we focus on recreational activity that requires you to use your large muscles and involves considerable movement.

Many types of vigorous recreation are done outdoors because participants feel that the beauty of the setting and the fresh air help rejuvenate them. Examples of vigorous recreation include the following.

Backpacking and Hiking

Hiking is particularly enjoyable because it takes place outdoors and can be done either independently or in a group. Most county, state, and national parks offer scenic trails for hikers of all levels of experience. Hiking usually involves a one-day trip, whereas backpacking often involves a multi-day venture that requires you to carry food, shelter, and other supplies on your back.

> "[Leave] all the afternoon for exercise and recreation, which are as necessary as reading; I will rather say more necessary, because health is worth more than learning."
>
> —Thomas Jefferson, U.S. president

Boating, Canoeing, Kayaking, and Rowing

Boating can be done in various forms that offer the enjoyment of water and the outdoors, free from the hassles of normal daily life. When done vigorously, these activities also help you build fitness and promote good health. Kayaking and rowing can be especially vigorous, and they require considerable skill to perform well and safely. Even when not done vigorously, boating activities can be relaxing and refreshing.

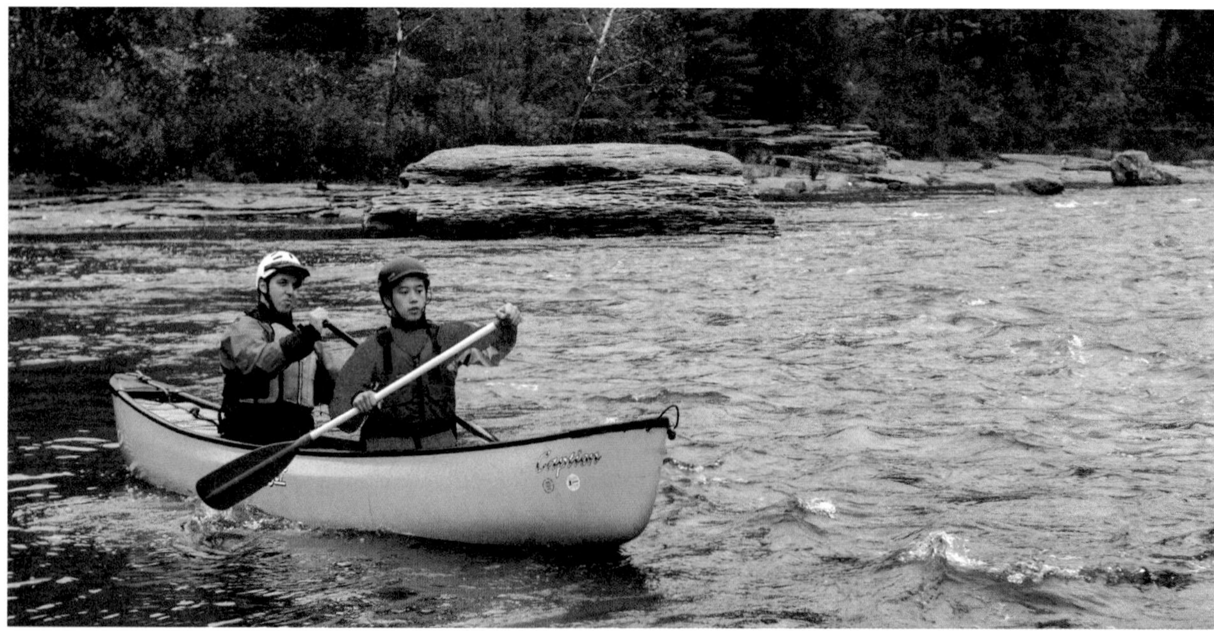

Boating can be a vigorous recreational activity that builds cardiorespiratory endurance and provides other health benefits.

SCIENCE IN ACTION: Anaerobic Physical Activity

Unlike aerobic activity that can be sustained for long periods of time, **anaerobic activity** is activity that is so intense your body cannot supply adequate oxygen to sustain performance for more than a few seconds. Very vigorous anaerobic activity, such as an all-out sprint, can be sustained for only about 10 seconds and relies on high-energy fuel stored in the muscles (ATP-PC). Some vigorous activities (also anaerobic) are not "all-out" but are still very intense (they can be sustained for 11 to 90 seconds), and for those activities, the glycolytic system is used. Glucose (glycogen) stored in the muscles and liver provides the energy. Anaerobic activities are typically done in short bursts followed by rest periods. During the anaerobic activities your body builds up an oxygen debt because it can't take in enough oxygen to replenish the fuel needed to continue performance. After the activity is completed, oxygen is available to replenish the fuel stores—it repays the oxygen debt.

Your ability to perform anaerobic activity is referred to as **anaerobic capacity**. One of the most common tests of anaerobic capacity is the Wingate Test, which is done on a bicycle ergometer (stationary bicycle) and requires an all-out effort to pedal as fast as possible. This test is typically reserved for people interested in high-level anaerobic performance.

Sports such as basketball, football, and soccer involve sprints up the court or down the field. These sprints are anaerobic because they often require short but maximal effort. Sports allow time for recovery after these anaerobic bursts. This pattern means that players' heart rates may exceed the target zone during anaerobic sprints, then drop below the threshold of training during rest intervals (for example, when a free throw is taken in basketball). In fact, vigorous sports are not true aerobic activities, but when they are done for similar amounts of time they can be considered similar to vigorous aerobics. This is because they provide health benefits and improve cardiorespiratory endurance.

These sports offer the added advantage of building anaerobic capacity (also called *anaerobic power* and *anaerobic fitness*). Anaerobic capacity allows you to recover more quickly from anaerobic bursts and therefore improve your performance in certain sport activities. Some vigorous recreation activities, such as kayaking, are similar to vigorous sport activities in that they require good cardiorespiratory endurance as well as anaerobic fitness.

People who train for vigorous sport and recreation activities often use special anaerobic training techniques, such as interval training. Interval training involves repeated high-intensity exercise alternated with rest periods or bouts of lower-intensity exercise. There are many different kinds of interval training, including high-intensity interval training (HIIT) that alternates bouts of exercise at various intensities and lengths. The FIT formula for the most commonly used type of interval training is as follows.

- **F**requency = three to six days a week
- **I**ntensity = upper level of the target heart rate zone (because your exercise bouts are short)
- **T**ime = multiple exercise bouts of 10 to 60 seconds alternated with 1- to 2-minute rest periods or bouts of moderate exercise (totaling at least 10 minutes of exercise)

Depending on your goal, your length of exercise may vary from the durations given in the preceding formula. This type of training is appropriate for people who have already achieved the good fitness zone for cardiorespiratory endurance and who have regularly been doing vigorous activity. Before beginning this type of training, consult your teacher or coach or other qualified expert in kinesiology.

Student Activity

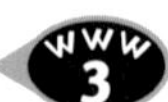

While participating in an intermittent activity—such as basketball, soccer, or tennis—count your heart rate right after several vigorous bursts of activity. Determine whether the intensity of the activity is near the upper level of your target heart rate zone for aerobic activity.

Orienteering

Orienteering combines walking, jogging, and skilled map reading. It is usually done in a rural area and might include hiking through rugged terrain. Participants depart from a starting point in staggered fashion every few minutes so that no participant can simply follow another. Each participant uses a compass and a map that describes a course up to 10 miles (16 kilometers) long. The compass is used to help locate several checkpoints marked by flags or other identifiers. At each checkpoint, the participant marks a card to indicate that he or she has located it. The activity can be competitive if the goal is to cover the course as fast as possible. Urban orienteering uses the same ideas and skills but in inner-city areas rather than rural settings.

Rock Climbing and Bouldering

Many schools now teach rock climbing on climbing walls. Learning on a climbing wall allows you to get proper instruction with good spotting (protection against falling). More advanced climbers are skilled in using special safety ropes and equipment. Beginners and intermediate climbers should always climb with the help of an expert. When rock climbing is done properly with proper equipment, it is a relatively safe activity. It's also a good type of activity for building muscle fitness.

Bouldering is a type of rock climbing in which the climber tries to reach the top of a boulder using only gloves and special shoes (no special ropes or other equipment). Bouldering is most often done outside, but some clubs have artificial boulders for indoor climbing. The height of climbs is typically limited to 30 feet (about 9 meters). As with rock climbing, bouldering requires specials skills, so instruction is recommended for beginners.

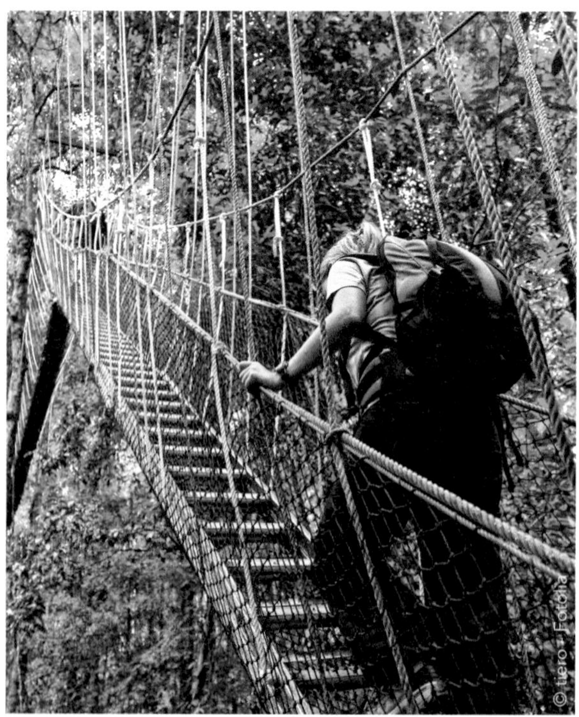

Outdoor vigorous recreational activities have health benefits and help you meet national activity guidelines.

Skateboarding

As you probably know, skateboarding is a popular recreational activity among teens. Competitive skateboarding is now considered an extreme sport. Therefore, it can be considered both a recreational activity and a sport (for high-level competitors). Like in-line skating, skateboarding is a risky activity, so you should use proper safety equipment and seek proper instruction. You also need to find a proper place to perform skateboarding. Many skate hangouts are unsafe, and they are sometimes located in places where skating is prohibited. But many cities offer planned skate parks to provide safe places to skate.

FIT FACT

Leisure time is more than free time. It is an attitude of declaring freedom from doing things you have to do. Similarly, the word *recreation* suggests refreshing or re-creating yourself. For this reason, a recreational activity is one that you do during your leisure or free time to refresh or re-create yourself. Recreational activities are done for fun and enjoyment. They need not be vigorous or purposeful. They can include watching TV, reading a book, playing chess, and doing many other relatively inactive pursuits. Some leisure activities—such as fishing, camping, and some forms of boating—can be considered moderate activities.

Skating

Types of skating include in-line, roller, and ice. In-line skating is one of the fastest-growing activities in the United States. It was originally developed as a method of training for cross-country skiers in the summer, but its popularity has grown, and in-line sports (for example, hockey) have been developed. One study by a sports medicine group found that in-line skating was the most risky of the many participation activities studied, possibly because people fail to use proper safety equipment or because they try advanced skills too soon. The risk involved in skating activities makes it especially important for you to follow the safety guidelines described later in this chapter.

Skiing

Kinds of skiing include cross-country skiing (a type of Nordic skiing), downhill skiing, snowboarding, and ski jumping. Cross-country skiing is typically done at a steady pace over a relatively long distance. For this reason, it could be considered a vigorous aerobic activity. Downhill skiing typically involves faster skiing, sometimes over moguls (bumps) and jumps. Snowboarding is like skateboarding on snow and has become extremely popular. It has joined the other forms of skiing as an Olympic sport, and some forms of snowboarding (halfpipe, superpipe, and slopestyle) can also be considered extreme sports. Ski jumping is also an Olympic sport, and it involves skiing down a ramp and jumping, trying to land as far down the hill as possible. All types of skiing could be considered sports, but they are included here because so many people do them just for fun and recreation, although ski jumping isn't typically a recreational activity for most people.

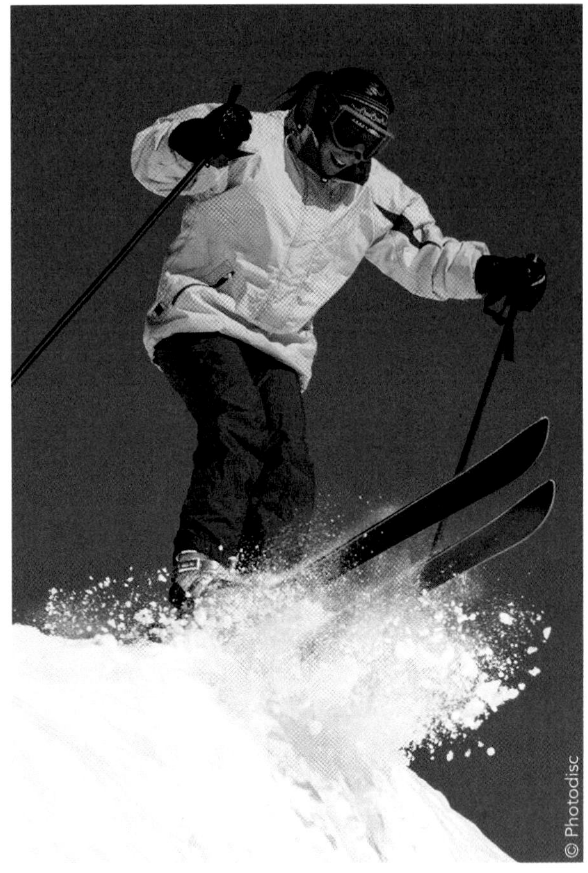

Skiing can be considered both a vigorous sport and a form of vigorous recreation.

Lesson Review

1. What is vigorous aerobic activity, and what are the two major categories of vigorous activity included in the Physical Activity Pyramid?
2. What are some types of vigorous aerobic activity?
3. How is *sport* defined, and what are some categories of sport? Give an example of each.
4. How is *vigorous recreation* defined, and what are some examples?

SELF-ASSESSMENT: Assessing Jogging Techniques

If you're looking for an excellent vigorous activity that requires little skill and no equipment—except for a good pair of running shoes and proper clothing—then jogging might be for you. Millions of people jog (that is, run recreationally and noncompetitively), and millions more run competitively (and are called runners rather than joggers). Learning to jog properly can help you make the activity safe and fun. Guidelines for jogging have been developed on the basis of the principles of biomechanics and exercise physiology. Look over the two sets of principles, then study table 9.1 to learn about jogging guidelines.

Biomechanical Principles

- Changing velocity (acceleration) is less efficient than maintaining a constant velocity.
- Applying force in the direction of movement is more efficient than moving to the side.
- Friction is necessary in order to apply force and to prevent slipping.
- Action (foot striking) results in a reaction (impact to the sole of the foot or heel).
- Stability requires a wide base of support.
- Proper leverage increases efficiency.
- Proper posture increases efficiency.

Exercise Physiology Principles

- Muscle contractions not used to produce movement are inefficient.
- You must do more than normal to improve (this is the overload principle).

Work With a Partner

- Jog about 100 yards (90 meters) while your partner stands behind you and checks your technique.
- Have your partner answer the questions in table 9.1 after watching you jog. Your instructor may provide a worksheet that contains the questions.
- Now have your partner jog while you evaluate his or her technique.
- Discuss the assessment with your partner.
- Both you and your partner can perform the jog a second time.
- Try to correct your technique and have your partner check you again. Do the same for your partner.

The self-assessment not only will help you jog more efficiently but also can reduce your risk of injury. Improper jogging technique can cause injuries such as sore shins, sore calves, and even a sore back. Having your feet and legs out of alignment can cause unnecessary strain on your joints and muscles.

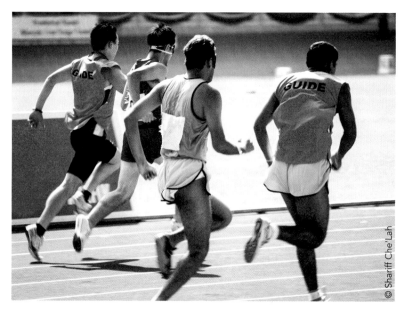

Proper technique is important for everyone, from beginning joggers to elite runners.

TABLE 9.1 Jogging Self-Assessment Guidelines and Checklist

Guideline	Principle	Checklist	✔
Use proper foot action. Land on your heel or your entire foot. Then rock forward and push off with the ball of your foot and your toes.	Leverage	Do you land on your heel or whole foot? Do you push off with the ball of your foot and toes?	
Swing your legs and feet forward. Do not let your feet turn out to the sides.	Force application	Do your legs and feet swing and land straight ahead?	
Swing your arms forward and backward. Do not swing them across your body or to the sides.	Force application	Do your arms swing straight forward and backward?	
Keep your trunk fairly erect. When jogging, do not lean forward as you would when starting to run fast. Keep your head and chest up.	Proper posture	Is your body erect or leaning forward only slightly? Are your head and chest up?	
Use a longer step than your normal walking step.	Leverage	Is your jogging stride longer than your walking stride?	
Keep your arms bent at the elbow and your hands relaxed. Try to keep your shoulders relaxed. Avoid jogging with a clenched jaw to allow your upper body to relax more.	Efficient muscle use	Are your elbows bent properly (90 degrees) with your hands relaxed? Is your jaw relaxed?	
Jog at a steady pace. Avoid speeding up and slowing down. Correct jogging pace can vary from person to person. Find your own pace that elevates your heart rate into your target zone. If you are panting or gasping for breath, you are jogging too fast.	Velocity Overload	Is your pace steady? Is your heart rate in your target zone after several minutes of jogging? Is your pace slow enough to prevent gasping for breath?	
Wear shoes with a wide sole and heel, good heel cushions, and outer soles designed for running.	Stability Friction	Do your shoes have a wide heel and sole and good tread?	

Beginner's Jogging Workout

This workout helps you learn about how fast to jog in order to get a fitness benefit (by reaching your target heart rate). Try this workout after you've practiced your jogging technique.

1. Determine your target heart rate.
2. Jog for five minutes, trying to get your heart to the target level. Keep track of how long you run—how long you run is more important than how far. By using time instead of distance, you can jog anywhere. Set your own course. Try to jog half the time moving away from your starting point and the other half returning to your starting point. If you are not near your starting point at the end of five minutes, walk the rest of the way back.
3. Focus on using the jogging techniques that you learned earlier in this self-assessment.
4. At the end of five minutes, determine your one-minute exercise heart rate. Determine whether your rate was in your target heart rate zone.
5. Jog for five minutes again. If your exercise heart rate was lower than your target heart rate on the first jog, jog faster this time. If your exercise heart rate was higher than your target rate on the first jog, jog slower this time. If your exercise heart rate was in the target zone on the first jog, jog at the same speed this time. After your second run, count your exercise heart rate again.
6. As directed by your teacher, record your results.

Lesson 9.2

Preparing and Performing a Safe and Vigorous Physical Activity Program

Lesson Objectives

After reading this lesson, you should be able to

1. describe several guidelines for participating safely in vigorous physical activity,
2. collect information about your personal needs and build a fitness and activity profile,
3. set goals for vigorous physical activity, and
4. select vigorous activities and write a plan for vigorous activity.

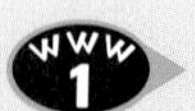

Lesson Vocabulary

compendium, over-exercising

Are you prepared to do regular vigorous physical activity? In this lesson, you'll learn why it's important to be well prepared before you begin. You'll also use the five steps of program planning to prepare your personal plan for vigorous physical activity. Creating your plan will help you meet national physical activity guidelines both now and later in life. Vigorous activities can be some of the most enjoyable, and they also offer many health benefits.

Fitness for Vigorous Aerobics, Sport, and Recreation

Just as vigorous physical activity contributes to good fitness, you also must stay fit in order to participate in vigorous activity. Some people mistakenly assume that fitness is not necessary for certain sports, especially if the sport itself does little to build fitness. For example, softball is not particularly good for developing fitness, but it does require good fitness. Similarly, some people snow-ski only once or twice a year and otherwise do not exercise regularly. Nevertheless, they believe they are fit enough to ski. In reality, these people should exercise regularly for at least several weeks before skiing in order to get ready for the activity and to reduce their chance of injury.

Participating in vigorous activity involves greater risk of injury than doing no activity or doing light or moderate activity. Even vigorous aerobics, which is relatively safe compared to other vigorous sport and recreational activities, can result in injury if overdone. Jogging (or running) is one of the top five activities in terms of injury to participants, and regular participants in high-impact and step aerobics are also often injured. Unlike common sport injuries such as ligament sprains and muscle strains, the injuries typically experienced by joggers and aerobic dancers involve overuse—for example, heel bruises, sore shins, stress fractures in the legs and feet, and sometimes knee or back injury. Long distance runners and aerobic dance instructors also have a higher-than-normal rate of injury. More generally, the people most prone to injury are those who train every day or who participate in several vigorous aerobic activity sessions in a day.

Safety Tips for Vigorous Physical Activity

- **Warm up before your workout.** Use a low- to moderate-intensity general warm-up for 5 to 10 minutes, a series of dynamic exercises, or a stretching warm-up, depending on the activity to be performed. For a stretching warm-up, remember to hold stretches no more than 30 seconds prior to strength, power, and speed activities.
- **Cool down after the workout.** A cool-down helps you recover more quickly.
- **Wear proper safety equipment.** For example, bikers and skaters should wear helmets, and skaters should also wear hand and knee pads. Dress appropriately for the weather.
- **Use safe equipment.** Bikes should have lights and reflectors. Backpacking equipment should

fit your body size, and loads should not be too heavy. Skis and other equipment should be in good repair, properly sized, and equipped with proper releases or other safety features. Boaters should wear life preservers. Rock climbers should use appropriate safety equipment. When doing any vigorous activity, especially in the heat, drink water regularly.

- **Get proper instruction.** Whether you're skiing, in-line skating, boating, rock-climbing, or doing some other activity, you should get proper instruction before participating. Performing an activity improperly has caused many people to get injured or have an accident.
- **Perform within the limits of your current skills.** Many injuries occur because people try to perform beyond their skill limits; for example, beginning skiers should not attempt to ski advanced slopes. For all activities, start with simple skills and then gradually attempt to perform more difficult skills as your abilities improve.
- **Don't overdo it.** Taking at least one day a week to rest can help you avoid injury, especially if you're participating in a vigorous aerobic activity such as aerobic dance or running. Most injuries can be prevented simply by not **over-exercising** (doing so much exercise that you increase your risk of injury or soreness).
- **Plan ahead.** If you're going on a hike, make sure that you have a map and know where you're going. Carry an emergency phone. If you're going skiing, make sure that the trail is open, and don't ski in restricted areas. When backpacking, carry enough food and water to supply you if you get lost. When traveling in an unfamiliar area, stay with your group.

For most vigorous sport and recreation activities, you must have good fitness in order to perform well. For example, a baseball player must sprint between bases, slide into bases, and jump to catch the ball. Each of these actions could result in an injury if the player is not physically fit. Good or high-performance fitness is especially necessary for activities with the following characteristics.

FIT FACT

Each year, participation in common recreational activities leads to two million medically treated injuries among youth in the United States. Medical groups state that you can dramatically decrease your risk of injury by following simple safety tips when participating in physical activity.

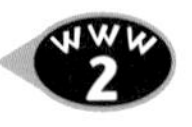

- Physical contact (football, rugby, wrestling, ice hockey)
- Sprinting (baseball, softball, soccer, ultimate)
- Sudden fast starts and stops (volleyball, racquetball, track, basketball)
- Vigorous jumping (basketball, high jumping, soccer)
- Danger of falling (skiing, skating, judo)
- Danger of overstretching muscles (tennis, football, squash)

Finding the Best Vigorous Activities for You

In this class, you'll get the opportunity to try many types of vigorous activity, such as aerobic dance, step

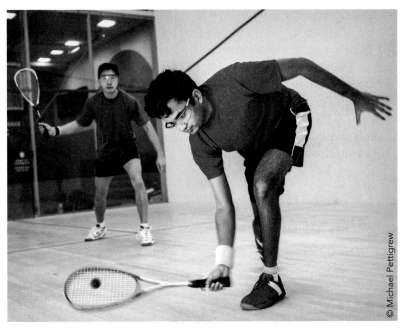

Exercise helps you get fit, but you must also be fit to perform physical activities safely.

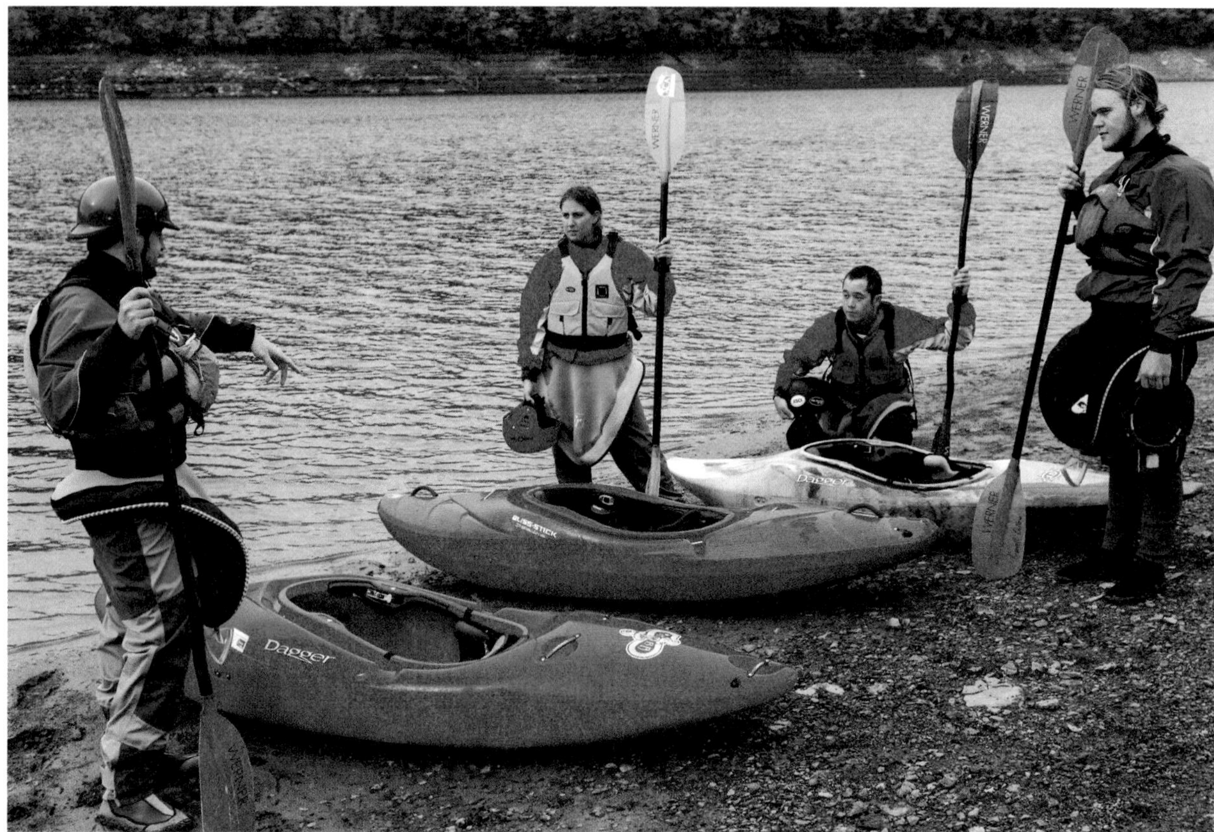

Important safety tips for vigorous physical activity include using safe equipment and getting proper instruction.

aerobics, line dancing, jogging, exercise circuits, and rope jumping. Try a variety of activities to discover which ones you like best. For any given activity, try it more than once before you decide whether to do it in the future. It takes time to decide what you like and don't like. If you're going to stick with an activity over the long term, it must be enjoyable. To help you enjoy an activity, consider finding good instruction, wearing appropriate clothing, getting good equipment (if necessary), and finding others with whom you can participate.

Preparing a Vigorous Physical Activity Plan

Lin Su used the five steps of program planning to prepare a vigorous physical activity program. She had been doing some regular moderate activity but wanted to do more vigorous activity. Her program is described in the following sections of this chapter.

FIT FACT

Teen boys are more likely than teen girls to be vigorously active at least three times a week, and high school girls are especially likely to become less active as they grow older. Health experts are interested in finding ways to help teen girls be more physically active.

Step 1: Determine Your Personal Needs

To get started, Lin Su wrote down her fitness test results that related to vigorous physical activity. She also made a list of the vigorous physical activities that she had performed over the past week. Her results are shown in figure 9.2.

Lin Su's cardiorespiratory endurance ratings showed that she was in the marginal category for each of the self-assessments that she performed. She

Physical fitness profile			
Fitness self-assessment	**Score**	**Rating**	
Walking test	Time: 18:30 Heart rate: 150	Marginal	
PACER	37 mL/kg/min	Marginal	
Step test	Heart rate: 104	Marginal	
One-mile (1.6 km) run	No score	No rating	
Physical activity profile			
Day	**Vigorous activity (min)**	**All activity (min)**	**Met 60 min guideline?**
Mon.	0	40	
Tues.	20	60	✔
Wed.	0	40	
Thurs.	20	60	✔
Fri.	20	40	
Sat.	0	20	
Sun.	0	20	

FIGURE 9.2 Lin Su's vigorous physical activity and fitness profiles.

met the national activity guideline of 60 minutes per day on two days of the previous week. She did vigorous activity for 20 minutes on Tuesday and Thursday in her physical education class. On Friday she jogged for 20 minutes with her friend Eric, but she didn't do that regularly. She had also walked to and from school (20 minutes each way), and this moderate activity combined with her physical education activities and jogging totaled 60 minutes. On the other days, she did only moderate activity (walking to and from school) totaling less than 60 minutes, except on Friday when she had physical education class. Lin Su knew that she needed to be more active and especially wanted to do more vigorous activity.

WWW 3

Step 2: Consider Your Program Options

Lin Su wanted to include activities that would help her build her cardiorespiratory endurance and that offered other health-fitness benefits. She also wanted to focus on activities that she thought she would enjoy. To select vigorous activities, she used table 9.2, which illustrates the health-related fitness benefits of a wide variety of vigorous activities. Even this list, however, includes only a sample of the most popular vigorous aerobics, sport, and recreation activities; it was adapted from a larger **compendium** of activities. A link to the compendium can be found in the student section of the Health Opportunities Through Physical Education website.

After reviewing the list of activities, Lin Su wrote down her preferred activity options.

Continue Current Activities

- Walking to and from school
- Jogging
- Physical education class activities

Vigorous Aerobics

- More jogging
- Aerobic dance

Vigorous Recreation

- Hiking
- In-line skating

Vigorous Sport

- Tennis
- Badminton

School

- Before-school recreation
- After-school sports

TABLE 9.2 Health-Related Benefits of Selected Vigorous Physical Activities

Activity	Develops cardiorespiratory endurance	Develops strength	Develops muscular endurance	Develops flexibility	Helps control body fat
Aerobic dance*+	Excellent	Fair	Good	Fair	Excellent
Aerobics machine+	Excellent	Fair	Good	Poor	Excellent
Backpacking+	Fair	Fair	Excellent	Poor	Good/Excellent
Badminton+	Fair	Poor	Fair	Fair	Fair/Good
Baseball/Softball*	Poor	Poor	Poor	Poor	Poor/Fair
Basketball, half-court*+	Fair	Poor	Fair	Poor	Poor/Fair
Basketball, full-court*+	Excellent	Fair	Good	Poor	Excellent
Biking+	Good	Fair	Good	Poor	Good/Excellent
BMX cycling	Good	Good	Excellent	Fair	Good
Canoeing+	Fair	Fair	Fair	Poor	Fair/Good
Circuit training+	Good	Good	Good	Fair	Good/Excellent
Football*	Fair	Good	Fair	Poor	Fair
Gymnastics	Fair	Excellent	Excellent	Excellent	Fair
Handball/Racquetball*+	Good/Excellent	Fair	Good	Poor	Good/Excellent
Hiking	Fair	Fair	Fair/Good	Poor	Good
Hip-hop dance	Good/Excellent	Fair	Good	Fair	Good/Excellent
Horseback riding+	Poor	Poor	Poor	Poor	Poor
Kayaking*+	Good	Good	Good	Fair	Good
Martial arts*+	Good	Fair	Fair	Fair	Fair
Mountain or rock climbing*+	Good	Good	Good	Poor	Good
Racquetball*+	Good/Excellent	Fair	Good	Poor	Good/Excellent
Rowing (crew)*	Excellent	Fair	Excellent	Poor	Excellent
Sailing+	Poor	Poor	Poor	Poor	Poor
Skating (roller or ice)*+	Good	Fair	Good	Fair	Good
Skiing (cross-country)*+	Excellent	Fair	Good	Poor	Excellent
Skiing (downhill)*+	Fair/Good	Fair	Good	Poor	Fair/Good
Snowboarding*+	Fair/Good	Fair	Good	Fair	Fair/Good
Soccer*	Excellent	Fair	Good	Fair	Excellent
Social dance+	Fair	Poor	Fair	Fair	Fair
Surfing*+	Fair	Poor	Good	Fair	Fair/Good
Swimming+	Good	Fair	Good	Fair	Good/Excellent
Table tennis*+	Poor	Poor	Poor/Fair	Poor	Poor/Fair
Tennis*+	Good/Excellent	Fair	Good	Poor	Good/Excellent
Volleyball*+	Fair	Fair	Good	Poor	Fair/Good
Waterskiing*+	Fair	Fair	Good	Poor	Fair/Good

*Fitness needed to prevent injury.

+Lifetime activity.

Step 3: Set Goals

For this vigorous activity plan, Lin Su chose a time period of two weeks. Since this was too short to accommodate long-term goals, she developed only short-term physical activity goals for the plan. Later, she will develop long-term goals, including some physical fitness goals, when she prepares a longer plan. For now, in developing her short-term goals for vigorous physical activity, she referred to her activity preferences decided in step 2. She also reviewed her work to be sure that she was setting SMART goals. She set the following goals.

1. Continue to jog one day a week for 20 minutes.
2. Continue to do vigorous activity in physical education class two days a week (20 minutes).
3. Play tennis for 60 minutes of moderate activity one day every other week.
4. Do aerobic dance for 30 minutes one day a week.
5. Go hiking for 60 minutes one day every other week.

Step 4: Structure Your Program and Write It Down

Lin Su's written two-week plan for vigorous physical activity is shown in figure 9.3. Lin Su included most of the activities from her list. She didn't include badminton or in-line skating, and she didn't participate in before-school recreation or after-school sports. Her plan met the national activity guideline of at least 20 minutes of vigorous activity three days a week. In fact, her plan called for more than 20 minutes of vigorous activity on six days of the week. Lin Su decided to take a break from vigorous activity on Sunday. She also kept walking to and from school daily. Although this was moderate activity, she planned to keep doing it to help her meet the national activity goal of 60 minutes of moderate to vigorous physical activity each day.

Step 5: Keep a Log and Evaluate Your Program

Over the next two weeks, Lin Su will self-monitor her activities and place a checkmark in her written plan beside each of the activities that she performs.

Week 1				Week 2			
Day	Activity	Time	✔	Day	Activity	Time	✔
Mon.				Mon.			
Tues.	Physical education class	10:30–11:15 a.m.*		Tues.	Physical education class*	10:30–11:15 a.m.*	
Wed.	Aerobic dance	4:00–4:30 p.m.		Wed.	Aerobic dance	4:00–4:30 p.m.	
Thurs.	Physical education class	10:30–11:15 a.m.*		Thurs.	Physical education class	10:30–11:15 a.m.*	
Fri.	Jog	4:00–4:20 p.m.		Fri.	Jog	4:00–4:20 p.m.	
Sat.	Tennis	9:00–10:00 a.m.		Sat.	Hiking	9:00–10:00 a.m.	
Sun.	No planned activity			Sun.	No planned activity		

*Only 20 minutes of the 45-minute class included vigorous activity.

FIGURE 9.3 Lin Su's written plan.

CONSUMER CORNER: Using the Web for Fitness, Health, and Wellness Information

One national health goal in the United States for the year 2020 is to increase the number of high-quality websites related to health. Health is the most common subject of web searches, and 75 percent of all teens and young adults seek health information on the web. But many websites, including popular web encyclopedias, contain incorrect information about health, which can result in injury, illness, failure to get adequate care, and loss of money spent on products and treatments that don't work. With all this in mind, one of the most important goals of *HOPE* is to help you become a critical consumer of fitness, health, and wellness information. Consider the following guidelines when you search the web.

- Consider using websites provided by government agencies. They contain information supplied by experts based on scientific research. Most government website addresses end with the extension .gov. One example of a good governmental source for information is the U.S. Centers for Disease Control and Prevention.
- Consider using websites provided by universities and professional organizations (such as the American Medical Association). Professional organizations' website addresses typically end with the extension .org, and universities' addresses typically end with the extension .edu.
- Beware of websites with names intended to fool you. When the web was first developed, only a few extensions (such as .gov, .org, .edu, and .com) were available for use at the end of a web address. Now, many more extensions are in use, and some people take advantage of this variety to create copycat websites intended to fool you into thinking you're choosing a reliable site when in fact you're not. They do this by using the same name as a reliable website (or a similar name) but a different extension—for example, reliablewebsite.xyz instead of reliablewebsite.gov.

At the end of two weeks, she will evaluate her activity to see whether she met her goals, then use the evaluation to help her create another activity plan.

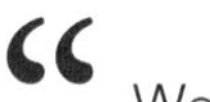

We are what we repeatedly do.

—Aristotle, Greek philosopher

In the Taking Action activity later in this lesson, you will get to use the same planning steps that Lin Su used to create a two-week personal plan for vigorous physical activity. Use tables similar to those used by Lin Su to help you in your planning. Then try out your program and see if you can meet your goals. The same steps can be used in the future to plan health goals or prepare for a special event, such as running a 10K race or participating on the cross-country team.

Lesson Review

1. What steps can you take to make vigorous activity safe and fun?
2. How can you assess personal needs and build a fitness and activity profile?
3. What are some factors to consider in setting goals for vigorous physical activity?
4. How can you best select vigorous activities and write a plan for vigorous activity?

TAKING CHARGE: Activity Participation

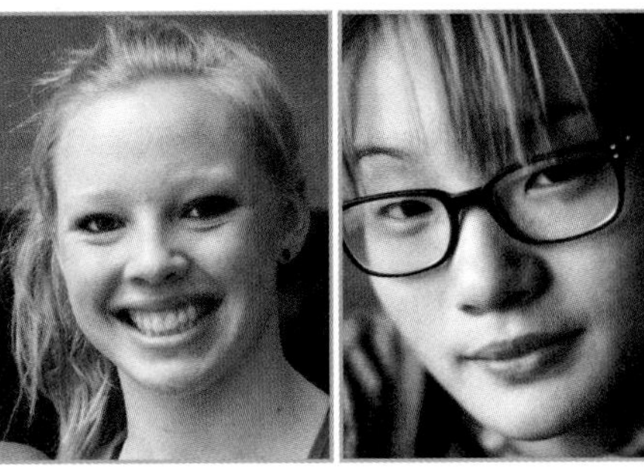

You can help yourself be active by choosing activities you're likely to do both now and throughout your life. One way to evaluate an activity is to find out the number of people who participate and how long they tend to stay involved. Here's an example.

At a recent high school reunion, the alumni enjoyed seeing their former classmates again. Everyone remembered Norma as an athlete. She had played soccer, basketball, and softball. What a surprise when her classmates discovered that 10 years later Norma was doing very little physical activity! The closest she got to participating in any sport was to watch her son's tee ball games. According to Norma, "It was just too hard to find people who wanted to play the team sports I used to enjoy."

Kim Lea was just the opposite. In high school, she had always gone to the games and cheered for the teams, but she had never dreamed of taking part in a sport. In fact, she would have been the first to admit that she was sedentary. Now, Kim Lea was biking with her two children and organizing her neighborhood aerobics class. She described it this way: "Every Tuesday and Thursday morning, we all get together and talk while we work out. No one cares how we dress or how good we are at doing the exercises. We all just seem to be energized as we go on to our next activities."

For Discussion

Why did Norma feel that it was no longer feasible to continue participating in the sports she played in high school? What might help her get involved in a physical activity again? Why do you think Kim Lea started to participate in activities? What advice would you have for other people who want to get active later in life? Consider the guidelines presented in the Self-Management feature as you answer the discussion questions.

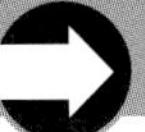

SELF-MANAGEMENT: Skills for Choosing Good Activities

Research shows that the most active people in society are those who have identified specific activities that they enjoy. For example, many people love tennis, golf, or running and participate in their chosen activity on a regular basis. Others prefer variety, so they choose several activities. In both cases, these people might not have become so active if they were not doing activities that they especially enjoy. Use the following guidelines to help you find a physical activity (or activities) especially good for you.

- **Consider your physical fitness.** How well you do in an activity depends on all parts of fitness—both health related and skill related. Choose activities that match your abilities in both kinds of fitness. Also consider activities that help you build health-related fitness (see table 9.2).
- **Consider your interests.** Don't avoid an activity that you really enjoy or have always wanted to do just because it doesn't match your fitness profile. Do be aware, however, that even with practice it may take you longer than others to learn the activity. But finding an activity that is fun for you is very important, so consider a variety of activities.
- **Consider an activity that you can do with others.** Try to find others of your own ability so that you won't be discouraged if you don't learn the activity as quickly as you'd like.
- **Consider the activity's benefits.** As you progress through this book, you'll learn about the benefits of various activities. If you want to get optimal fitness, health, and wellness benefits, select activities

from each area of the Physical Activity Pyramid.

- **Practice, practice, practice.** Becoming skilled in a sport or activity increases your enjoyment. If you choose an activity that is new to you, there is no substitute for practice. To make your practice more productive, consider taking lessons.
- **Consider activities that do not require high levels of skill.** Some activities do not require high levels of any part of skill-related fitness. Of the activities included in the Physical Activity Pyramid, sport provides the most benefit for skill-related fitness, but it also *requires* relatively high levels of both sport skill and skill-related fitness in order to play. Sport skills such as throwing, catching, hitting, and kicking are different from skill-related fitness abilities such as agility, balance, and coordination—though these do help you learn sport skills more easily. Learning sport skills requires a lot of practice in order to perform them well. Generally speaking, fewer skills are required for moderate and vigorous aerobic activities than for sport. As a result, even people with relatively low scores on most or all parts of skill-related fitness can find a moderate or aerobic activity to enjoy—for example, jogging, walking, or cycling. Because these activities don't require high skill levels, they also tend not to require extensive practice. Therefore, you might want to consider one of these activities if you're not willing to put in the necessary time to learn a more complicated one.

ACADEMIC CONNECTION: Figurative Language

Part of meeting standards for English language arts is being able to describe the meaning of words and phrases, including figurative and literal meanings. Figurative language describes a person or thing by comparing it to another thing. Literal language describes people and things as they actually are (in real terms).

When studying fitness, health, and wellness, you might have come across figurative language. It has several categories. Following are some examples of the use of figurative language from various categories.

- She is strong as an ox (a simile—compares two things using the words *like* or *as*).
- He is a couch potato (metaphor—a phrase that doesn't make sense literally but uses similarities between two things to make a connection that is meaningful).
- He ran at the crack of the bat (onomatopoeia—uses words that mimic sounds or sound like their meaning).
- I was so tired you could have knocked me down with a feather (hyperbole—exaggerating to emphasize a point).
- The team's bright uniforms screamed for attention (personification—things or ideas are described as if they had human characteristics).

Try to think of other examples of figurative language associated with fitness, health, or wellness.

TAKING ACTION: Your Vigorous Physical Activity Plan

Prepare a vigorous physical activity plan using the five steps described in the second lesson in this chapter. Like Lin Su, consider activities from all three categories: vigorous aerobics, vigorous sport, and vigorous recreation. Your goal should be to accumulate at least 20 minutes of vigorous physical activity on at least three days each week.

Prepare a written plan and carry out it over a two-week period. Your teacher may give you time in class to do some of the activities included in your plan. Consider the following suggestions for **taking action**.

- Before you do vigorous physical activity, perform a dynamic warm-up.
- Consider the tips presented in this chapter for safe vigorous activity.
- Consider the guidelines presented in this chapter for making good activity selections.
- Progress gradually. Don't try to do too much too soon.
- After your workout, perform a cool-down.

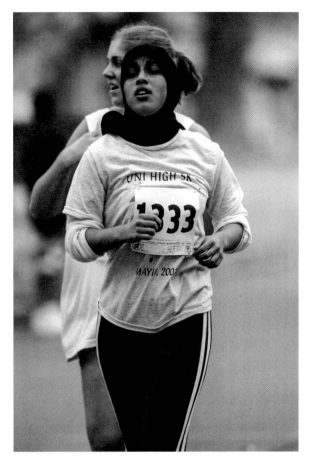

Take action by performing your vigorous physical activity plan.

Reviewing Concepts and Vocabulary

As directed by your teacher, answer items 1 through 5 by correctly completing each sentence with a word or phrase.

1. Vigorous activity is exercise that raises your heart rate above the ______________.
2. Activities that are competitive and have rules are called ______________.
3. Activities so intense that you can perform them for only a few seconds are called ______________ activities.
4. Free time, or time free from work, is called ______________.
5. A ______________ is a list that tells you the intensity of various activities.

For items 6 through 10, as directed by your teacher, match each term in column 1 with the appropriate phrase in column 2.

6. water aerobics	a. aqua dynamics
7. orienteering	b. several exercise stations
8. in-line skating	c. done for fun during free time
9. recreational activity	d. uses map-reading skills
10. circuit training	e. has relatively high injury risk

For items 11 through 15, as directed by your teacher, respond to each statement or question.

11. What is the difference between individual and dual sports?
12. What are some examples of outdoor, challenge, and extreme sports? Why are these sports popular?
13. What is interval training and what are the best frequency, intensity, and time for performing it?
14. What are several safety tips for vigorous physical activity?
15. What are some guidelines for making good physical activity selections?

Thinking Critically

Write a paragraph to answer the following question.

You have a friend who wants to avoid vigorous physical activity because of suffering frequent injuries in the past. What advice would you give your friend to help him or her avoid such problems in the future?

Project

Create a vigorous aerobics exercise routine. Choose music paced at about 100 to 120 beats per minute and plan for the routine to last two to three minutes. You can do an aerobic dance routine, a hip-hop routine, or some other form of continuous exercise. Work with a group to perform a routine (yours or another group member's) in class.

UNIT IV

Muscle Fitness and Flexibility

Healthy People 2020 Goals

- Increase the percentage of teens who do regular muscle fitness exercises.
- Increase the percentage of adults who meet national guidelines for muscle fitness exercise.
- Reduce the percentage of teens who do no leisure physical activity.
- Increase out-of-school physical activity by teens.
- Decrease steroid use among teens.
- Reduce incidence of back problems.
- Reduce incidence of osteoporosis.
- Reduce sport and recreation injuries.
- Reduce overweight and obesity.

Self-Assessment Features in This Unit

- Muscle Fitness Testing
- Healthy Back Test
- Arm, Leg, and Trunk Flexibility

Taking Charge Features in This Unit

- Preventing Relapse
- Finding Social Support
- Overcoming Barriers

Self-Management Features in This Unit

- Skills for Preventing Relapse
- Skills for Finding Social Support
- Skills for Overcoming Barriers

Taking Action Features in This Unit

- Resistance Machine Exercises
- Your Muscle Fitness Exercise Plan
- Your Flexibility Exercise Plan

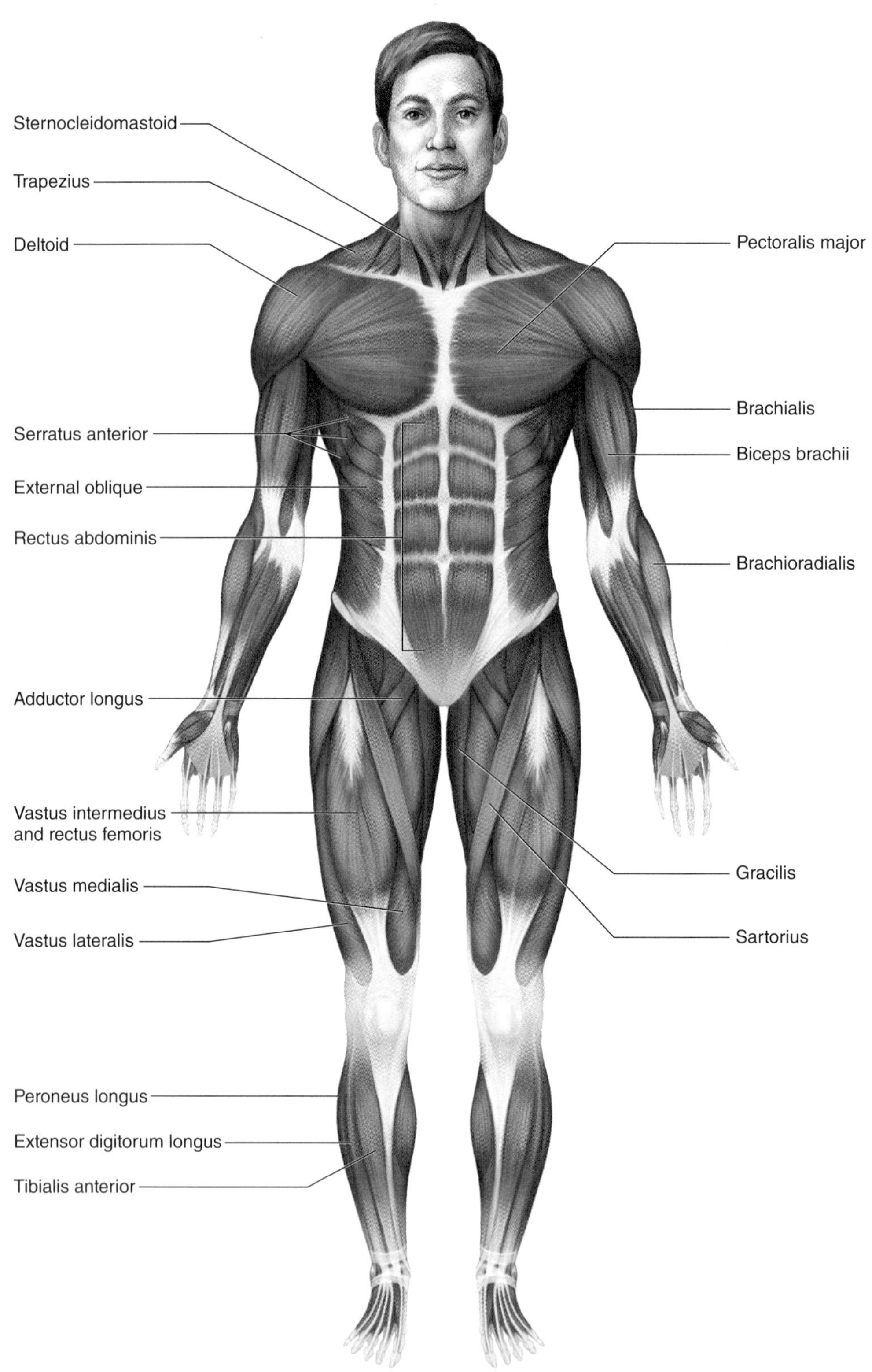

The major muscles of the body. The specific muscles addressed in the chapters that follow are described with each exercise. Refer to these two illustrations for exact muscle locations.

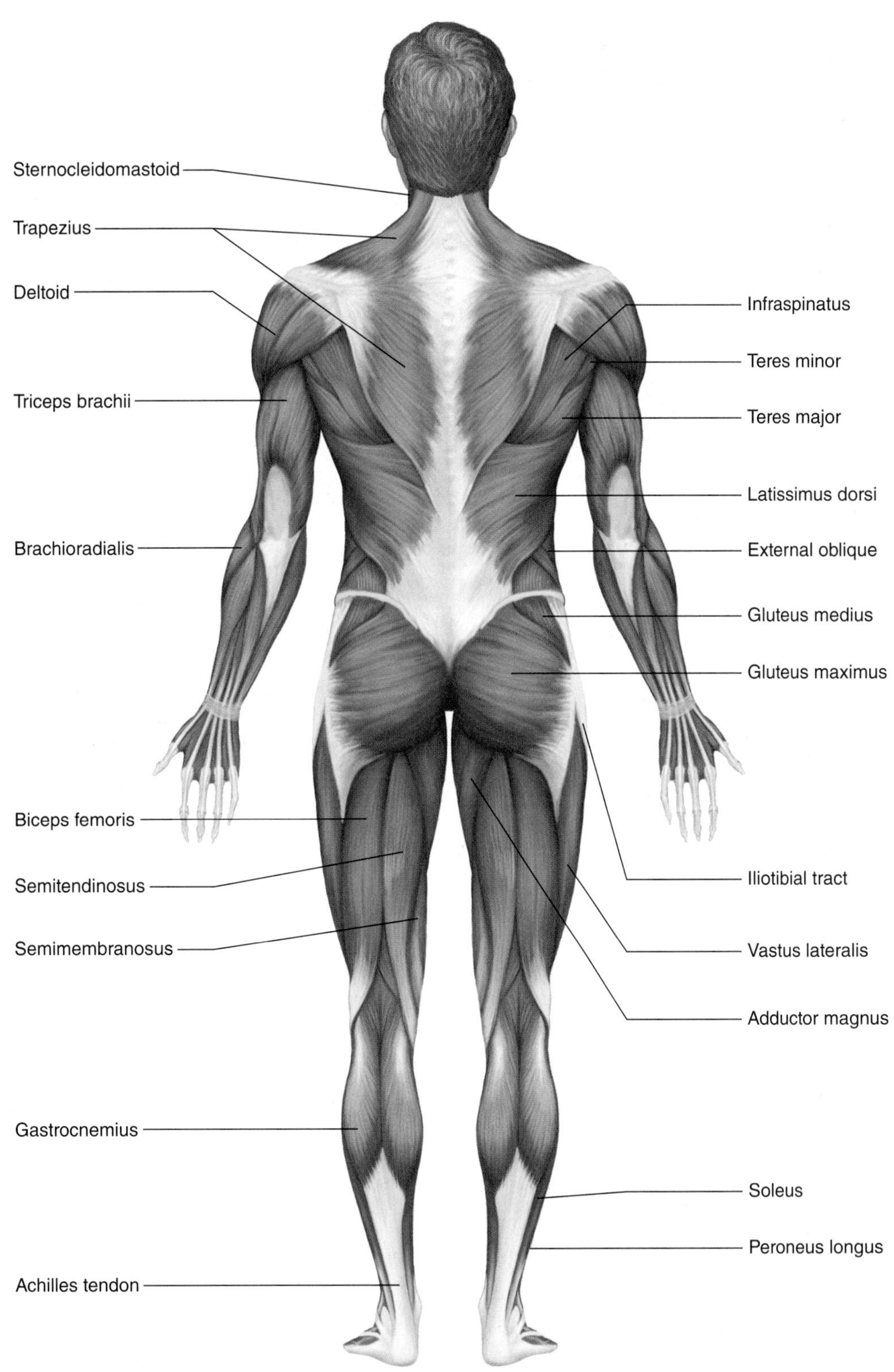
Sternocleidomastoid
Trapezius
Deltoid
Triceps brachii
Brachioradialis
Biceps femoris
Semitendinosus
Semimembranosus
Gastrocnemius
Achilles tendon
Infraspinatus
Teres minor
Teres major
Latissimus dorsi
External oblique
Gluteus medius
Gluteus maximus
Iliotibial tract
Vastus lateralis
Adductor magnus
Soleus
Peroneus longus

10

Muscle Fitness Basics

In This Chapter

Student Web Resources

www.HOPEtextbook.org/student

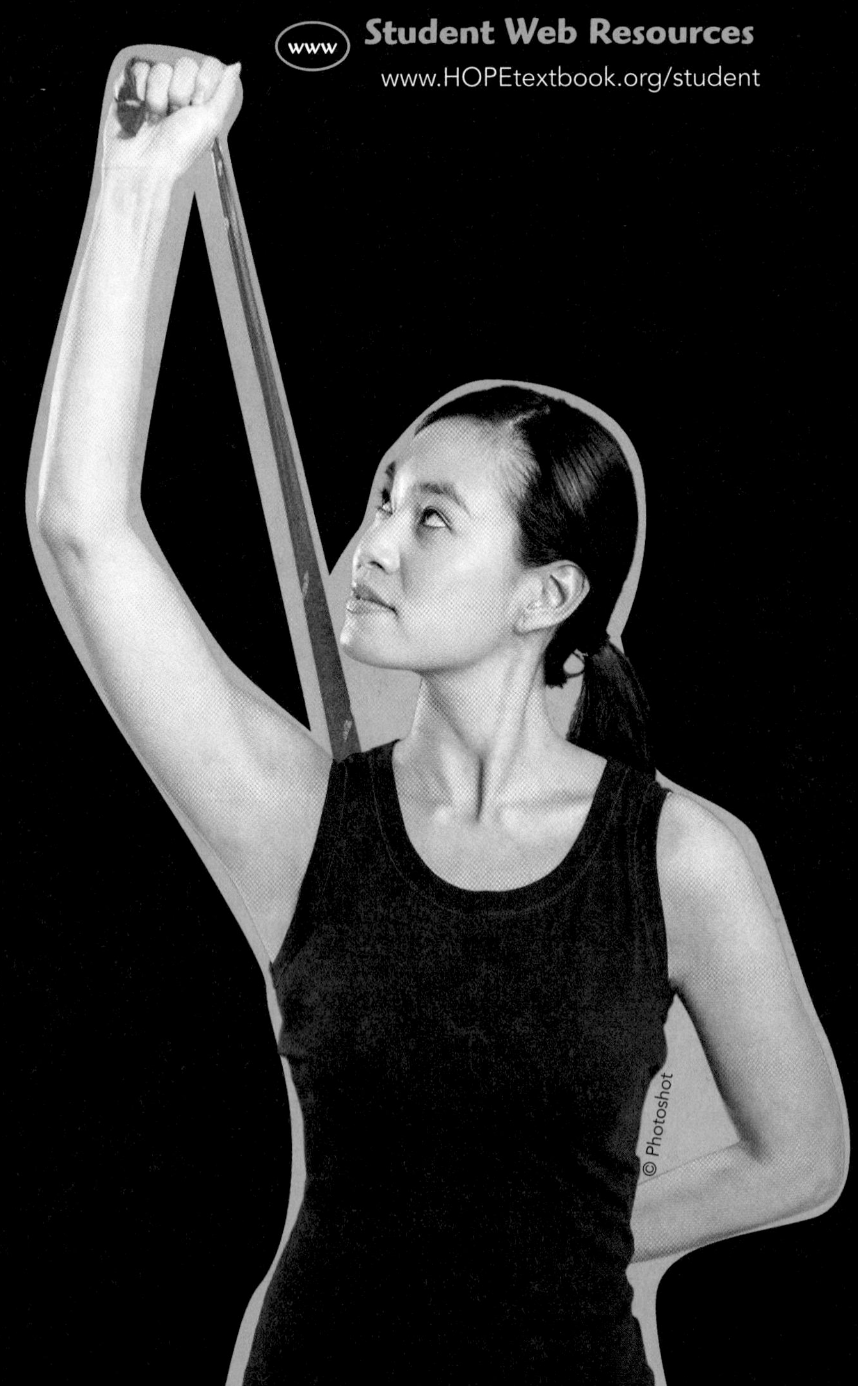

© Photoshot

Lesson 10.1

Muscle Fitness Facts

Lesson Objectives

After reading this lesson, you should be able to

1. explain the differences between strength, muscular endurance, and power;
2. describe how exercise principles apply to muscle fitness;
3. describe the types of muscle fitness exercise; and
4. describe several methods for assessing muscle fitness.

WWW 1

Lesson Vocabulary

absolute strength, calisthenics, concentric, dynamometer, eccentric, fast-twitch muscle fiber, hypertrophy, intermediate muscle fiber, isokinetic exercise, isometric contraction, isometric exercise, isotonic contraction, isotonic exercise, 1-repetition maximum (1RM), plyometrics, principle of rest and recovery, progressive resistance exercise (PRE), relative strength, reps, set, slow-twitch muscle fiber

Does your favorite activity require muscle fitness? Do you have enough muscle fitness? Muscle fitness is made up of three health-related parts of physical fitness: strength, muscular endurance, and power.

FIT FACT

Together strength, muscular endurance, power, and flexibility are referred to as *musculoskeletal fitness* because all four of these parts of fitness are associated with the muscular and skeletal systems. In this book, *muscle fitness* is used as a general term to describe the three parts of musculoskeletal fitness that require the muscles to produce force (strength, muscular endurance, and power).

Strength is the amount of force that a muscle can exert. The amount of weight that a group of muscles can lift one time is called a **1-repetition maximum (1RM)**, which is a good indicator of force exerted. This is considered the best measure of strength. Having good strength enables you to apply effective force in sports (such as football) and in tasks that require heavy lifting (figure 10.1*a*).

Muscular endurance is the ability to contract muscles many times without tiring or to hold a muscle contraction for a long time without fatigue. Muscular endurance allows you to resist muscle fatigue in recreational activities such as backpacking and to persist in work activities such as carrying a mailbag for hours at a time (figure 10.1*b*).

The third part of muscle fitness is power. Power is the ability to use strength (produce force) quickly; thus it involves both strength and speed. It is often referred to as explosive strength. Examples of power include jumping high or far and throwing objects a great distance. Research has shown that power is especially important to bone health and that bone health built in the teen years provides lifelong benefits (figure 10.1*c*).

All three components of muscle fitness—strength, muscular endurance, and power—are important to both health and good performance. This chapter includes exercises from step 4 of the Physical Activity Pyramid (figure 10.2) to develop muscle fitness.

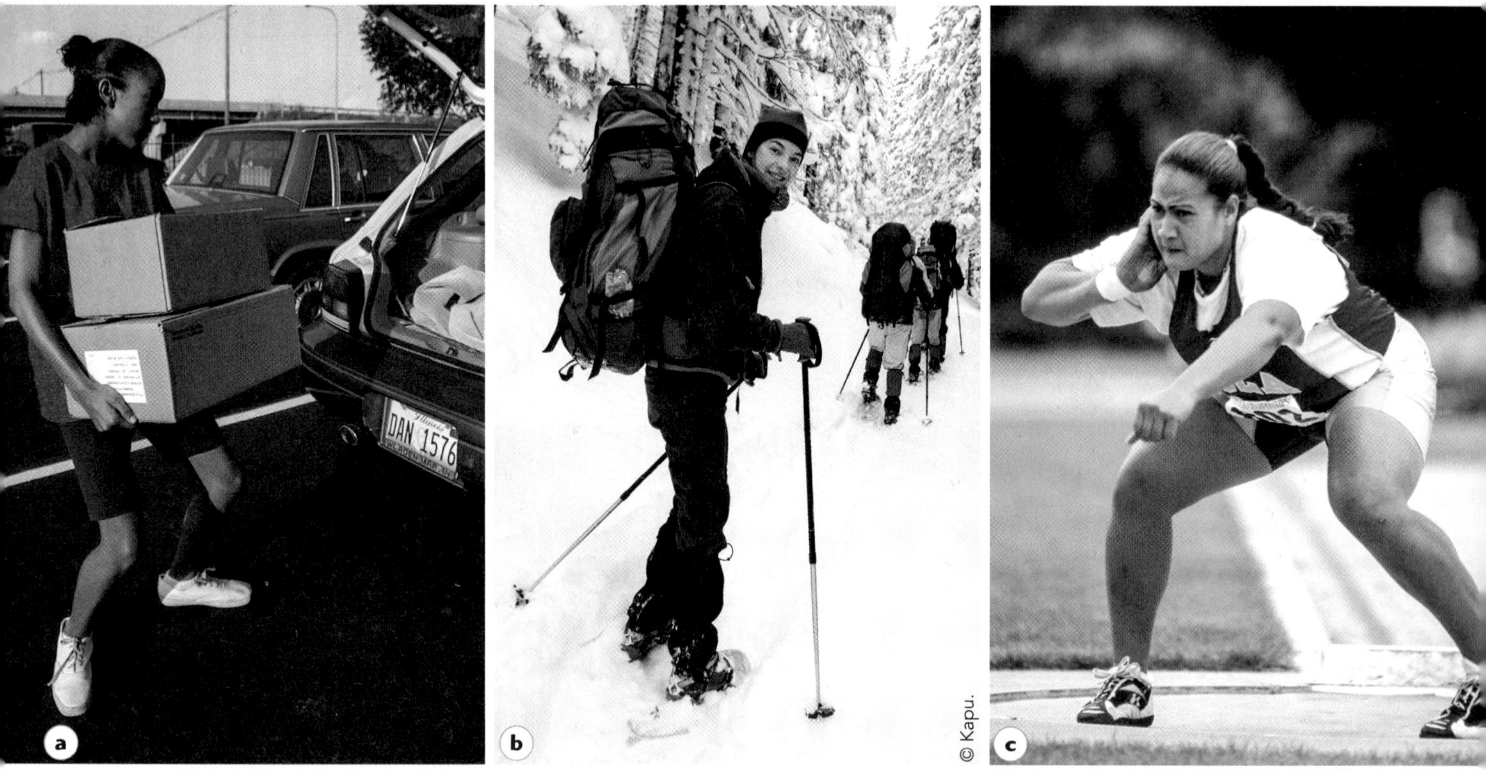

© Kapu.

FIGURE 10.1 The parts of muscle fitness: *(a)* Lifting a heavy object requires strength; *(b)* using your muscles for a long time requires muscular endurance; and *(c)* doing activities that involve fast application of force requires power.

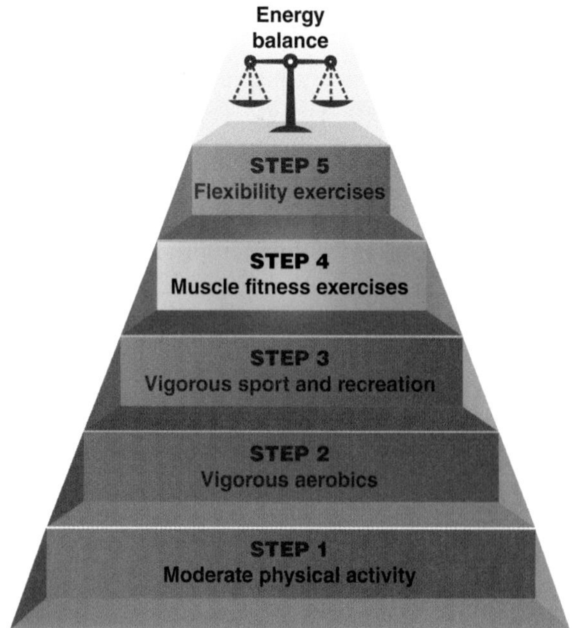

FIGURE 10.2 Activities from step 4 of the Physical Activity Pyramid build muscle fitness.

Muscle Fitness Terminology

You may have heard the terms *reps* and *sets* in relation to muscular fitness, and figure 10.3 can help you understand them. The term **reps** (short for *repetitions*) refers to the number of consecutive times you do an exercise. A **set** is one group of repetitions. For example, suppose you do an exercise 8 times, then rest; repeat it 8 times, then rest again; and repeat it another 8 times. You have just done 3 sets of 8 repetitions each.

The Muscular Endurance–Strength Continuum

The exercises used to develop muscular endurance and strength differ only in the number of repetitions and the amount of resistance. The relationship between endurance and strength can be represented on a continuum such as the one shown in figure 10.4, which presents pounds of resistance on one edge and number of repetitions on the other.

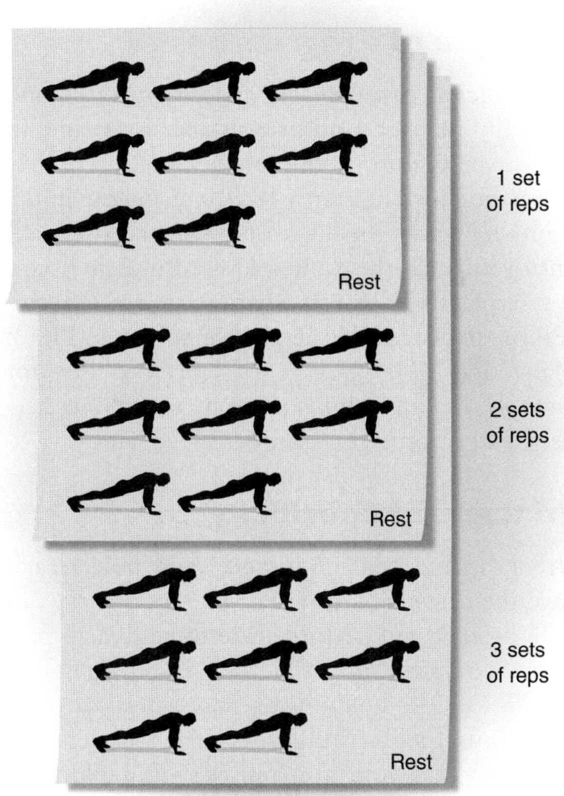

FIGURE 10.3 Muscle fitness exercises are typically done in reps and sets.

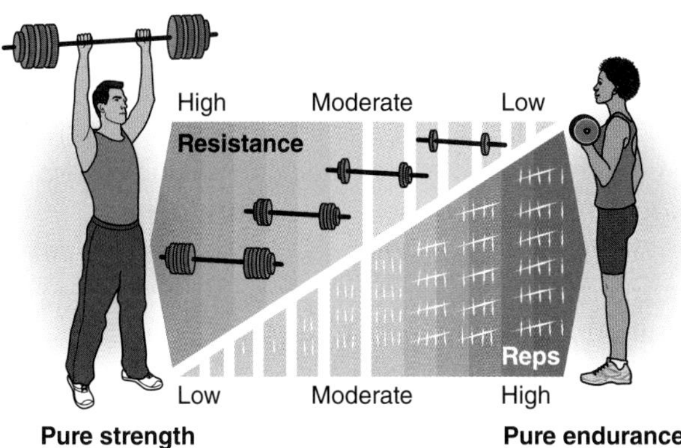

FIGURE 10.4 Muscular endurance–strength continuum.

The continuum shows the resistance and repetitions that a person might use to build muscle fitness. To develop strength, you would use high resistance with fewer repetitions; to develop endurance, you would use low resistance with more repetitions; and to develop both strength and endurance, you would use the resistance and repetitions shown in the middle of the continuum. This continuum also shows that usually when you train for strength you will also develop some endurance, and when you train for endurance you will also develop some strength.

Cardiorespiratory Endurance and Muscular Endurance

Muscular endurance is one part of muscle fitness, and it is different from the other parts (strength and power). It is also different from cardiorespiratory endurance, which depends on your cardiovascular and respiratory systems to supply oxygen. Cardiorespiratory endurance is general (not specific to one area of the body), and good cardiorespiratory endurance allows your entire body to function.

Muscular endurance, on the other hand, is the ability to contract your muscles many times without tiring or to hold one contraction for a long time. Muscular endurance depends on the ability of your muscle fibers to keep working without getting tired. You can have good muscular endurance in one part of your body (such as your legs) without having it in another part of your body (such as your arms).

Strength and Power

For years, power was considered to be a skill-related part of fitness. Sometimes it was referred to as a combined part of fitness because it involves both strength (the ability to exert force) and speed (the ability to cover a distance in a short time). Because it involves a strength component, power is often referred to as explosive strength. There is no doubt that both power and strength are important for performance, but today we understand that both are also important for your health. The Institute of Medicine reports that adults who lack power have a higher-than-normal risk of chronic disease, reduced lifespan, and poor functional health as they grow older. Exercise physiologists have also demonstrated that power—and activities that produce power—are very important in building healthy bones in youth. Because of these links to health, power is now classified as a health-related part of fitness.

Fitness Principles and Muscle Fitness

The three basic fitness principles can be applied to muscle fitness exercise. These principles—overload, progression, and specificity—have been covered elsewhere in part 1 of this book. They are discussed again in this chapter to show how they relate specifically to muscle fitness.

Principle of Overload

To improve muscle fitness, a muscle must contract harder than normal. In other words, the muscle must work against a greater load than it normally bears in regular daily activity. High overload (high resistance) builds strength, whereas more moderate overload repeated many times builds muscular endurance. Exercises for power require overload for speed and strength. The reverse of the overload principle also applies—if you don't use your muscles, you'll lose muscle fitness. "Use it or lose it!"

Principle of Progression

The principle of progression holds that you should gradually increase load or resistance over time in order to best improve your muscle fitness. If you try to use too much resistance too soon, you can injure yourself. Exercise that increases resistance (overload) until you reach the desired level of muscle fitness is referred to as **progressive resistance exercise (PRE)** or progressive resistance training (PRT). Many kinds of progressive resistance exercise—for example, weight training, resistance machine exercises, and plyometrics—are described later.

Principle of Specificity

Strength, muscular endurance, and power each have their own FIT formula. The specific type of training that you perform determines which part of muscle fitness you build. In addition, you build specific muscles by doing exercises specifically for those muscles. To build your arm muscles, you must overload your arm muscles. To build your

SCIENCE IN ACTION: Resistance Exercise Among Youth

Exercise scientists have developed recommendations to help youth, including preteens and teens, use PRE to build their muscle fitness. The guidelines were developed by a variety of experts—including exercise physiologists, medical doctors, and exercise professionals (such as athletic trainers and strength coaches)—who worked with the National Strength and Conditioning Association (NSCA).

Not so long ago, some experts felt that muscle fitness exercises were unsafe and inappropriate for preteens and teens. NSCA experts now provide evidence that, when done properly, PRE provides health benefits for teens similar to those for adults. These benefits include reduced risk of chronic disease, reduced risk of injury and muscle pain or soreness, improved muscle fitness and sport performance, and psychological well-being. Muscle fitness exercise also builds bone fitness, reduces the risk of osteoporosis (porous and weak bones), reduces the risk of back pain, enhances posture, and increases your ability to work and play without fatigue. In addition, well-developed muscles help you look your best. Muscle is more dense than fat, so it takes up less space. Muscle also uses more calories than fat, so increasing muscle mass helps the body to burn calories.

Keys to keeping PRE safe for youth include using proper technique and safe and appropriate equipment, following sound exercise principles, and seeking and accepting good supervision. Much of this chapter focuses on giving you the information you need in order to meet the safe exercise recommendations for PRE.

Student Activity

PRE can be safe for teens when done properly but carries risks when done improperly. Create a list of the most important ways to make PRE safe for teens. Consider making a sign to be posted in a fitness room used by teens.

leg muscles, you must overload your leg muscles. Examples of types of PRE for each part of muscle fitness and the basic exercises for specific muscle groups are discussed later in this chapter.

Principle of Rest and Recovery

The **principle of rest and recovery** holds that you need to give your muscles time to rest and recover after a workout. This is why muscle fitness exercises are typically performed on only two or three days per week. Because you need to perform exercises to build all of the important muscles of your body, some people choose to work out every day but do exercises for different muscle groups on different days. For example, they might perform upper body exercises one day and lower body exercises the next. For optimal results, you should also rest between sets of exercise (more information about rest is given throughout this chapter).

> "Where there is no struggle, there is no strength."
>
> —Oprah Winfrey, media personality

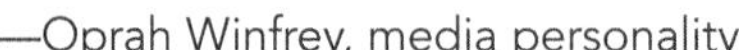

Muscles and Muscle Biomechanics

Your body's muscles create the movement that allows you to do the activities described in this book. There are hundreds of muscles in the human body. Some of the most frequently used muscles in physical activity are illustrated in figure 10.5. This section helps you learn more about how your muscles work.

Muscle Contraction and Joint Movement

Your skeletal muscles are attached to your bones and make your movements possible. You use these muscles to do physical activity. They are called voluntary muscles because you consciously control them. Your muscles work together to allow your body parts to function efficiently and effectively. For example, when you contract your biceps muscle (see figure 10.6*a*), your arm bends at the elbow, bringing your hand closer to your shoulder. At the same time, your triceps muscle relaxes to allow your biceps to do its work.

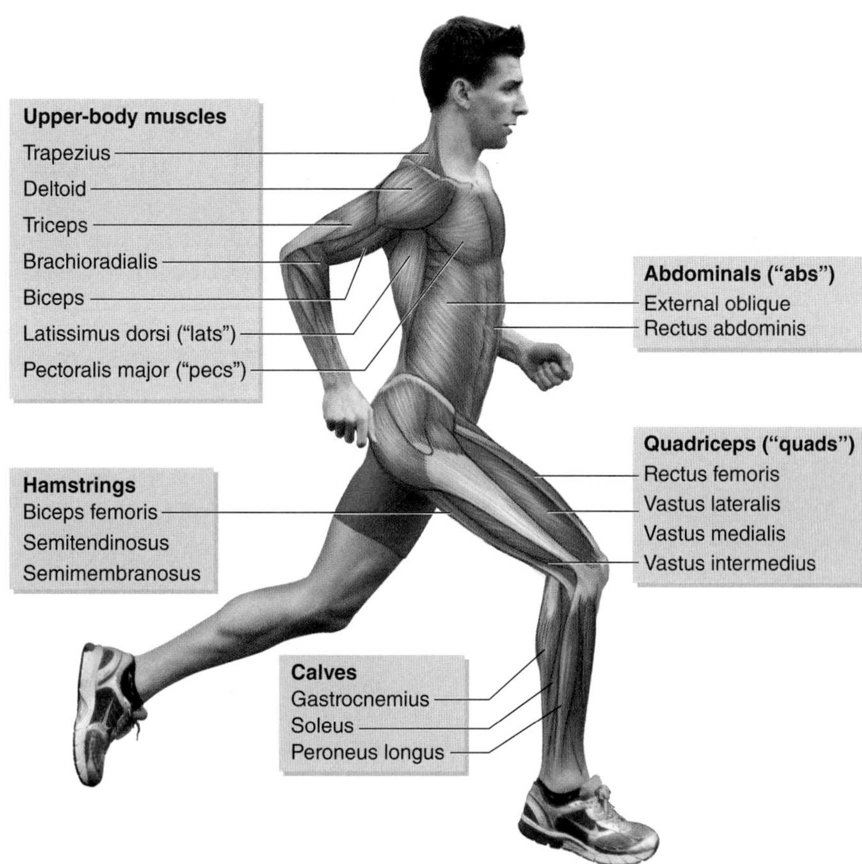

FIGURE 10.5 Some of the major muscles used in physical activity.

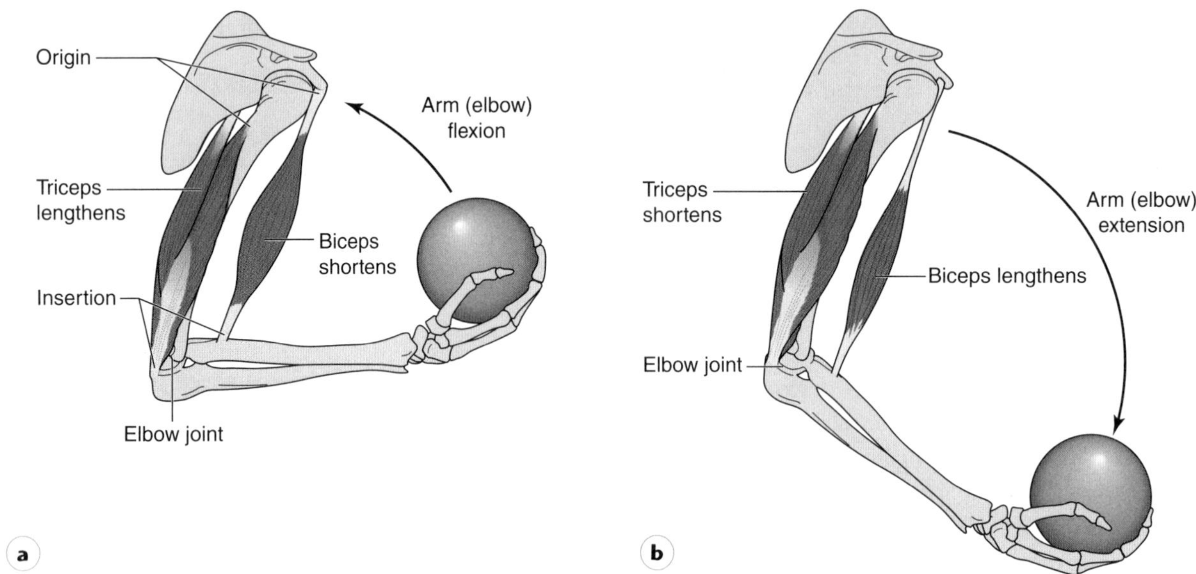

FIGURE 10.6 The origin, insertion, and action of the arm muscles: *(a)* flexion; *(b)* extension.

The tendons of each muscle connect with bone in two places, the origin and the insertion. The origin is typically connected to the bone that is stationary during a movement, and the insertion is typically connected to the bone that moves. In figure 10.6, the origin of the biceps is at the shoulder, and the insertion is on the bone of the lower arm that moves during flexion and extension.

Type of Muscle Fitness Exercise

As figure 10.6 shows, your skeletal muscles are attached to your bones on either side of a joint; your bones act as levers to which your muscles apply force. When stimulated by a nerve, muscle fibers are activated to apply force. Muscle contractions can be isotonic or isometric. **Isotonic contractions** pull on your bones to produce movement of your body parts. **Isotonic exercises** are those that use muscle contractions to move body parts. The two types of isotonic muscle contractions are **concentric** (shortening contraction) and **eccentric** (lengthening contraction). Figure 10.6*a* shows the biceps muscle doing a concentric contraction in which the muscle shortens to cause the elbow to flex. In figure 10.6*b*, as the arm is slowly straightened, the biceps is doing an eccentric, or lengthening, contraction that causes the elbow to extend.

In contrast, an **isometric contraction** (sometimes called a static contraction) occurs when muscles contract and pull with equal force in opposite directions so that no movement occurs. **Isometric exercises** involve isometric contractions, and body parts do not move in these exercises. One example of an isometric contraction involves pushing your hands and arms together in front of your body. You push hard with each hand, applying force against the other, but no movement occurs. You can also do isometric calisthenics, such as holding your body still in the push-up position.

Plyometrics is a type of muscle fitness exercise that is especially useful in building power. This type of activity involves doing isotonic muscle contractions explosively (as in jumping). You'll learn more about all forms of muscle fitness exercise later in this chapter.

FIT FACT

An eccentric contraction is sometimes called a braking contraction because the lengthening of a muscle works against gravity to slow the lowering of a weight (see figure 10.6). For example, in a biceps curl after using a concentric contraction to flex the elbow and lift a weight, you lower the weight using an eccentric contraction. The lengthening of the biceps slows the weight down (or "puts on the brakes") so that the weight does not drop too quickly.

Isokinetic exercise is a type of isotonic exercise in which the velocity of movement is kept constant through the full range of motion. As noted in the Fitness Technology feature, isokinetic exercise requires special machines.

Muscle Fibers

Muscle fibers are long, thin, cylindrical muscle cells. Skeletal muscles (such as those in your arms and legs) are made of many muscle fibers (figure 10.7). The strength and endurance of skeletal muscles depend on whether the muscles are made of slow, fast, or intermediate fibers and on how much exercise they get.

Slow-twitch muscle fibers contract slowly and are usually red because they have a lot of blood vessels delivering oxygen to the muscle. These fibers generate less force than **fast-twitch muscle fibers** but are able to resist fatigue. For this reason, a muscle with many slow-twitch fibers has good muscular endurance, and slow-twitch fibers are involved in activities such as running for distance. Fast-twitch muscle fibers contract quickly and are white because they have less blood flow delivering oxygen. They generate more force when they contract, and for this reason muscles with many fast-twitch fibers are important for strength activities.

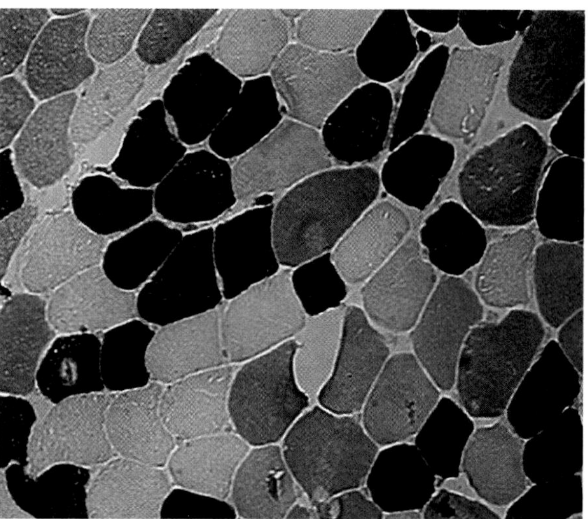

FIGURE 10.7 This photomicrograph shows slow-twitch (black) and fast-twitch (gray and white) muscle fibers.

Reprinted, by permission, from W.L. Kenney, J.H. Wilmore and D.L. Costill, 2004, *Physiology of sport and exercise*, 5th ed. (Champaign, IL: Human Kinetics), 37.

Intermediate muscle fibers have characteristics of both slow- and fast-twitch fibers. You use them for activities involving both types of muscle fitness and cardiorespiratory endurance.

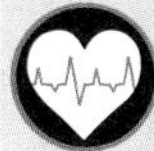

FITNESS TECHNOLOGY: Isokinetic Exercise Machines

In recent years, tremendous technological advances have been made in resistance exercise machines. Innovations include adjustable benches and chairs so that machines fit people of all sizes, systems for changing resistance that make the machines easier to use, and the creation of isokinetic resistance machines. These machines use special hydraulics or electronics to regulate movement velocity and allow full exertion at all angles of joint movement during an exercise. In contrast, with traditional free weights or resistance machines, resistance is often greater during the first part of a movement than at the end of the movement, and the speed of the movement may also be greater at one point than at another. Isokinetic exercise allows the muscle to be developed equally at all joint angles and can be used to develop power by using fast (high speed) movements. Isokinetic machines are considered quite safe and are often used by researchers and people who are rehabilitating injuries. Their disadvantages include being expensive and often not allowing eccentric contractions, which are used frequently in sport performance.

Using Technology

If your school has an isokinetic machine, ask for a demonstration and try it out. If not, see if you can find a machine locally or on the Internet (for a visual demonstration).

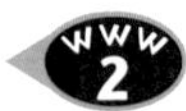

Your muscle capabilities are determined in part by heredity. People who inherit a large number of fast-twitch muscle fibers are especially likely to be good at activities requiring sprinting and jumping, whereas people who inherit a large number of slow-twitch muscle fibers are likely to be good at activities requiring sustained performance such as distance running and swimming. Although heredity and genes play an important role, we now know that training can also affect muscle fiber function. So, regardless of your genes, you can increase your muscle strength, endurance, and power with proper training.

FIT FACT

Birds, like humans, have both fast-twitch and slow-twitch muscle fibers. The flying muscles (breast muscles) of a duck or goose are dark colored because they contain many slow-twitch fibers (which are typically red) that are needed for long-distance flights. In contrast, the breast of a chicken is made up of mostly fast-twitch fibers (typically white) because the chickens typically don't fly long distances.

Muscle Hypertrophy

Muscle **hypertrophy** refers to growth in the size of muscles and muscle fibers. Hypertrophy is affected not only by overloading but also by several other factors. You've already learned that we each inherit a unique pattern of muscle fiber types and that this inheritance makes a difference in how your body responds to training. But age, maturation, and sex also play a role.

As we age, our muscles grow, as do other tissues in the body. For preteens and young teens, who are not yet fully mature, the body does not produce enough hormones to build big muscles (hypertrophy), even with PRE. These hormones are not fully present until a person reaches full maturity, which occurs at various ages for various people, though typically earlier for girls than for boys. Prior to maturity, PRE can improve strength but may not noticeably increase muscle size; in fact, the strength gains are typically due to increased skill in performing the exercises or an increase in the number of muscle fibers called upon for a movement during exercise. In most exercises, only some of the available muscle fibers contract to cause a movement, but with regular PRE more fibers are called upon, increasing the number of exercises you can perform.

Because preteens and older teens who are late developers may not see big gains in muscle size with training, they may get discouraged and feel that PRE doesn't work. They may want to focus instead on gains in performance skills and accept the fact that noticeable muscular changes will occur when the body begins to produce more of the hormones that stimulate growth in muscle size.

Some people think that only males can build muscle fitness and increase muscle hypertrophy. This notion is false. Both males and females need strength in order to be healthy, avoid injury, look good, and be able to save themselves or others in an emergency.

Some girls and women fear that strength training will cause their body to look masculine. However, the hormones that promote muscle hypertrophy are not as prevalent in the bodies of females. In addition, females at maturity have a lower relative percent of muscle as compared with total body weight than males do. For this reason, most girls and women find it difficult to develop large, bulky muscles even when their exercise amounts are similar to those described in part 1 of this book. Even so, women and girls who perform strength exercises do develop strong muscles. And both men and women look more attractive with strong muscles because they are more likely to have good posture and a firm body. Building good strength can also help build your self-confidence.

Muscle Fitness Assessment

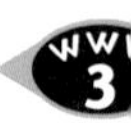

You can assess muscle fitness in many ways. The best test for strength is generally agreed to be the 1-repetition maximum (1RM) test (see the Self-Assessment at the end of this lesson). The 1RM test requires you to determine the amount of weight you can lift or the resistance you can overcome in 1 repetition. For example, if a person can lift 100 pounds once, but not twice, 100 pounds is the 1RM for the muscle group being tested. You can use the 1RM test for each of your major muscle groups, and you can use the results both to get a good idea of your strength and to determine how much weight or resistance to use when you perform exercises.

The true 1RM test is commonly used by athletes and adults. Done properly, it can also be safe for teens, but most experts recommend that teens use a modified self-assessment. The modified 1RM self-assessment gives you a good estimate of your true 1RM but does not require you to lift maximal weight or use maximal resistance. Teens are advised to use only a percentage of 1RM, both in testing their strength and in performing strength exercises. In the Self-Assessment feature included in this chapter, you'll estimate your 1RM by performing the modified 1RM test that uses multiple repetitions and lower than maximal weight (or resistance). This self-assessment is safe for teens when performed properly. You can do a 1RM test for many muscle groups, but two are used most often—one for the upper body (arm press) and one for the lower body (leg press).

Another 1RM test is the grip dynamometer test (figure 10.8), which tests isometric rather than isotonic strength. This grip test is easy to do but does require a grip **dynamometer**. People who score well on the isotonic 1RM test often score well on the grip test as well. This test is used in national fitness assessments in Canada, Japan, and Poland and in the ALPHA-FIT battery that is often used in Europe. Dynamometers are also available for testing other muscle groups, such as leg muscles, but they are more expensive and harder to use than grip dynamometers and thus are used less frequently.

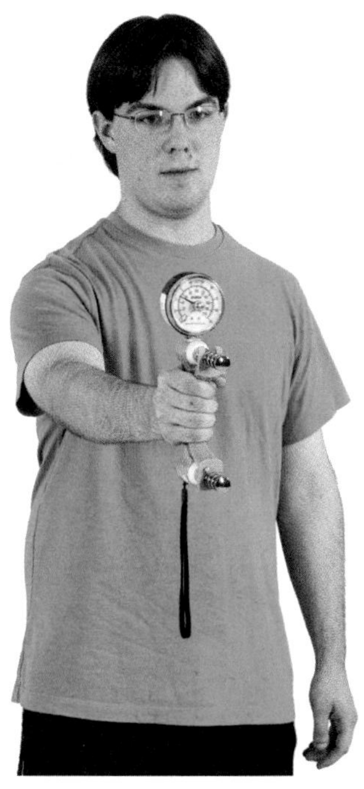

FIGURE 10.8 The grip dynamometer test measures isometric strength.

You've already tried several self-assessments for muscular endurance and power that are used in common fitness test batteries. Muscular endurance tests typically require you to repeat the performance of **calisthenics**; examples include push-ups, curl-ups, and trunk lifts. Common tests of leg power include the long jump and vertical jump, and one common test of upper body power is the medicine ball throw. In the Self-Assessment feature in this lesson, you'll learn how to do tests of strength, muscular endurance, and power beyond those you've already tried.

Absolute Versus Relative Strength

Your 1RM score is an example of **absolute strength**, which is measured by how much weight or resistance you can overcome regardless of your body size. Big people typically have more absolute strength than smaller people, and since males are generally larger than females, their average absolute strength is higher. **Relative strength**, on the other hand, is adjusted for body size. The most common method for determining relative strength is to divide your weight into your absolute strength score to get a score for your strength per pound of body weight. Relative strength scores are considered to be fairer assessments of strength for those who do not have large bodies; thus relative strength is used for the ratings in this chapter's Self-Assessment feature.

Lesson Review

1. What are the differences between strength, muscular endurance, and power?
2. What are the basic exercise principles of muscle fitness, and why are they important?
3. What are the types of muscle fitness exercise?
4. What are some methods for assessing muscle fitness?

SELF-ASSESSMENT: Muscle Fitness Testing

Self-assessment of any part of fitness—including muscle fitness—is important because it allows you to establish your baseline level of fitness, determine your fitness needs, set goals, and determine whether you've met your goals. Certified personal trainers who know their stuff have their clients perform a baseline fitness test (a pretest) and, after they go through a fitness program, a follow-up fitness test (a post-test) to see if the program was effective. In this class, you are learning to become your own personal trainer.

Before performing these tests, consider doing a general and dynamic warm-up. If the 1RM test causes fatigue that keeps you from doing your best on the muscle fitness tests in part 3 of this sequence, repeat that assessment on another day. As directed by your instructor, record your scores and ratings for the three parts of this self-assessment. If you're working with a partner, remember that self-assessment information is personal and considered confidential. It shouldn't be shared with others without the permission of the person being tested.

Part 1: Estimating Your 1RM

To review, 1RM means 1-repetition maximum—the maximum weight a muscle or group of muscles can lift (or the maximum resistance they can overcome) one time. Because beginners should start gradually (without heavy lifting), a modified method has been developed that allows you to determine your 1RM without overexerting. Your results indicate how strong you are.

The modified 1RM can be done with free weights or machines, but the instructions that follow are for machine use. Resistance machines are recommended for these self-assessments, especially for beginners, because they are safer. Two tests are used most often, and the ones performed in this self-assessment activity are for your upper body (arm press) and your lower body (leg press).

Use the following directions for each of the two self-assessments.

- Choose a weight (resistance) that you think you can lift (move) 5 to 10 times. Do not use a weight that you can lift fewer than 5 times or more than 10 times.
- Using correct technique, lift the weight as many times as you possibly can. Count your lifts and write the total on your record sheet. If you were able to do more than 10 lifts, wait until another day before you try a heavier weight for that assessment. Go to the next muscle group assessment.
- If you can tell that you will not be able to lift the weight at least 5 times, stop and choose a lighter weight.
- If you were able to do 5 to 10 lifts (no fewer and no more), refer to table 10.1 and find the weight you lifted. Now find the number of reps you did. Your 1RM score is the number in the box where your horizontal weight row and your vertical rep column intersect.
- Divide each of your two 1RM scores (arm press and leg press) by your body weight to get your score for strength per pound of body weight. This score adjusts for body size to indicate your relative strength. For example, a person who weighs 150 pounds and has a 1RM of 100 pounds on the arm press has a score of 0.67 pound lifted per pound of body weight. After figuring your relative strength score, use tables 10.2 and 10.3 to determine your fitness rating. Record your 1RM scores, relative strength scores, and ratings.
- Tables 10.2 and 10.3 do not show high performance ratings for the 1RM. For now, focus on getting into the good fitness zone. Athletes should consult coaches in their sport to get more information about appropriate 1RM scores.

Safety tip: Proper form is essential for safety. Before you do the 1RM test, read the descriptions of the exercises and the directions that follow. Before performing each assessment, practice the exercise and have a teacher check your form. Work with a partner to get feedback about proper lifting technique.

TABLE 10.1 Predicted 1RM Based on Reps to Fatigue

Weight (lb)	Repetitions						Weight (lb)	Repetitions					
	5	6	7	8	9	10		5	6	7	8	9	10
30	34	35	36	37	38	39	**140**	157	163	168	174	180	187
35	40	41	42	43	44	45	**145**	163	168	174	180	186	193
40	46	47	49	50	51	53	**150**	169	174	180	186	193	200
45	51	53	55	56	58	60	**155**	174	180	186	192	199	207
50	56	58	60	62	64	67	**160**	180	186	192	199	206	213
55	62	64	66	68	71	73	**165**	186	192	198	205	212	220
60	67	70	72	74	77	80	**170**	191	197	204	211	219	227
65	73	75	78	81	84	87	**175**	197	203	210	217	225	233
70	79	81	84	87	90	93	**180**	202	209	216	223	231	240
75	84	87	90	93	96	100	**185**	208	215	222	230	238	247
80	90	93	96	99	103	107	**190**	214	221	228	236	244	253
85	96	99	102	106	109	113	**195**	219	226	234	242	251	260
90	101	105	108	112	116	120	**200**	225	232	240	248	257	267
95	107	110	114	118	122	127	**205**	231	238	246	254	264	273
100	112	116	120	124	129	133	**210**	236	244	252	261	270	280
105	118	122	126	130	135	140	**215**	242	250	258	267	276	287
110	124	128	132	137	141	147	**220**	247	255	264	273	283	293
115	129	134	138	143	148	153	**225**	253	261	270	279	289	300
120	135	139	144	149	154	160	**230**	259	267	276	286	296	307
125	141	145	150	155	161	167	**235**	264	273	282	292	302	313
130	146	151	158	161	167	173	**240**	270	279	288	298	309	320
135	152	157	162	168	174	180	**245**	276	285	294	304	315	327

To convert from pounds to kilograms, multiply by 0.45.

Adapted, by permission, from M. Brzyck, 1993, "Strength testing - predicting a one-rep max from reps-to-fatigue," *JOPERD* 64(1): 89. www.informaworld.com

Seated Arm Press

1. Sit on the stool of a seated press machine and position yourself so that the handles are even with your shoulders. Grasp the handles with your palms facing away from you. Tighten your abdominal muscles.
2. Push upward on the handles, extending your arms until your elbows are straight.
   Caution: Do not arch your back. Do not lock your elbows.
3. Lower the handles to the starting position.

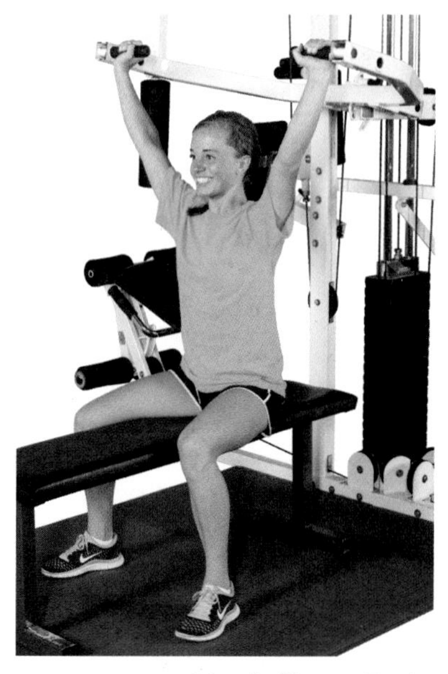

This test evaluates the strength of your triceps and pectoral muscles.

TABLE 10.2 Rating Chart: Relative Strength for Arm Press

	15 years or younger		16 or 17 years old		18 years or older	
	Male	Female	Male	Female	Male	Female
Good fitness	≥0.80	≥0.60	≥1.00	≥0.70	≥1.10	≥0.85
Marginal fitness	0.67–0.79	0.50–0.59	0.75–0.99	0.60–0.69	0.80–1.09	0.67–0.84
Low fitness	≤0.66	≤0.49	≤0.74	≤0.59	≤0.79	≤0.66

Relative strength is calculated by dividing 1RM by body weight.

Seated Leg Press

1. Adjust the seat position on a leg press machine for your leg length. Sit with your feet resting on the pedal.
2. Push the pedal until your legs are straight.
   Caution: Do not lock your knees.
3. Slowly return to the starting position.

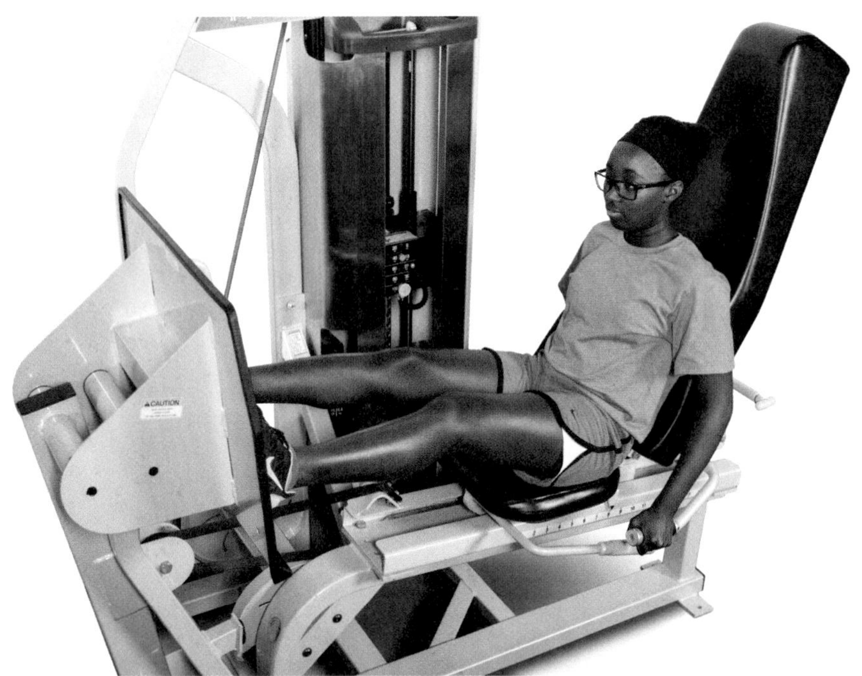

This test evaluates the strength of your quadriceps, gluteal, and calf muscles.

TABLE 10.3 Rating Chart: Relative Strength for Leg Press

	15 years or younger		16 or 17 years old		18 years or older	
	Male	Female	Male	Female	Male	Female
Good fitness	≥1.50	≥1.10	≥1.75	≥1.30	≥1.90	≥1.40
Marginal fitness	1.35–1.49	0.95–1.09	1.50–1.74	1.10–1.29	1.65–1.89	1.30–1.39
Low fitness	≤1.34	≤0.94	≤1.49	≤1.09	≤1.64	≤1.29

Relative strength is calculated by dividing 1RM by body weight.

Part 2: Muscular Endurance Tests

Many tests can help you evaluate muscular endurance, but the best ones assess your body's large muscles. In this self-assessment, you'll perform several isotonic and some isometric tests. For each, check "yes" if you could do the test as long or as many times as indicated. Check "no" if you could not. Look up your rating in table 10.4. As directed by your teacher, record your results.

TABLE 10.4 Rating Chart: Muscular Endurance

Fitness rating	Number of tests passed
Good fitness	5
Marginal fitness	3 or 4
Low fitness	0–2

Side Stand (isometric)

1. Lie on your side.
2. Use both hands to get your body in position so that it is supported by your left hand and the side of your left foot. Keep your body stiff.
3. Raise your right arm and leg in the air. Hold this position. Record 1 point if you meet the standard (30 seconds if you are male or 20 seconds if you are female).
4. Return to the starting position and repeat the test on your right side.

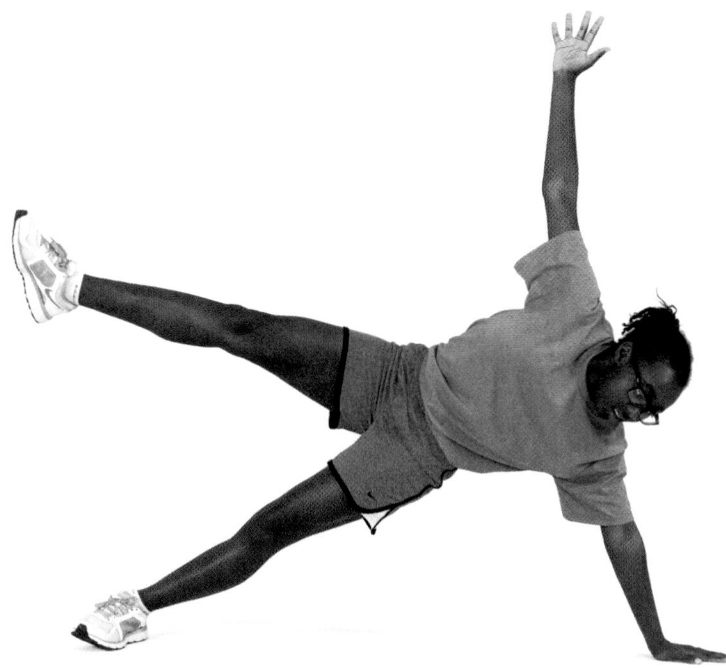

This test evaluates the isometric muscular endurance of some of your leg and arm muscles as well as your trunk-stabilizing muscles.

Trunk Extension (isotonic)

1. Lie facedown on a stable weight bench or the end of a bleacher that is 15 to 20 inches (38 to 51 centimeters) high. The top of your hips should be even with the end of the bench, and your upper body should hang off the end of the bench. If the surface is hard, cover it with a mat or a towel.
2. Have a partner hold your calves using one hand on each leg 12 inches (30 centimeters) above your ankles. Overlap your hands and place them (palms away) in front of your chin.
3. Start with your upper body bent at the hip so that your chin is near the floor with the palm of your lower hand against the floor. Place a small mat on the floor below your hands and chin.
4. Keeping your head and neck in line with your upper body, slowly lift your head and upper body off the floor until your upper body is in line with your lower body.

   Caution: Do not to lift your upper trunk higher than horizontal (in line with your lower body).
5. Lower to the starting position so that the palm of your lower hand touches the floor.
6. Perform one lift every three seconds. You may want to have a partner say "up, down" to help you. Record 1 point if you can meet the standard (20 reps if you are male or 15 reps if you are female).

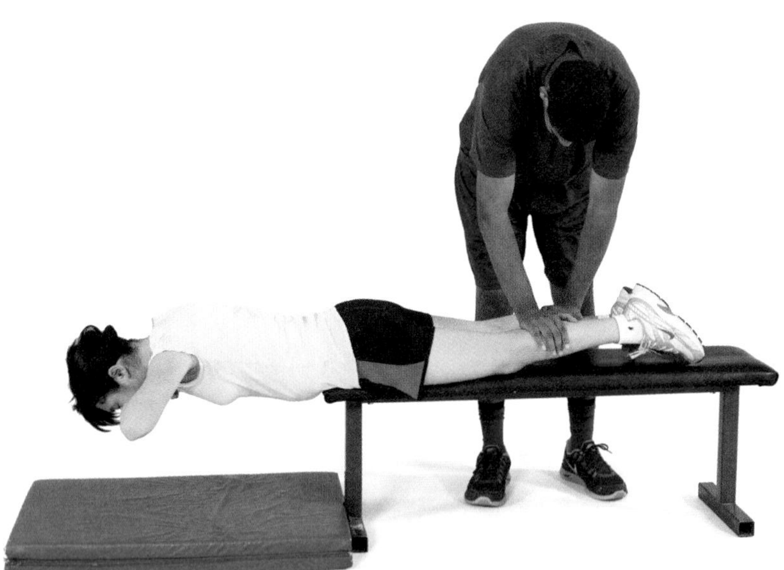

This test evaluates the isotonic muscular endurance of your upper back muscles.

Sitting Tuck (isotonic)

1. Sit on the floor with your knees bent and your arms outstretched.
2. Lean back (to about a 45-degree angle) and balance on your buttocks. Keep your knees bent near your chest (feet off the floor).
3. Straighten your knees so your body forms a V. You may move your arms sideways for balance.
4. Bend your knees to your chest again. Repeat the exercise as many times as you can. Count each time you push your legs out. Record 1 point if you can meet the standard (25 reps if you are male or 20 reps if you are female).

Safety tip: Avoid arching your lower back repetitively.

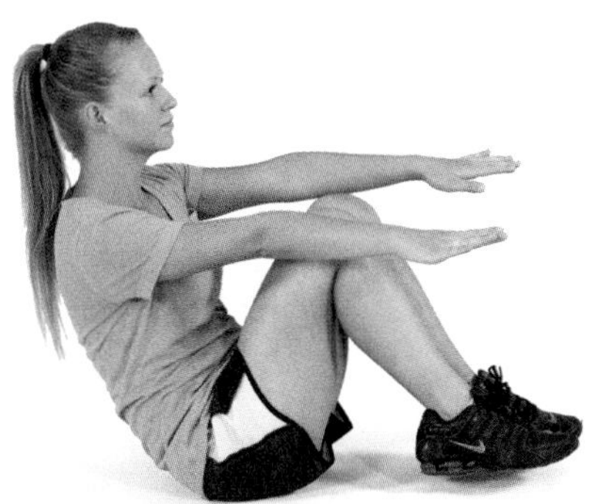

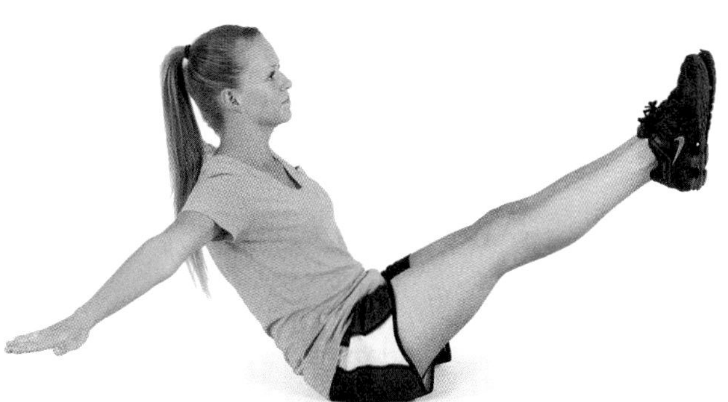

This test evaluates the isotonic muscular endurance of your abdominal muscles and some of your hip and leg muscles.

Leg Change (isotonic)

1. Assume a push-up position with your weight on your hands and feet.
2. Pull your right knee under your chest, and keep your left leg straight.
3. Change legs by pulling your left leg forward and pushing your right leg back.

   Caution: Do not let your lower back sag.
4. Continue changing legs (about one change with each leg every 2 seconds).
5. Count the number of leg changes performed in 1 minute. Record 1 point if you can meet the standard (25 changes for both males and females).

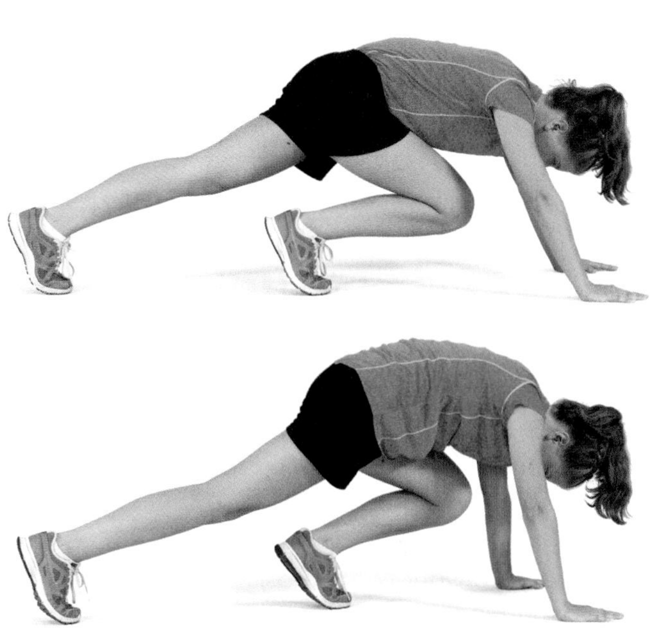

This test evaluates the isotonic muscular endurance of your hip and leg muscles.

Flexed-Arm Hang (isometric)

1. Hang from a chinning bar with your palms facing away from your body.
2. Standing on a chair, or with help from a partner, lift your chin above the bar.
3. At the start signal, your partner lets go or removes the chair so you are hanging by your own power. Count how long you can hang. The time count begins when the support is removed and ends when your chin touches or goes below the bar or your head tilts backward. Record 1 point if you can meet the standard (hold for 16 seconds if you are male or 12 seconds if you are female).

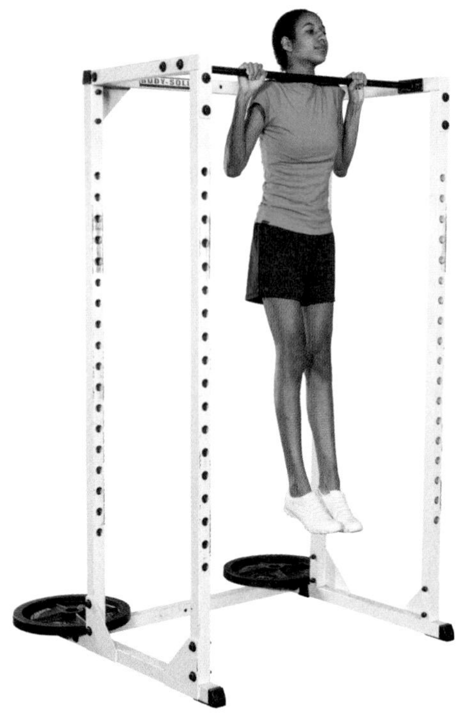

This test evaluates the muscular endurance of your arm, shoulder, and chest muscles (isometric).

Part 3: Tests of Power

In this self-assessment, you'll test the power of your lower body by performing the standing long jump and the upper body by performing the medicine ball throw.

Standing Long Jump

1. Use masking tape or another material to make the necessary line on the floor.
2. Stand with your feet shoulder-width apart behind the line on the floor. Bend your knees and hold your arms straight in front of your body at shoulder height.
3. Swing your arms downward and backward, then vigorously forward as you jump forward as far as possible, extending your legs.
4. Land on both feet and try to maintain your balance on landing. Do not run or hop before jumping.
5. Perform the test two times. Record the better of your two scores, then find your rating in table 10.5 and record it.

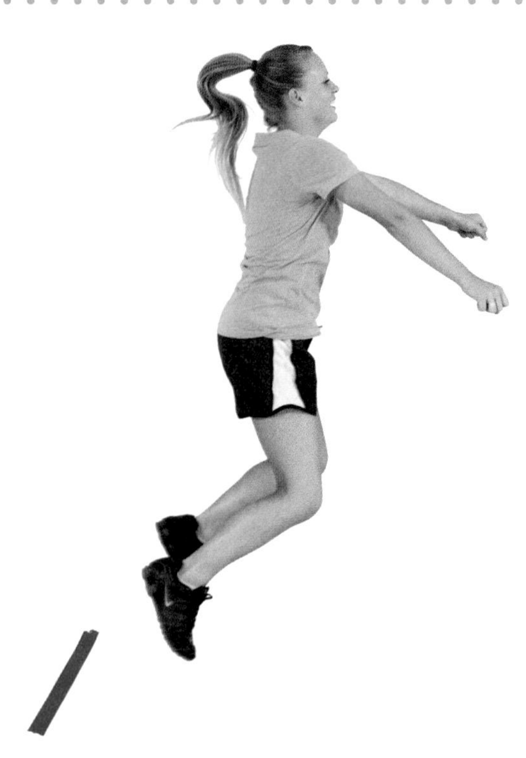

This test evaluates the power of the lower body.

TABLE 10.5 Rating Chart: Standing Long Jump in Inches

	13 years old		14 years old		15 years old		16 years old		17 years or older	
	Male	Female	Male	Female	Male	Female	Male	Female	Male	Female
High performance	≥73	≥59	≥80	≥60	≥85	≥61	≥88	≥62	≥91	≥68
Good fitness	67–72	57–58	73–79	58–59	78–84	59–60	82–87	60–61	86–90	63–67
Marginal fitness	61–66	54–56	67–72	55–57	73–77	56–58	77–81	57–59	80–85	58–62
Low fitness	≤60	≤53	≤66	≤54	≤72	≤55	≤76	≤56	≤79	≤57

To convert inches to centimeters, multiply by 2.54.

Medicine Ball Throw

1. Sit on a chair positioned against a wall. Sit back as far as possible so that your lower and upper back are against the back of the chair.
2. Hold a 14-pound (about 6.5-kilogram) medicine ball with both hands so that it rests against the middle of your chest.
3. Push with both hands to throw the medicine ball as far as possible. Throw as you would in a basketball chest pass. Keep your back against the chair.
4. Measure the distance from the wall (behind the chair) to the spot on the floor where the ball landed. Measure in inches (or centimeters).
5. Measure the distance from the wall to the end of your fingers (that is, your arm length) in inches (or centimeters). Your score is the distance that the ball was thrown minus the length of your arm.
6. Perform the test two times and use the better of your two scores.

Based on your better score, use table 10.6 to determine your rating. As directed by your instructor, record your score and your rating.

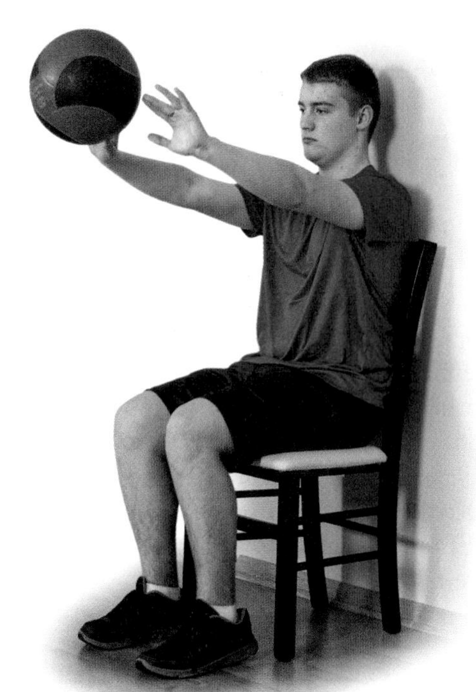

The medicine ball throw test evaluates power in your upper body.

TABLE 10.6 Rating Chart: Medicine Ball Throw in Inches

	15 years or younger		16 or 17 years old		18 years or older	
	Male	Female	Male	Female	Male	Female
Good fitness	≥145	≥98	≥155	≥102	≥165	≥108
Marginal fitness	130–144	90–97	140–154	94–101	150–164	98–107
Low fitness	≤129	≤89	≤139	≤93	≤149	≤97

To convert inches to centimeters, multiply by 2.54.

Lesson 10.2

Building Muscle Fitness

Lesson Objectives

After reading this lesson, you should be able to

1. explain the FIT formula for developing muscle fitness with isotonic PRE,
2. describe the double progressive system for using PRE,
3. describe several free weight and resistance machine exercises and their advantages and disadvantages,
4. describe several other forms of exercise for building muscle fitness,
5. describe basic guidelines for doing PRE safely, and
6. describe some myths about strength and explain why they are wrong.

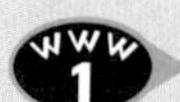

Lesson Vocabulary

bodybuilding, body dysmorphia, double progressive system, interval training, muscle bound, powerlifting, weightlifting

Do you know the health benefits of PRE and muscle fitness? Have you ever wanted to increase your muscle fitness? Are you familiar with the types of resistance training? In this lesson, you'll learn some of the health benefits associated with achieving muscle fitness through PRE. You'll also learn how to apply the FIT formula for the most popular methods of building muscle fitness. And you'll learn about recommended guidelines for properly performing progressive resistance exercise (PRE) and about some common misconceptions concerning muscle fitness.

Health Benefits of PRE and Muscle Fitness

Many of the health benefits described throughout this book are associated with doing muscle fitness exercises and achieving good muscle fitness. Most people know that muscle fitness helps reduce back problems, improves posture, reduces risk of muscle injury, and increases working capacity. They may not know that muscle fitness exercises are very important to bone health (preventing osteoporosis), prevention of heart disease and diabetes, and rehabilitation from chronic diseases such as cancer. Muscle fitness exercises can also reduce your risk of becoming overweight or obese. In addition, they provide mental health benefits such as looking and feeling your best and experiencing a high quality of life. Among older people, muscle fitness also helps reduce the risk of falling and improves a person's ability to do tasks of daily life.

Building Muscle Fitness With Isotonic PRE

In this section, you'll learn about the FIT formula for isotonic PRE. You'll also learn some of the advantages and disadvantages of resistance machine and free weight exercises and some general guidelines for performing isotonic PRE.

The FIT Formula for Isotonic PRE: Resistance Machines and Free Weights

Table 10.7 provides FIT formula information for isotonic exercises using resistance machines and free weights, such as those described later in this lesson. The same FIT formula can be used for isokinetic exercises. As indicated in the table, beginners use lower resistance, do more reps, and perform fewer sets than people who are more advanced.

The American College of Sports Medicine (ACSM) recommends a two- or three-minute rest between sets. In general, you should use longer rests between high-resistance exercises and shorter rests between low-resistance exercises. To make your workout more efficient, you can alternate arm and

TABLE 10.7 Fitness Target Zones for Muscle Fitness (Isotonic)

	Beginner		Intermediate		Advanced	
	Threshold	Target	Threshold	Target	Threshold	Target
Frequency (days per week)	2	2 or 3	2	2 or 3	3	3 or 4
Intensity (% of 1RM)	50	50–70	60	60–80	70	70–85
Time	1 set of 10–15 reps	1 or 2 sets of 10–15 reps	2 sets of 8–12 reps	2 or 3 sets of 8–12 reps	3 sets of 6–10 reps	3–4 sets of 6–10 reps

leg exercises. That way, when your arms are working, your legs are resting, and vice versa.

The FIT formula for muscle fitness for teens differs somewhat from the formula for adults, especially for exercise intensity. ACSM recommends a FIT formula similar to the one shown in the table for teens. For adults, beginners can start at 60 percent of 1RM rather than 50 percent for teens, and advanced exercisers can use 80 to 90 percent of 1RM rather than 70 to 85 percent. Adult beginners can start with two sets rather than one set, which is what is recommended for teens.

The Double Progressive System of PRE

You already know that in order to achieve optimal development of your muscle fitness, you need to progress gradually. The most commonly used method for applying the principle of progression to muscle fitness is the **double progressive system**. The first part of the system involves increasing repetitions (reps). For example, as shown in table 10.7, a beginner starts with one set of 10 reps at 50 percent of 1RM, then gradually increases the number of reps until he or she can easily perform 15 reps.

The second part of the system involves increasing resistance or weight. The number of reps is dropped back to 10, and the resistance is increased by 5 to 10 percent of 1RM; for teens, this often means an increase of about 2 to 5 pounds (0.9 to 2.3 kilograms). This double progression—increasing reps and resistance—continues until the person can do the maximum percent of 1RM in the beginner category. At that point, he or she can add a second set. It may be necessary to drop back to a lower number of reps and a lower percent of 1RM to perform two full sets of 10 to 15 reps.

When doing multiple sets, longer rest intervals between sets allow you to lift a higher percent of 1RM than shorter rest intervals. So it is important to use rest intervals of a consistent length of time.

Once a person can perform two sets of 15 reps at 70 percent of 1RM (a goal that may take several months to attain), he or she is ready to move to the intermediate stage. Here, the double progression sequence begins again. The person follows the double progressive system at the moderate stage until he or she can perform three sets of 8 to 12 reps at 80 percent of 1RM. It may take a year or longer to progress to this point.

Some exercisers choose to stay at the intermediate level because many health benefits can be achieved using the FIT formula for this stage (moderate sets and reps and moderate resistance). Because the FIT formula for advanced exercisers focuses more on low reps and higher resistance, it builds more pure strength than the FIT formula for beginners and intermediates. Therefore, the advanced FIT formula offers benefits for people who plan to do sports or jobs requiring high levels of strength and for people especially interested in muscle hypertrophy. However, the FIT formula for intermediates provides many benefits and is appropriate for regular use by most teens.

Resistance Machines Versus Free Weights

Resistance machine and free weight exercises require considerable equipment but are among the most popular forms of isotonic PRE because they are two of the most effective methods for building muscle fitness. They allow you to build both strength and muscular endurance and isolate most of the major muscle groups in your body with specific exercises.

To help you consider these forms of PRE, compare their advantages and disadvantages as outlined in table 10.8. Some basic exercises using free weights and resistance machines are described at the end of this lesson; for each exercise, the muscles used are listed and illustrated.

Mens sana in corpore sano (a sound mind in a sound body).

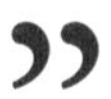

—Juvenal, Roman poet

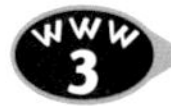

FIT FACT

In addition to the National Strength and Conditioning Association (see the first lesson in this chapter), several other groups of experts have now prepared statements indicating that resistance training can be safe for teens when performed properly. These groups include the American College of Sports Medicine, the American Academy of Pediatrics (medical doctors who specialize in treating children and youth), and the American Orthopaedic Society of Sports Medicine (medical doctors who specialize in bone problems associated with sport and activity). The self-assessments and muscle fitness exercises described in this book follow the guidelines of these organizations.

PRE

When performed correctly, resistance training is safe and improves your muscle fitness while helping you feel and look your best. Stick to the following guidelines created especially to help teens use PRE safely and effectively.

- **Warm up** with recommended dynamic exercises or perform low-resistance sets before doing your regular workout.
- **Learn proper technique.** From the beginning, get good instruction from an expert. Start with little or no weight as you're learning the fundamentals. Use the following tips for good technique.
    - **Use moderate-velocity movements**—not too slow and not too fast.
    - **Use both concentric and eccentric contractions through a full range of motion.** For example, when doing the biceps curl, lift the weight all the way up (this uses a concentric contraction) and lower the weight all the way down (this uses an eccentric contraction).
    - **Avoid sudden or quick movements.** Stop briefly at the beginning and end of each repetition. Use your muscles, not the movement of your body, to do the exercise (for example, don't rock forward and backward with the upper body during a biceps curl).

TABLE 10.8 Resistance Machines Versus Free Weights

	Resistance machines	Free weights
Safety	Safer because weights cannot fall on lifter Spotter often not needed	Greater chance of injury from falling weights Easy to lose control of—spotter needed
Cost	Very expensive to own If not owned, club membership required to use	Relatively inexpensive
Versatility	Easy to isolate specific muscle groups	More balance, muscle coordination, and concentration required More muscles used, movements more like moving heavy loads in daily life
Convenience	Much floor space needed Must be used where installed	Little space needed Some weights small enough to carry around Easily scattered, lost, or stolen

- **Do not hold your breath when you exercise.** Holding your breath can cause you to black out. Some resistance trainers recommend exhaling when applying resistance and inhaling on the return movement.
- **Use good biomechanics.** Avoid body positions and movements that cause your joints to move in ways for which they are not intended or that put your muscles at risk of injury.

- **Make sure that your workout area is safe.** Use equipment in good working order. Keep free weights on weight racks rather than scattered on the floor. Clean the machine after you're done by wiping it with a towel—or even before you use it, if it wasn't cleaned by the previous user.
- **When working with free weights, always use spotters.** You might be tempted to work on your own, but working with a partner is much safer.
- **Progress gradually.** Young teens, and all teens with little PRE experience, should exercise with the FIT formula for beginners for several months before moving to the intermediate level. Do not let the word *beginner* be a reason for violating the principle of progression. And remember that the advanced FIT formula is typically reserved for people with at least one year of experience and for older teens who have reached physical maturity.
- **Select exercises for all major muscle groups.** Experts recommend that you perform 8 to 10 muscle fitness exercises to be sure that you build all of the major muscle groups. Performing only a few exercises can lead to unbalanced muscle development. In part 1 of this book, 8 to 10 exercises are provided for many types of PRE.
- **Rest between sets.** For building pure strength, allow two to three minutes between sets; for muscular endurance, allow one to two minutes between sets.
- **Allow rest days between exercise sessions.** For best results, do not perform PRE for the same muscle group on consecutive days. You can, however, exercise daily if you alternate muscle groups to avoid exercising the same muscle group on consecutive days.
- **Vary your program to keep it interesting.** ACSM points out the importance of progression and volume when exercising. Using the double progressive method to progress gradually provides variety while helping you get optimal benefits. You can also get variety while keeping your volume (total amount of exercise) constant by varying repetitions and resistance (for example, many reps with low resistance can result in the same volume of exercise as fewer reps with higher resistance).
- **Avoid overhead lifts with free weights.** If possible, use machines for these lifts. If you must use free weights, always use a trained spotter.
- **Master single-joint exercises before attempting multiple-joint exercises or sport movements.** For example, a biceps curl is a single-joint exercise because the only joint it moves is the elbow. Most of the exercises needed to build good health, as shown in part 1 of this book, are single-joint exercises. Multiple-joint lifts, such as the clean and jerk in the sport of **weightlifting**, require

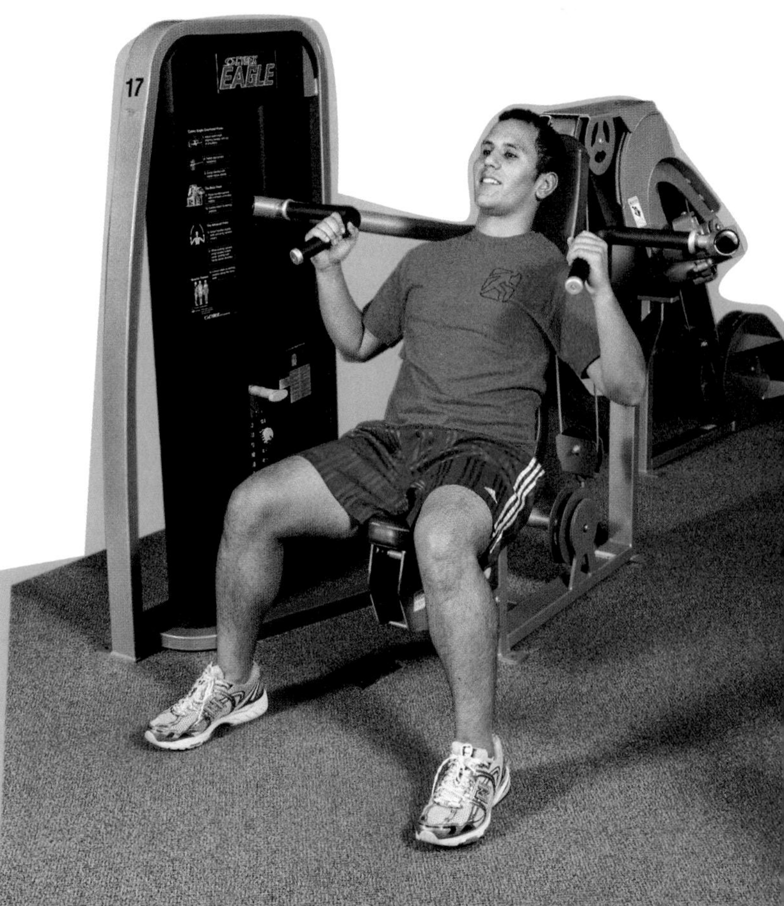

good muscle fitness that results from PRE consisting of single-joint exercises. Multiple-joint exercises also involve a high level of skill that requires special training to ensure good technique.

- **Never use weights carelessly.** Concentrate on your technique and on what you're doing. Use care when changing free weights and put them away properly when you're finished.
- **Never compete when you do resistance training.** For example, do not have a contest to see who can lift the most weight. Genetic differences have a lot to do with how strong a person can be. Concern yourself only with trying to improve your own strength gradually and enjoying the exercise—not lifting more than someone else.

PRE Using Resistance Machines and Free Weights

Experts recommend doing 8 to 10 basic exercises to build all of your major muscle groups. At the end of this lesson, 9 free weight exercises and 10 resistance machine exercises are described. Before performing these exercises, practice each exercise and the spotting techniques described in the next section. Spotting means supporting a partner by being ready to help if he or she loses control of the weight or gets off balance. Your instructor will help you practice these techniques.

Practicing Proper Exercise and Spotting Technique

Performing and spotting exercises properly require practice. Before you begin your PRE program, practice by moving through the four levels described in this section. Start with level 1 *for each exercise* until you achieve mastery. Then move to the next level. The specific techniques for performing exercises and spotting properly are described in this lesson in the individual descriptions of exercises using free weights and resistance machines. Some experts use the phrase "feel is not real" to emphasize that just feeling that you're doing an exercise properly does not necessarily mean that you really are. In many facilities, mirrors are provided so that you can check your form. A partner can also help you determine whether you're using correct spotting and lifting techniques (figure 10.9).

- **Level 1.** Focus on lifting technique, not weight. Perform each exercise without any weight by using a wand or stick instead of a barbell. When you're practicing a lift, concentrate on correct form (placement of your body parts). When you're watching a partner, give useful coaching.
- **Level 2.** Focus on spotting technique, not weight. While your partner performs the rep with the wand, you and another partner practice correct spotting technique. Pay particular attention to your leg and hand positions.
- **Level 3.** At this level, you combine lifting and spotting with light weights. Perform each exercise by doing five repetitions with light weight. Practice your lifting and spotting techniques and continue to give each other coaching about both lifting and spotting.
- **Level 4.** At this level, you perform a normal workout using free weights. Select the appropriate percentage of your 1RM and the appropriate number of sets and repetitions (see table 10.7). Perform each of the basic exercises.

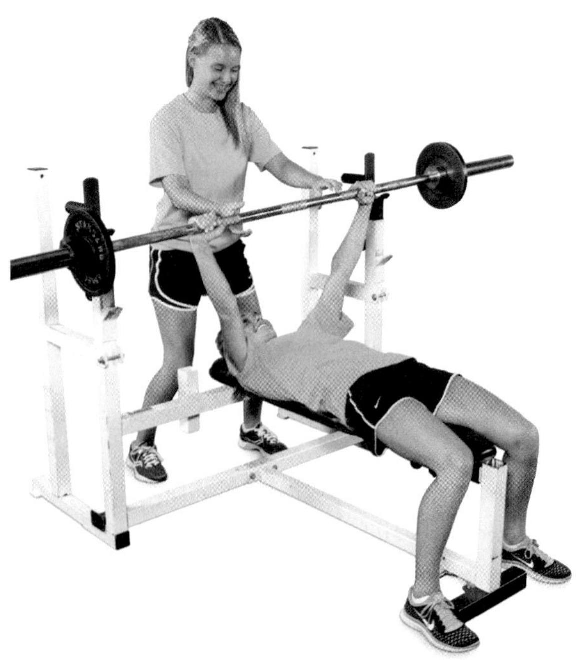

FIGURE 10.9 Having a spotter is essential when using free weights.

Clarifying Progressive Resistance Training Terms

As you now know, PRE is a method of building muscle fitness. It differs from three sports that use similar names or terminology.

Olympic-Style Weightlifting

In this Olympic sport, athletes use free weights to try lifting a maximum load. The sport includes only two lifts: the snatch and the clean and jerk. For those who train with weights but do not participate in Olympic-style weightlifting, the preferred term is *weight training*.

Powerlifting

Powerlifting is another competitive sport using free weights. It includes only three exercises: the bench press, the squat, and the dead lift. Athletes in this sport try to make one maximal lift for each type of lift.

Bodybuilding

Bodybuilding participants are concerned primarily with the appearance of their body, and judges rate them based on how large and well defined their muscles are rather than how much they can lift. This sport can also be done competitively.

Other Types of Isotonic PRE

Resistance machine and free weight exercises are popular and effective, but they are not the only types of isotonic PRE. The following entries describe some other frequently used forms, including calisthenics, elastic band exercises, and exercise with homemade equipment.

FIT FACT

An electromyograph (EMG) is a machine used by researchers to determine how hard a muscle contracts. In EMG results, smaller contractions (such as those used for muscular endurance) show a low muscle action wave, whereas harder contractions (such as those used for strength) show a larger muscle action wave.

Calisthenics

Calisthenic exercises use all or part of your body weight to provide resistance; examples include push-ups and curl-ups. Because only your body weight is used for resistance, this type of PRE is better for building muscular endurance than for building strength. The lower resistance also means that you can do calisthenics more frequently. The FIT formula for isotonic calisthenics is shown in table 10.9. Calisthenics are good for both home use and travel because you can do them almost anywhere with little equipment.

Exercising With Elastic Bands, Homemade Weights, Partner Resistance, and Balls

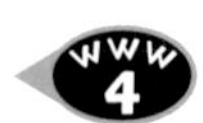

These types of PRE are similar to resistance machine and free weight exercises but use various other means to provide resistance. Like calisthenics, elastic band exercises require little equipment and are easy to do both at home and when traveling. Exercises using a stability ball can also be effective in building core fitness. All of these types of PRE use the FIT formula described in table 10.7. Some exercises using partner resistance and homemade weights are described in the student section of the Health Opportunities Through Physical Education website.

TABLE 10.9 Target Zone for Calisthenics (Isotonic)

	Threshold	Target zone
Frequency (days per week)	3	3–6
Intensity	Moving the weight of parts of the body	Moving the weight of parts or all of the body
Time	1 set of 10 reps	1–4 sets of 11–25 reps

Rest for 2 minutes between sets.

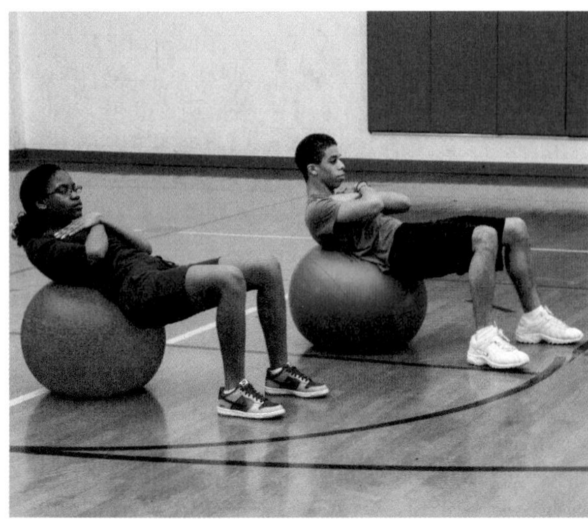

Stability ball exercises can help you build core fitness.

Building Muscle Fitness With Isometric PRE

Isometric exercises can be done easily at home or when you travel because they require little or no equipment and can be done in a confined space—even a space as small as an airplane seat. A disadvantage of isometric PRE is that it's sometimes hard to tell when you're doing a maximum contraction, and this uncertainty can affect your motivation to work hard. In isotonic exercise, on the other hand, you can see your movement and you know how much effort you're giving. In addition, experts do not consider isometric exercise to be as effective in building muscle fitness as isotonic PRE. As with all PRE, when doing isometric exercise, breathe rather than hold your breath while you're performing exercises. The FIT formula for isometric exercises is included in table 10.10. Some basic isometric exercises are illustrated and described at the end of this lesson. The muscles used in each exercise are also listed and illustrated.

Building Power

As you may recall, power is a combination of strength and speed. Exercise physiologists have shown that power is related to bone development in children and teens and offers health benefits similar to those provided by other parts of muscle fitness. It's also important for good performance in various sports, including track and field (as in putting the shot or throwing the discus), baseball (hitting the ball a long way), and football (rushing the passer). For this reason, athletes often want to improve their power not only for their health but also for improved performance.

One of the most frequently used methods of building power is plyometrics (plyometric exercise). Plyometrics was pioneered by Olympic track-and-field coaches from the former Soviet Union. Plyometric exercise involves a rapid eccentric contraction of a muscle followed by a concentric contraction of the muscle. For example, one common low-resistance form of plyometric exercise is rope jumping. Landing after a jump requires your calf muscle to do an eccentric, or lengthening, contraction, and the next jump into the air requires a concentric contraction of the calf muscle. Resistance is provided by body weight. Plyometrics often uses more vigorous jumping activities.

Like other forms of muscle fitness exercise, plyometrics was previously thought to be dangerous for teens. However, recent evidence suggests that when performed properly and progressively with good supervision, plyometrics can be safe for teens, enhance athletic performance, increase both power and speed, and actually reduce athletic injuries. Nevertheless, plyometric and other power-building techniques have resulted in injury when performed excessively. The FIT formula for plyometrics is described in table 10.11; the formula, developed by experts, shows a progression based on age and fitness level. Fit athletes may do advanced plyometrics or

TABLE 10.10 Target Zone for Isometric PRE

	Threshold	Target zone
Frequency (days per week)	3	3–6
Intensity	Contracting muscle as tightly as possible or holding part or all of body weight	Contracting muscle as tightly as possible or holding part or all of body weight
Time	3 reps (1 rep = hold for 7 sec)	3–4 reps (1 rep = hold for 7–10 sec)

TABLE 10.11 Target Zone for Plyometrics

	Threshold	Target zone
Frequency (days per week)	2 (nonconsecutive)	2 or 3 (nonconsecutive)
Intensity (jumps of varying intensity based on age)	Age 12: low intensity (in place) Age 13: medium intensity (moving jumps and hops) Ages 14 and 15: medium intensity (box and obstacle jumps) Age ≥16: high intensity (bounding—multiple jumps over distance and drop jumping)	Same as threshold
Time	1 set of 6–10 repetitions Rest for 1–3 minutes between sets.	1–3 sets of 6–10 repetitions Rest for 1–3 minutes between sets.

Beginners should start at low intensity and progress to higher intensity regardless of age. Youth who have been regularly active and have high fitness may move to more advanced levels at ages lower than suggested with proper supervision by a qualified expert who has evaluated the maturational and fitness status of the exerciser.

other forms of training, but you should consult with a parent or guardian and an instructor or certified exercise leader before performing them.

Interval Training

Interval training uses bouts of high-intensity exercise followed by rest periods. For example, runners and swimmers often use a series of high-intensity sprints (exercise intervals) followed by rest intervals. This type of training was developed to improve anaerobic performance in activities such as sprinting and fast swimming and in the short bursts of vigorous activity typical of soccer, hockey, football, and basketball. Now, interval training is regularly used by endurance athletes as well. For more information about interval training, check with your physical education teacher or coach.

Myths and Misconceptions

The amount of muscle fitness you need in order to stay healthy and do what you want depends on your personal situation and interests. For example, people who do jobs requiring a lot of lifting need more strength than people who work at a desk. Despite the fact that muscle fitness exercise offers many benefits, many people still hold misconceptions about them.

No Pain, No Gain

Some people still cling to the myth that exercise must hurt in order to be effective. Some of the worst offenders are people who are hooked on strength-building exercises. In reality, you should listen to your body. If you feel pain, your body is telling you something. When doing PRE, it's true that you'll become quite fatigued and feel a sensation sometimes called the exercise "burn," and you need to learn the difference between this feeling and pain. If in doubt, back off to avoid injury.

Muscle Bound

Some people think that strength training will cause them to be **muscle bound**—to have tight, bulky muscles that prevent them from moving freely. However, inflexibility is caused not by resistance training but by incorrect training. Two kinds of incorrect exercise that *can* cause a muscle-bound condition are training muscles on only one side of a joint and failing to stretch muscles. Another example of incorrect training is failure to move the joints through their full range of motion when lifting weights or doing other resistance exercises. For example, your elbow joint can bend to allow your hand to reach your shoulder and to let your arm straighten completely. Therefore, when you do a biceps curl with weight, bring the weight all the way to your shoulder, then straighten your elbow each time you lower the weight. *Caution: Do not bend your elbow or any other joint backward beyond its full range of motion. You can damage a joint if you move it in a way in which it was not designed to move.* Recent research suggests that when done properly, PRE can actually enhance flexibility.

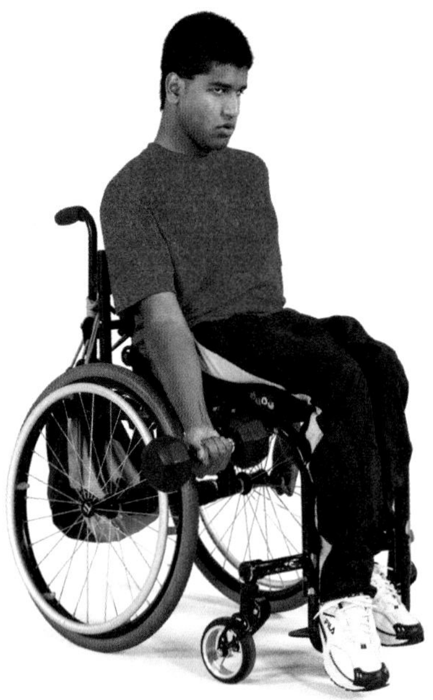
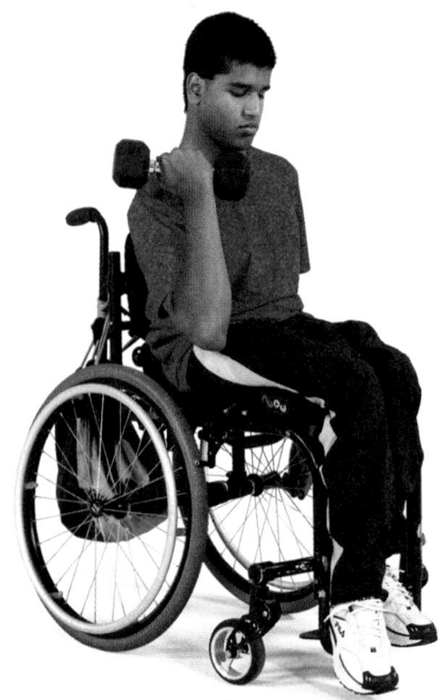

Moving a joint through the full range of motion is important for optimal functioning.

Muscle Fitness for Females

As noted earlier, some people think that girls and women cannot build muscle fitness. Others think that PRE will cause girls and women to look masculine. Both of these statements are false.

Muscle Tone

Advertisers often promise that a product or program can build something they call muscle tone. However, "tone" in this usage is considered to be a quack word because it does not refer to anything that can be measured in the same way as strength, muscular endurance, or power. Inspecting or feeling a muscle cannot objectively measure it; therefore, "tone" is not a good word to use to define muscle fitness, and any claim based on it is suspect.

Body Dysmorphia

The term **body dysmorphia** refers to a condition in which a person becomes obsessed with building muscle. This psychological disorder, sometimes referred to as "reverse anorexia," often begins with a reasonable amount of exercise to build muscle fitness. At some point, however, a person with this problem gets carried away in wanting to build more and more muscle. The disorder is an obsessive-compulsive one and often requires treatment by a professional. In more than a few cases, people with this disorder have done unhealthy behaviors, such as taking drugs and doing unhealthy exercises. People with this condition experience high injury rates. Doing reasonable PRE can enhance your health. Becoming obsessed with fitness can hurt it.

Lesson Review

1. What is the FIT formula for developing muscle fitness with isotonic PRE?
2. What is the double progressive system, and how is it helpful in using PRE?
3. What are some basic free weight and resistance machine exercises, and what are their advantages and disadvantages?
4. What are several other forms of exercise for building muscle fitness?
5. What are some of the basic guidelines for doing PRE safely?
6. What are some muscle fitness myths?

FREE WEIGHT EXERCISES

The following basic exercises use free weights to work the major muscle groups. The exercises that use barbells (bar and weights) can also be performed with dumbbells (small bar and weights or fixed weight dumbbells). The last two exercises require dumbbells. You can determine your 1RM for the various muscle groups using some of these exercises, but because resistance machines exercises are safer, they are the preferred method.

SEATED OVERHEAD PRESS

Weights: barbell

This exercise requires two spotters, who stand by the lifter's shoulders on either side of the bench. If you are serving as a spotter, keep your hands under the bar with your palms up. Be ready to take the bar if the lifter loses control (especially at the top of the lift), if the barbell begins to move backward, or if the lifter begins to tremble.

1. Sit on the end of a bench in front stride (split-foot) position.
2. Hold the barbell at chest height in preparation for pushing the bar vertically. Grasp the barbell with your hands facing away from your body and positioned slightly more than shoulder-width apart.
3. Tighten your abdominal, back, and arm muscles. Tip your head back slightly.
4. Push the bar straight up, directly overhead.

Caution: Do not let the bar go forward or backward. Do not lock your elbows. Do not arch your back.

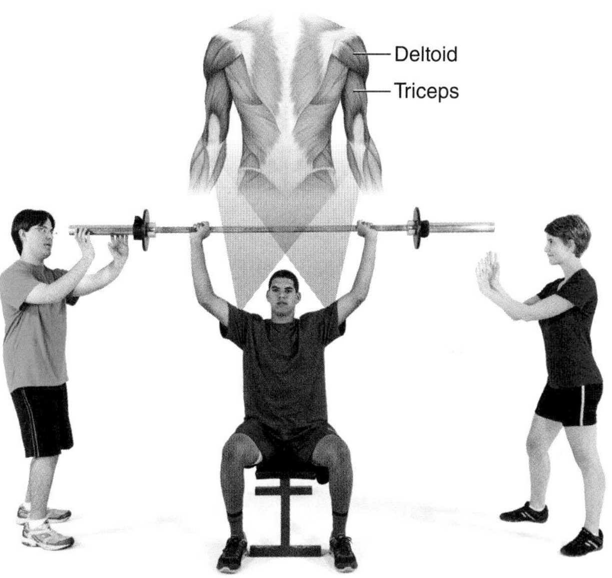

This exercise uses the muscles at the top of your shoulders, between your shoulder blades, and on the back of your arms.

BENCH PRESS

Weights: barbell

This exercise requires two spotters, who stand by the lifter's shoulders on either side of the bench. If you are serving as a spotter, place the bar into the lifter's hands. During the exercise, keep your hands under the bar with your palms up. Be prepared to take the bar if the lifter loses control.

1. Lie on your back on a bench with your feet on the floor and your lower back flat. Extend your arms into the up position (perpendicular to the floor).
2. Grasp the bar with a palms-up grip and your hands slightly farther than shoulder-width apart, your elbows straight, and the bar approximately over your collarbones.
3. Lower the bar until it touches your chest just below your armpits. When the bar touches your chest, your forearms should be perpendicular to the floor and your elbows should point neither toward your feet nor out to the sides but halfway between (at 45 degrees).

4. Tighten your abdominal, back, and arm muscles. Tip your head back slightly.
   Caution: Do not lock your elbows.
5. Push the bar up to the starting position with your arms perpendicular to the floor. The bar follows a slightly curved path.
   Caution: Do not lock your elbows or bounce the bar off of your chest. Do not arch your back or lift your hips. If the weight gets in front of or behind your arms, you may lose control.

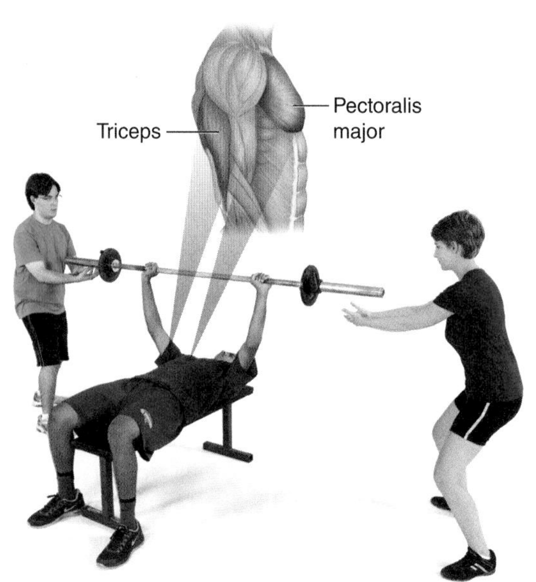

This exercise uses the muscles on the front of your chest (pectoral) and the back of your upper arms (triceps).

KNEE EXTENSION

Weights: weighted boot or ankle weight

One person can help the lifter put on the boot or ankle weight.

1. Put the weight on one foot or ankle. Sit on a bench with your lower leg hanging over the edge. Grasp the bench with your hands.
2. Lift the weighted boot by extending your knee until your leg is straight.
   Caution: Lift slowly. Do not lock your knee when you extend and do not kick your leg upward.
3. Repeat the exercise with your other leg.

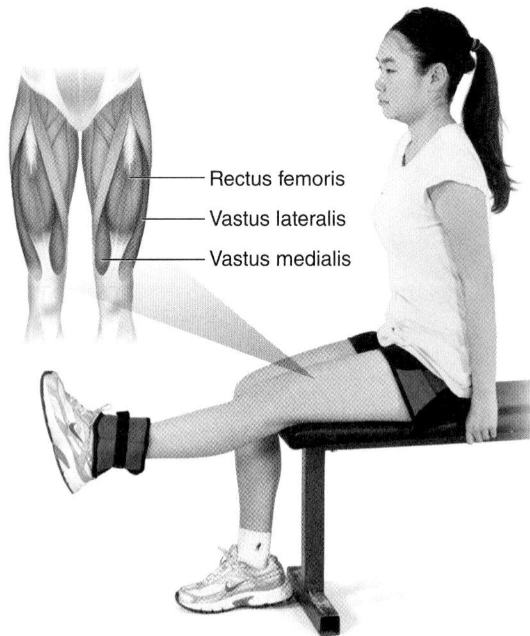

This exercise uses the muscles at the top of your thighs (quadriceps). The fourth quadriceps muscle, the vastus intermedius, lies beneath the rectus femoris and therefore is not shown in the illustration.

HALF SQUAT

Weights: barbell

Note: This exercise can be done only if a squat rack is available.

1. Stand in a side-stride position with your feet shoulder-width or slightly farther apart. Your toes should point straight ahead or be slightly turned out. Keep your head up and your back straight.
2. Hold the barbell across the back of your shoulders at the base of your neck with your hands slightly farther than shoulder-width apart and your palms facing away from your body. Point your elbows toward the floor with your forearms perpendicular to the floor.
3. Squat until your knees are at a right angle, then rise. Keep your heels flat on the floor. Do not let your knees get in front of your toes. Focus on a spot on the wall slightly higher than your standing height. Look at this spot for the duration of the lift—when lowering and when straightening.

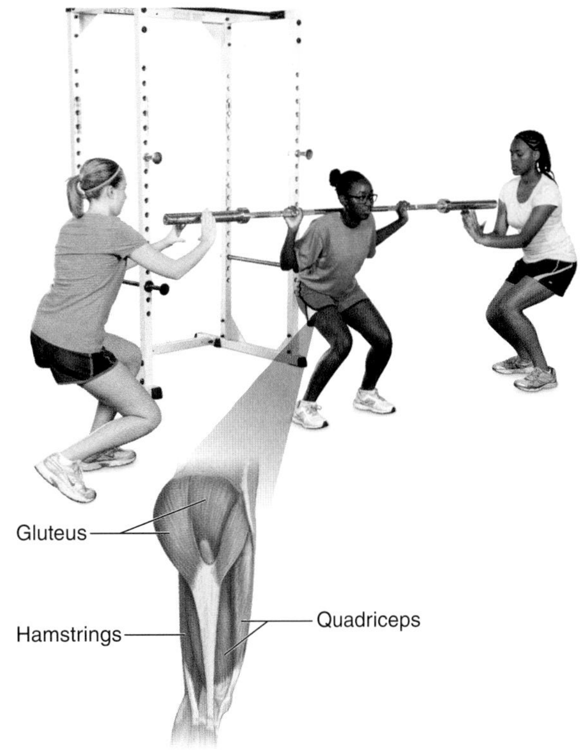

This exercise uses the muscles on the front of your thighs (quadriceps) and your buttock muscles (gluteal).

Caution: Do not round your back. Do not lean too far forward at your hips or let your knees get in front of your toes. Do not squat too deeply.

HAMSTRING CURL

Weights: weighted boot or ankle weight

One person can help the lifter put on the boot or ankle weight.

1. Put the weight on one foot or ankle. Lie facedown on a bench, with your kneecaps hanging over the edge. Grasp the bench with your hands.
2. Lift the weighted boot by flexing your knee to a right angle.
   Caution: Do not lock your knee when you extend.
3. Repeat the exercise using your other leg. To determine your 1RM for this exercise, use the hamstring curl on the resistance machine.

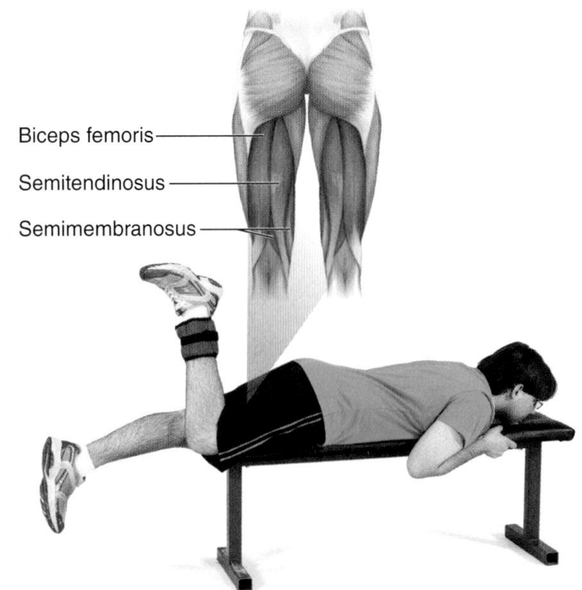

This exercise uses the muscles on the back of your thighs (hamstring).

BICEPS CURL

Weights: barbell

Spotters are not required, but they can place the barbell in the lifter's palm-up hands.

1. Stand erect with your feet in side-stride position. Tighten your abdominal and back muscles.
2. Grasp the bar with your palms up and your hands slightly more than shoulder-width apart. The arms are fully extended.
3. Keep your elbows close to your sides and lift the weight by bending your elbows only. Raise the weight to near your chin, then return to the starting position.
   Caution: Do not move other joints, especially in your back.
4. You can also perform this exercise with your palms down.

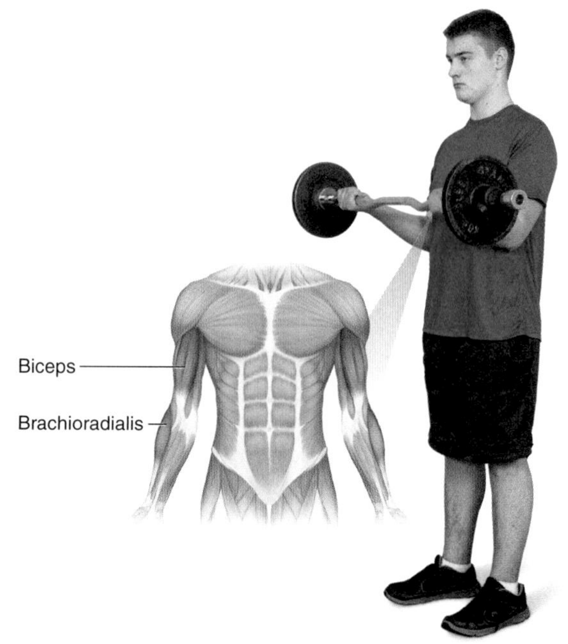

This exercise uses the muscles on the front of your upper arms (biceps) and other elbow flexor muscles.

HEEL RAISE

Weights: barbell

This exercise requires two spotters, who stand by the lifter's shoulders, one on each side.

1. If weight is manageable, lift the bar above your head like you would in an overhead press (with spotters). Then lower the bar to your shoulders. If the weight is heavier than you can easily press, have spotters lift the weight to your shoulders.
2. Once the bar is on your shoulders, stand with the balls of your feet on a 2-inch (5-centimeter) board and your toes turned in slightly.
3. Rise onto your toes, then lower to the starting position.
   Caution: Keep your spine straight.
4. Advanced lifters may also try this exercise with their toes pointing straight ahead (more difficult) or with their toes turned outward (even more difficult). To determine your 1RM for this exercise, use the heel raise on the resistance machine.

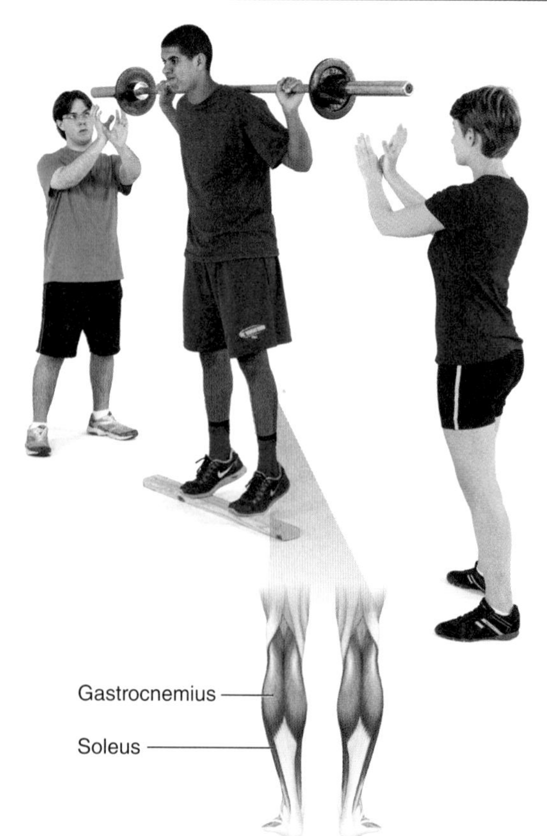

This exercise uses your calf muscles.

SEATED FRENCH CURL

Weights: dumbbell

This exercise requires one spotter.

1. Sit on the end of a bench with your arms extended overhead and your palms facing up.
2. Hold one end of a dumbbell in both hands above and behind your head. Tighten your abdominal and back muscles. Slowly lower the weight toward the back of your neck until your arms are fully flexed at the elbows. Keep your elbows high.
3. Slowly return to the starting position, moving only your elbow joints. To determine your 1RM for this exercise, use the triceps press.

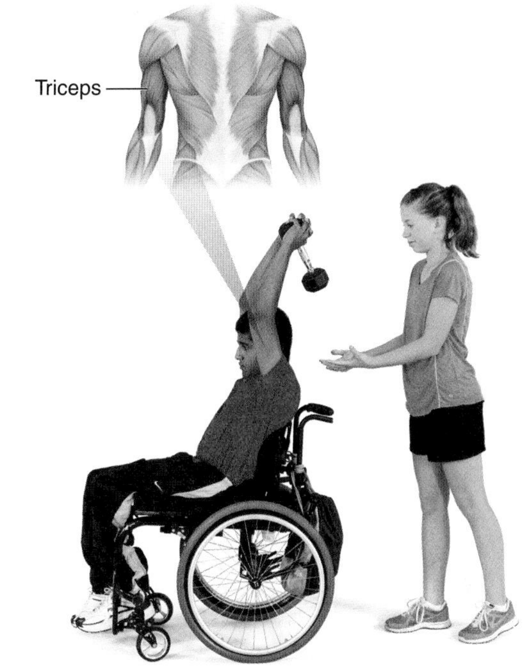

This exercise uses the muscles on the back of your upper arms (triceps).

BENT-OVER DUMBBELL ROW

Weights: dumbbell

This exercise requires no spotters.

1. Hold the dumbbell in one hand and rest your opposite hand and knee on a bench to support the weight of your trunk and protect your back.
2. Pull the dumbbell upward until it touches the side of your chest near your armpit and your upper arm is parallel to the floor.
3. Slowly lower the weight.
4. Repeat the exercise with your other arm. To determine your 1RM for this exercise, use the seated row.

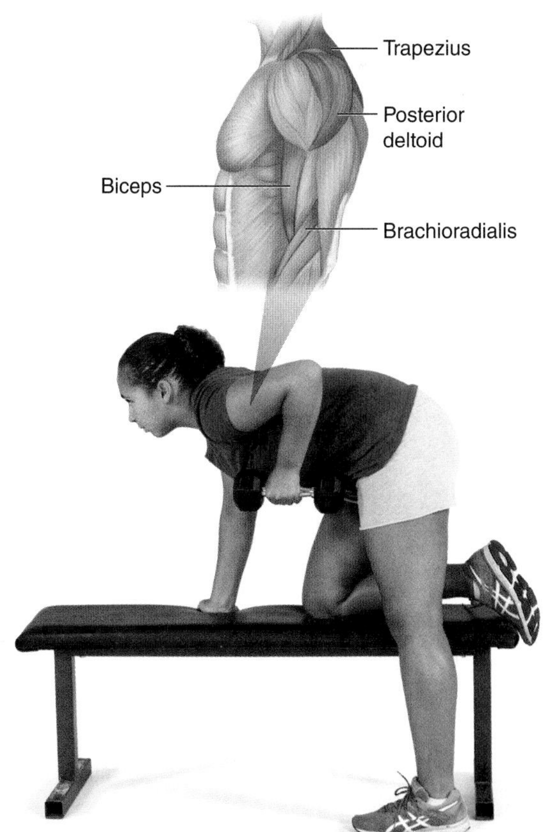

This exercise uses your biceps muscles, your shoulder muscles, and the muscles between your shoulder blades.

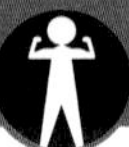

RESISTANCE MACHINE EXERCISES

The following basic exercises use resistance machines to work the major muscle groups. They can be used to determine your 1RM for each muscle group just as you determined your 1RM for the seated arm press and leg press in the Self-Assessment.

SEATED ARM PRESS

1. Sit on the stool of a seated press machine and position yourself so that the handles are even with your shoulders. Grasp the handles with your palms facing away from you. Tighten your abdominal muscles.
2. Push upward on the handles, extending your arms until your elbows are straight.
   Caution: Do not arch your back. Do not lock your elbows.
3. Lower the handles to the starting position.

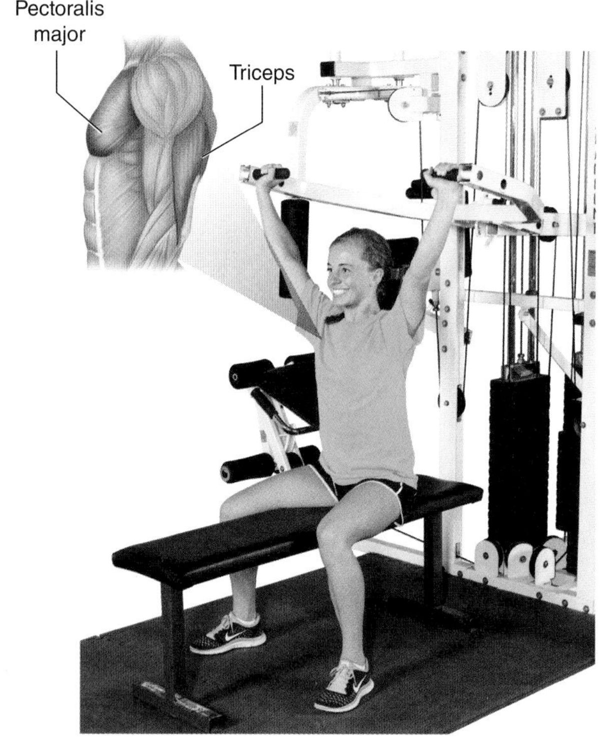

This exercise uses your pectoral and triceps muscles.

BENCH PRESS

1. Lie on your back on the bench with your feet flat on the floor. Grasp the handles with your palms facing away from your body. Flatten your back. If possible, place your feet on the floor to help flatten your back and avoid arching it. If your feet do not reach the floor easily, bend your knees and place your feet on the bench to accomplish the same purpose.
   Caution: Do not place your feet on the bench if it so narrow that your feet might slip off the bench or if the bench is unstable.
2. Push upward on the handles, extending your arms completely.
   Caution: Do not lock your elbows. Do not arch your back.

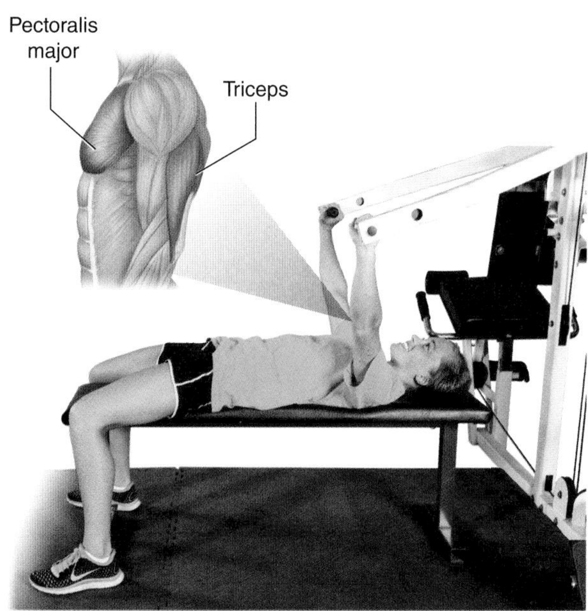

This exercise uses your pectoral and triceps muscles.

3. Return to the starting position.
4. You may choose either this exercise or the seated arm press. You may substitute this exercise in the self-assessment if you have a bench press machine and do not have a seated press machine.

SEATED LEG PRESS

1. Adjust the seat position on a leg press machine for your leg length. Sit with your feet resting on the pedal.
2. Push the pedal until your legs are straight.
   Caution: Do not lock your knees.
3. Slowly return to the starting position.

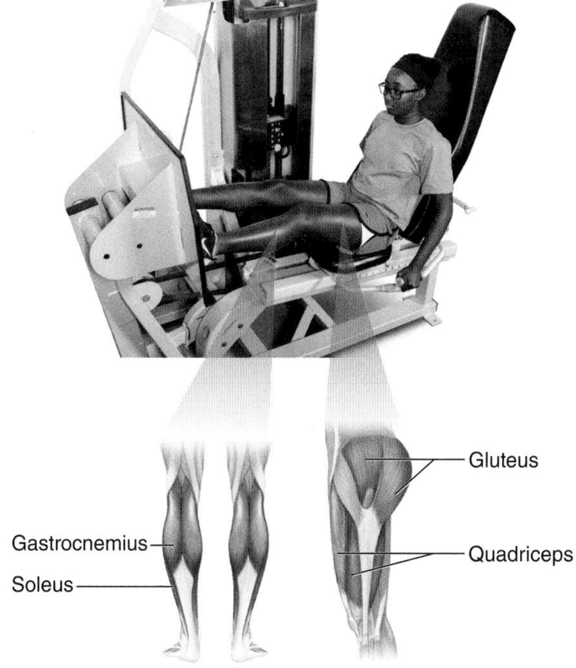

This exercise uses the quadriceps, gluteal, and calf muscles.

KNEE EXTENSION

1. Sit on the bench and hook one of your ankles under the pad. Grasp the handles on the bench.
2. Extend your knee through its full range of motion.
3. Return to the starting position. Repeat the exercise with your other leg.
4. You may choose either this exercise or the seated leg press.

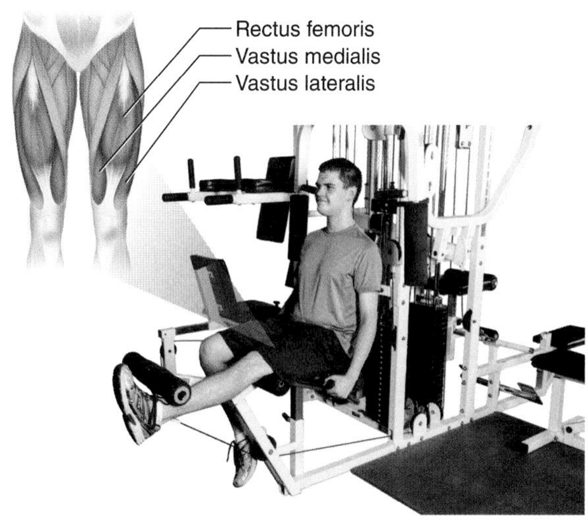

This exercise uses the muscles at the top of your thighs (quadriceps). The fourth quadriceps muscle, the vastus intermedius, lies beneath the rectus femoris and therefore is not shown in the illustration.

HAMSTRING CURL

1. Lie facedown on the bench with your kneecaps extending over the edge of the bench. Hook your heels under the cylindrical pads. Grasp the handles on the bench.
   Caution: Do not lock your knees when putting your heels under the pads. If necessary, have a partner lift the pads so that you can avoid locking.
2. Bend your knees so that you can lift the cylindrical pads. Bend your knees through their full range of motion. At the top of the lift, the pads will almost touch your buttocks.
3. Lower to the starting position.

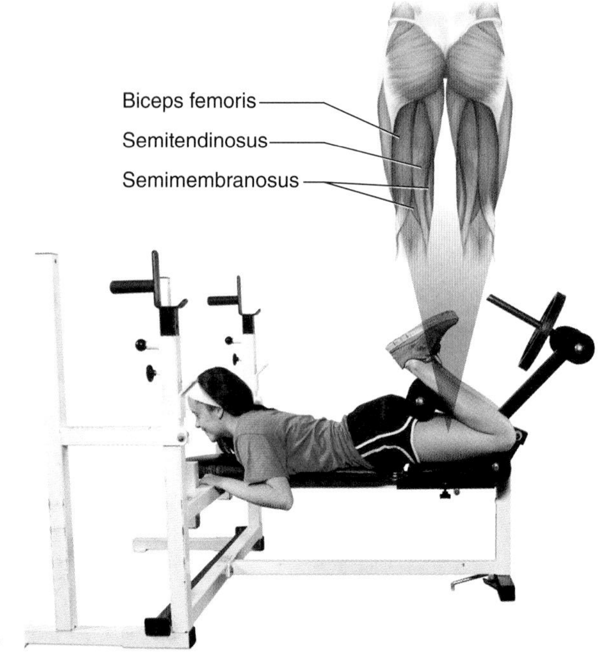

This exercise uses your calf muscles.

BICEPS CURL

1. Stand in front of the station and grasp the handle of the low pulley with your palms up. Tighten your abdominal muscles and buttocks (gluteal muscles).
2. Pull the handle from thigh level to chest level. Bend your elbows but keep them close to your sides.
   Caution: Do not move other body parts.
3. Return to the starting position.

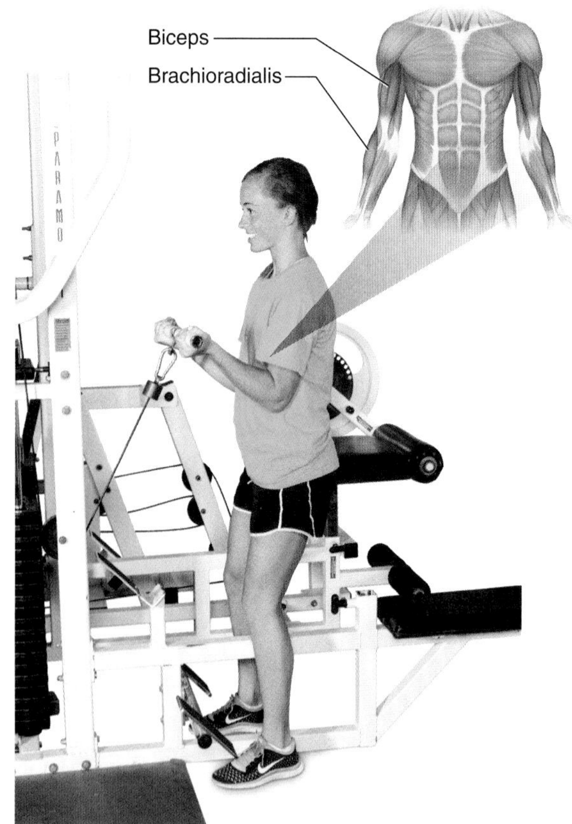

This exercise uses muscles in your back.

HEEL RAISE

1. Place a board that is 2 inches (5 centimeters) thick on the floor. Stand with the balls of your feet on the board and the handles even with your shoulders.
2. Grasp the handles with your palms facing away from your body. Keep your hands and arms stationary during the lift.
3. Rise onto the balls of your feet, then lower to the starting position.

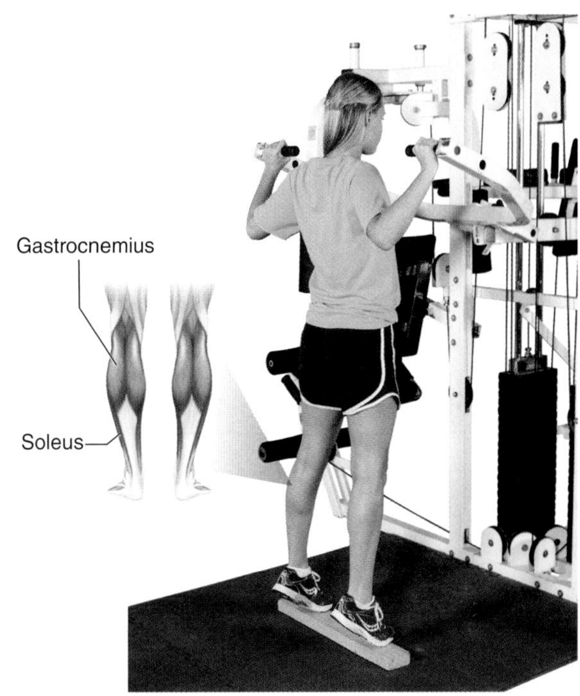

This exercise uses your hamstring muscles.

LAT PULL-DOWN

1. Sit on the bench (or floor, depending on the machine). Adjust the seat height so that your arms are fully extended when you grab the bar.
2. Grab the bar with your palms facing away from you. Your arms should be at least shoulder-width apart.
3. Pull the bar down to chest level.
4. Return to the starting position.

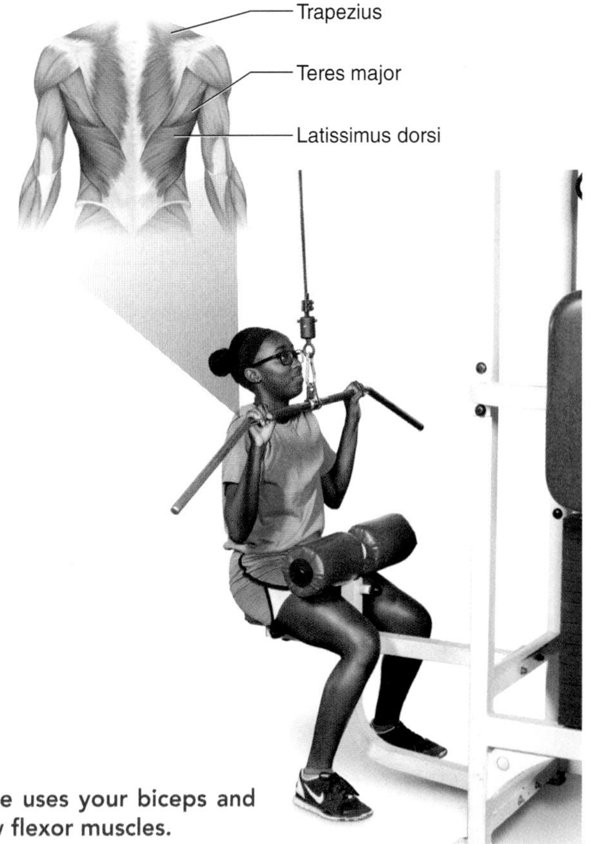

This exercise uses your biceps and other elbow flexor muscles.

TRICEPS PRESS

1. With your palms facing away from you, grab the handles.
   Note: If performed while sitting, adjust the seat height so that your hands are on the handles just above shoulder height.
2. Keep your elbows by your sides, and avoid leaning forward with your body.
3. Keeping your back straight, push forward and down with your arms until they are straight.
4. Return to the starting position.

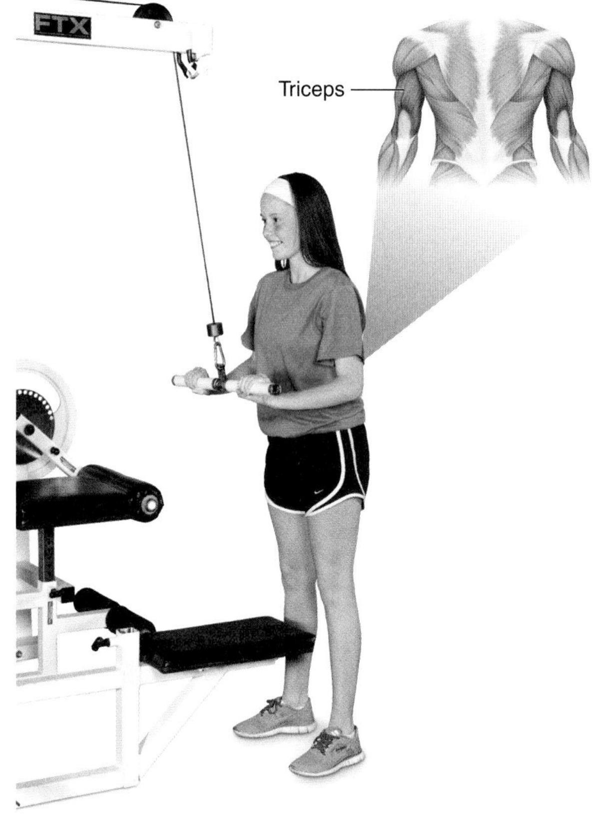

This exercise uses the muscles on the back of your arms (triceps).

SEATED ROW

1. Adjust the machine so that your arms are almost fully extended and are parallel to the ground.
2. Grab the handles with your thumbs up.
3. Keeping your back straight, pull straight back toward your chest.
4. Return to the starting position.

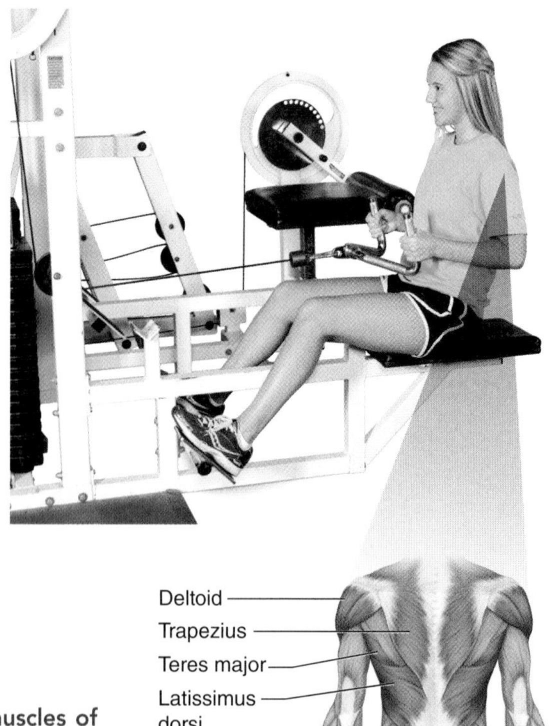

This exercise uses the muscles of your back and shoulders.

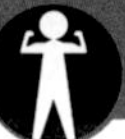

ISOMETRIC EXERCISES

The following basic isometric exercises work your major muscle groups.

HAND PUSH

1. Sit in a sturdy chair, on a bench, or on the floor with your back straight. You may cross your legs if you prefer. Place the palms of your hands together.
2. Raise your hands and elbows to shoulder-height. Push your hands against each other as hard as you can. Hold the position for 7 seconds; rest for 30 seconds.
3. Do 2 or 3 reps as time allows.

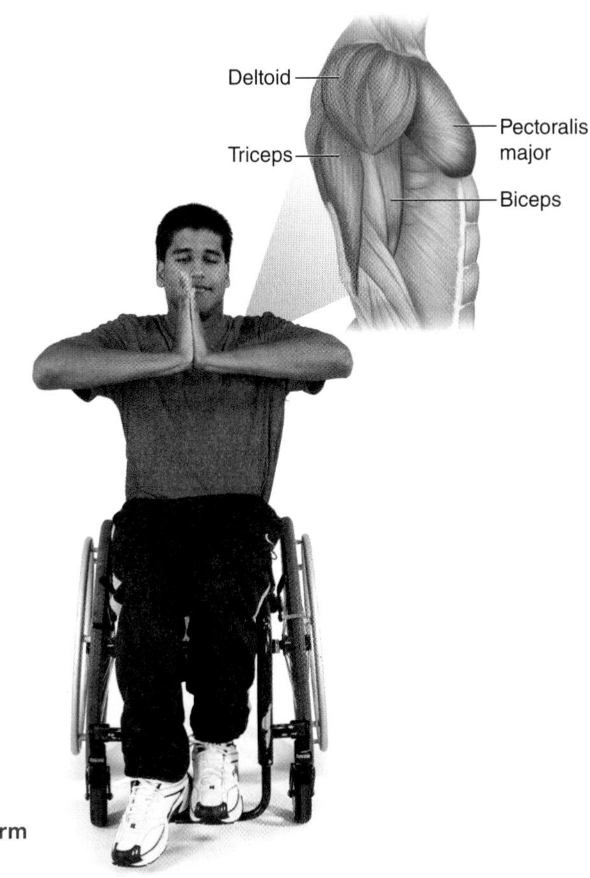

This exercise uses your arm and shoulder muscles.

BACK FLATTENER

1. Lie on your back with your knees bent.
2. Pull in your abdomen by contracting your abdominal muscles as tightly as possible. Flatten your lower back against the floor. Hold the position for 7 seconds; rest for 30 seconds.
3. Do 2 or 3 reps as time allows.

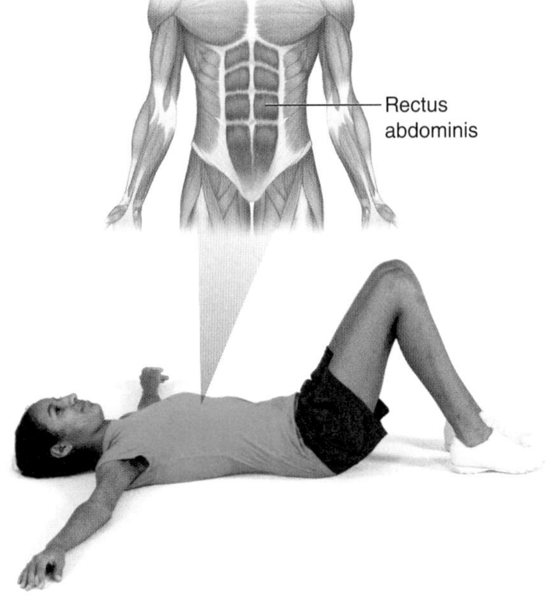

This exercise uses your abdominal muscles.

KNEE EXTENDER

1. Hold onto something for support and stand on your left foot. Lift your right foot behind you, bending your knee to a 90-degree angle.
2. Loop a towel under your right ankle; hold the ends of the towel in your right hand.
3. Push downward with your foot, trying to straighten your leg against the resistance of the towel.
4. Repeat the exercise 2 or 3 times with each leg as time allows.

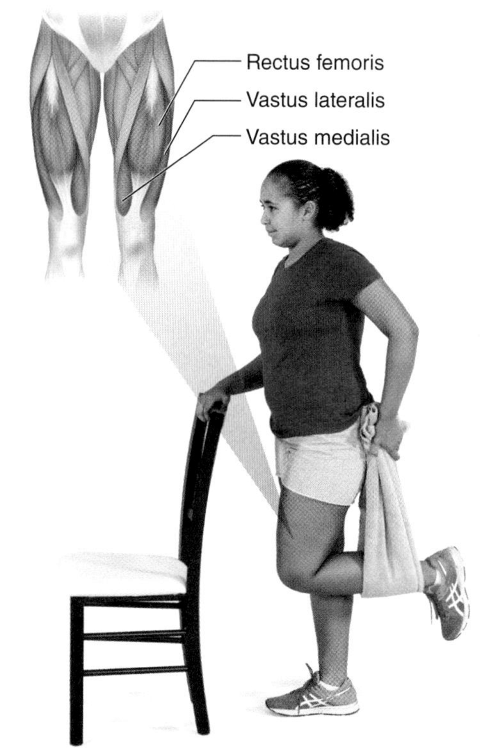

This exercise uses the muscles on the front of your thighs (quadriceps). The fourth quadriceps muscle, the vastus intermedius, lies beneath the rectus femoris and therefore is not shown in the illustration.

WALL PUSH

1. Stand with your back against a wall.
2. Move your feet out as you lower yourself into a half squat. Keep your thighs parallel to the floor.
3. Push your back against the wall by pushing with your legs as hard as you can. Hold the position for 7 seconds; rest for 30 seconds.
4. Do 2 or 3 reps as time allows.

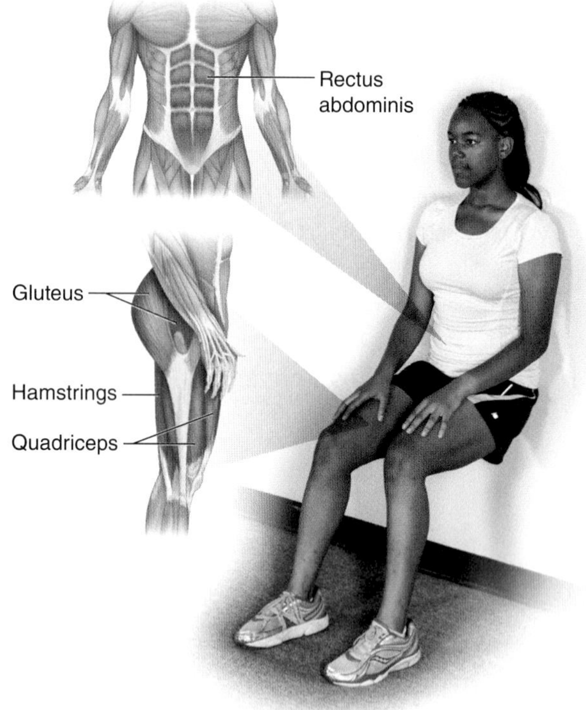

This exercise uses the muscles of your legs and abdomen.

BICEPS CURL WITH TOWEL

1. Stand with your back straight and your knees slightly bent.
2. Loop a towel under the back of your thighs.
3. Grasp the towel ends with your palms up. Keep your elbows against your sides.
4. Pull up on the towel as hard as possible. Hold the position for 7 seconds; rest for 30 seconds.
5. Do 2 or 3 reps as time allows.

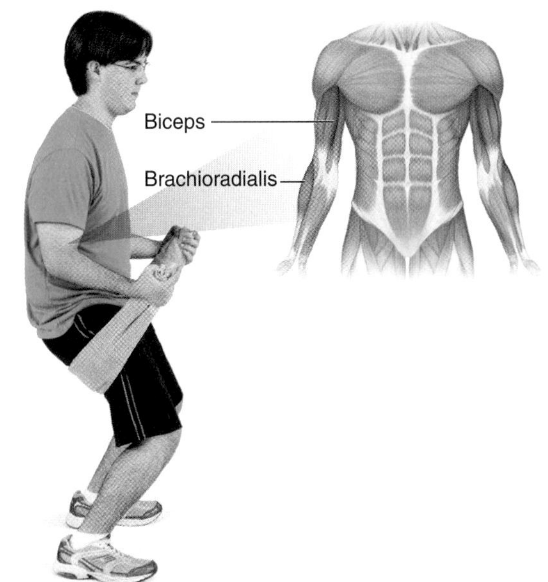

This exercise uses the muscles on the front of your upper arms (biceps).

TOE PUSH

1. Sit on the floor using good posture.
2. Hold the end of a jump rope or towel in each hand. Loop it over the balls of your feet so that it is tight against your soles.
3. Push with the balls of your feet as you pull on the rope or towel. Keep your back straight. Hold the position for 7 seconds; rest for 30 seconds.
4. Do 2 or 3 reps as time allows.

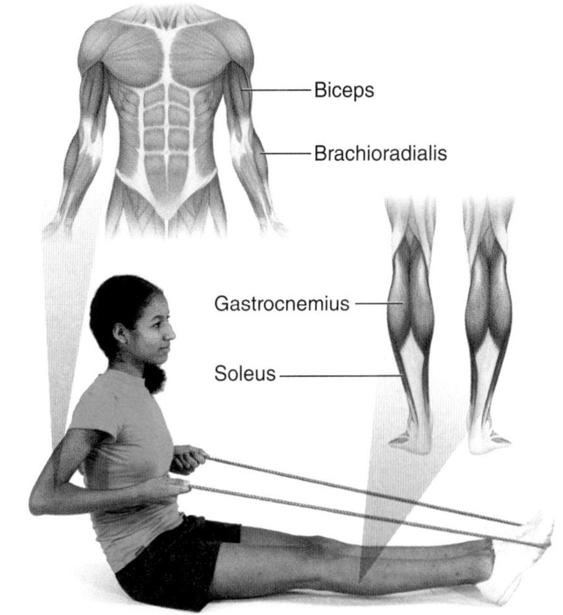

This exercise uses the muscles of your arms and lower legs.

LEG CURL

1. Stand on your left leg. Hold on to a chair or wall for balance.
2. Loop a towel behind your right ankle and stand on the ends of the towel with your left foot.
3. Keeping your posture erect and your back straight, try to bend your knee against the resistance of the towel. Hold the position for 7 seconds; rest for 30 seconds.
4. Do 2 or 3 reps with each leg as time allows.

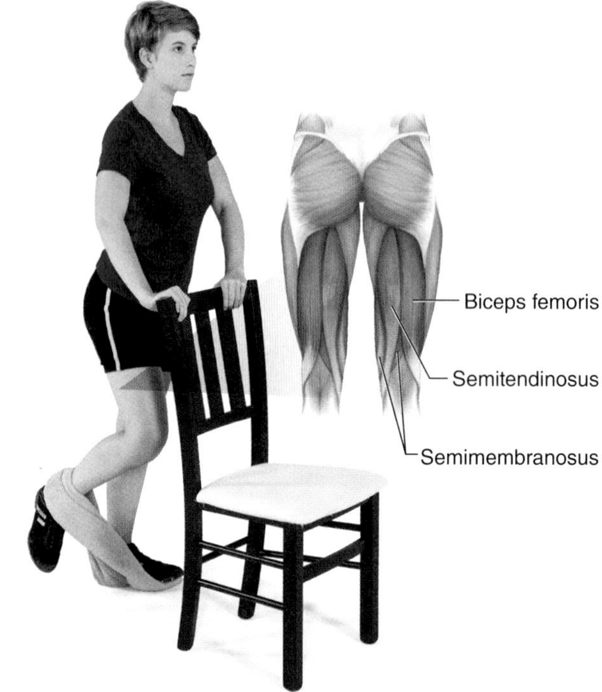

This exercise uses your hamstring muscles.

BOW EXERCISE

1. Stand in a position that an archer would take when shooting a bow.
2. Hold a towel with your right arm as if you were holding a bow.
3. Hold the other end of the towel with your left hand near your chin as if you are holding the string of the bow.
4. Push with your right hand and pull with your left hand. Hold the position for 7 seconds; rest for 30 seconds.
5. Do 2 to 3 reps with each arm forward as time allows.

Safety tip: Breathe normally while doing these exercises. Do not hold your breath. Holding your breath can cause dizziness and possibly a blackout.

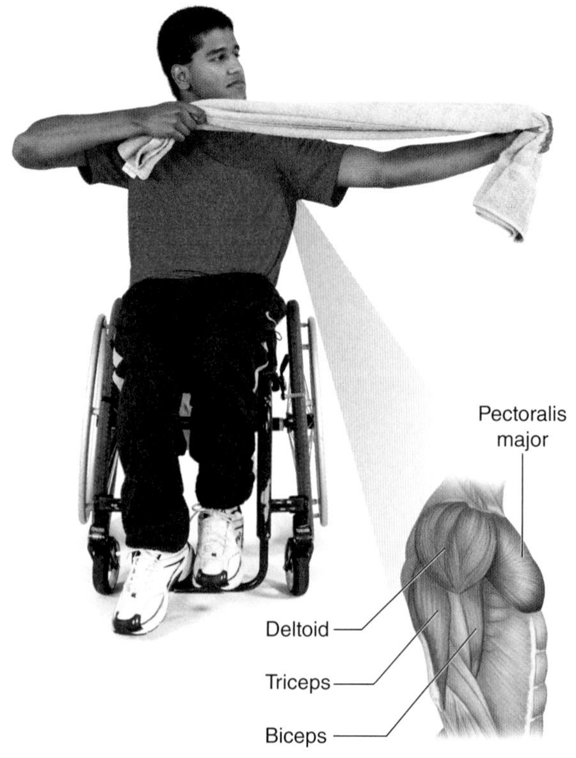

This exercise uses the muscles of your arms and shoulders.

TAKING CHARGE: Preventing Relapse

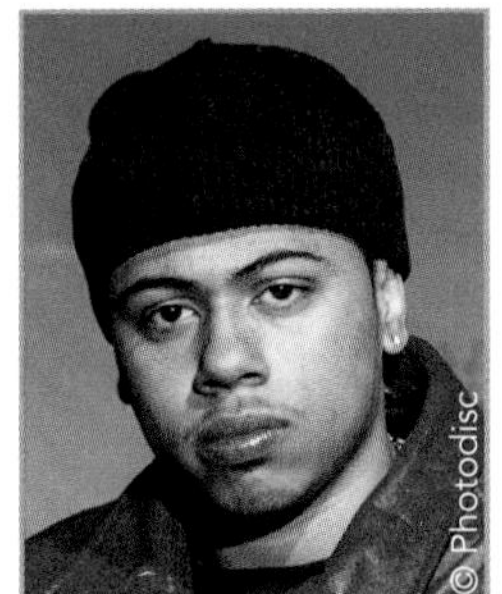
© Photodisc

Anyone can begin a program to increase physical fitness, but just beginning a program is not enough. Some people are active for a while, then drop out for a while. This behavior is called a relapse. Those who stay active all of their lives learn how to avoid relapses that can lead to becoming sedentary.

Luis missed his old school, especially his old friends. Now he usually came straight home after school instead of heading for the neighborhood court to play a little three-on-three basketball with his buddies. For the first month after he moved, Luis ate dinner, did his homework, and then clicked on the television to fill the time.

Early one evening, his mom said, "Luis, why are you lying around? You like to be active. Get up and get moving!"

Luis yawned and said, "Where am I going to go? Who am I going to go with? I don't have any friends here."

"What about that boy who lives down the hall? I saw him leave with a gym bag the other day. He must have been going somewhere you'd like to go."

"Well, maybe," Luis said. "But maybe he was going to do weight training or something like that—something I don't know how to do."

"Maybe it wouldn't kill you to learn more about weight training. It might help you be better in basketball, right?"

Luis smiled up at his mom. "Maybe. What's his apartment number?"

"3B—and while you're there, ask his mom whether she knows about any exercise classes around here for old people like me, okay?"

For Discussion

What caused Luis to relapse into inactivity? What could he do if it turns out that the boy down the hall hates basketball? What are some other things that cause relapse? What can be done to avoid them? What other suggestions do you have to help Luis? Consider the guidelines presented in the Self-Management feature as you answer the discussion questions.

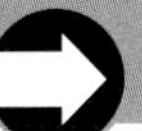

SELF-MANAGEMENT: Skills for Preventing Relapse

A person who relapses stops doing something that they want to keep doing or think they should keep doing. For example, you might start a PRE program but then stop doing it because you feel you can't take the time. Use the following guidelines to help you stick with something once you've started it.

- **Do a self-assessment.** It may help you see whether you're likely to stick with an activity, and it may give you ideas for how to stick with it if you've had relapse problems in the past.
- **Use the information from your self-assessment to determine areas in which you can improve.** Self-assessments help you learn about your current status (for fitness, activity, or nutrition, for example). If you are to improve, you first need to know where you need improvement.
- **Write down your goals for doing the activity.** Put them on the refrigerator or another place where you'll see them every day. You have good reasons to accomplish these goals or you would not have started to make a change in the first place. Stay focused on your goals.
- **Monitor your behavior by keeping a log or chart, then use it to reinforce or reward yourself.** Tell yourself that you've stuck with it so far and you can keep it up.
- **Tell other people what you're trying to accomplish.** Ask them to encourage you regularly.
- **Select a regular exercise time.** If you're trying to stick with exercise or another similar behavior, select a time of day and try to do the behavior at the same time every day.
- **Do not let one setback be a reason for a long-term relapse.** If you miss a day, tell yourself, "It's okay to take a day off once in a while." Repeat this saying to yourself periodically.
- **Consider a variety of activities.** Consider trying different physical activities from time to time.

TAKING ACTION: Resistance Machine Exercises

If you're just starting a muscle fitness program, you may want to begin by using resistance machines at your school or local recreation center. Developing muscle fitness through resistance training will build your muscle mass and bone density and can help you develop a healthy body composition. Muscle fitness can also help you look your best and make it easier for you to perform everyday tasks, such as climbing stairs, opening food jars, and carrying your backpack. In addition, developing muscle fitness through resistance training helps you perform your best at your favorite sport and other physical activities.

Take action by trying some resistance machine exercises that you've learned in this chapter. Be sure to follow the guidelines for PRE described in the chapter.

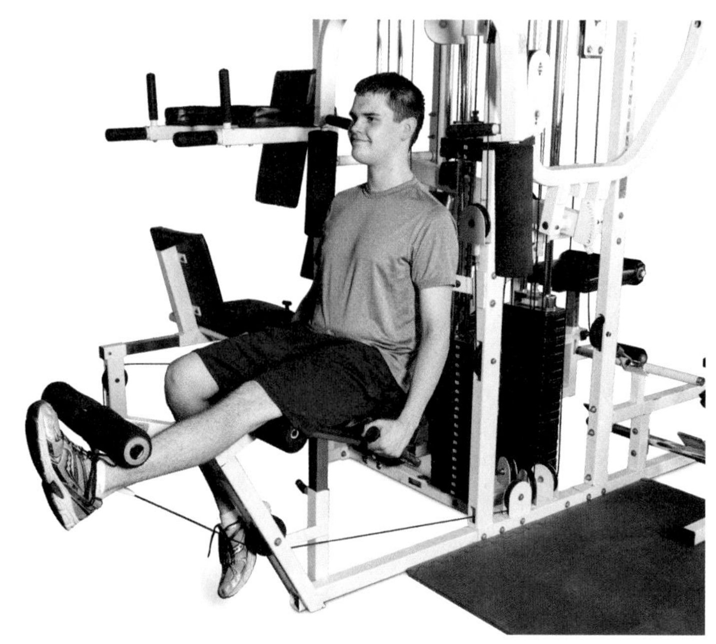

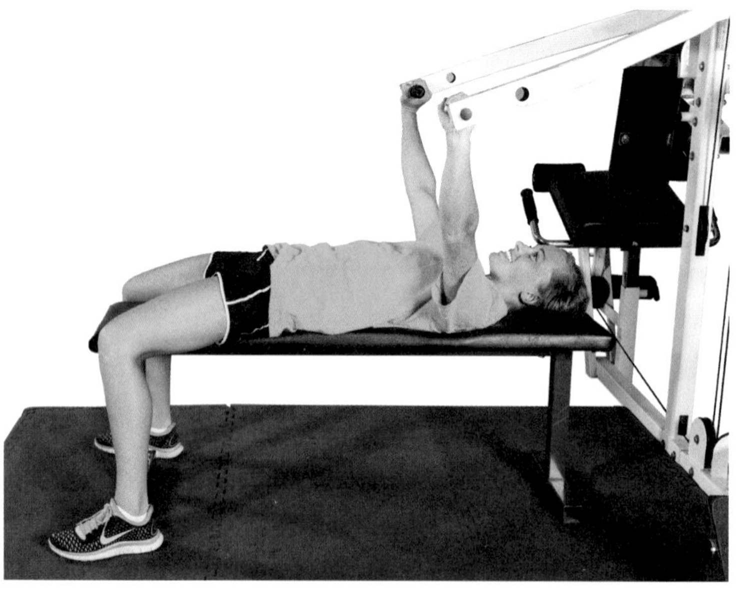

You can take action by doing PRE on resistance machines.

CHAPTER REVIEW

Reviewing Concepts and Vocabulary

As directed by your teacher, answer items 1 through 5 by correctly completing each sentence with a word or phrase.

1. _______________ is the amount of force a muscle can exert.
2. _______________ refers to an increase in muscle fiber size.
3. A person can become _______________ if he or she does strength training improperly by developing some muscles while ignoring others.
4. When you do calisthenics to develop strength, you use your body weight as the _______________.
5. The _______________ system refers to altering reps, sets, and weight as muscle fitness improves.

For items 6 through 10, as directed by your teacher, match each term in column 1 with the appropriate phrase in column 2.

6. isokinetic exercise	a. sport, not an exercise program
7. Olympic-style weightlifting	b. the maximum weight that a person can lift once
8. 1RM	c. exercise that requires a special machine
9. plyometrics	d. muscle fitness exercise that involves movement
10. isotonic exercise	e. exercise that builds power

For items 11 through 15, as directed by your teacher, respond to each statement or question.

11. How do strong muscles help you look better and prevent health problems?
12. Describe several methods for testing muscle fitness discussed in this chapter.
13. Describe two myths about muscle fitness exercise.
14. Describe several guidelines for preventing relapse.
15. Discuss the guidelines for using PRE effectively and safely.

Thinking Critically

Go to the student section of the Health Opportunities Through Physical Education website for this chapter. The address is on the first page of this chapter. Using information provided there and in this chapter, write a short article about muscle fitness for high school students. You can find additional information on the websites of NSCA, ACSM, and the President's Council on Fitness, Sports, and Nutrition. Share your article with your class or submit it to the school newspaper for publication.

Project

Some schools provide wellness programs for teachers and other school employees. Typical offerings include exercise classes before and after school, fitness assessments, and classes in nutrition and stress reduction. Plan a special activity for teachers addressing one of these topics as it relates to muscle fitness. Prepare a written plan and work with other students to carry it out.

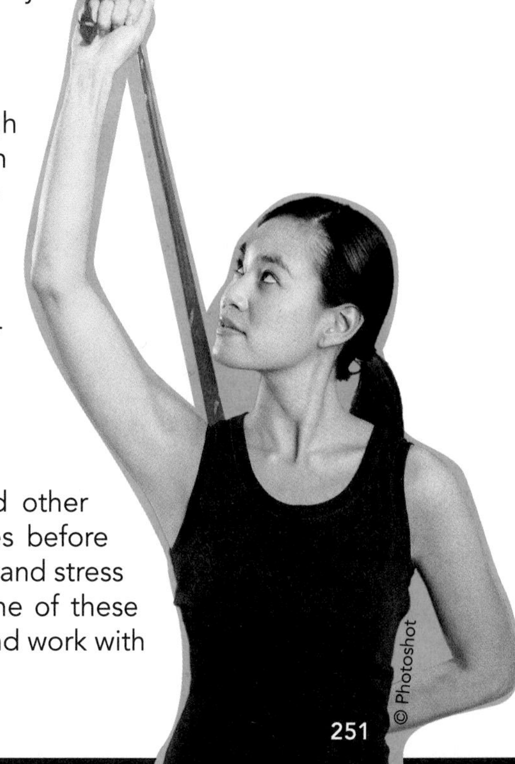

11

Muscle Fitness Applications

In This Chapter

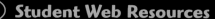

www **Student Web Resources**
www.HOPEtextbook.org/student

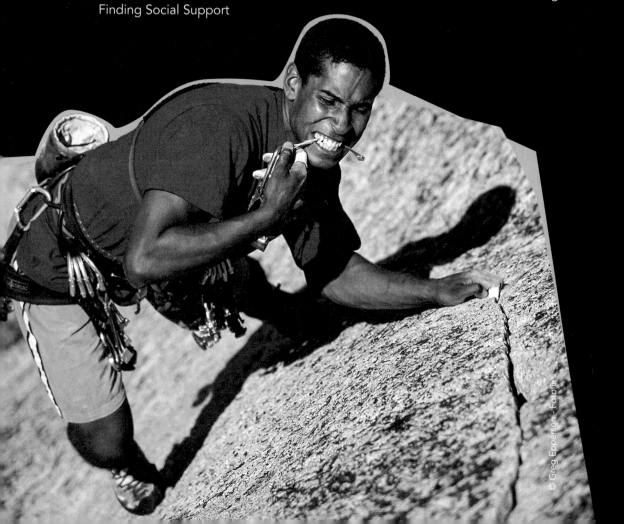

Lesson 11.1

Core Fitness, Posture, and Back Care

Lesson Objectives

After reading this lesson, you should be able to

1. name several core muscles and types of core muscle exercises and explain why they are important,
2. describe some common back and posture problems, and
3. list some biomechanical principles that can help you improve your posture and avoid back problems.

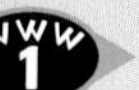

Lesson Vocabulary

force, kyphosis, laws of motion, lordosis, Pilates, ptosis

Do you know what core fitness is? Do you have it? In this lesson, you'll learn about your core muscles and why they are important for good health and functioning. You'll also learn about exercises, including core muscle exercises, that you can perform to improve your posture and reduce your risk of back pain and other muscle injuries.

Core Muscles

Your core muscles support your spine, keep your rib cage and pelvis stable, and help you maintain a healthy posture while standing, sitting, and moving in a variety of body positions. They also are the muscles that connect the upper and lower parts of your body. They include the muscles of your back, hips and pelvis, and abdominal area (see figure 11.1).

It's not uncommon for people to neglect their core muscles and focus more on muscles in their arms, legs, and shoulders because these muscles are easily seen and are considered to be important especially by young people. But you need fit core muscles—not only for healthy living and performing the tasks of daily life but also for performing sport and work-related activities and preventing injury. Core fitness allows you to keep your trunk stable while performing lifting and movements of all types. Some basic core exercises are presented at the end of this lesson.

Exercises that use resistance machines or free weights often do not build your abdominal muscles and some other core muscles. Since core exercises are an important part of a total muscle fitness program, they are performed in addition to other progressive resistance exercises (PRE).

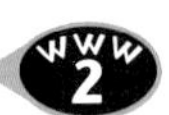

Many core exercises can be done without special equipment, and others can be done with inexpensive equipment. For example, you can improve core muscle fitness by exercising with large balls inflated with air. Exercises done with these balls are sometimes called stability ball exercises because physical therapists use them to help people build muscles that stabilize the body. You can also build your core muscles by doing medicine ball exercises.

FIT FACT

Pilates is a form of training designed to build core muscle fitness that has become quite popular in recent years. It is named for Joseph Pilates, who described core exercises and developed special exercise machines for building the core muscles. However, a recent U.S. court ruling declared that the term "Pilates" is a generic name like yoga and karate, which means that anyone can call himself or herself a Pilates expert even without special training. As a result, although many Pilates instructors may be quite knowledgeable about exercises, others may not. Some Pilates programs have been modified in ways that are inconsistent with Pilates' original principles. When done properly, Pilates is a good way to build core muscles.

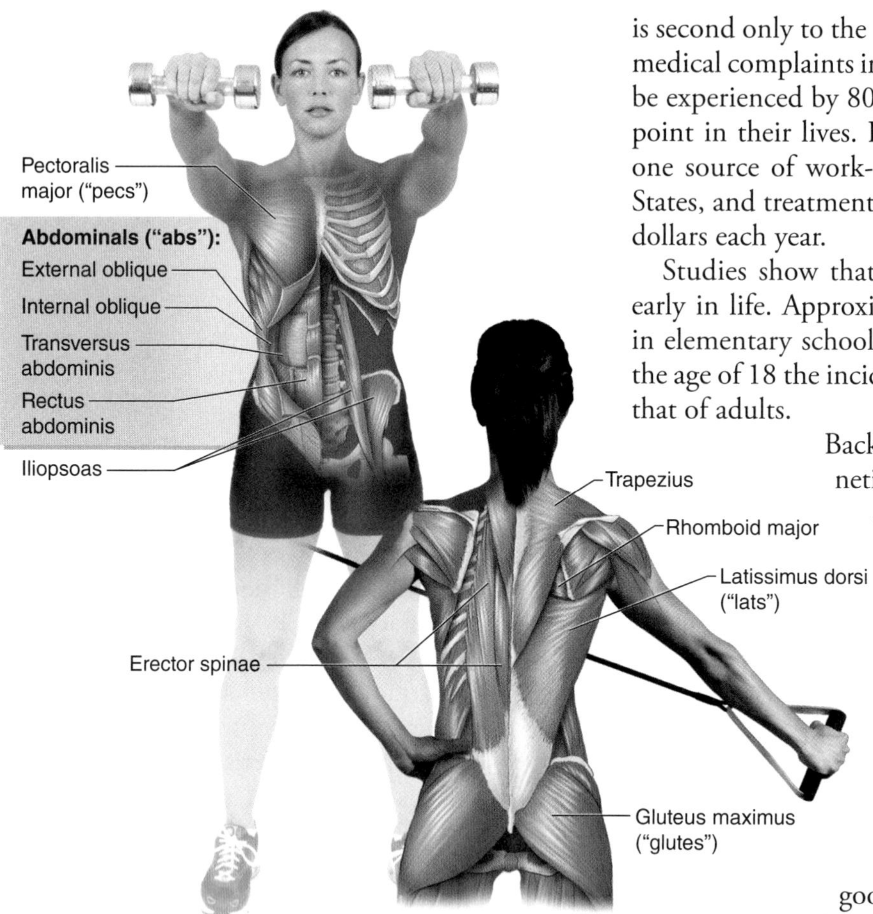

FIGURE 11.1 The core muscles.

Back Problems

Have you ever had a sore back after sitting for a long time or lifting heavy objects? Each year, as many as 25 million Americans seek a doctor's care for backache. According to some experts, back pain is second only to the common cold among leading medical complaints in the United States, and it will be experienced by 80 percent of all adults at some point in their lives. Back injuries are the number one source of work-related injury in the United States, and treatment of back pain costs billions of dollars each year.

Studies show that back problems often begin early in life. Approximately one-third of children in elementary school have had back pain, and by the age of 18 the incidence rate of back pain is near that of adults.

Backache is considered a hypokinetic condition because weak and short muscles are linked to some types of back problems. Poor posture is also associated with muscles that are not strong or long enough. By building fit muscles to improve your posture, you can help reduce your risk of back pain and look your best. Even if you never experience back pain, a healthy back and good posture help you function more efficiently in your daily activities.

How does good fitness help your back operate efficiently? Good biomechanics are important. Your body parts are balanced like blocks on your legs. Your chest hangs from your spine and is balanced over your pelvis. Your head sits on top of your spine, balanced over the other blocks in the stack. Because your spine is flexible and can move back and forth, the pull of your muscles keeps your

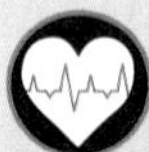

FITNESS TECHNOLOGY: Exercise Machines With Memory

Computer technology now allows exercise machines at fitness clubs to "memorize" your exercises. The machine stores your resistance amount for each exercise, making it easy to quickly prepare for each exercise. The machine also stores the number of sets and repetitions you perform for each exercise. You can also install fitness apps on a smartphone, tablet, or other personal computer to help you keep your own record of your exercises that do not require machines (for example, core exercises).

Using Technology

Identify and describe an exercise machine or app that can be used to self-monitor muscle fitness exercise.

body parts balanced. If your muscles on one side are weak and long, but your muscles on the opposite side are strong and short, your body parts are pulled off balance.

One back problem that often occurs among teens is **lordosis**, in which the lower back has too much arch. Also called swayback, lordosis results when the core muscles, particularly the abdominal muscles, are weak and the hip flexor muscles (iliopsoas) are too short (see figure 11.2). Lordosis can lead to backache.

Even people who are relatively fit in other areas can lack fitness in the muscles related to back problems. One reason for this lack of fitness is that sports and games often overdevelop some muscles and neglect others. As a result, it is not unusual for basketball players, gymnasts, band members, and other active people to have weak back and abdominal muscles (core muscles) and short hamstrings and hip flexors.

Posture Problems

Figure 11.2*a* illustrates some of the common posture problems associated with poor core fitness. Some of the most common are lordosis, **ptosis** (protruding abdomen), and **kyphosis** (rounded back and shoulders). You might recognize these problems in your own posture or that of someone you know. In figure 11.2*b*, you can see which muscles contribute to posture problems if they are too short or weak. Figure 11.2*c* shows you what good posture looks like and illustrates how it depends on long, strong muscles. Just as strong, long muscles contribute to a healthy back, they also are important for good posture.

Knowing what constitutes good posture can help you improve your own posture. And good posture helps you look good, helps prevent back problems, and helps you work and play more efficiently.

Back and Posture Improvement and Maintenance

You can take several steps to help yourself enjoy good back health. First, you can perform self-assessments to determine your current back health and posture status. You can then identify exercises that will help you develop or maintain the muscle fitness and flexibility necessary for good back health and good posture. You can also use key principles of biomechanics to prevent back pain and injury.

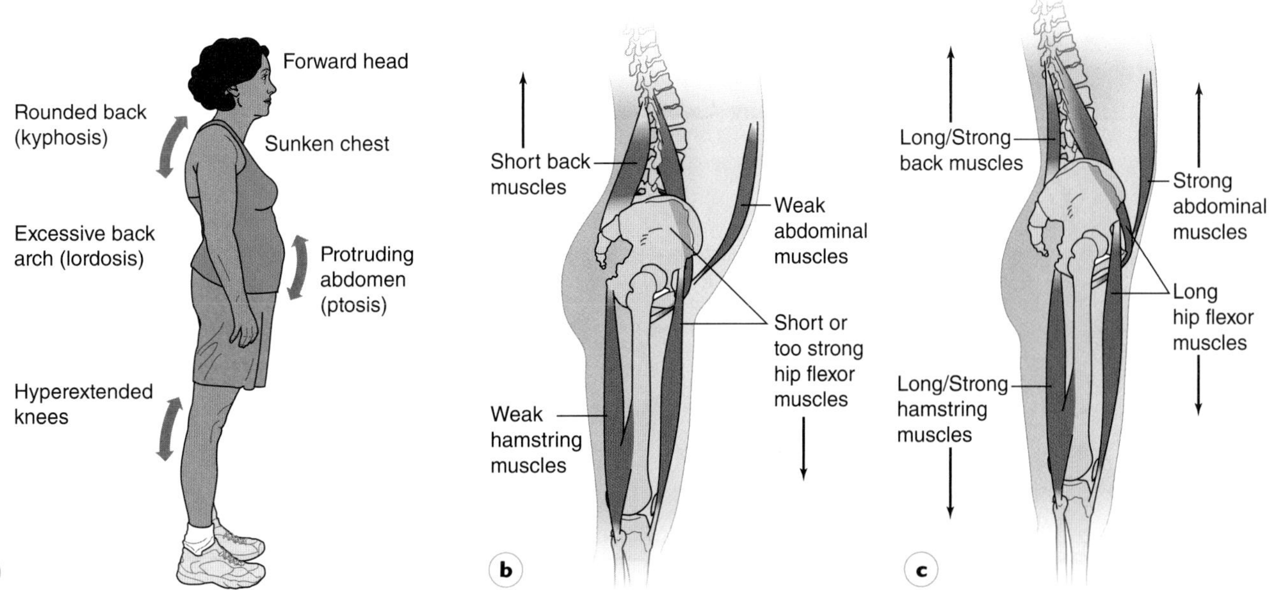

FIGURE 11.2 *(a)* Problems associated with poor posture; *(b)* core muscles in poor posture; *(c)* core muscles in good posture.

FIT FACT

Many teens wear backpacks. To carry a backpack effectively, you need adequate strength and muscular endurance. In a typical year, the U.S. Consumer Product Safety Commission reports more than six thousand backpack-related injuries, mostly among youth. Improving your muscle fitness can help you reduce your risk of injury from wearing a backpack.

Healthy Back Test

In the Self-Assessment feature at the end of this lesson, you'll get the opportunity to take the healthy back test. This will help you determine what you can do to keep your back fit and healthy. Core exercises are especially good for back health and for maintaining good posture. Stretching exercises are also commonly recommended.

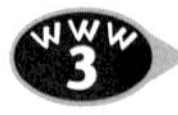

As shown in figure 11.2*c*, strong and long muscles help you avoid posture problems. The problems shown in figure 11.2*a* and 11.2*b* are not present in a healthy posture. The head is centered over the shoulders, the shoulders are back and balanced, the low back has a gentle curve, the abdomen does not protrude, and the knees do not bend backward. Working with a partner, you can evaluate posture to see whether problems exist and whether the body is in proper alignment. See the chapter titled Making Good Consumer Choices.

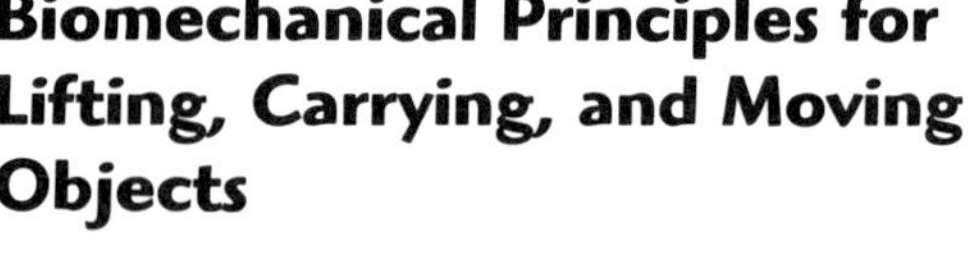

Biomechanical Principles for Lifting, Carrying, and Moving Objects

For good health and safety, avoid exercises that violate the principles of biomechanics. As shown in the Science in Action feature, these principles and **laws of motion** apply when you use your body's levers—the bones of your arms and legs—to apply **force** in lifting, carrying, and moving objects. The most frequent use of these levers occurs when you walk or run or perform skills such as throwing, jumping, kicking, and striking. Using your body levers efficiently is also important in applying force when performing resistance exercises. Use the following biomechanical principles to help you avoid injury and back problems.

- **Use your large muscles when lifting.** Let your strong leg muscles—not your relatively weak back muscles—do the work.
- **Keep your weight (hips) low.** To make lifting safer, keep your weight low by squatting (bending your knees) with your back straight and your hips tucked.
- **Keep your core muscles firm when lifting.** Tighten your abdominal and back muscles to stabilize your body.
- **Use a wide base of support for balance.** Keep your feet spread about shoulder-width apart for stability when lifting.
- **Avoid a bent-over position when sitting, standing, or lifting.** Your body's levers, such as your spine, do not work efficiently when you are bent over. When sitting in a chair, sit back in the seat and lean against the backrest. Do not work for long periods of time in a bent-over position.
- **Divide a load to make it easier to carry.** For example, carrying two small suitcases, one in each hand, is easier than carrying one larger suitcase in one hand. A backpack is an efficient way to carry books. It's best to carry the backpack using both straps rather than over one shoulder. Avoid overloading your backpack or book bag. If you must carry your books in your arms, carry some in each arm. If you do carry your books in one arm, change arms from time to time.

SCIENCE IN ACTION: The Mechanics of Lifting

Kinesiology experts who study biomechanics have shown that lifting with your back rather than with your legs is inefficient and can be dangerous. The most efficient way to lift is to use your leg muscles and keep the weight near your body (see figure 11.3*a*). When you bend at your waist while lifting, you use your back muscles rather than your stronger leg muscles, and you greatly increase the amount of force necessary to lift the object (figure 11.3*b*). The same is true when you reach while lifting (figure 11.3*c*). These points are illustrated in the following example.

In figure 11.3*a*, a weight is held near the body. When the weight is lifted by using the leg muscles with the back straight, the force needed to do the lifting is only slightly more than the weight of the load itself because the load is held near the body. In figure 11.3*b*, lifting the same weight requires up to 50 times as much force because the lifter has to lift the weight of the upper body and because the necessary force is magnified when the weight is positioned at the end of a long lever. The longer the lever, the more the force is magnified. If a person reaches to lift (figure 11.3*c*), the necessary force is even greater because of the increased length of the lever.

The extra force needed for incorrect lifting puts unnecessary stress on the muscles and causes compression of the discs and bones, especially in the lower back. Incorrect lifting (figure 11.3, *b* and *c*) also requires the lifter to use the back muscles, rather than the stronger leg muscles, thus increasing the risk of injury. To reduce your risk of injury due to incorrect lifting, follow the principles described in the section about biomechanics.

As previously mentioned, it is best to use the stronger leg muscles rather than the weaker back muscles when lifting. It's also important to avoid bending at the waist when lifting. However, you need to improve fitness of the back muscles (back extensors) for back health and normal functioning in daily life. To build the back muscles, exercises such as the trunk lift and some forms of the leg lift are appropriate even though they use inefficient movements. The key is to perform the exercises in a controlled manner with appropriate resistance. To remind you how to perform these exercises safely, caution statements are provided for these exercises.

Student Activity

What are some real-life actions that could put you at risk of injury due to movements that use your body's levers poorly?

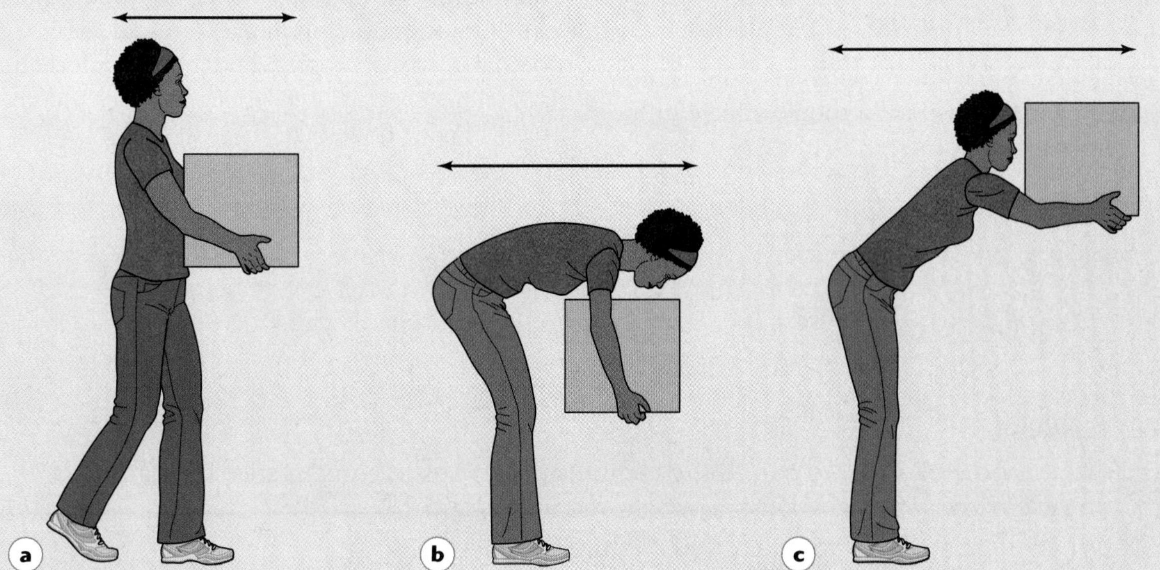

Figure 11.3 For efficiency, *(a)* lift with the weight close to the body. *(b)* Avoid bending forward at the waist or *(c)* reaching while lifting because the longer levers increase stress on the back.

- **Avoid twisting while lifting.** If you have to turn while lifting, change the position of your feet. It's especially important to avoid twisting your spine as you are straightening or bending it.
- **Push or pull heavy objects.** Heavy lifting can cause injury. Pushing or pulling an object is more efficient than lifting it.

Stretching

Healthy back care and good posture also depend on flexibility. Several good exercises are the knee-to-chest, the single-leg hang, the hip and thigh stretch, the back-saver sit-and-reach, and the back and hip stretch. Your instructor can show you these exercises when you study flexibility.

Calisthenics

Calisthenics are exercises that use all or part of your body weight to provide resistance—for example, the core exercises discussed earlier in this lesson. Calisthenics for muscle fitness in your limbs are presented at the end of this lesson. Calisthenics build strength, and because they use body weight and typically involve multiple repetitions, they also build muscular endurance. The FIT formula for calisthenics is

- **F:** three to six days a week,
- **I:** lift part or all of the body weight, and
- **T:** 1 to 3 sets of 10 to 25 reps.

Calisthenics that involve explosive movement such as jumping build power and should adhere to the FIT formula for plyometrics.

PRE and Injury

Experts have now determined that when PRE is performed properly and with good supervision, it is safe for teens. However, even when done properly, there is a risk of injury when performing both PRE and lifting sports such as weightlifting. The most frequent injury among school athletes performing PRE is back injury, especially in the low back. However, the National Strength and Conditioning Association indicates that "this risk is no greater than [the risk in] many other sports and recreational activities in which children and adolescents regularly participate." For example, studies show that the average injury rate in youth sports, especially contact sports, is much higher than for PRE. The risk of injury from PRE performed at home is much higher than the risk of PRE done in schools, primarily because of better supervision, better equipment, and required use of spotters at school.

> "Preventing a back injury is much easier than repairing one."
>
> —U.S. Occupational Safety and Health Administration (OSHA)

Some injuries associated with PRE are not immediately noticeable. As a result, when cautioned about improper lifting or using incorrect biomechanics, some people might say, "I've done that before and it didn't cause a problem." But we know that repeated small injuries (microtraumas) can lead to big injuries later. Many people who ignore biomechanical guidelines eventually experience injuries and say, "I wish I hadn't done that."

Lesson Review

1. Name some of the core muscles, describe some types of exercises for building core muscle exercises, and explain why they are important.
2. What are some common back and posture problems?
3. What are some biomechanical principles that can help you improve your posture and avoid back problems?

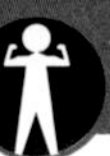

CORE MUSCLE FITNESS EXERCISES

CURL-UP

The curl-up is considered to be among the best abdominal exercises because it isn't risky like some abdominal exercises. The curl-up is sometimes referred to as the crunch, and it's a good substitute for the straight-leg sit-up and hands-behind-the-head sit-up.

1. Lie on your back with your knees bent at 90 degrees and your arms extended.
2. Curl up by rolling your head, shoulders, and upper back off the floor. Roll up only until your shoulder blades leave the floor.

   Caution: Do not hold your feet while doing a trunk curl. Do not clench your hands behind the head or neck.
3. Slowly roll back to the starting position.

Variations

- **Arms across chest or hands by face (more difficult):** Fold your hands across your chest rather than keeping them straight, or place your hands on your face by your cheeks (not behind your head or neck).
- **Twist curl (builds oblique muscles):** Fold your arms across your chest, turn your trunk to the left, and touch your right elbow to your left hip. Repeat to the opposite side.

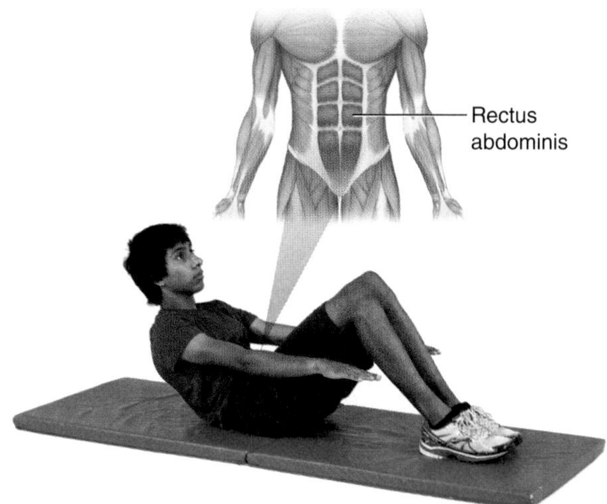

This exercise uses your abdominal muscles.

TRUNK LIFT (BENCH)

1. Lie facedown on a padded bench (or a bleacher with a towel on it) that is 16 to 18 inches (41 to 46 centimeters) high. Your upper body (from your waist up) should extend off the bench.
2. Have your partner hold your calves just below the knees.
3. Place one hand over the other on your forehead with your palms facing away and your elbows held to the side at the level of your ears.
4. Start with your upper body lowered. Lift slowly until your upper body is even with the bench (in line with your legs).

   Caution: Do not lift the trunk higher than horizontal.
5. Lower to the beginning position.

Safety tip: As you do these exercises, lift slowly and move only as far as the directions specify. This exercise is appropriate when performed properly, but as noted earlier, using the trunk muscles for lifting or carrying is not recommended.

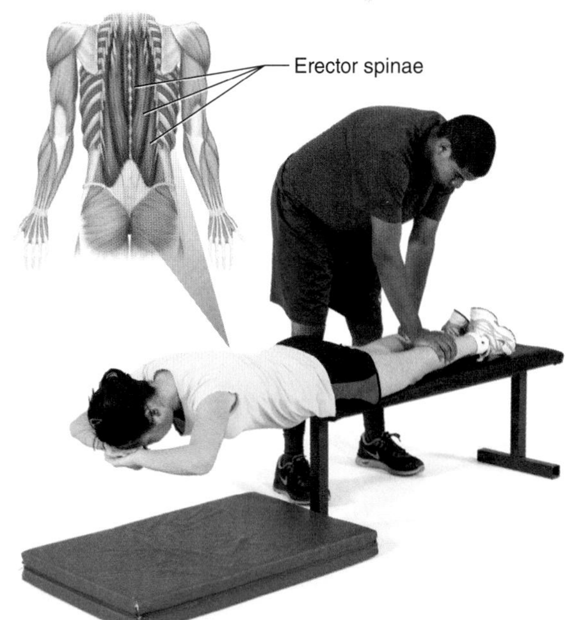

This exercise uses your back extensor muscles.

TRUNK LIFT (FLOOR)

1. Lie facedown with your hands clasped behind your neck.
2. Pull your shoulder blades together, raise your elbows off the floor, and then lift your head and chest off the floor. Arch your upper back until your breastbone (sternum) clears the floor. You may need to hook your feet under a bar or have someone hold your feet down.

   Caution: Do not lift your chin more than 12 inches (30 centimeters) off the floor. This exercise is appropriate when performed properly but as noted earlier, using the trunk muscles for lifting or carrying is not recommended.
3. Lower your trunk and repeat the exercise.

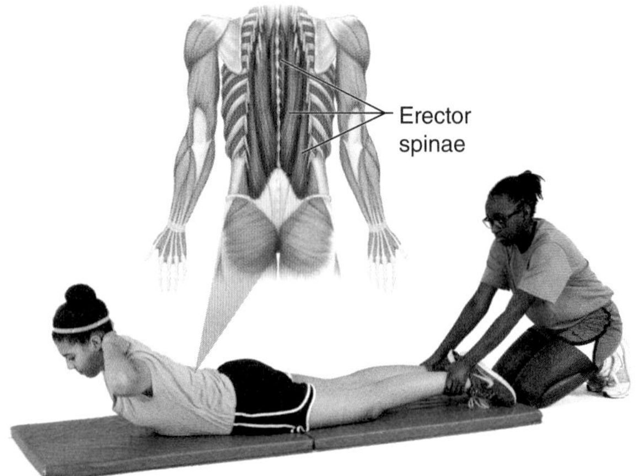

This exercise develops the muscles of your upper back and helps prevent "hump back."

ARM-AND-LEG LIFT

1. Lie facedown with your arms stretched in front of you.
2. Raise your right arm, then lower it. Raise your left arm, then lower it. Finally, raise both arms, then lower them.
3. Raise you right leg, then lower it. Raise your left leg, then lower it.
4. Raise your right arm and right leg, then lower them. Raise your left arm and left leg, then lower them.
5. Raise your left arm and right leg, then lower them. Raise your right arm and left leg, then lower them.

Caution: Do not arch your back during this exercise.

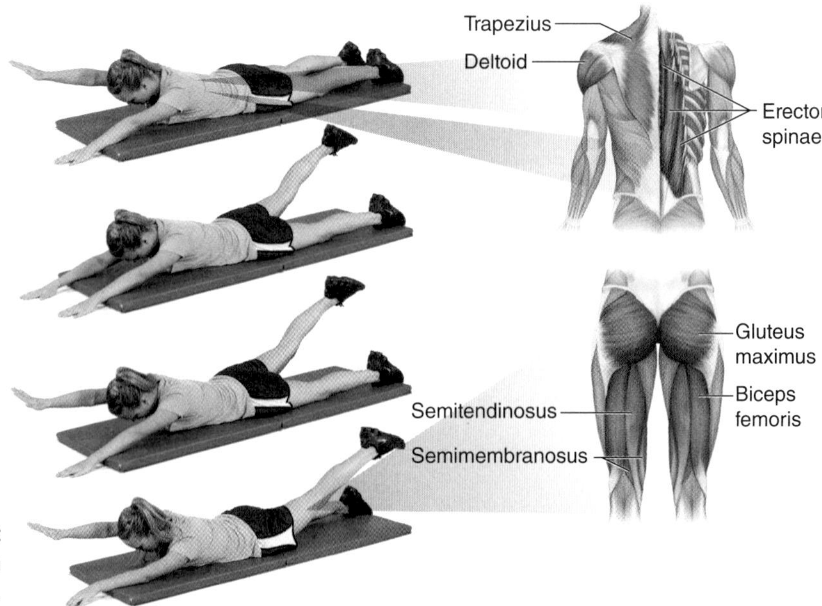

This exercise helps prevent rounded shoulders, sunken chest, and rounded upper back.

BRIDGING

1. Lie on your back with your knees bent and your feet close to your buttocks.
2. Contract your gluteal muscles. Lift your buttocks and raise your back off the floor until your hip joint has no bend.
   Caution: Do not overarch your lower back.
3. Lower your hips to the floor and repeat the exercise.

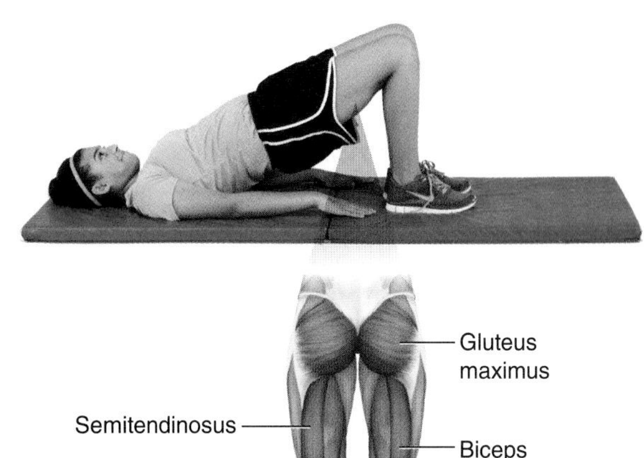

This exercise develops the muscles of your buttocks (gluteal) and the muscles on the back of your thighs (hamstring).

SIDE PLANK

1. From a right-facing, side-lying position on a mat or carpet, lift your body into a side support position, supporting your body weight on your right forearm and your feet. Your left is arm bent and on your left hip. Tighten your abdominal and back muscles.
2. Keep your hips in line with your body. Hold this position for 7 to 10 seconds.
3. Repeat facing to the left.

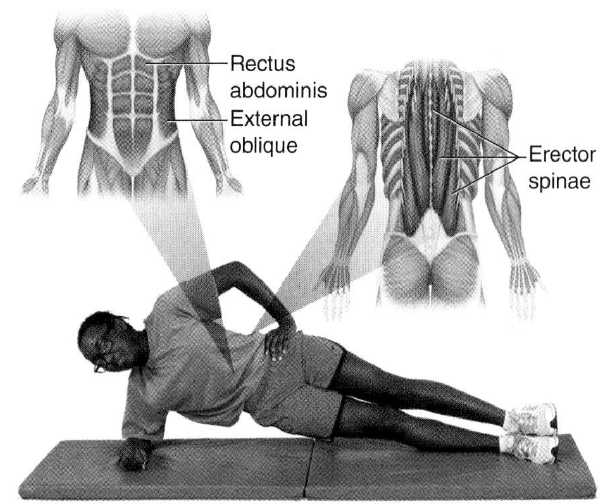

This exercise develops the abdominals and back muscles.

REVERSE CURL

1. Lie on your back. Bend your knees, placing your feet flat on the floor. Place your arms at your sides.
2. Lift your knees to your chest, raising your hips off the floor.
3. Return to the starting position. Repeat the exercise up to 10 times.

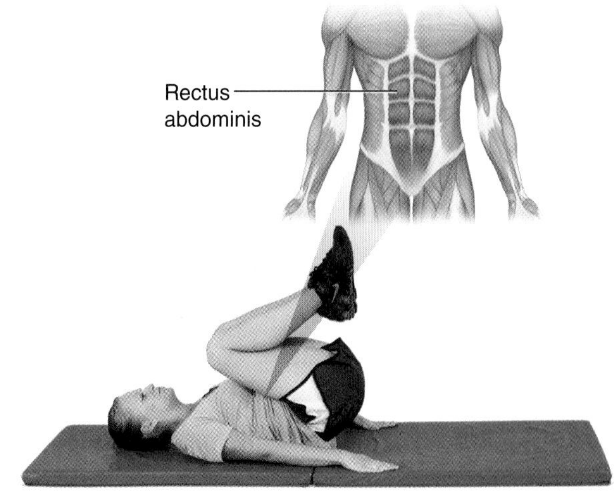

This exercise develops your abdominal muscles.

FRONT PLANK

1. On a mat or carpet, support your body with your forearms and toes.
2. Keep your head in line with your body. Hold this position for 7 to 10 seconds.

Variations

- **Less difficult:** Support your body with your knees rather than your feet.
- **More difficult:** Perform the same exercise in the full push-up position.

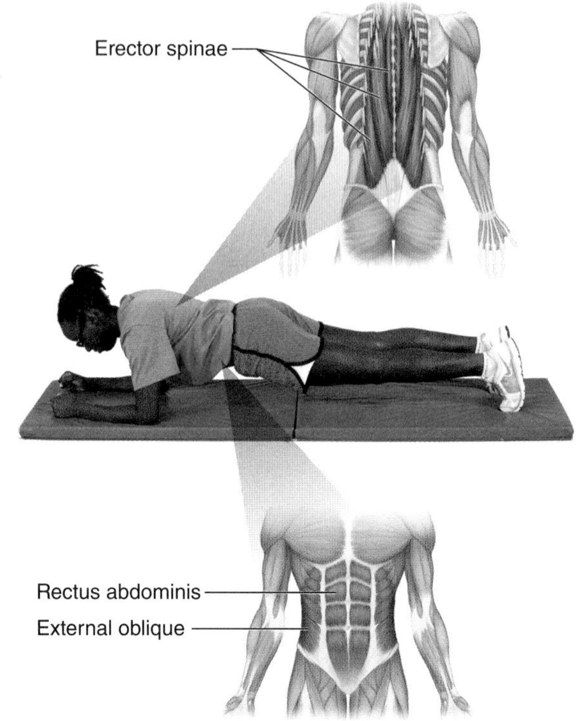

This exercise develops the abdominals, buttocks, and back muscles.

DOUBLE-LEG LIFT (BENCH OR TABLE)

1. Lie facedown on a table (or bench) with your legs extending off the end. With a partner holding your upper body, lower your legs to the ground. If you have no partner, grasp under the edge of the table.
2. Lift your legs slowly until they are even with the top of the table.

   Caution: Do not lift any higher. If necessary, lift one leg at a time until you are able to lift both legs at once.
3. Lower to the starting position.

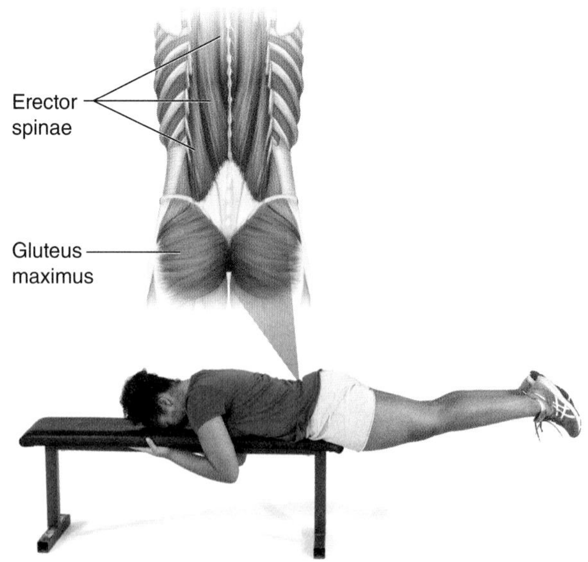

This exercise strengthens your lower back and gluteus muscles.

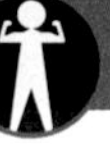

CALISTHENICS: Exercises for Muscle Fitness in Your Limbs

PUSH-UP

1. Lie facedown on a mat or carpet with your hands under your shoulders, your fingers spread, and your legs straight. Your legs should be slightly apart and your toes should be tucked under.
2. Push up until your arms are straight. Keep your legs and back straight. Your body should form a straight line.
3. Lower your body by bending your elbows until your upper arms are parallel to the floor (elbows bent at a 90-degree angle). Then push up until your arms are fully extended. Repeat, alternating between the fully extended and the 90-degree arm positions.

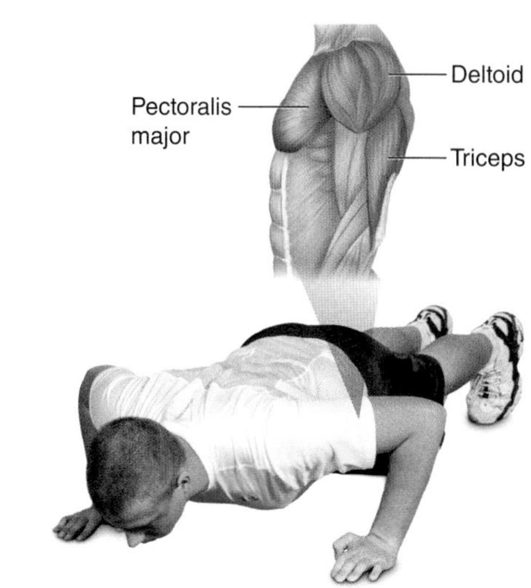

This exercise develops your chest muscles (pectorals) and the muscle (triceps) on the back of your upper arms.

KNEE PUSH-UP

1. If you cannot complete 20 reps of the 90-degree push-up, try this version. Lie facedown with your hands placed under your shoulders.
2. Push up, keeping your body rigid, until your arms are straight, but keep your knees on the floor.
3. Keep your body rigid, and lower it until your chest touches the floor.

This exercise develops your chest muscles (pectorals) and the muscle (triceps) on the back of your upper arms.

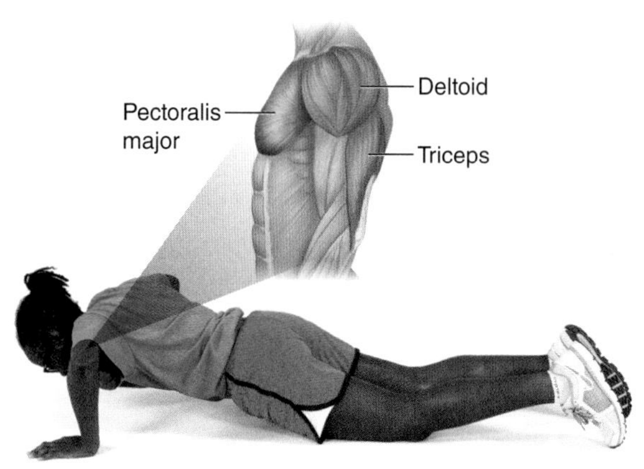

PRONE ARM LIFT

1. Lie facedown on the floor with your arms extended and held against your ears.
2. Keep your forehead and chest on the floor and lift your arms so that your hands are 6 inches (15 centimeters) off the floor.
3. Lower your arms, then repeat the exercise. Keep your arms touching your ears and keep your elbows straight.

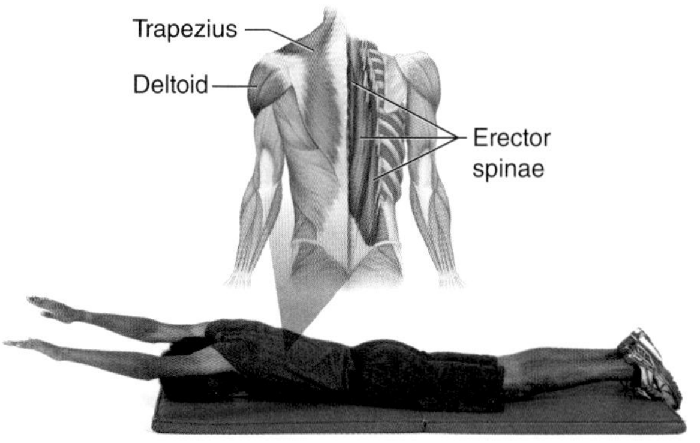

This exercise develops the muscles of your back and shoulders.

STRIDE JUMP

1. Stand with your left leg forward and your right leg back. Hold your right arm at shoulder height straight in front of your body and your left arm straight behind you.
2. Jump and move your right foot forward and your left foot back. As your feet change places, your arms switch position. Keep your feet 18 to 24 inches (about 45 to 60 centimeters) apart.
3. Continue jumping, alternating your feet and arms. Count 1 rep each time your left foot moves forward.

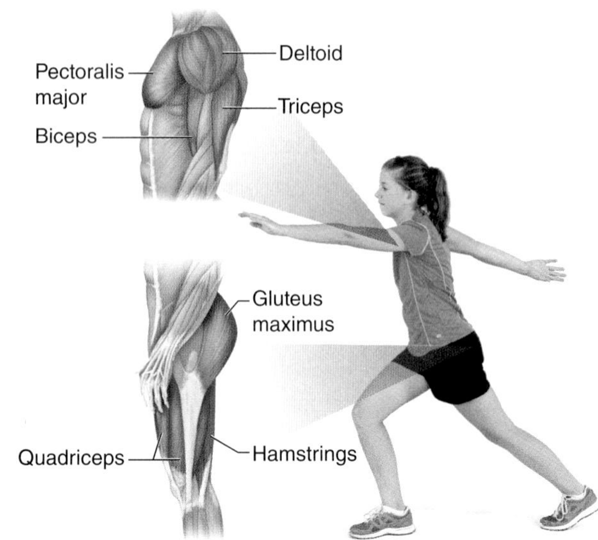

This exercise develops the muscles of your legs and arms as well as cardiorespiratory endurance and power.

SIDE LEG LIFT

1. Lie on your right side. Use your arms for balance.
2. Lift your top (left) leg 45 degrees. Keep your kneecap pointing forward and your ankle pointing toward the ceiling. If your leg rotates so that your knee points upward, you will work the wrong muscles.
3. Lower your leg. Repeat the movement. To increase intensity, you can use an ankle weight.
4. Roll over and repeat the exercise with your right leg.

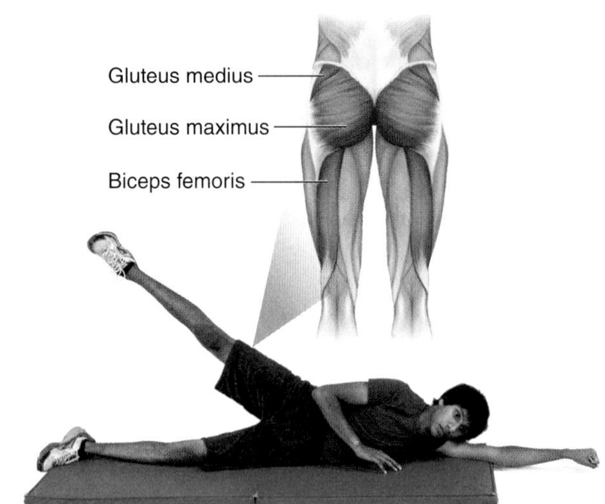

This exercise develops your hip and thigh muscles.

KNEE-TO-NOSE

1. Kneel on all fours.
2. Pull your right knee toward your nose.
3. Extend your right leg until it is in line with the back and shoulders (parallel to the floor). Keep your head in line with the shoulders, back, and extended leg.
   Caution: Do not lift your leg higher than your hips. Do not hyperextend your neck or lower back.
4. Return to the starting position. Repeat the exercise with your left leg.

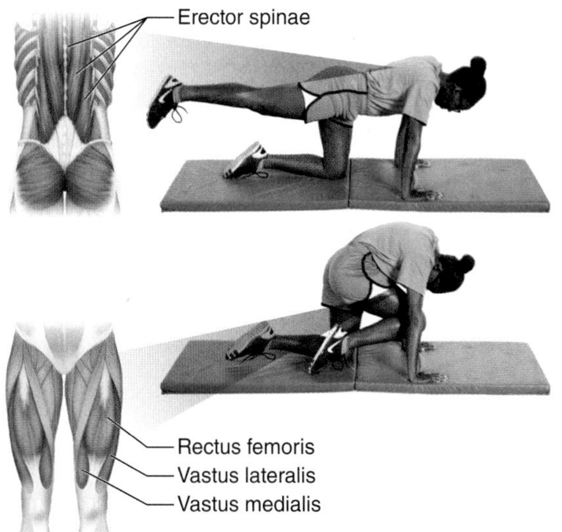

This exercise develops the gluteal, lower back, and quadriceps muscles. The fourth quadriceps muscle, the vastus intermedius, lies beneath the rectus femoris and therefore is not shown in the illustration.

HIGH-KNEE JOG

1. Jog in place. Try to lift each knee so that your upper leg is parallel with the floor.
2. Count 1 rep each time your right foot touches the floor. Try to do one or two jog steps per second.

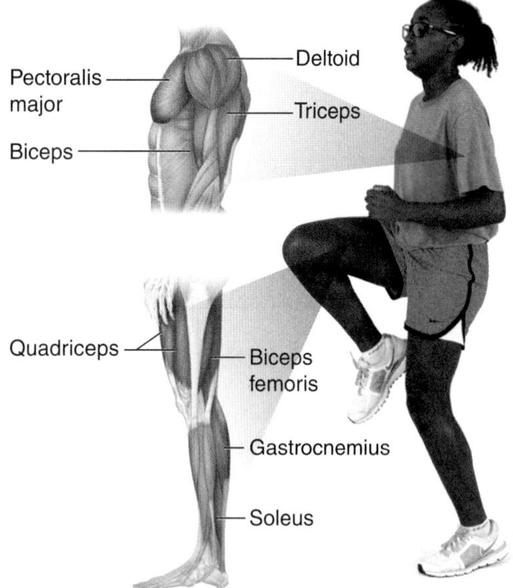

This exercise develops the muscles of your arms and legs and is also good for cardiorespiratory endurance.

SELF-ASSESSMENT: Healthy Back Test

Backache is often caused by weak muscles and by muscles that are too short. Test your back muscles by using the following self-assessment. Each part focuses on a certain muscle group. If you do well on this assessment, you're likely to have a healthy back. If not, it's especially important that you do exercises to improve your back health. In doing the test, work with a partner. Your partner will anchor your body for certain tests and can help in recording scores. Add your scores for the individual test item to get your total score. Then use table 11.1 to determine your risk of back problems. Record your results as directed by your instructor. Remember that self-assessment information is personal and considered confidential. It shouldn't be shared with others without the permission of the person being tested.

Test Item 1: Single-Leg Lift (supine)

1. Lie on your back on the floor. Lift your left leg off the floor as high as possible without bending either knee.
2. Repeat using your right leg. Score 1 point if you can lift your left leg to a 90-degree angle with the floor. Score an additional point if you can lift your right leg to a 90-degree angle.

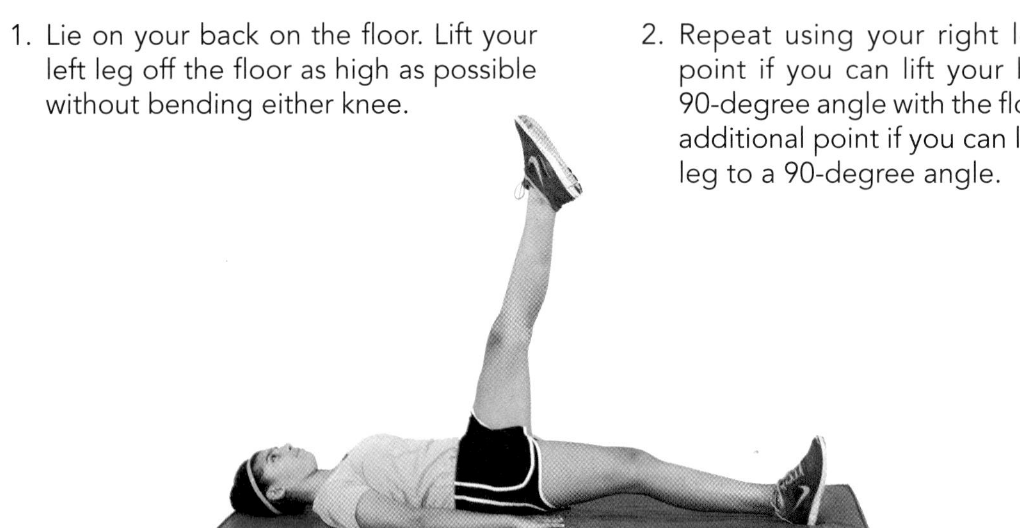

Test Item 2: Knee-to-Chest

1. Lie on your back on the floor. Make sure your lower back is flat on the floor.
2. Grasp the back of your thigh to bring your right knee up until you can hold it tightly against your chest. Keep your left leg straight. The left leg may lift off the floor to allow the right knee to reach your chest.
3. Repeat using your left leg.
4. Score 1 point if you can keep your left leg touching the floor while holding your right leg against your chest. Score an additional point if you can keep your right leg touching the floor while holding your left leg against your chest.

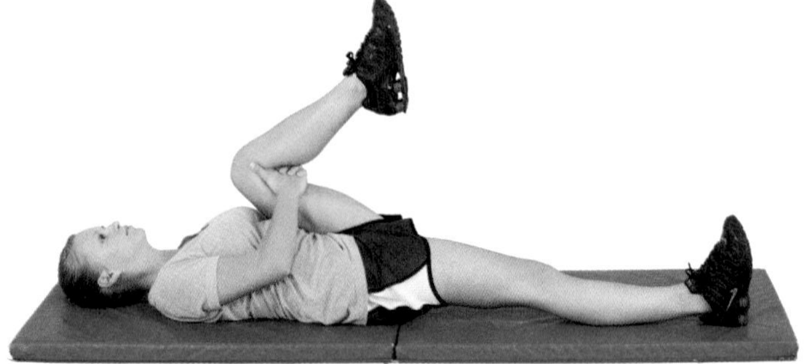

Test Item 3: Single-Leg Lift (prone)

1. Lie facedown on the floor. Lift your straight right leg as high as possible. Hold the position for a count of 10. Then lower your leg.
2. Repeat using your left leg.
3. Score 1 point if you can hold your right leg 12 inches (30 centimeters) off the floor for a count of 10. Score an additional point if you can do the same with your left leg.

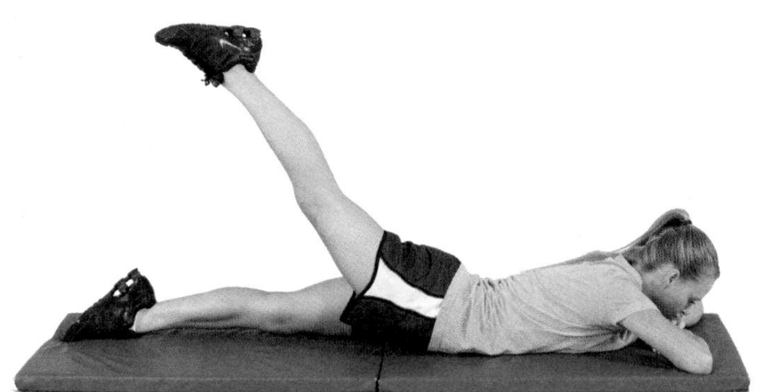

Test Item 4: Curl-Up

1. Lie on your back with your knees bent at 90 degrees and your arms extended.
2. Curl up by rolling your head, shoulders, and upper back off the floor. Roll up only until your shoulder blades leave the floor.
3. Score 1 point if you can curl up with your arms held straight in front of you and hold the position for 10 seconds without having to lift your feet off the floor.
4. Score an additional point if you can curl up with your arms across your chest and hold the position for 10 seconds without your feet leaving the floor.

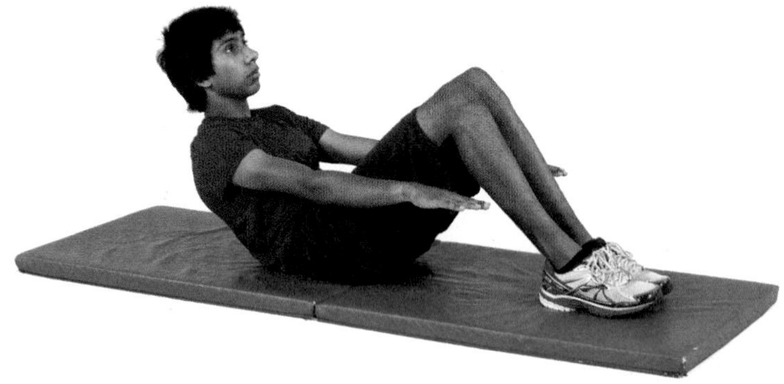

Test Item 5: Trunk Lift and Hold

1. Lie facedown on a padded bench (or a bleacher with a towel on it) that is 16 to 18 inches (41 to 46 centimeters) high. Your upper body (from your waist up) should extend off the bench.
2. Have your partner hold your calves just below the knees.
3. Place one hand over the other on your forehead with your palms facing away and your elbows held to the side at the level of your ears.
4. Start with your upper body lowered. Lift slowly until your upper body is even with the bench. Hold the position for a count of 10.
5. Score 1 point if you can lift your trunk even with the bench. Score an additional point if you can hold your upper body even with the bench for a count of 10.

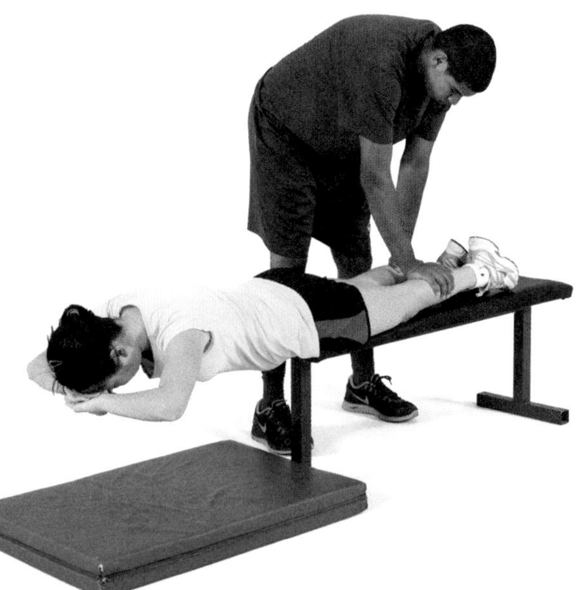

Test Item 6: Front Plank

1. On a mat or carpet, support your body with your forearms and toes.
2. Keep your head in line with your body and hold this position for 10 seconds.
3. Score 2 points if you can hold your body straight for the full 10 seconds.

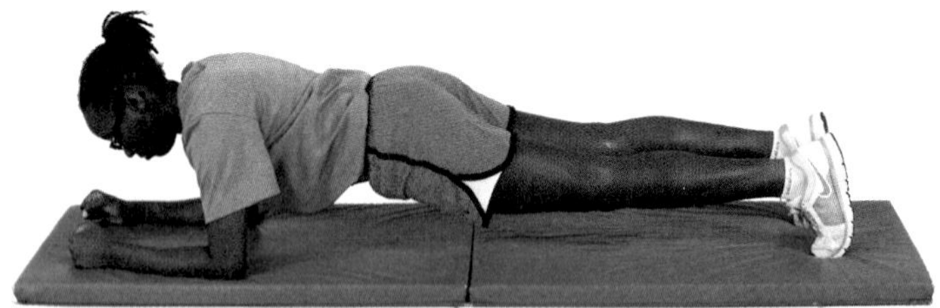

TABLE 11.1 Rating Chart: Healthy Back Test

Rating	Score
Good fitness	11 or 12
Marginal (some risk)	9 or 10
Low (greater risk)	6–8
High risk	≤5

Lesson 11.2

Ergogenic Aids and Muscle Fitness Exercise Planning

Lesson Objectives

After reading this lesson, you should be able to

1. list several ergogenic aids and supplements and the risks associated with their use,
2. collect information about your personal needs and build a muscle fitness and activity profile,
3. set goals for muscle fitness exercise,
4. select muscle fitness exercises and prepare a written muscle fitness exercise plan, and
5. describe periodization and explain why it is used.

Lesson Vocabulary

anabolic steroid, androstenedione, creatine, ergogenic aid, ergolytic, human growth hormone (HGH), periodization, rhabdomyolysis

Do you know someone who takes pills with the hope of finding an easy way to get muscle fitness? Do the pills really work? Would you like to improve your muscle fitness? Are you among the nearly 50 percent of teens who do no regular muscle fitness exercise? In this lesson, you'll learn about products advertised as muscle builders—and the problems associated with them. You'll also learn how to prepare a personal muscle fitness exercise plan that is safe and effective. Carrying out a good plan is the surest way to build your muscle fitness, which will help you meet national guidelines for physical activity both now and later in your life.

> “Fitness—if it came in a bottle, everyone would have a great body. 
>
> —Cher, singer and actress

Ergogenic Aids

For centuries, people, especially those interested in high-level performance, have tried to find methods of enhancing performance—including methods other than the exercise training presented in part 1 of this book. *Ergo* relates to work, and *genic* relates to the word *generate*. Thus an **ergogenic aid** helps you generate work or increases your ability to do work, including performing vigorous exercise. Some ergogenic aids, or products thought to be ergogenic aids, are classified as drugs, whereas others are classified as food supplements. In the United States, a drug must be approved by the Food and Drug Administration (FDA) before it can be sold by prescription or over the counter. Supplements, however, are not subject to FDA approval, so there is no assurance that they are what they appear to be or that they are as effective as advertisements indicate.

Many ergogenic aids can be dangerous. Others are not ergogenic at all because they do not work as advertised. Some are detrimental to health and performance and are better referred to as **ergolytic** (*ergo* again meaning work and *lytic* meaning destruction). Examples of ergolytic substances include alcohol, tobacco, and marijuana. Some of the products marketed as ergogenic aids are described in the following pages.

Anabolic Steroids and Their Dangers

Many types of steroid are used by doctors to treat disease. **Anabolic steroids** are synthetic drugs that resemble the male hormone testosterone and produce lean body mass, weight gain, and bone maturation. For certain diseases, doctors legally prescribe anabolic steroids in small doses. However, some people illegally buy and use anabolic steroids to increase muscle size and strength. Anabolic steroids are not only illegal when used without a doctor's prescription but also dangerous. For this reason, their use is prohibited by the United States Olympic Committee (USOC) and most other athletic associations. Some of their harmful effects are illustrated in figure 11.4.

Teenagers are at high risk for harm from steroids because their bodies are still growing. Anabolic steroids can damage the growth centers of bones, causing the long bones of the body to stop growing. This condition can prevent a person from growing to his or her full height. Many side effects do not go away when use of the drug is discontinued; examples include hair loss, acne, deepening voice, and dark facial hair growth in women. For athletes, another major problem is the increased risk of injury to tendons and ligaments, which become less elastic with steroid use.

Some athletes also use certain drugs in an attempt to enhance their performance, and sport officials develop tests to detect these drugs. Like steroids, they can be dangerous, and most are banned by sport groups and may also be illegal.

Steroid Precursors

A precursor is a substance from which another substance is formed; thus a steroid precursor is a nonsteroid substance that leads to the formation of a steroid. Some supplements are marketed as precursors, and they can cause the body to form its own anabolic steroids. Examples are **androstenedione**, DHEA, and androstenediol.

Androstenedione, often referred to as "andro," is considered to be a steroid precursor because it is converted into anabolic steroids such as testosterone (male hormone) after it enters the body. In some countries, it is viewed as a food supplement. It was formerly considered to be a food supplement in the

FIT FACT

Rhabdomyolysis is a condition in which muscle fibers break down, causing the bloodstream to absorb muscle fiber elements (such as myoglobin), which can damage the kidneys. Symptoms include muscle weakness and aching, fatigue, joint pain, and, in severe cases, seizure. Causes of this condition include exercising in the heat, lack of water replacement, and severe exertion. In several reported instances, high school and college athletes have been hospitalized for rhabdomyolysis due to excessive calisthenics and training drills. Some athletes push beyond healthy limits after taking supplements that they think will give them the ability to do extreme training. This practice can result in problems such as rhabdomyolysis.

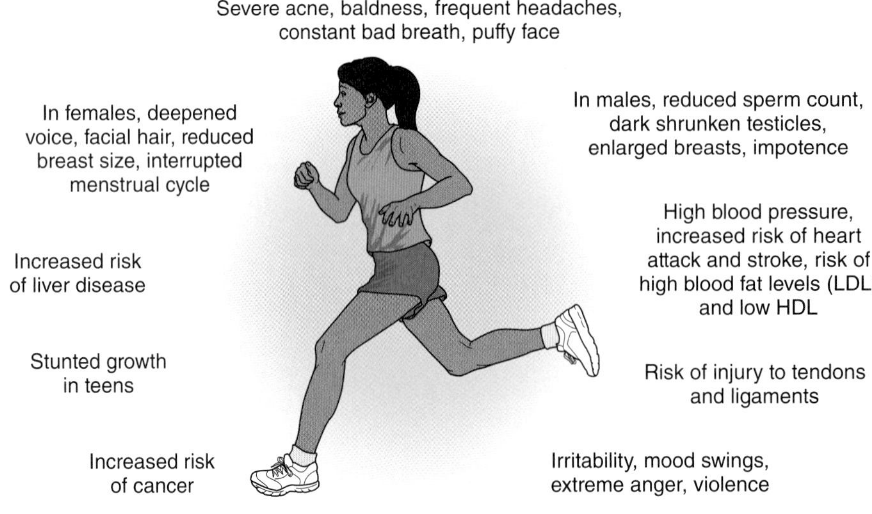
Severe acne, baldness, frequent headaches, constant bad breath, puffy face
In females, deepened voice, facial hair, reduced breast size, interrupted menstrual cycle
In males, reduced sperm count, dark shrunken testicles, enlarged breasts, impotence
High blood pressure, increased risk of heart attack and stroke, risk of high blood fat levels (LDL) and low HDL
Increased risk of liver disease
Stunted growth in teens
Risk of injury to tendons and ligaments
Increased risk of cancer
Irritability, mood swings, extreme anger, violence

FIGURE 11.4 The dangers of using anabolic steroids.

CONSUMER CORNER: Health and Fitness in a Bottle

WWW 2

Many products sold as ergogenic aids are classified as food supplements. Most people in the United States think that the Food and Drug Administration (FDA) tests food supplements to make sure that they are safe. This assumption is false. Unlike medicines, which must be tested before they are approved for safe use, food supplements are unregulated by the government. The law does *not* require that they be tested for effectiveness or safety before they are sold. And unlike foods, which must be labeled with nutrition information, food supplements are not required to carry a label. As a result, there is great variation in the content of different products with the same name. Be aware of the following facts about food supplements.

- **Regulation.** Manufacturers are supposed to regulate their products, but many do not.
- **Claims.** Manufacturers are not supposed to make unsubstantiated health claims for their products, but many do it anyway. Although the FDA does not test products, it can investigate claims and has taken action against some companies for making false claims. However, because there are few investigators, many false claims do not get caught. Beware of health claims made for supplements.
- **Contents.** Many supplements do not contain what their makers claim they do. Some contain too little or too much of the key substance they are supposed to contain. Some have been shown to contain substances that they are *not* supposed to contain. These problems have led to health risks for some users.
- **USP.** The U.S. Pharmacopeial Convention (USP) is a nonprofit organization that tests supplements on store shelves to see whether they meet advertised standards for purity, strength, and quality. Products with the USP label are more likely than other products to be what they claim to be.
- **Recall.** Although the FDA does not regulate or test supplements, it does maintain a registry of side effects experienced from use of a supplement. You can report side effects to the FDA, and user reports have resulted in FDA bans on several supplements.
- **Dose or amount.** Because research is not required for supplements, as it is for medicines, very little is known about appropriate doses (amounts) for most supplements.

United States, but because manufacturers failed to meet marketing requirements it can no longer be sold in the country as a supplement. In fact, the FDA has sent letters to companies that sell it indicating that "enforcement action" can be taken against them. The FDA took this action after concluding that use of androstenedione "may increase the risk of serious health problems."

The use of steroid precursors such as androstenedione results in side effects similar to those associated with steroid use. As a result, just as USOC and other sport organizations banned steroid use, they now also ban the use of androstenedione, androstenediol, DHEA, and other steroid precursors. Cautions against the use of steroid precursors have also been issued by several medical associations, including the American Medical Association and the American Academy of Pediatrics.

Human Growth Hormone (HGH)

Human growth hormone (HGH) is an illegal drug that is exceptionally dangerous, especially for teens. It causes the bones to stop growing properly, and its effects can be deforming and even life threatening. Like anabolic steroids, HGH is banned by virtually all high school, college, national, and international sport groups. Testing is now possible to detect HGH, and many sport groups now do mandatory testing. Many high-profile athletes have destroyed their reputations and careers by using HGH and other substances described in this lesson.

Creatine

Creatine is a natural substance manufactured in the bodies of meat-eating animals, including humans. It is needed for the body to perform anaerobic exercise, including many types of progressive resistance exercise. Creatine can also be taken as a food supplement. Taking extra creatine as a supplement allows your body to store more of it. Medical and kinesiology experts who have studied creatine indicate that it may be effective in improving performance in high-intensity exercise, such as sprinting, possibly because it allows training with shorter rest periods. It does not seem to improve aerobic or endurance performance or to improve performance among older people or highly trained athletes. Doctors use it to treat some medical conditions.

There is some evidence that creatine "loading"—using 20 grams daily for five days—may be more effective than continuous use. But remember, there is still some uncertainty about exactly who can benefit from creatine and at what dose. Studies to date have included only a small number of people (all have involved fewer than 40 participants), and it is not possible to draw firm conclusions from such small numbers.

In addition, because creatine is a supplement, it is not regulated by the FDA, and for this reason some products marketed as creatine may not be creatine or may contain substances other than creatine. Little or no information exists about potential long-term dangers of using creatine. Short-term use of appropriate amounts has not been linked with serious health effects, but the U.S.-based Institute of Medicine indicates that high doses are possibly unsafe. There is also some concern about possible increased risk of dehydration among athletes who use creatine. Experts agree that before teens consider using any supplement, including creatine, they should consult with their parents or guardians and a qualified expert such as a medical doctor.

Other Supplements

Athletes and bodybuilders hoping to enhance their appearance or sport performance sometimes use one or more of many other supplements as well. Sport organizations and the FDA have banned more than a few of these substances due to health problems associated with them. Ephedra is one example of a substance that was included in many supplements alleged to improve athletic performance and aid in weight loss. It was shown to cause several problems, including irregular heart rate and other potentially dangerous effects on the heart and the nervous system. For this reason, it is considered to be an ergolytic substance.

Protein supplements are also used very commonly among athletes because they are legal and easy to obtain. Indeed, your body needs protein for growth and development of most tissues. Because protein is a major part of the muscles, many people believe that taking extra protein builds extra muscle. However, most people eat more protein in their regular diet than they really need. The United States government suggests that a healthy diet should contain about 12 to 15 percent of calories as protein. A more liberal recommendation of 10 to 35 percent of the diet as protein was recently presented by the Institute of Medicine to allow for dietary differences among individuals.

Athletes and very active people do need to consume more calories of protein than inactive people, but because they take in many more total calories, experts agree that 12 to 15 percent of their diet is adequate to meet their body's protein need. Taking more than 15 percent of the diet as protein does not result in greater gains in muscle. If not taken in excess, extra protein in the diet is relatively safe, but too much protein can cause kidney problems. Protein supplements in the form of pills, powders, and protein bars are very expensive, costing as much as 50 cents per gram of protein. In contrast, the

FIT FACT

Approximately 27 percent of adults say they do muscle fitness exercise. The percentage of men who do muscle fitness exercise decreases from nearly 50 percent among young men (18 to 24 years old) to only 16 percent at age 75. The percentage of women decreases from 28 percent among young women to only 11 percent at age 75.

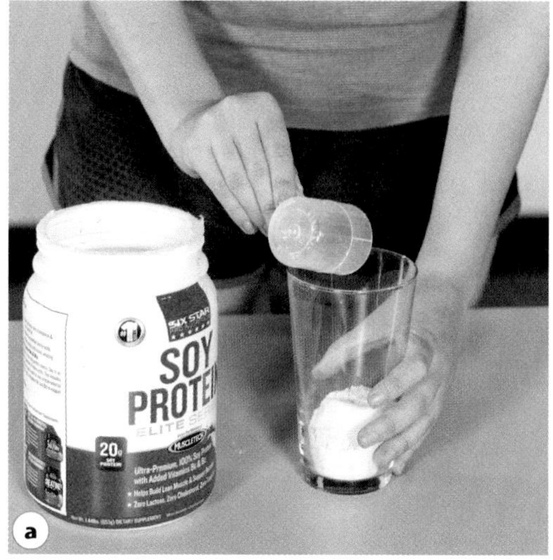

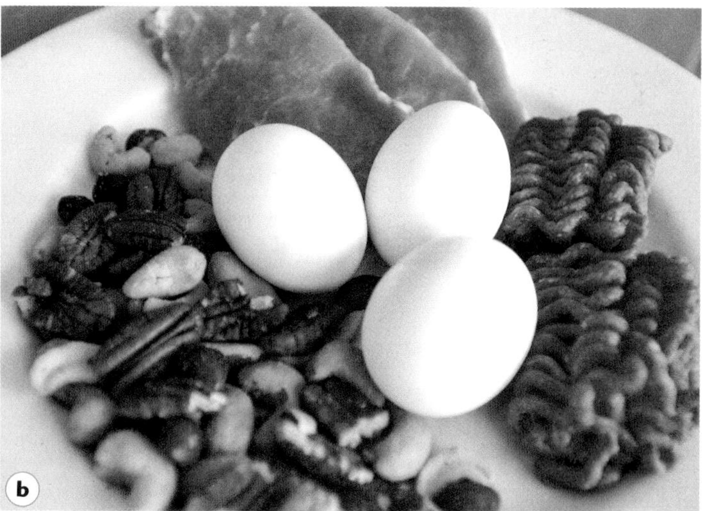

FIGURE 11.5 *(a)* Protein supplements can be expensive; *(b)* foods with protein are generally less expensive than supplements.

protein in foods such as meat, poultry, fish, beans, and eggs is much cheaper, costing only a few cents per gram (figure 11.5). The calories in extra dietary protein (in excess of body needs) are stored as fat, as are calories from extra dietary fat and carbohydrate.

Planning a Muscle Fitness Exercise Program

Molly is 15 years old and has used the five steps of program planning to prepare a muscle fitness exercise program. Her program is described here.

Step 1: Determine Your Personal Needs

To get started, Molly made a list of the muscle fitness exercises and activities she had performed over the last week. She also wrote down her fitness test results that related to vigorous physical activity. Her results are shown in figure 11.6.

Molly met the national activity guideline for muscle fitness (exercising on two days a week). But when she was not in physical education class, she did no muscle fitness exercise. In addition, Molly's fitness test scores were mostly in the marginal zone, indicating that she needed improvement. Molly wanted to try out for the softball team, and she now knew that she needed to improve her fitness in order to be the best player she could be.

Step 2: Consider Your Program Options

Molly wanted to consider all of the various types of muscle fitness exercise, so she made a list of the types of PRE that she had to choose from. Her list is included here.

- Resistance machine exercises
- Free weight exercises
- Core exercises
- Calisthenics
- Elastic band exercises
- Ball exercises
- Homemade weights
- Isometric exercises
- Isokinetic machine exercises
- Pilates
- Plyometric exercises (jump rope)

Step 3: Set Goals

For this muscle fitness plan, Molly set a time period of two weeks—too short for long-term goals—so she developed only short-term physical activity goals. Later, she'll develop long-term goals, including some muscle fitness improvement goals, when she prepares a longer plan. For now, she wanted to

Physical activity profile		
Day	Muscle fitness exercise(s)	How much?
Mon.	Curl-up Knee push-up	1 set, 10 reps 1 set, 10 reps
Tues.	None	
Wed.	Curl-up Knee push-up	1 set, 10 reps 1 set, 10 reps
Thurs.	None	
Fri.	Curl-up Knee push-up	1 set, 10 reps 1 set, 10 reps
Sat.	None	
Sun.	None	
Physical fitness profile		
Fitness self-assessment	**Score**	**Rating**
1RM arm press (score divided by body weight) 1RM leg press (score divided by body weight)	0.55 (strength per pound of body weight) 1.10 (strength per pound of body weight)	Marginal Good fitness
Grip strength	105 lb	Marginal
Muscle endurance test	4 points	Marginal
Back test	9 points	Marginal
Standing long jump	59 in.	Marginal
Medicine ball throw	95 in.	Marginal

FIGURE 11.6 Molly's muscle fitness exercise (physical activity) and fitness profiles.

try some new exercises to get started and improve her chances of making the softball team.

Molly used the information she put together in step 2 to help develop her short-term goals for muscle fitness exercise (PRE). She had many choices but decided on resistance machines, core exercises, and plyometrics (jump rope). Before writing down her goals, Molly made sure that she chose SMART goals. Here they are:

1. Continue to perform two calisthenics in physical education class (1 set of 10 reps).
2. Perform five resistance machine exercises two days a week (1 set of 10 reps at 50 percent of 1RM).
3. Perform four core exercises three days a week (hold 10 seconds or do 1 set of 10 reps).
4. Perform jump rope two days a week (5 minutes).

Step 4: Structure Your Program and Write It Down

Molly's fourth step was to write down her two-week muscle fitness plan (see figure 11.7). Molly chose resistance machine exercises because she could use the school's exercise room on Tuesdays and Thursdays after school and she thought these exercises would be good for preparing for softball. She decided to do them just two days a week because she was just beginning this type of exercise. She decided to do her jump rope (plyometrics) on Tuesday and Thursday as well. She scheduled core exercises because they were good for back health and good posture and she could do them at home. She listed the exercises she did in physical education class because she expected to keep doing them for the two weeks of her plan. Molly's plan met the national guideline of performing muscle fitness exercises on at least two to three days a week.

	Week 1			Week 2		
Day	**Exercises**	**Time, sets, reps**	**✔**	**Exercises**	**Time, sets, reps**	**✔**
Mon.	Curl-up* Knee push-up* **Core exercises** Front plank Side plank (left) Side plank (right) Reverse curl	1 set, 10 reps 1 set, 10 reps Hold 10 sec Hold 10 sec Hold 10 sec 1 set, 10 reps		Curl-up* Knee push-up* **Core exercises** Front plank Side plank (left) Side plank (right) Reverse curl	1 set, 10 reps 1 set, 10 reps Hold 10 sec Hold 10 sec Hold 10 sec 1 set, 10 reps	
Tues.	Jump rope **Resistance machine** Arm press Knee extension Hamstring curl Biceps curl Heel raise	3:30–3:35 p.m. 3:35–4:30 p.m. 1 set 10 reps 50% 1RM for each exercise		Jump rope **Resistance machine** Arm press Knee extension Hamstring curl Biceps curl Heel raise	3:30–3:35 p.m. 3:35–4:30 p.m. 1 set 10 reps 50% 1RM for each exercise	
Wed.	Curl-up* Knee push-up* **Core exercises** Front plank Side plank (left) Side plank (right) Reverse curl	1 set, 10 reps 1 set, 10 reps Hold 10 sec Hold 10 sec Hold 10 sec 1 set, 10 reps		Curl-up* Knee push-up* **Core exercises** Front plank Side plank (left) Side plank (right) Reverse curl	1 set, 10 reps 1 set, 10 reps Hold 10 sec Hold 10 sec Hold 10 sec 1 set, 10 reps	
Thurs.	Jump rope **Resistance machine** Arm press Knee extension Hamstring curl Biceps curl Heel raise	3:30–3:35 p.m. 3:35–4:45 p.m. 1 set 10 reps 50% 1RM for each exercise		Jump rope **Resistance machine** Arm press Knee extension Hamstring curl Biceps curl Heel raise	3:30–3:35 p.m. 3:35–4:45 p.m. 1 set 10 reps 50% 1RM for each exercise	
Fri.	Curl-up* Knee push-up* **Core exercises** Front plank Side plank (left) Side plank (right) Reverse curl	1 set, 10 reps 1 set, 10 reps Hold 10 sec Hold 10 sec Hold 10 sec 1 set, 10 reps		Curl-up* Knee push-up* **Core exercises** Front plank Side plank (left) Side plank (right) Reverse curl	1 set, 10 reps 1 set, 10 reps Hold 10 sec Hold 10 sec Hold 10 sec 1 set, 10 reps	
Sat.						
Sun.						

*Performed in physical education class

FIGURE 11.7 Molly's written plan.

Step 5: Keep a Log and Evaluate Your Program

Over the next two weeks, Molly will self-monitor her activities and place a checkmark on her plan beside each activity she performs. Then she'll evaluate to see whether she met her goals.

Periodization

Variety and enjoyment are important because they can help you stick with your exercise plan. Experts have found that if you change your program from time to time, you'll find it more interesting and feel more motivated to continue. **Periodization** is a systematic approach to scheduling your muscle fitness training and is used for long-term fitness programs (months to years). When you periodize a training program, you use variations in your exercise routines based on your needs for that phase of training.

For example, over 15 weeks of training, a person might do three periods of 5 weeks each. In one period, you might focus on muscular endurance exercises with relatively high repetitions and relatively low resistance. In another period, you might focus more on strength using higher resistance and fewer repetitions. Your third period might focus on combining strength and muscular endurance training or on using plyometrics to develop power. Many periodization options exist, so the three periods might look different for different people.

WWW 3

Periodization is used by athletes to gradually increase performance so that they peak, or reach their best performance level, at the right time. For example, an Olympic athlete would want to reach peak performance at the Olympic games, whereas a high school athlete might want peak performance for a key game or meet. Nonathletes use periodization more to provide variety and continued interest than peaking to prepare for a specific sporting event.

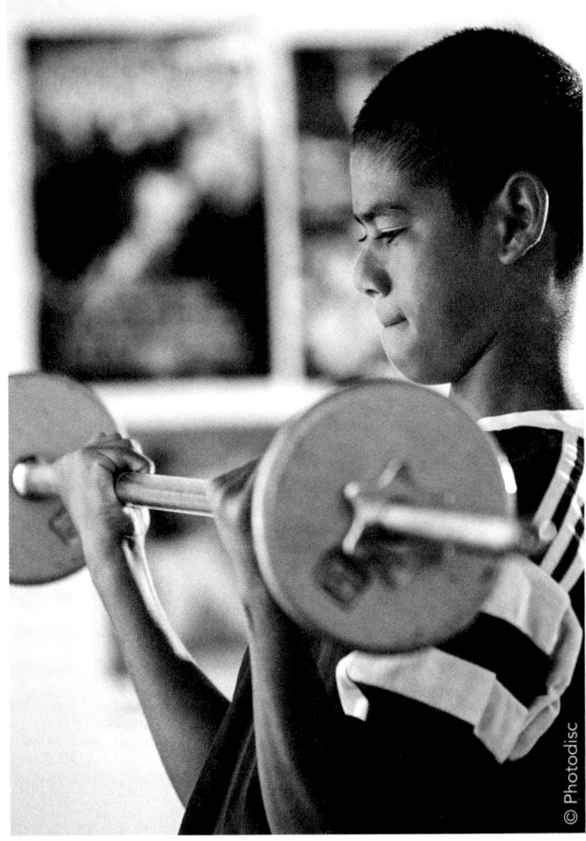

Varying your schedule for resistance training can help keep it interesting.

Lesson Review

1. What are some ergogenic aids and supplements, and what risks are associated with using them?
2. How do you assess your personal needs and build a muscle fitness and activity profile?
3. What should you consider in setting goals for muscle fitness exercise?
4. How do you select muscle fitness exercises and prepare a written muscle fitness exercise plan?
5. What is periodization, and why is it used?

TAKING CHARGE: Finding Social Support

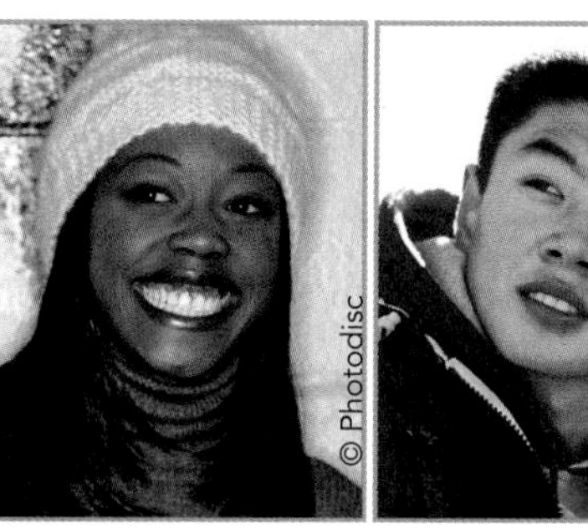
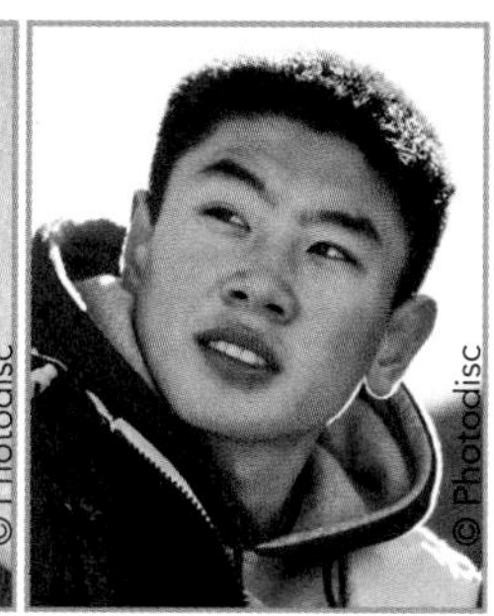

© Photodisc

© Photodisc

Social support involves your family members, friends, teachers, and community members encouraging your physical activities or participating with you. You're more likely to begin or continue an activity if the people you associate with also do it.

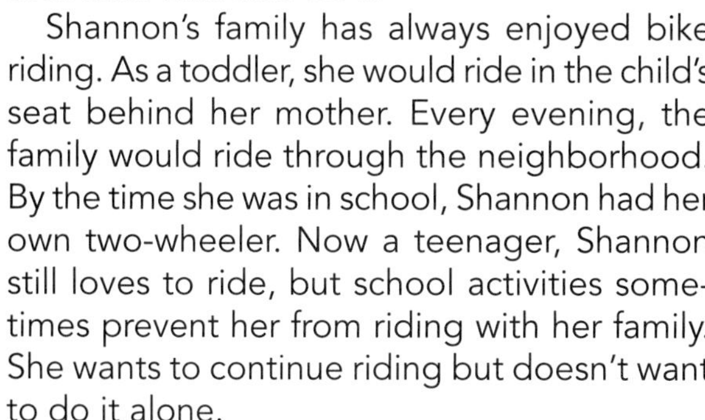

Shannon's family has always enjoyed bike riding. As a toddler, she would ride in the child's seat behind her mother. Every evening, the family would ride through the neighborhood. By the time she was in school, Shannon had her own two-wheeler. Now a teenager, Shannon still loves to ride, but school activities sometimes prevent her from riding with her family. She wants to continue riding but doesn't want to do it alone.

Jim's family has never been very active. Most of his friends tend to watch television, play video games, or just hang out rather than do anything active. Sometimes, Jim watches while a group of his classmates plays a quick game of volleyball after school. They often invite him to join the game. He has been tempted to join but has hesitated because he is not friends with any of the players. He has enjoyed the activities he has tried in the past but has never continued them for very long.

Both Shannon and Jim need social support. Shannon needs it to continue an activity she already enjoys. Jim needs it to begin an activity and then reinforce his participation.

For Discussion

Who might Shannon ask to go riding with her? What could Jim do to become involved in physical activity? What other suggestions can you offer for finding social support? What groups might Shannon and Jim identify with to get social support? Consider the guidelines presented in the Self-Management feature when you answer the discussion questions.

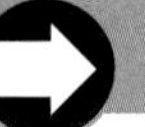

SELF-MANAGEMENT: Skills for Finding Social Support

Experts indicate that people who experience support from others are more likely to participate in regular physical activity, especially over the course of a lifetime. Social support is also helpful to people in losing weight, building muscle fitness, and improving their eating habits. Consider the following guidelines to help you gain others' support for your physical activity.

- **Do a self-assessment of your current level of social support.** Ask your teacher about the social support worksheet that can help you do this assessment. Use the self-assessment to determine areas in which you can improve your social support.
- **Birds of a feather flock together.** Find friends who are interested in the activities that interest you, or encourage your current friends to support you or join you in your participation.
- **Join a club or team.** If no club or team exists for your chosen activity, talk to a teacher, family member, or community recreation leader about starting one.
- **Discuss your interests with family and teachers.** Ask them for their support. Ask them to help you learn the activity.
- **If possible, get lessons.** In addition to formal lessons, you can also ask teachers and others to support you by helping you learn to perform an activity properly.
- **Family matters.** Encourage your family members to try the activity.
- **Get proper equipment.** Ask for equipment for your birthday or other special occasion.

TAKING ACTION: Your Muscle Fitness Exercise Plan

Prepare an exercise plan for muscle fitness using the five steps described in the second lesson of this chapter. Like Molly, consider activities from a variety of types of PRE. The goal is to perform the exercises on at least two days per week (for beginners) and as many as three days per week for more advanced exercisers. Carry out your written plan over a two-week period. Your teacher may give you time in class to do some of the activities included in your plan. Consider the following suggestions for **taking action**.

- Before your PRE, perform a dynamic warm-up.
- Follow the tips for safe PRE.
- Progress gradually—don't try to do too much too soon.
- After your workout, perform a cool-down.

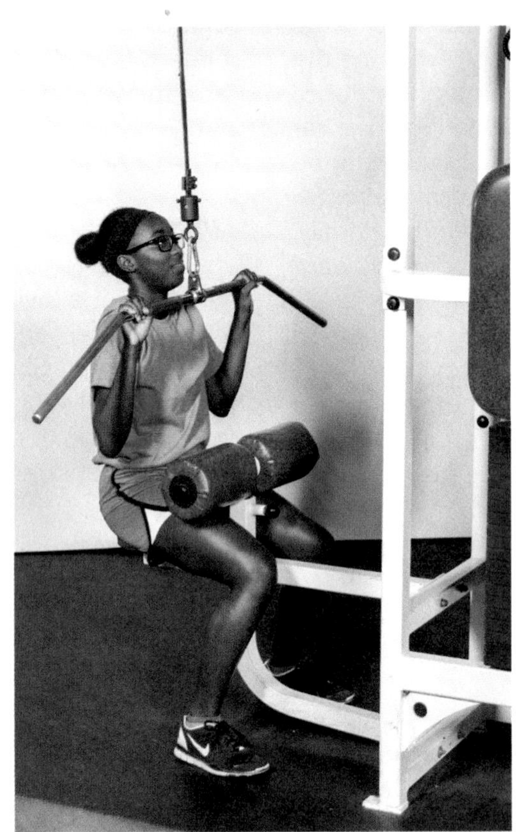

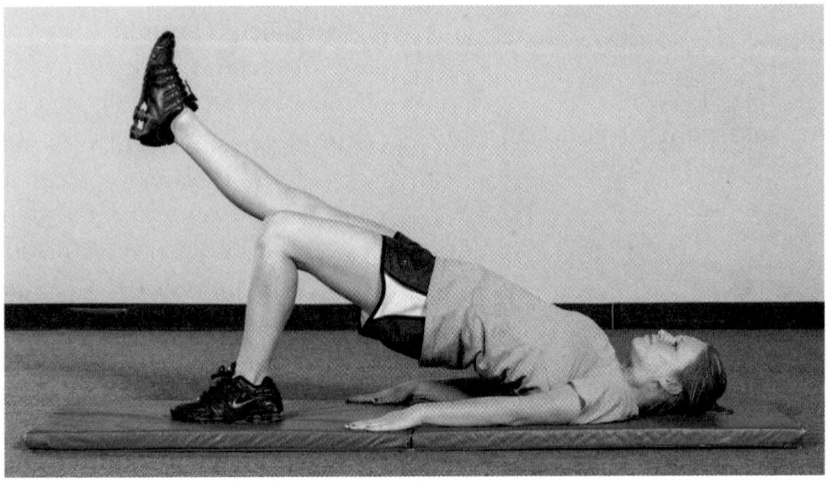

Take action by performing your muscle fitness plan.

Reviewing Concepts and Vocabulary

As directed by your teacher, answer items 1 through 5 by correctly completing each sentence with a word or phrase.

1. The muscles that support your spine and keep your rib cage and spine stable are referred to as your ______________ muscles.
2. About ______________ percent of adults experience back pain at some point.
3. ______________ are exercises that use all or part of your body weight to provide resistance.
4. ______________ is the real name of the supplement sometimes called andro.
5. The full name for the substance called HGH is ______________.

For items 6 through 10, as directed by your teacher, match each term in column 1 with the appropriate phrase in column 2.

6. rhabdomyolysis	a. swayback
7. periodization	b. rounded shoulders
8. lordosis	c. breakdown of muscle fiber
9. kyphosis	d. varying your program schedule for muscle fitness
10. ptosis	e. protruding abdomen

For items 11 through 15, as directed by your teacher, respond to each statement or question.

11. What are some of the best exercises for building your core muscles?
12. Describe three guidelines for properly lifting, carrying, and moving objects.
13. What self-assessments can you do to determine whether you are at risk for back pain?
14. What are some harmful effects of steroids?
15. What are some good strategies for finding social support?

Thinking Critically

Write a paragraph to answer the following question.

A friend of yours is excited about an advertisement in a muscle magazine. The ad describes a pill that is "guaranteed to add size to your muscles in two weeks without exercise." What advice would you give your friend?

Project

Assume that you've been hired as a reporter for a local newspaper. Write an article about preventing back pain or injury. Interview relevant people, such as a physical therapist, a physical education teacher, an athletic trainer, and a person who has experienced back pain or injury. Present your article in class or submit it to a newspaper for publication.

12

Flexibility

In This Chapter

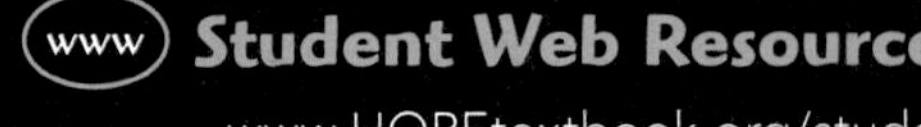

Student Web Resources

www.HOPEtextbook.org/student

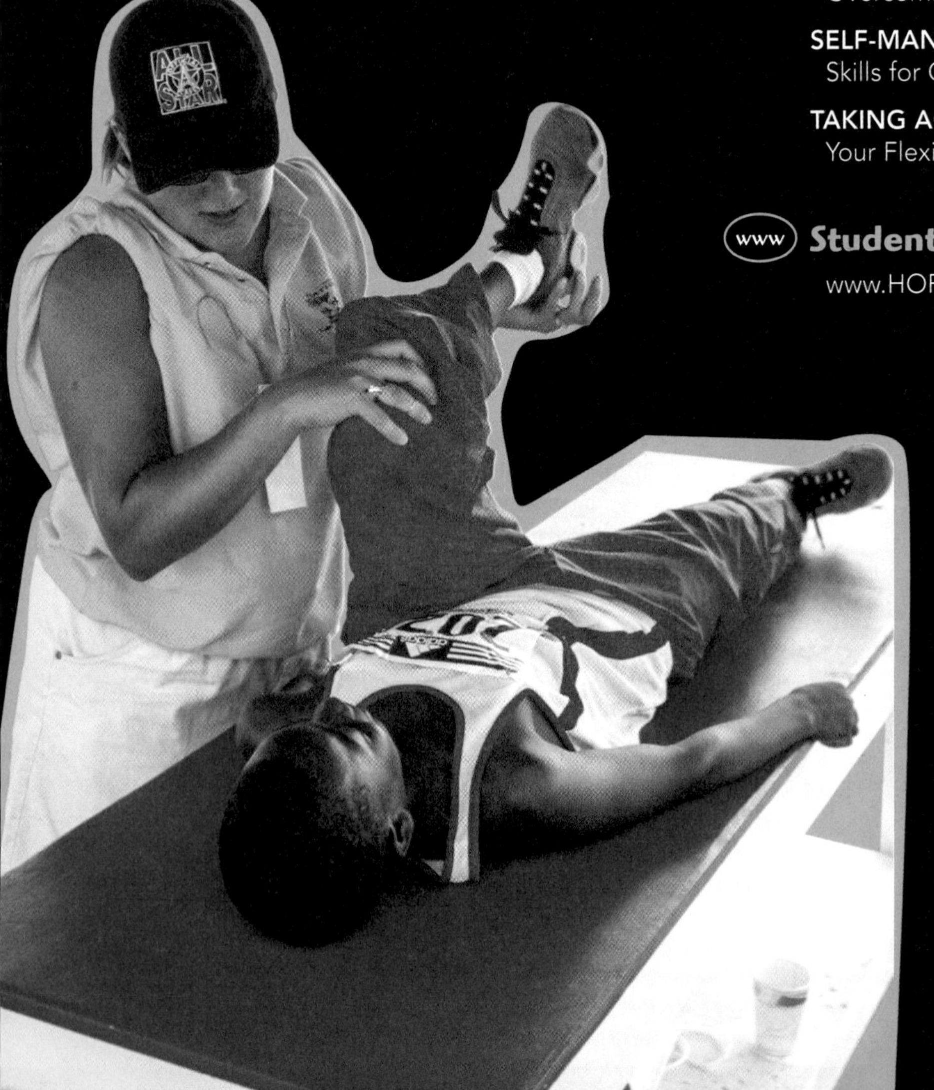

Lesson 12.1

Flexibility Facts

Lesson Objectives

After reading this lesson, you should be able to

1. explain the difference between a warm-up and a flexibility workout,
2. describe flexibility and some of the factors that influence it,
3. explain the benefits of good flexibility,
4. describe types of flexibility exercise and the FIT formula for each, and
5. explain why it is important to balance strength and flexibility exercise.

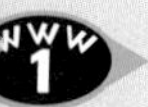

Lesson Vocabulary

active stretch, antagonist, ballistic stretch, CRAC, dynamic movement exercise, dynamic stretching, hypermobility, muscle-tendon unit (MTU), passive stretch, PNF stretch, range of motion (ROM), range-of-motion (ROM) exercise, static stretch

Do you have good flexibility? Do you do any regular stretching to improve your flexibility? In this lesson, you'll learn about the importance of being flexible and how to improve your flexibility by applying fitness principles. You'll also learn to evaluate your flexibility.

Sometimes people confuse a warm-up with a flexibility workout, but they are two different things. A warm-up is a group of exercises done to get ready for a specific workout or competition. A flexibility workout is a group of exercises done to build flexibility. Stretching exercises are now used less frequently in warm-ups than in the past, especially when preparing for certain types of activity, such as those involving strength, speed, and power. But this does not mean that flexibility exercises, including stretching, are not important. Flexibility is a key component of health-related physical fitness.

What Is Flexibility?

Flexibility is the ability to move your joints through a full **range of motion (ROM)**. A joint is a place in your body where bones come together. The best-known joints include the knees, ankles, elbows, wrists, knuckles, shoulders, hips, and the joints between the vertebrae in the spine. Some joints, such as your knees and elbows, work like a hinge, permitting movement in only two directions. Other joints, such as your hips and shoulders, work like a ball and socket, allowing movement in all directions. ROM is the amount of movement you can make in a joint (figure 12.1).

Your bones are connected at your joints by nonelastic bands called ligaments; as you'll see later, they should not be stretched. Your bones are connected to your muscles by tendons. When your muscles contract, they pull on your tendons to cause your bones to move. Unlike ligaments, muscles and tendons need to be stretched in order to maintain a healthy length. Together, muscles and tendons are called a **muscle-tendon unit (MTU)** (figure 12.1). Both parts of the MTU are stretched when performing flexibility exercises, but we frequently refer only to "stretching the muscle" for simplicity. If your muscles and tendons are too short, they restrict a joint's ROM.

Benefits of Good Flexibility

Flexibility is sometimes referred to as the forgotten part of health-related fitness because many people focus exclusively on the other parts. We know, however, that good flexibility provides many benefits, including health benefits, especially when you grow older.

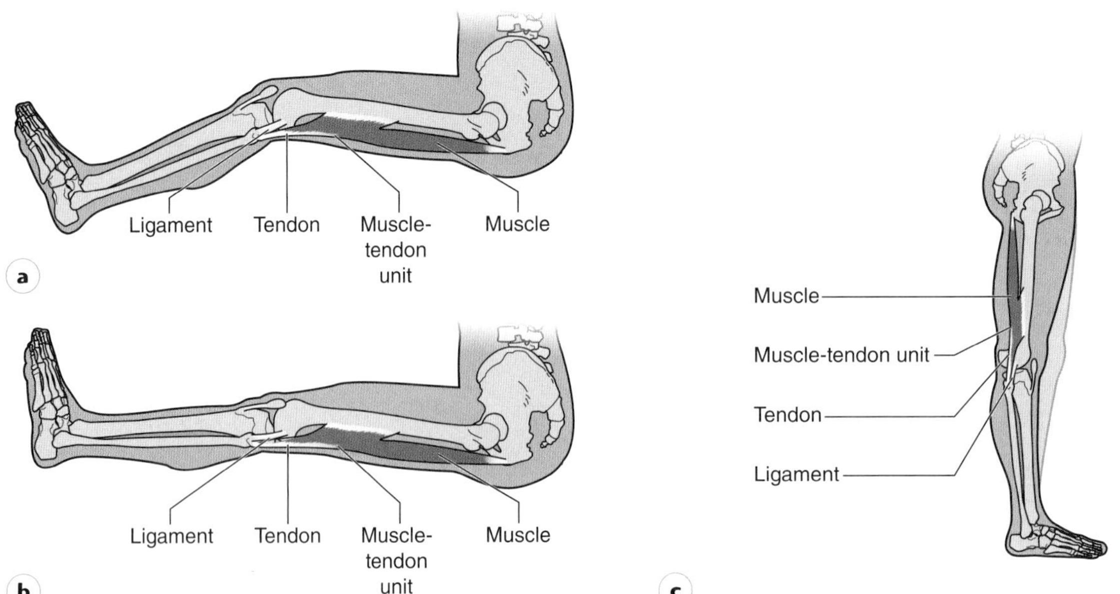

FIGURE 12.1 *(a)* Poor joint range of motion—knee does not fully extend because of short hamstring muscles; *(b)* good range of motion—knee fully extends because of long hamstrings; *(c)* too much range of motion—knee bends backward.

Improved Function

Everyone needs at least some flexibility in order to maintain health and mobility. The exact amount of flexibility needed for normal daily function depends on the demands of the activities that you perform. For example, plumbers, painters, and dentists often need to bend and stretch, and some musicians need very flexible fingers and wrists. As people grow older, their flexibility tends to decrease, which can limit simple movements such as looking over the shoulder while driving. Therefore, it's especially important for older people to do exercises that build and maintain a full range of motion.

Flexibility is also important to many athletes, especially in certain sports. Dancers and gymnasts must be very flexible to perform their routines. Swimmers need good flexibility to get maximum performance, as do kickers in football. Good flexibility also allows a longer backswing—and therefore a faster forward swing—in the throwing and striking movements that are crucial in golf, tennis, and baseball pitching. While some research has questioned the value of stretching right before a competition or performance, muscles of adequate length can be beneficial even in such activities as weightlifting and the shot put.

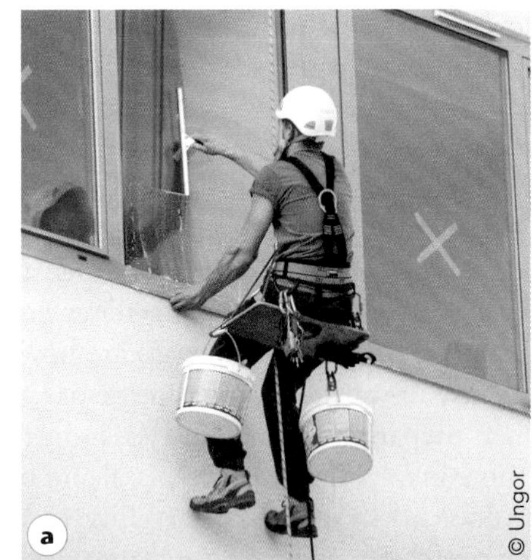

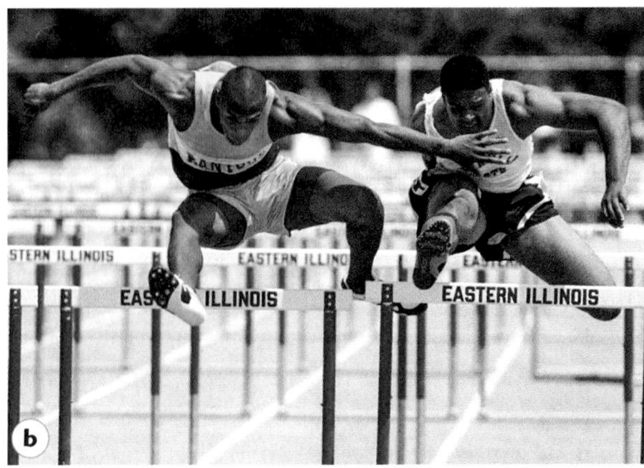

Good flexibility is needed *(a)* for some jobs and *(b)* by most athletes.

Improved Health and Wellness

Good flexibility is important for your back health and your posture. For example, back pain and poor posture are associated with short hamstring and hip flexor muscles. More generally, very short muscles are at risk of being overstretched and injured. Stretching exercises also have a beneficial effect on a number of conditions. Flexible musicians are less likely to have pain in their joints. Stretching exercises can often alleviate menstrual cramps in women. They can prevent or provide relief from leg cramps and shin splints (pain in the front of the shins caused by overuse). Stretching a muscle can also help it relax, and some forms of stretching can help you manage stress.

Rehabilitation From Injury and Medical Problems

Flexibility exercises are used for rehabilitation from a variety of injuries and medical problems. Both physical therapists (PTs) and athletic trainers (ATs) use a variety of techniques, including stretching and muscle fitness exercises, in their work. PTs treat patients after surgery and patients with medical conditions such as arthritis, back pain, stroke, and osteoporosis. ATs help athletes train to prevent injury and help them recover when injury does occur.

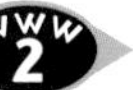

FIT FACT

Physical therapists (PTs) are health care professionals who treat patients with medical problems or who have had surgery. They help patients manage pain and improve their mobility. They also help people perform regular exercises to prevent muscle-related problems and to maintain or regain their ability to function normally. PTs have many years of advanced education and, in the United States, must be licensed in the state in which they practice. They work in many settings, including private practices, hospitals, nursing homes, outpatient clinics, schools, and sport and fitness facilities. More than 75,000 PTs belong to the American Physical Therapy Association, a professional group whose goal is to help people improve their health and quality of life.

> I want to get old gracefully. I want to have good posture, I want to be healthy and be an example to my children.
>
> —Sting, musician

Factors Influencing Flexibility

You already know that short muscles and tendons reduce flexibility and that they can be stretched to improve flexibility. Your flexibility is also influenced by the following factors.

Heredity

Inherited anatomical differences in our bodies help determine what we can and cannot do. Some people inherit joints that do not favor a large a range of motion. These people will have to exercise regularly in order to develop a healthy range of motion. Other people have an unusually large range of motion in certain joints—a condition sometimes referred to as being double jointed but officially called **hypermobility**. People with hypermobility score better on flexibility tests and can extend the knee, elbow, thumb, or wrist joint past a straight line, as if the joint could bend backward. Some people who have hypermobile joints are prone to joint injury and may be more likely to develop arthritis, a disease in which the joints become inflamed. For the most part, however, those with hypermobile joints do not have problems, other than a slight disadvantage in some sports. For example, when doing push-ups, the elbows of a hypermobile person might lock when the arms straighten, making it difficult to unlock the elbows to begin the downward movement.

Body Build

Can short people touch their toes more easily than tall people? In most cases, this is not true, because a shorter person tends to have not only shorter legs and trunk but also shorter arms (though there are exceptions). In contrast, a taller person tends to have longer legs and trunk and longer arms. Some people do have exceptionally long arms or legs, and these characteristics may make it easier or harder for them to score well on flexibility tests, but this is the exception rather than the rule.

Sex and Age

Generally, females tend to be more flexible than males. About twice as many females as males are hypermobile, and at most ages more females than males meet minimum fitness standards for flexibility. Similarly, younger people tend to be more flexible than older people. As people grow older, their muscles typically grow shorter because they are used less, and their joints tend to allow less movement due to conditions such as arthritis. With this in mind, one important reason for doing regular flexibility exercises when you're young is to reduce your risk of joint problems when you're older. Good flexibility also enhances performance in a variety of tasks for people of all ages.

Different Types of Flexibility Exercise

The following discussion presents methods of building and maintaining flexibility. For best results, perform exercises especially designed to improve your flexibility (step 5 of the Physical Activity Pyramid; figure 12.2). The four major types of exercise for building flexibility are range-of-motion exercise, static stretching, ballistic stretching, and dynamic stretching.

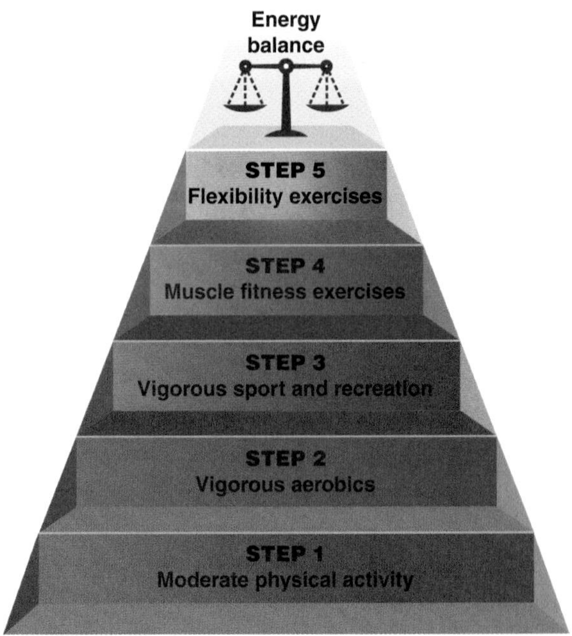

FIGURE 12.2 Exercises for building flexibility are represented by step 5 of the Physical Activity Pyramid.

Range-of-Motion (ROM) Exercise

Technically, all flexibility exercises are range-of-motion exercises because they are all designed to help allow a healthy ROM in the joints. More specifically, the term **range-of-motion (ROM) exercise** refers to exercise that requires a joint to move through a full ROM, powered either by the body's own muscles or by assistance from a partner or therapist. Such exercises are commonly used in physical therapy for people who have lost ROM or who want to avoid loss of ROM associated with an injury or medical problem. The exercise movement is typically continuous and performed at a slow to moderate pace.

Each joint has its own normal or healthy range of movement, so exercises are designed specifically for each joint. Examples include shoulder rotation exercises for people with shoulder injuries (for example, baseball pitchers) and knee flexion and extension of the fingers for people with arthritis. The weight of the body part and the momentum of the movement do cause some stretch in the muscles and connective tissues, but these exercises typically do not use the same intensity of stretch as those described in the next section; therefore, ROM exercises are not as good as stretching exercises for improving flexibility.

Muscles often work as **antagonists**—meaning they perform opposite functions—to allow multiple movements and full range of motion. For example, if you're lying down and contract the quadriceps muscles on the front of your thigh, they lift your leg off the floor; at the same time, the muscles on the back of your thigh, which are the antagonists, relax to allow the quadriceps to lift your leg.

Static Stretching

A **static stretch** involves stretching slowly as far as you can without pain, until you feel a sense of pulling or tension. For best results, static stretches are held for 10 to 30 seconds. The FIT formula for static stretching is described in table 12.1. Done correctly,

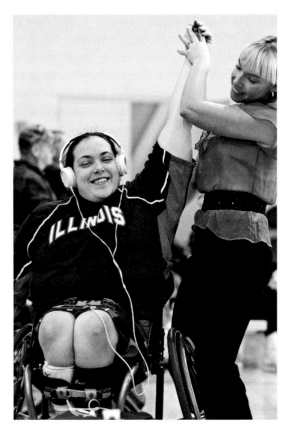

ROM exercises are commonly used in physical therapy for people who have lost range of motion associated with an injury or medical condition.

static stretching increases your flexibility and can help you relax. Some experts think that static stretching exercises are safer than ballistic stretching exercises because you're less likely to stretch too far and injure yourself.

Static stretching can be performed using either **active stretch** or **passive stretch**. A static stretch requires an assist from an external source, such as gravity, a partner (as in figure 12.3*b*), or some other source. Active static stretch is caused by contracting your own antagonist muscles—for example, contracting your shin muscle to move your toes upward, thus causing a stretch in your calf muscles (figure 12.3*a*). Passive static stretch is achieved without use of an antagonist muscle. The calf stretch, for example, can be done by having a partner push gently on your foot or by using your own arms to pull your foot upward (figure 12.3*b*).

Some experts consider active static stretch to be safer than other types of stretch because you don't have to worry about the external force overstretching your muscle (for example, if a partner pushes too hard). The advantage of passive static stretch is that makes it easier to create adequate stretch in order to improve the length of the muscle.

PNF Stretching

PNF stretching (PNF stands for proprioceptive neuromuscular facilitation) is a stretching technique originally used by physical and occupational therapists to help soldiers who had been injured. It is now widely used by many people interested in improving their flexibility, including athletes. PNF stretching is a variation of static stretching. Some experts believe that it is the most effective type of exercise for improving flexibility, though it may cause more soreness than static stretching. PNF involves contracting the muscle before you stretch it to help the muscle relax so that it can be more easily stretched. Active stretch is sometimes called active isolated stretch because the contraction

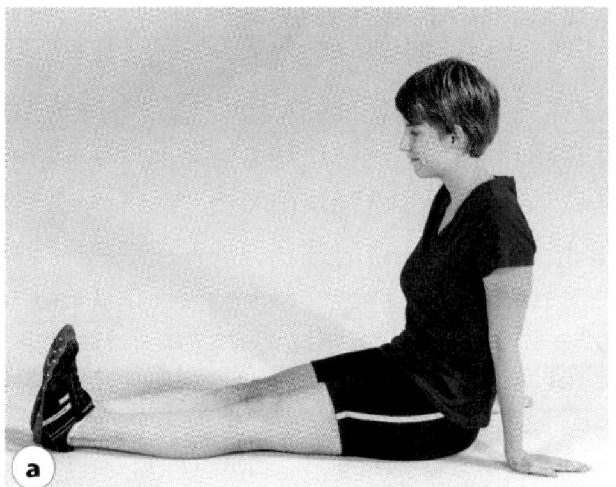

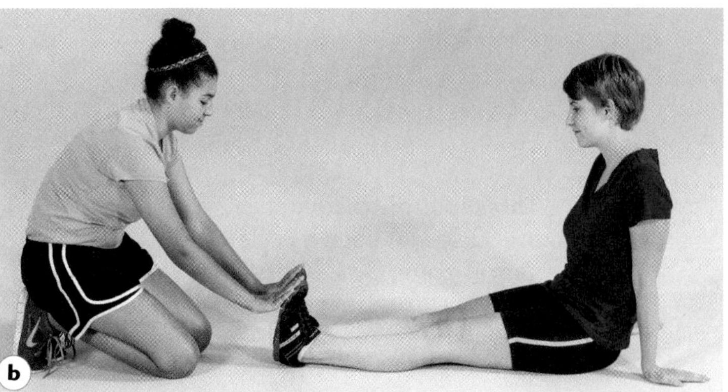

FIGURE 12.3 Stretching the calf: *(a)* active stretch; *(b)* passive stretch (with a partner assisting).

before the stretch isolates, or identifies, the muscle to be stretched. One popular form of PNF is called **CRAC** (contract-relax-antagonist-contract). After you contract a muscle that you want to stretch, the muscle automatically relaxes. Contracting the opposing (antagonist) muscles during the stretch also makes the muscle you're stretching relax. CRAC does both of these actions.

The static stretch exercise shown in figure 12.3*b* can be made into a CRAC form of PNF exercise by contracting the calf muscles by pushing the toes against the partner's hands before doing the stretch.

The FIT formula for PNF stretch is described in table 12.1.

Ballistic Stretching

Ballistic stretching involves a series of gentle bouncing or bobbing motions that are not held for a long time. The FIT formula for ballistic stretch is described in table 12.1. Like static stretching and PNF, ballistic stretching exercises are designed to use the joints through a full range of movement and cause the muscles and tendons to stretch beyond their normal length. Most of the static stretching exercises shown in this chapter can be made into ballistic stretching exercises. For example, the hamstring stretch can be made into an active ballistic stretch by using the thigh muscles to bob the upper leg forward. It can be made into a passive ballistic stretch by having a partner alternately push forward and pull backward to produce a bobbing movement of the upper leg.

Sport movement stretching uses movements that closely mimic those of a specific sport. Examples include baseball batters who swing with a weighted bat and golfers who swing the club several times before beginning a round of golf. This type of warm-up has also been referred to as sport-specific ballistic stretching. Regardless of the name preferred, it involves using the muscles to initiate a sport-specific movement that causes the muscles to be used beyond their normal ROM. Consult with

TABLE 12.1 FIT Formula and Fitness Target Zones for Stretching Exercise

	Static and PNF	Ballistic
Frequency	**Threshold of training:** Stretch each muscle group on 2 or 3 days each week. **Target zone:** Stretch each muscle group on 2–7 days each week.	**Threshold of training:** Stretch each muscle group on 2 or 3 days each week. **Target zone:** Stretch each muscle group on 2–7 days each week.
Intensity	**Threshold of training:** Stretch the muscle beyond its normal length until you feel tension, then hold. **Target zone:** Stretch the muscle beyond its normal length, from first point of tension to point of mild discomfort (not pain). Hold.	**Threshold of training:** Stretch the muscle beyond its normal length until you feel tension. Use slow, gentle bounces or bobs. Use the motion of your body part to stretch the specific muscle. **Target zone:** Stretch the muscle beyond its normal length, from first point of tension to point of mild discomfort (not pain). Use the same gentle bouncing stretch as for threshold. *Caution: No stretch should cause pain, especially sharp pain. Be especially careful when doing ballistic stretching.*
Time	**Threshold of training:** Do 2 stretches of 10–30 sec for each muscle group. **Target zone:** Do 2–4 stretches with a goal of 60 sec (total) of stretching for each muscle group (6 × 10, 4 × 15, or 2 × 30 sec). Rest for 15 sec between stretches.	**Threshold of training:** For each muscle group, perform 2 sets. Bounce against the muscle slowly and gently. Perform 15 reps. Rest for 10 sec between sets. **Target zone:** For each muscle group, perform 2–4 sets of 15 reps. Rest for 10 sec between sets. Start with 2 sets and progress to 4.

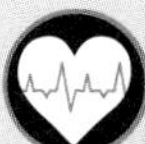

FITNESS TECHNOLOGY: Goniometers

When you perform flexibility self-assessments, you use low-tech aids such as a yardstick or ruler. In some cases, you may use a flexibility box that includes a built-in measuring stick. When experts do research on flexibility, they use more sophisticated instruments, such as a goniometer, which measures joint angles. Some goniometers are electronic. Your school may have an inexpensive goniometer, such as the one shown, that you can use when assessing the range of motion in your joints.

Using Technology

Do some investigation to learn more about goniometers and other devices for measuring flexibility.

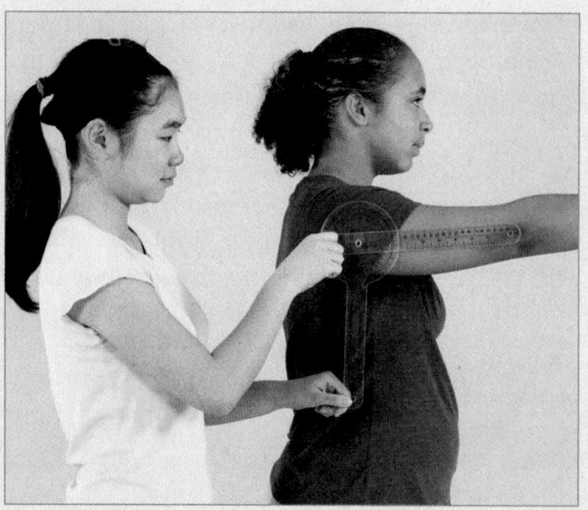

A goniometer can be used to assess range of motion and flexibility.

your instructor or coach to find out about recommended exercises for a given sport.

FIT FACT

ACSM refers to dynamic stretching exercises as an additional way to build flexibility. They are similar to static stretching exercises, but the stretch is slow, gradual, and continuous until the muscle is fully stretched. Developmental stretching is another type of flexibility exercise recommended by some experts. It is performed slowly like dynamic stretching, and the stretch is held for 10 to 30 seconds (the same as static stretching). The difference is that in developmental stretching you stretch until you feel slight tension and then reduce the stretch for 3 to 5 seconds. The stretch is then increased slightly beyond the previous stretch. You repeat these steps (stretch, reduce stretch, stretch) until you reach a full stretch as outlined in table 12.1. Both dynamic and developmental stretching exercises are good alternatives for people who have been injured or who are just beginning a stretching program.

Some teachers and coaches have concerns about ballistic stretching because of the possibility of overstretching and injuring muscles if it is not done carefully. However, studies show that, if performed properly, ballistic stretching can be safe and does not cause as much muscular soreness as static stretching. Therapists do caution against ballistic stretching after a muscle or tendon injury, and they recommend consulting an expert to determine the best method of stretch for rehabilitation.

Balancing Muscle Fitness and Flexibility

You should do muscle fitness and flexibility exercises together. We now know that muscle fitness exercises, when properly performed, need not limit flexibility. In fact, when done through a full range of motion, they can even help you build flexibility. But muscle fitness exercises are best for building muscle fitness, and flexibility exercises are best for building flexibility.

Therefore, a balanced exercise program includes both muscle fitness and flexibility exercises for all of your muscles so that they can apply equal force on all sides of a joint. People commonly use the flexors (muscles on the front of the body) a great

SCIENCE IN ACTION: Dynamic Movement Exercise

Dynamic movement exercises include jumping, skipping, and calisthenics such as those used in a warm-up. They move the joints beyond normal resting ROM and cause the muscles and tendons to stretch. The stretch caused by dynamic movement exercise is followed by a contraction of the stretched muscle. For example, jumping stretches the calf muscle; after the stretch caused by landing from a jump, the muscle contracts again to provide the force for the next jump. This type of exercise is also referred to as dynamic calisthenics. Dynamic movement exercises should not be confused with dynamic stretching exercises (see the Fit Fact on dynamic stretching).

Experts who pioneered the use of dynamic movement exercises point out that they are not the same as ballistic stretching exercises because they do not involve bobbing or bouncing against the muscle. Dynamic movement exercise routines use many kinds of movement, including muscle fitness calisthenics (such as push-ups, curl-ups, and half squats) and some other types of muscle fitness exercise (such as elastic band exercise).

Whereas dynamic *stretching* exercises are done primarily to build flexibility, that is not the primary intent of dynamic *movement* exercises (calisthenics). For this reason, a specific FIT formula is not provided for this type of exercise. However, it is often included in a warm-up and as part of other exercise circuits, and it does provide flexibility benefits and improve muscle fitness and power. Typically, when dynamic movement exercises are included in a warm-up, exercises are chosen for different muscle groups, and the total time for the exercise is 5 to 10 minutes.

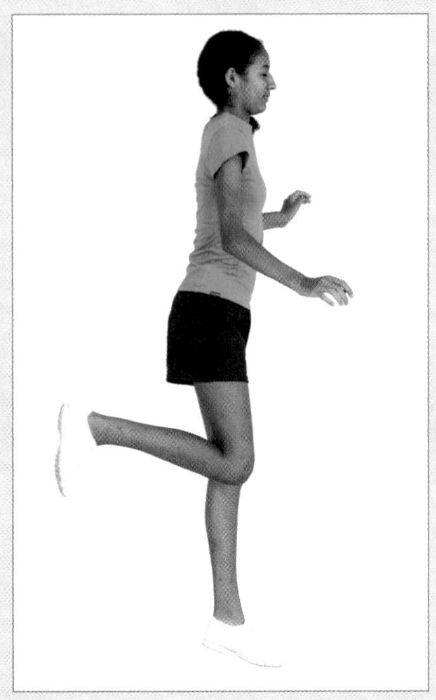

Dynamic movement exercises, such as the backward hop, stretch muscles and tendons.

Student Activity

Prepare a brochure explaining dynamic movement exercise and the reasons for doing it.

deal because many daily activities emphasize the use of those muscles. For example, the majority of people have strong biceps muscles (on the front of the arms), pectoral muscles (on the front of the chest), and quadriceps muscles (on the front of the thighs). The pull of these strong muscles results in the body hunching forward. To avoid becoming permanently hunched over, you need to make certain that these strong, short muscles on the front of your body get stretched. At the same time, you must strengthen the weak, relatively unused muscles on the back of your body. Table 12.2 lists the muscles for which most people need the most flexibility exercise.

Specificity of Stretching

Are there any muscles that do not need stretching? For many people, the answer is yes. For example, some people eventually begin to develop a hunched-over posture often called humpback at some point in life. Because the upper back muscles become overstretched in people with this postural problem, they should avoid further stretching of those muscles.

TABLE 12.2 Muscles That Need the Most Stretching

Muscle(s)	Reason for stretching
Chest	Prevent poor posture
Front of shoulders	Prevent poor posture
Front of hip joints	Prevent swayback posture, backache, pulled muscle
Back of thighs (hamstring)	Prevent swayback posture, backache, pulled muscle
Inside of thighs	Prevent back, leg, and foot strain
Calf	Avoid soreness and Achilles tendon injury (may result from running and jumping)
Lower back	Prevent soreness, pain, back injury

The abdominal muscles are another example. You do need to keep your abdominal muscles strong, but most people don't need to stretch them, In fact, if they're stretched, they begin to sag, and the abdomen protrudes, leading to poor posture.

Each person must evaluate his or her own needs to avoid stretching already-overstretched muscles and avoid strengthening muscles that are already so strong that they are out of balance with their opposing muscles. Keeping muscles on opposites sides of a joint in balance helps them pull with equal force in all directions. This balance helps align your body parts properly, ensuring good posture.

Lesson Review

1. How does a stretching warm-up differ from a flexibility (stretching) workout?
2. What is flexibility, and what factors influence it?
3. What are the benefits of good flexibility?
4. What are the types of flexibility exercise, and what is the FIT formula for each?
5. Why is it important to balance strength and flexibility exercise?

✓ SELF-ASSESSMENT: Arm, Leg, and Trunk Flexibility

In this self-assessment, you'll evaluate the flexibility in several areas of your body. Use these general directions for the tests that follow. Then score yourself using table 12.3.

- Perform each exercise as described and illustrated here.
- Stretch and hold the position for two seconds while a partner checks your performance.
- Score one point for each test for which you meet the standard. Total your score for all tests.
- Determine your rating using table 12.3. Record your results as directed by your instructor.

You are expected to do these tests in class only once, unless your instructor tells you otherwise. However, you may want to retest yourself periodically. A retest helps you to see progress and can also be used to help set new goals. If you're working with a partner, remember that self-assessment information is personal and considered confidential. It shouldn't be shared with others without the permission of the person being tested.

Safety tip: Before taking a flexibility test, do a general warm-up and try each movement two or three times.

TABLE 12.3 Rating Chart: Flexibility

Fitness rating	Score (items passed)
Good	8–11
Marginal	5–7
Low	0–4

Arm Lift

1. Lie facedown. Hold a ruler or stick in both hands. Keep your fists tight and your palms facing down.
2. Raise your arms and the stick as high as possible. Keep your forehead on the floor and your arms and wrists straight.
3. Hold this position while your partner uses a ruler to check the distance of the stick from the floor.
4. Record one point if you meet the standard: 10 inches (25 centimeters) or more.

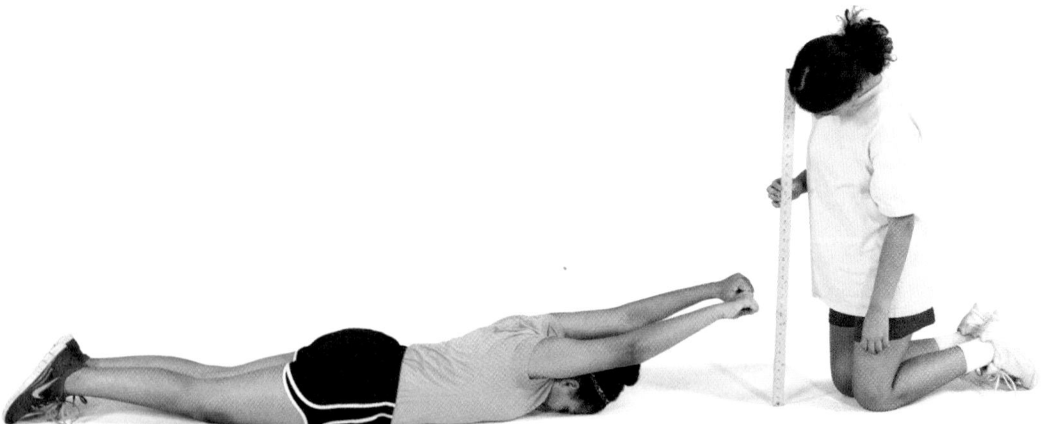

This test evaluates your chest and shoulder flexibility.

Zipper

1. Reach your left arm and hand over your left shoulder and down your spine, as if you were going to pull up a zipper.
2. Hold this position while you reach your right arm and hand behind your back and up your spine to try to touch or overlap the fingers of your left hand.
3. Hold the position while your partner checks it.
4. Repeat, this time reaching your right arm and hand over your right shoulder and your left arm and hand up your spine.
5. Record one point for each side on which you meet the standard: touching or overlapping fingers.

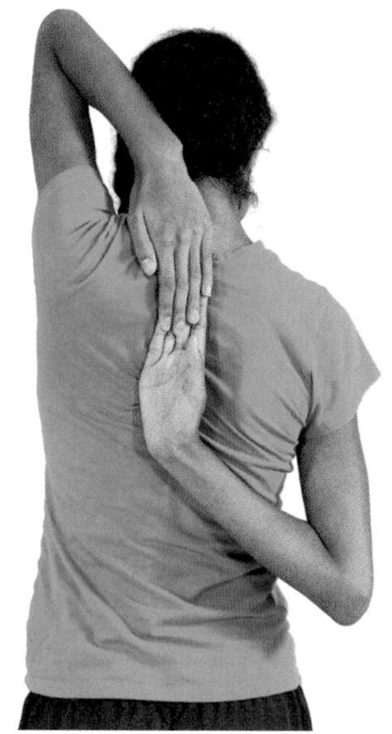

This test evaluates your shoulder, arm, and chest flexibility.

Trunk Rotation

1. Stand with your toes on the designated line. Your left shoulder should be an arm's length (with fist closed) from the wall and directly on a line with the target spot located on the wall.
2. Drop your left arm and extend your right arm to your side at shoulder height. Make a fist with your palm down.
3. Without moving your feet, rotate your trunk to the right as far as possible. Your knees may bend slightly to permit more turn, but don't move your feet. Try to touch the target spot or beyond with a palm-down fist.
4. Hold the position while your partner checks it.
5. Repeat, rotating to the left.
6. Record one point for each side on which you meet the standard: touch the center of the target or beyond.

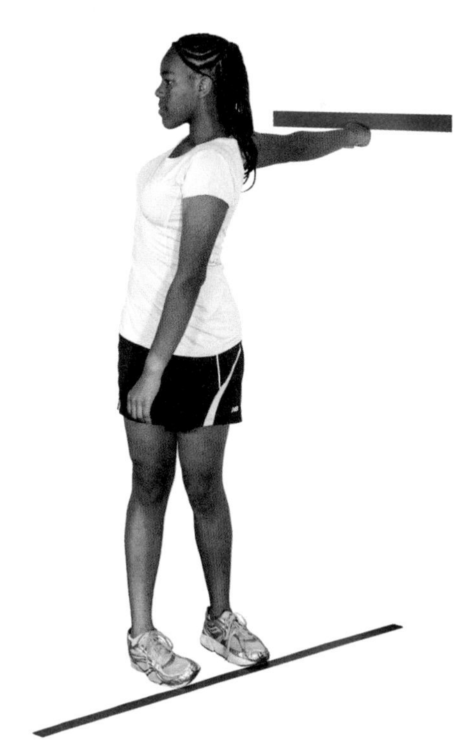

This test evaluates your spine, shoulder, and hip flexibility.

Wrap-Around

1. Raise your right arm and reach behind your head. Try to touch the left corner of your mouth. You may turn your head and neck to the left.
2. Hold the position while your partner checks it.
3. Repeat with your left arm.
4. Record one point for each side on which you meet the standard: touching the corner of the mouth.

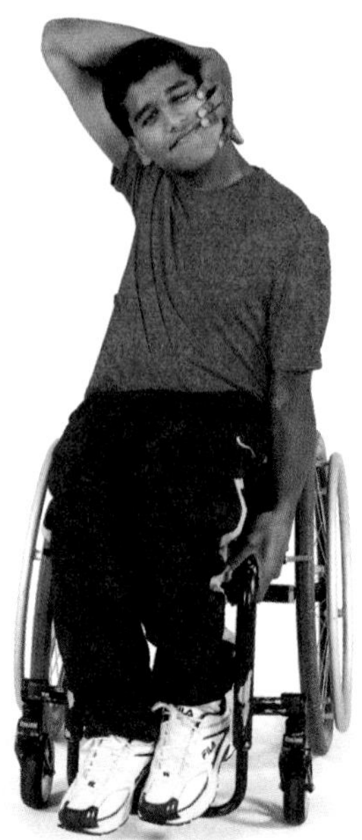

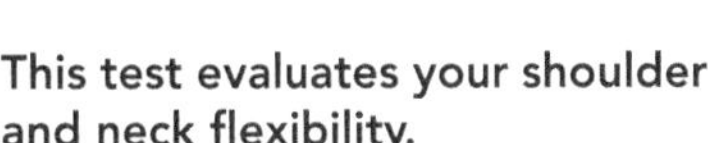

This test evaluates your shoulder and neck flexibility.

Knee-to-Chest

1. Lie on your back and extend your right leg. Place your hands on the back of your left thigh and pull toward you to draw the knee closer to the chest. Do not place your hands on top of the knee.
2. Keep your right leg straight and on the floor if possible. Keep your lower back flat on the floor.
3. Hold the position. Have your partner check to see if your upper left thigh and knee are against your chest and your right leg is straight and on the floor.
4. Repeat with the opposite leg.
5. Record one point for each side on which you meet the standard: thigh and knee against the chest and calf on the floor.

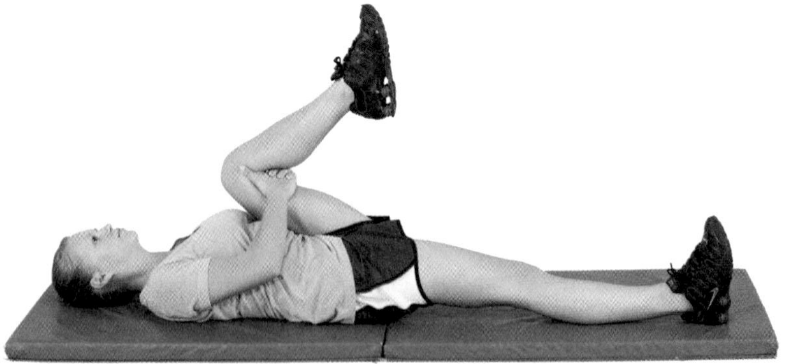

This test evaluates the flexibility of your hamstrings, your lower back, and the hip flexor muscles.

Ankle Flex

1. Sit erect on the floor with your legs straight and together. You may lean backward slightly on your hands if necessary.
2. Start with the soles of your shoes at 90 degrees (perpendicular) to the floor.
3. Flex your ankles by pulling your toes toward your shins as far as possible. Hold this position while your partner checks whether the angle that the sole of each foot makes with the floor is 75 degrees. (You can use a protractor to make a 75-degree angle on a sheet of paper.).
4. Record one point for each ankle for which you meet the standard: soles angled 75 degrees or more.

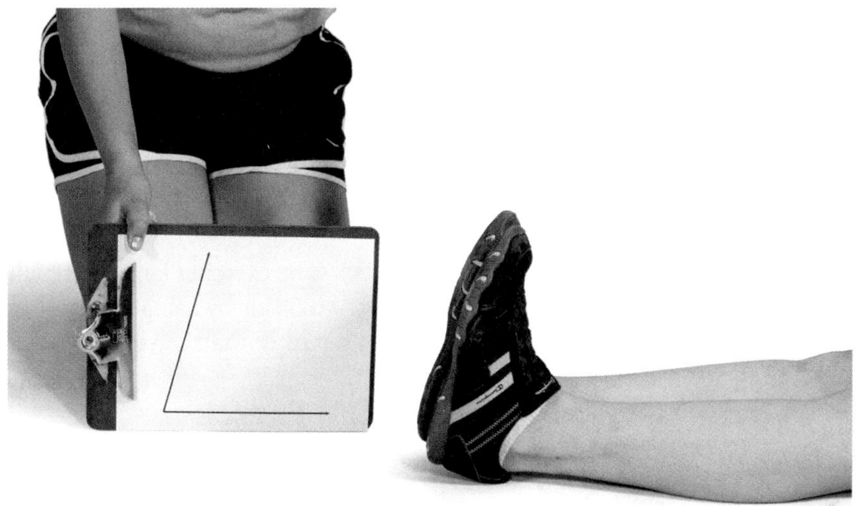

This test evaluates the flexibility of your calf muscles and your range of ankle movement.

Lesson 12.2

Preparing a Flexibility Exercise Plan

Lesson Objectives

After reading this lesson, you should be able to

1. describe several basic flexibility (stretching) exercises,
2. describe other forms of activity that build flexibility,
3. describe and explain how to apply basic guidelines for stretching, and
4. select flexibility exercises and prepare a written flexibility exercise plan.

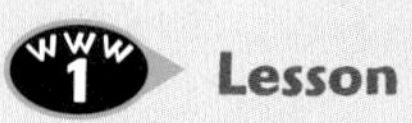

Lesson Vocabulary

tai chi, yoga

Do you know which specific exercises are best for developing flexibility using the different types of stretching? Have you ever considered safety issues when performing flexibility exercise? In the previous lesson, you learned about several types of flexibility exercise. In this lesson, you'll learn some of the most common exercises used to build flexibility; you'll also learn how to plan a personal flexibility exercise program.

Exercise Choices for Building Flexibility

The type of exercises that you choose for building flexibility depends on your personal goals. The following sections describe some of the most popular flexibility exercises.

Basic Flexibility Exercises

The American College of Sports Medicine recommends that you perform exercises to stretch all of your major muscle groups. The 12 exercises described at the end of this lesson allow you to do so by choosing 8 to 10 exercises. As you'll see, all of these exercises can be done using static stretching, and some can also be done using PNF or ballistic stretching. The following guidelines will help you perform these exercises effectively.

- Consider the FIT formula information in table 12.1. Also consider the recommendations for the appropriate number of reps, sets, and time that accompany each of the exercises described in this lesson.
- The exercises labeled as PNF include a contraction of the muscle before stretching. To perform them as static stretches, omit the contraction phase.
- The exercises labeled as ballistic can be made ballistic by using a gentle bobbing movement rather than a static stretch.

ROM Exercises

As noted in this chapter's first lesson, ROM exercises are commonly used in physical therapy and can be performed daily to help retain a healthy ROM. Dynamic and developmental stretching exercises can also be used by people recovering from injury and by beginners. Specific details for these types of exercises are not provided here because the static, PNF, and ballistic exercises are better choices for healthy teens. However, most of the basic exercises listed here can be done using dynamic or developmental stretching.

Yoga, Tai Chi, and Pilates

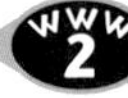

In addition to the static, PNF, and ballistic stretching exercises described in this chapter, there are other popular activities that can be good for building flexibility. ACSM refers to these types of activities as functional fitness training because they help people (especially older people) perform tasks of daily living effectively. They also have health benefits (see Fit Fact). Tai chi and yoga are sometimes called neuromotor exercises because they build components of skill-related fitness such as agility and balance that require the nerves (neuro) and muscles to work together.

Tai chi is an ancient form of exercise that originated in China. It is considered to be a martial art and has many different forms. Tai chi is now practiced worldwide as a form of exercise rather than a martial art, and its basic movements have been shown to increase flexibility and reduce symptoms of arthritis in some people. When practiced regularly, it can help in developing muscle fitness, preventing back pain, and improving posture and balance.

FIT FACT

Research studies show that tai chi provides a variety of benefits, including improved bone health, improved functional fitness, better quality of life, and, among older people, reduced risk of falls.

Yoga was introduced centuries ago in India. Traditional forms include meditation as well as the exercises and breathing techniques that are common in modern forms. Yoga poses, called asanas, are similar to many flexibility exercises and can contribute to improved flexibility and provide other health benefits similar to those for tai chi. Yoga is practiced by millions of young adults as a method of relaxing and training, and many schools now have yoga clubs. However, yoga should be undertaken with care. Physical therapists and other health experts caution against performing certain yoga poses because they are considered to be risky exercises. In addition, beginners are cautioned to progress gradually; it can be more harmful than helpful to try advanced poses without weeks or even months of practice.

Pilates was originally developed as a form of therapy but is now practiced as a method of building muscle fitness and flexibility. It focuses on core muscle fitness but also includes exercises for building flexibility. When practiced properly, it helps prevent back pain, improves posture, and aids functional capacity in daily life.

If you're considering tai chi, yoga, or Pilates, you should seek qualified instruction and follow the guidelines outlined in this chapter for building flexibility.

Guidelines for Flexibility Exercise

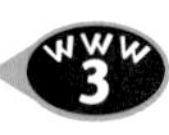

To get the most benefit and enjoyment from your exercise program, perform the exercises correctly and exercise caution to avoid injury. Before you begin stretching, follow these guidelines and cautions to help you safely achieve and maintain flexibility.

- **Before stretching, do a general warm-up.** Warm muscles respond better than cold ones, and ACSM recommends doing a general warm-up of 5 to 10 minutes before performing stretching exercise.
- **Make flexibility exercises part of your workout.** Don't rely on warm-up exercises to build flexibility. Select an appropriate type of exercise and follow the FIT formula for that type.
- **Choose exercises for all major muscle groups.** Twelve different exercises for all muscle groups are described later in this lesson.

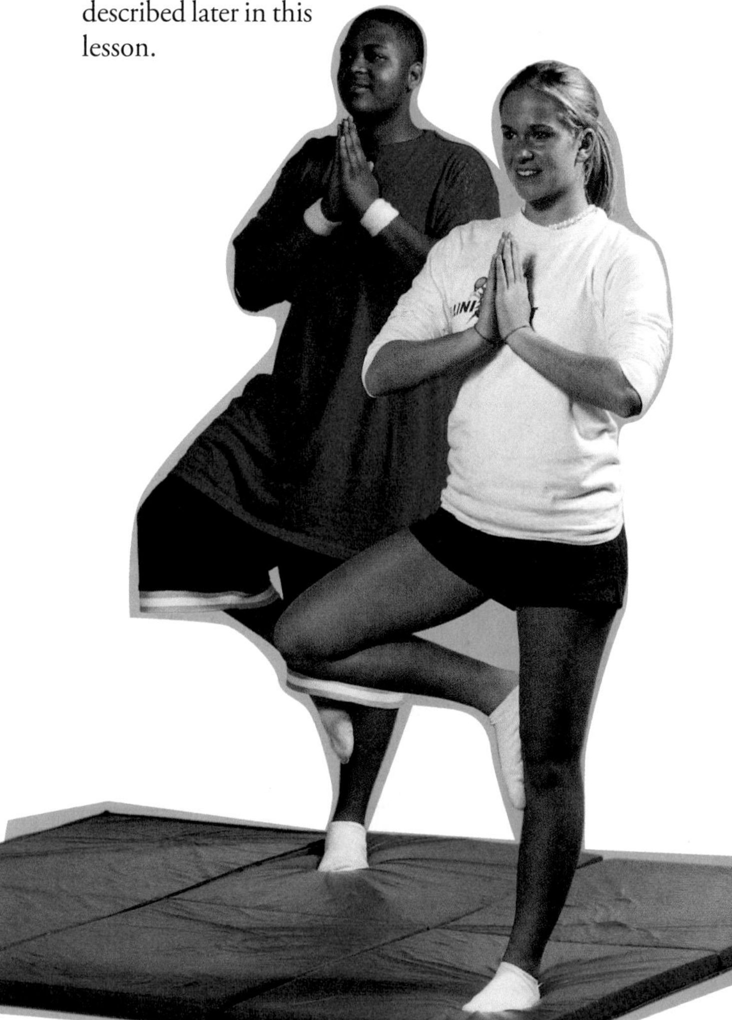

- **When beginning (or for general health), use static stretching or PNF.** Consider ballistic stretching after achieving the good fitness zone. Dynamic and developmental stretching may also be beneficial.
- **Progress gradually.** Regardless of the type of flexibility exercise you choose, progress gradually. Some flexibility exercises may seem easy, but, as with muscular endurance exercise, it does not take much to make your muscles sore. Gradually increase the time and number of repetitions and sets.
- **Avoid risky exercises.** Exercises that hyperflex or hyperextend a joint should be avoided as should exercises that cause joint twisting and compression.
- **Do not stretch joints that are hypermobile, unstable, swollen, or infected.** People with these conditions or symptoms are at risk of injury from overstretching.
- **Do not stretch to the point of feeling pain.** The old saying "no pain, no gain" is wrong. Stretch only until your muscle feels tight and a little uncomfortable.
- **Avoid stretching muscles that are already overstretched from poor posture.** The abdominal muscles, for example, typically do not need to be stretched.
- **Avoid stretches that last 30 seconds or more before performing strength and power activities.** Research suggests that stretches lasting longer than 30 seconds may have a negative effect on performances of strength and power in sport and other activities. As a result, some experts recommend doing dynamic movement exercises rather than stretching before strength and power performances.

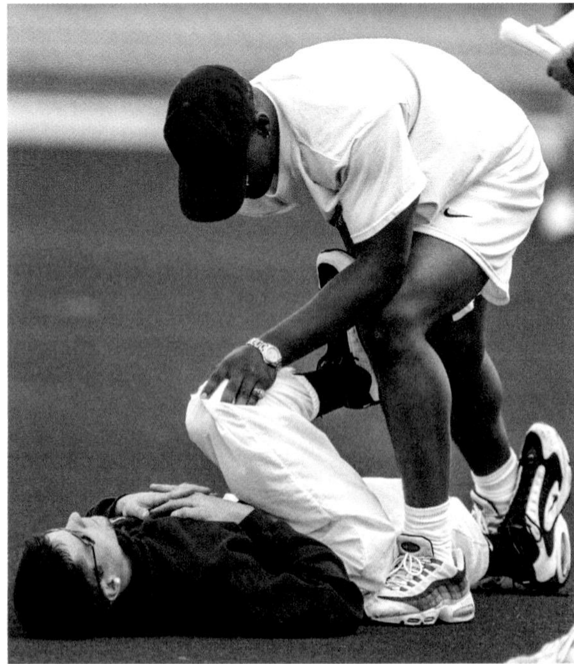

Stretching works best after a 5- to 10-minute general warm-up.

> "I never struggled with injury problems because of my preparation—in particular my stretching."
>
> —Edwin Moses, Olympic gold medalist

FIT FACT

Once you've reached an acceptable level of muscle flexibility, you must continue to move all of your joints and muscles through this new and improved range of motion on a regular basis. If you don't, your muscles will begin to shorten again, and you'll lose that flexibility. All types of exercise described in this lesson help maintain flexibility.

Planning a Flexibility Exercise Program

Elijah is a 16-year-old who used the five steps of program planning to prepare a flexibility exercise program. His program is described here.

Step 1: Determine Your Personal Needs

To get started, Elijah prepared a table summarizing his flexibility activity (or lack thereof) over the past two weeks and his flexibility scores. (He wrote his plan during the summer when he was not in school.) As you can see in figure 12.4, he did no flexibility exercise during that two-week period. He also had

Day	Flexibility exercises	Amount
Mon.	None	None
Tues.	None	None
Wed.	None	None
Thurs.	None	None
Fri.	None	None
Sat.	None	None
Sun.	None	None
Fitness self-assessments	**Score**	**Rating**
Arm lift	8 in. (20 cm)	Need improvement
Zipper		
Right	Fingers touch	Met standard
Left	Fingers do not touch	Need improvement
Trunk rotation		
Right	Reached target	Met standard
Left	Did not reach target	Need improvement
Wrap-around		
Right	Touched mouth	Met standard
Left	Touched mouth	Met standard
Knee-to-chest		
Right	Calf lifted >1 in. (2.5 cm)	Need improvement
Left	Calf lifted >1 in. (2.5 cm)	Need improvement
Ankle flex		
Right	75 degrees	Met standard
Left	80 degrees	Need improvement
Total score	6 items passed	Marginal fitness
Back-saver sit-and-reach	5 in. (13 cm)	Low fitness

FIGURE 12.4 Elijah's flexibility exercise (physical activity) and fitness profiles.

not done any recent flexibility tests, but he did have scores from tests he had done in school during the previous semester.

Elijah obviously did not meet the ACSM recommendation of performing flexibility exercise for the major muscle groups on at least two days a week. Even so, he had passed several of his recent flexibility tests (and he had been doing some flexibility exercises at that time).

Step 2: Consider Your Program Options

Elijah listed seven types of flexibility exercise that he wanted to consider. He reviewed many types of exercises before preparing a list of exercises that he thought would be good for him and that he would be most likely to perform.

- Static stretching exercises
- PNF exercises
- Ballistic stretching exercises
- Yoga
- Tai chi
- Pilates
- Dynamic movement exercises (for warm-up)

Step 3: Set Goals

For his flexibility exercise plan (see figure 12.5), Elijah chose a time period of two weeks. This was too short a time for setting long-term goals, so he developed only short-term physical activity goals for this plan. Later, he'll develop long-term goals, including some flexibility improvement goals, when he prepares a longer plan. For now, he just wanted

Day	Exercise type	✔	Time, sets, reps
Mon.	**Static Stretch** Back-saver sit-and-reach Knee-to-chest Side stretch Sitting stretch Zipper Hip stretch Chest stretch Calf stretch		3:00 p.m. after daily jog One set of two repetitions for each exercise. Hold each exercise 15 seconds.
Tues.	**Dynamic Movement Exercise Warm-Up** High-knee march Standing flutter Quarter-turn cha-cha Shutter Grapevine Frankenstein Knee-high skip Jump-and-tuck Slow jog, fast sprint		1:00 p.m. before soccer Approximately 10 minutes. Perform each exercise five times, then continue on to the next exercise. Exercises followed by a slow jog for 30 seconds and a fast sprint for 10 seconds repeated three times.
Wed.	**Static Stretch** Back-saver sit-and-reach Knee-to-chest Side stretch Sitting stretch Zipper Hip stretch Chest stretch Calf stretch		3:00 p.m. after daily jog One set of two repetitions for each exercise. Hold each exercise 15 seconds.
Thurs.	**Dynamic Movement Exercise Warm-Up** High-knee march Standing flutter Quarter-turn cha-cha Shutter Grapevine Frankenstein Knee-high skip Jump-and-tuck Slow jog, fast sprint		1:00 p.m. before soccer Approximately 10 minutes. Perform each exercise five times, then continue on to the next exercise. Exercises followed by a slow jog for 30 seconds and a fast sprint for 10 seconds repeated three times.
Fri.	**Static Stretch** Back-saver sit-and-reach Knee-to-chest Side stretch Sitting stretch Zipper Hip stretch Chest stretch Calf stretch		3:00 p.m. after daily jog One set of two repetitions for each exercise. Hold each exercise 15 seconds.
Sat.	Yoga class		10:00–10:30 a.m. with sister
Sun.	None		None

FIGURE 12.5 Elijah's written flexibility exercise plan.

to get started by trying some new exercises. Besides, it was summer, and he didn't have access to school facilities, nor was he a member of a fitness club. So he chose SMART goals for his specific situation and wrote them down.

1. Perform one set of eight static stretching exercises on three days a week, including back-saver sit-and-reach, knee-to-chest, side stretch, sitting stretch, zipper, hip stretch, chest stretch, and calf stretch.
2. Perform a dynamic movement exercise warm-up for 10 minutes including nine basic exercises before playing sports.
3. Perform yoga for 30 minutes on one day a week.

Step 4: Structure Your Program and Write It Down

Elijah's next step was to write down his two-week flexibility exercise plan (see figure 12.5). He chose static stretching that he could do at home three days a week. Since he played soccer two days a week, he also decided to do a dynamic movement exercise warm-up prior to his matches. He didn't expect the warm-up to be his main source of flexibility development, but he thought it would supplement his other flexibility exercise. He also agreed to go to yoga class with his sister Nicole, who was allowed to bring a guest for two free sessions.

Step 5: Keep a Log and Evaluate Your Program

Over the next two weeks, Elijah will self-monitor his activities and place a checkmark beside each activity he actually performs. At the end of the two weeks, Elijah will evaluate his activity to see whether he met his goals. He can then use the evaluation to help him write a future activity plan.

Lesson Review

1. Describe several basic flexibility (stretching) exercises.
2. What are some other forms of activity that build flexibility?
3. What are the basic guidelines for stretching?
4. What flexibility exercises should you include in your written flexibility exercise plan? Why?

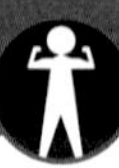

BACK-SAVER SIT-AND-REACH (PNF OR STATIC)

1. Assume the back-saver sit-and-reach position with your right knee bent and your left leg straight.
2. Bend your left knee slightly and push your heel into the floor as you contract your hamstrings hard for 3 seconds. Relax.

   Note: For static stretch, omit step 2.
3. Immediately grasp your ankle with both hands and gently pull your chest toward your knee. Hold the position for 15 seconds.
4. Repeat the exercise on the other leg.

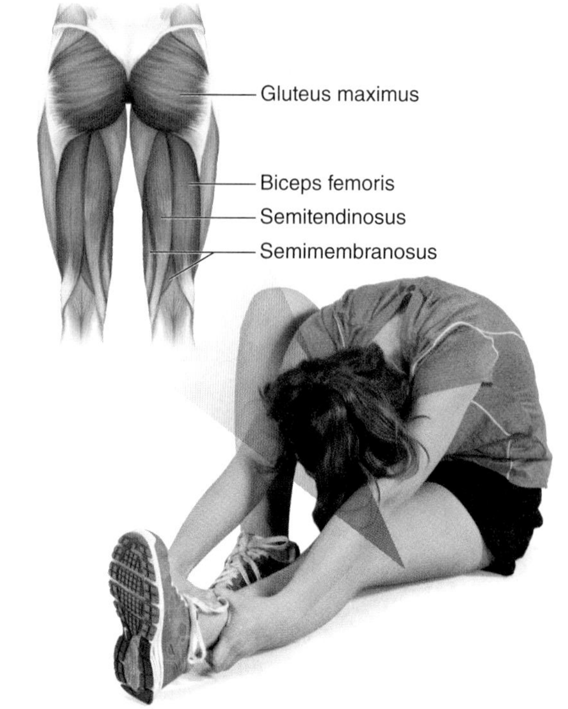

This exercise stretches your hamstrings and lower back muscles.

KNEE-TO-CHEST

1. Lie on your back and extend your right leg. Place your hands on the back of your left thigh and pull toward you to draw the knee closer to the chest. Do not place your hands on top of the knee.
2. Keep your right leg straight and on the floor if possible. Keep your lower back flat on the floor.
3. Hold the position for 15 seconds.
4. Repeat with the opposite leg.

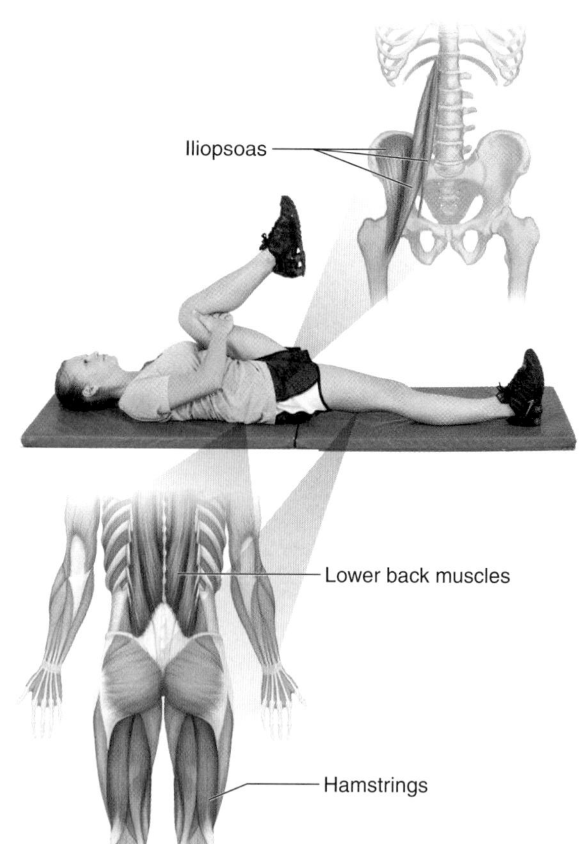

This exercise stretches your hamstrings, your lower back, and the hip flexor muscles.

BACK AND HIP STRETCH (PNF OR STATIC)

1. Lie on your back with your knees bent and your arms at your sides.
2. Lift your hips until there is no bend at the hip joint. Squeeze the buttocks muscles hard for 3 seconds. Relax by lowering your hips to the floor.
   Note: For a static stretch, omit step 2.
3. Immediately place your hands under your knees and gently pull your knees to your chest. Hold the position for 15 seconds or more.

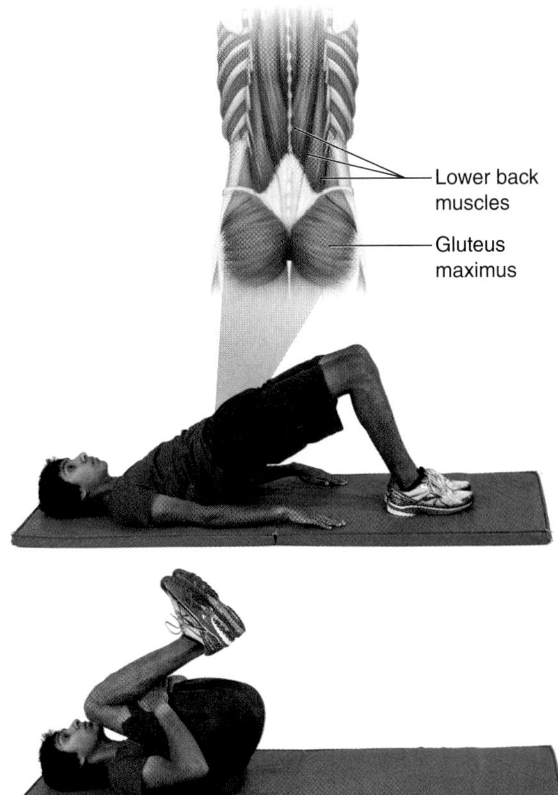

This exercise stretches your lower back and gluteal muscles.

SIDE STRETCH (STATIC OR BALLISTIC)

1. Stand with your feet slightly wider than shoulder-width apart.
2. Lean to your left.
3. Reach down to your left foot with your left hand. Reach over your head with your right arm. Hold for a count of 10 to 30 seconds.
   Caution: Do not twist or lean your body forward.
4. Repeat the exercise on your right side.
   Note: For a ballistic stretch, do a gentle bouncing stretch.

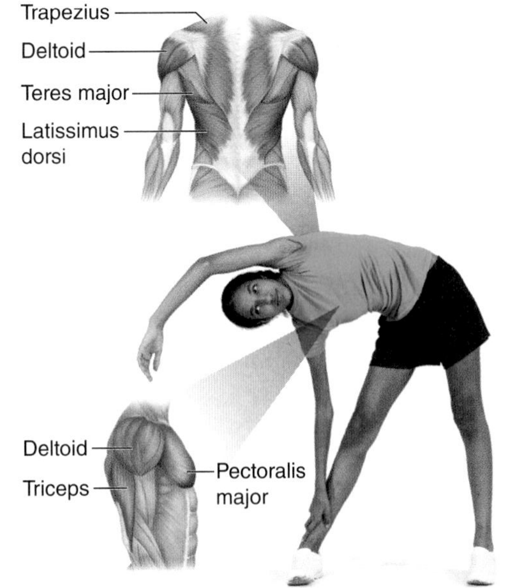

This exercise stretches the muscles of your arms and shoulders and the sides of your body.

TRUNK AND HIP STRETCH (STATIC)

1. Lie on your back with your knees bent and your arms extended at shoulder level.
2. Cross your left leg over your right leg.
3. Keep your shoulders and arms on the floor as you rotate your lower body to the left and touch your right knee to the floor. Stretch and hold the position for 10 to 30 seconds.
4. At the end of the stretch, reverse the position of your legs (cross your right leg over your left), then rotate to the right and hold the position.

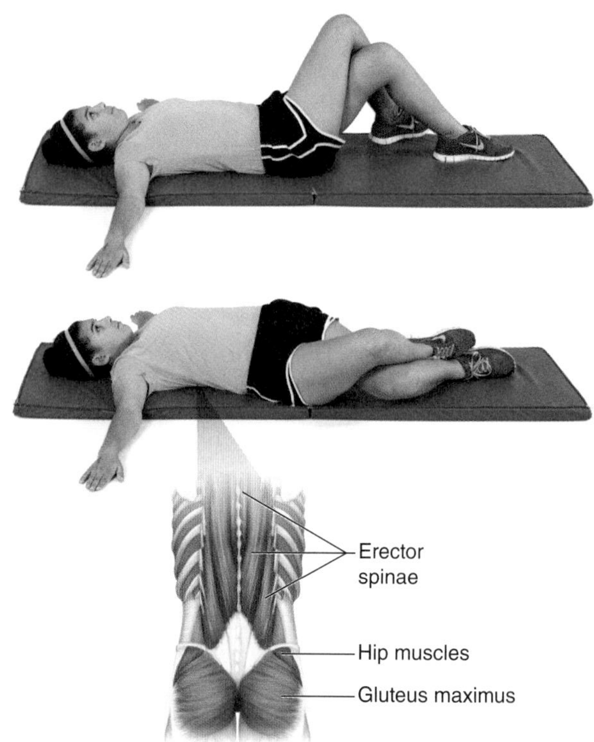

This exercise stretches the muscles of your hips and lower back.

SITTING STRETCH (PNF OR STATIC)

1. Sit with the soles of your feet together and your elbows or hands resting on your knees.
2. Contract the muscles on the inside of your thighs, pulling up as you resist with your arms pushing down. Hold the position for 3 seconds. Relax your legs.
   Note: For a static stretch, omit step 2.
3. Immediately lean your trunk forward and push down on your knees with your arms to stretch your thighs. Hold the position for 10 to 30 seconds.

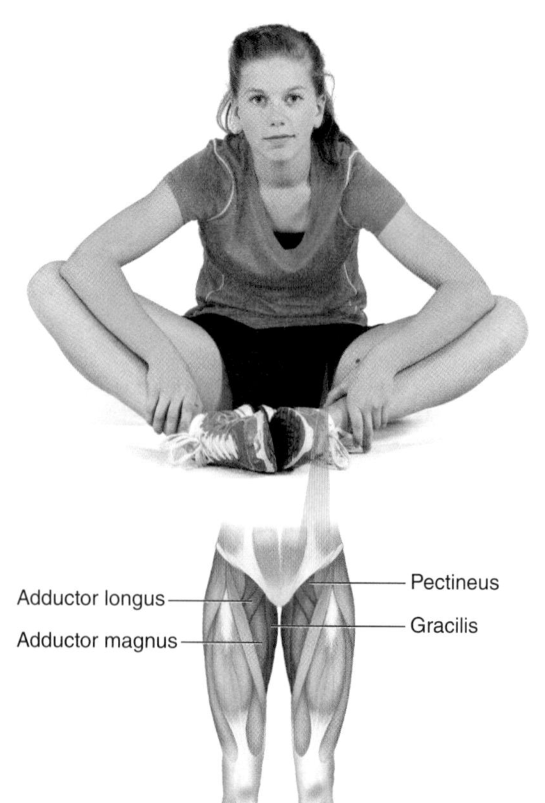

This exercise stretches the muscles of the inside of your thighs.

ZIPPER (PNF OR STATIC)

1. Stand or sit. Lift your right arm over your right shoulder and reach down your spine.
2. With your left hand, press down on your right elbow. Resist the pressure by trying to raise that elbow, contracting the opposing muscles. Hold the position for 3 seconds. Relax.

   Note: For a static stretch, omit step 2.
3. Immediately stretch by reaching down your spine with your right arm as your left arm assists by pressing on your elbow. Hold the position for 10 to 30 seconds.
4. Repeat the exercise with your other arm.

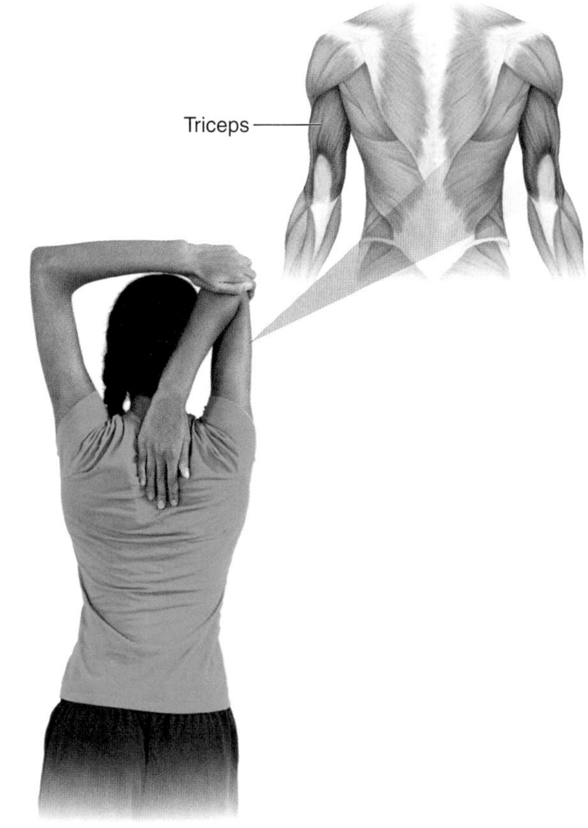

This exercise stretches your triceps and latissimus muscles.

ARM PRETZEL (STATIC OR BALLISTIC)

1. Stand or sit. Bend your elbows and hold both hands as if shaking hands. Cross your right hand over your left so that the backs of the two hands are facing each other about two inches apart. Turn your right palm upward and point your thumb down over the left hand.
2. Grasp your right thumb with your left hand and pull down gently. Stretch and hold the position for 10 to 30 seconds.
3. Reverse arm positions and stretch your left shoulder.

   Note: For a ballistic stretch, do a gentle bouncing stretch.

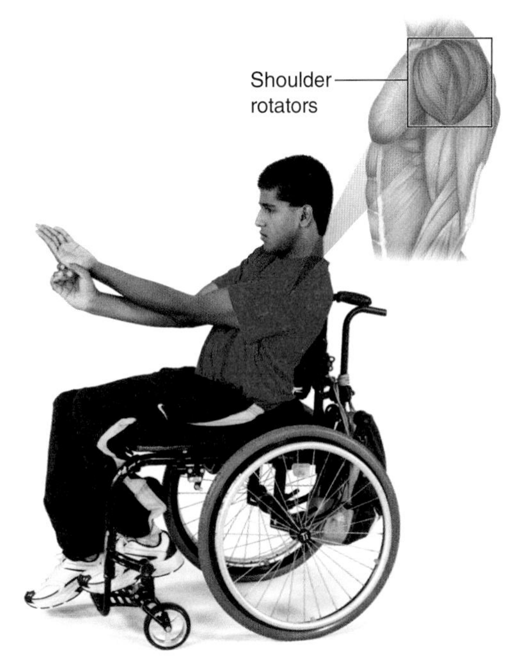

This exercise stretches your shoulder rotator muscles.

HIP STRETCH (STATIC OR BALLISTIC)

1. Take a long step forward on your right foot and kneel on your left knee. Your right knee should be directly over your ankle and bent at a right angle.
2. You should feel a stretch across the front of your left hip joint and in the front of your thigh muscles.
3. Place your hands on your right knee for balance. Stretch by shifting your weight forward as you tilt your pelvis and trunk backward slightly. Keep your back knee in the same spot to stretch your hip and thigh muscles. Hold the position for 10 to 30 seconds.
4. Repeat the exercise with your other leg.
   Note: For a ballistic stretch, do a gentle bouncing motion forward as you tilt your pelvis back.

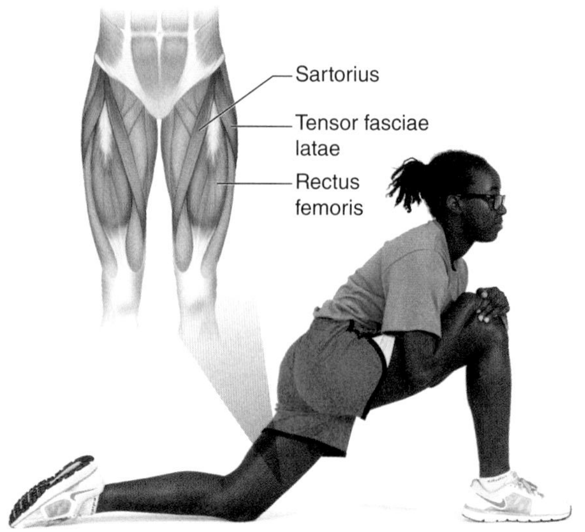

This exercise stretches the quadriceps muscles on the front of your thighs and the muscles on the front of your hips.

ARM STRETCH (STATIC)

1. Sit or stand and cross your right arm over your left (just above your head) with your palms facing. Lace your fingers together.
2. Straighten your elbows to raise your arms overhead as high as possible (your upper arms should touch your ears). Hold the position 10 to 30 seconds.

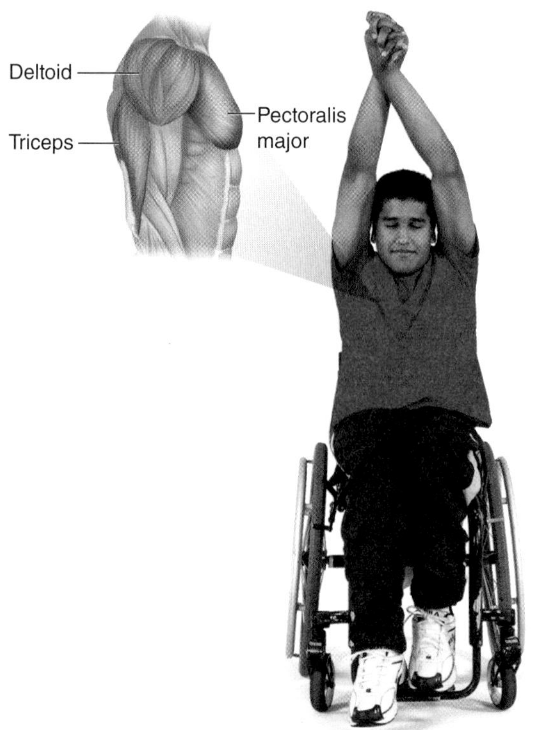

This exercise stretches the muscles of your shoulders, arms, and chest.

CHEST STRETCH (PNF, STATIC, OR BALLISTIC)

1. Stand in a forward stride position in a doorway. Raise your arms slightly above shoulder-height. Place your hands on either side of the doorway.
2. Lean your body into the doorway. Resist by contracting your arm and chest muscles. Hold the position for 3 seconds. Relax.
3. Immediately lean further forward, letting your body weight stretch your muscles. Hold the position for 10 to 30 seconds.
4. For a ballistic stretch, gently bounce your body forward.

   Note: For a static stretch, omit steps 2 and 4.

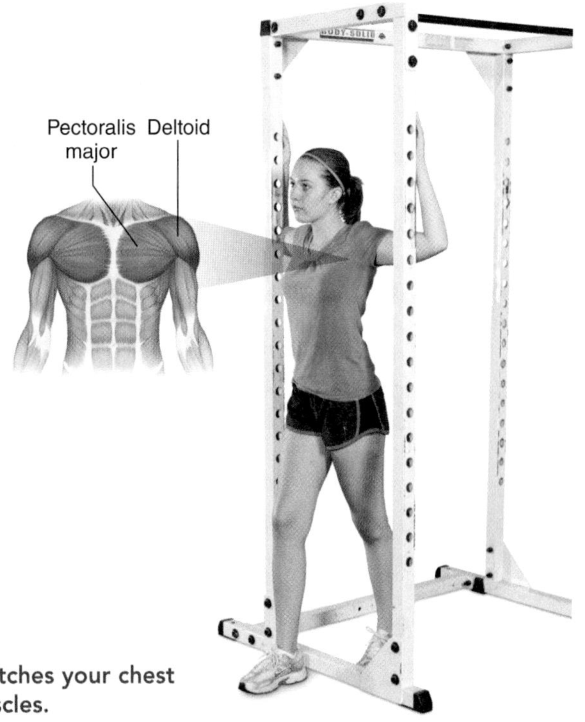

This exercise stretches your chest and shoulder muscles.

CALF STRETCH (STATIC OR BALLISTIC)

1. Step forward with your right leg in a lunge position. Keep both feet pointed straight ahead and your front knee directly over your front foot. Place your hands on your right leg for balance.
2. Keep your left leg straight and the heel on the floor. Adjust the length of your lunge until you feel a good stretch in your left calf and Achilles tendon. Hold the position for 10 to 30 seconds.
3. Repeat the exercise with your other leg.

   Note: For a ballistic stretch, gently bounce your heel toward the floor.

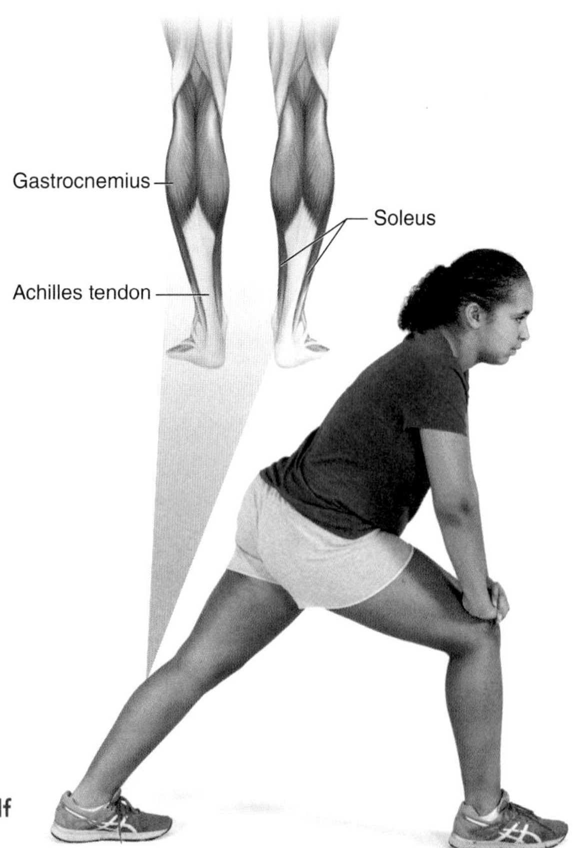

This exercise stretches your calf muscles and Achilles tendons.

TAKING CHARGE: Overcoming Barriers

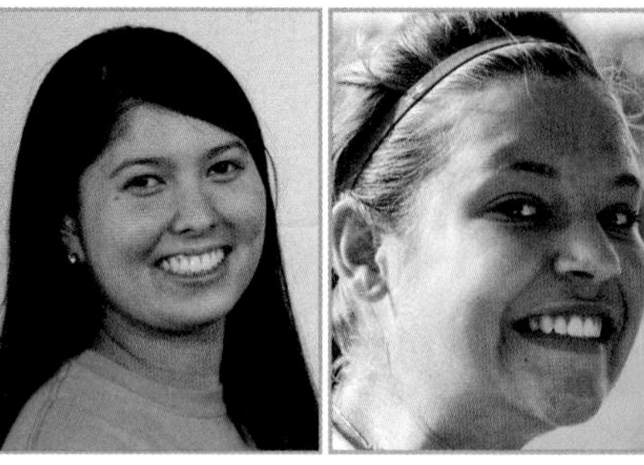

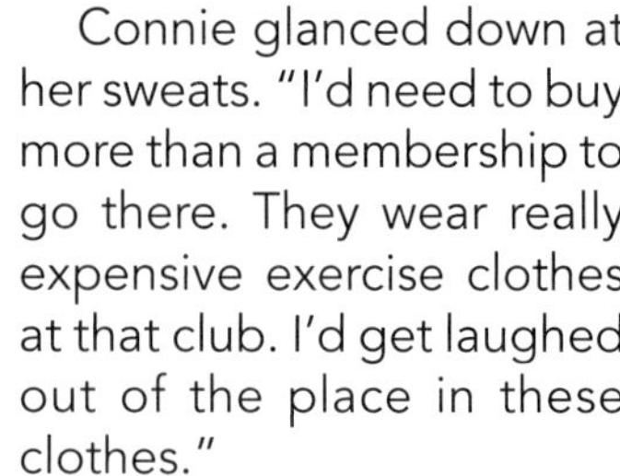

When some people face a problem beyond their control, they use it as an excuse for not being physically active. Someone might say, "I'm too short to be a basketball player, so I'm not going to try out for any sports." To be physically active, focus not on what you can't change but on what you *can* do.

Connie stood at the window. "It's pouring out there! How can we go hiking?"

Bridgette sighed. "I guess we're stuck spending the afternoon here."

Yesterday it was too hot to go hiking; now it was too rainy. It seemed as if they were never going to have good weather. But the weather was not the only problem. The last time they tried hiking at the state park, it was sunny, but the paths were too crowded.

"I bet Alanzo is at the athletic club right now," Bridgette said. "He can exercise no matter what the weather is. I wish we could afford to go there!"

Connie glanced down at her sweats. "I'd need to buy more than a membership to go there. They wear really expensive exercise clothes at that club. I'd get laughed out of the place in these clothes."

Bridgette smiled. "You don't look so bad—and the rain's starting to let up now. What if we put on older clothes, take rain gear, and hike around the park for a while?"

"You're right! So what if we get a little damp?"

For Discussion

What reasons do Connie and Bridgette give for not being active? Which of these problems can they control? They eventually decide not to let the weather stop them; what other strategies could they use to cope with the problems they've identified? Consider the guidelines in the Self-Management feature when answering the discussion questions.

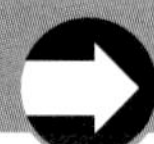

SELF-MANAGEMENT: Skills for Overcoming Barriers

People face many barriers to becoming and staying active. Some barriers involve the environment (such as areas unsafe for exercise, lack of nearby exercise facilities, bad weather, expense), some involve personal physical characteristics (lack of physical size or skill), and some are psychological (low self-confidence, perceived lack of time). People who are active throughout life overcome such barriers, and programs have been developed to help people overcome barriers. Use the following strategies to overcome the barriers you face.

- **Find a way to exercise at home or at school.** If parks, fitness clubs, and other places for exercise are too expensive, too far away, or unsafe, find another way to exercise. Buy some equipment that you can use at home. If possible, use school facilities to exercise before or after school. Start a fitness club at school and ask school officials to help you find facilities and equipment.
- **Develop alternate plans.** Make multiple plans for activity. That way, for example, if you plan to play tennis and it rains, you can switch to your alternate plan, which might be an indoor activity. If something interferes with your planned exercise time, find another time.
- **Get active in community or school affairs.** Many communities have developed community centers; trails for biking, walking, and jogging; and other recreational facilities, such as tennis courts, basketball courts, and sport fields. If these options are not available in your community, write to your city or county officials or contact school officials and see what you can help create.
- **Use self-management skills to develop realistic plans that you will stick with.** Practice skills such as goal setting, program planning, self-monitoring, and time management.
- **Develop a new way of thinking.** Accept yourself as you are. If negative self-talk is an issue, use the strategies presented in this book to adjust your self-perceptions and boost your self-confidence.

TAKING ACTION: Your Flexibility Exercise Plan

Prepare a two-week muscle fitness flexibility exercise plan. As directed by your teacher, prepare tables similar to those used by Elijah and use the five steps of program planning. Try out your program and see if you can meet your goals. The goal is to perform flexibility exercises three days a week. Carry out it over a two-week period. Your teacher may give you time in class to do some of the activities in your plan. Consider the following suggestions for **taking action**.

- Before performing stretching exercises, do a general warm-up.
- Consider the guidelines for flexibility exercise presented in lesson 2 of this chapter.
- If you're already participating in organized sport or physical activity, consider doing your flexibility exercise during the cool-down portion of your workout.

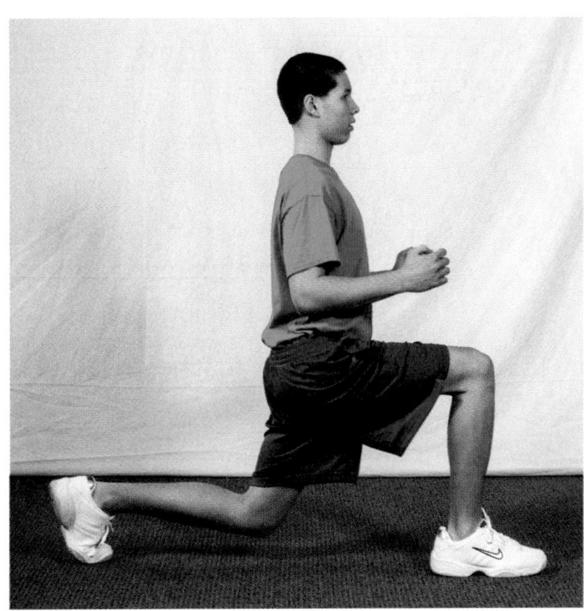

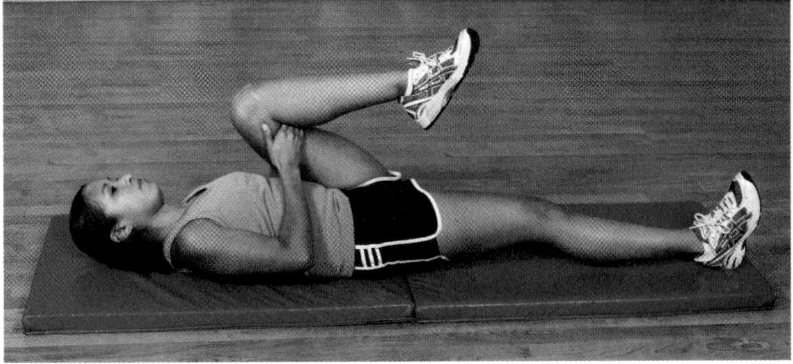

Take action by performing your flexibility exercise plan.

CHAPTER REVIEW

Reviewing Concepts and Vocabulary

As directed by your teacher, answer items 1 through 5 by correctly completing each sentence with a word or phrase.

1. The amount of movement you can make in a joint is called your ______________.
2. Exercises including jumping, skipping, and calisthenics (such as those used in a warm-up) are called ______________ exercises.
3. Being able to move beyond a typical healthy range of motion is called ______________.
4. ______________ is an ancient form of exercise that originated in China.
5. Gentle bouncing motions are part of ______________.

For items 6 through 10, as directed by your teacher, match each term in column 1 with the appropriate phrase in column 2.

6. zipper	a. stretch created by gravity or an outside force
7. passive stretch	b. form of exercise from India
8. active stretch	c. stretch created by an antagonist muscle
9. PNF	d. stretch after muscle contraction
10. yoga	e. arm stretching exercise

For items 11 through 15, as directed by your teacher, respond to each statement or question.

11. What are some benefits of good flexibility?
12. What are some factors that influence flexibility other than stretching?
13. What are some good tests of flexibility described in this chapter?
14. What are some good basic flexibility (static stretching) exercises for the major muscle groups?
15. What are some guidelines for overcoming barriers?

Thinking Critically

Write a paragraph to answer the following question.

Sean's father went to a physical therapist to get treatment after a hip injury. The therapist recommended static stretching with a passive assist. Sean's dad asked him to help with the exercises. What safety concerns should Sean have in helping his father?

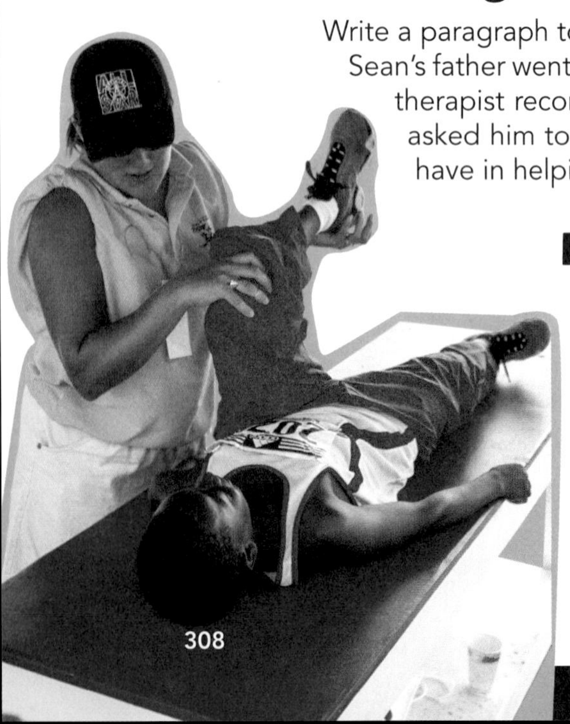

Project

Young people typically have better flexibility than older people. For this reason, parents and grandparents are likely to be less flexible than their children or grandchildren. Interview a parent or grandparent. Prepare a list of five questions related to current flexibility, past flexibility (at an earlier age), steps taken to maintain flexibility, and future plans for flexibility exercise. Prepare a report presenting your findings.

UNIT V

Healthy Choices

Healthy People 2020 Goals

- Reduce teen overweight and obesity.
- Prevent inappropriate weight gain among teens.
- Increase body mass index (BMI) measurement by physicians.
- Reduce disordered eating among adolescents.
- Reduce the percentage of teens who do no leisure-time physical activity.
- Increase the percentage of adults who meet guidelines for aerobic and muscle fitness activity.
- Increase teen participation in daily physical education.
- Increase participation in adolescent extracurricular and out-of-school activities.
- Increase number of schools with activity spaces that can be used during nonschool hours.
- Increase the number of trips made by walking and biking.
- Reduce the percentage of teens who get too much screen time.
- Improve health literacy.
- Increase web access and wise use of health information available on the web.
- Increase the number of high-quality websites presenting health-related information.
- Increase the percentage of teens who have had a wellness checkup in the past 12 months.
- Increase the percentage of people who have good social support.

Self-Assessment Features in This Unit

- Body Measurements
- Your Personal Fitness Test Battery
- Assessing Your Posture

Taking Charge Features in This Unit

- Improving Physical Self-Perception
- Changing Attitudes
- Learning to Think Critically

Self-Management Features in This Unit

- Skills for Self-Perception
- Skills for Building Positive Attitudes
- Skills for Thinking Critically

Taking Action Features in This Unit

- Elastic Band Workout
- Your Physical Activity Plan
- My Health and Fitness Club

13

Body Composition

In This Chapter

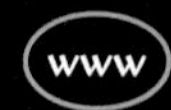

Student Web Resources

www.HOPEtextbook.org/student

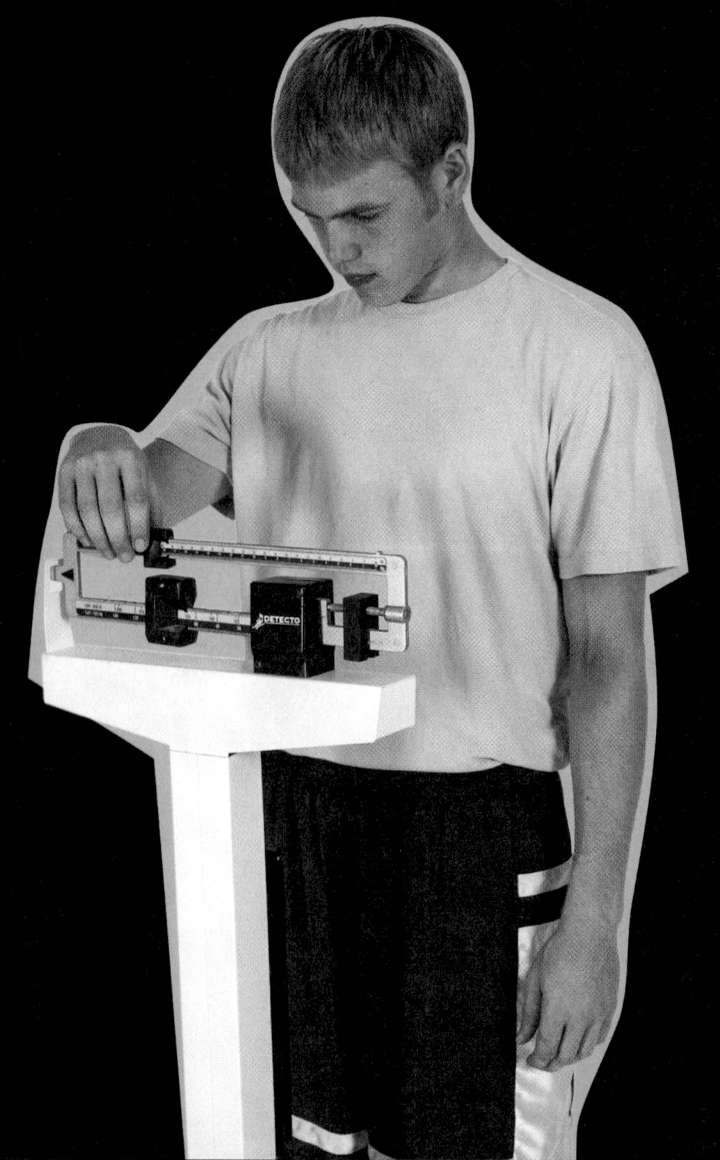

Lesson 13.1

Body Composition Facts

Lesson Objectives

After reading this lesson, you should be able to

1. define *body composition*, *overweight*, and *obesity*;
2. describe some factors that influence body composition;
3. define *anorexia nervosa*, *bulimia*, and *anorexia athletica*;
4. explain how body composition and body fat level are related to good health; and
5. describe several laboratory and nonlaboratory tests for measuring body composition.

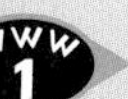

Lesson Vocabulary

anorexia athletica, anorexia nervosa, basal metabolism, body composition, body fat level, bulimia, essential body fat, lean body tissue, metabolic syndrome, obesity, overweight, skinfold, underweight

Body composition is a part of health-related physical fitness. It refers to all the tissues that make up your body. In this lesson, you'll learn about the types of tissue that make up your body and about key terms related to body composition. You'll also learn how to assess your current body composition and determine whether it is optimal for good health.

Body Composition Definitions

Your body is made up of two major types of tissue. In a healthy person, the great majority of the body consists of **lean body tissue**, including muscle, bone, skin, and body organs such as the heart, liver, kidneys, and lungs. All of the types of physical activity included in the Physical Activity Pyramid build lean body tissue, but muscle fitness exercises are especially good because they both build muscle and enhance bone development.

The other major type of body tissue is fat. Your **body fat level** refers to the percentage of your body that is fat tissue. A fit person has the right amount of body fat—neither too much nor too little.

About half of your body fat is located deep within your body. The remaining fat is located between your skin and your muscles. People who do regular physical activity typically have a larger percentage of lean body weight (especially from muscle and bone) and less body fat than people who do not do such activity. It's good if fat accounts for a relatively low percentage of your total body weight. However, for good health, you do need some body fat. Determining your body fatness requires special equipment and expertise. Later, you'll learn how to measure the fat between your skin and muscles to estimate your total body fatness.

The terms **underweight** and **overweight** are commonly used to describe a body weight that is outside the healthy weight range—either below the range or above it. These terms have limitations because weight, or the combination of weight and height, does not always accurately reflect the amount of fat and lean tissue in the body. You'll learn more about underweight and overweight later in this chapter. The term **obesity** refers to the condition of being especially overweight or high in body fat.

FIT FACT

More than two-thirds of all American adults are considered overweight or obese. Fewer children and teens are considered overweight or obese, and the percentage varies by age, sex, and ethnic group. Obesity is high among Hispanic, African American, and Native American youth. For all ethnic groups combined, about 18 percent of youth and teens are considered obese. This is more than three times the rate of 30 years ago.

Factors Influencing Body Fatness

Many factors influence a person's level of body fat. Some are described in the following sections.

Heredity

You inherit your body type from your parents. Some people are born with a tendency to be lean, or muscular, or heavy. Inherited tendencies make it easier for some people and harder for others to keep their body fat level in the good fitness zone. You can't control your heredity, but you can be aware of tendencies in your family.

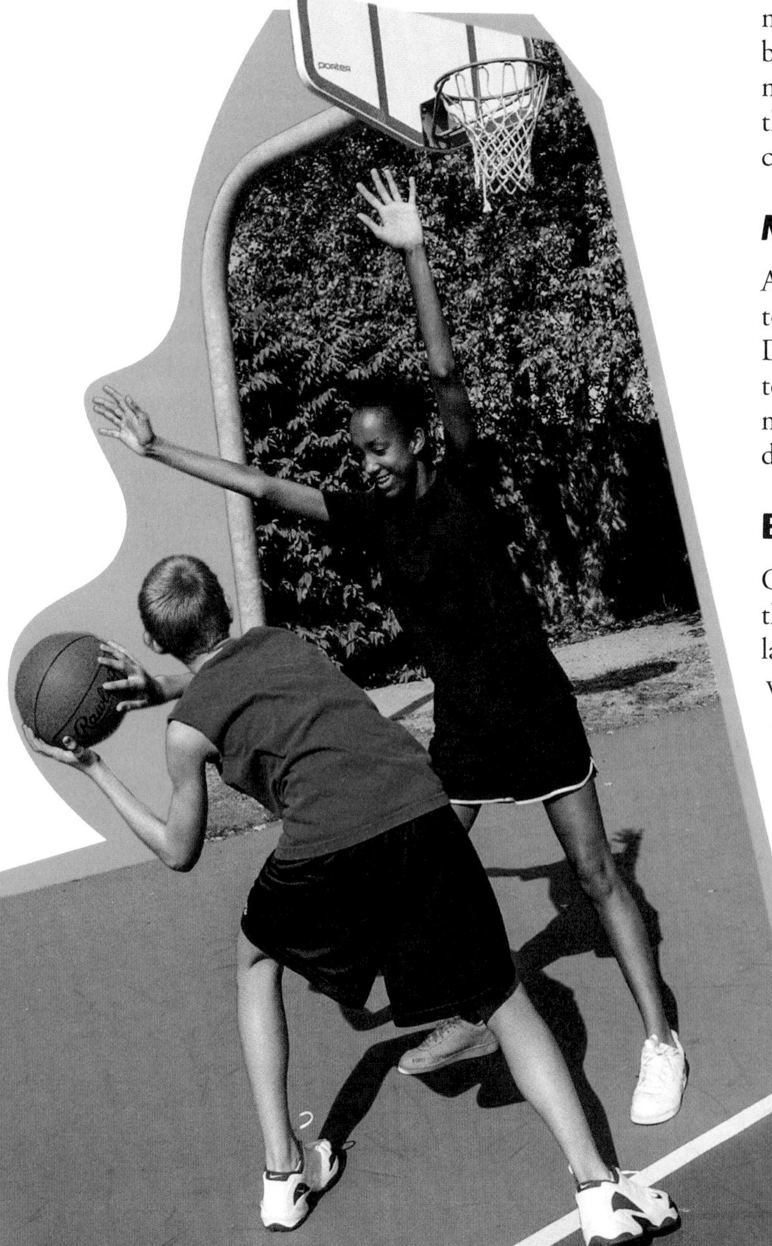

Metabolism

Your **basal metabolism** is the amount of energy (calories) your body uses just to keep you living. Your basal metabolism does not include the calories you burn while working, enjoying recreation, studying, or even sitting and watching television. Some people have a higher basal metabolism than others. This means that their bodies, at complete rest, burn more calories than the bodies of people with a lower metabolism. People with more muscle mass have a higher metabolism than people with less muscle mass. People with a higher metabolism can consume more calories than others can without increasing their level of body fat.

Your metabolism is affected by your heredity, age, and maturation. Most young people have a high metabolism because their bodies are growing and building muscle. As you grow older and lose muscle mass, your metabolism typically slows, which means that most people need to reduce the number of calories in their diet in order to avoid gaining fat.

Maturation

As you grow older and your hormone levels begin to change, your level of body fat also changes. During the teen years, female hormones cause girls to develop more body fat than boys. Because of male hormones, teenage boys have greater muscle development than girls.

Body Fat Levels Early in Life

Children who are too fat develop extra fat cells that make it more difficult to control their fat level later in life. Therefore, keeping your body fat level within the good fitness zone during your childhood and teen years will help you keep it in check throughout life.

Diet

The amount of energy contained in foods is measured in calories. Teens typically need more calories than adults. A typical teen male needs to consume about 2,500 to 3,000 calories a day to maintain an ideal level of body fat. A typical teenage female needs about 2,000 to 2,500 calories a day. Most males need more calories than most females because they are larger and have more muscle mass.

Physical Activity

Your body burns calories for energy. Therefore, the more vigorous activity you do (the more energy your body uses), the more calories you need. An inactive person uses less energy each day than an active person and thus needs to consume fewer calories. As a result, teens who participate in sports need to consume more calories than less active teens.

Body Fatness, Health, and Wellness

Having too much fat can be unhealthy. Scientists report that people who are high in body fat have a higher risk of heart disease, high blood pressure, diabetes, cancer, and other diseases. Until recently, type 2 diabetes was considered to be an adult disease, but it has become more common among youth primarily because of increases in body fat levels among youth. High levels of body fat are also associated with a condition called **metabolic syndrome**. This syndrome occurs when a person has a high level of body fat, large waist girth, and other health risks, such as high blood pressure, high blood fat, and high blood sugar.

In addition, health costs for obese people total thousands of dollars a year more than for people with healthy levels of body fat, and being high in body fat reduces a person's chances of successful surgery. A person with too much body fat also tires more quickly and easily than a lean person and therefore might be less efficient in both work and recreation. Many experts believe that the reason so many adults have too much body fat is that they try to achieve an unrealistic weight or fat level. For example, many people try to be as lean as a movie star or an athlete shown in a commercial. When they cannot attain or maintain such an exceptionally low level of body fat, they give up and gain body fat. Instead, experts recommend setting less extreme goals that are achievable, which helps people maintain a healthy level of body fat throughout life.

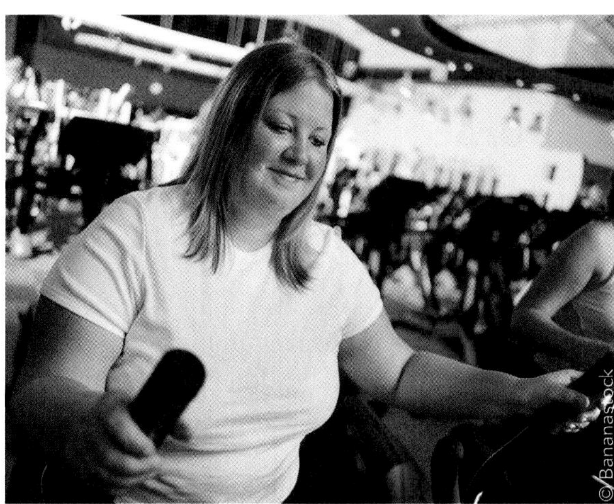

Regular exercise expends calories.

> "We have to make sure that our kids still feel good about themselves no matter what their weight, no matter how they feel. We need to make sure that our kids know that we love them no matter who they are, what they look like."
>
> —Michelle Obama, First Lady of the United States

Too Little Body Fat

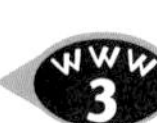

Having too little body fat is also a health risk. Eating disorders such as **anorexia nervosa**, **anorexia athletica**, and **bulimia** have many negative health consequences and can even be fatal. It is extremely important to identify the symptoms of an eating disorder as early as possible. An excessive desire to lose fat or maintain a very low fat level can lead to serious health problems.

The minimum amount of body fat required for healthy body functioning is called **essential body fat**. Having too little body fat can cause abnormal functioning of various organs. In fact, exceptionally low body fat can result in serious health problems, particularly among teenagers. Females with especially low body fat experience health problems related to their reproductive system and risk losing bone density. The following list summarizes several reasons your body needs some fat.

The Importance of Body Fat

- Fat is an insulator; it helps your body adapt to heat and cold.

- Fat acts as a shock absorber; it can help protect your organs and bones from injury.
- Fat helps your body use vitamins effectively.
- Fat is stored energy that is available when your body needs it.
- In reasonable amounts, fat helps you look your best, thus increasing your feelings of well-being.

Anorexia Nervosa

Anorexia nervosa is a serious eating disorder. A person who has this disorder severely restricts the amount of food that he or she eats in an attempt to be exceptionally low in body fat. In addition, many people with anorexia do extensive physical activity, thus further lowering their body fat to extremely dangerous levels.

Anorexia is most common among teenage girls, but it is becoming increasingly common among teenage boys. People with this disorder are usually very hard workers and high achievers. They have a distorted view of their body and see themselves as being too fat even when they are extremely thin. Persons with this disorder often fear maturity and the weight gain associated with adulthood. They often try to hide their condition by wearing baggy clothing, pretending to eat, and exercising in private. Anorexia is a life-threatening condition, and people who have it need immediate professional help.

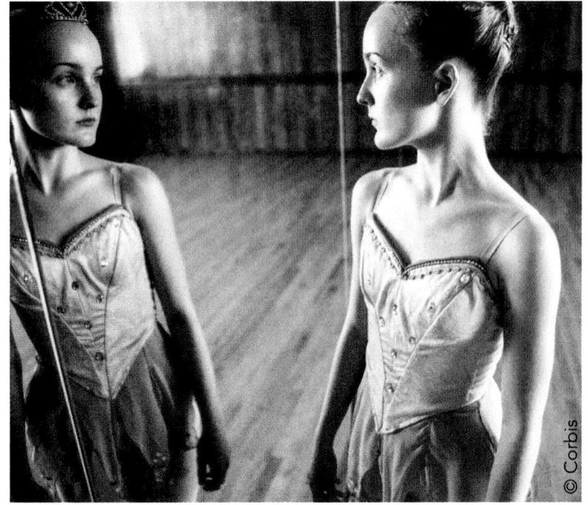

People with eating disorders may be obsessed with their body weight even if they're already thin.

Anorexia Athletica

Anorexia athletica has many symptoms similar to those of anorexia nervosa. It is most common among athletes involved in sports—such as gymnastics, wrestling, and cheerleading—in which low body weight is desirable. This disorder can lead to anorexia nervosa. It is thought to be related to the pressure to maintain low weight and an excessive preoccupation with dieting and exercising for weight loss.

Bulimia

Bulimia is an eating disorder in which a person engages in binge eating—eating a very large amount of food in a short time. Bingeing is followed by purging, perhaps by vomiting or by the use of laxatives to rid the body of food and prevent its digestion. Bulimia can result in severe digestive problems and other health problems such as tooth loss and gum disease.

FIT FACT

Studies show that the number of teens who think they are overweight is four to five times the number who really are. At the same time, interviews with teens who actually are overweight show that 44 percent either have been or currently are teased about their body weight. Getting teased for being overweight—or just feeling like one is overweight—can result in low physical self-perceptions. Teens can help other teens improve their self-perceptions by being supportive rather than critical.

Laboratory Measurements for Assessing Body Composition

The most accurate methods for measuring body composition require special equipment and trained people. They are typically done in a laboratory. Three of the best methods are DXA, underwater weighing, and the Bod Pod (figure 13.1). All three are useful in determining how much of the body weight is fat and how much is lean tissue.

SCIENCE IN ACTION: Media Misrepresentation

Over the years, both exercise psychologists and nutrition scientists have conducted research about physical self-perceptions. They have found that people of all ages are self-conscious about the way they look. In fact, most people are far more critical of their own body than other people are. One reason is that we often compare ourselves with movie stars and other celebrities. Experts point out that the pictures we see of these people have been designed specifically to make them look as glamorous as possible and are touched up to enhance appearance. For example, computer programs can be used to make a female movie star's waist smaller and a male star's muscles larger. Some magazines have promised to limit changes in photos, but there are no regulations, and each magazine can do as it pleases.

Websites also use fake or altered pictures. Advertisements frequently show supposed before-and-after pictures to promote a product. The "before" photos often are taken with bad lighting and in unflattering conditions. The "after" photos are taken with better lighting and are sometimes altered. Video games also present unrealistic images of the human body. For example, body proportions for some male and female video game figures are literally impossible for real-life people.

Many experts believe that the misrepresentation of the human body in the media results in an obsession with leanness. Statistics indicate that many teens, especially girls, set unrealistic standards in judging their body composition. Many feel that they have more fat than they really do, and they try to lose weight unnecessarily.

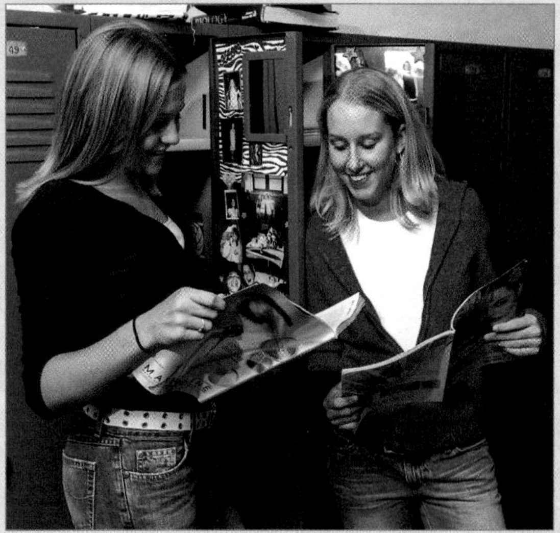

Magazines and websites often alter photos of models and celebrities to make their bodies look unrealistically thin.

Because we are all a bit self-conscious, it is easy to overreact when others make comments about the way we look. For this reason, experts point out the importance of not making critical comments about others. It is also important to keep personal information, such as self-assessment results, confidential. You'll learn more about self-perceptions in the Taking Charge feature in the next lesson of this chapter.

Student Activity

Explore a variety of media sources to find examples of misrepresentation of the human body.

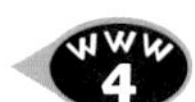

Dual-Energy X-Ray Absorptiometry

Dual-energy X-ray absorptiometry (DXA) is now considered the best method of assessing body composition (figure 13.1*a*) because it can accurately detect body fat, bone, muscle, and other body tissues. First, a high-tech X-ray machine takes a three-dimensional picture of the entire body. Then a computer analyzes the picture to determine the amounts of different kinds of tissue, including fat, bone, and muscle.

Underwater Weighing

Until recently, underwater weighing was considered the best way to assess body fat level, and it is still a very good laboratory method. With this technique, you are weighed on land, then immersed in a tank of water and weighed again (figure 13.1*b*).

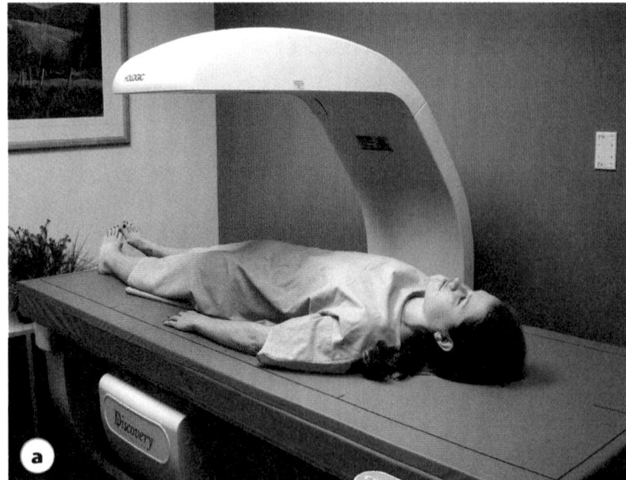

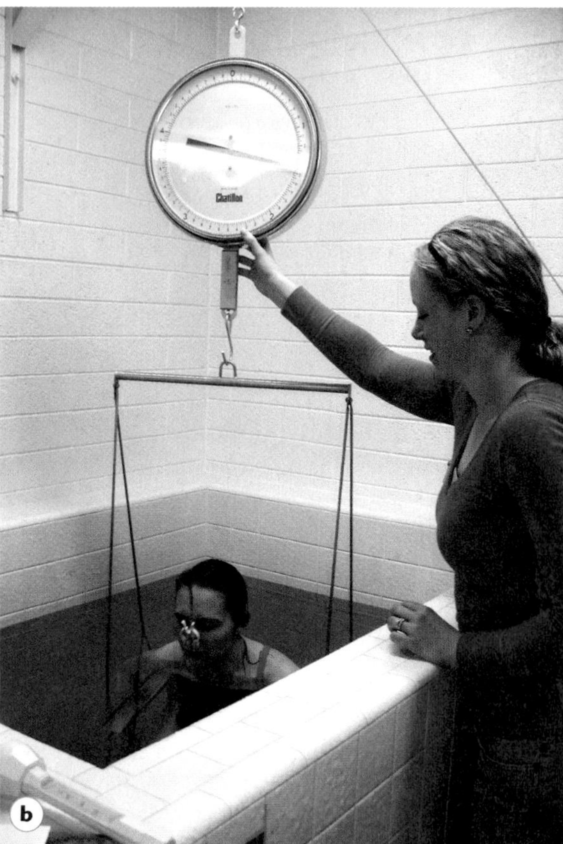

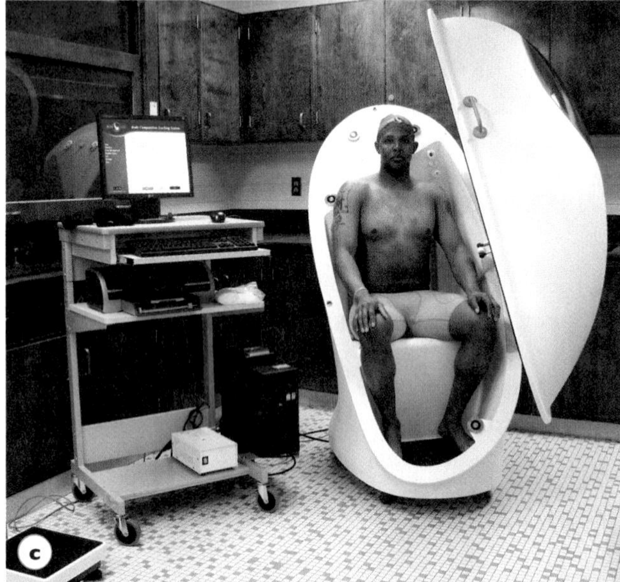

FIGURE 13.1 Laboratory methods for assessing body composition: *(a)* DXA; *(b)* underwater weighing; *(c)* Bod Pod.

Measurements of your lung capacity are also taken because the amount of air in your lungs influences your weight in water. A formula is then applied to determine your body fat level based on your land weight, your underwater weight, and your lung capacity.

Bod Pod

A third type of laboratory assessment of body composition uses a machine called the Bod Pod. In this method, the person being tested sits in an egg-shaped chamber or pod (figure 13.1*c*). The person's body, of course, takes up space in the pod, thus causing air to be moved from the pod. Information gained from changes in the pod's air is then plugged into a special formula to determine the person's body fatness.

Nonlaboratory Measures

Because laboratory measures require special equipment and special training, they are rarely used in schools. For school and home use, nonlaboratory measures are available. Several practical methods of assessment are described here. However, not all of these measures accurately predict the amount of fat and lean body tissue; for this reason, they are typically referred to as body measurements. Body measurements are easier to use than laboratory measures and can be performed at school and often at home. Because you will probably encounter all of these measures at some time in your life, you should try each one of them.

Skinfold Measurements

Your body fat level can also be determined by measuring **skinfold** thickness (the amount of fat under your skin). Skinfold thickness is measured by means of a special instrument called a caliper (see figure 13.2). Skinfold measurements can be used to provide an estimate of the total amount of fat in the body. As noted earlier, a high level of body fat is associated with a variety of health problems, including diabetes, heart disease, and other chronic diseases. You'll learn to do skinfold measurements in this chapter's Self-Assessment feature.

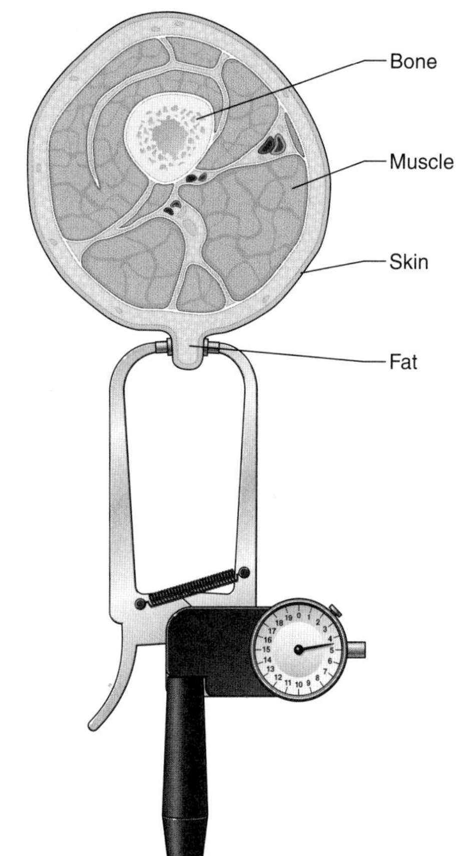

FIGURE 13.2 A caliper measures skinfolds.

Height–Weight and BMI

Height and weight are commonly used in two ways. One method uses height–weight tables that show "normal" weight ranges for people according to age, height, and sex. These tables indicate what the average person of a given sex weighs at a given height. However, because nearly two-thirds of adults in the United States are overweight or obese, many people who are classified as "normal" or "average" are still overweight or obese. For this reason, height–weight tables are considered less useful than some other methods presented in this chapter. You'll get a chance to use height–weight charts in the self-assessment that follows this lesson.

Height and weight are also used to calculate a person's body mass index (BMI). This index is considered to be a better measure than height and weight alone, but it still does not give as accurate an assessment of body fatness as DXA, underwater weighing, Bod Pod analysis, or skinfold measurement. Both the BMI and the height–weight charts can provide inaccurate measurements for people who have a lot of muscle (athletes, for example) because muscle weighs a lot more than fat. As a result, a very muscular person could be high in weight but not too fat. Similarly, a person who appears normal according to height–weight and BMI charts could actually have an unhealthy level of body fat. This is why skinfolds and laboratory techniques are often considered to be better measures.

In spite of the BMI index's limitations, however, high BMI has been associated with a variety of health problems among both teens and adults. In addition, BMI is often used because it's easy to measure, especially in large groups.

Body Measurements: Waist-to-Hip Ratio

The waist-to-hip ratio is used not to determine body fatness but to assess health risk. Scientists now know that people who carry more weight in the middle of the body have a higher risk of disease than people who carry more weight in the lower body (legs and hips). People who carry too much weight in their midsection are said to have an apple body type, whereas people who carry more weight in their hips are said to have a pear body type. In general, women are more likely to be the pear type, and men are more likely to be the apple type.

The waist-to-hip ratio is a simple method for assessing the risk associated with body type. As you'll see when you do the self-assessment for this chapter,

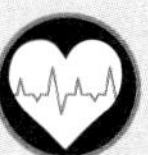

FITNESS TECHNOLOGY: Bioelectrical Impedance Analysis

Computers and other machines have been developed to test body fat levels. For example, bioelectrical impedance analysis (BIA) requires a special machine and expertise in using the machine, but in recent years BIA machines have become more common in schools because of lower prices and improved ease of use. Used properly, they can provide reliable and accurate estimates of body fatness. One limitation is that different machines can give different results, so it is important to use the same machine and to be sure that the machine is properly calibrated (tested for accuracy). In addition, testing should be done under similar conditions each time you are tested—for example, at the same time of day and not at times when you might be dehydrated. Some health and fitness clubs and doctors' offices now have BIA machines. Results of a BIA test can help determine the accuracy of measurements made using other techniques described in this chapter.

Using Technology

If possible, arrange to have a BIA test done. Compare your BIA results with the results of other self-assessments performed in this chapter. If a BIA test is not available, do some research about BIA testing and report your findings.

this ratio is determined by using a tape to measure your waist circumference and your hip circumference. It is desirable to have a waist circumference smaller than your hip circumference.

Body Measurements: Waist Girth (Circumference)

Waist girth (also called waist circumference) can be used by itself as an indicator of health risk. Evidence indicates that people with a very large waist are at risk for health problems. As people grow older, their waist size often increases, thus exposing them to greater health risk. Thus waist girth is a useful health risk indicator that you can use throughout your life.

What Is My Ideal Body Weight?

Even after learning about the various forms of assessment, many people wonder what their ideal body weight is. Experts agree that there is no such thing as one ideal body weight for all people; that is, there is no single table or test that provides a best number for everyone. The best advice is to set a long-term goal of achieving a body fat level in the good fitness zone. Once you have achieved a body fat level that you are comfortable with and that puts you in the good fitness zone, weigh yourself and maintain that weight (this is sometimes referred to as target weight). It's a desirable lifetime goal to maintain this weight and a fat level in the good fitness zone.

If you're in the marginal or low fitness zone, develop a plan that will gradually move you to the next zone. Trying to achieve the good fitness zone when you're too far from it is unrealistic. Instead, people in the low fitness zone should try to move to the marginal zone. Those in the marginal zone should try to move to the good fitness zone. If you're already in the good fitness zone, a reasonable goal for you is simply to stay there.

Some athletes and people in careers that require high levels of fitness may be in the very lean zone, and some people can be very lean because of hereditary factors. While it is possible to be fit and healthy and be in the very lean zone, exceptional leanness is not necessarily a sign of good health and may not be a realistic goal for all people. As noted earlier in this chapter, your body needs a certain amount of body fat (essential body fat), and having too little can cause health problems. Too little body fat can also indicate an eating disorder. If you already have too little fat, increase your weight by gaining body fat. People with eating disorders often try to reduce body fat even when they already have too little for good health. It is important for all people to eat well, especially people who want to be athletes or perform jobs that require high levels of fitness.

As part of a lifelong self-assessment plan, you may choose to monitor your hip-to-waist ratio and your waist girth, especially if you find it difficult to get a good assessment of your body fat level. These measurements are good indicators of health risk. You may also choose to track your BMI over time because physicians often use this measure. High scores are associated with health risks, but because BMI does not estimate body fat levels or lean body mass, it may misclassify some people as overweight or obese when they are not. Similarly BMI may classify a person as "normal" in weight when the person has a higher than healthy level of body fat. The same is true for height–weight charts.

Assessment Confidentiality

Self-assessments are done to gain information that will help the person build an accurate personal profile and plan for healthy active living. The results of self-assessments are personal information. In many assessments, you'll work with a partner, and you and your partner must agree to keep test results private. Information may be submitted to an instructor or a parent or guardian but always with the expectation that the information is private. Assessment-related information should not be shared with others without permission from the person being tested.

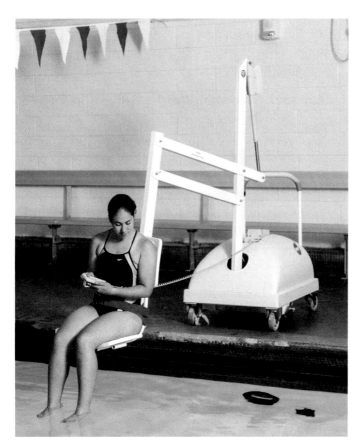

Body fat helps buoyancy in water, so people with disabilities can do exercises in water that they can't do on land.

Lesson Review

1. What do the terms *body composition*, *overweight*, and *obesity* mean?
2. What are some factors that influence body composition?
3. What do the terms *anorexia nervosa*, *bulimia*, and *anorexia athletica* mean?
4. How are body composition and body fat level related to good health?
5. What are some laboratory and nonlaboratory tests for measuring body composition?

SELF-ASSESSMENT: Body Measurements

Earlier in this chapter, you learned about ways to determine body composition. Laboratory measures are the most accurate, but they typically require expensive equipment and people who know how to use the equipment correctly. Height and weight are the most commonly used nonlaboratory measures because they can be determined easily and do not require a lot of equipment.

In addition, body circumferences (such as waist-to-hip ratio and waist girth) can be used to determine health risks, and skinfold measurements can be used both to estimate body fat and to assess health risk. Your fitness scores are your personal information and should be kept confidential. You should also be sensitive to the feelings of others when body fat measurements are being taken; it may be appropriate to take measurements privately. Record your results as directed by your instructor.

Height–Weight Charts

1. Locate the appropriate part of table 13.1 for your sex. Next, find your height (to the nearest inch) at the left and your age at the top of the table. The "normal" weight range for your sex, height, and age is shown in the box where your height row and your age column intersect.
2. Record the weight range for your sex, age, and height.

TABLE 13.1 Normal Weight Ranges in Pounds

Male					Female				
Height		Age (years)			Height		Age (years)		
Ft	In.	13 or 14	15 or 16	17–20	Ft	In.	13 or 14	15 or 16	17–20
4	6	69–72			4	6	73–76		
4	7	73–76			4	7	76–79		
4	8	78–81			4	8	79–82		
4	9	82–85	82–85		4	9	86–89	91–94	
4	10	87–90	87–90		4	10	91–94	98–101	99–102
4	11	88–91	88–91		4	11	96–99	102–105	104–107
5	0	89–92	97–100	101–104	5	0	104–107	106–109	109–112
5	1	97–100	101–104	106–109	5	1	105–108	109–112	113–116
5	2	100–103	106–109	114–117	5	2	106–109	112–115	116–119
5	3	106–109	111–114	121–124	5	3	110–113	115–118	120–123
5	4	113–116	115–118	124–127	5	4	115–118	120–123	125–128
5	5	116–119	120–123	129–132	5	5	119–122	124–127	129–132
5	6	120–123	126–129	134–137	5	6	126–129	128–131	134–137
5	7	126–129	132–135	137–140	5	7	127–130	131–134	137–140
5	8	130–133	135–138	140–143	5	8	128–131	135–138	143–146
5	9	135–138	139–142	147–150	5	9	129–132	137–140	148–151
5	10	141–144	142–145	149–152	5	10	130–133	139–142	153–156
5	11	146–149	149–152	152–155	5	11		142–145	158–161
6	0	151–154	152–155	156–159	6	0		146–149	163–166
6	1		158–161	162–165					
6	2		160–163	167–170					
6	3			177–180					

To convert inches to centimeters, multiply by 2.54 (1 ft = 12 in.). To convert pounds to kilograms, multiply by 0.45.

Waist-to-Hip Ratio (Male and Female)

1. Measure your hips at the largest point (the largest circumference of your buttocks). Make sure that the tape is at the same level (horizontal to ground) in the front, in the back, and on your sides. The tape should be snug but not so tight as to cause indentations in your skin (do not use an elastic tape). Stand with your feet together when making the measurement.
2. Measure your waist at the smallest circumference (called the natural waist). If there is no natural waist, measure at the level of the umbilicus. Measure at the end of a normal inspiration (just after a normal in-breath). Do not suck in to make your waist smaller. This measurement is slightly different from the one used to measure waist girth by itself.
3. To calculate your waist-to-hip ratio, divide your waist girth by your hip girth.
4. Find your ratio in table 13.2 to determine your rating.
5. Record your hip and waist measurements and rating.

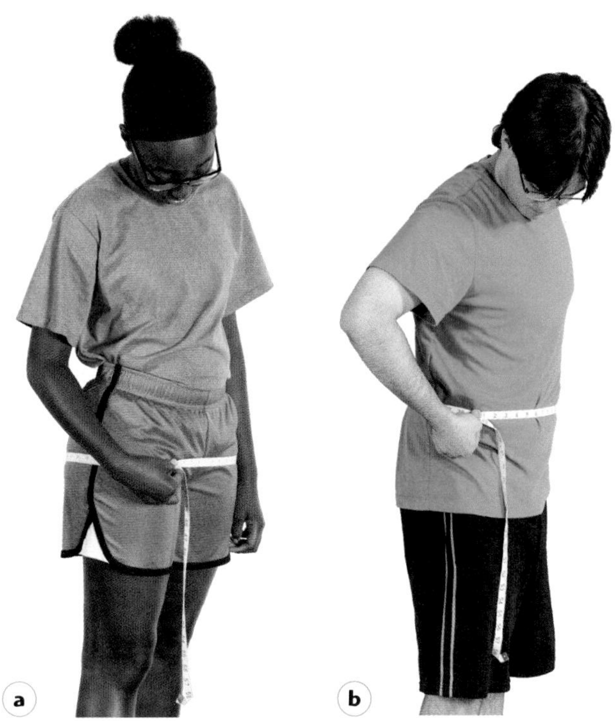

To determine your waist-to-hip ratio, measure *(a)* your hips and *(b)* your waist.

TABLE 13.2 Rating Chart: Waist-to-Hip Ratio

	Male	Female
Good fitness zone	≤0.90	≤0.79
Marginal	0.91–1.0	0.80–0.85
Low fitness zone	≥1.1	≥0.86

Waist Girth (Circumference)

1. Measure your waist at a level just above the top of your hipbones. Mark the top of your hipbone on each side and hold the tape just above the marks.
2. Measure after a normal inspiration (at the end of a normal in-breath). Do not suck in to make your waist smaller. Keep the tape horizontal to the ground when making the measurement.
3. Use table 13.3 to determine your rating.
4. Record your waist girth and rating.

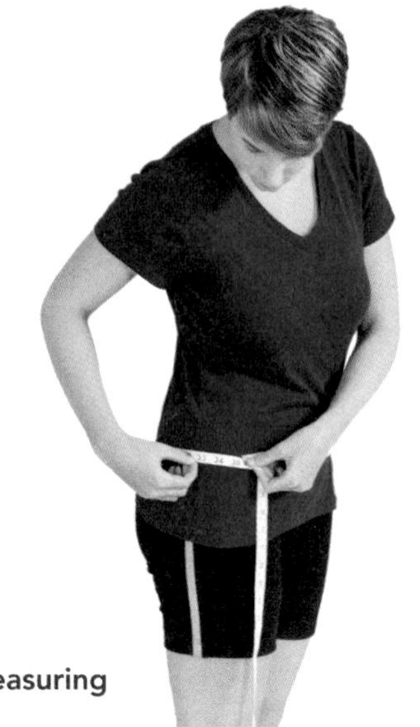

Waist girth is determined by measuring your waist above the hipbone.

TABLE 13.3 Rating Chart: Waist Girth in Inches

Age (years)	12	13	14	15	16	17	≥18
Male							
Good fitness zone	≤28.9	≤29.9	≤30.9	≤31.9	≤32.9	≤33.9	≤34.9
Marginal	29.0–33.4	30.0–34.4	31.0–35.9	32.0–37.4	33.0–38.4	34.0–39.9	35.0–41.4
Low fitness zone	≥33.5	≥34.5	≥36.0	≥37.5	≥38.5	≥40.0	≥41.5
Female							
Good fitness zone	≤28.9	≤29.9	≤30.9	≤31.9	≤32.4	≤33.4	≤34.4
Marginal	29.0–32.4	30.0–33.9	31.0–34.9	32.0–35.9	32.5–38.4	33.5–38.4	34.5–39.9
Low fitness zone	≥32.5	≥34.0	≥35.0	≥36.0	≥38.5	≥38.5	≥40.0

To convert inches to centimeters, multiply by 2.54 (1 ft = 12 in.).

Skinfold Measurements

Skinfold measurements require a special caliper, and using the caliper requires special training. But when done properly by a trained expert, skinfold measurements can provide a good estimate of body fatness. For best results, an expensive caliper is used, but research has shown that inexpensive plastic calipers, such as those shown in the photos here, can be quite accurate if used properly by a trained person who practices the measurement technique. Various measurements can be used; in part 1 of this book, the calf and triceps are used because of their ease of measurement.

Use the following procedures to complete the various measurements and determine your ratings for each assessment. You can use skinfold measurements to estimate your body fat percentage and determine your target weight. For teenagers, upper arm (triceps) and calf measurements provide a good estimate of body fat percentage. If possible, have the measurements done by an expert. If not, work with a partner to take each other's measurements. With practice, you and your partner will improve your measurement skills. Comparing your measurements to those done by an expert will help you determine the accuracy of the measurements. If you're working with a partner, remember that self-assessment information is personal and considered confidential. It shouldn't be shared with others without the permission of the person being tested.

For the triceps skinfold, pick up a skinfold on the middle of the back of the right arm, halfway between the elbow and the shoulder. The arm should hang loose and relaxed at the side.

For the calf skinfold, the person being tested should stand and place his or her right foot on a chair. Pick up a skinfold on the inside of the right calf, halfway between the shin and the back of the calf, where the calf is largest.

1. Use your left thumb and index finger to pick up the skinfold. Do not pinch or squeeze the skinfold.
2. Hold the skinfold with your left hand while you pick up and use the caliper with your right hand to get a reading.
3. Place the caliper over the skinfold about 0.5 inch (1.3 centimeter) below your finger and thumb. Hold the caliper on the skinfold for 3 seconds, then note the measurement. If possible, read the caliper measurement to the nearest half-millimeter.
4. Make three measurements each for the triceps and the calf skinfolds. Allow at least 10 seconds between measurements. Use the middle of the three measures as the score. For example, an 8, 9, and 10 give a score of 9. If your three measurements differ by more than 2 millimeters, take a second, or even third, set of three measurements.
5. Now determine your percent body fat and your body fatness rating. Add your triceps and calf scores to get your sum in millimeters, then use table 13.4 to estimate your body fat percentage based on your sum. Use the appropriate table for your sex and find your skinfold sum. Your percent body fat is the number just to the right. For example, if you're male and your skinfold sum is 26, your percent body fat is 21.
6. Once you have determined your percent body fat, use table 13.5 to determine your body fatness rating.

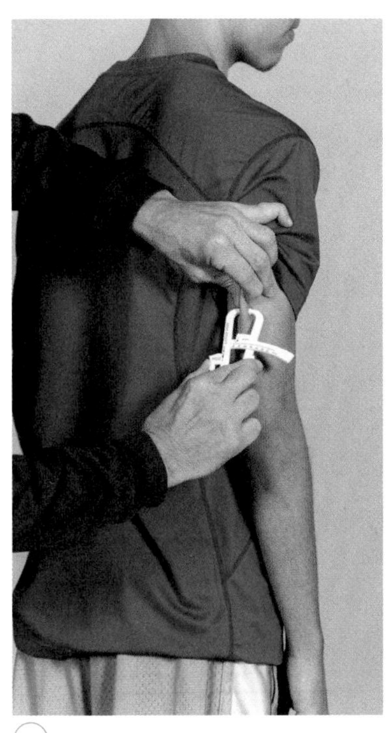
a

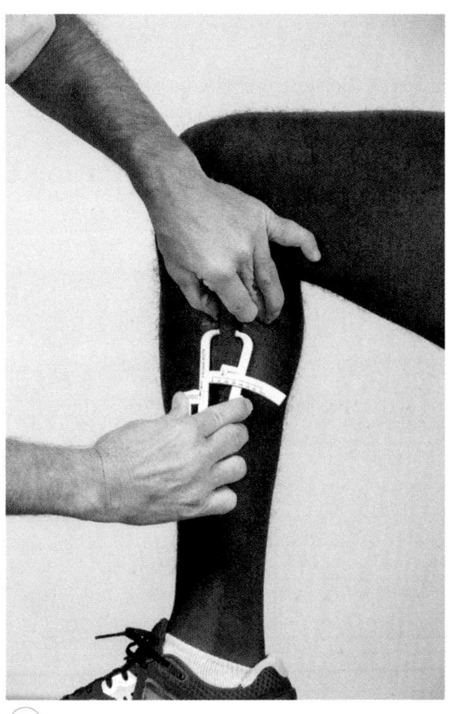
b

Skinfold measurements: *(a)* triceps; *(b)* calf.

TABLE 13.4 Percent Body Fat From Skinfolds

Sum (mm)	% fat	Sum (mm)	% fat	Sum (mm)	% fat	Sum (mm)	% fat	Sum (mm)	% fat	Sum (mm)	% fat
Male											
5	6	15	13	25	20	35	28	45	35	55	42
6	7	16	14	26	21	36	28.5	46	36	56	43
7	7.5	17	14.5	27	21.5	37	29	47	36.5	57	43.5
8	8	18	15	28	22	38	30	48	37	58	44
9	9	19	16	29	23	39	30.5	49	37.5	59	44.5
10	10	20	17	30	24	40	31	50	38	60	45
11	10.5	21	17.5	31	25	41	32	51	39		
12	11	22	18	32	26	42	33	52	39.5		
13	11.5	23	18.5	33	26.5	43	33.5	53	40		
14	12	24	19	34	27	44	34	54	41		
Female											
5	7	15	14	25	21	35	29	45	36	55	43
6	8	16	15	26	22	36	29.5	46	37	56	44
7	8.5	17	15.5	27	22.5	37	30	47	37.5	57	44.5
8	9	18	16	28	23	38	30.5	48	38	58	45
9	10	19	17	29	24	39	31	49	38.5	59	45.5
10	11	20	18	30	24.5	40	32	50	39	60	46
11	12	21	18.5	31	25	41	33	51	40		
12	12.5	22	19	32	26	42	34	52	40.5		
13	13	23	19.5	33	27	43	34.5	53	41		
14	13.5	24	20	34	28	44	35	54	42		

Reprinted by permission, from Dr. Tim G. Lohman, Department of Exercise and Sport Sciences, University of Arizona.

TABLE 13.5 Rating Chart: Body Fatness

	Age (years)					
Rating	13	14	15	16	17	18 or older
Male						
Very lean	≤7.7	≤7.0	≤6.5	≤6.4	≤6.6	≤6.9
Good fitness	7.8–22.8	7.1–21.3	6.6–20.1	6.5–20.1	6.7–20.9	7.0–22.2
Marginal	22.9–34.9	21.4–33.1	20.2–31.4	20.2–31.5	21.0–32.9	22.3–35.0
Low fitness	≥35.0	≥33.2	≥31.5	≥31.6	≥33.0	≥35.1
Female						
Very lean	≤13.3	≤13.9	≤14.5	≤15.2	≤15.8	≤16.5
Good fitness	13.4–27.7	14.0–28.5	14.6–29.1	15.3–29.7	15.9–30.4	16.6–31.3
Marginal	27.8–36.2	28.6–36.7	29.2–37.0	29.8–37.3	30.5–37.8	31.4–38.5
Low fitness	≥36.3	≥36.8	≥37.1	≥37.4	≥37.9	≥38.6

Lesson 13.2

Energy Balance

Lesson Objectives

After reading this lesson, you should be able to

1. explain how to use the FIT formula for fat control,
2. describe how many calories are expended in doing various physical activities,
3. explain how physical activity helps a person maintain a healthy body fat level, and
4. describe some common myths about fat control.

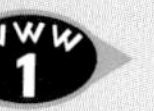

Lesson Vocabulary

calorie, calorie expenditure, calorie intake, energy balance

Do you know how many **calories** you expend in a typical day? Do you know how many calories you consume in a typical day? One major health goal is to achieve and maintain an acceptable level of body fat throughout your life. To do this, you must balance the calories you consume and the calories you expend. In this lesson, you'll learn the FIT formula for fat control and appropriate activities for gaining weight and losing body fat.

Balancing Calories

The term *calorie* is commonly used to describe the amount of energy in a food. The true term is *kilocalorie* (a unit of energy or heat), but when talking about diet and nutrition, *calorie* is typically used. **Energy balance** refers to balancing **calorie intake** and **calorie expenditure** (figure 13.3; also see figure 13.4 and notice the energy balance scale at the top of the Physical Activity Pyramid). Calorie intake is the number of calories or total energy in the foods you eat. Calorie expenditure is the number of calories (energy) you expend in physical activity. If you take in (eat) more calories than you expend (in activity), you will gain weight because extra energy is stored in the body as fat. If you expend more calories than you take in, you will lose weight. If you balance the calories you consume and expend, you will maintain your current weight.

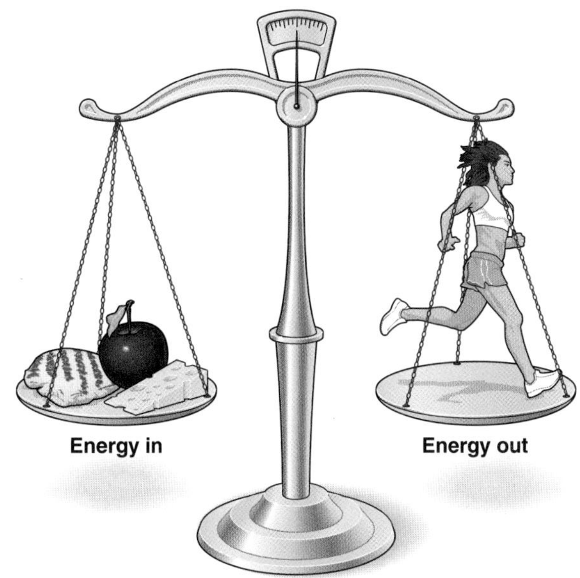

FIGURE 13.3 Balancing energy (calorie) intake with energy (calorie) output is essential for healthy weight maintenance.

FIT FACT

One pound of fat contains 3,500 calories. Therefore, you can lose 1 pound (about 0.5 kilogram) of fat by eating 3,500 calories fewer than you normally eat in a given time or by burning 3,500 calories more than normal in physical activity. Eating food that provides more calories than your body uses will cause you to gain weight. Therefore, you can gain a pound of fat by eating 3,500 calories more than you usually eat within a given time or by expending 3,500 calories fewer than usual in physical activity within a given time.

The FIT Formula

Both diet and physical activity are important for fat control. For this reason, each has a target zone, as shown in table 13.6.

Gaining Weight

Combining proper physical activity and diet is the best way to gain weight. In terms of activity, strength and muscular endurance exercises can help you gain weight. Resistance exercises that help build muscle are especially effective because muscle weighs more than fat.

Remember that every physical activity burns calories. Therefore, when you're active, you need to increase your intake of calories in order to gain weight. You do not, however, need to eat a special diet or take protein supplements; you need only eat a well-balanced diet that contains more calories.

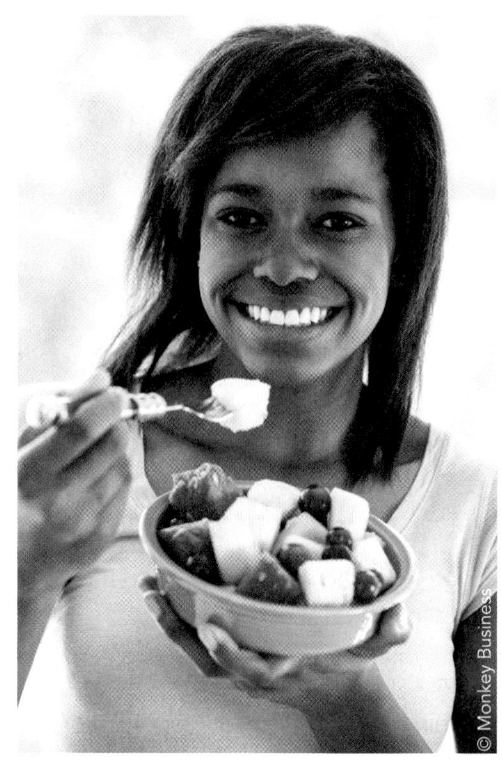

Eating a healthy diet is an essential component of maintaining a healthy weight.

Physical Activity and Calories

You might wonder how many calories are burned by different activities. Table 13.7 shows the approximate number of calories burned each hour during selected vigorous recreational activities. To use the table, find the weight value nearest to your own weight. If you weigh more than the nearest weight,

TABLE 13.6 FIT Formula for Fat Control

	Diet*	Physical activity**
Frequency	Eat three regular meals or four or five small meals daily. Regular, controlled eating is best for losing fat. Skipping meals and snacking is usually not effective.	Participate in physical activity daily. Regular physical activity is best for losing fat. Short or irregular physical activity does little to control body fat.
Intensity	To lose 1 pound (about 0.5 kg) of fat, you must eat 3,500 fewer calories than normal over a given span of time. To gain 1 pound (0.5 kg) of fat, you must eat 3,500 more calories than normal over a given span of time. To maintain your weight, you must keep eating the same number of calories over a given span of time.	To lose 1 pound (0.5 kg) of fat, you must use 3,500 more calories than normal over a given span of time. To gain 1 pound (0.5 kg) of fat, you must use 3,500 fewer calories than normal over a given span of time. To maintain your weight, you must keep your level of physical activity the same over a given span of time.
Time	Neither dietary change nor physical activity results in quick fat loss. Medical experts recommend that a person lose no more than 2 pounds (1 kg) per week without medical supervision.	Together diet and physical activity can be used to safely lose 1 or 2 pounds (0.5–1.0 kg) per week.

*Assumes physical activity is constant.

**Assumes that diet is constant.

TABLE 13.7 Energy Expenditure

	Calories used per hr based on weight				
	100 lb (45 kg)	120 lb (54 kg)	150 lb (68 kg)	180 lb (82 kg)	200 lb (91 kg)
Backpacking/Hiking	307	348	410	472	513
Badminton	255	289	340	391	425
Baseball	210	238	280	322	350
Basketball (half-court)	225	240	300	345	375
Bicycling (normal speed)	157	178	210	242	263
Bowling	155	176	208	240	261
Canoeing (4 mph [6.5 kph])	276	344	414	504	558
Circuit training	247	280	330	380	413
Dance (ballet/modern)	240	300	360	432	480
Dance (aerobic)	300	360	450	540	600
Dance (social)	174	222	264	318	348
Fitness calisthenics	232	263	310	357	388
Football	225	255	300	345	375
Golf (walking)	187	212	250	288	313
Gymnastics	232	263	310	357	388
Horseback riding	180	204	240	276	300
Interval training	487	552	650	748	833
Jogging (5.5 mph [9 kph])	487	552	650	748	833
Judo/Karate	232	263	310	357	388
Racquetball/Handball	450	510	600	690	750
Rope jumping (continuous)	525	595	700	805	875
Running (10 mph [16 kph])	625	765	900	1,035	1,125
Skating (ice or roller)	262	297	350	403	438
Skiing (cross-country)	525	595	700	805	875
Skiing (downhill)	450	510	600	690	750
Soccer	405	459	540	575	621
Softball (fastpitch)	210	238	280	322	350
Swimming (slow laps)	240	272	320	368	400
Swimming (fast laps)	420	530	630	768	846
Tennis	315	357	420	483	525
Volleyball	262	297	350	403	483
Walking	204	258	318	372	426
Weight training	352	399	470	541	558

add 5 percent to the number of calories for each 10 pounds (4.5 kilograms) you weigh above the listed weight value. If you weigh less than the nearest weight, subtract 5 percent from the number of calories for each 10 pounds you weigh below the listed weight value. Use this table to determine which physical activities are best for burning calories, then see which activities appeal to you.

> "Choice, not chance, determines your destiny."
>
> —Aristotle, Greek philosopher

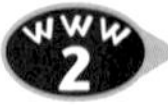

Physical Activity and Fat Loss

The best way to lose fat is to combine regular physical activity with a healthy diet. Research shows that a person who reduces calorie intake without increasing activity will lose both fat and muscle tissue, whereas a person who increases physical activity and reduces calorie consumption loses mostly body fat. Notice that physical activities from all steps of the Physical Activity Pyramid (figure 13.4) are appropriate for helping to control body fat level and provide energy balance.

Moderate Physical Activity

Moderate physical activity is especially effective in long-term fat control. In fact, studies indicate that moderate activity is just as effective as organized sports and games for losing fat—and more effective for permanent fat loss. You can do moderate activities for relatively long periods of time, thus burning many calories.

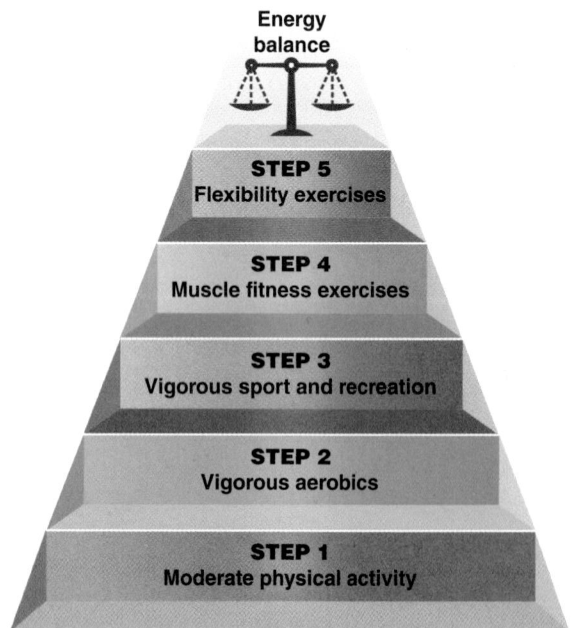

FIGURE 13.4 All activities in the Physical Activity Pyramid result in calorie expenditure and aid in energy balance.

Vigorous Aerobics

Because vigorous aerobic activity is more intense than moderate activity, you can burn more calories in a shorter time with this type of activity. It is most often continuous, thus allowing you to expend calories for the full duration of the activity. Vigorous aerobic activities can be sustained for a relatively long time and therefore have potential for considerable calorie expenditure.

Vigorous Sport and Recreation

Like vigorous aerobics, vigorous sport and recreational activities are more intense than moderate activities. Therefore more calories are expended per unit of time than in moderate activities. The way you perform these activities makes a difference in the number of calories you expend. For example, shooting baskets typically expends fewer calories than playing a game of full-court basketball. The greater the intensity of the activity, the greater the number of calories expended over a similar length of time.

Muscle Fitness Exercises

Muscle fitness exercise expends considerable calories and is therefore beneficial in maintaining a healthy level of body fat. In addition, the extra muscle tissue you build with these exercises provides a second benefit by helping you expend more calories even when you're resting.

Flexibility Exercises

Flexibility exercises do not expend as many calories as the other four types of activity represented in the Physical Activity Pyramid. They do, however, expend more calories than resting, and any calories expended above normal can help you control body fatness.

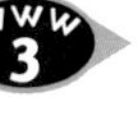

Calculating Your Daily Calorie Expenditure

If you keep a record of all the activities you perform in a day, you can determine the total calories you expended. As directed by your teacher, keep a daily record. After recording your activities for a full day, you can calculate your daily calorie expenditure and compare it with your daily calorie intake. To maintain weight, you must expend as much energy as you take in. To lose weight, you must expend more energy than you take in. To gain weight, you must take in more calories than you expend.

Myths About Fat Loss

Some people hold incorrect ideas about physical activity and fat loss. Read table 13.8 to identify some mistaken ideas and learn some facts about losing body fat. No matter what your body is like now, regular physical activity and proper diet will help you control body fatness. When you're fit, you look better, feel better, and have fewer health problems than people who have a high level of body fat and are unfit.

FIT FACT

If you maintain your normal calorie intake and increase your activity by playing 30 minutes of tennis daily, you will lose 16 pounds (about 7 kilograms) in a year. If you walk briskly for 15 minutes a day instead of watching TV, you will lose 5 or 6 pounds (about 2.5 kilograms) in a year. On the other hand, if you sit for 15 minutes instead of taking a regular 15-minute walk each day, you will gain 5 to 6 pounds in a year.

TABLE 13.8 Myths and Facts About Fat Loss

Myth	Fact
Exercise cannot be effective for fat loss because it takes many hours of exercise to lose even 1 pound (0.5 kg) of fat.	You can lose body fat over time with regular physical activity if your calorie intake remains the same. Fat lost through physical activity tends to stay off longer than fat lost through dieting alone.
Exercise does not help you lose fat because it increases your hunger and encourages you to overeat.	If you are moderately active instead of inactive, your hunger should not increase. Even moderate to vigorous activity will not cause hunger to increase so much that you overeat. People who overeat usually do so for other reasons (habit, anxiousness, presence of empty calories, large portion sizes, and so on).
Most people with too much body fat have glandular problems.	While some people do have glandular problems, most people who are high in body fat eat too much, do too little physical activity, or both.
You can spot-reduce by exercising a specific body part to lose fat in that area.	Any exercise that burns calories will cause the body's general fat deposits to decrease. A given exercise does not cause one area of fat to decrease more than another.

Lesson Review

1. How can you use the FIT formula to control your body fat level?
2. How many calories are expended in the five most common physical activities that you perform?
3. How can physical activity help you maintain a healthy body fat level?
4. What are some common myths and facts about fat control?

TAKING CHARGE: Improving Physical Self-Perception

Each person has a mental picture of himself or herself. If you think you do well in a certain activity, you'll probably take part in that type of activity. If you feel embarrassed about your appearance or ability level while doing an activity, you'll probably avoid that activity. Here are two very different examples of physical self-perception.

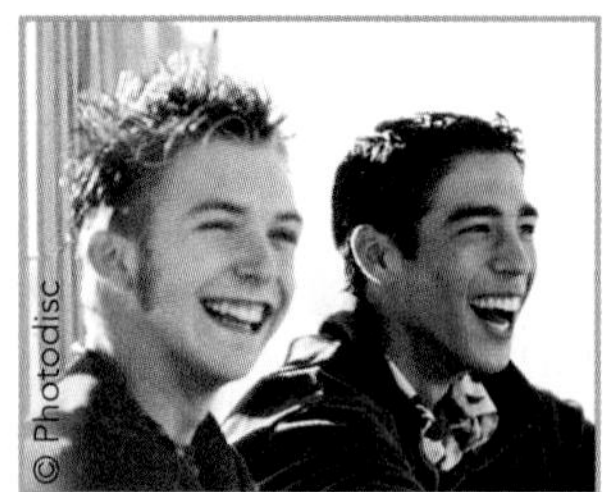
© Photodisc

Michael was not sure that he wanted to go back to school after the summer break. It seemed as if all of his friends had grown taller in the last few months, but he had stayed the same height. Michael felt embarrassed and a little jealous, even though none of his friends seemed to notice. His height certainly did not alter his ability to play tennis. In fact, his friends still called him "King of the Court" because he usually won.

Raul was one of the shortest people in his class, but his height did not stop him from being involved in activities. He realized that he had never been a great basketball player, but he still liked to play with his friends from school. He also discovered that height had nothing to do with his ability to go hiking, nor did it prevent him from being a good wrestler.

For Discussion

Michael had a negative self-perception because of his height. What can he do to change his negative perception? How does Raul keep a positive self-perception? What else can a person do to develop a positive self-perception? Consider the guidelines presented in the Self-Management feature as you answer the discussion questions.

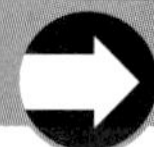

SELF-MANAGEMENT: Skills for Self-Perception

A self-perception is an idea you have about your own thoughts, actions, or appearance. It is influenced by how you think other people view you. Some of the many kinds of self-perception are academic, social, and artistic. In part 1 of this book, the focus is on physical self-perceptions—the way you view your physical self.

Four aspects of physical self-perception are strength, fitness, skill, and physical attractiveness. People with good physical self-perceptions are happy with their current strength and fitness levels; they also feel that their skills are adequate to meet their needs, and they like the way they look. We know that people who have positive physical self-perceptions are more likely to be physically active than those who do not. The following list provides guidelines you can use to maintain or improve your physical self-perceptions.

- **Assess your physical self-perceptions.** You may use the worksheet provided by your teacher.
- **Consider your self-assessment results.** Use the self-assessment worksheet to determine whether you have any areas in which your physical self-perceptions are especially low (strength, fitness, skill, or physical attractiveness).
- **Perform regular physical activity to improve your physical fitness or practice regularly to improve your physical skills.** Regular physical activity can help you look your best, and learning skills can help you perform your best.
- **Consider a new way of thinking about yourself.** People often set unrealistic standards for themselves, such as looking like someone they see on television or in the movies. Understand that in real life these people do not look the way they look on the screen. In fact, their appearance is often enhanced by special cameras and computers programs. You also do not know whether a movie

star has an eating disorder or practices healthy habits. Consider your heredity and set realistic standards for yourself.

- **Think positively.** Almost all people have a physical characteristic that they would like to change. But studies show that the things people don't like about themselves are rarely seen as problems by other people. You're often your own worst critic, and thinking positively can help you present yourself in a positive way.
- **Do not let the actions of a few insensitive people cause you to feel negatively about yourself.** There will always be some people who are insensitive to others' feelings. These people often have low self-perceptions and try to build themselves up by tearing other people down. Recognize that criticism from these people is their problem, not yours.
- **Consider how your behavior and actions influence the way other people view you.** Acting cheerful and friendly has as much to do with how others perceive you as your physical characteristics.
- **Realize that all people have some imperfections.** Try to build on your strengths and improve your areas of weakness.
- **Find a realistic role model and be a role model for others.** Instead of trying to be like someone who is totally unlike you, find someone you admire who has characteristics you can realistically achieve. And, just as you look to others for models, remember that others may look to you as a model. Providing a positive model for others can help you think positively about yourself.

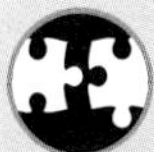

Academic Connection: Quartiles

Various statistics can be used to describe scores for a group of people. The term *quartile* is used to describe the scores for each quarter of a distribution. In the following example, each number represents a score (in inches) on the waist girth test for 36 15-year-old females. The distribution is divided into quartiles (25 percent of scores per quartile, listed in different colors).

A good fitness rating for waist girth for 15-year-old females is 32 inches or less. Which color of quartile includes scores for the good fitness range? What percentage of girls were in the good fitness zone for waist girth? What percentage of girls had scores that did not qualify them to be in the good fitness zone?

Distribution of Waist Girth Scores (Inches) for 15-Year-Old Females

						34									
					33	34	35								
				32	33	34	35	36							
	28		30	**32**	33	34	35	36	37	38	39	40			
27	28	29	30	**32**	33	34	35	36	37	38	39	40	41	42	43

Check Your Answers

The red quartile includes scores in the good fitness range, so 25 percent of the girls were in the good fitness zone. That also means that 75 percent, or three quartiles, of the girls were not in the good fitness zone.

TAKING ACTION: Elastic Band Workout

Muscle fitness exercises provide a triple benefit in helping you maintain a healthy body composition. First, they build muscles that help you look your best. Second, they expend energy, thus helping you to achieve a good energy balance. Finally, the extra muscle that you build through resistance exercise causes you to burn extra calories even at rest.

You can **take action** by completing an elastic band resistance circuit. Elastic bands are beneficial because they are affordable, travel well, and allow you to easily exercise many muscles. They are appropriate for people of all fitness levels, and they will help you improve your overall coordination and your muscular fitness. Consider the following guidelines for performing resistance band (elastic band) exercises.

- When choosing bands, make sure they are the right length for you and that they do not have cracks or other signs of wear.
- Choose a band that provides the proper resistance that allows you to perform the recommended number of sets and reps.
- You can also do resistance exercises that use your body weight to add variation and create a good workout circuit.

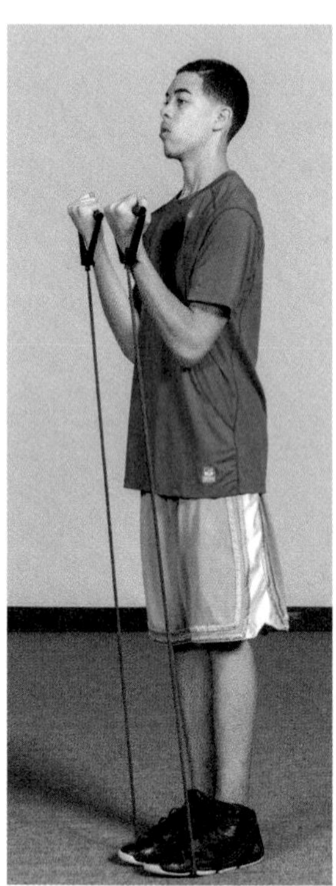

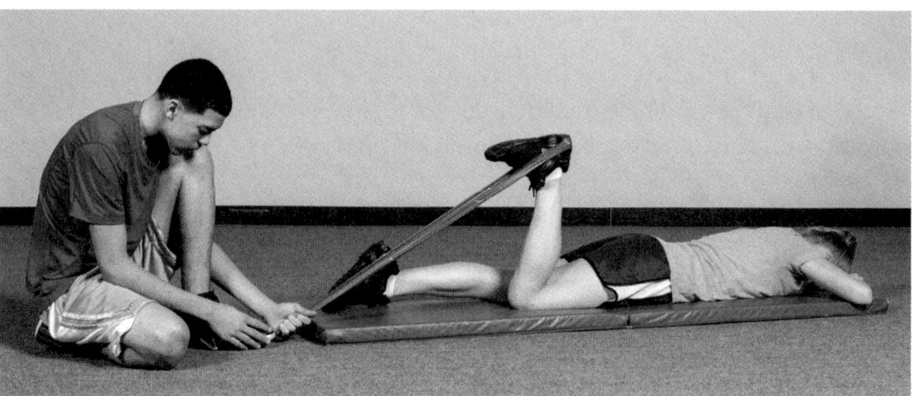

Take action by performing elastic band exercises.

CHAPTER REVIEW

Reviewing Concepts and Vocabulary

As directed by your teacher, answer items 1 through 5 by correctly completing each sentence with a word or phrase.

1. A term used to describe a person who has a high body fat level is _______________.
2. An eating disorder characterized by bingeing and purging is called _______________.
3. The minimum amount of body fat needed for good health is _______________.
4. People with _______________ see themselves as too fat even when they are extremely thin.
5. Keeping your calories consumed equal to your calories expended is called _______________.

For items 6 through 10, as directed by your teacher, match each term in column 1 with the appropriate phrase in column 2.

6. metabolic syndrome	a. best measure of body composition
7. caliper	b. used to measure skinfolds
8. DXA	c. condition associated with health risk factors
9. anorexia athletica	d. energy your body uses just to keep you living
10. basal metabolism	e. eating disorder most common among performers

For items 11 through 15, as directed by your teacher, respond to each statement or question.

11. Discuss why 3,500 calories is an important number for maintaining a healthy body composition.
12. Why is confidentiality so important when making body composition assessments?
13. Why is it important to maintain essential body fat?
14. Describe one myth about fat loss and explain how it is incorrect or misleading.
15. What are some guidelines for improving physical self-perceptions?

Thinking Critically

Each year, people spend billions of dollars on weight loss and muscle-building products that do not work. Look at a newspaper, popular magazine, or website and find an advertisement for a weight loss product. Read the ad and make a list of its claims. Place a checkmark by the claims that are consistent with the information presented in this chapter. Place an X by those that appear to be false or questionable. Write a paragraph evaluating the advertisement.

Project

The U.S. government provides annual ratings of obesity for each state and for some cities. Prepare a poster showing how your city or state compares with the U.S. average obesity rate. List five factors that you think may cause your state to rank as it does.

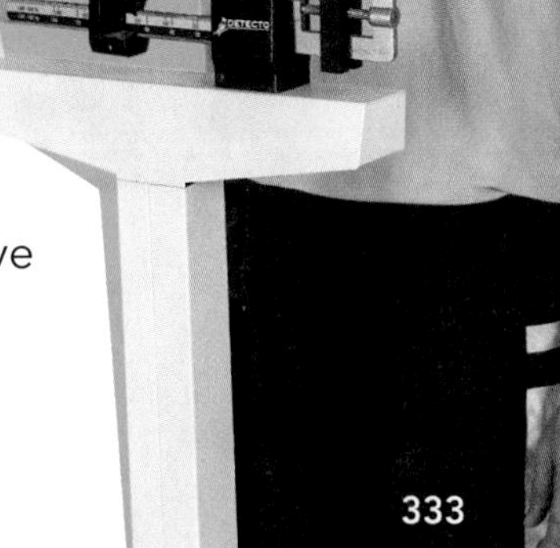

14

Physical Activity Program Planning

In This Chapter

LESSON 14.1
Physical Activity and Fitness Assessment

SELF-ASSESSMENT
Your Personal Fitness Test Battery

LESSON 14.2
Maintaining Active Lifestyles

TAKING CHARGE
Changing Attitudes

SELF-MANAGEMENT
Skills for Building Positive Attitudes

TAKING ACTION
Your Physical Activity Plan

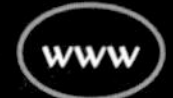

Student Web Resources
www.HOPEtextbook.org/student

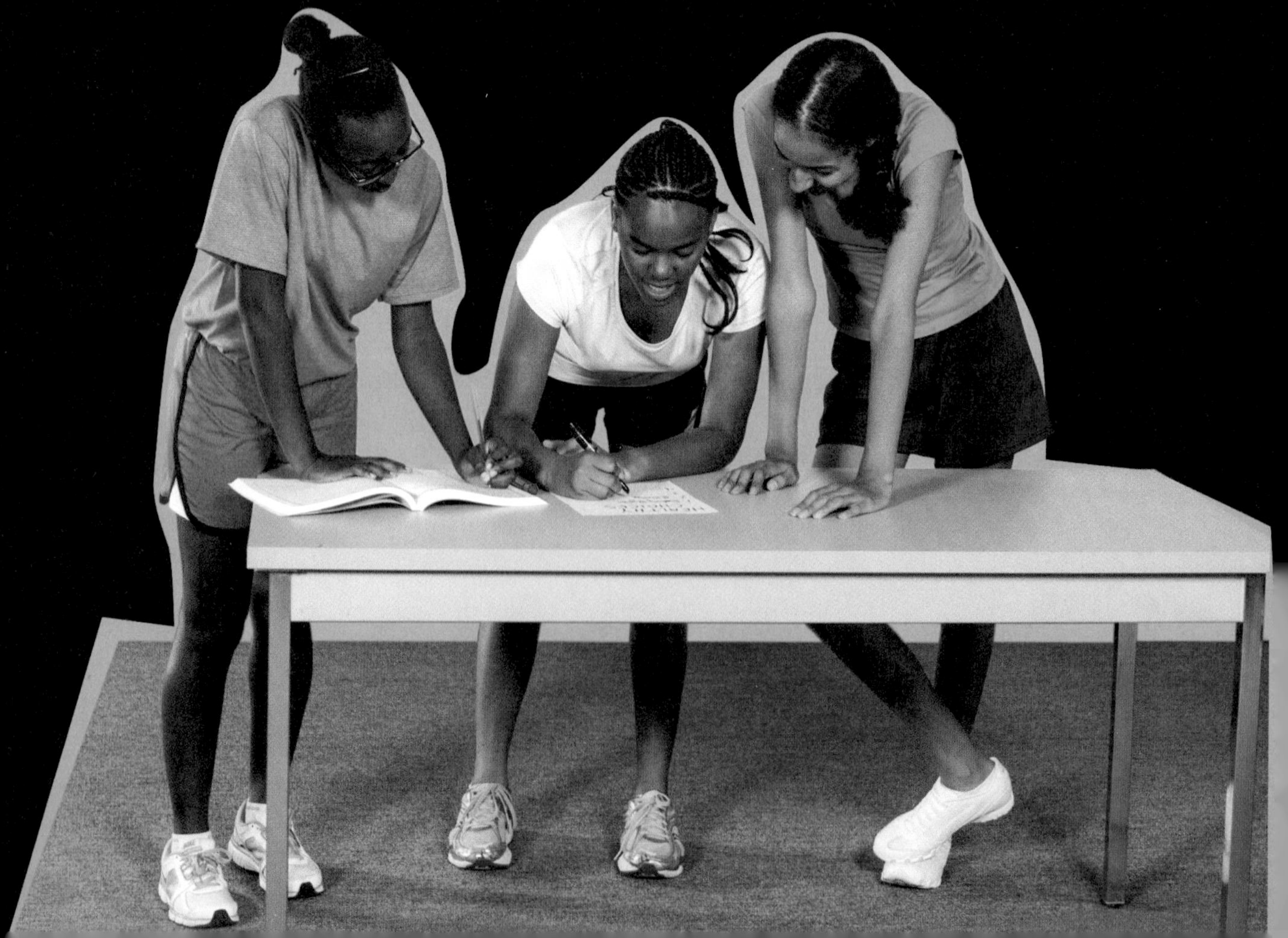

Lesson 14.1

Physical Activity and Fitness Assessment

Lesson Objectives

After reading this lesson, you should be able to

1. explain how to use a fitness profile to plan a personal fitness program,
2. describe the five steps in planning a comprehensive personal fitness program, and
3. describe some ways in which physical activity enhances academic performance.

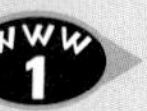

Lesson Vocabulary

cognitive skills, fitness profile

Do you have a personal fitness and physical activity plan? In other chapters, you've been introduced to the five steps of program planning, learned which types of activity are most appropriate for building each part of health-related physical fitness, and planned a program for each of the five types of activity included in the Physical Activity Pyramid. In the first part of this chapter, you'll use the plans you've previously developed to create a comprehensive personal physical activity program. First, read about the comprehensive program that Alicia developed, then plan your own program. To help you create your plan, your teacher will provide you with worksheets.

Step 1: Determine Your Personal Needs

As you know from your previous program planning, collecting information is the first step toward making good decisions and preparing a good plan. In this case, construct a comprehensive fitness profile and an activity profile to help you determine your needs and interests. Use the many self-assessments that you've performed throughout this class.

A **fitness profile** is a brief summary of your self-assessment results that helps you determine your areas of personal need. You can see a sample for Alicia, a 15-year-old, in figure 14.1. To create a fitness profile, first make a list of all of the fitness self-assessments that you have performed. Then record your scores and ratings for each of the self-assessments. Your profile should look similar to the one that Alicia prepared.

She determined that she met the national physical activity goals for moderate and vigorous physical activity and placed a checkmark by those goals (figure 14.2). Her walks to school and jogs on two days a week helped her meet these goals. Alicia did not do any exercises for muscle fitness and flexibility on a regular basis and did none for the last week. Alicia did not meet the national goals for muscle fitness and flexibility exercises, so she did not place a check by those. Alicia was not enrolled in physical education class, so she did not get any physical activity at school that lasted at least 10 minutes at a time. Prepare a written activity profile using a chart similar to the one used by Alicia. List the activities that you regularly perform and answer the questions related to national physical activity goals.

FIT FACT

Each year high school students are surveyed to determine their activity levels. Teens are asked if they meet national goals for moderate activity, vigorous activity, and muscle fitness. The questions are similar to those that you ask yourself when you prepare a physical activity profile.

Step 2: Consider Your Program Options

Alicia prepared a list of several activities to consider for her activity plan. She was already doing some walking and jogging, but she was not doing any muscle fitness or flexibility exercise. She prepared

Self-assessment	Rating
Cardiorespiratory endurance	
PACER	Good fitness
Step test	Good fitness
Walking test	Good fitness
One-mile run	Marginal
Muscle fitness	
Curl-up	Good fitness
Push-up	Marginal
1RM arm press (per lb of body weight)	Good fitness
1RM leg press (per lb of body weight)	Marginal
Muscular endurance	
Grip strength (left)	Marginal
Grip strength (right)	Good fitness
Standing long jump	Marginal
Medicine ball throw	Good fitness
Body composition	
Body mass index (BMI)	Good fitness
Height–weight	Good fitness
Skinfold measures	Good fitness
Waist-to-hip ratio	Good fitness
Waist girth	Good fitness
Flexibility	
Back-saver sit-and-reach	Low fitness
Trunk lift	Marginal
Arm, leg, and trunk flexibility	Marginal

FIGURE 14.1 Alicia's fitness profile.

the following list that included her current activities and additional activities from the Physical Activity Pyramid that she thought she might enjoy and was likely to perform regularly.

Moderate Physical Activity

- Walking to and from school
- Additional walking
- Yardwork
- Biking

Vigorous Aerobics

- Continue her current jogging
- Additional jogging
- Aerobic dance class

Vigorous Sport and Recreation

- Volleyball club
- Tennis

Muscle Fitness Exercise

- Elastic band exercises
- Jump rope

Flexibility Exercises

- Static stretching exercises
- Yoga

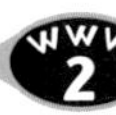

Make a list similar to the one that Alicia made. Consider activities that you currently perform, as well as other types of moderate activity, vigorous activity (including vigorous aerobics, sports, and recreation), muscle fitness exercise, and flexibility exercise. As you choose activities, consider the health benefits and health-related fitness benefits provided by each.

Step 3: Set Goals

Setting SMART goals can help you build a complete fitness and physical activity program that meets your personal needs. First, consider the reasons for doing your program. Are you primarily interested in fitness and physical activity for health and wellness, or are you interested in building a higher level of fitness necessary for playing a sport?

For example, Alicia is interested in health but also wants to try out for the volleyball team. First, however, she's going to participate in the volleyball club to develop skills that will help her make the team when volleyball season comes.

Next, consider your fitness and activity profiles. If you're low in one part of physical fitness, you may want to work on it. If you did not meet national activity guidelines for one type of physical activity, you might want to do more of that type. Alicia had marginal ratings in flexibility and muscle fitness and did not meet the national guidelines for muscle fitness and flexibility exercises.

In your earlier plans, you've focused only on physical activity goals because you were just learning to plan and were doing a short-term plan with short-term goals. Now that you're more experienced in planning, you can build a plan for a longer time that addresses long-term goals, including physical *fitness* goals.

As you can see in figure 14.3, Alicia chose physical activity (process) and fitness (product) goals designed to improve her weaknesses—specifically, flexibility exercise to improve her flexibility and muscle fitness exercise to improve her muscle fitness and volleyball performance. Alicia wanted to keep walking to school because she wanted to do a moderate activity that she can continue to do later in life. She decided to drop her jogging two days a week so that she could attend volleyball club on Tuesdays and Thursdays. She felt that the vigorous activity in volleyball club would serve the same purpose. She decided to include tennis just for fun. She also included jump rope as a warm-up before her muscle fitness exercise and to build power in her legs.

Alicia set some of her activity goals for eight weeks (long-term). She did this because she had been walking to school on a regular basis so she felt confident that she could continue to do it regularly. She also set eight weeks for her volleyball club meetings. She felt that she could stick with it for eight weeks

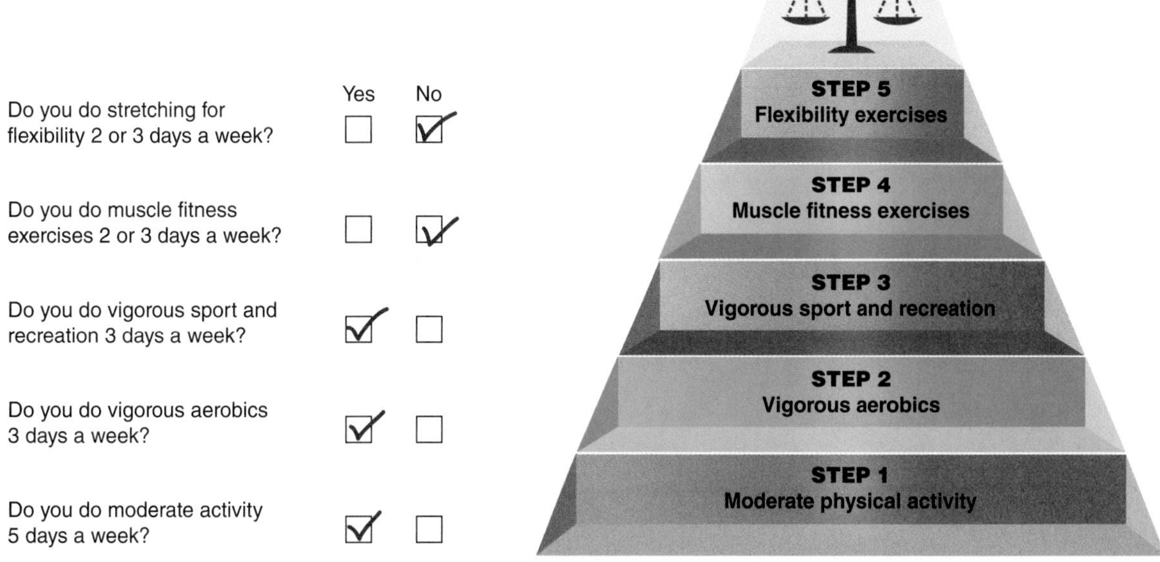
Yes
No
Do you do stretching for flexibility 2 or 3 days a week?
Do you do muscle fitness exercises 2 or 3 days a week?
Do you do vigorous sport and recreation 3 days a week?
Do you do vigorous aerobics 3 days a week?
Do you do moderate activity 5 days a week?
Energy balance
STEP 5
Flexibility exercises
STEP 4
Muscle fitness exercises
STEP 3
Vigorous sport and recreation
STEP 2
Vigorous aerobics
STEP 1
Moderate physical activity

FIGURE 14.2 Alicia's physical activity profile.

Physical activity goals	Days	Amount	Weeks
		Long-term goals	
1. Brisk walk to and from school	3	30 minutes a day (15 minutes each way)	8
2. Volleyball club	2	60 minutes after school	8
3. Stretching exercises	2	2 sets of 2 reps of each exercise, hold stretch 30 seconds (performed after volleyball club when the muscles are warm)	8
		Short-term goals	
1. Jump rope warm-up	3	5 minutes, alternate jumping 30 seconds, walking 15 seconds	2
2. Resistance machine exercises	3	2 sets of 10 reps, 60% of 1RM	2
3. Cool-down	3	5-minute walk	2
4. Jump rope warm-up	1	5 minutes, alternate jumping 30 seconds, walking 30 seconds	2
5. Tennis	1	60 minutes	2
6. Cool-down	1	5-minute walk	2
Physical fitness component	**Goal**		**Completion date**
1. Improve push-up score.	8 reps		Nov. 15 (8 weeks)
2. Improve leg press score.	1.75 lb (0.8 kg) per lb (kg) of body weight		Nov. 15 (8 weeks)
3. Improve back-saver sit-and-reach score.	12 in. (30 cm)		Nov. 15 (8 weeks)
4. Improve arm, leg, and trunk flexibility score.	Score of 8 points		Nov. 15 (8 weeks)

FIGURE 14.3 Alicia's activity and fitness goals.

because it was important for improving her skills for making the volleyball team. She set two-week goals (short-term) for her muscle fitness, flexibility, and tennis goals. She wanted to try her plan for these new activities to see if it was reasonable. If necessary, she planned to modify her short-term activity goals after two weeks. She added jump rope to her plan as a warm-up for her muscle fitness exercises. Alicia did not use all of the activities from her list of possible activities because she wanted to be realistic. She set fitness goals for two muscle fitness self-assessments and two flexibility self-assessments. She hoped to achieve these fitness goals in eight weeks (long-term goals) because she knew that improving fitness takes weeks to achieve. Using a chart similar to Alicia's (figure 14.3), prepare your own SMART physical activity and physical fitness goals, including both short-term and long-term goals.

> "A good plan is like a road map: it shows the final destination and usually the best way to get there."
>
> —H. Stanley Judd, author

Step 4: Structure Your Program and Write It Down

Once Alicia had established her goals, she built a schedule. Her schedule included all of the activities that she listed as goals in step 3 (figure 14.4). Alicia chose the days of the week that made exercise most convenient for her. She chose Monday, Wednesday, and Friday for her jump rope and muscle fitness exercise because the school fitness center was open after school on those days. Volleyball club met on Tuesdays and Thursdays and she planned to do her flexibility exercises after volleyball club when the muscles were warm. The flexibility exercises also served as a good cool-down after volleyball club. She chose to do tennis on Saturday morning and planned no activities on Sunday.

In a separate chart, she listed her flexibility and muscle fitness exercises (see figure 14.5). Since they were the same exercises each time, she needed to list them only once to help her remember them.

FIT FACT

Walking or biking to school increases the amount of activity that teens accumulate by an average of 16 minutes a day. According to a report by the Surgeon General of the United States, approximately 200,000 lives could be saved each year if adults were more physically active.

Step 5: Keep a Log and Evaluate Your Program

The Taking Action feature in this chapter allows you to perform your plan, but you won't have time to complete your entire plan in this class. Therefore, you'll need to put your program into action on your own. In the weeks ahead, try out your plan and use a log to keep a record of your activities. A log will help you see if you met your goals.

After you've tried your program for some time (the specific time depends on your goals), evaluate

Day	Activity	Time of day	How long?
Mon.	Walk to school Jump rope warm-up Muscle fitness exercises Walking cool-down	7:15–7:30 a.m. 3:35–3:40 p.m. 3:40–4:25 p.m. 4:25–4:30 p.m.	15 min 5 min 45 min 5 min
Tues.	Walk to school Volleyball club Cool-down and flexibility exercises	7:15–7:30 a.m. 3:45–4:45 p.m. 4:45–5:00 p.m.	15 min 60 min 15 min
Wed.	Walk to school Jump rope warm-up Muscle fitness exercises Walking cool-down	7:15–7:30 a.m. 3:35–3:40 p.m. 3:40–4:25 p.m. 4:25–4:30 p.m.	15 min 5 min 45 min 5 min
Thurs.	Walk to school Volleyball club Cool-down and flexibility exercises	7:15–7:30 a.m. 3:45–4:45 p.m. 4:45–5:00 p.m.	15 min 60 min 15 min
Fri.	Walk to school Jump rope warm-up Muscle fitness exercises Walking cool-down	7:15–7:30 a.m. 3:35–3:40 p.m. 3:40–4:25 p.m. 4:25–4:30 p.m.	15 min 5 min 45 min 5 min
Sat.	Jump rope warm-up Tennis Walking cool-down	9:00–9:05 a.m. 9:05–10:05 a.m. 10:05–10:10 a.m.	5 min 60 min 5 min
Sun.	None		

FIGURE 14.4 Alicia's schedule for her physical activity plan.

Cool-down and flexibility exercises	Repetitions	Time
Back-saver sit-and-reach	2 sets of 2 reps	15 sec
Knee-to-chest	2 sets of 2 reps	15 sec
Sitting stretch	2 sets of 2 reps	15 sec
Zipper	2 sets of 2 reps	15 sec
Hip stretch	2 sets of 2 reps	15 sec
Calf stretch	2 sets of 2 reps	15 sec
Muscle fitness exercises	**Repetitions**	**Resistance**
Bench press	2 sets of 2 reps	60% of 1RM
Knee extension	2 sets of 2 reps	60% of 1RM
Hamstring curl	2 sets of 2 reps	60% of 1RM
Biceps curl	2 sets of 2 reps	60% of 1RM
Triceps press	2 sets of 2 reps	60% of 1RM

FIGURE 14.5 Alicia's muscle fitness and flexibility exercises.

SCIENCE IN ACTION: Exercise and Academics

The U.S. Centers for Disease Control and Prevention (CDC) is a government agency created to help people and communities "protect their health through health promotion; prevention of disease, injury, and disability; and preparedness for new health threats." The CDC recognizes the importance of regular physical activity as one means of achieving its goal of good health for all people and all communities. CDC scientists reviewed more than 400 studies and found that in addition to providing health benefits, regular physical activity can "help improve academic achievement, including grades and standardized test scores." The CDC also concluded that physical activity improves **cognitive skills** such as concentration and attention, as well as academic behavior (including classroom behavior).

The conclusion that physical activity helps students concentrate on academic tasks is supported by research conducted by kinesiologists at the University of Illinois. They found, for example, that walking stimulates brain areas that increase concentration and attention in the classroom. The images show brain activation after 20 minutes of sitting and 20 minutes of walking. The red and yellow areas (after exercise) indicate activation of the brain.

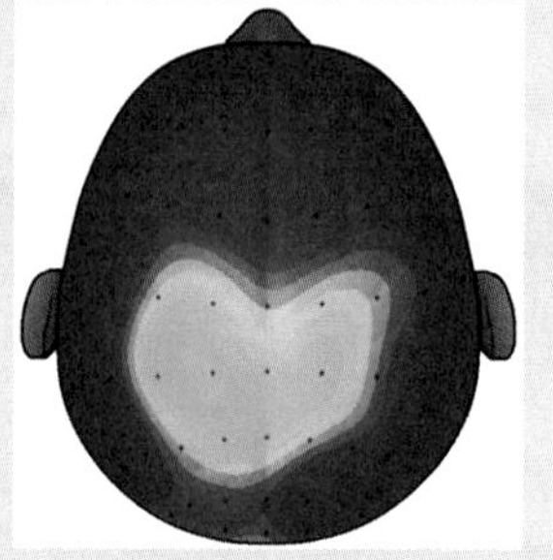

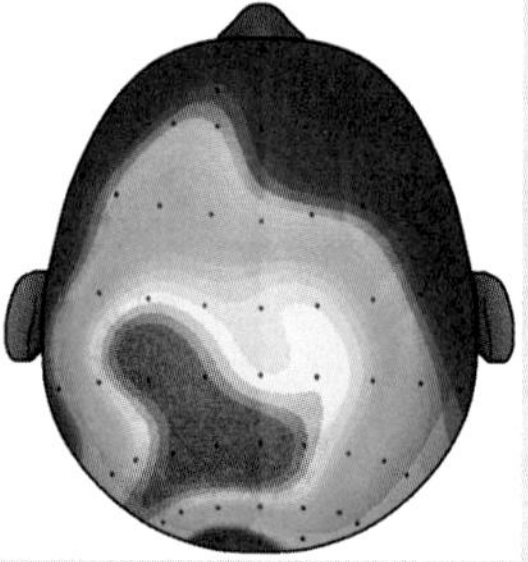

Brain activation: *(a)* after 20 minutes of sitting; *(b)* after 20 minutes of walking.

Reprinted from *Neuroscience*, Vol. 159, C.H. Hillman et al., "The Effect of acute treadmill walking on cognitive control and academic achievement in preadolescent children," pgs. 1044-1054, copyright 2009, with permission of Elsevier.

The CDC report and the University of Illinois research suggest that classroom-based physical activity, including exercise breaks, can help students perform well both on tests and in academics in general.

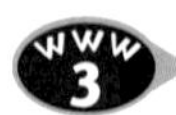

Student Activity

Given the evidence concerning physical activity and academic achievement, create a plan for introducing physical activity in your high school classrooms.

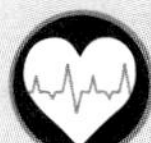

FITNESS TECHNOLOGY: Swim Watches

One good option for your personal physical activity program is swimming, which is an excellent total body activity. It can also be done by most people, including those who have joint problems, who are recovering from an injury, or who are high in body fat and have a hard time with other forms of exercise. To help you self-monitor your swimming activity, consider using a swim watch. These waterproof devices are worn on the wrist and have a built-in accelerometer similar to the technology used in activity watches to monitor steps in walking or running. Most swim watches provide information about total time for a swim session, laps completed, pace and total time per lap, total distance covered, stroke type, and stroke length. You can download the information to your computer and store or print records of each workout. The watch can also estimate the number of calories you expend in a swim session.

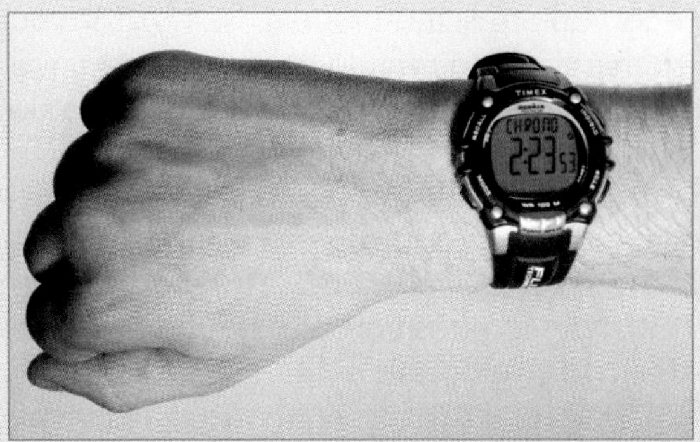

A waterproof swim watch can help you self-monitor swimming activity.

Using Technology

Investigate different types of swim watches and prepare a review. Submit your review to the school newspaper or a school blog.

it. List the activities in your plan that you did complete and those that you didn't complete. For the part of your plan that you didn't complete, list your reasons why not (for example, bad weather or homework). Perform tests of fitness to see if you met your fitness goals. Next, prepare a written evaluation of your program. To help you with this evaluation, answer the following questions.

- Do you think your daily plan is one you can regularly complete?
- Do you think you need to make any changes in your program?
- What changes would you make in your program and why?

Evaluating your program will help you determine how well it's working for you. If you're not meeting your goals, revise your program so that you can perform activities that will meet them.

Lesson Review

1. How do you build a fitness and physical activity profile?
2. What are the five steps in planning a personal fitness program? Describe each step.
3. How does physical activity enhance academic performance?

SELF-ASSESSMENT: Your Personal Fitness Test Battery

As you've worked your way through part 1 of this book, you've had the opportunity to take many physical fitness tests. The tests available to you are listed in table 14.1. After you finish this class, you would be wise to continue assessing your fitness, but it's not reasonable to perform all the tests you've done here. To simplify things, you can prepare your own fitness test battery that includes tests from each of the four categories (cardiorespiratory endurance, body composition, muscle fitness, and flexibility) listed in table 14.1. A test battery refers to several tests designed to measure all parts of fitness. Use the following guidelines in choosing tests for your test battery.

- For cardiorespiratory endurance choose at least one test.
- For flexibility choose at least two of the three tests available.
- For body composition choose at least one test.
- For muscle fitness choose at least one test for the arms and upper body, one test for the trunk and abdominals, and one test for the lower body. Consider including tests for different parts of muscle fitness (muscular endurance, strength, power).
- Choose tests for which you have adequate equipment.
- Choose tests that you think you're likely to actually do.
- Use a chart similar to table 14.1 to select tests for your battery.

Perform the tests in class, then retest yourself from time to time to see how you're doing and to help you set future fitness and physical activity goals. If you're working with a partner, remember that self-assessment information is personal and considered confidential. It shouldn't be shared with others without the permission of the person being tested.

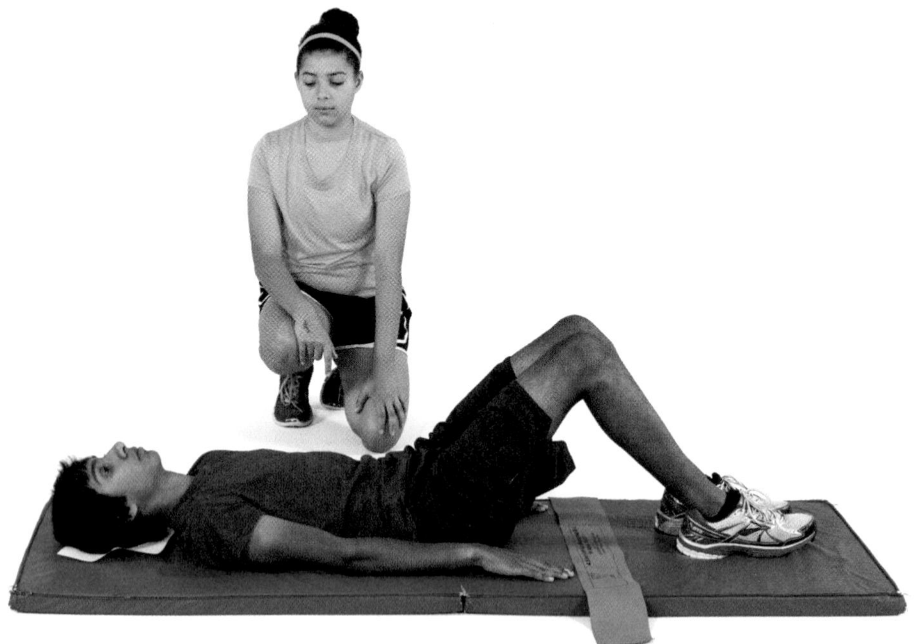

Create your own fitness test battery to track your fitness over time and help you prepare future personal plans.

TABLE 14.1 Choices for Your Personal Fitness Test Battery

Self-assessment	Place a ✔ to select a test
Cardiorespiratory endurance	
PACER	
Step test	
Walking test	
One-mile run	
Muscle fitness	
Curl-up	
Push-up	
Side stand	
Sitting tuck	
Arm press 1RM (per lb of body weight)	
Leg press 1RM (per lb of body weight)	
Grip strength (right)	
Grip strength (left)	
Standing long jump	
Medicine ball throw	
Body composition	
Height–weight (based on BMI)	
Skinfold measures	
Waist-to-hip ratio	
Waist girth	
Flexibility	
Back-saver sit-and-reach	
Trunk lift	
Arm, leg, and trunk flexibility tests	

Lesson 14.2

Maintaining Active Lifestyles

Lesson Objectives

After reading this lesson, you should be able to

1. list and describe several self-management skills that help you maintain physical activity throughout life,
2. define *attitude* and describe several positive and negative attitudes about physical activity, and
3. explain ways to create positive attitudes about physical activity and reduce negative ones.

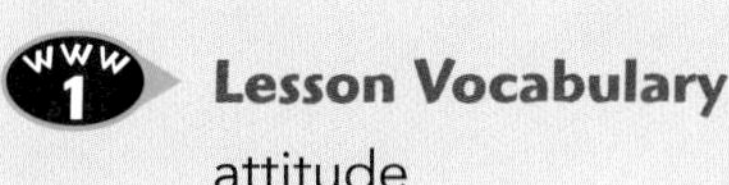

Lesson Vocabulary

attitude

Now that you have learned how to plan your comprehensive physical activity program, do you think you will be able to perform your plan on a regular basis? Consider the information that follows to help you stick with your plan.

Stages of Change and Self-Management Skills

As you learned earlier, there are five stages of change that people go through in adopting healthy lifestyles such as being regularly active. By now, you have probably moved well past the first three stages of change (see table 14.2) and are either at the stage of action or maintenance. The goal is to reach the stage of maintenance and stay there. There are several things that you can do to increase the likelihood that you will maintain your active lifestyle throughout life. One thing that you can do is use the self-management skills that you learned about in each of the chapters of part 1 of this book. Table 14.3 provides a review of the different self-management skills. Research shows that people who use self-management skills are more active and stay in the top stage of change (maintenance) over the long haul.

Strengthening Positive Attitudes and Avoiding Negative Attitudes

Another important thing that you can do is to adopt positive attitudes about physical activity. A physical activity plan is worthwhile only if you carry it out, and that is determined in large part by your attitudes. The word **attitude** refers to your feelings about something. We all have attitudes about food, subjects of study, music, clothing, and many other topics—including physical activity. Active people have more positive attitudes toward physical activity

TABLE 14.2 Five Stages of Physical Activity

Stage of physical activity	Description
5. Active exerciser (maintenance)	Active on a regular basis. Can overcome obstacles that may discourage others.
4. Activator (action)	Active but participates inconsistently.
3. Planner (planning to change)	Has taken steps to get ready to be active, such as buying special clothing or equipment.
2. Contemplation (thinking about change)	Not active but thinking about becoming active.
1. Precontemplation (not thinking about change)	Sedentary living; does no regular activity.

TABLE 14.3 Self-Management Skills for Fitness, Health, and Wellness

Skill	Description
Self-assessment	This skill helps you see where you are and what to change in order to get where you want to be.
Building knowledge and understanding	You can use a modified form of the scientific method to solve problems—such as how to make healthy changes in your life.
Identifying risk factors	Identifying your health risks enables you to assess and then reduce them.
Positive attitude	This skill helps position you to succeed in adopting healthy lifestyles.
Self-confidence	This skill helps you build the feeling that you're capable of making healthy changes in your lifestyles.
Goal setting and self-planning	These skills create a foundation for developing your personal plan by setting goals that are SMART (specific, measurable, attainable, realistic, and timely) and preparing a written schedule.
Time management	This skill helps you be efficient so that you have time for the important things in your life.
Choosing good activities	This skill involves selecting the activities that are best for you personally so that you will enjoy and benefit from doing them.
Learning performance skills	This skill helps you perform well and with confidence. For example, learning motor skills helps you become active, learning stress-management skills helps you avoid or reduce stress, and learning nutrition skills helps you eat well.
Improving self-perception	This skill helps you think positively about yourself so that you're more likely to make healthy lifestyle choices and feel that they will make a difference in your life.
Stress management	This skill involves preventing or coping with the stresses of daily life.
Self-monitoring	This skill involves keeping records (logs) to see whether you are in fact doing what you think you're doing.
Overcoming barriers	This skill helps you find ways to stay active despite barriers, such as lack of time, temporary injury, lack of safe places to be active, inclement weather, and difficulty in selecting healthy foods.
Finding social support	This skill enables you to get help and support from others (such as your friends and family) as you adopt healthy behaviors and work to stick with them.
Saying "no"	This skill helps keep you from doing things you don't want to do, especially when you're under pressure from friends or other people.
Preventing relapse	This skill helps you stick with healthy behaviors even when you have problems getting motivated.
Thinking critically	This skill enables you to find and interpret information that helps you make good decisions and solve problems in living a healthy lifestyle.
Resolving conflicts	This skill helps you solve problems and avoid stress.
Positive self-talk	This skill helps you perform your best and make healthy lifestyle choices such as being active by thinking good thoughts rather than negative ones that detract from success.
Developing good strategy and tactics	This skill helps you focus on a specific plan of action and successfully execute the plan.
Finding success	Finding success is technically not a skill. Finding success is something that comes from using a variety of self-management skills to change behavior. If you use the self-management skills described in this table, and believe that they will help you to succeed, your chances of success improve dramatically.

than negative ones. If you follow certain guidelines, you can strengthen your positive attitudes and get rid of any negative ones (see the Self-Management feature later in this chapter).

FIT FACT

Active teens have more positive attitudes than negative attitudes. This state of mind is called a positive balance of attitudes.

Active people have more positive than negative attitudes. Here's a list of reasons that people like to be physically active. Think about these attitudes and how you might make some of them your own.

- **"Physical activities are a great way to meet people."** Many activities provide opportunities to meet people and strengthen friendships. For example, aerobic dance and team sports are good social activities.
- **"I think physical activity is really fun."** Many teenagers do activities simply because they're fun. Participating in activities you enjoy also helps you reduce stress.
- **"I enjoy the challenge."** When the famous mountain climber George Mallory was asked why he climbed Mount Everest, he replied, "Because it's there." Helen Keller was deaf and blind but became a famous author. She said in one of her books that "life is either a daring adventure or nothing at all." Some people just enjoy a challenge. Are you one of them?
- **"I like the rigor of training."** Some people enjoy intense training. For these people, competition and winning can be secondary to training.
- **"I like competition."** If you enjoy competition, sport and other physical activities provide ways to test yourself against others. You can even compete against yourself by trying to improve your score or time in an activity.
- **"Physical activity is my way of relaxing."** Physical activity can help you relax mentally and emotionally after a difficult day—for example, a day of demanding schoolwork.
- **"I think physical activity improves my appearance."** Physical activity can help you build muscle and control body fat. Remember, however, that regular activity cannot completely change your appearance.
- **"Physical activity is a good way to improve my health and wellness."** As you are learning from this book, regular physical activity helps you resist illness and improves your general sense of well-being.
- **"Physical activity just makes me feel good."** Many people just feel better when they exercise, and many have a sense of loss or discomfort when they don't exercise.

> "The greatest discovery of my generation is that human beings can alter their lives by altering their attitudes."
>
> —William James, American philosopher

Changing Negative Attitudes

WWW 3

The following list shows you some negative attitudes, along with suggestions for turning them into positive ones. To decrease any negative attitudes you may have, give some thought to the suggested alternative.

Negative: "I don't have the time."

Positive: "I will plan a time for physical activity." If you planned time for physical activity, you would feel better, function more efficiently, and therefore have more time to do other things that you want to do.

Negative: "I don't want to get all sweaty."

Positive: "I'll allow time to clean up afterward." Sweating is a natural by-product of a good workout. Allow yourself time to change before exercising and to shower and change afterward. Focus on how good you will feel.

Negative: "People might laugh at me."

Positive: "When they see how fit I get, they'll wish they were exercising too." Find friends who are interested in getting fit. Anyone who does laugh may simply be jealous of your efforts and results.

Negative: "None of my friends work out, so neither do I."

Positive: "I'll ask my friends to join me, and maybe we'll work out together." Talk with your friends. Some of them may be interested in working out or doing lifestyle activities together.

Negative: "I get nervous and feel tense when I play sports and games."

Positive: "Everyone gets nervous. I'll stay as calm as I can and do the best I can." Many athletes learn techniques to reduce their stress levels. You can learn them too.

Negative: "I'm already in good condition."

Positive: "Physical activity will help me stay in good condition." Use the self-assessments in this book, then take an honest look at yourself. Are you as fit as you thought? Physical activity can help you get in shape and stay in shape.

Negative: "I'm too tired."

Positive: "I'll just do a little to get started, then as I get more fit I'll do more." You'll probably find that once you get started, physical exertion gives you *more* energy. Begin realistically, then gradually increase the amount of activity you do.

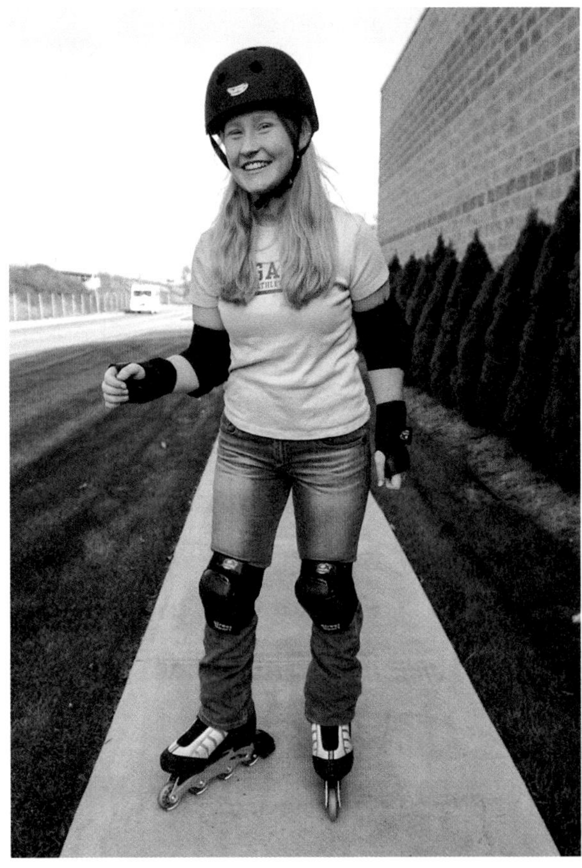

Physical activity can be fun and challenging.

FIT FACT

The U.S. guideline for teens calls for doing 60 minutes of physical activity on each day of the week. This goal is met by only 29 percent of high school students, and 14 percent don't do 60 minutes of physical activity on any day of the week.

Lesson Review

1. What are some self-management skills that you can use to maintain physical activity throughout life?
2. What is an attitude, and what are some common positive and negative attitudes about physical activity?
3. What are some things you can do to build positive attitudes and reduce negative ones?

TAKING CHARGE: Changing Attitudes

Allen and Matt are friends who often do things together, including sport activities. Sometimes they play tennis together on the weekend. Lately, Allen has been winning most of their matches.

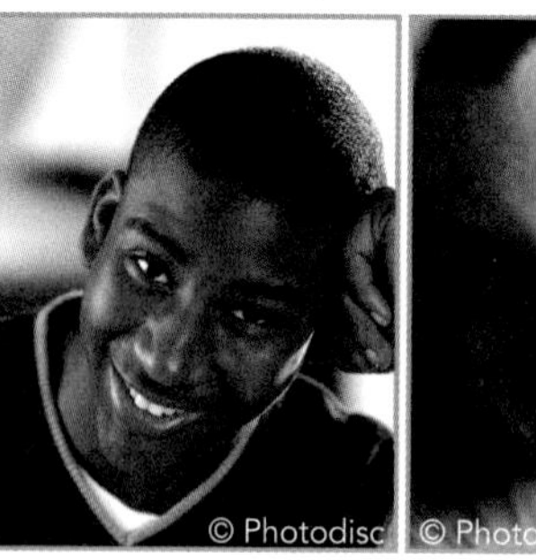

© Photodisc

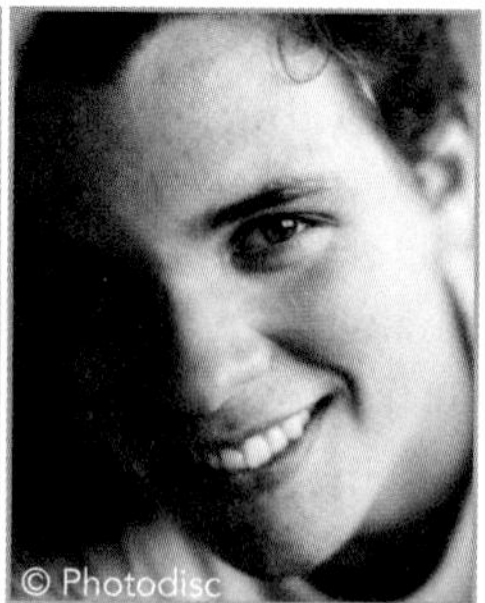

© Photodisc

"You ready to hit the court?" Allen asked Matt as he grabbed his tennis racket.

"I don't feel like playing today," Matt said. "Anyway, there's a good show on TV." He walked into the family room and sat on the couch.

Allen followed him. "I think you just don't want to lose again."

"You're right," Matt admitted. "I hate losing."

"You win sometimes, Matt. The competition is what makes tennis fun."

"Not when I lose," Matt replied.

Allen thought for a minute. "How about taking a jog around the block?" he asked. "There'll be no winner or loser that way."

"I don't want to get all sweaty," Matt replied. "I'd rather relax watching TV."

"Oh, come on, Matt. Jogging will help you relax. We need to stay in shape."

Matt looked at Allen and said, "I'm thinking about it."

For Discussion

What does Allen like about being physically active? What does Matt like—and not like—about physical activity? How could Matt change his negative attitudes and become more active? What are some other negative attitudes that keep people from being active, and how can they be changed? What are some positive attitudes that help people stay active? Consider the information in the Self-Management section when answering the discussion questions.

SELF-MANAGEMENT: Skills for Building Positive Attitudes

Most of us have had both positive and negative attitudes about physical activity at one time or another. Experts have shown that people with more positive attitudes toward physical activity than negative ones are likely to be active. Use the following guidelines to build positive attitudes and get rid of negative ones.

- **Assess your attitudes.** Make a list of your positive and negative attitudes. You can use the attitudes listed in this lesson to help you.
- **Identify your reasons for any negative attitudes.** Your self-assessment will help you identify any negative attitudes you hold. Ask yourself why you feel negative about physical activity. If you can find the reason, it may help you change. For example, you may not have liked playing a sport when you were young because you didn't like a particular coach or player. Maybe you can now find a situation that will make an activity more fun. Consider the alternatives to negative attitudes described earlier in this chapter.
- **Find activities that bring out fewer negative attitudes.** People have different attitudes and feelings about different activities. For example, maybe you don't like team sports but you do enjoy recreational activities. List your negative attitudes, then ask yourself whether there are activities you don't dislike. If so, consider trying them.
- **Choose activities that accentuate the positive.** If you really like certain activities and feel good about them, focus on these activities rather than ones you don't like as much.
- **Change the situation.** You may feel negatively about an activity because of things unrelated to the activity. For

example, if you hated playing basketball because you had too little time to get dressed and groomed after participating, maybe you can find a situation in which you can do the activity and also have more time to shower and dress.

- **Be active with friends.** Activities are often more fun when you do them with friends. Sometimes participating with other people you like is enough to change your feelings about an activity.
- **Discuss your attitudes.** Just talking about your attitudes can sometimes help. People sometimes think they're the only ones who have problems in certain situations. Talking about it with others can help you change the situation to make it more fun for everyone concerned.
- **Help others build positive attitudes.** The ways in which others react can affect a person's feelings about physical activity. Your positive reactions can help others change negative feelings about physical activity. Consider the following suggestions when you interact with others in physical activity.
    - **Instead of laughing, provide encouragement.** Do you remember how difficult it is to start something new or different? You can encourage others by making statements such as, "Good to see you exercising. Way to go!"
    - **Try to make new friends through participation in physical activities.** Introduce yourself to others and offer to help others when appropriate.
    - **Don't hesitate to ask for help from others.** Start or join a sport or exercise club at school. An activity club can be a great way for you and your friends to combine socializing with physical activity. If you're thinking about starting a club, check with your school's activity coordinator first.
    - **Be sensitive to people with special needs.** Some people need certain accommodations or modifications when performing physical activity. People with no special needs can help by participating with those who do have special challenges and by being sensitive to their needs.
    - **Be considerate of differences.** The popularity of physical activities varies from culture to culture. What is popular in one culture is not necessarily popular in another. For example, field hockey and curling are not popular in the United States but are very popular in other countries. Similarly, what one person enjoys may not be so enjoyable to another. Learning to accept cultural and personal differences helps all people enjoy activity and contributes to better interpersonal understanding.

TAKING ACTION: Your Physical Activity Plan

You've learned how to prepare a physical activity plan and have already done some planning for certain types of activity included in the Physical Activity Pyramid. Now you'll prepare a comprehensive written plan for personal physical activity that includes many types of physical activity. You will not be able to perform your full program in class, but you can start trying it out in class. **Take action** by performing one day of your personal physical activity plan in class. Choose a day from your program that includes enough activities to fill a full class period. If no single day's activities last as long as one class period, supplement your program for that day with activity planned for another day. If needed equipment is not available for your chosen activity, select a different activity that offers similar benefits and is one that you're likely to enjoy.

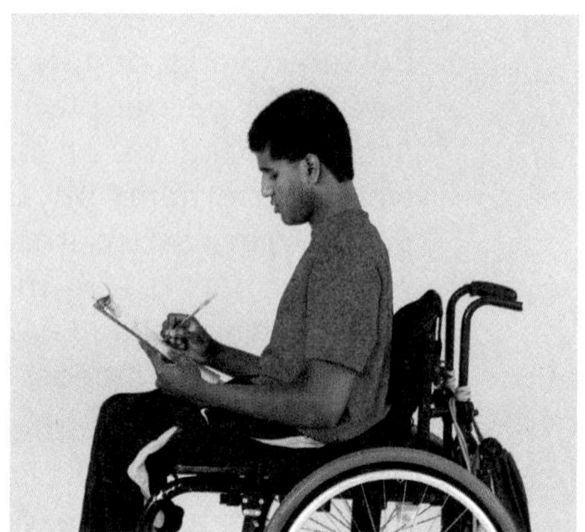

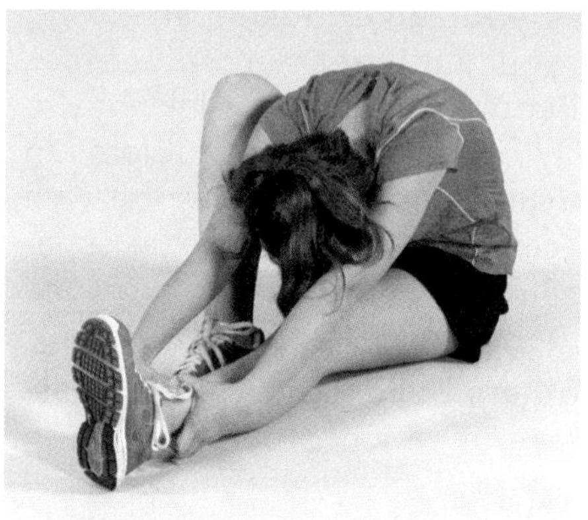

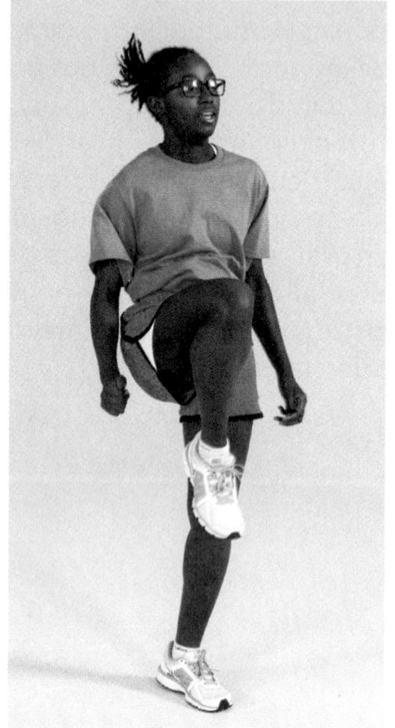

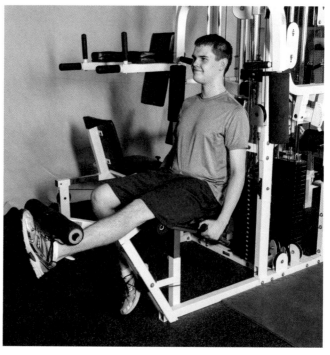

Take action by performing your physical activity plan.

Reviewing Concepts and Vocabulary

As directed by your teacher, answer items 1 through 5 by correctly completing each sentence with a word or phrase.

1. A _______________ is a brief summary of your fitness self-assessment results.
2. _______________ is an acronym used to characterize good goals for your program.
3. A device that can be used in the water to monitor physical activity is called a _______________.
4. A self-management skill that helps you see where you are and what you need to change is called _______________.
5. A/An _______________ refers to how you feel about something.

For items 6 through 10, as directed by your teacher, match each term in column 1 with the appropriate word or phrase in column 2.

6. Stage of change 1 for physical activity	a. sometimes active
7. Stage of change 2 for physical activity	b. sedentary
8. Stage of change 3 for physical activity	c. thinking about it
9. Stage of change 4 for physical activity	d. maintenance
10. Stage of change 5 for physical activity	e. planner

For items 11 through 15, as directed by your teacher, respond to each statement or question.

11. Explain why constructing a fitness profile is an important part of collecting information for program planning.
12. Explain the link between academic performance and regular physical activity.
13. Describe the steps in preparing a personal physical fitness test battery.
14. Describe some of the most common positive attitudes about physical activity.
15. Describe several guidelines for turning negative attitudes into positive attitudes.

Thinking Critically

Write a paragraph to answer the following question.

Why is it important to develop your own fitness program and not just use one developed for someone else?

Project

Fitnessgram is the national youth fitness test for the President's Youth Fitness Program. Many of the self-assessments you performed in this book are derived from Fitnessgram.

Build a fitness profile by summarizing your results on all of the Fitnessgram self-assessments. Use the worksheet provided by your teacher or enter your results on the Fitnessgram website (your school must be enrolled for you to use the site). If you choose, you can share your fitness profile with your parents or guardians. You may also want to encourage them to perform health-related fitness assessments of their own.

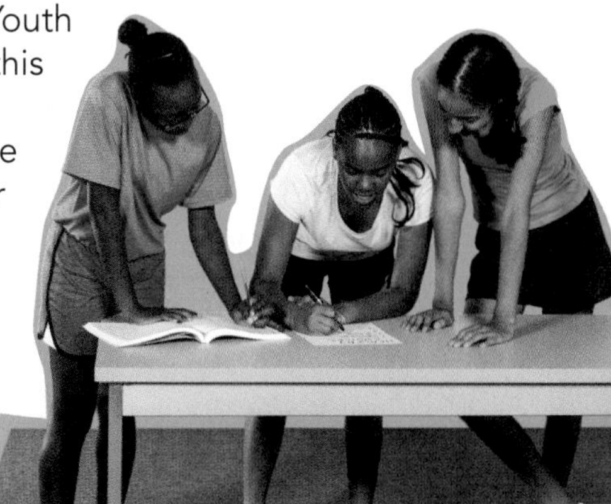

15

Making Good Consumer Choices

In This Chapter

www **Student Web Resources**
www.HOPEtextbook.org/student

Lesson 15.1

Health and Fitness Quackery

Lesson Objectives

After reading this lesson, you should be able to

1. explain the difference between quackery and fraud;
2. explain the importance of being an informed consumer in the area of fitness, health, and wellness;
3. name some reliable sources of health- and fitness-related information; and
4. describe some examples of health and fitness misconceptions and quackery.

Lesson Vocabulary

con artist, electrolyte, fraud, passive exercise, quack, quackery

You've probably come across ads for health and fitness products and services in newspapers and magazines and on radio, television, and the web. Is a product or service effective simply because it is advertised? Would you buy the product advertised in figure 15.1? In this lesson, you'll learn how to become a wise consumer (purchaser) of health and fitness products.

What Is Quackery?

Some people are in a hurry to lose body fat or gain muscle. Often, people who want quick results are persuaded to purchase useless health or fitness products or services. In other words, they become victims of **quackery**—a method of advertising or selling that uses false claims to lure people into buying products that are worthless or even harmful. Some people who practice quackery actually believe their products work; thus they may have good intentions but still do harm. A person who practices quackery is sometimes referred to as a **quack**.

Some people who practice quackery are guilty of **fraud**. People who practice fraud try to deceive you and get you to buy products or services that they *know* are ineffective or harmful. A person who practices fraud is called a **con artist**. Because what they do is often illegal, con artists may be convicted of a crime.

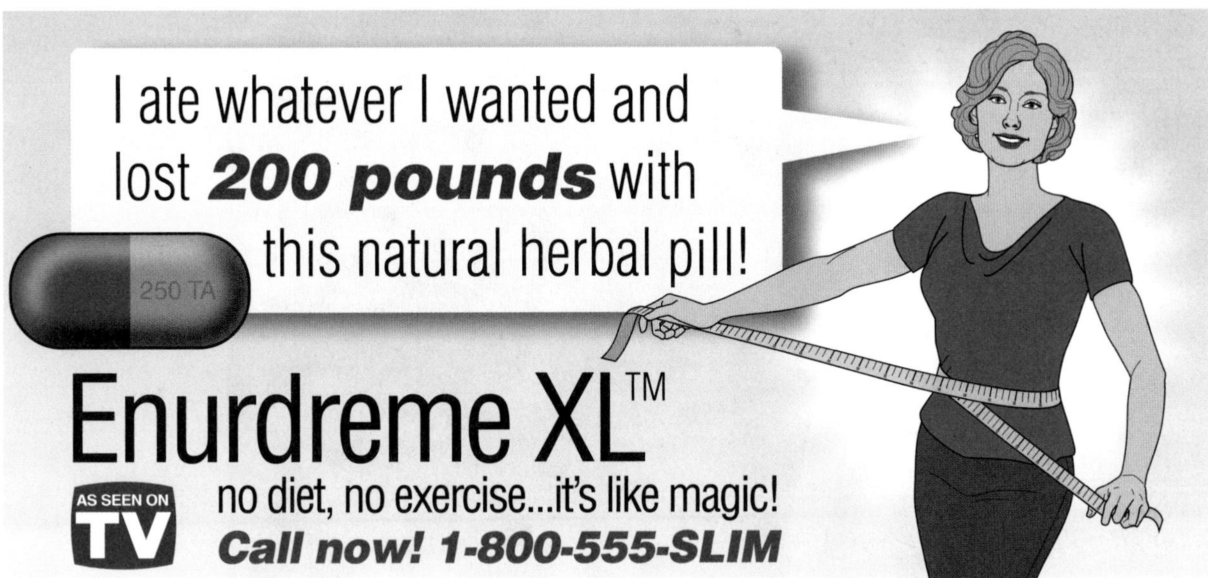
I ate whatever I wanted and lost 200 pounds with this natural herbal pill!
250 TA
Enurdreme XL™
AS SEEN ON TV
no diet, no exercise...it's like magic!
Call now! 1-800-555-SLIM

FIGURE 15.1 Some advertisements make false claims about fitness products and supplements.

The common saying, "If it seems too good to be true, it's probably untrue!" cautions buyers that con artists are good at making you believe they're offering you a good deal. But deals that seem exceptionally good are often not as good as the con artist makes them seem.

> "Modern health quacks are super-salesmen. They play on fear. They cater to hope. And once they have you, they'll keep you coming back for more . . . and more . . . and more."
>
> —Stephen Barrett and William T. Jarvis of the Quackwatch website

Detecting Quackery and Fraud

People who commit quackery and fraud use a variety of deceptive practices to get you to buy their products or services or use products they endorse. Separating fact from fiction can be difficult. Use the guidelines presented in the following sections to help you spot health and fitness quackery and fraud.

Check Credentials

Be sure that the person you think is an expert really is an expert. A con artist might claim to be a doctor or to have a college or university degree. However, the degree might be in a subject unrelated to health and physical fitness. It might also come from a nonaccredited school; it might even be falsified. You can verify credentials by checking with your local or state health authorities or with professional organizations.

If you have questions about health or fitness, ask a real expert's advice. For example, physical education teachers have a college degree that requires them to study all branches of kinesiology. Some other fitness leaders are certified by a group such as the American College of Sports Medicine. For medical advice, talk to a physician (MD or DO) or a registered nurse (RN). For questions about general health, ask a certified health education teacher. For questions about using exercise to rehabilitate from injury, consult a registered physical therapist (RPT). All of these experts have college degrees and relevant training in their area of specialization.

For questions about diet, food, and nutrition, consult a registered dietitian (RD). Be aware that a person who uses the title of nutritionist is not necessarily an expert. Similarly, staff members in health clubs are often not required to hold college degrees. Practitioners certified by a well-respected organization are more qualified than those without certification, but certification without a degree is not adequate to be considered an expert. Neither nutritionists nor health club employees are considered

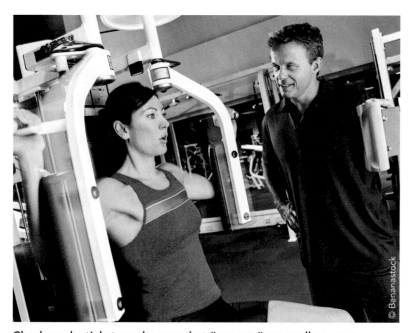
© Bananastock

Check credentials to make sure that "experts" are really experts.

reliable sources of health or fitness information unless they hold the credentials described here.

FIT FACT

Caveat emptor is a Latin phrase that means "let the buyer beware." People who commit fraud make promises that they know they cannot or will not keep, and buyers must beware of people trying to sell fraudulent products. However, if a seller makes a promise (warranty) for a product, it must be fulfilled.

Check the Organizations of the Experts You Consult

Quacks and con artists sometimes try to get you to believe that they know more than experts from well-known organizations such as those listed in the Consumer Corner feature. Be wary of people who claim they know more than well-known experts or who try to discredit respected organizations.

Quacks and con artists also use names and initials of phony organizations with important-sounding names that are similar to the names of well-known organizations. But anyone can form an organization and use it to try to impress you. Check the background of anyone who claims to be a member of an organization whose name you've never heard.

As a consumer, you need to be informed about the products and services you use. Do not assume that every advertised product is safe and effective. Corporations do not always live up to their claims for their products. For example, the Federal Trade Commission (FTC) recently stopped two famous shoe companies from making untrue claims (for details, see the relevant Fit Fact in the second lesson of this chapter). In another example, a study by the American Council on Exercise found so-called "hologram bracelets," commonly worn by many famous athletes, to be ineffective. The bracelets' maker falsely claimed that they improved fitness in areas such as strength, flexibility, and balance.

So remember: The fact that a famous person uses a product does not mean that it is safe or effective. Agencies such as the ones named in the Consumer Corner feature can provide accurate information, but they do not police all products. In many cases, *you* are the one who has to make the final decision about buying a product or service. Being informed can help you stay safe and avoid spending money on worthless products.

Guidelines for Preventing Quackery and Fraud

Consider the following guidelines before purchasing a product or service.

Be Wary of Advisors Who Sell Products

People who sell products make money by selling them, and salespeople often have little training in

CONSUMER CORNER: Reliable Consumer Groups

Many organizations work to protect consumers from misleading advertising and quackery. U.S. governmental agencies that do this type of work include the Centers for Disease Control and Prevention, the Consumer Product Safety Commission, the Federal Trade Commission, the Food and Drug Administration, the Department of Agriculture, and the U.S. Postal Service. Some reputable private organizations include the Society of Health and Physical Educators, the American College of Sports Medicine, the American Medical Association, the American Dental Association, the Academy of Nutrition and Dietetics, the Better Business Bureau, Consumer Reports, the Cooper Institute, the Mayo Clinic, and the National Council Against Health Fraud.

The groups listed here maintain websites that provide reliable health information. However, some other popular websites are unreliable. As a consumer, you need to be able to accurately evaluate potential sources of health and fitness information, as well as the quality of products and services offered for purchase.

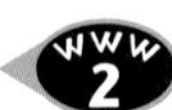

health, fitness, and wellness. For example, people who sell exercise equipment or food supplements may know less about their products than their customers do. In addition, salespeople are often willing to stretch the truth in order to make a sale. With this in mind, consult a true expert before you make a purchase.

Be Suspicious of Sales Pitches That Promise Results Too Good to Be True

Look for words and phrases such as *miracle*, *secret remedy*, *scientific breakthrough*, and *endorsed by movie stars*. A quack or con artist is likely to use these or similar terms in a sales pitch for an item that is useless. Be suspicious if a salesperson promises immediate, effortless, or guaranteed results.

Be Cautious About Mail-Order and Internet Sales

You cannot examine mail-order and Internet-marketed products before buying them. Money-back guarantees may seem to protect you, but a guarantee is only as good as the company that backs it. Unlike a brick-and-mortar store, where you can take a product back and talk to someone in person, mail-order and Internet-based companies may not offer this opportunity. Some have staff members to help you with returns and questions, but many do not. Some also require you to pay return mail costs. Before buying from any source, know the company's return policy. Internet-based companies are usually rated for reliability and quality of service, and you should check a company's rating before buying from it.

SCIENCE IN ACTION: Sport and Energy Drinks

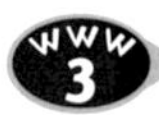

Exercise physiologists, dietitians, and medical scientists work together to investigate heat-related conditions that can result from physical activity, especially during hot weather. In fact, regardless of the weather, you need to keep your body hydrated during exercise to prevent conditions such as heat stress and heatstroke. To replenish the body, researchers have developed flavored "sport drinks" that contain important minerals called **electrolytes**. When appropriate ingredients are used, these drinks can help adults keep their body hydrated during exercise. "Energy drinks" are also popular, but they are not intended primarily to replace fluids lost during exercise. They may contain ingredients similar to those in sport drinks, but they often also contain large amounts of sugar and relatively large amounts of caffeine.

The American Academy of Pediatrics (AAP) has expressed concern about sport and energy drinks because they are often marketed to children and teens via TV, magazines, and the web. The AAP discourages use of these drinks by children and teens and notes that high-caffeine energy drinks have "no place in the diet of children and adolescents." The group further states that sugars in these drinks may be linked to increases in weight and even obesity. The AAP indicate that sport drinks (not energy drinks with caffeine) can be helpful to young athletes who are engaged in "prolonged, vigorous physical activity, but in most cases they are unnecessary on the sport field or in the school lunch room." For most teens who perform the amount of activity recommended by national guidelines, plain water is best.

A separate group of medical doctors has asked the U.S. Food and Drug Administration (FDA) to restrict the amount of caffeine in energy drinks to protect youth from medical problems. Indeed, each year more than 20,000 ER visits involve health problems in which energy drink consumption was a contributing factor. Common problems caused by too much caffeine include fast heart rate, inability to sleep, stomach upset, anxiety, and headache. The FDA has issued warnings indicating that mixing alcohol and caffeine is especially dangerous.

Student Activity

Research a sport or energy drink. Find out about its key ingredients and prepare a report about the possible benefits and dangers associated with the drink.

Be Wary of Product Claims

A favorite trick of some con artists is to claim that a product is "brand new" or is just now being offered for the first time. Others may claim to be "available in the United States for the first time." They try to make you think that you're getting something special. Quacks and con artists may also try to get you to believe their product is popular in Europe, Asia, or some other location. This technique is usually used to impress you. It does not provide any useful information.

Be Wary of Untested Products

Using untested products can be risky. Quacks do not subject their products to thorough scientific testing. Their products are often rushed to market in order to make money as quickly as possible. One way to tell whether a product or service is a good one is to see whether information about it has been published in a respected journal. If so, the study was conducted by a qualified expert.

Health Quackery

The market is flooded with health products, many of which are useless. Although some of these products may not be harmful, false advertising claims give people unrealistic expectations about the benefits they can provide. Indeed, many advertisers promote myths about health and fitness.

FIT FACT

Cellulite is a term often used for fat that causes the skin to look rippled or bumpy. Con artists would have you believe that cellulite is a special kind of fat that can be eliminated with creams or other special products. In fact, cellulite occurs when fat cells become enlarged. It is best reduced by expending more calories than you consume.

Food Supplements

A food supplement is a product that is not part of the typical diet. Supplements are often produced as syrups, powders, or tablets (figure 15.2). Generally, they are sold in health food stores or through the mail. Common supplements include protein (amino acids), vitamins, minerals, and herbs. Packaged food—such as canned goods, boxed goods, and frozen foods—must carry a label that informs you of the product's ingredients. Such labels are *not* required on food supplements.

Most Americans believe that food supplements are regulated by the government in the same way as drugs and foods. This is not true. A law passed in 1994 changed the regulation of supplements from government control to manufacturer control. Manufacturers do not have to prove that a supplement works before they sell it, and the law does not regulate the contents of a supplement. For

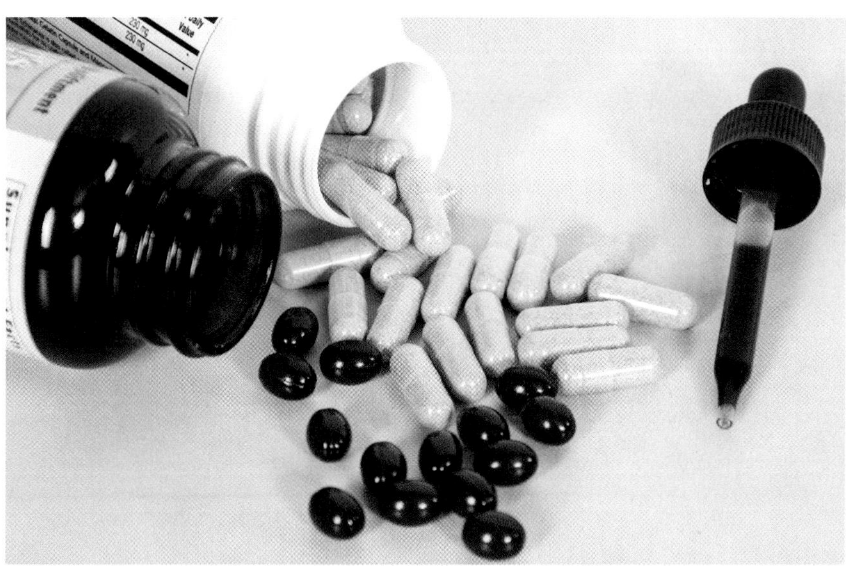

FIGURE 15.2 Food supplements are not regulated by the government.

this reason, you cannot be sure that you're buying what you think you are buying when you purchase a supplement. More than a few people have died from taking supplements that were contaminated or contained ingredients that were not supposed to be in the supplement. Many people have also suffered illness and even death as the result of taking supplements marketed as causing fat loss or enhancing performance. While food supplements are not regulated, the FDA will investigate if enough complaints are received for a specific supplement. The supplement ephedra, for example, has been implicated in several deaths. After an FDA investigation, ephedra was banned by the U.S. Food and Drug Administration.

Some other supplements are not harmful but simply do not provide the benefits promised by those who sell them. Since the regulation of supplements was changed in 1994, the sale of supplements has increased dramatically. Many people are wasting money on products that don't work.

Some supplements can be beneficial if used according to a physician's recommendation. For example, a vitamin B_{12} supplement is recommended for strict vegetarians (vegans), and a folic acid supplement is recommended for expectant mothers. But even vitamins can be dangerous if taken in amounts that are too large. Before you take any supplement, consult with your parent or guardian, as well as your family physician.

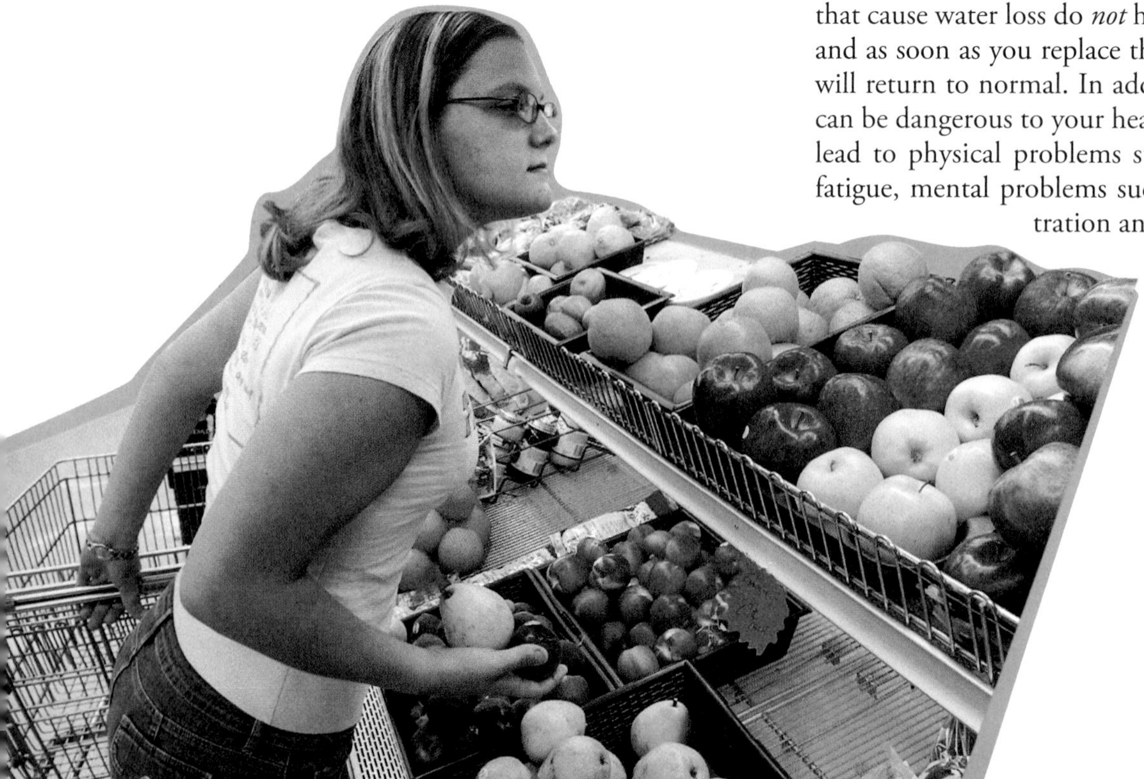

Sport Supplements

One current fad involves the use of sport supplements or sport vitamins—products sold to enhance athletic performance. These supplements are also called ergogenic aids. Many supplements sold as ergogenic aids are actually quack products. Many supplements can also be harmful to your health.

Fad Diets

"Lose pounds a day on the ice cream diet!" "The rice diet works wonders!" "Fruit diet dissolves fat!" How many similar weight-loss claims have you seen? Each of these claims is false and serves as an example of a fad diet. Although fad diets are popular because they usually promise fast results, nearly all are nutritionally unbalanced. They often restrict eating to only one or two food groups, or even one specific food. As you've learned, the only safe and effective way to reduce body fatness and lose weight is to combine physical activity with eating fewer calories. Eating healthy, low-calorie foods can help you control your calorie intake.

Restricting Fluids

It is possible to lose weight in a short time as a result of dehydration. If you do not drink enough fluid, or if you lose excessive water through sweating, you will become dehydrated, thus losing water weight. Some people think this weight loss is permanent. It is not! Restricting fluid intake and taking products that cause water loss do *not* help you lose body fat, and as soon as you replace the fluids, your weight will return to normal. In addition, these practices can be dangerous to your health. Dehydration can lead to physical problems such as headache and fatigue, mental problems such as lack of concentration and mood changes, and heat illnesses such as heat exhaustion and heatstroke.

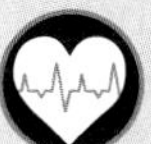

FITNESS TECHNOLOGY: Quack Machines

You've learned in other chapters of part 1 about many technological innovations that can make our lives better. However, not all technological devices are safe and effective. Some unscrupulous people sell devices that not only are ineffective but also can be quite dangerous.

One example is a device with electrodes that are placed on the abdominal muscles. Electrical current is sent through the electrodes, thus stimulating the muscles. People who advertise these devices claim that you can use them to build strong abdominal muscles without doing any regular abdominal exercises, such as crunches or curl-ups. But studies show that these devices do not build fitness. In addition, because the electrodes are placed on the abdomen, they can cause the heart to beat irregularly and result in serious health problems.

Physical therapists do use muscle stimulators to help restore normal muscle function in people who have been injured or who are recovering from illness. These machines can be effective when used by experts for very specific therapeutic purposes. They are not the same as muscle stimulators sold with claims of building abdominal muscle. Be wary of sellers who promise fitness without exercise.

Using Technology

Check with a physical therapist to see how a muscle stimulator works and how it helps people with injury or illness. Also ask for more information about the dangers of using an abdominal muscle stimulator.

Fitness Quackery

Many useless products claim to improve fitness and reduce body fat. Claims for these products are false. Be alert for the following worthless fitness devices and methods.

Passive Exercise Machines

Passive exercise refers to the use of machines or devices that move your body for you and supposedly promote fat reduction and weight loss. Examples include machines with rollers that roll along your hips or legs; vibrating machines that shake certain body areas and are said to "break up" fat cells; and motorized belts, cycles, tables, and rowing machines. The claims made for these products are false. These passive exercise programs are ineffective because your body is moved by outside forces rather than your own muscles.

Figure Wrapping

Figure wrapping involves the use of bandages or nonporous garments to compress body parts. The wraps are sometimes soaked in fluid, or the person may soak in a bath after being wrapped. The wraps are advertised for weight loss or as a method of losing "inches" from the body. In reality, they are not effective for either fat loss or size reduction. They can, however, cause overheating and dehydration and can be extremely dangerous to your health.

An unqualified fitness instructor might recommend that you perform "spot" fat loss exercises. Those who promote spot fat loss claim that fat can be removed from specific spots in the body by performing exercises in a specific location. Research shows, however, that no type of exercise causes fat loss at one specific location.

Lesson Review

1. What are quackery and fraud, and how do they differ?
2. Why is it important to be an informed consumer in the area of fitness, health, and wellness?
3. What are some of the more reliable sources of health-related and fitness-related information?
4. What are some examples of health and fitness misconceptions and quackery?

SELF-ASSESSMENT: Assessing Your Posture

Assessing your posture can help you achieve and maintain good posture and prevent problems that could make you susceptible to quackery.

You can use the following self-assessment to determine whether your posture is as good as it should be. If you find that improvements are needed, you can work at applying proper biomechanics when sitting, standing, and walking.

For this self-assessment, wear exercise clothing or a swimsuit. Work with a partner to determine each other's scores. Record your results as directed by your instructor.

1. Stand sideways next to a string hanging from a point at least 12 inches (30 centimeters) above your head. The string should be weighted at the bottom so that it hangs straight and reaches nearly to the floor. Position yourself so that the string aligns with the side of your ankle bone.
   - Head: Is the ear in front of the line?
   - Shoulders: Are the shoulders rounded? Are the tips of the shoulders in front of the chest?
   - Upper back: Does the upper back stick out in a hump?
   - Lower back: Does the lower back have excessive arch?
   - Abdomen: Does the abdomen protrude beyond the pelvic bone?
   - Knees: Do the knees appear to be locked or bent backward?
2. Now stand with your back to the string so that the string is aligned with the middle of your back.
   - Head: Is more than half of the head on one side of the string?
   - Shoulders: Is one shoulder higher than the other?
   - Hips: Is one hip higher than the other?
3. Add the number of yes answers to get a total score. Then determine your rating on table 15.1.

TABLE 15.1 Rating Chart: Posture Test

Score (yes answers)	Rating
0 or 1	Good posture
2–4	Can use some improvement
≥5	Needs considerable improvement

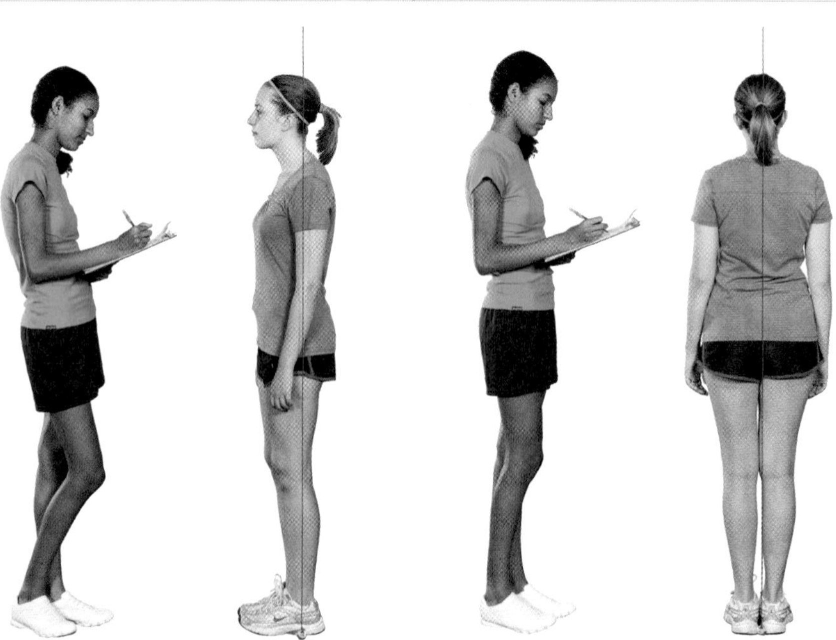

The posture test can help you achieve and maintain good posture.

Lesson 15.2

Evaluating Health Clubs, Equipment, Media, and Internet Materials

Lesson Objectives

After reading this lesson, you should be able to

1. evaluate health-related and fitness-related facilities,
2. describe the proper clothing and equipment for physical activity,
3. evaluate printed materials and video resources related to health and fitness, and
4. describe the guidelines for choosing a good website for health and fitness information.

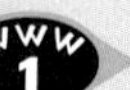

Lesson Vocabulary

spa, web extension

Where do you get your health, fitness, and wellness information? Have you ever considered how that information is created? People in developed countries are more interested in health and fitness now than at any other time in history, and they look to many sources to get it. As a result, many magazines are now totally dedicated to health and fitness, but the leading source of health information throughout the world is the web. In fact, there has been an explosion of health and fitness information, but not all of it is accurate. In this lesson, you'll learn how to evaluate printed material and web resources. First, however, you will learn about health and fitness clubs, where many people seek information delivered in person, as well as exercise clothing and equipment.

Evaluating Health Clubs

You do not need to join a health club, **spa**, or gym to attain or maintain fitness. Health clubs do offer their members special equipment and personnel, and modern spas offer saunas, whirlpool baths, and other services such as massage and hair and skin care. In addition, some people find that joining a club helps motivate them to exercise and remain physically active. But these services are expensive, and well-educated people can save money and still get the benefits of regular exercise by designing their own fitness and activity programs without using special facilities or equipment.

Many low-cost programs are offered through community centers, universities, churches, and other groups. In addition, your school may be among the many that have built their own fitness centers, sometimes called wellness centers. Such programs can give you the same benefits and motivation as more expensive clubs. Still, if you feel that it would help you stay active, you may be interested in joining a commercial club, spa, or gym at some point. Some schools have made cooperative arrangements with fitness clubs that allow their students to work out at special rates or allow school classes to use club facilities. Use the following guidelines when deciding whether to join a health club.

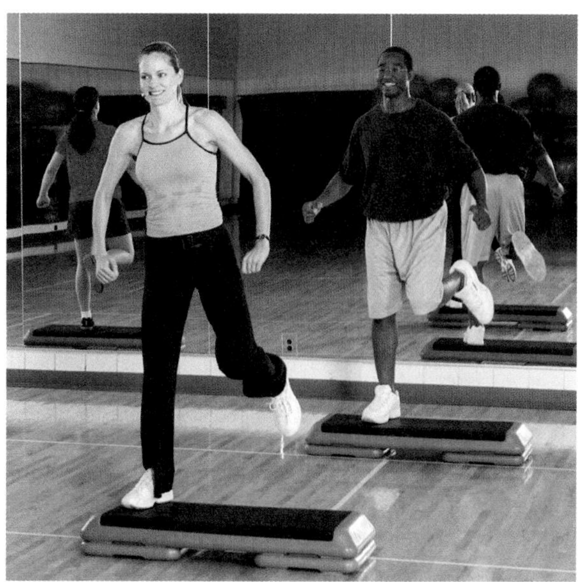

When choosing a club, be sure to pick a well-established club that includes activities you enjoy.

- **If possible, join on a pay-as-you-go basis.** If you sign a contract, make it a short-term one. Read the fine print carefully. Do not sign a contract right away. Too often, people pay a lot for a long-term contract, then stop using the facility. It's best to pay for a short membership until you're sure that you'll stick with it. The fine print may contain special clauses that will cost you money. For example, do you still have to pay if you move? Often, the salesperson pressures you to sign a contract on your first visit, but it's best to think about it for a while before signing.
- **Choose a well-established club.** Such a club is less likely to go out of business. Make sure the facility employs qualified fitness experts such as those described in this chapter. Be alert for signs of fitness quackery; if you see them, consider choosing a different club.
- **Make a trial visit to the club.** Visit at a time when you would normally use the club. Make sure you feel comfortable with the employees and other patrons. Also make sure that the equipment and facilities are available for you to use at that time.
- **Choose a club that meets your personal needs.** For example, a person with joint pain might prefer to avoid harsher activities such as jogging and decide instead to swim for cardiorespiratory endurance. Such a person, of course, should choose a facility that includes a swimming pool.
- **Avoid clubs that cater primarily to bodybuilding for adults.** Research shows that clubs frequented mostly by adults interested in bodybuilding are more likely to sell unproven supplements and even illegal products. Some people who frequent these places subscribe to their own theories and reject scientific evidence developed by experts. Furthermore, practices that may be acceptable for adults are often not appropriate for teens. Find a club that is appropriate for families and teens and employs qualified experts on its staff. Avoid advice from so-called experts with theories that are not consistent with the information provided in part 1 of this book.
- **Consider any medical needs.** If weight loss is your primary goal, consider joining a program recommended by your physician or sponsored by a hospital rather than joining a health club. If you have a special medical need, you may need the help of a physical therapist.

FIT FACT

The U.S. Federal Trade Commission (FTC) reached settlements with two major shoe companies after it was determined that they deceived consumers with their advertisements. The FTC required Reebok and Skechers to refund money to customers because of unsupported claims. Reebok made unsupported claims for its "toning shoes," and Skechers made unsupported claims for its "shape-up" and "tone-up" shoes.

Exercise Equipment

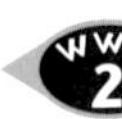

Some people choose not to join a club but to buy home exercise equipment instead. If you're considering home exercise equipment, use the following guidelines.

- **Consider inexpensive home equipment.** For resistance exercise, you can use homemade weights, inner tubes, or rubber or latex bands. To build cardiorespiratory endurance, you can use jump ropes, stepping benches, or stairs. If you're interested in fitness for health and wellness, this equipment may be all you need.
- **Consider your personal needs before buying equipment.** If you're interested in a higher level of fitness for sport or a high-performance job, you might choose to purchase machines or other equipment for use at home. For building muscle fitness, you can use free weights and home exercise machines. For cardiorespiratory endurance, you can use home exercise machines such as treadmills, bicycles, and stair steppers. A regular bicycle is also a good choice if you have a safe place to ride. Exercise equipment is often quite expensive, so it's important to choose well. Rather than depending on the advice of a salesperson, consult an expert, the website of the American College of Sports Medicine, or Consumer Reports. Buy from a well-established company that honors the warranty, services the product, and sells replacement parts.
- **Be sure before you buy.** Avoid investing money in exercise equipment until you're sure you'll use it. Many people buy equipment, then don't use it after the first few months. You can see evidence of this behavior in the many ads for

slightly used equipment. Some of the high-tech equipment described in part 1 of this book, such as pedometers and heart rate watches, can be useful. However, some equipment can be quite expensive, and you may find that you won't use it regularly. See if you can try equipment owned by a friend or by your school before deciding to buy the product. In addition, some high-tech products simply are not worth the cost. For example, expensive electrical devices for measuring body fat level are not worth the personal investment when an inexpensive caliper can give you accurate fat measurements.

- **Make sure you have enough space for the equipment.** One of the main reasons people fail to use the exercise equipment they buy is that they don't have a good place to keep it. If you have to get the equipment out each time you use it or move it from place to place, you're less likely to use it than if you have a room or a place where you can set it up permanently.

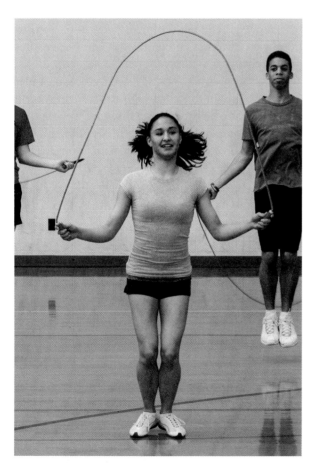

Equipment does not need to be expensive to be helpful in promoting fitness.

> "Spending money is easy. Spending money wisely is another thing altogether."
>
> —U.S. Federal Trade Commission

Evaluating Books and Articles

The growing emphasis on health and fitness has led to the publication of many books and articles on weight control and exercise. Unfortunately, much of the information presented through the media is misleading or incorrect. How can you evaluate health and fitness information that you read, view, or hear? Use the following guidelines to help you decide which information sources are worthwhile.

- **Consider the author's credentials.** The author or consultant should be a registered dietitian, should have completed advanced study in nutrition, or should hold an advanced degree in an exercise-related field such as exercise science, kinesiology, or physical education.
- **Check for sound information.** The book or article should provide information about a balanced diet and physical activity that is consistent with the information presented in part 1 of this book. Books that promise quick and easy fitness or fat loss are not good sources. The information in the book or article should not support techniques used by quacks and con artists (see the first lesson in this chapter). Exercise discussions should address the principles of overload, progression, and specificity, in addition to the FIT formula for each type of physical fitness.
- **Recommended exercises should be safe and effective.** The exercises should require you to use your own muscles (they should not recommend effortless devices). Make sure that the exercises are performed with proper biomechanics.

Evaluating Exercise Videos

You've probably noticed exercise videos for sale and television shows featuring exercises you can perform. Exercise videos are also available for web viewing. Use the following guidelines to help you evaluate an exercise video or show.

- **Check the creator's credentials.** The creator is the person who prepares the exercises, which may then be performed by someone other than the creator. Check to see that the creator has a degree or certification from a reputable institution or organization. Check to see that the person performing the exercises is doing them properly.
- **Choose a video that includes appropriate warm-up and cool-down exercises.** The warm-up and cool-down should be consistent with guidelines provided in part 1 of this book.
- **Make sure the video contains only safe exercises.** Part 1 of this book provides you with information about safe exercises, as well as dangerous exercises to avoid.
- **Choose a video that rotates muscle groups and addresses all parts of fitness.** For example, use arms, then legs, then back, then abdominal muscles, and so on. If the video claims to be a total fitness program, make sure it includes activities for all parts of fitness and rotates them appropriately.
- **Choose a video that is appropriate for you.** Make sure that the activities on the video are appropriate for your skill and fitness level. For example, if it says it is for beginners, are the exercises really for beginners?
- **Make sure the exercises start gradually and progress in intensity.** If the first part of the exercise program is moderate in intensity, it may serve as the warm-up.
- **Choose a video with a fun and interesting routine.** Review the video to see if it includes exercises that you would enjoy doing on a regular basis.
- **If the video does not meet all of these guidelines, modify it.** For example, change the order of the routine to make it better.

Evaluating Internet Resources

We depend on the web more than any other source for health and fitness information. Yet research shows that many web sources provide incorrect information. If you use the web to locate information about health, fitness, and wellness, ask yourself the following questions.

- **Who developed the website?** Websites with the best information are developed by government agencies, professional organizations, and educational institutions. Governmental health agencies' web addresses end with .gov, professional organizations' web addresses end with .org, and education institutions' web addresses end with .edu. Choose websites presented by well-known agencies, organizations, and institutions such as those listed in the Consumer Corner feature in this chapter or the student section of the Health Opportunities Through Physical Education website. Sites with an address ending in .gov, .org, or .edu often provide you with more reliable

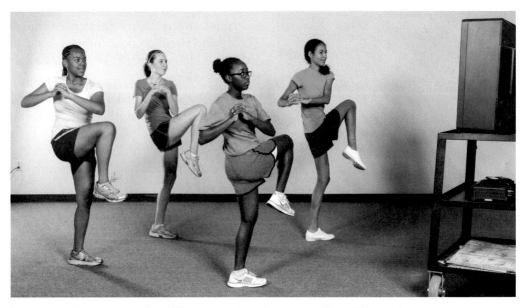

Video exercise routines should be appropriate for your skill and fitness level.

information than sites with an address ending in .com or .net. Remember, however, that any organization can now obtain a .org web address, so that alone does not guarantee that the information on the site is reliable. At the same time, some websites with an address ending in .com or .net do provide good information.

- **Did you reach the website you intended to reach?** In 2013, the Internet Corporation for Assigned Names and Numbers was authorized to offer new **web extensions** (web address endings). As a result, extensions other than the most common ones (.gov, .org, and .com) are now available. Some examples of the newer extensions are .book, .movie, and .app. These are only a few of the 2,000 new extensions that will ultimately be developed. This variety makes it even more difficult to know which websites offer good information. An unscrupulous company may use a web address similar to that of a legitimate company but with a different extension. For example, the website for Health Opportunities Through Physical Education is www.HOPEtextbook.org, and another organization could set up a site with a similar address but a different extension (for example, www.HOPEtextbook.xyz) and thus pretend to be the Health Opportunities Through Physical Education website. Some quacks or con artists use websites with names very similar to legitimate ones in hopes that some people will reach them by accident if they type the intended web address incorrectly. Make sure that you avoid errors when typing health-related web addresses. For more information about good web sources for health and fitness, visit the student section of the Health Opportunities Through Physical Education website.
- **Is the web article a research document, or is it really an advertisement?** The U.S. Federal Trade Commission has cracked down on companies that post web articles falsely appearing to be scientific research. These "fake news" articles are really advertisements. They are not based on real science, and they advertise products that do not work as claimed. Examples include dietary supplements, products that supposedly provide fitness without exercise, and weight loss products. Several companies have paid fines for deceptive practices and have been banned from mounting future promotions. Unfortunately, such companies often make a lot of money before they are caught, and the fines they pay are much smaller than their profits. In light of these practices, you need to make sure that you use information from reliable news sources and scientific journals rather than the fake news articles that often appear in ads and pop-up screens on your computer. You can also visit the FTC's website to see which companies have been caught posting fake news.

FIT FACT

Be wary of advertisements for lotions or creams to improve muscle tone. *Tone* is a term created by advertisers and cannot be easily measured. For this reason, it's easy to claim that creams or lotions can improve tone, but it's very hard to prove. There are no creams or lotions that can improve muscle fitness as measured by legitimate tests of muscle fitness. Place your trust in experts who help you build muscle fitness using sound exercises programs rather than quack products.

To reduce your chances of being deceived by a website, ask yourself the following questions.

- **Does the website sell products?** Websites that sell products are more likely to provide false information than those that do not.
- **Do you recognize any techniques that seem suspicious?** Be wary of websites using the techniques associated with quacks and con artists as described in this chapter.
- **Do experts find the website credible?** The site should be recommended or highly regarded by genuine health and fitness experts.

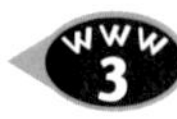

Lesson Review

1. What are some guidelines for evaluating health and fitness clubs?
2. What should you consider before buying exercise equipment?
3. What are the guidelines for evaluating exercise videos and books and articles about health and fitness?
4. What are the guidelines for choosing a good website for health and fitness information?

TAKING CHARGE: Learning to Think Critically

A misconception is a belief based on incorrect or misunderstood information or lack of facts. The best way to counter a misconception is to increase your knowledge so that you can recognize and interpret facts correctly. Here's an example.

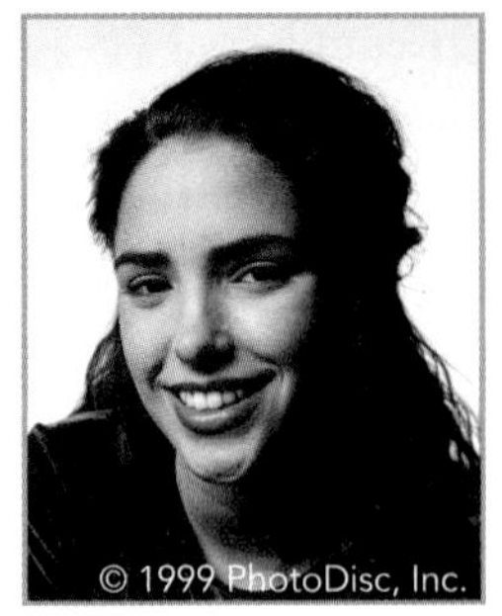

Mary Lou had tried several exercise programs but had not found one that she felt would help her meet her goal of developing muscle fitness. She had never even considered progressive resistance exercise (PRE) because she believed it would cause her to develop big, bulky muscles.

One day, Mary Lou's physical education teacher took her class to the fitness room. There, the teacher explained how to use the free weights and resistance machines for the best benefit. Over the next several weeks, the class practiced the correct use of the PRE equipment. As a class assignment, Mary Lou's teacher had each member of the class find one news article about PRE and write a report on it. In doing her report, Mary Lou learned that muscles do not become bulky if weight training is done properly.

With this new knowledge, Mary Lou realized that the correct PRE program would give her exactly what she was looking for. She began working out with PRE on three days each week. The knowledge she gained about PRE dispelled her original misconceptions. Now Mary Lou is trying to help others change their irrational beliefs about PRE. When friends ask her why she is trying to build big muscles, she tells them, "If muscle fitness is what you're after, you should give resistance training a try."

For Discussion

What misconception did Mary Lou have? How was she able to build knowledge to dispel her misconception? What are some other misconceptions people have about physical activity? Why do you think people have misconceptions about PRE? Consider the guidelines provided in the Self-Management feature when answering the discussion questions.

SELF-MANAGEMENT: Skills for Thinking Critically

Thinking critically means using a problem-solving process before making important decisions. You can use several steps to solve problems and make good choices. These steps are similar to those used in applying the scientific method. The steps are listed here with examples for using each one to help you select exercise equipment. You can use the same steps to solve problems and make decisions about other important topics.

- **Step 1: Identify the problem to be solved or clarify the decision that must be made.** If you know that you want to improve your muscle fitness but are not sure how to do it, you have to define the problem more clearly. Do you want to do your exercises at school, join a health and fitness club, buy exercise equipment, or use inexpensive equipment? You also need to clarify your reasons for wanting to build muscle fitness. Do you want to improve your health, improve your appearance, or get fit for sport performance? For this discussion, let's assume that you want to decide what equipment to use in order to build your muscle fitness for good health. Thus the problem has been clearly defined.
- **Step 2: Collect information and investigate.** One way to collect information relevant to the defined problem is to perform self-assessments for muscle fitness. Knowing your current status will help you to know about areas of personal need so that you can select exercises to meet your needs. You can also consult experts and explore reliable websites, such as those described in this chapter's Consumer Corner feature or in the student section of the Health Opportunities

Through Physical Education website. In this case, you would also want to try out several equipment options, perhaps by using the school exercise room, visiting local health and fitness clubs, or trying out machines on display at a sporting goods store. You could also try several of the inexpensive equipment options you've learned about in part 1 of this book. Focus on finding information that will help you solve the specific problem you've identified in step 1.

- **Step 3: Develop a plan of action.** Use the information gained from your investigation to formulate a plan. For example, your results from step 2 might indicate that the school exercise room is not open when you are free to use it, and perhaps the health and fitness clubs are too far from your home and cost too much. In addition, exercise equipment available in stores can be quite expensive. After rejecting these options, then, you might decide to do elastic band exercises. The equipment is inexpensive, and you can do all the exercises necessary to meet your goal. You might decide to choose several of the exercises described in part 1 of this book. You could then make a written plan specifying the days of the week on which you'll do each exercise and how many sets and reps you'll do each day.
- **Step 4. Put your plan into action.** For a plan to be effective, you must use it. The sooner you begin to act after preparing your plan, the more likely you are to change your behavior. In this example, you would use the plan developed in step 3 to get started with the elastic band exercises.
- **Step 5. Evaluate the effectiveness of your plan.** Use self-monitoring to keep records and use self-assessments (reassessments) to chart your progress. As you go forward, you can continue using the five critical thinking steps presented here to solve problems that arise and make effective decisions about your health, fitness, and wellness.

ACADEMIC CONNECTION: Critical Thinking Skills

Preparing for a career or for college requires critical thinking skills. Education experts have described learning standards for the English language arts that help you prepare. Following are some of the skills needed for success in the workplace and in college:

- **Demonstrating independence.** In addition to being able to understand ideas presented by others, independence requires a person to add to others' ideas and express his or her own thoughts and views.
- **Building strong knowledge of subject matter.** Research and study are required to develop knowledge in different subject matter areas, including health and physical education. This requires extensive reading and attentive listening.
- **Comprehending as well as knowing facts.** Knowing refers to possessing information or facts. Comprehending refers to grasping the significance of information or facts.
- **Valuing evidence.** Evidence refers to something tangible or visible. One step in the scientific method is collecting data (tangible evidence). This evidence can be used to help make decisions or solve problems.
- **Using technology capably.** Modern technology makes a considerable amount of information available in an instant. Capable use of technology requires the ability to evaluate the quality of information acquired from online and other technical sources and the thoughtful use of that information.

Practice the self-management skills in this chapter to help you meet these important standards.

TAKING ACTION: My Health and Fitness Club

You've learned how to plan a personal physical activity program, and by now you're performing it regularly on your own. But you may also enjoy being active with others. Using school facilities and equipment, you can create your own health and fitness club for use during class time. Work with the other students in class to survey the types of activity that class members enjoy.

When putting together a workout for others, consider their current fitness, their skill levels, and their interests. Prepare several exercise stations for which equipment is available. Balance the workout so that a variety of activities are offered and all the parts of health-related fitness are addressed. Have a class member describe the purpose of each exercise station to the rest of the class in a way similar to what a fitness instructor would do at a commercial health or fitness club. **Take action** by having all class members use the health and fitness club to perform a physical activity workout that meets their personal goals. Evaluate the effectiveness of your health and fitness club.

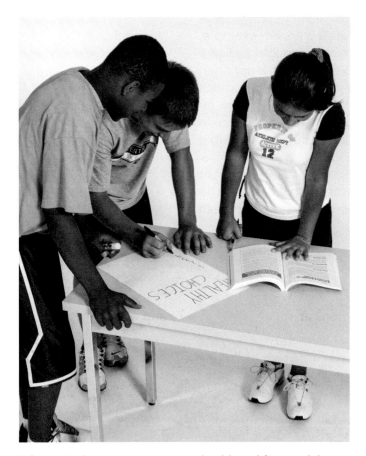

Take action by creating your own health and fitness club.

CHAPTER REVIEW

Reviewing Concepts and Vocabulary

As directed by your teacher, answer items 1 through 5 by correctly completing each sentence with a word or phrase.

1. A method of advertising or selling a health product or service that uses false claims is called ______________.
2. Selling a health product you know to be worthless is called ______________.
3. A ______________ is a product added to the diet rather than being part of the regular diet.
4. ______________ exercise uses machines or outside forces to move your muscles.
5. The extension .gov indicates that a website is associated with the ______________.

For items 6 through 10, as directed by your teacher, match each term in column 1 with the appropriate phrase in column 2.

6. medical doctor	a. may not be an expert
7. certified health education teacher	b. provides medical advice
8. registered physical therapist	c. offers advice about diet and nutrition
9. dietitian	d. has information about exercises
10. nutritionist	e. provides general health information

For items 11 through 15, as directed by your teacher, respond to each statement or question.

11. Describe three ways to recognize quackery.
12. Describe the posture test and why it is important.
13. Describe three guidelines for selecting a fitness or health club.
14. Describe three guidelines for finding good health information on the web.
15. Describe the five steps for critical thinking that you can use to solve problems and make decisions about physical activity and good health.

Thinking Critically

Write a paragraph to answer the following question.

Your friend Lee visited a health food store and got interested in taking a supplement. He says that he can make his own decision because the products must be safe and must work or they wouldn't be on the shelves of the store. What advice would you give your friend? Explain your reasons.

Project

Choose one of the following: Visit a local health club, choose an article about exercise from a popular magazine, view an exercise video, or visit a health or fitness website. Use the guidelines presented in this chapter to evaluate its quality. Write a brief report of your evaluation.

UNIT VI

Moving Through Life

Healthy People 2020 Goals

- Increase the percentage of teens who meet physical activity guidelines for teens.
- Reduce time spent watching television and playing computer games.
- Increase biking to school.
- Improve community facilities to promote activity.
- Increase physical education in schools.
- Increase education to promote health-enhancing behaviors and reduce health risks.
- Increase education designed to prevent inactivity.
- Reduce overweight and obesity among teens.
- Improve teens' comprehension of health promotion and disease prevention concepts.
- Increase the number of people who achieve high-quality, longer lives by reducing preventable disease, injury, and early death.
- Create environments that promote health, fitness, and wellness for all.

Self-Assessment Features in This Unit

- Assessing Game Strategy and Tactics
- Analyzing Basic Skills
- Modifying Rules in Games

Taking Charge Features in This Unit

- Developing Tactics
- Positive Self-Talk
- Conflict Resolution

Self-Management Features in This Unit

- Skills for Developing Tactics
- Skills for Positive Self-Talk
- Skills for Conflict Resolution

Taking Action Features in This Unit

- Cooperative Games
- Applying Principles
- Team Building

16

Strategies for Active Living

In This Chapter

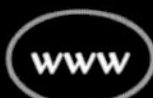

Student Web Resources

www.HOPEtextbook.org/student

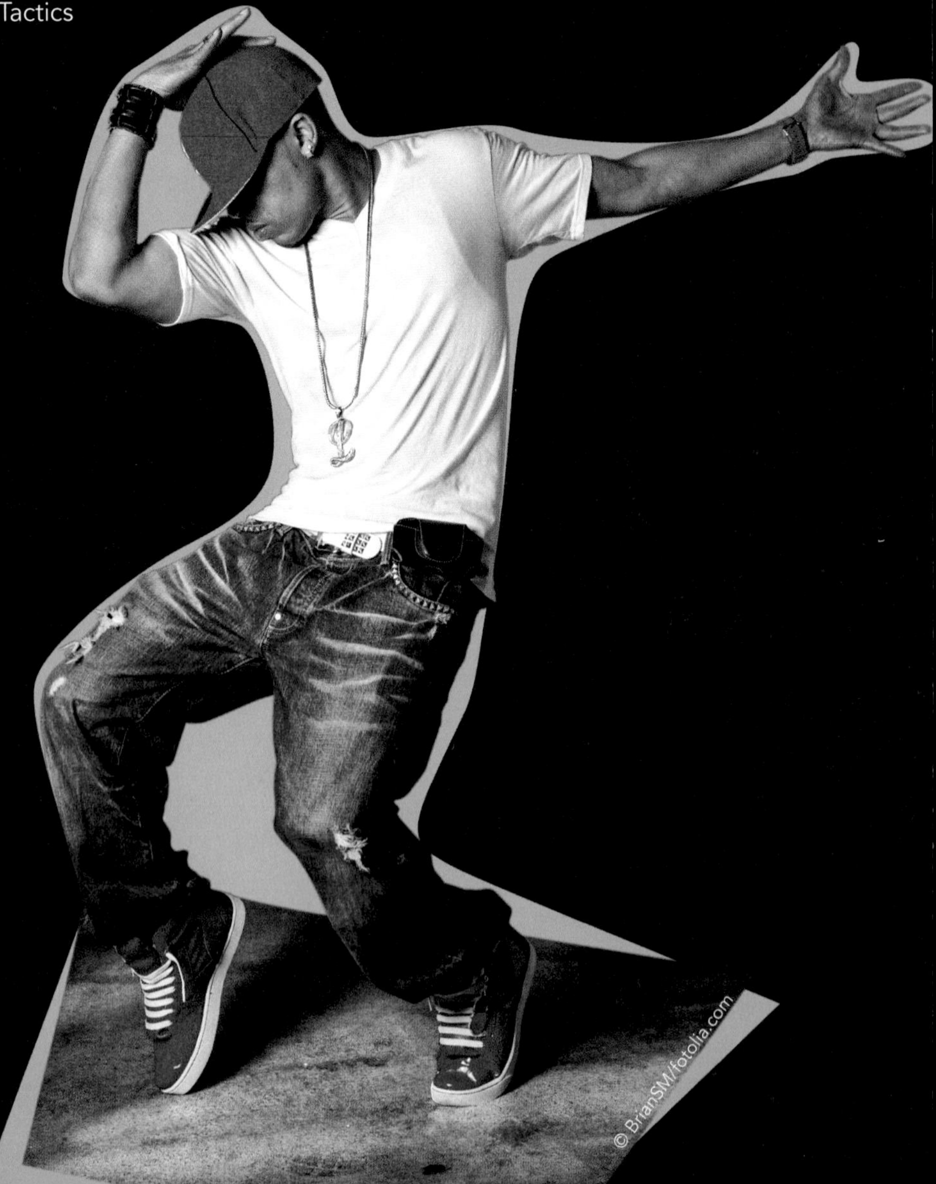

Lesson 16.1

Opportunities in Physical Education

Lesson Objectives

After reading this lesson, you should be able to

1. name the five characteristics of a physically educated person,
2. describe the top 10 reasons that high-quality physical education is needed, and
3. describe several approaches to physical education.

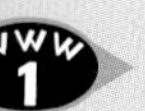

Lesson Vocabulary

adventure education, cooperative game, dance education, fitness education, outdoor education, physical literacy, sport education

Are you physically literate? Do you know what **physical literacy** is? Physical literacy refers to being physically educated. A physically literate (or physically educated) person has the knowledge, skills, and confidence to enjoy a lifetime of healthful physical activity. According to the Society of Health and Physical Educators (SHAPE America), a person who achieves these five goals is considered to be a physically literate or physically educated person. Specifically, a physically literate person

- participates regularly in physical activity,
- is physically fit,
- has learned skills necessary to perform a variety of physical activities,
- values physical activity and its contribution to healthy living, and
- knows the implications and benefits of being involved in physical activities.

Adapted from SHAPE America.

FIT FACT

Literacy refers to being educated or "cultured." Early definitions of literacy referred only to the ability to read and write (prose and document literacy). Literacy has been expanded to include other skills, such as oral, quantitative, computer and technical, problem-solving, and physical. The types of literacy apply to all subject matter areas, including the sciences, the humanities, the arts, math, health, and physical education (physical literacy).

Physical Education Units

Virtually all schools conduct physical education classes that help teens learn to perform a variety of physical activities included in the Physical Activity Pyramid. Classes are normally organized in units, each of which typically focuses on one type of activity from the pyramid. A unit can last a few weeks or as long as a full semester. It isn't possible to show all of the activities that can be included in the units, but some examples are illustrated in figure 16.1. Learning more about different programs and units within physical education can help you to make choices both in future physical education classes and about participation in physical activity programs after you graduate.

Physical Education Program Approaches

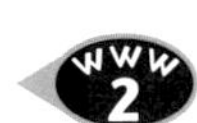

Within physical education, several approaches have gained popularity in high schools in recent years. All of these are part of the regular physical education program, but each focuses on achieving certain physical education objectives in certain ways. Some examples are described in the following discussion.

Fitness Education

Fitness education refers to physical education classes or units that focus on teaching fitness and activity concepts and learning self-management skills that can help you be active for a lifetime. Fitness education classes often use a text such as *Health Opportunities*

FIT FACT

A survey from the Harvard School of Public Health found that more than 90 percent of parents believe schools should provide physical education, particularly for fighting obesity.

Through Physical Education and include some classroom study and some participation in activities either in the gym or on the playing field. Fitness education can be mixed in a variety of units or taught as an independent class. One key feature of fitness education is to help students learn to be independent thinkers capable of solving problems and making informed decisions. One example of a desired outcome of fitness education is for students to plan personal programs based on self-assessment and sound personal goals. Teens who complete a fitness education class are more likely to be active several years after they graduate from high school than those who don't.

Sport Education

Sport education is an approach to teaching physical education that is designed to make playing sport fun, interesting, and authentic. In sport education, as in the sporting world itself, the year is divided into several "seasons" (for example, baseball season or soccer season). During a season in sport education, several different activities are performed, including sport, recreational, and fitness activities. Early in each season, three to five teams are formed within the class, and members remain with the same team throughout the season. Teams practice together to learn skills and compete against other teams in the class. An effort is made to balance teams to make competition fair. Games are modified to accommodate team size, equipment, and rules.

In sport education, team members develop a sense of belonging (or team affiliation). During a season, members play different roles such as coach, fitness trainer, statistician, publicist, equipment

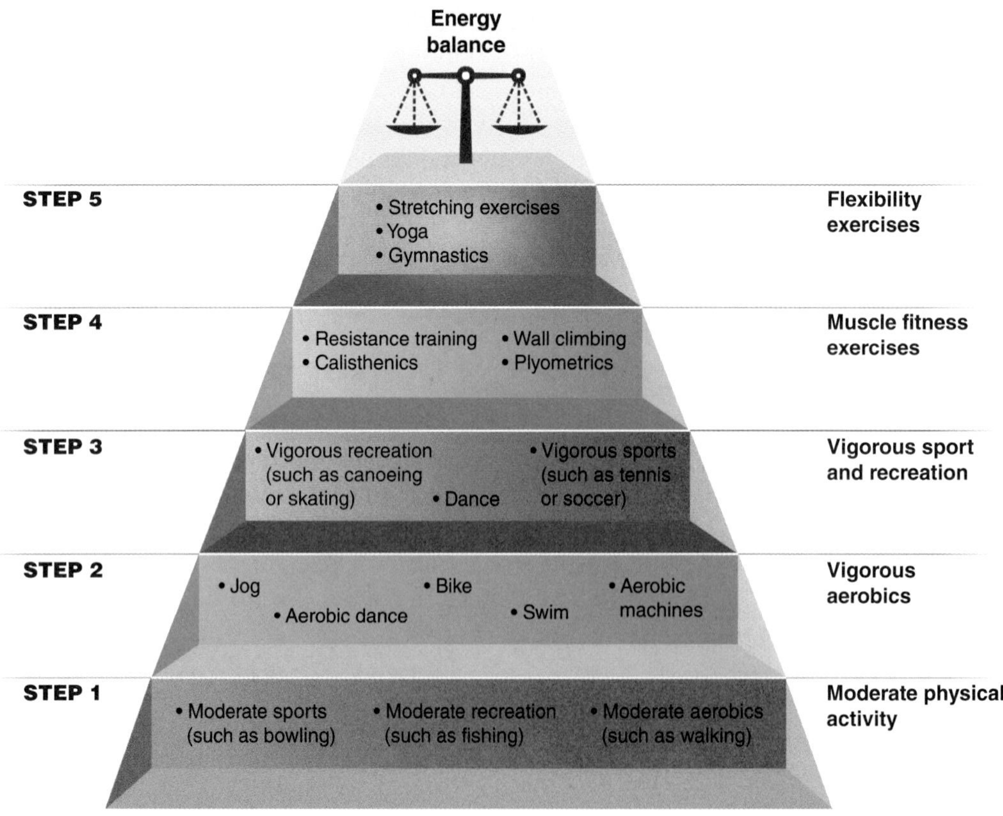

FIGURE 16.1 Examples of physical education units from the Physical Activity Pyramid. All of the units shown contribute to energy expenditure and aid in energy balance.

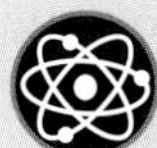

SCIENCE IN ACTION: Top 10 Reasons for High-Quality Physical Education

Scientists from several areas of kinesiology have identified 10 research-based reasons that high-quality physical education (HQPE) is important. HQPE programs offer the opportunity for *all* students to learn, provide meaningful content, provide quality instruction by trained teachers, and offer student and program assessments.

1. **Regular physical activity helps prevent disease.** Regular physical activity reduces risk of hypokinetic diseases, including heart disease, cancer, diabetes, and osteoporosis.
2. **Regular physical activity promotes lifetime wellness.** Health involves more than freedom from disease. Being regularly active improves wellness (quality of life, sense of well-being).
3. **HQPE provides unique opportunities for activity.** Physical education, including dance education, is the primary subject that provides an opportunity to be active during school hours. Teens who do physical education meet national activity goals more often than those who do not.
4. **HQPE helps fight obesity.** About one-third of youth and two-thirds of adults are overweight or obese. Being active in physical education classes and at other times during the school day helps expend calories to reduce the risk of overweight and obesity.
5. **HQPE helps promote lifelong physical fitness.** Regular physical activity using the FIT formula for each type of physical activity helps build all parts of health-related physical fitness. This enhances health and increases your ability to function effectively in work and play.
6. **HQPE teaches self-management and motor skills.** Teens who learn self-management skills are more likely to be active after they graduate from school. They know how to plan personal activity programs and avoid quackery. Students who learn a variety of motor skills are more active later in life.
7. **HQPE and regular physical activity promote learning in other academic areas.** Teens who are active and fit score better on academic tests than those who are inactive. Evidence shows that physical activity is necessary for the brain to function optimally. Active students are less likely to miss school or have discipline problems.
8. **HQPE and regular physical activity make good economic sense.** The annual cost of sedentary living in the United States exceeds $150 million. Worksite wellness programs enable many companies to save money, reduce absenteeism, and increase job satisfaction. High-quality physical education promotes the same benefits.
9. **HQPE is widely endorsed.** More than 50 organizations in the U.S. support the value of HQPE in schools, including the American Academy of Pediatrics (AAP); the American College of Sports Medicine (ACSM); the American Heart Association (AHA); the U.S. Centers for Disease Control and Prevention (CDC); and the President's Council on Fitness, Sports, and Nutrition.
10. **HQPE helps educate the total person.** As President John F. Kennedy said, "physical fitness is the basis of all the activities in our society. And if our bodies grow soft and inactive, if we fail to encourage physical development and prowess, we will undermine our capacity for thought, for work, and for the use of those skills vital to an expanding and complex America."

Adapted from Le Masurier and Corbin 2006.

Student Activity

Interview at least one teacher who is not a physical education teacher. Ask questions to see if he or she is aware of the 10 reasons for high-quality physical education.

manager, scout, scorekeeper, or referee. Game results are posted, and standings are updated regularly. Each season concludes with postseason playoffs and an award ceremony. A key aspect of sport education is that team members provide leadership and assume responsibility for activities conducted during each season.

Adventure Education

Adventure education typically focuses on challenging recreational activities such as rock climbing, orienteering, boating, rafting, and ropes courses. Adventure education units are sometimes taught as part of physical education and sometimes used in camp settings, recreational programs, and even programs designed to train business executives. Among the principal goals of adventure education are trust building, problem solving, and enhancement of self-confidence. This approach often uses teams, and it emphasizes placing trust in team members and working together to overcome risks. While adventure education is often conducted in outdoor and wilderness settings, it can also be conducted indoors using trust-building activities and cooperative games. Like fitness education and sport education, adventure education is really a way of teaching physical education.

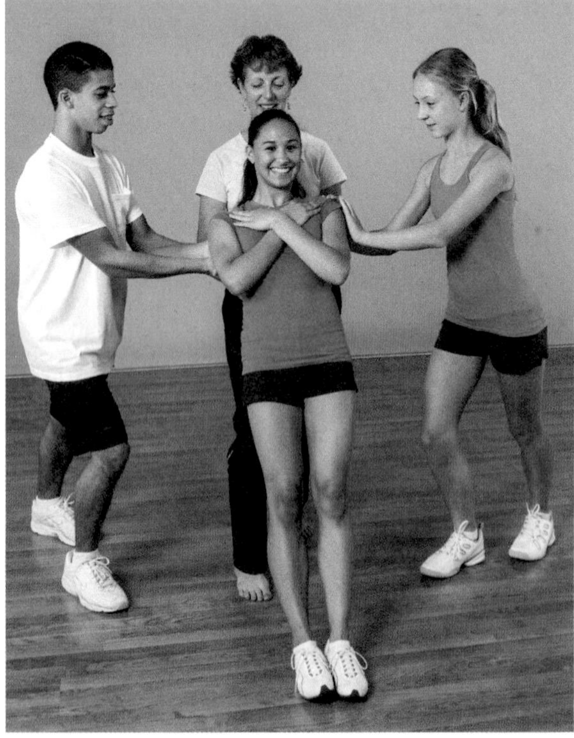

Trust-building activities can be part of the adventure education curriculum.

Outdoor Education

Outdoor education is education that occurs in an outdoor classroom. One type of outdoor education is adventure education that is conducted outside. Like adventure education, outdoor education uses activities such as camping, fishing, and hiking to develop physical literacy. Some schools conduct camps where students participate for several days and learn in outdoor settings.

Cooperative Games

Like sport education, **cooperative games** use teams to help students learn cooperation, have fun, and overcome challenges. But cooperative games focus on working *together* in teams rather than competing or winning. Some physical education programs include units focused on cooperative games; as previously mentioned, cooperative games are also sometimes part of adventure education. Many books describe cooperative games that keep all people active and emphasize working together to solve problems. Cooperative games are sometimes used to help people get to know each other (through "icebreakers") and build trust. You can try some cooperative games in this chapter's Taking Action feature.

Dance Education

Dance education can be part of a physical education program or a separate program that focuses on teaching various forms of dance both in and out of school. Dances are performed in many cultures and can be done individually, with a partner, or in a group. For example, ballet is a form of classical dance that is often performed by accomplished dancers as a form of art. Modern dance is a more contemporary form of dance. Dance education can include classes or units focused on these forms or others, ranging from social dances of moderate intensity to more vigorous options such as ballroom dance. Traditional types include ballroom dances such as the waltz, foxtrot, and quickstep. Latin dances include the samba, cha-cha, and rumba. Hip-hop is a vigorous type of dance popular among

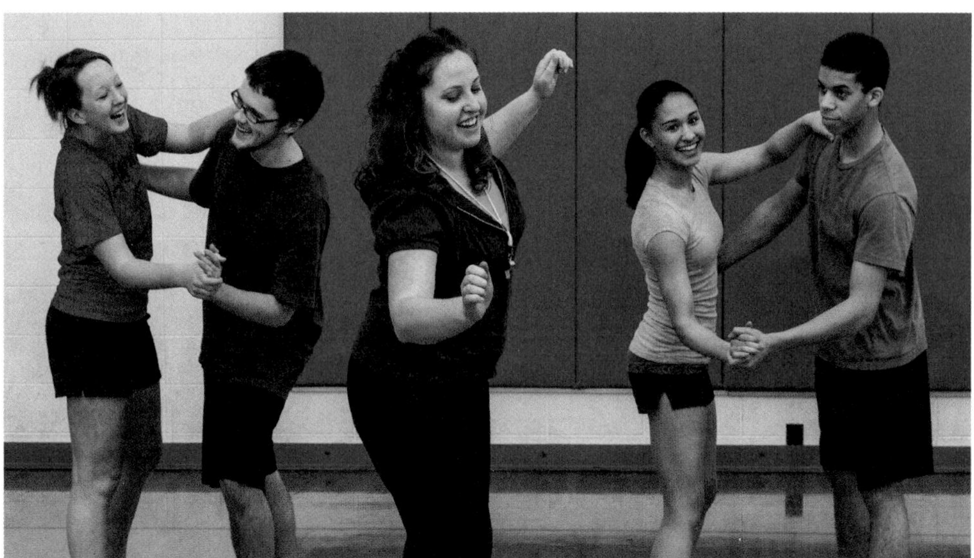

Dance in many forms can be included in physical education units or separate dance education classes.

youth. Other currently popular types include jazz, country and western, line dance, swing dance, and the jitterbug. Dance education classes often include various dances strongly associated with a particular culture, such as square dance, Irish dance, and African dance. Aerobic dance and other types of fitness dance such as Zumba may be included as part of dance education or fitness education units.

> "I do not try to dance better than anyone else. I only try to dance better than myself."
>
> —Mikhail Baryshnikov, professional dancer

Lesson Review

1. What are the five characteristics of a physically literate (educated) person?
2. What are the top 10 reasons for conducting high-quality physical education?
3. Describe several approaches to conducting physical education.

SELF-ASSESSMENT: Assessing Game Strategy and Tactics

In this chapter's second lesson, you'll learn several steps for developing strategy and tactics in various situations. In this self-assessment, you'll do an experiment to determine the effectiveness of different game strategies and tactics. As directed by your instructor, record your results and report on the effectiveness of the various options. Remember that self-assessment information is personal and considered confidential. It shouldn't be shared with others without the permission of the person being tested.

Directions

1. Form teams of 2 to 4 players. Each team must have the same number of players.
2. Place four hoops on flat ground such as a gym floor or outdoor field. The hoops are placed at the following distances from a throwing line: 10 feet (3 meters), 20 feet (6 meters), 30 feet (9 meters), and 40 feet (12 meters). See figure 16.2.
3. Each team member throws three beanbags at each hoop target.
4. Record the number of beanbags that land inside each hoop for each team (more than half of the bag must be in the hoop). Score 1 point for every beanbag that lands inside the first target (the one that is 10 feet, or 3 meters, from the throwing line), 2 points for each bag in the second target, 3 points for each bag in the third target, and 4 points for each bag in the fourth target. Total your team's points and record your team score.
5. After completing step 4, each team decides on a short- or long-toss strategy for achieving the highest possible team score. In the short-toss strategy, only targets 1 and 2 can be used. In the long-toss strategy, only targets 3 and 4 can be used.
6. Each player on each team tosses three beanbags at the chosen targets (short or long toss). All players must throw only at the two targets chosen based on team strategy.
7. At least one player on each team must throw at each target. For example, if you have three players on a team, two can throw at the same target, but the third must choose the other target.
8. Decide tactics as a team. Who will throw at which target? How many players will throw at the shorter of the two targets?
9. After all players have completed their throws, calculate your team's score by adding the scores of all team members' throws (see step 4 for scoring). Record individual and team results.
10. Play again using the same procedures, but use the opposite strategy (if your team used the long-toss strategy the first time, use the short-toss strategy this time, or vice versa). As noted in item 7, at least one player on each team must throw at each target.
11. Using the same scoring procedure, calculate your team's score for the second strategy. Record your individual and team results.
12. Based on previous scores, determine which of the two strategies gives your team the better probability of success.
13. Prepare a brief report that includes the results of all trials. If more time was provided to practice the task, how might the probability of success change for each strategy? Comment on whether the group would use the same strategy after having time to practice.

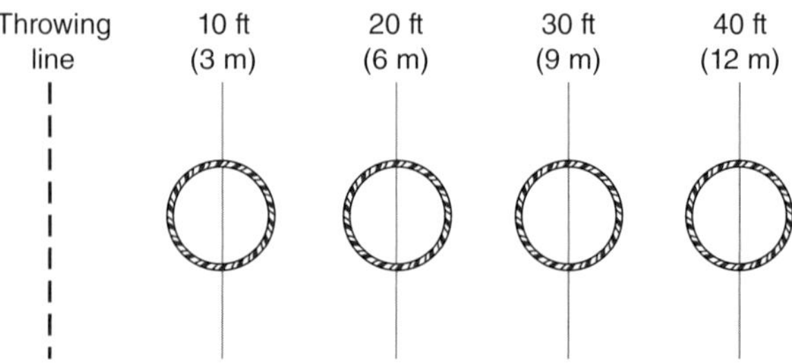

Figure 16.2 Setup for the strategy and tactics assessment game.

Lesson 16.2

Strategy and Tactics

Lesson Objectives

After reading this lesson, you should be able to

1. define *strategy* and provide examples that relate to physical activity and healthy lifestyle choices,
2. define *tactic* and explain its role in implementing a strategy, and
3. explain the five steps for planning strategy and tactics.

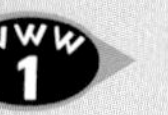

Lesson Vocabulary

strategy, tactic

Success in sport and other physical activities requires certain physical abilities, including good fitness and good motor skills. People who train properly can achieve fitness and, with good practice, can master skills. But physical abilities are not the only requirements for success. You also need a good strategy and sound tactics.

Strategy

A **strategy** is a master plan for achieving a goal. The word *strategy* comes from the Greek word *strategos*, which refers to the general or leader of an army. Consistent with its origin, many early uses of the word *strategy* were associated with military planning. Today, the word *strategy* is still often used in military contexts, as when referring to a war strategy. In modern times, however, it is also used in business and organizational contexts. Marketing, for example, is an aspect of business that helps companies develop strategies for selling their products. Strategies are also useful in sport and other physical activities. In sport, for example, coaches develop strategies or master plans for winning games, and players use strategies to be effective team members.

> "A strategy lays out a plan for reaching your goals; tactics help you carry out your strategy."
>
> —Phil Abbadessa, teacher and coach

Tactics

A **tactic** is a specific method for carrying out a strategy. The word *tactic* derives from the Greek *taktikos*, which refers to arranging forces in a battle formation. As with strategy, tactics were first used in the military, in this case to carry out a fighting strategy. Generals first developed a master plan or strategy, then developed specific tactics or procedures to carry out the strategy or battle plan.

Similarly, in marketing a product or service, companies first develop a strategy, then use specific

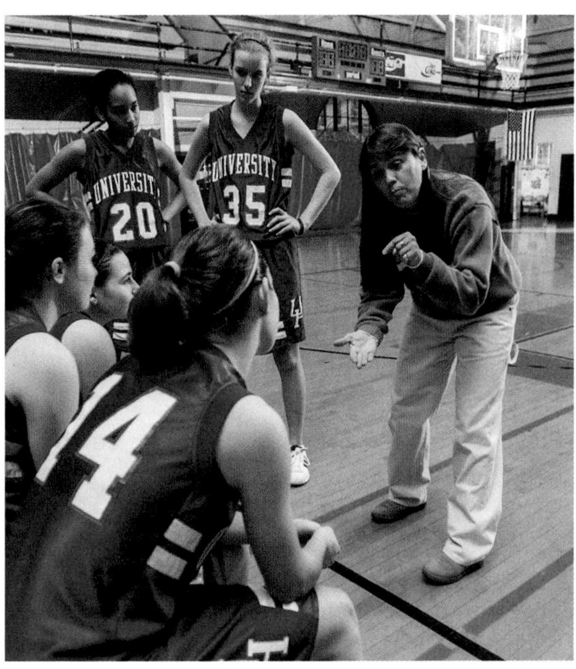

Strategies and tactics are used in sports, and they are also important in other areas of life.

tactics to carry it out. For example, a food manufacturer might adopt a strategy of selling cereals high in sugar and low in nutrients. In this example, the strategy is to convince children that they want the cereal. Even though adults buy the cereal, children have a big influence on what adults buy. Specific tactics might include placing ads for the cereal on Saturday morning TV shows aimed at children or placing toys in cereal boxes. Children see the ad or want the toy and beg a parent to buy the cereal.

In sports and games, a coach, team leader, or (in an individual sport or game) individual competitor develops the strategy. For example, a basketball team might decide to adopt a defensive strategy—that is, to emphasize defense in order to force the other team to make errors. Within this strategy, one specific tactic would be to use a full-court press, in which players guard their opponents at both ends of the court. Another defensive tactic might be to double-team the other team's best shooter (that is, to have two players guard one very good player on the other team).

You can also use strategy and tactics in other areas of your life. Some examples are provided in table 16.1.

FIT FACT

The game of chess requires both strategy and specific tactics. In fact, many coaches and military leaders use the game to sharpen their ability to use tactics to carry out a strategy.

Planning a Strategy and Developing Tactics

As shown in table 16.1, a strategy and accompanying tactics can be useful in many areas of your life. But how do you develop a strategy and tactics? You can use steps similar to those in the scientific method and those used in program planning. Since tactics are used to implement a strategy, the strategy is planned first.

Step 1: Use Existing Information

Much is already known about strategies for various sports and activities. Therefore, a good first step is to read books and articles about the strategies that have been used successfully in your chosen sport

TABLE 16.1 Examples of the Use of Strategies and Tactics

Situation	Strategy example	Tactic examples
Healthy eating Person consumes more calories than expended each day.	Eat less food with empty calories.	Remove food with empty calories from house. Learn to say no. Eat healthy snacks. Avoid buying food from vending machines.
Physical activity Person does not meet national activity guidelines.	Prepare a written physical activity plan.	Follow the five steps for writing a plan. Log daily activity.
Managing stress Person has too many things to do and not enough time to do them.	Reduce commitments and spend more time on important things.	Self-assess current time use. Rank current commitments from high to low importance. Focus on high-importance commitments. Learn to say no to unimportant commitments.
Playing a team sport Person's intramural team wants to do well in the soccer league.	Focus on defense.	Assign more players to defense. Use zone defense because some players lack skills. Use long defensive kicks to clear ball and reduce shots on goal.
Preventing back pain Person wants to reduce risk of back pain.	Focus on good posture in standing, sitting, and moving.	Assess current posture and core fitness. Perform core exercises. Practice good posture.

CONSUMER CORNER: TV Tactics—Creating Needs

You've now learned about developing a strategy and using tactics to achieve a goal. Companies also develop strategies and tactics. Sometimes their strategies help them but are not good for you. For example, a company's strategy may be to get you to buy something you don't really want or need. To help them carry out their strategies, companies buy advertising in various media—such as television, the web (pop-up ads), magazines, radio, and newspapers. The money these companies pay for advertisements is what allows media outlets to survive. So both the companies that sell the products and the media outlets who sell the ads are trying to influence your consumer behavior in order to make money. In fact, marketers create media messages that flood our senses every day. Of course, not all advertisements are deceptive, but many are. It takes a very critical eye to detect the messages being conveyed in ads and to distinguish between good and bad information.

As you're exposed to media advertisement, try to determine the strategy and tactics being used. Ask the following questions: What is this ad trying to get me to do? Is the product they're selling something I really need? Is the product likely to work as advertised? In this chapter, you learn how to develop a strategy and identify tactics to carry out that strategy. You can use this knowledge to help you analyze marketing strategies and become an informed consumer.

WWW 2

or activity. You can also consult with experts and others who have succeeded in the sport or activity. For example, if you're playing tennis, you can learn about successful tennis strategies used by others—or by yourself in past matches. Keeping notes about successful strategies can help you carry out steps 2 through 5.

Step 2: Collect New Information

One way to decide which available strategy will work best for you is to conduct a self-assessment of your strengths and weaknesses (for planning a sport performance) or of your personal needs (for planning a lifestyle change). If you're planning to play a sport, let's say tennis, it would also be helpful to assess your opponent's strengths and weaknesses. Coaches do this by means of "scouting reports" that describe other teams' strengths and weaknesses and identify strategies and tactics they have been known to use. To help you plan, write down what you learn about your own strengths and weaknesses and about the strengths and weaknesses of an opponent. Even the pros collect information. For example, professional basketball player LeBron James, who has excellent physical abilities and skills, also studies video of opponents and reads the full scouting report of other teams. He does this to implement a strategy and use tactics that keep him one step ahead of opponents.

Step 3: Prepare a Plan

After considering available strategies and collecting information about yourself and your opponent, prepare a written plan. In competitive sport, you consider how you or your team can use your strengths and take advantages of your opponent's weaknesses. For example, if your strength in tennis is your serve and your opponent's weakness is return of serve, you might consider an offensive strategy. On the other hand, if you're quite fit and your opponent is not so fit, you might consider a strategy of trying to tire out your opponent so that you could take advantage later in the match.

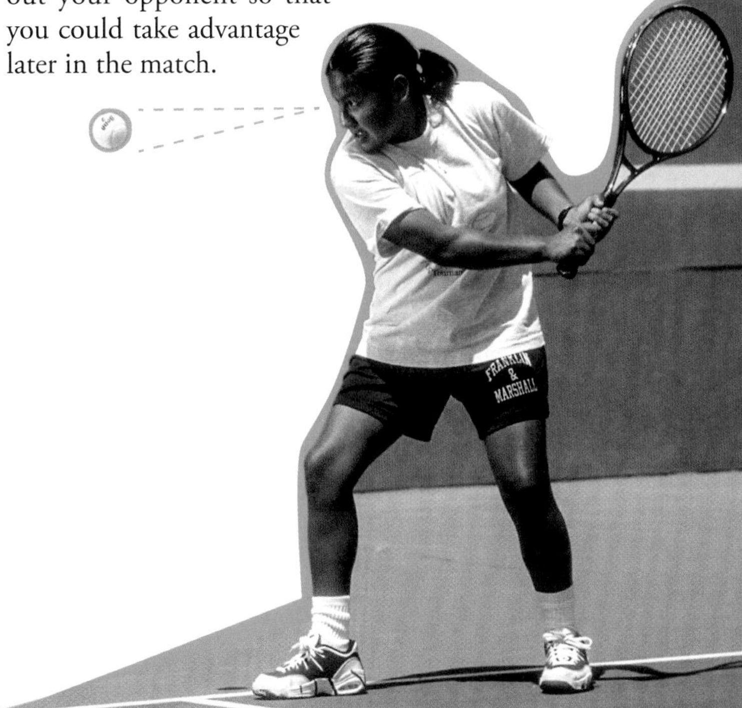

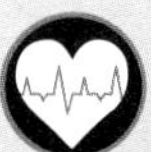

FITNESS TECHNOLOGY: Computers Keep Getting Smarter

New technology allows large amounts of information to be stored in the tiny chips that make up a computer's "brain." It has also allowed computers to process information much faster than in the past. In this light, perhaps it's no surprise that a computer (named Watson) used its "artificial intelligence" to beat two human competitors on the TV game show *Jeopardy*. Watson was developed by researchers at IBM and is named after the company's founder, Thomas Watson. The two human competitors were the biggest winners in the show's history, Ken Jennings and Brad Rutter. Watson won the million-dollar prize by using information stored in its computer memory. It was able to quickly retrieve and analyze information in ways similar to those of the human brain. Watson also performed some physical tasks in ways similar to or better than those of humans. For example, it had better reaction time and thus was able to respond to the buzzer more quickly than the human contestants. Watson was also immune to psychological strategies employed by some contestants. Watson did have some problems interpreting clues provided by the show's host.

Using Technology

Prepare a report to answer this question: How can computers be used to help people who have physical disabilities?

FIT FACT

Preparing a written plan is a commitment to action. People who make a formal commitment are more likely to act than those who do not make a commitment.

Step 4: Include Tactics in Your Plan

To carry out your strategy, plan to use specific tactics. For example, if you want to implement an offensive strategy in tennis, you might consider coming to the net after each of your serves to take advantage of your good serve and your opponent's poor service return. If your opponent is out of shape, you might use the tactic of making him or her move around a lot by hitting the ball first to one side of the court and then to the other.

When deciding on tactics, you can use the same steps as in planning a strategy. First, become familiar with existing information (study known tactics), then collect information, and then make a list of the tactics to consider. Rank the possible tactics and decide which ones are best for implementing your strategy.

Step 5: Practice

When most people think of practice, they think of practicing skills to get better at performance. Doing that is indeed very important, but so is practicing your strategy and tactics. Once you've chosen a strategy and tactics, practice them. For the tennis player in our example, this practice would involve serving, coming to the net, and volleying. It would also include hitting the ball from side to side to make the opponent move.

As with any plan, you should also evaluate the success of the strategy and tactics you implement. What you learn will become part of step 1 when you plan your next strategy. The examples used here are for playing a sport, but you can use the same steps for making lifestyle changes as well (for examples, see table 16.1).

Lesson Review

1. Define *strategy* and explain how it is relevant to physical activity and healthy lifestyle choices.
2. Define *tactic* and explain its role in implementing a strategy.
3. What are the five steps for planning strategy and tactics?

TAKING CHARGE: Developing Tactics

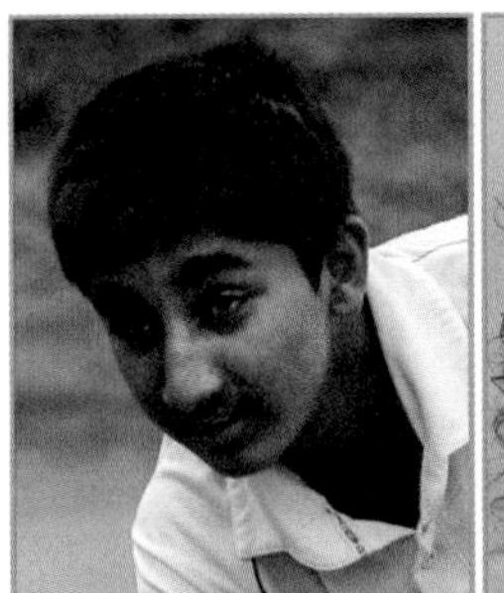

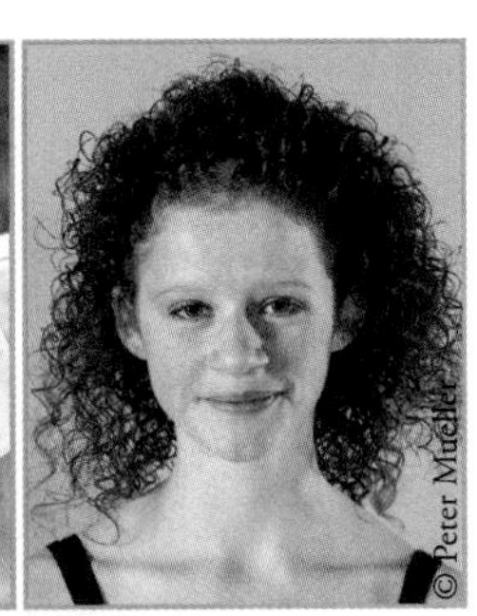

© Peter Mueller

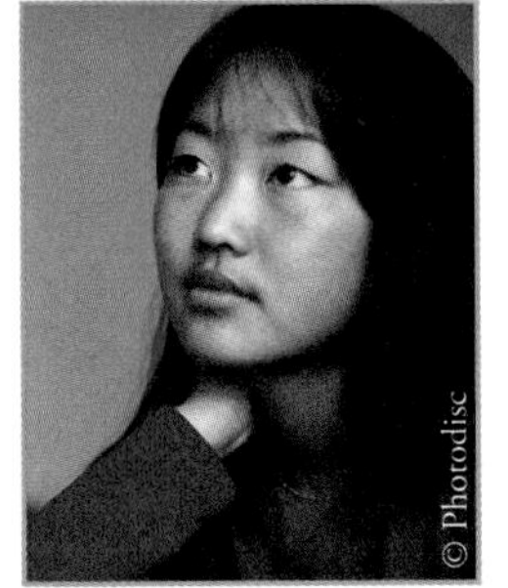

© Photodisc

Jason, Ali, Lucy, and Katie have been friends since elementary school. When Ali's mother was diagnosed with breast cancer, the friends wanted to do something to show Ali and his family how much they cared. Jason, Lucy, and Katie got together to plan a strategy. First, they considered what they already knew. They knew the dangers of breast cancer. They also knew that they were not qualified to help medically. After collecting information and considering all options, the group decided on a strategy. They would raise money for breast cancer by entering a Relay for Life event in their local community.

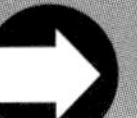

The Relay for Life is an annual event that takes place in communities throughout the world. This American Cancer Society event raises money for the fight against cancer. People from communities form relay teams that camp out overnight. Team members walk or run around a track or a predetermined course. Cancer survivors run or walk the first lap, caregivers perform the second lap, and team members take turns walking or running additional laps over a predetermined amount of time, often 24 hours. Contributions are made for laps completed by team members. The funds raised from the Relay for Life are used to make a difference in the fight against cancer. The three friends needed to find other team members, ask supporters for pledges, and take care of other details such as arranging for an overnight stay.

For Discussion

Is the friends' strategy a good one for people in their situation? What other strategies might they have considered? What tactics should they consider to carry out their strategy? How can they best recruit other team members, get the most pledges, and arrange for the details of the event? Consider the skills in the Self-Management feature when answering the discussion questions.

SELF-MANAGEMENT: Skills for Developing Tactics

You will have opportunities to use strategies and tactics in the future. Use the following guidelines to help you succeed.

- **Plan your strategy.** Use the five steps described in this lesson. Plan tactics after you adopt a strategy.
- **Learn about and list available tactics.** Read, consult with others who have expertise, and observe. Make a list and rate tactics in terms of their likely effect on your strategy's success.
- **Collect information about yourself (or your team or group).** Choose tactics that emphasize your strengths and minimize your weaknesses.
- **Collect information about others who are involved.** If you're competing against another team or individual, collect information about your opponent. If you're planning an event, collect information from others who've been successful and find out as much as you can about the event (for example, Race for the Cure).
- **Choose the best tactics.** If you're working with others, consult with your group when making decisions about which tactics to use. If someone else decides the tactics (for example, a coach or team leader), provide input.
- **Commit.** Once you've decided, commit to your strategy and tactics.

TAKING ACTION: Cooperative Games

You're more likely to be active and lead a healthy lifestyle if you have friends and family members who are also active. Sometimes it's fun to be active with friends without the competition that's typical in many sports and games. You can do this by playing cooperative games, such as footbagging, throwing a flying disc, and participating in a volleyball circle. Activities that enable everyone to participate and succeed are also great for social events such as cookouts, work parties, and group gatherings at a park or beach. Cooperative activities are relaxing because the emphasis isn't on winning. You can also have a lot of good laughs when people are encouraged to fool around while playing. **Take action** by trying several cooperative games.

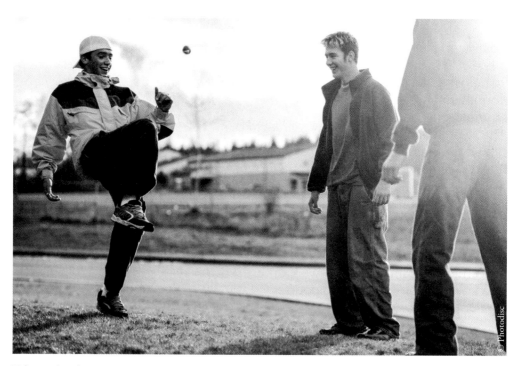

Take action by trying cooperative games.

CHAPTER REVIEW

Reviewing Concepts and Vocabulary

As directed by your teacher, answer items 1 through 5 by correctly completing each sentence with a word or phrase.

1. A ______________ person does regular activity, is fit, has skills, values activity, and knows the benefits of activity.
2. Activities that use teams to teach cooperation and overcome challenges are called ______________.
3. A ______________ is a master plan for achieving a goal.
4. ______________ are specific methods for carrying out a strategy.
5. Watson is the name of a computer that uses ______________ to solve problems and answer questions.

For items 6 through 10, as directed by your teacher, match each term in column 1 with the appropriate phrase in column 2.

6. sport education	a. uses challenging recreational activities
7. adventure education	b. uses seasons and teams to educate
8. outdoor education	c. uses cultural movement activities
9. dance education	d. teaches concepts and self-management skills
10. fitness education	e. may use camps to teach activities

For items 11 through 15, as directed by your teacher, respond to each statement or question.

11. Discuss 2 of the top 10 reasons for providing high-quality physical education in schools.
12. Describe adventure education. Why can it be an important part of physical education?
13. Describe dance education. Why can it be an important part of physical education?
14. Describe how the five steps for developing strategy and tactics can be used in a sport of your choice.
15. Describe several guidelines for developing tactics.

Thinking Critically

Choose a member of your family that you would like to encourage to be more active or eat better. Write a paragraph to devise a strategy for helping that person change.

Project

Media outlets—such as newspapers and radio and television networks—are major news and information sources. But in recent years, blogs and podcasts have become more prominent in providing information. Prepare a blog (a written article that could appear on a blog) or podcast (a recording that could appear on a podcast) describing reasons why high-quality physical education is important.

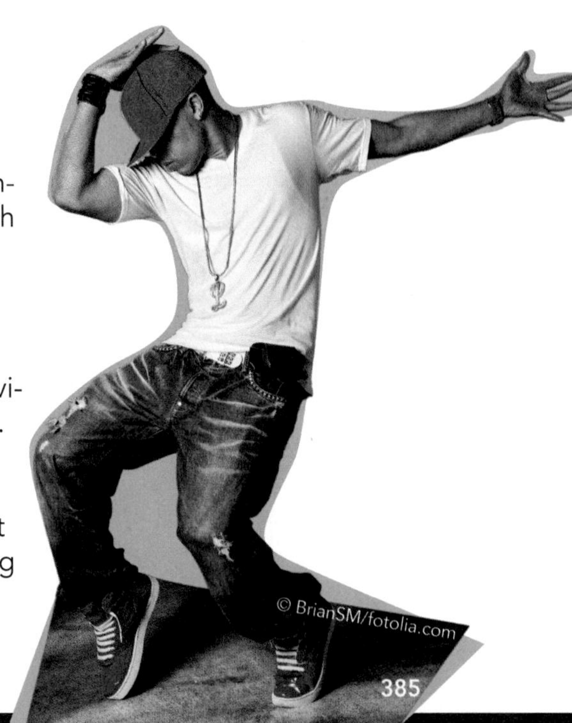

17

The Science of Active Living

In This Chapter

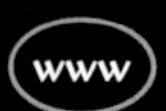

Student Web Resources

www.HOPEtextbook.org/student

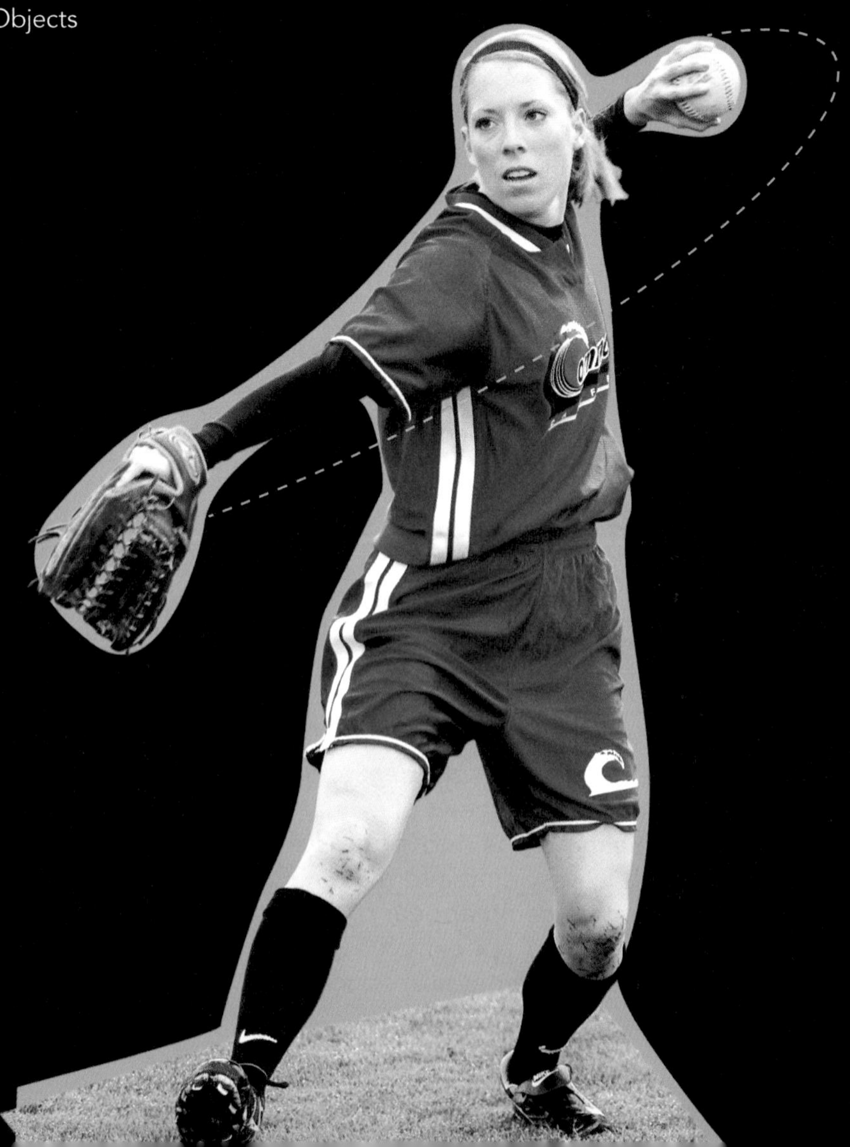

Lesson 17.1

Moving Your Body

Lesson Objectives

After reading this lesson, you should be able to

1. describe nine key biomechanical principles of motor skill learning,
2. describe the two stances commonly used in physical activity,
3. describe several forms of locomotion, and
4. explain the meaning of the term *biomechanical analysis*, and describe how it is used to aid motor skill performance.

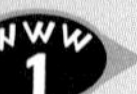

Lesson Vocabulary

acceleration, aerodynamics, biomechanical principles, center of gravity, deceleration, force, hydrodynamics, locomotion, stance, velocity

Why do some people let themselves go and become out of shape and unhealthy as they move into adulthood while others continue to be active? For example, when Gretchen was a teen she played softball and basketball. During her 20s and 30s, her job and home responsibilities kept her from playing these team sports, but she stayed active by doing aerobic dance and muscle fitness and flexibility exercises at the local fitness club. During her 40s, Gretchen had more time to get back into sports, so she joined a slow-pitch softball league with some friends at work. She also kept up her aerobic dance and other exercises at the gym. In her 50s, she decided to try tennis at the urging of a friend who needed a doubles partner. Today, at 74, she walks, does her muscle fitness and flexibility exercises, and plays doubles tennis in a local league. Thus, while her activities have changed, she's never been inactive, and along the way she's developed some great friendships and had a lot of fun.

Early in life, Gretchen was fortunate to have a physical education teacher and coach who taught her the principles of movement. As her life changed, her activities also changed, but she could apply those principles of movement to them. In addition, knowing some movement basics enabled her to have fun participating in activities with friends.

Throughout part 1 of this book, you've learned various principles and how you can apply them in various situations. In this chapter, you'll review some of these principles and learn about others that can help you move efficiently throughout your life.

When performing activities from the Physical Activity Pyramid, you use motor skills, which range from simple to complex. Successful performance of motor skills requires you to apply principles of human movement. Experts in biomechanics study human movement and help us understand and apply the principles in all types of activity.

> Excellence is the gradual result of always striving to do better.
>
> —Pat Riley, basketball coach

Biomechanical Principles

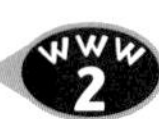

The principles of biomechanics are based on the basic laws of physics and are complex enough to be the subject of college courses and even college degrees. Physical education teachers and other exercise professionals typically take at least one class in biomechanics, and the **biomechanical principles** summarized here are only a few of the many. Those that were chosen for this discussion relate directly to the motor skills described in this chapter.

1. Stability

Stability of the body, at rest or in movement, is related to the location of the body's **center of gravity** and the base of the body's support. Stability while standing is increased by a wide base of support and a low center of gravity.

2. Force

To get a body or object moving, or to make a moving body or object stop, **force** must be applied. Many forces are involved, but the contraction of muscles provides the primary force that moves the body (or an object such as a thrown ball). External forces such as gravity and air resistance slow a body in motion. Applying force in one direction results in the production of force in the opposite direction (for every action there is an equal and opposite reaction).

3. Acceleration, Deceleration, and Velocity

Velocity is speed of movement. **Acceleration** (increase in velocity) occurs when a force is applied to a body or object. The bigger the object's mass, the more force must be applied to cause acceleration. **Deceleration** (a decrease in velocity) occurs when resistance is applied to an object.

4. Accumulation of Forces

Greater force can be applied to an object or body if each new force is added sequentially. For example, when a person throws a ball effectively, the lower body moves first, the trunk moves second, the upper body moves third, and then finally the arm and hand move (see the Self-Assessment later in this chapter). Force production is greatest if each movement is added after the previous movement has reached its greatest acceleration.

5. Resistance

Resistance is opposition to a force or movement. One source of resistance is friction. Friction is a force caused by one surface rubbing against another. Factors such as the air (including wind) and water offer resistance. Gravity is a source of resistance in motions such as jumping and throwing an object for distance. Resistance can also be applied by an opposing force such as another player pushing you in football or by a weight on a barbell in progressive resistance training.

6. Levers

A lever is a very basic machine—a bar or stiff, straight object that can be used to lift weight or increase force. Levers can be used to increase force for producing movement. The body has three types of lever: first, second, and third class. Third-class levers are the most common. Bones act as levers, and muscle contractions create the force that moves the levers.

7. Angles

An angle is defined as a figure formed by two lines originating in the same place. Angles are important for successful physical performance. For example, when you throw a ball, the angle of release affects the distance it travels. The ground is one line in the angle, and the trajectory of the ball is the other line. The size of an angle is measured in degrees—for example, a right angle is a 90-degree angle.

8. Aerodynamics

In physics, the study of dynamics addresses the causes of motion, including factors that cause changes in motion. **Aerodynamics** includes the study of motion in the air (represented in the term by *aero*). Performance is influenced by various factors associated with motion in the air; examples include spin (on a ball, for example), wind (air resistance in running, for example), and other factors (such as turbulence, humidity, and altitude).

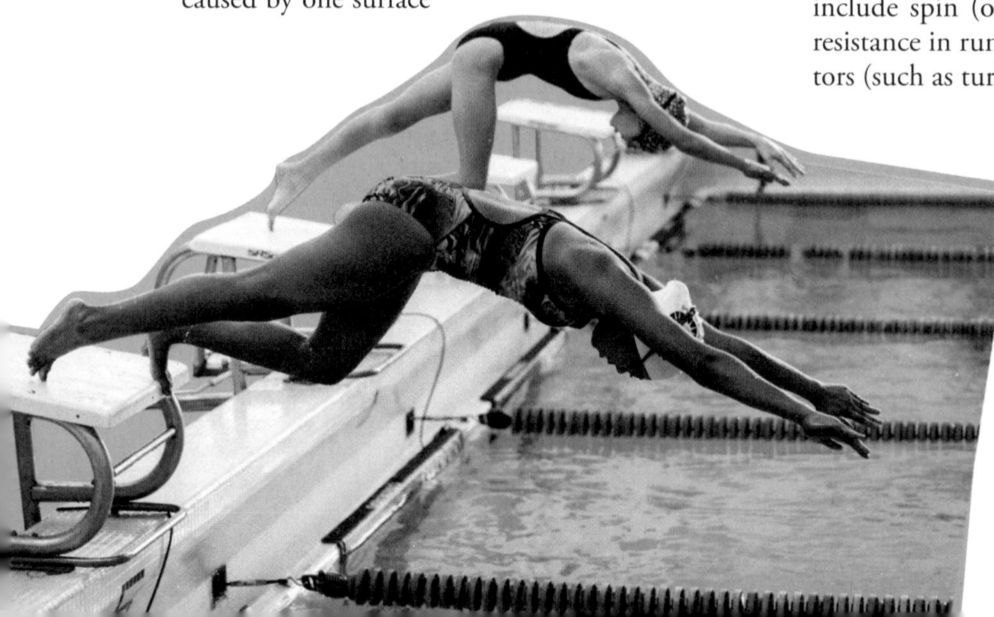

9. Hydrodynamics

Hydrodynamics refers to the study of motion in fluids. Factors that affect movement in water include water resistance, turbulence (water movement patterns), and temperature.

FIT FACT

Some garments are made from special materials that reduce resistance to air and water when running, biking, or swimming. To further reduce resistance, some bikers also shave their legs, and some swimmers shave their entire bodies.

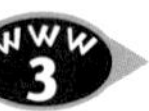

Fundamental Skills: Stance and Locomotor Skills

Fundamental skills are those that are common to many activities. If you understand and learn to apply the principles of biomechanics when performing fundamental skills, you can use them to help you learn new skills. Virtually all skills are affected in some way by every one of the nine biomechanical principles.

Balanced (Athletic) Stance

Stance is a way of standing, and the most basic stance is standing with good posture and stability. When performing in sport and other physical activities, you need to use a stance that prepares you for action. For this reason, the balanced stance is basic to many sport and other physical activities. The balanced stance, sometimes called the ready stance or athletic stance, allows you to be stable when standing and prepares you to move in any direction. Figure 17.1 shows the balanced stance. Some of its characteristics include a wide base (feet shoulder-width apart or slightly more), lowered center of gravity (knees bent), and center of gravity located within the body (body is not leaning backward, forward, or to either side).

Variations of the balanced stance are used, for example, by baseball and softball players when playing in the field, basketball players when playing defense, tennis players when getting ready to receive a serve, and many other participants in a wide variety of physical activity situations. Balance and stability are needed in these cases because the performer doesn't know in which direction he or she will need to move—forward, backward, right, or left.

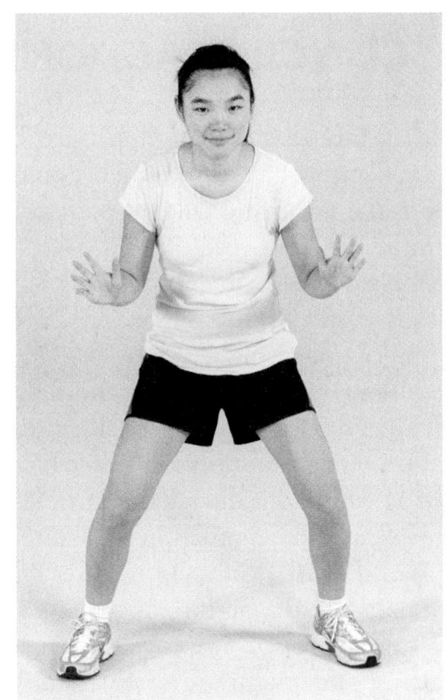

FIGURE 17.1 The balanced stance.

Unbalanced Stance

The unbalanced stance (figure 17.2) is used when a performer anticipates moving in a certain direction. This stance is used, for example, by sprinters and swimmers at the start of a race and by football players lined up for the start of a play. Rather than being stable, a performer using an unbalanced stance leans in the direction of anticipated movement, thus allowing the body to get moving more quickly.

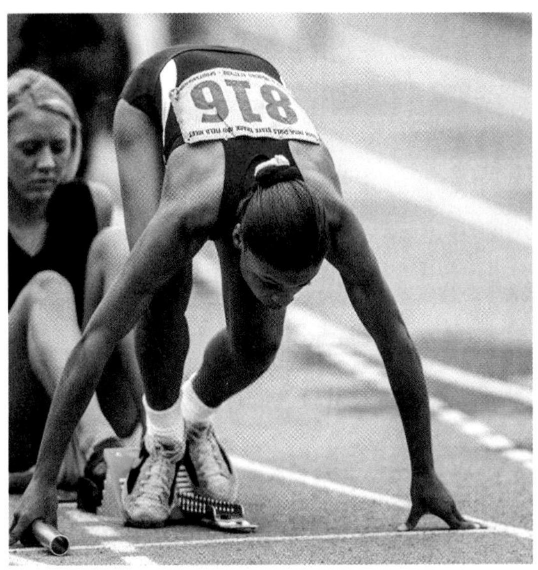

FIGURE 17.2 The unbalanced stance.

SCIENCE IN ACTION: Biomechanical Analysis

Before the invention of motion pictures or video recording, scientists depended on live observation of sport and occupational skill performance to determine the most efficient and effective ways for people to perform motor skills. The first motion pictures were developed by the Frenchman Louis Lumière in the late 1800s. The American Thomas Edison invented the first movie projector that was a commercial success. This invention allowed motion pictures to be used for analyzing work skills during the early 1900s. As sport became more popular in the United States after World War II, moving pictures were also used to analyze the performance of sport skills by baseball players to improve their mechanics in batting and pitching. Researchers such as John Cooper at Indiana University and Richard Nelson at Pennsylvania State University used special high-speed cameras to perform slow-motion analysis of very fast movements recorded on film.

In the early 1950s, the magnetic video tape recorder replaced film as the most popular method of recording and analyzing movements in physical activity. Digital photography was used by the U.S. National Aeronautics and Space Administration for space exploration in the 1960s but did not become commercially available until 1981, when Sony introduced the first mass-produced digital (filmless) camera. In 1995, Sony introduced the first digital video camera. Now, digital cameras are used with computers to analyze movement. The software was originally developed for use in research laboratories and by sport teams but is now available for use by people who participate in leisure-time sport and recreational activities. For example, many golf stores use special cameras and software to offer motion analysis of a person's golf swing. Programs are also available to help individuals use a home computer to analyze their own sport performance.

Student Activity

Investigate motion analysis systems. If your school has one for student athletes, ask for a demonstration. If not, check with a local golf or tennis store to get a demonstration, or investigate the motion analysis systems found in the student section of the Health Opportunities Through Physical Education website. Write a brief report summarizing your investigation.

FIT FACT

It takes 30 times as much force to lift an object as to push it. Pushing is also more efficient than pulling.

Lifting

Lifting is a motor skill used in resistance training and in sports such as weightlifting, powerlifting, and wrestling. Principles 1 through 7 as described earlier are particularly relevant in lifting.

Locomotion (Walking, Running, and Sprinting)

Locomotion refers to moving the body from place to place. The most basic forms of locomotion (that is, using locomotor skills) are walking and running. In walking, one foot or the other is in contact with the ground at all times. In running (or jogging), both feet are off the ground for a short time during each stride. Biomechanical principles 1 through 8 are especially important to apply when performing walking, running, and other locomotor skills. Sprinting, or fast running, is used in track and field for events such as the 100-meter dash and the run-up to a long jump and in sports such as soccer (for example, sprinting to get to a loose ball).

Locomotion (Jumping and Leaping)

Two other common forms of locomotion in sport and other physical activities are jumping and leaping. In jumping, a person leaves the ground with both feet and lands on both feet (see figure 17.3). For example, in the standing jump you push against the ground with both feet and land on both feet. The standing jump can be forward, as in the standing long jump, or upward, as in the vertical jump (figure 17.3). Both the standing long jump and the vertical jump are used as tests of leg power. In leaping, a person leaves the ground on one foot and lands on the opposite foot (see figure 17.4). Leaps are common in ballet and gymnastics. Leaping is different from hopping. In hopping, one foot leaves the ground and the landing is on the same foot. Elements of jumping and leaping are often combined in physical activities. For example, in the running long jump, the performer leaves the ground on one foot and lands on two feet (see figure 17.5). Although this type of movement is a combined movement, it is commonly referred to as a jump. Plyometrics uses jumping and leaping to build power and muscle fitness.

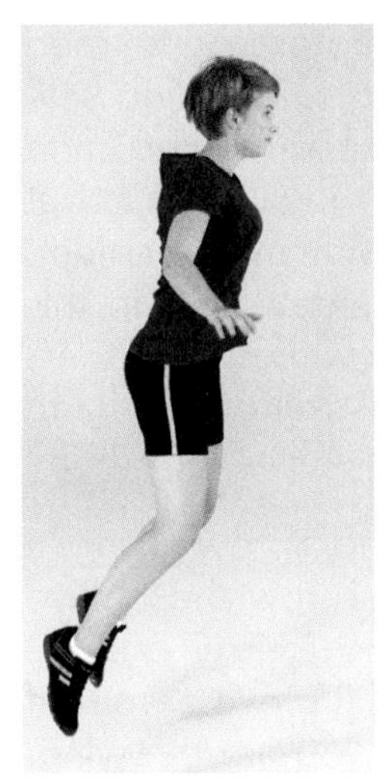

FIGURE 17.3 Vertical jump.

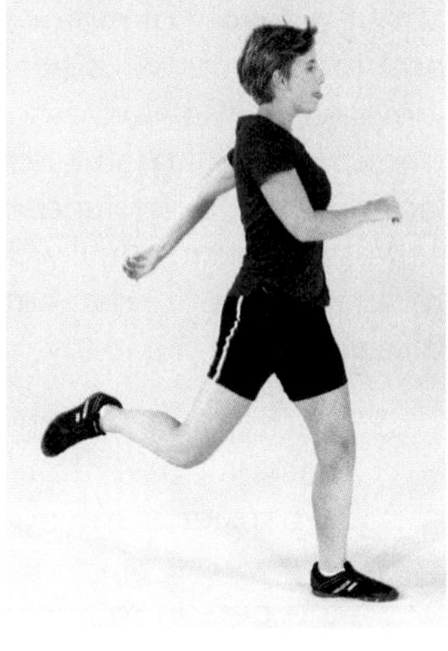

FIGURE 17.4 Leap.

Other Locomotor Movements

Space constraints do not allow for discussion here of all forms of locomotor movement. Some examples of other forms are skipping, hopping, galloping, and skating. Shuffle and crossover running are also common in many sports, and there are many variations of moving in water.

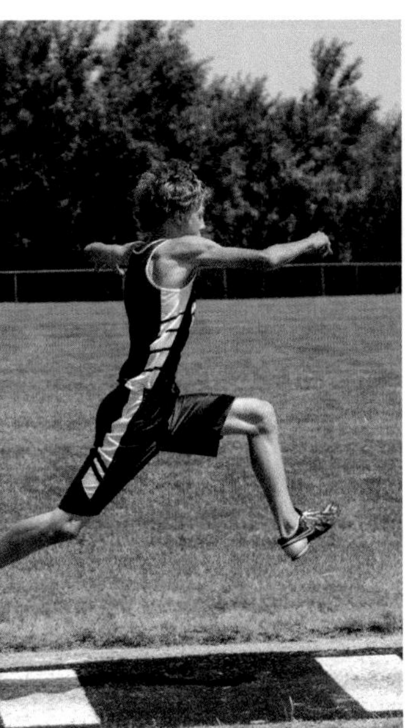

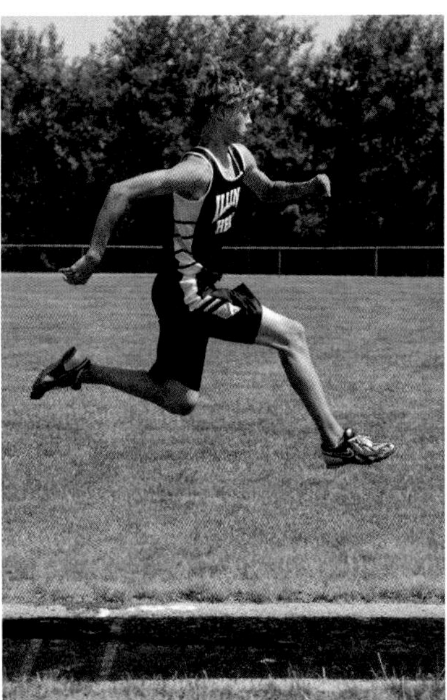

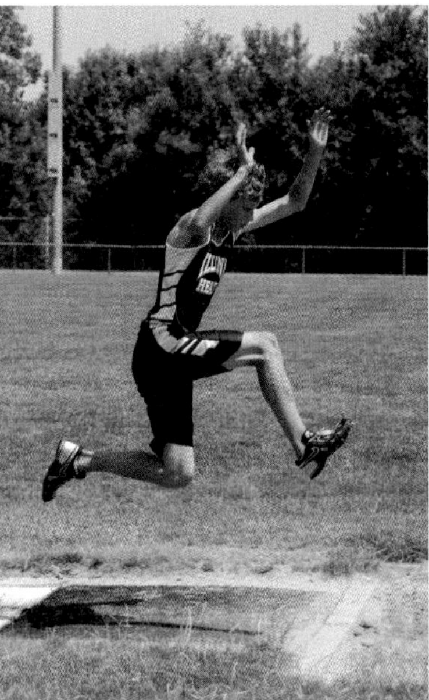

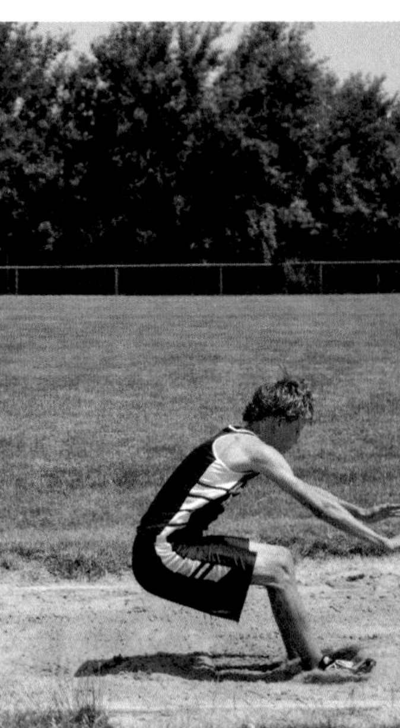

FIGURE 17.5 Running jump.

Lesson Review

1. What are nine biomechanical principles? How are they important to learning motor skills?
2. What are the two basic stances, and when should each be used?
3. What are some examples of locomotor skills? Describe them.
4. What is biomechanical analysis, and how can it be used to improve motor skills?

✓ SELF-ASSESSMENT: Analyzing Basic Skills

In the first lesson of this chapter, you learned about a variety of motor skills, including several locomotor skills (walking, running, and jumping). In the next lesson, you'll learn about throwing, striking, striking with an implement, kicking, and other fundamental skills. In this self-assessment, you'll work with two partners to analyze the fundamental skill of overhand throwing. Use the following steps.

1. Perform an overhand throw using a baseball or softball. Throw the ball to a partner standing 30 feet (9 meters) away. Your target is the glove or mitt of the person to whom you are throwing. Repeat the throw several times.
2. Have a second partner watch your throws and rate them using table 17.1. This partner should record the results. For each element of the throw listed in table 17.1, indicate whether you used good mechanics or need improvement in that area. Figure 17.6 in the next lesson may be useful as you make your assessment.
3. Rotate your duties so that each member of your team gets a chance to throw and rate.
4. When your ratings are done, use the information you gained to practice throwing properly. You can use peer teaching to help each other improve where needed.

Remember that self-assessment information is personal and considered confidential. It shouldn't be shared with others without the permission of the person being tested.

TABLE 17.1 Rating Chart: Overhand Throwing

Throwing mechanics	Needs improvement	Good mechanics
Preparation phase: Stands with the side pointing in the direction of the throw.		
Force production phase 1: Reaches backward with the throwing arm and hand, and the elbow is at or above shoulder height.		
Force production phase 2: Makes a long step forward with the foot opposite of the throwing arm.		
Force production phase 3: Turns the lower body toward the target, and the upper body lags behind.		
Force production phase 4: The shoulders turn toward the target, and the upper arm lags behind.		
Force production phase 5: The upper arm moves forward, and the elbow remains high.		
Force production phase 6: Flexes the wrist prior to follow through.		
Critical instant: Releases the ball at an angle that is appropriate for reaching the target.		
Recovery phase: Follows through across the body with the throwing arm after ball release.		

Lesson 17.2

Moving Implements and Objects

Lesson Objectives

After reading this lesson, you should be able to

1. describe three methods (and the related principles) of moving objects with body parts;
2. describe how striking with an implement (and the related principles) can be used in physical activity;
3. define *aerodynamics*, *hydrodynamics*, and *complex skills*, and explain how each is important to human movement; and
4. define *motor learning* and describe some factors that help you learn motor skills.

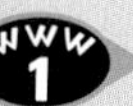

Lesson Vocabulary

complex skill, implement, jai alai, object, pelota, tracking

Do you ever think about the large number of physical skills you use every day? It's amazing to consider how many actions we perform without even thinking about them. In many things we do, whether work or play, we use an **implement**—a device or tool that helps us perform a task. For example, we use a rake to clean up leaves in the yard, a shovel to dig holes, brushes and rollers to apply paint, and hammers to pound nails. We also use implements in sport—for example, bats, rackets, clubs, and paddles to hit balls and birdies; paddles and oars to propel boats and canoes; sticks to play pool; and mallets to play croquet and polo. Of course, we can also use the body alone (most often a hand, arm, foot, or leg) to move an **object** without the aid of an implement. For example, we kick footballs and soccer balls, throw baseballs and softballs, and strike volleyballs. In all of these examples—those using an implement and those using only body parts—we are producing force to move an object.

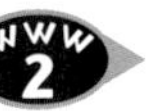

Skills That Move Objects

Too many skills involve moving implements and objects for us to consider them all here. However, the sections that follow describe some of the more basic skills that use body parts to move objects (for example, throwing and kicking). The descriptions also identify the principles related to performing each skill.

Throwing

The word *throw* means to propel an object through the air using a forward motion of the arm and hand. A throw can be underhand (as in bowling and softball pitching), sidearm (as in some baseball pitches), or overhand (as in most baseball pitches). The focus in throwing is sometimes on accuracy and sometimes on speed or velocity (how hard or fast you throw).

When learning a skill such as throwing, you go through three stages. In the first (cognitive) stage, you have to think about what you're doing, which slows you down. In this stage, you may have to sacrifice speed for accuracy (this is sometimes called the speed–accuracy trade-off). As you move through the second (associative) stage, you get better as you automatically associate your knowledge about throwing with the physical skill itself. You can now move more quickly and still be accurate. In the final

FIT FACT

The angle of a thrown object's release differs depending on the purpose of the throw. To throw a ball as far as possible, use a release angle of about 45 degrees. For hitting a target, especially one close to you, use a much lower angle of release (see principle 7 in lesson 1).

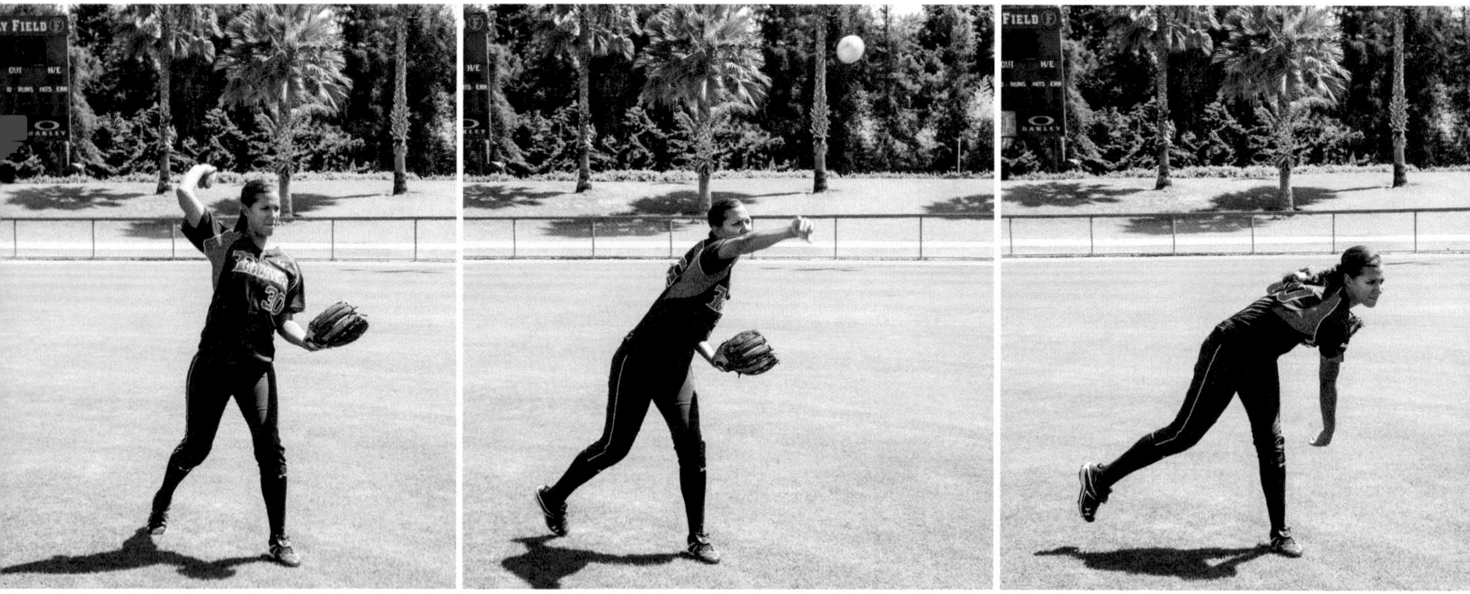

FIGURE 17.6 Overhand throwing.

(autonomous) stage, your performance becomes automatic. You can perform the skill, in this case throwing, with both speed and accuracy.

All types of throwing are used in a variety of settings, but only overhand throwing is described here (see figure 17.6). The photos show (1) force production (levers moved by muscles to produce force in proper sequence), (2) ball release (at the critical instant and at the appropriate angle), and (3) follow through (during the recovery phase).

Striking (With a Body Part)

Striking involves delivering a blow or making contact forcefully. It can be done with a body part, as in using a hand to spike a volleyball or deliver a karate blow. Like throwing, striking can be done at many arm angles, and contact can be made with the hand (open hand or fist), the heel of the hand, the forearms (as in a volleyball dig), or the elbows. Figure 17.7 shows one form of striking—the

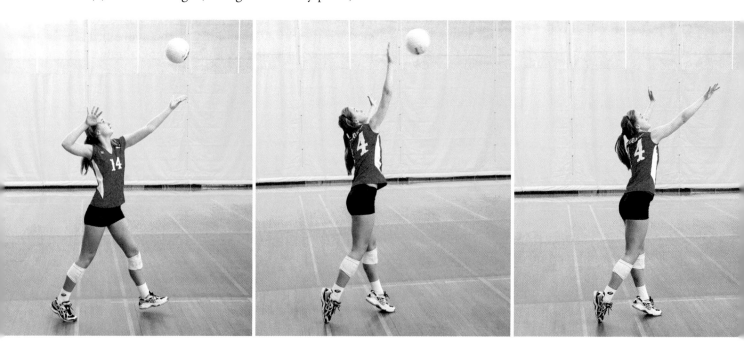

FIGURE 17.7 Striking for a volleyball serve.

volleyball serve—which uses a motion very similar to the standard throwing motion. The photos show (1) force production (levers moved by muscles to produce force in proper sequence), (2) ball strike (at the critical instant and at the appropriate angle), and (3) follow through (during the recovery phase). The strike can be done from a standing jump or a running jump. In this example, the focus is on the mechanics of striking the ball with the arm and hand, but, as discussed in a later section, striking can also be done with an implement.

Kicking (Striking With a Foot or Leg)

Kicking, which involves striking with a foot or leg, is used in various sports, including football (in punting and place-kicking), rugby, and soccer, and in games such as footbagging. Various kicks are also used in martial arts such as judo and karate. Kicking often involves contact, as when a foot hits the ball in soccer or strikes an object in karate, but some kicks do not make contact. In dance, for example, many types of kick are performed without striking. Kicked objects may be still at the time of contact (as in a soccer corner kick) or moving (as when the ball is rolling toward you in soccer). Kicking is often preceded by running, as in a football kickoff, and the performer sometimes alternates kicking and running (as in soccer dribbling). Figure 17.8 shows a soccer kick.

Catching

The skills described in this section allow you to receive objects that have been thrown, kicked, or propelled by an implement, such as a bat. For each skill, the discussion also identifies the related biomechanical principles.

The word *catch* carries many meanings. In sport and other physical activities, it means to grasp and hold onto an object, such as a ball. You can catch with one hand, two hands, or an implement. Several kinds of catching are shown in figure 17.9.

Both one-hand and two-hand catches can be performed either bare-handed (as when catching a bouncing tennis ball or a soccer shot on goal) or with the assistance of a glove (as in baseball and softball). Sometimes a two-hand catch also requires the use of the arms; for example, a football player catching a punt or kickoff might use arms as well as hands.

Some sports require you to use an implement to catch an object. For example, a lacrosse stick is used to catch and throw a ball. In **jai alai** (pronounced hi' lie), a wicker basket glove is used to catch and throw the **pelota** (ball; pronounced puh low' tuh).

Certain steps in catching are typical regardless of the type of catching. Specifically, you need to track the object, receive it, and absorb its force. Before you can catch an object, you must locate it and track it. **Tracking** involves keeping track of the object to be caught from the time it is thrown or projected (for example, kicked) until it gets close enough to

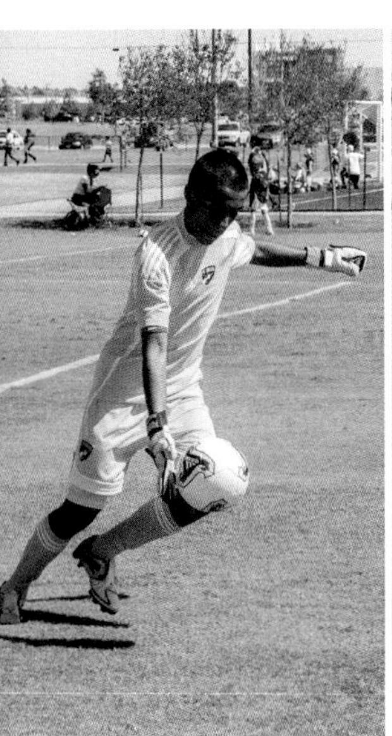
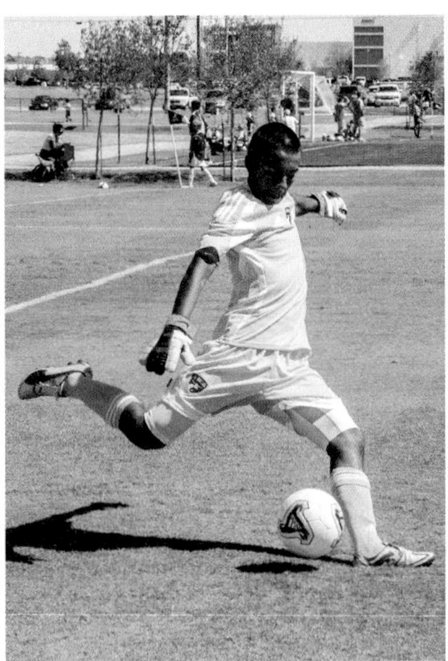
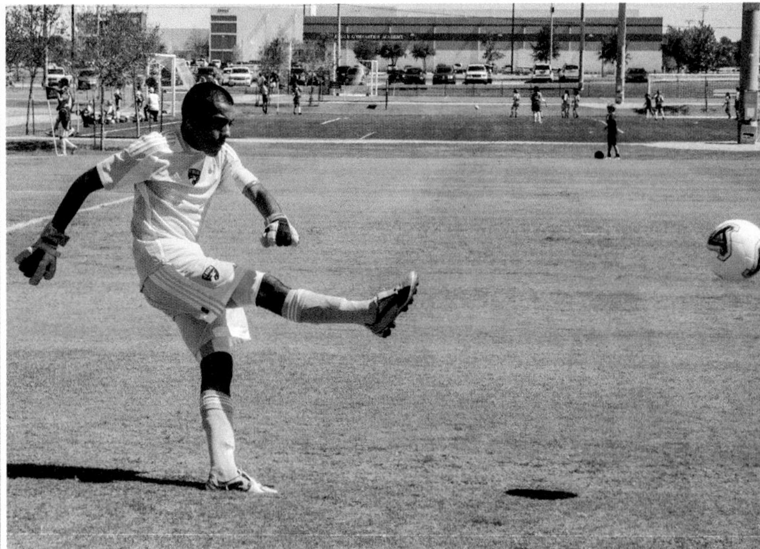

FIGURE 17.8 Kicking.

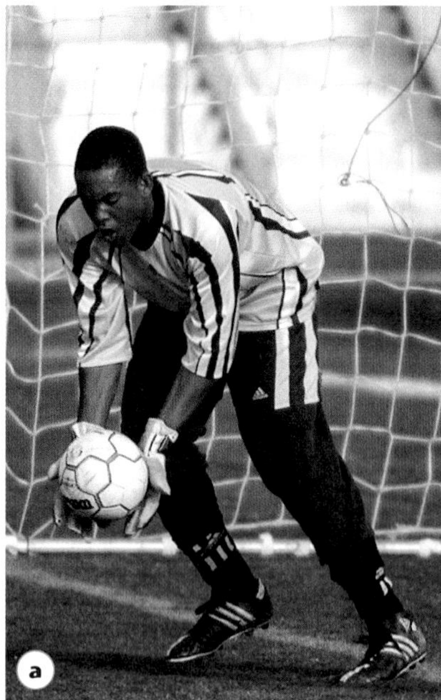
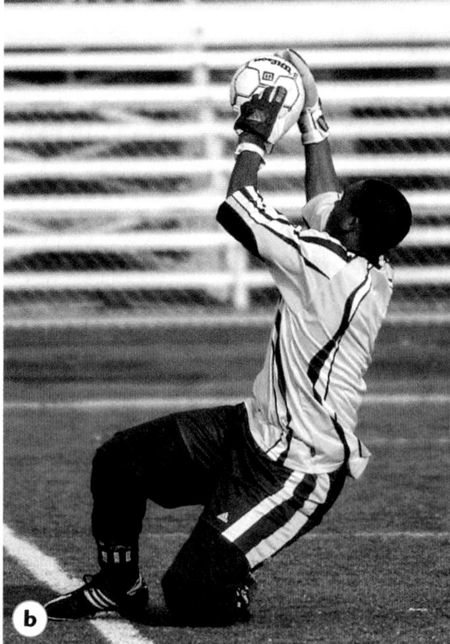
 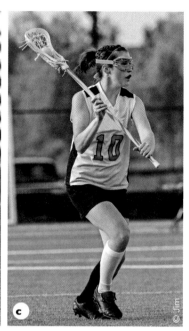

FIGURE 17.9 Examples of different kinds of catching: *(a)* two hands, below the waist; *(b)* two hands, above the waist; *(c)* with an implement.

catch. One key to catching, then, is expressed in the adage "keep your eye on the ball."

In football, players who catch passes are called receivers because catching really is a form of receiving an object. After tracking the ball, you must move your hands, arms, glove, or other catching implement to a location that makes the object easy to receive. The exact positioning depends on where you will receive the object. For example, when catching a ball below your waist, your palms should face away from your body, but your thumbs should face away from each other (figure 17.9*a*). For a catch above your waist, the palms of your hands should face away from your body with your thumbs together (figure 17.9*b*). When making an over-the-shoulder catch in football, your palms should face up with your thumbs facing away from each other.

In many types of catching, the object is moving very fast. As a result, once the object hits your hands, glove, or other implement, you should "give" with the blow to absorb the force by allowing the object to continue moving a bit before totally stopping it (figure 17.9*c*). For this reason, people who are good at catching are said to have "soft" hands.

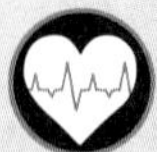

FITNESS TECHNOLOGY: Movement Analysis Apps

In this chapter's Science in Action feature, you learned about motion analysis systems that use special cameras and software to analyze physical performance. Coaches and athletes use these systems to study sport skill performance and identify areas for improvement. For example, softball pitchers study their pitching mechanics to see if changes are needed. Similarly, a batter can make a video when performing well and compare it with a video of his or her performance when not hitting well. Specialized apps even allow you to record and analyze your performance with a computer tablet or smartphone.

Using Technology

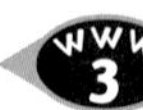

Visit the Health Opportunities Through Physical Education website and read about sport performance apps. If possible download a free app and use a tablet or smartphone to analyze a sport performance. If a download is not possible, read about the app. Prepare a brief report.

FIT FACT

Some sport and work skills require both hands to control an implement—for example, swinging an ax, digging with a shovel, hitting a two-hand tennis backhand, and swinging a baseball bat.

Striking (With an Implement)

As you may recall, an implement is a tool or piece of equipment used to accomplish a specific task. Examples of using an implement to apply force in sport include serving a tennis ball and hitting a baseball. Implements are typically used as levers to create a force greater than could be created by the body alone. For example, the most powerful major league pitchers can throw a baseball about 100 miles (160 kilometers) per hour, whereas the most powerful tennis players can serve a ball more than 150 miles (240 kilometers) per hour. Because a tennis racket provides greater leverage (longer lever), it creates greater ball speed.

The process of striking is typically referred to as the swing (as in swinging a hammer or a softball bat). Some implements are used to strike a moving object, as in tennis, whereas others are used to strike a still object, as in golf and croquet. Both kinds of striking are complex skills, but striking a moving object requires the ability to track it (figure 17.10)—and, in some cases, to toss it so that it can be struck properly, as in a tennis serve. Objects are struck at different angles depending on the sport. For example, a tennis serve goes from high to low, a golf swing from low to high, and a softball swing from front to back at about waist height.

Complex Skills

Walking and running are examples of basic motor locomotor skills. The basic skills described in this chapter are the most often used in sport and physical activity. Many activities, however, require **complex skills**. Some complex skills require the use of several basic skills in sequence. For example, in softball an outfielder must run, catch, and quickly throw the ball. Dance involves a wide range of intricate sequential steps, including ballet movements, Latin dance moves, and complex hip-hop maneuvers. Other complex skills require the coordination of several different movements. For example, swimming uses virtually all body parts at the same time, and the levers of the upper and lower body must be used in the proper sequence. Even the trunk must move to produce optimal movement through the water.

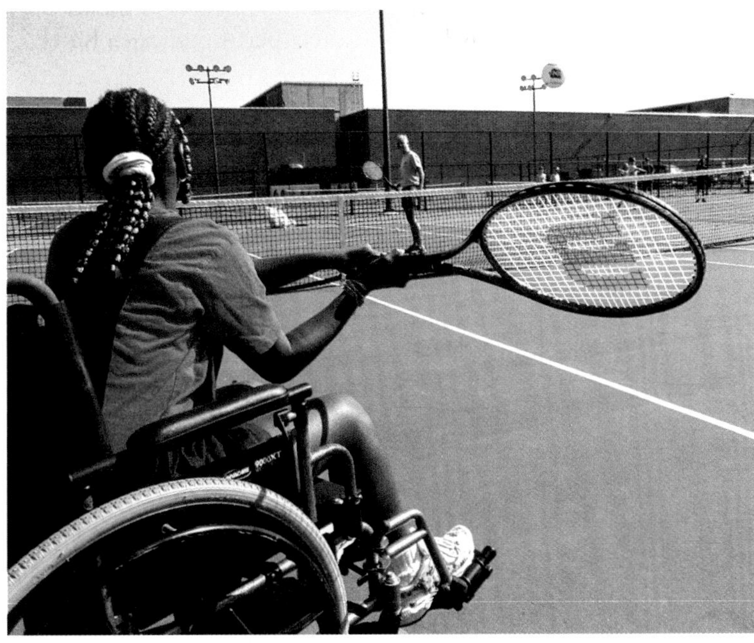

FIGURE 17.10 To strike a moving object with an implement, you must first track it visually.

Aerodynamics and Hydrodynamics

Aerodynamics refers to the study of motion in the air. When you use skills at work or play, air can affect your performance. Spin, for example, affects the motion of an object that has been thrown or struck by an implement. Here are some examples from softball in which spin is imparted by the use of the body without an implement.

- Forward spin (topspin) causes the ball to drop faster than normal.
- Backward spin (backspin) creates lift so that the ball appears to rise (does not drop as fast as normal).
- Sidespin causes the ball to "break" or curve from its normal path.

Spin can also be imparted to an object by means of an implement. For example, tennis players swing from low to high to create topspin, which allows them to hit the ball hard and still keep it in bounds because the spin causes the ball to come down faster than normal. As with a pitched baseball, sidespin causes a tennis ball to curve. Spin on a football causes it to spiral and stay stable in the air. Spin on a pool or billiard ball causes it to curve or even jump.

Wind (a type of air movement) can cause resistance to movement; a headwind, for example, slows a runner. Wind can also exaggerate the effect of spin on a ball. For example, if a ball is curving because of spin, the wind may either cause more spin or cause resistance to the curving caused by the spin. In sailing, the wind is essential to the boat's movement, and skilled sailors can use it to move a boat in all directions.

Moving objects, including your body, can also be affected by humidity, temperature, and altitude. Dry air, for example, provides less resistance than humid air. Very cold air cools an object, which may limit the distance it travels when struck or kicked. The air at high altitude is thinner and therefore provides less resistance than air at lower altitudes.

Hydrodynamics refers to the study of motion in fluid. It's especially important to swimmers and people who do other water activities, such as surfers, boaters, kayakers, and rowers. Water causes resistance to movement and therefore affects the movement of swimmers and boaters. In fact, pushing against the resistance of water is what propels you forward when swimming or using an oar. Water itself moves because of various forces, including wind and gravitational pull, which can cause waves. Swimmers' movements also cause the water to move, as does splashing of water against the side of a pool. Waves and other water movements affect performance in water.

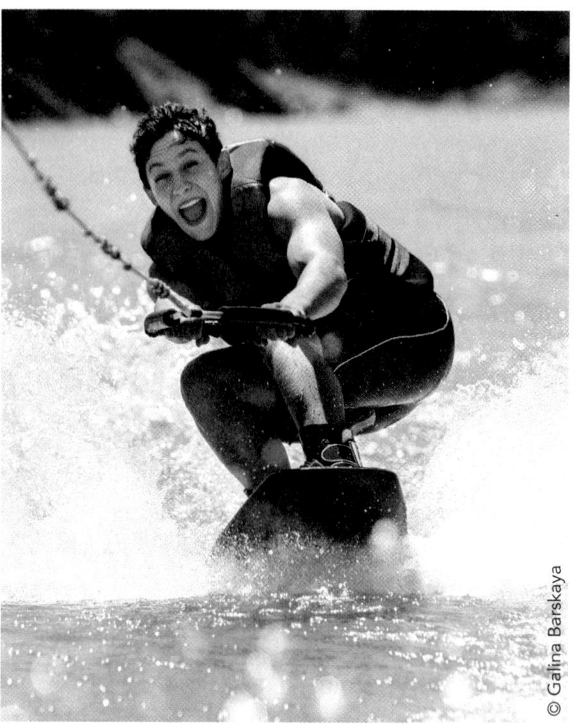

Water resistance affects a variety of water activities.

Motor Learning

Motor learning involves practicing movements in order to improve motor skills. Some movements are voluntary; others are involuntary. Involuntary movements occur when a reflex initiates the movement. A reflex is an automatic movement that does not require your brain to directly stimulate your nerves to cause your muscles to contract. One example is the knee jerk reflex that occurs when a doctor taps your knee with a small hammer during a physical exam.

Most movements involved in motor skills are voluntary. When you perform a voluntary movement, such as throwing a ball, your brain signals your nerves, which signal your muscles to contract. The contraction of your muscles then moves your bones (in throwing, the bones or levers of your arm). The movement of the levers provides the force to throw the ball. Some principles of motor learning are described in this section.

Practice

With good practice, you can improve your motor skills. You can get the most out of your practice by getting specific feedback from an instructor or using a video that teaches you about specific things to practice.

Skill Transfer

Once you learn the basics of a motor skill, you can transfer it—that is, use it when learning a similar skill. For example, if you use practice to become good at throwing a baseball, it will be easier for you to learn to throw a football and even to strike a ball as in volleyball spiking.

Skill Change

If you learn a skill very well and then try to change your technique, it will take some time before you see improvement. For example, if you practice for a long time to learn to bowl using a straight ball, then decide to change your delivery to a hook, you may not see immediate improvement. It took a lot of practice for you to learn the first delivery, and it will take time and practice to "forget" it and learn the new one. Allow yourself time to learn the new delivery before expecting improvement in your performance. It's also advisable to avoid making big changes in the way you perform a skill right before you compete or have a test of performance. Change when you have time to practice before performing.

> "Just keep going. Everybody gets better if they keep at it."
>
> —Ted Williams, Hall of Fame baseball player

Mental Practice

Mental practice involves rehearsing a skill in your mind without moving the relevant body parts. It is useful for rehearsing the biomechanics of a movement and has been shown to help people learn skills.

Lesson Review

1. What are three methods (and the related principles) of moving objects with body parts?
2. How can striking with an implement (and the related principles) be used in physical activity?
3. What are aerodynamics, hydrodynamics, and complex skills? How is each important to human movement?
4. What is motor learning, and what factors help you learn motor skills?

TAKING CHARGE: Positive Self-Talk

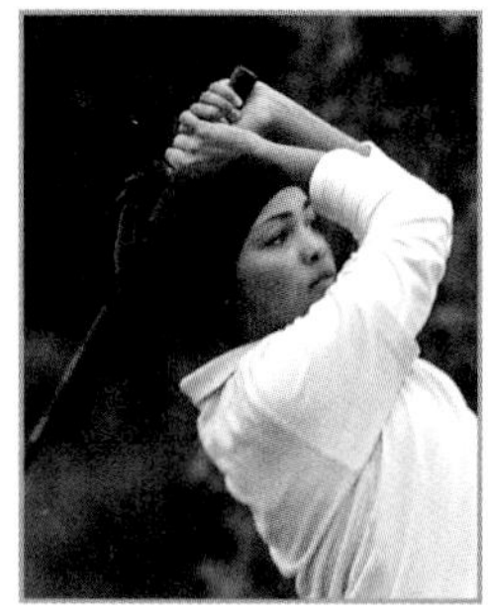

Alexis was not on the school golf team, but she did like to play golf. She thought about trying out for the team, but she wasn't sure that she was good enough. When she played with her family, she did well, but when she played with people she didn't know, she didn't do as well. Sometimes she talked to herself while playing, saying things like, "Why did you do that, dummy?" or "Oh, no—I'm starting to play badly again." Sometimes she even talked to herself out loud, saying things like, "I got a 7 on that hole? Now I don't even have a chance for a good score!"

After one particular round in which she didn't play as well as she would have liked, Alexis asked her mother, "Why do things always go wrong when I play with people I don't know?" Her mother said that she had read a book by a sport psychologist who recommended avoiding negative self-talk (saying negative things to yourself, which affects your self-confidence and leads to poor play). The key is to replace the negative self-talk with positive self-talk. As Alexis' mom said, "If you expect bad things to happen, they probably will. Next time you play, try to cut the negative talk and focus on positives. If you have a bad hole, say to yourself, 'It's just one hole—I'm going to do better on the next one.'"

For Discussion

What are some examples of negative self-talk common in sport and other activities? What are some examples of positive self-talk that can be used to replace negative self-talk? What other suggestions do you have for Alexis and other people who are in sporting situations? In crafting your advice, consider the guidelines presented in the Self-Management feature.

SELF-MANAGEMENT: Skills for Positive Self-Talk

You know that some people are considered pessimists and others optimists. A pessimist thinks bad things are going to happen, and an optimist believes good things are sure to come. Experts in exercise and sport psychology have found that with practice, you can develop "learned optimism." Specifically, you can replace negative thoughts and negative self-talk with positive thoughts and positive self-talk. Follow these guidelines to use positivity to improve your performance.

- **Learn the ABCs.** A stands for adversity, which can lead to negative thoughts and negative self-talk. Learn to recognize when you're facing adversity. B stands for beliefs. If you believe that you're going to do poorly when you face adversity, you probably will. Learn to recognize negative beliefs when you face adversity. C is for consequences. Learn to recognize your feelings about the consequences of adversity. A pessimist might say, "If I do poorly on one hole in golf, I have no chance to get a reasonable score." Learning to reassess consequences and be more realistic can help you become more optimistic.
- **Accept adversity as a challenge rather than a sure cause of failure.** Adversity causes negative self-talk only if you let it.
- **Alter your beliefs about adversity.** If you accept adversity as a challenge, you can tell yourself to avoid negative thoughts and replace them with positive ones. Experts suggest that replacing negative comments (such as "That was a dumb decision!") with positive ones (such as "I know I can do it!") leads to better performance. So when you're faced with adversity, respond with positive self-talk. Tell yourself, "I believe I can do this!"
- **Don't overdramatize the consequences of adversity.** Think realistically about adversity. Ask yourself if your view of the potential consequences is pessimistic. If so, replace it with a more realistic or even positive view.

- **Put the past behind you.** Failing at a task or doing less well than you'd like doesn't necessarily mean you'll fail next time. For example, in golf, don't let one bad hole get you down. You can't change the past—only the future. Worrying about the last hole leads to negative thoughts when you play the next one. Playing a hole badly creates adversity, but positive thinking and positive self-talk can turn the last bad hole into the next good one.
- **Practice creating a positive circle of success.** Pessimists think negatively when faced with adversity. Negative beliefs lead to poor performance, which contributes to more negative thoughts, thus creating a negative circle. Work instead to create a positive circle of success. Every time you face adversity, remember the ABCs (recall the first item in this list) and practice them. Recognize adversity when it arises and establish positive beliefs ("I know I can do this"). This can lead to positive consequences (improved performance).
- **Be realistic.** In learning about SMART goals, you've learned that being realistic is important to setting effective goals. Setting unrealistically high goals can lead to feelings of failure even when you're doing quite well. Remember that practice is necessary for success.

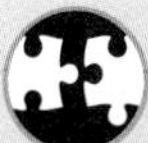

ACADEMIC CONNECTION: Multiple Meanings

Meeting standards for English language arts requires an understanding of the multiple meanings of words. The word *force* has many meanings. For example, there is military force (troops and ships), violent force (a physical attack), and mechanical force (energy exerted). In this chapter, *force* refers to energy exerted by the muscles to cause tension or to cause the body or an object to move. Force can also be used to stop a body or object from moving (resistance force). The definition in the box is the one included in the glossary.

> **force**—In physical activity, it is energy exerted by the muscles to cause movement or resist movement; other uses include military force (ships and troops), violent force (a physical attack), or resistance force (stopping a moving body or object).

Identify other words used in part 1 of this book that have multiple meanings. An example is the word *power*, which refers to a part of health-related fitness (strength × speed) in part 1 of this book. But *power* can also refer to possession of influence or control (political power) or a source of energy (electric or solar power). You may want to use the glossary to assist you.

TAKING ACTION: Applying Principles

In this chapter, you've learned nine biomechanical principles that are important for performing motor skills. These principles apply to skills used in a variety of work and play situations.

Take action by trying several different skills and describing the principles that apply to the performance of each one.

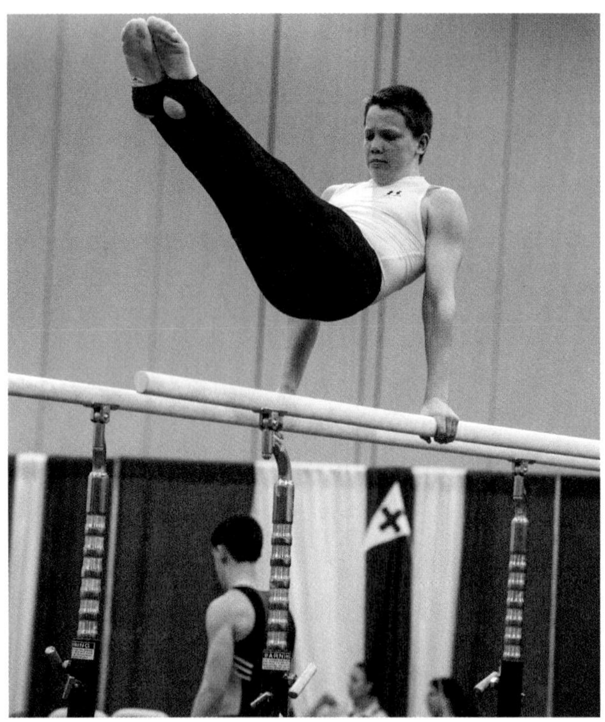

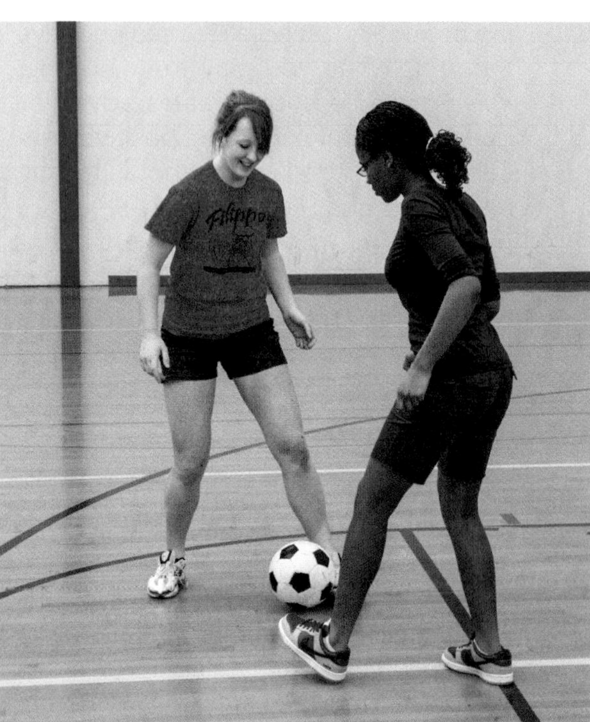

Take action by applying biomechanical principles as you perform different skills.

CHAPTER REVIEW

Reviewing Concepts and Vocabulary

As directed by your teacher, answer items 1 through 5 by correctly completing each sentence with a word or phrase.

1. A _______________ refers to a way of standing.
2. Moving your body from place to place is called _______________.
3. _______________ is the study of motion in fluids.
4. Delivering a blow or making contact forcefully is called _______________.
5. When you perform the skill of _______________, you must track the object before receiving it.

For items 6 through 10, as directed by your teacher, match each term in column 1 with the appropriate phrase in column 2.

6. transfer	a. study of motion in the air
7. mental practice	b. using one skill to perform another
8. motor learning	c. practicing to improve a skill
9. aerodynamics	d. rehearsing a skill in your mind
10. striking with an implement	e. tennis serve

For items 11 through 15, as directed by your teacher, respond to each statement or question.

11. Describe three different principles of biomechanics.
12. Describe biomechanical analysis and how it uses technology.
13. Give examples of striking a ball with an implement.
14. What are some aerodynamic factors that influence the flight of a ball?
15. What are some guidelines for eliminating negative self-talk?

Thinking Critically

Write a paragraph to answer the following question.

A friend has been selected to kick a 15-yard field goal at your school's next home football game. If she succeeds, she wins a prize. When she was younger she played soccer, but she has not played in a while. Now she would like your help to improve her kicking. How would you help her win the prize?

Project

To improve academic performance, many schools perform three- to five-minute exercise breaks in the classroom. The breaks include by-the-desk exercises that can be performed in a small space and often include dance steps (thus also involving motor skills). Plan an exercise break for one of your classes. You can use video or music or just lead the group in an exercise. Show it to one of your teachers and ask to present it to the class.

18

Lifelong Activity

In This Chapter

Student Web Resources
www.HOPEtextbook.org/student

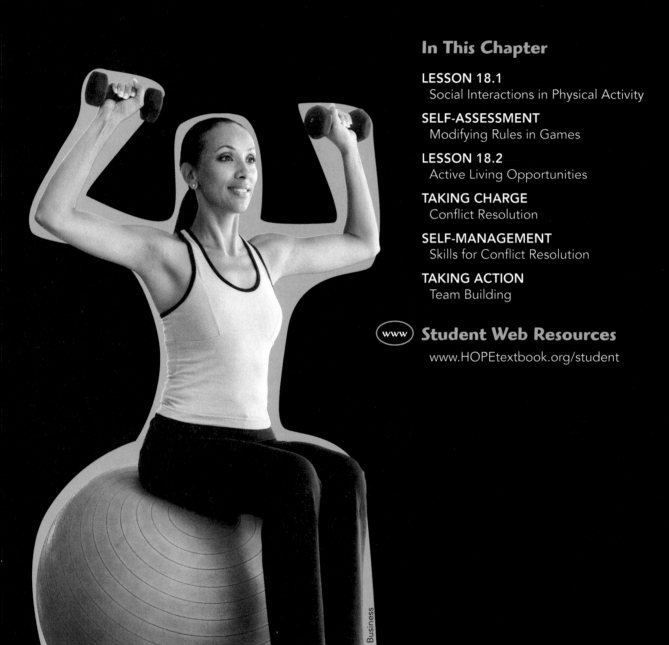

Lesson 18.1

Social Interactions in Physical Activity

Lesson Objectives

After reading this lesson, you should be able to

1. describe five leadership skills,
2. define *teamwork* and describe five guidelines for becoming an effective team member,
3. define *group cohesiveness* and factors that develop it,
4. define *rule* and *etiquette* and explain how they are important in sport and physical activity, and
5. describe *sportsmanship*, *diversity*, and *bullying* and explain how they are important in sport and physical activity.

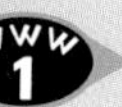

Lesson Vocabulary

etiquette, group cohesiveness, leadership, rule, sportsmanship, teamwork

Have you ever played on a sport team? Have you been part of a different kind of team? If you answered yes to either question, what role did you play on the team, and how comfortable were you in that role? Did the team have good chemistry, or were there issues that kept team members distant from each other?

One goal of this book is to help people move from dependence to independence, whether in working out to get fit or in making decisions about what to eat. This growth involves not only engaging in positive social interactions in school but also developing skills that will help you in the future. In school, teachers and coaches often appoint leaders, and rules are often made and enforced by others. This chapter provides guidelines for helping *you* make responsible choices, especially in physical activity settings.

> "If your actions create a legacy that inspires others to dream more, learn more, do more, and become more, then you are an excellent leader."
>
> —Dolly Parton, singer and actor

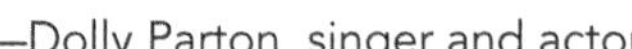

Leaders and Leadership

A leader guides or directs a group of people, such as a sport team or club. **Leadership** involves actively assuming the role of a leader. You can't be a leader just because you want to. Becoming a leader requires leadership skills that can be developed, and some of the most important are presented in table 18.1. Like all skills, leadership skills must be practiced in order to be mastered.

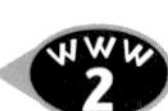

One way to get leadership experience is to play sports and games. Another way is to participate in physical education class; for example, in the physical education approach known as sport education, students are grouped into teams whose members serve as leaders, team members, and referees. In the workplace, companies often use cooperative games to train their leaders (in this case, managers and executives).

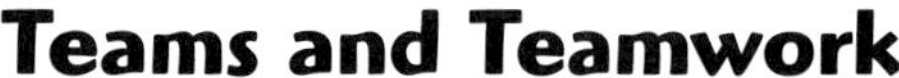

Teams and Teamwork

A team is a group of people who band together or are assigned to work together. Ideally, team members work together to achieve a common goal. Sometimes, however, not all team members are committed to the team's goal; in fact, some members may even work to subvert the team's efforts. **Teamwork** is effective, combined work by all team members toward achieving the common goal. In order to experience teamwork, group members often have to sacrifice personal recognition in favor of team goals. For this reason, sport teams often use the slogan "There is no I in TEAM" to emphasize that individual goals are secondary to team goals (figure 18.1).

TABLE 18.1 Leadership Skills

Skill	Description	How to build
Integrity	Integrity means being fair; for a leader, it means directing while adhering to rules and standards of the group. Not all leaders have integrity, but good leaders do.	Integrity is built over time. You establish a reputation based on your actions.
Communication	Good leaders are good listeners. They listen in order to understand the group's needs, then speak clearly to be understood. Good leaders also inspire and persuade.	Practice listening even when you have much to say. Keep track of what others say. Ask whether what you think they said is what they meant. Ask what they heard you say to see if they got your message. Get the facts to help you make good arguments.
Strategy and planning	Creating a strategy requires creating a clear vision of your goals. It also involves developing tactics for carrying out the plan.	Practice using the steps for developing a strategy and carrying out a plan. Get the facts before planning.
Management	Leaders help group members work together to meet goals. Keys include building teamwork (group unity) and building trust based on integrity. Relevant skills that can be learned include directing and supervising others, resolving conflicts, and negotiating.	Study the information presented in this chapter about teamwork and conflict resolution.
Other	Other characteristics of a good leader include self-confidence, optimism, enthusiasm, decisiveness, and being proactive. Good leaders can also accept criticism and are willing to learn better ways to reach group goals.	Most of these characteristics are built through experience. It also helps to practice the self-management skills presented in part 1 of this book.

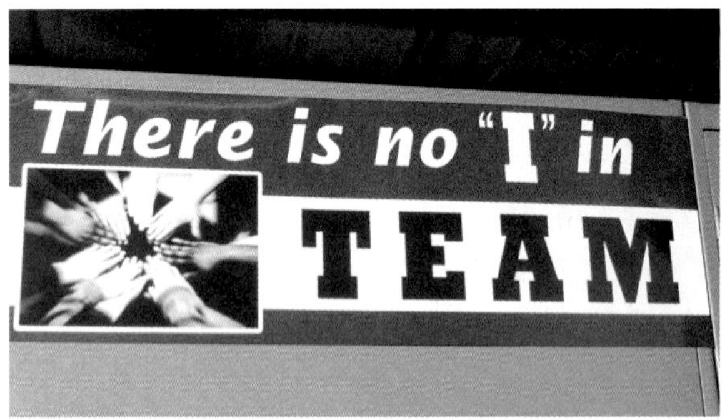

FIGURE 18.1 Motivational slogans are sometimes used to promote teamwork.

Aristotle, the Greek philosopher, stated, "the whole is greater than the sum of its parts." The implication is that if people work together, they can accomplish things that they could not accomplish working independently. Consider the following guidelines about teamwork. They can be useful in helping groups to function effectively.

- **Learning your role.** What tasks are you best able to perform that will help the team? A team has a few common goals but many different roles. While some roles are more prominent (for example, pitcher on a softball team), all roles must be performed well for the team to succeed.
- **Accepting your role.** The role you want may not be the role you get. A person who accepts an assigned role is more likely to help the team than one who does not. In addition, carrying out a role that you don't prefer can lead to more desirable roles in the future. As illustrated in this chapter's Science in Action feature, teams can function effectively even if a member does not like his or her role—and even when team members don't get along well—as long as members *accept* their roles. Of course, being on

a team is more fun if team members like each other and work well together.

- **Practicing your role.** As with being a leader, being an effective team member requires practice. Every role requires specific skills. For example, the pitcher on a softball team must have motor skills suited to that position but may not be an especially good hitter. For this reason, the pitcher may be called on to perform a sacrifice bunt to move a runner into scoring position. This pitcher will practice bunting more than other players because this is an assigned role. Of course, roles are often assigned by leaders on the basis of special skills that individuals possess. In an example from a school setting, one sophomore class president, named Hideko, sought artists to make posters, computer specialists to prepare websites, and other people with special skills for special roles.
- **Carrying out your role.** It's one thing to practice your role but another to carry it out effectively.

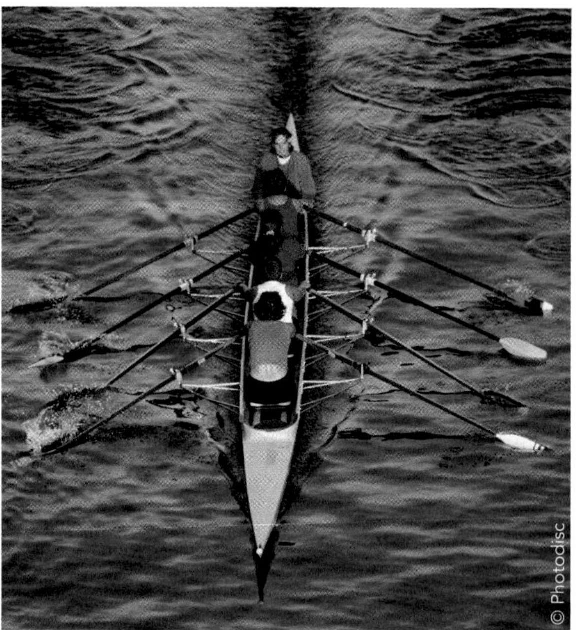

Group cohesiveness occurs when team members work together toward a common goal.

SCIENCE IN ACTION: Group Cohesiveness

Cohesion means sticking together tightly. In chemistry, it means uniting particles to form a single mass. When applied to groups of people, cohesion is referred to as **group cohesiveness,** which occurs when group or team members stick together in working toward common goals. Scientists have studied group cohesiveness in a variety of sports and found that several factors help groups stick together; they include small group size, friendship among members, commitment to the group's goals, group success or failure, and competitiveness of group members.

It's easier to achieve group cohesiveness in small groups because fewer people have to coordinate their efforts. For example, it's easier for 5 people on a basketball team to work together than for 11 people on a football team to do so. It's also easier for small groups to agree on goals.

In addition, if team members know and like each other, it's easier for them to agree on goals and work together. However, studies also show that some teams win championships despite dissension among their members because team members are strongly committed to the group's goals. Several studies of rowers, for example, show that personal feelings can be overcome if team members want strongly enough to win. Thus competitiveness is also a factor that creates desire among team members to work together, though it can cut both ways: Winning a competition can help members get along, but losing sometimes leads to disagreements between team members (see this chapter's Taking Charge feature).

Research also shows that it's important for group members to recognize that everyone makes mistakes sometimes. This acknowledgment reduces blaming when the team does poorly and increases the chances for achieving group cohesiveness in the future. It's crucial to support fellow team members when they're down.

Student Activity

Search websites, magazines, or newspapers to find a true story about group cohesiveness. Describe how the group members worked together to achieve a common goal.

Even when everyone does his or her job as practiced, success may not follow. For example, the opposing team may use a tactic that overcomes your team's tactic. Or the other team may simply have players who are very good. Thus, carrying out your role may not always get the desired result, but it does give your team the best chance for success. For this reason, it's important not to get discouraged if you and your team are not successful every time that you perform your role well.

- **Adapting as necessary.** Again, even if all team members work hard and perform their roles well, success may not follow. If the team's strategy and tactics are not working, adjustments need to be made, and those adjustments could mean a change in some team members' role.

Making and Enforcing Rules

A **rule** is a guideline or regulation for conduct or action. Rules help bring order and fairness to sports and games. They can be very formal—for example, the official rules of baseball. They can also be informal, as is the case for conduct of friends in an informal group.

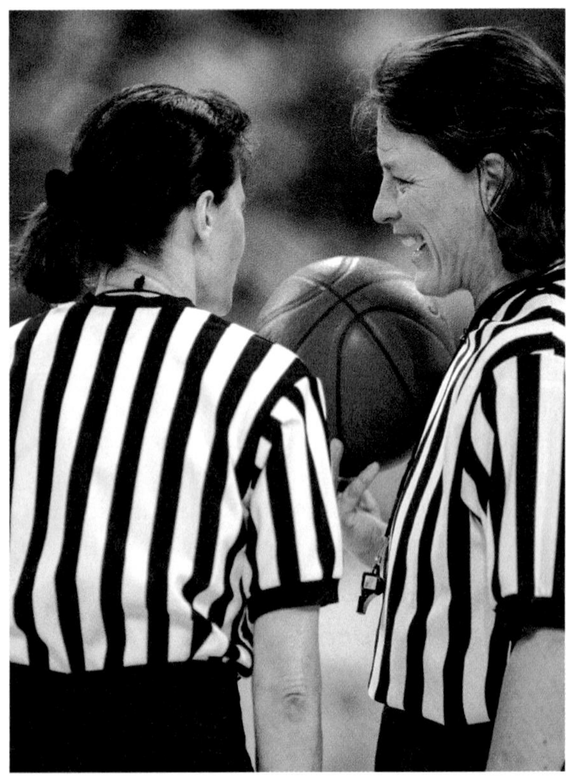

For rules to be effective, they must be consistently enforced.

There are many kinds of rules, ranging from societal laws (for example, the rules of the road for driving) to math and science laws and principles. Classrooms have rules, as do business meetings. Sport teams have rules for remaining in good standing with the team, and religions have rules of moral conduct. Violating a rule typically results in some sort of punishment, whereas regular adherence to rules is usually rewarded. Rules are enforced in a variety of ways; for example, police officers enforce laws, referees enforce sport rules, and coaches and team leaders enforce team rules.

FIT FACT

A recent national survey found that nearly 85 percent of American adults agree that bending or breaking the rules in sport is cheating and should not be tolerated. A similar percentage agree that bending or breaking the rules is cheating even if no one notices. Despite the high number of people who feel that cheating is wrong and makes games less fun and fair, one in five admits to breaking rules in sports, and nearly half say they know someone who has bent or broken rules.

Experts agree that for rules to be effective, they must be consistently enforced. They should also be appropriate for the situation, and punishment should be consistent with the violation. Rules must be fair to all members of the group.

In some cases, not much can be done to change rules, at least not quickly. In sport, for example, teams are bound by existing rules as they are enforced by officials. Team and school rules, however, can be changed more quickly if they are not serving their intended purpose. Teams and team members can modify bad rules by using a version of the scientific method. After identifying the rules that seem to need changing, the group can collect information, then use it to articulate clear reasons (evidence) for changing the rules. Group members should consult with each other and debate the evidence, after which either the group as a whole or its leaders can make a decision. Once the decision is made, the group's effectiveness depends on whether group members comply with the new rules. A group member who finds the rules unacceptable can opt out; that is, he or she doesn't have to continue to be a member.

Etiquette in Physical Activity

Etiquette involves acting in a way that is consistent with the typical or expected behavior of a social group. In Western society, for example, etiquette for eating indicates when to use a knife, a fork, or a spoon. In Eastern culture, however, etiquette for eating often calls for using chopsticks in particular ways. Sport also involves social situations subject to a code of etiquette. The code may not be written, but it is present nevertheless.

Some rules of sport etiquette are informal. In golf, for example, it is considered poor etiquette to talk while another player is swinging. Other rules of etiquette are more formal and may even be written. For example, tennis often involves a dress code, and many clubs and tournaments used to consider any color other than white to be inappropriate. In addition, for many years, female tennis players were expected to wear skirts rather than shorts. Over time, however, etiquette can change, and today it is common for women to wear shorts on the court. Clothing colors other than white are also now common.

Most people agree that following rules of etiquette, whether formal or informal, generally helps make social situations more fun and enjoyable. Knowing the etiquette of a particular sport or social group can also help you feel more comfortable in the group, whereas not knowing it can make you quite uncomfortable.

Diversity: Respect for Others

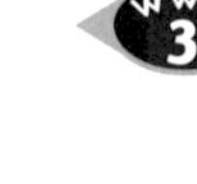

The word *society* refers to a large group of people who have a history of working and living together. It can refer to a neighborhood, a community, a nation, or an even larger group (for example, Western society). Characteristics of a society include traditions, organized laws and rules, and standards for living and conduct (social etiquette).

Societies provide for the common interests of their members and protect them from outside threats. One common interest in a society is that of providing for all members of the group, not just the biggest and strongest. Diversity in a society refers to the inclusion of different types of people, and the great diversity in many modern societies makes social sensitivity and responsibility necessary. Specifically, it requires sensitivity to others regardless of race, ethnicity, age, disability, culture, socioeconomic status, sex, or gender identity. To achieve the goal of treating all members equally and fairly, it is helpful to consider all people when selecting

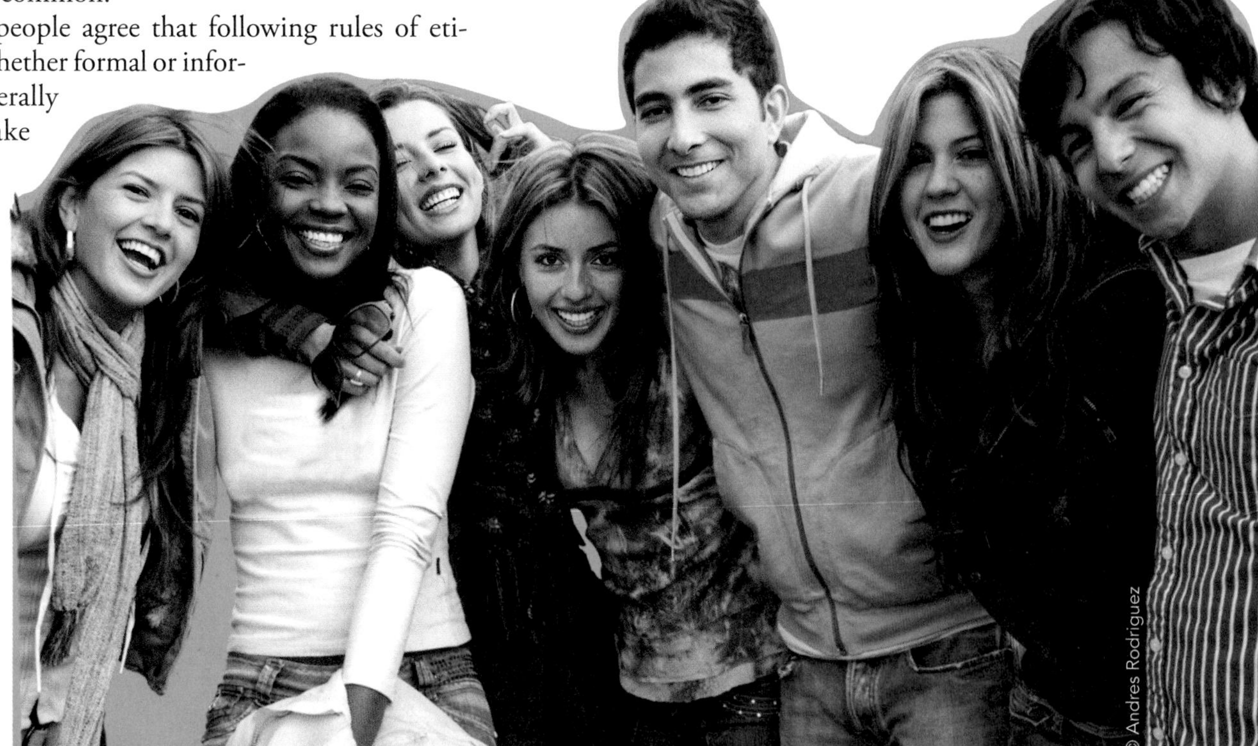

leaders; to follow the rules of the social group (such as a team or school); and to practice good etiquette in daily activities.

FIT FACT

Two-thirds of American adults believe that winning is overemphasized, and more than half believe that unethical behavior is common in certain sports, particularly football, hockey, wrestling, and baseball.

Sportsmanship

Sportsmanship is a term used to describe respect for opponents and grace in winning or losing when participating in a game or sport. A good sport exhibits good ethical conduct and plays by the rules. An overemphasis on winning can sometimes result in acts of poor sportsmanship, such as attempting to hurt an opponent or intentionally violating the rules to gain an advantage. You'll find that if you participate in games and sports for fun, health benefits, stress reduction, and social interaction you'll enjoy yourself much more than if you focus only on winning.

Sensitivity, Trust, and Respect

Sensitivity refers to paying attention to the feelings and concerns of others. Ways to build sensitivity include listening (for example, hearing what others have to say rather than only telling others what to do) and communicating in nonthreatening language (for example, giving positive comments rather than harsh criticism). Trust refers to the belief that others are honest and reliable. Demonstrating honesty and reliability in your actions helps others learn to trust you. Trustworthy people keep their promises and are sensitive to the needs of others. People who are trustworthy and sensitive (including leaders) typically have the respect of others.

Bullying

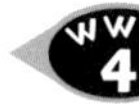

Bullying is a serious problem among teens. Experts in sport sociology indicate that half of all teens say they have been bullied, and nearly as many say they have bullied someone else. A U.S. government website (StopBullying.gov) describes several types of bullying, including verbal (name calling, teasing), social (spreading rumors, leaving people out, breaking friendships), physical (hitting, punching, shoving), and cyber (using the web and tech devices to do harm). Bullying shows disrespect for individual people and for the rules of the social group.

Lesson Review

1. What are the five leadership skills?
2. What is teamwork, and what are the five guidelines for becoming an effective team member?
3. What is group cohesiveness, and what are some factors that develop it?
4. What are rules and etiquette, and how are they important in sport and physical activity?
5. How are *sportsmanship*, *diversity*, and *bullying* defined, and how they are important in sport and physical activity?

SELF-ASSESSMENT: Modifying Rules in Games

This self-assessment will give you insight into the importance of fair rules when playing games. Perform the activity as described, then, as directed by your instructor, record information concerning the activity. Remember that self-assessment information is personal and considered confidential. It shouldn't be shared with others without the permission of the person being tested.

1. Each person in the class writes his or her name on a small piece of paper. Place the names in a box or bag. One member of the class draws the names of six people.
2. The people whose names are drawn come to the front of the class. Two teams are formed—the first three drawn are on one team, and the second three are on the other. Members of each team spread out in a defined game area in front of the class. They may stand wherever they want within the game area, but once their location is determined they cannot move from that spot (the right foot may not move).
3. The name of an additional person is drawn. This person is the referee. He or she tosses a small ball into the air within the playing area. When a player on either team touches the ball, the referee awards a point to one team. The referee decides which team gets the point and does not have to explain why the point was given. Points do not have to be awarded for the same reason for each throw. The referee retrieves the ball and continues to throw it and award points arbitrarily until the ball is thrown 10 times. The team with the most points is the winner. If the score is tied, the team that scores the next point wins.
4. Ask team members to explain how they felt about the game and its rules.
5. After the discussion, draw names for additional teams and referees, so that several games are played at the same time (all members of the class are involved). Before each group plays the game, both teams must agree on two or three rules for awarding points. The referee writes down the rules and uses them when throwing the ball and awarding points.
6. After all teams have finished playing their game, each group comes up with ideas for improving the game.
7. Each group then presents and justifies its list of rules to the rest of the class.
8. If time allows, play the game using rules created by one of the groups.

Adapted from an activity developed by the College of Education at the University of North Carolina.

Lesson 18.2

Active Living Opportunities

Lesson Objectives

After reading this lesson, you should be able to

1. define *autonomy* and explain how it relates to decision making about healthy lifestyles,
2. describe five or more sources of information about opportunities for physical activity,
3. explain three guidelines for organizing for participation in physical activity, and
4. define *extrinsic motivation* and *intrinsic motivation* and explain the difference between them.

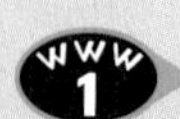

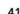

Lesson Vocabulary

autonomy, extrinsic motivation, intrinsic motivation, optimal challenge, self-reward system

Do you feel like you have the power to make your own decisions in life? How do you feel when you have a choice compared with when you don't? Consider the following scenario.

Two years after graduating from high school, a group of friends gathered at a social. Hal hosted the party at his house. He was now married and worked full-time. He'd gained a few pounds since high school and wasn't as active as he had been when he played football in school. His wife, Fatima, had been a cheerleader in school but was also less active now because she also had a full-time job. Hal and Fatima stayed in touch with their friends, but some were off at college, and others were busy working.

Other people attending the social event included Kris, who had also played on the football team. He was now attending a local community college and working part-time. Like Hal, he knew he was less active than he should be. Jennifer was attending the local university, where she played on the soccer team. She was very active but missed interacting with her friends. Will was also attending the university, where he played some intramurals and worked out at the campus recreation center. Coretta and Josh had not gone to school with the others but were now neighbors of Hal and Fatima. Josh played slow-pitch softball, and Coretta used some home exercise videos. They had a four-year-old daughter named Clara.

The seven friends decided that it would be good if they could all be more active (except, of course, for Jennifer, the soccer player). They also wanted to spend more time together socially. They decided to do some type of physical activity together to help them be more active and have fun at the same time. The rest of this lesson describes some of the steps that the friends used to investigate opportunities for their group.

FIT FACT

Self-determination theory is one theory of human motivation. It places high importance on autonomy and intrinsic motivation. It is often used in the study of sport and physical activity. Students report that physical education classes are more enjoyable when they are given an opportunity to choose (to have autonomy in) some of the activities in their classes.

Autonomy

Autonomy refers to self-direction or the ability to make decisions for yourself. One goal of this book is to help teens move from having others make decisions for them (dependence) to making decision for themselves (independence). Hal, Fatima, and their friends are at a stage of life where they make their own decisions. In elementary school, and even in middle school, many decisions had been made for them. Even in high school, they were somewhat dependent on others (such as parents, teachers, and coaches) for many things. Now, however, they have the autonomy to make their own decisions.

The friends applied some of the self-management skills they had learned in high school to their search for active living opportunities in their community.

For example, they had learned about the self-management skill of finding social support from friends, but they did have some barriers to overcome. For one thing, to be active together they would have to find activities that they were all interested in and find times when they would all be available. To solve this and other problems, they used elements of the scientific method and critical thinking skills. Like Hal, Fatima, and their friends, you can practice self-management skills and use the scientific method to become more autonomous in making decisions about healthy lifestyles.

Finding Opportunities to Participate

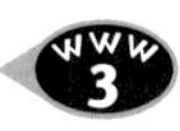

One of the first steps in finding ways to be active is to find out what's available. Options in most communities include government agencies, community organizations, worksite programs, commercial options, and places of worship. Table 18.2 summarizes multiple types of opportunity for being active in your local area.

TABLE 18.2 Finding Opportunities for Physical Activity in the Community

Type	Examples	How to contact
• Government agencies • Youth programs • Sport leagues • Facilities (tennis courts, bike trails, golf courses, hiking trails, parks) • Community centers • Zoos and cultural centers • Museums	• Local parks and recreation department • State parks and recreation department • Local public school programs	Use a phone book or do a web search to locate the agency. Search for a specific department or facility.
National sport organizations	• U.S. Olympic Committee (TeamUSA) • United States Tennis Association • Amateur Softball Association of America • National Senior Games Association • Special Olympics • U.S. Paralympics	Do a web search to locate the organization. For sites such as TeamUSA.org, use the pull-down menu to find specific sport pages.
Community organizations	• YMCA and YWCA • Boys & Girls Clubs of America • Activity-specific clubs (for example, walking, jogging, and tennis clubs) • Sport organizations (for example, Little League baseball)	Do a web search for the organization name and your town or city name (for example, YMCA and Los Angeles). Contact the organization by phone or in person.
Worksite programs	• Company wellness programs • Company fitness centers • Company sport leagues and teams	Check with the human resources office at your worksite to see what's available.
Commercial options	• Health and fitness clubs and spas • Private sport facilities (sport fields, ice rinks, skating rinks or parks, golf courses, leagues) • Dance and yoga studios • Martial arts studios • Youth activity centers • Physical therapy centers	Do a web search for the activity and your town or city name (for example, yoga and Detroit). Contact the facility by phone or in person.
Places of worship (for example, church, synagogue, mosque)	• Sport leagues • Exercise groups • Social groups	Check with your religious organization's office or look for listings in the bulletin or newsletter.

Organizing for Participation

After investigating opportunities, Hal and his friends decided to join a co-rec volleyball league sponsored by their community's parks and recreation department. They needed at least 10 people because a team requires 6 people every time it plays and they knew that not everyone would be able to make every game due to their busy schedules. They also needed their group to be evenly split between men and women because three of each had to be on the court during every game. The group elected Hal as captain and coach and recruited another couple (Nancy and Cole) who lived nearby. Jennifer also asked her friend Jasmine to join, which brought their total 10—5 women and 5 men.

Not all people have such a ready-made social group. Here are some good guidelines for finding or forming a group for physical activity participation.

- **Consider nonleague participation as a start.** Joining a club or league can be quite intimidating for some people. If you're just learning an activity, you may first want to join in recreational sessions or take a class at a local club before joining a league. For example, Coretta had not played much volleyball, so she joined with others in the group to practice at the park before the league started. Will went to the rec center at his university and played in some pick-up volleyball games to get some practice.
- **Check with friends at school or work.** Start with a few people, then each can recruit others with similar interests to participate. You might want to start with noncompetitive games before moving on to league play.
- **Check out your work wellness program or school recreation center.** See if there's a list of people interested in the same activity that you can recruit to join you. There might even be an existing club or exercise group that you can join. Club members often get to know each other and then form teams for leagues after starting with recreational play.
- **Check with the organizations listed in table 18.2.** See if they have opportunities for individuals or small groups to join larger teams.

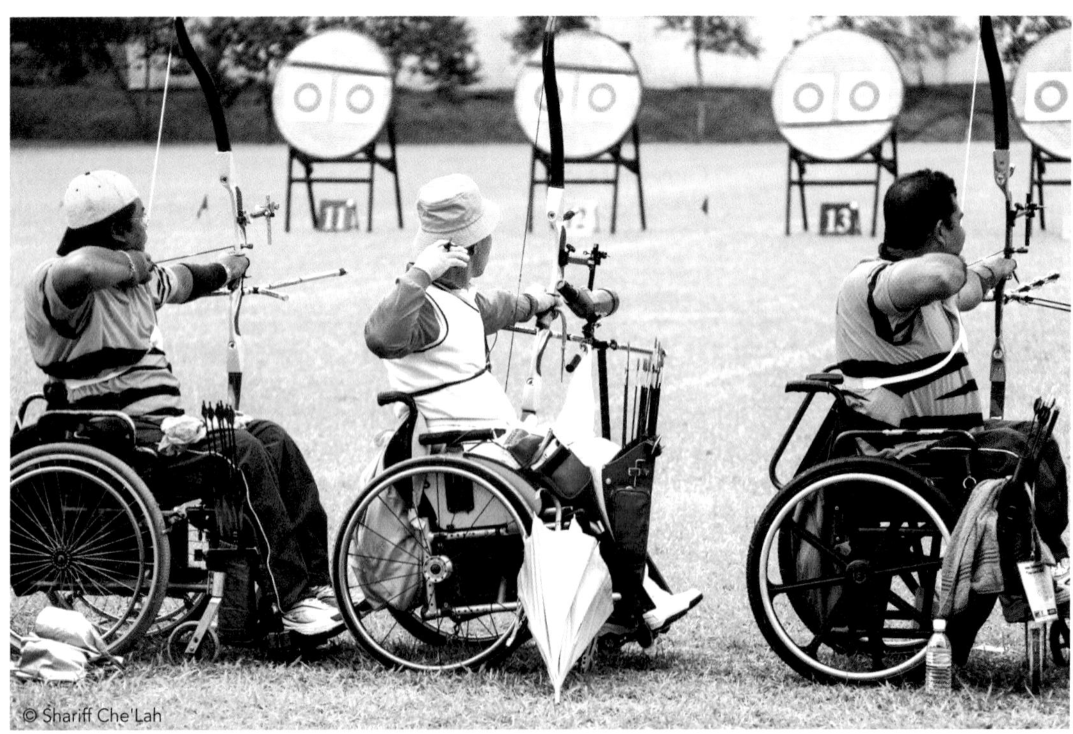

© Shariff Che'Lah

Community recreation, commercial, and worksite wellness programs provide good opportunities for lifelong participation.

Daring to Try

Sometimes one of the hardest things to do is simply to dare to try. This can be especially true when you're starting something new and don't have others to do it with. Coretta had friends to support her, so joining them on a volleyball team was not as threatening as it might have been. Still, she lacked confidence, so before the volleyball league began she joined with others to practice. She was initially motivated by her desire to please her friends in the group; she didn't want to let them down.

Coretta's initial motivation for playing is called **extrinsic motivation**. Extrinsic motivation is motivation that comes from outside the individual (for example, pressure from others, external rewards). In this case, Coretta wanted to be on the team not because she particularly enjoyed volleyball but because the team needed another player. Even after trying recreational volleyball, she felt very nervous when she first played on the competitive team. As she practiced, however, she found success in serving and digging, which encouraged her to keep trying. As she got better, she started to look forward to the games. She was not playing to please someone else (extrinsic motivation); she was now playing because she enjoyed it (**intrinsic motivation**). Intrinsic motivation comes from within the individual; the rewards for participation are personal and internal (for example, fun, joy of participation).

In school, Coretta had learned about **optimal challenge** (see figure 18.2). In her practice group, she tried to do things that were neither too easy nor too hard. Because the challenge was reasonable, she found success rather than failure. In turn, this success encouraged her to keep trying. Gradually, she started to enjoy herself, and that made her want to keep participating.

Coretta also learned to reward herself for her performance rather than rely on praise from others. If she had gone right into the volleyball league without practicing first, she might have become frustrated and quit trying.

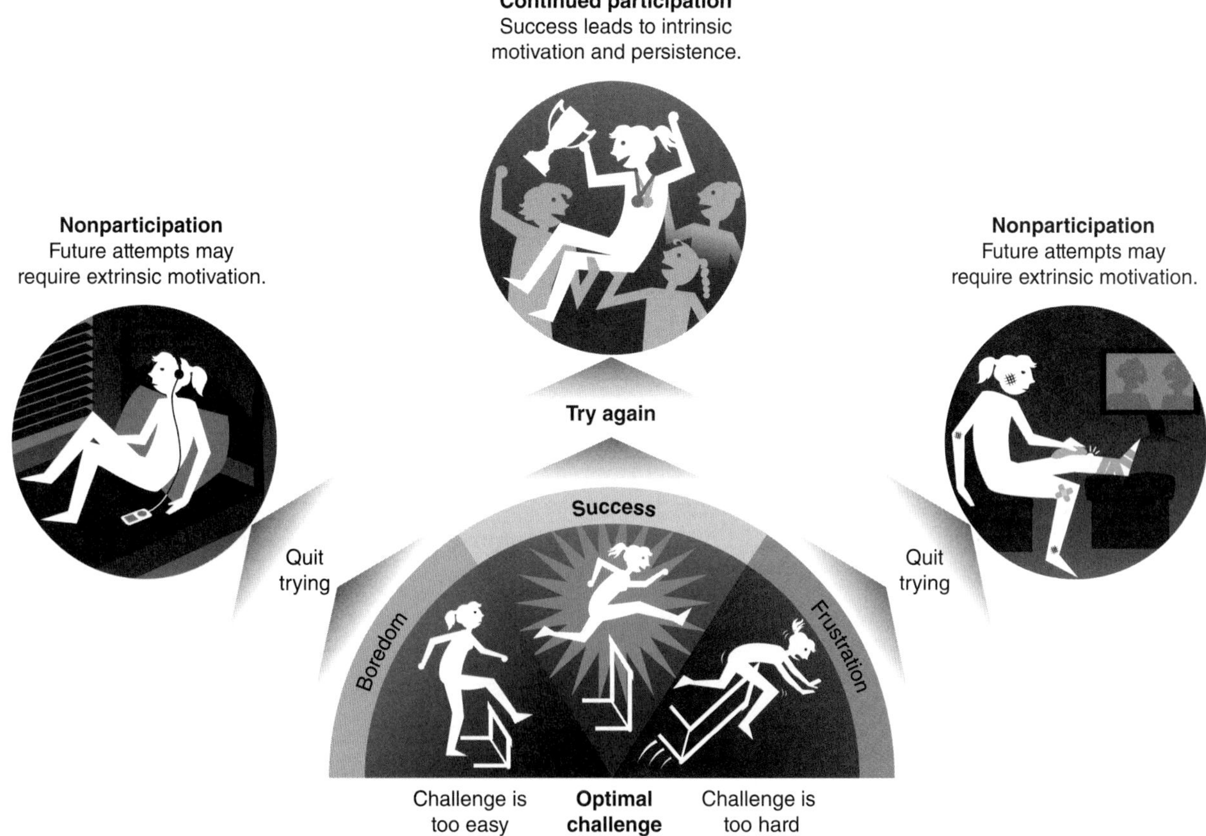

FIGURE 18.2 Finding an optimal challenge helps you achieve success and intrinsic motivation.

FIT FACT

Video game creators use the concept of optimal challenge. To ensure success, they design games that start players at a low level. This success creates intrinsic motivation that keeps players' interest high and encourages them to keep participating. Indeed, evidence shows that gamers play for hours with no extrinsic rewards.

Kris had a very different experience. He became bored with the volleyball team. Although he liked being with his friends, his volleyball skills were better than his friends' skills, and he lost interest in the games. It took encouragement and even pleading from his friends (extrinsic motivation) to keep him coming to the games. Ultimately, he dropped out of the league, and the team finished with nine players.

Sometimes you need a little extrinsic or external motivation to get you going. But researchers have shown that long-term participation requires intrinsic motivation. People who have intrinsic motivation (such as Coretta) are more likely to stick with participation than people who are extrinsically motivated (such as Kris). Being able to gradually build your skills and find success and ultimately intrinsic motivation is called having a **self-reward system**. You reward yourself rather than expecting others to reward you for your efforts.

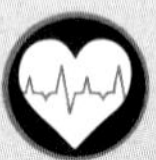

FITNESS TECHNOLOGY: Social Support

Social support is important in helping people adopt and stick with healthy lifestyle changes. Weight Watchers is an organization that uses social support to help people maintain a healthy weight throughout life. Meetings allow group members to support each other and receive support from program leaders. Weight Watchers also uses the web to provide social support through interactive tools that help members self-monitor their eating and activity habits. Optimal challenges are provided to encourage success and intrinsic motivation. Even people who are intrinsically motivated benefit from the support of others, and Weight Watchers messages are sent periodically to provide support and encouragement. Some doctors now also provide messages to encourage patients.

You can use the web and social media to encourage others and help them be successful in making healthy lifestyle choices. You can do this through e-mail messages and tweets to support group members with similar goals. For example, Hal and his friends could use e-mails, text messages, phone calls, or tweets to encourage each other to come to practice and games.

Messages from others can also be harmful if not done properly. You've learned that autonomy is important and that we all want to make decisions for ourselves. Messages that encourage a person to stick with his or her plan encourage autonomy. On the other hand, messages or comments that treat a person as if you're trying to control his or her behavior do not encourage autonomy and may be ignored. For example, if a person misses a practice, a good message of support might be, "Missed you at practice—hope to see you next time." A not-so-good message might be, "If you keep missing, you will never get better." This message suggests that the person should attend to please someone else.

Appropriately supportive personal messages delivered via phone or the web have been shown to help people who are trying to stop smoking, maintain a healthy weight, or be active for health and fitness.

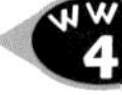

Using Technology

Work with a group of friends to form a support network. Outline ways in which the group will use social support technology to help members meet their goals.

Helping Others in Physical Activity

In part 1 of this book, you've learned many self-management skills designed to help you be active for the rest of your life. In the years ahead, you'll find that having active people around you helps you be more active. You'll also have the opportunity to help others be physically active. A few of these opportunities are described in the following list.

- **Family activities.** A popular slogan says, "Families that play together stay together." You can use the skills you've learned in this class to help family members be active. Examples include family outings (such as camping, fishing, and biking trips), family exercise sessions (such as walks and hikes), and family activity nights (such as bowling or skating night). Since not all family members will always like the same activities, you can also support each other's activities. Family support is a type of social support that can help family members stick with their exercise—for example, watching a family member's team play or praising the jogger in the family for sticking with it over time.
- **Coaching.** When you were younger, you may have played a sport such as soccer or tee ball. If so, someone coached your team. You can give back by volunteering to coach children in your neighborhood or your own children. Training for volunteer coaches is provided by many organizations.

> "You can motivate by fear, and you can motivate by reward. But both those methods are only temporary. The only lasting thing is self-motivation."
>
> —Homer Rice, football coach

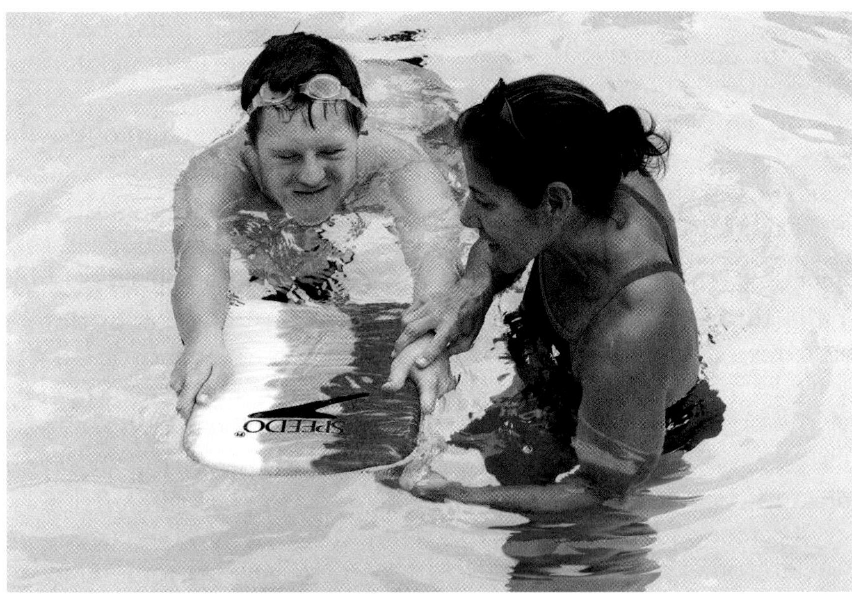

Helping others learn skills can be very rewarding.

Lesson Review

1. What is autonomy, and how does it relate to decision making about healthy lifestyles?
2. What are some sources of information about opportunities for physical activity?
3. What are some guidelines for organizing for participation in physical activity?
4. What are extrinsic and intrinsic motivation, and how do they differ?

TAKING CHARGE: Conflict Resolution

Conflict can be a barrier to participation; it can be the reason that a person doesn't stick to a physical activity plan. Here's an example. Monica and Juana developed a plan to walk to school five days a week for one month. Unfortunately, their friend Miguel kept offering them a ride to school. The third time Miguel offered, Monica accepted and left Juana to walk alone. Juana did not accept because she wanted to walk as planned. Juana then felt mad at both Monica and Miguel and didn't speak to them at school. The next day, Monica didn't stop by to walk with Juana—she just rode with Miguel. The friends did not speak at school. In fact, Monica said something to other friends about Juana that upset her.

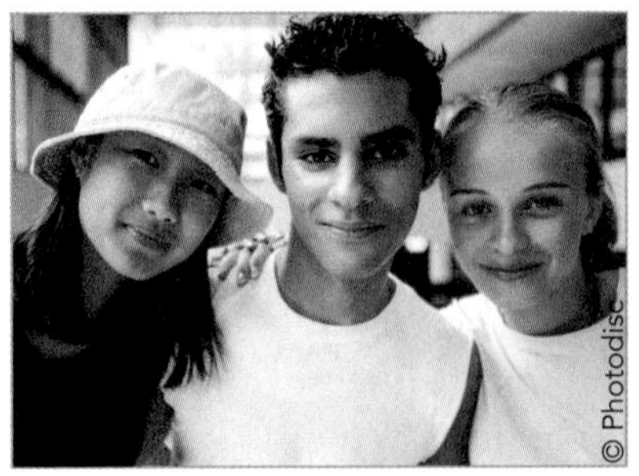

© Photodisc

For Discussion

What could the friends have done to avoid the conflict? What steps should they take to resolve it? List possible solutions. Consider the skills in the Self-Management feature when answering the discussion questions.

SELF-MANAGEMENT: Skills for Conflict Resolution

At times, all of us have disagreements with our friends. The disagreements are usually over small things and can be easily resolved. A conflict is typically bigger than a disagreement. When a conflict occurs, one or more of the people involved come to feel threatened, whether physically or emotionally. In sport, for example, one player may get angry with another, and strong emotions may lead to angry words. In extreme cases, the anger can result in fighting. Whether the conflict occurs in sport or daily life, the following steps can help you resolve it.

- **Consider the three Bs.** When working with others to resolve conflict, remember to *be calm*, *be patient*, and *be respectful*. Keeping emotions under control is essential.
- **Communicate.** To resolve a conflict, you need good communication. Be willing to listen to what the other person has to say. Watch what you say. Words can hurt, and it's crucial not to make the conflict worse.
- **Recognize that there is a conflict.** Don't ignore it. Avoiding a conflict can cause it to get worse.
- **Consider a meeting.** While a conflict can sometimes be resolved on the phone, by e-mail, through social media, or in other ways, it's often best to meet face to face. Meeting in person makes harsh words less likely. The meeting should be held in a neutral and safe setting for all involved.
- **Set the scene.** Define the problem, and restate it if necessary. Using the three Bs, each person should describe the problem without interruption. After each person has done so, the parties can try to find a statement of the problem that all can agree to.
- **List possible solutions.** Make a list of possible solutions based on ideas from people on all sides of the conflict.
- **Consider the options.** Once options have been proposed, communicate respectfully to find the options that best meet the needs of all parties concerned.
- **Compromise.** If the people involved have very different ideas about the conflict, it may be necessary for each person to give up something in order to find a resolution.
- **Seek help.** Another way to resolve a conflict is through arbitration. If the parties involved cannot resolve the conflict on their own, an independent arbitrator may be used. In sport, a coach or referee can resolve some conflicts, and others may be resolved with the help of a common friend, but difficult conflicts may call for a professional arbitrator.

TAKING ACTION: Team Building

The TEAM concept (Together Everyone Achieves More) can help you succeed in all aspects of your life. It's an exciting challenge to build a team of individuals who work well together in pursuit of a common goal. **Take action** by performing a team-building activity in your physical education class.

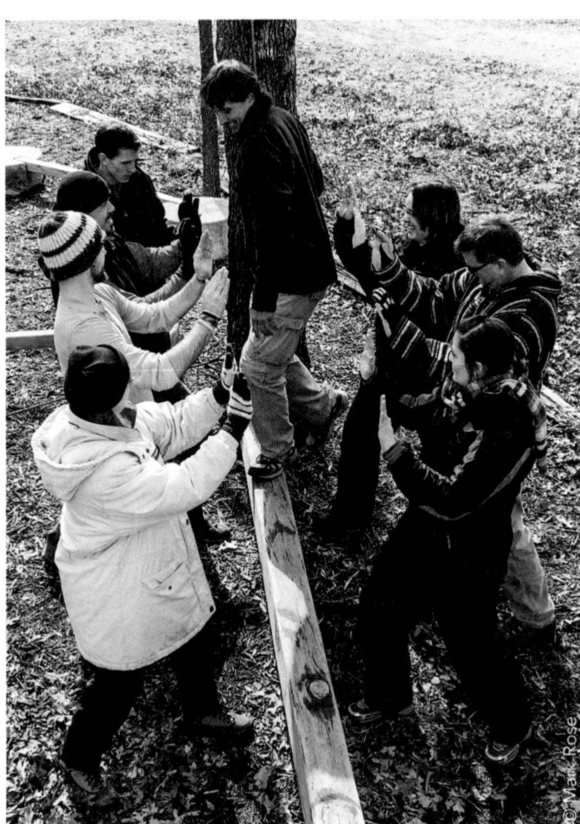

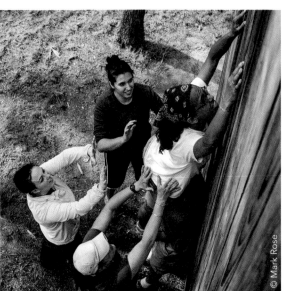

Take action by trying team-building activities.

Reviewing Concepts and Vocabulary

As directed by your teacher, answer items 1 through 5 by correctly completing each sentence with a word or phrase.

1. _______________ involves being fair and following the rules.
2. Sticking together when working toward a common goal is called _______________.
3. _______________ involves acting in a way that is consistent with expected behavior in a group.
4. People who have _______________ are self-directed and make their own decisions.
5. People who need an external reward to do a behavior have _______________ motivation.

For items 6 through 10, as directed by your teacher, match each term in column 1 with the appropriate phrase in column 2.

6. self-determination theory	a. places importance on autonomy
7. diversity	b. respect for others
8. optimal challenge	c. person who guides or directs
9. leader	d. comes from within
10. intrinsic motivation	e. neither too hard nor too easy

For items 11 through 15, as directed by your teacher, respond to each statement or question.

11. List and describe several leadership skills.
12. Explain some factors that contribute to good teamwork.
13. Discuss rules and their importance.
14. Describe groups that provide opportunities for physical activity in a community.
15. Describe the guidelines for resolving conflict.

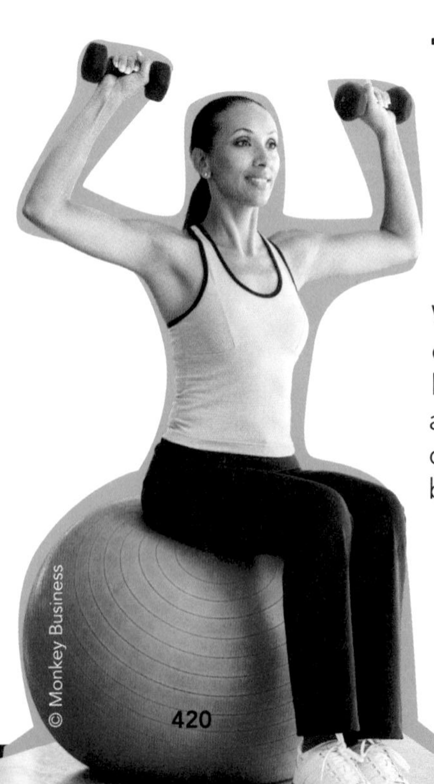

© Monkey Business

Thinking Critically

You've been asked to form an intramural team for a school league. Write a paragraph to describe the steps you would take to get a team organized.

Project

Work with a group to develop a directory of physical activity for your community. Include a list of agencies and businesses offering various kinds of physical activity. Consider the following categories and list the activities they provide: local government agencies, community sport organizations, worksite activity programs, commercial options (local businesses), places of worship, and other types. Use table 18.2 for ideas.

PART 2

Health for Life

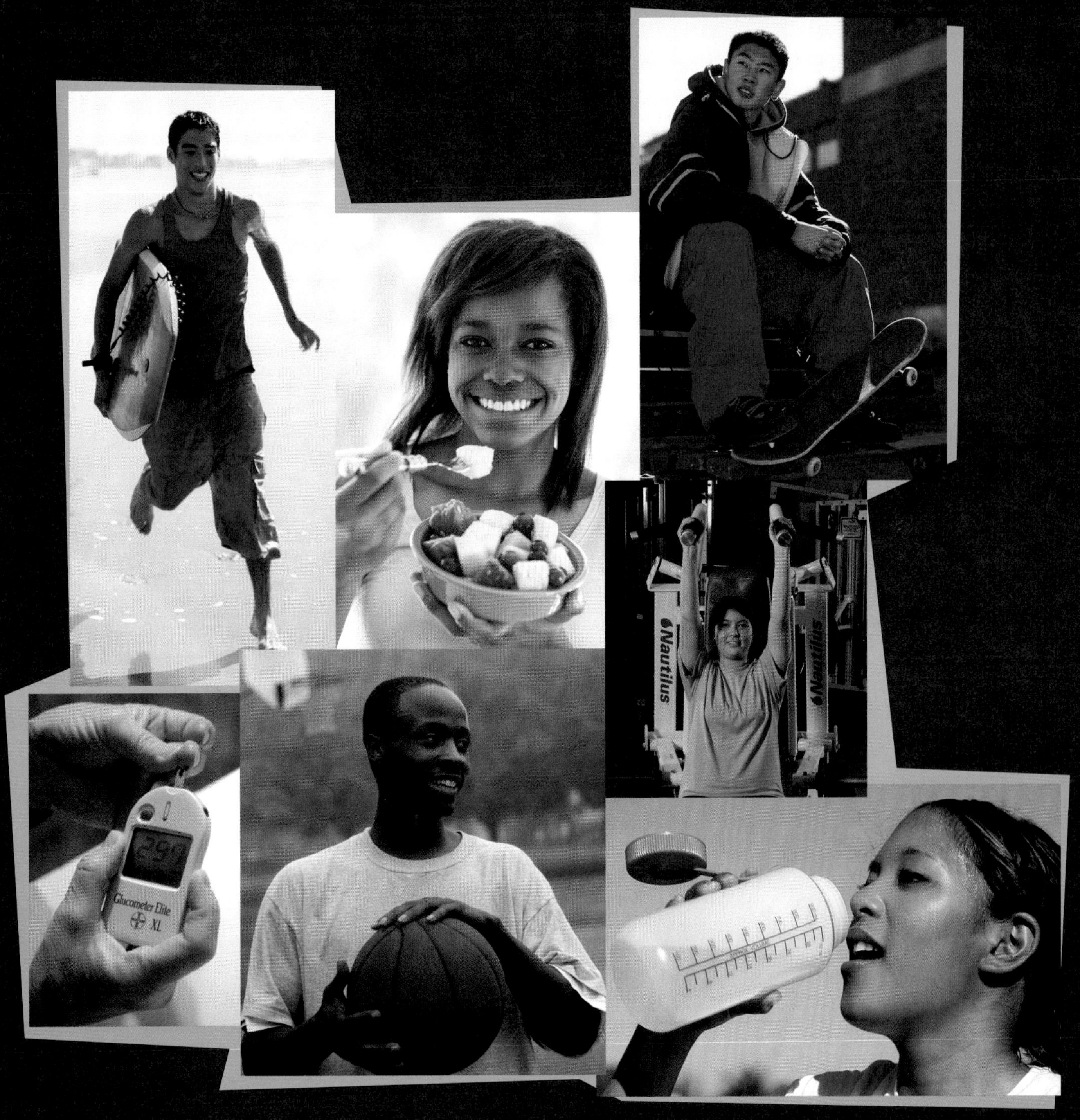

Touring Part 2

Do you want to be healthy and well? Do you want to look your best and feel good? In part 2 of this book, you'll study all aspects of health, including wellness. You'll see that, although your health and wellness are not totally under your control, the choices you make and the way you live can make a big difference in both your health and your wellness. By learning about the skills for healthy living and assessing your current health status you'll be able to develop a plan for healthy living to either maintain or improve your healthy behaviors. Two lessons are included in each chapter to help you learn key concepts relating to health and wellness. *Health Opportunities Through Physical Education* will help you meet your fitness and physical activity goals. Take this guided tour to learn about all of the features of this part.

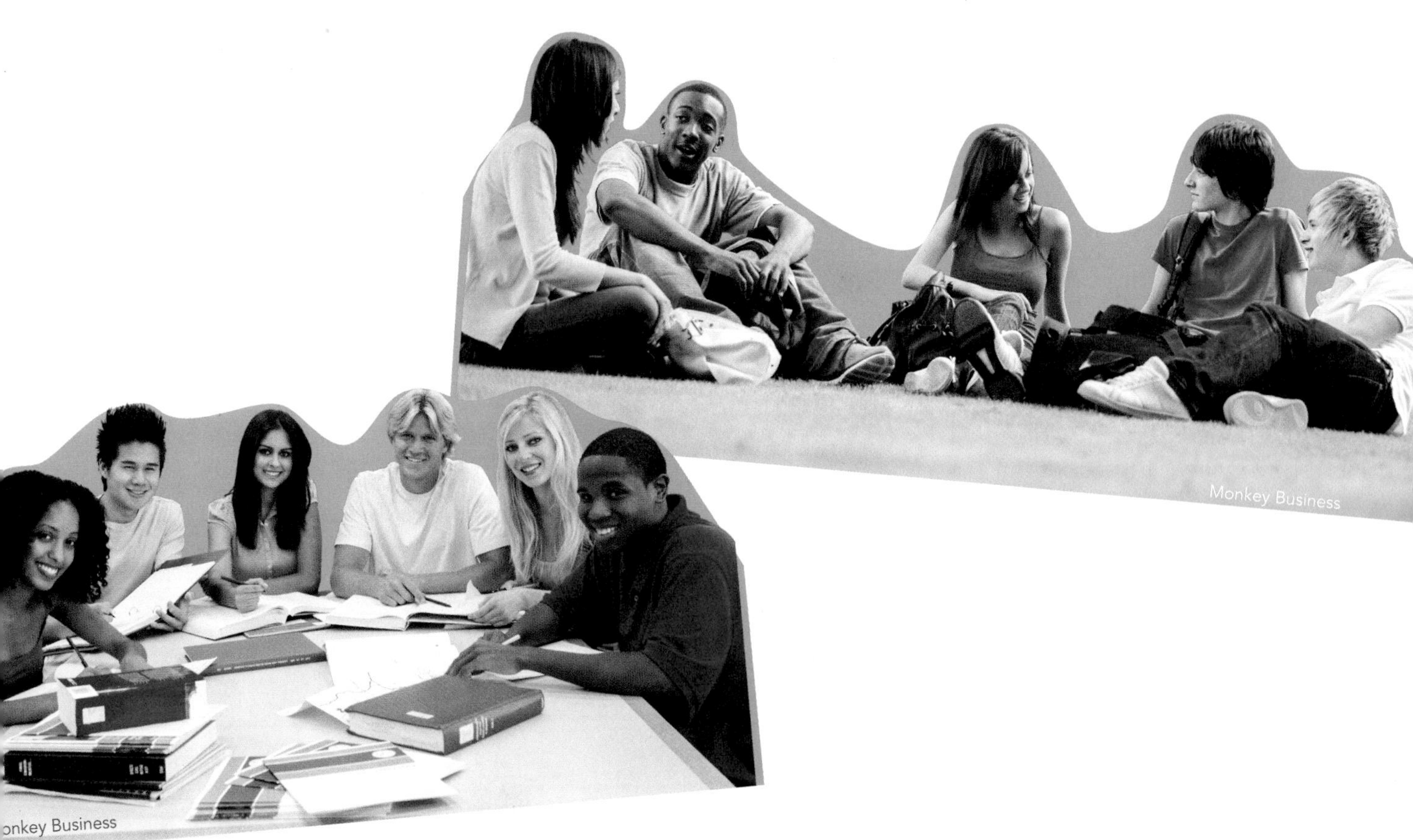
Monkey Business

Monkey Business

UNIT OPENER: Provides a brief overview of the content in each unit.

HEALTHY PEOPLE 2020 GOALS: Lists national health goals covered in each unit.

FEATURES: Lists the Self-Assessment, Making Healthy Decisions, Skills for Healthy Living, Living Well News, and special features in each unit.

STUDENT WEB RESOURCES: Provides the web addresses for finding additional information in each lesson.

CHAPTER OPENER: Provides a brief overview of the content of the chapter.

IN THIS CHAPTER: Lists the main elements of each chapter.

UNIT VII

Understanding Health and Wellness

Healthy People 2020 Goals

- Help people live high-quality, longer lives.
- Reduce preventable disease, injury, and early death.
- Increase awareness and understanding of what determines good health.
- Help people adopt a healthy lifestyle in order to achieve lifetime health, fitness, and wellness.
- Create environments that promote health, fitness, and wellness for all.
- Increase health literacy.
- Live high-quality, longer lives free of preventable diseases, injury, and early death.
- Increase the percentage of people who receive risk factor information.

Self-Assessment Features in This Unit

- The Wellness Questionnaire
- Stages of Health Behavior
- Healthy Living Skills

Making Healthy Decisi

- Self-Assessment
- Goal Setting
- Self-Planning

Special Features in Th

- Diverse Perspectives
- Consumer Corner: D
- Advocacy in Action:

Living Well News Fe

- The State of Youth
- Do the Rich Get to
- Can You Make a C

20

Health Behavior Change and Personal Health

In This Chapter

LESSON 20.1
Personal Health and Wellness

SELF-ASSESSMENT
Stages of Health Behavior

LESSON 20.2
Changing Health Behaviors

MAKING HEALTHY DECISIONS
Goal Setting

SKILLS FOR HEALTHY LIVING
Goal Setting

Student Web Resources
www.HOPEtextbook.org/student

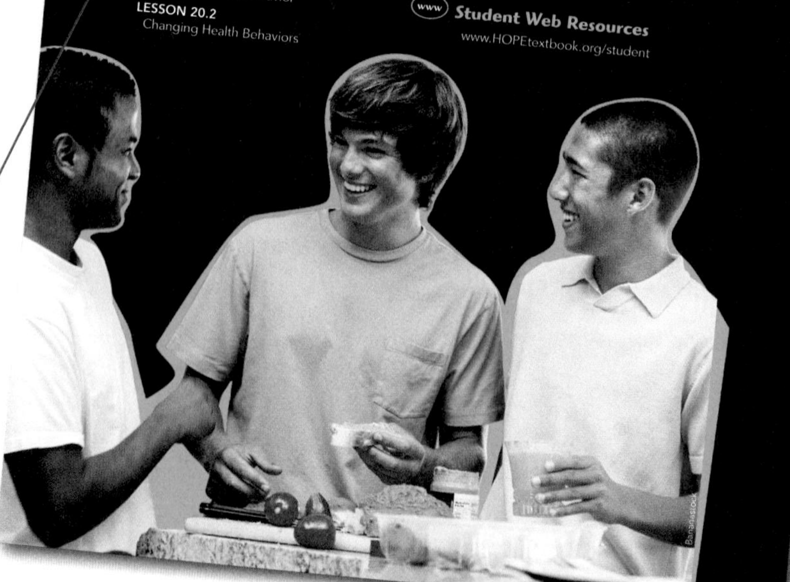

WEB ICONS: Indicate that additional information is available on the student website.

LESSON OBJECTIVES: Describes what you will learn in each lesson.

LESSON VOCABULARY: Lists key terms in each lesson, which are defined in the glossary and on the student website.

HEALTH TECHNOLOGY: Helps you become aware of new technological information related to health and wellness.

DIVERSE PERSPECTIVES: Helps you understand another's point of view.

CONNECT: Asks you to reflect on family, peer, media, or technology influences related to a specific topic in a chapter.

CONSUMER CORNER: Helps you to become a good consumer of health and wellness information and to avoid quackery.

COMPREHENSION CHECK: Helps you review and remember the information you learned in the lesson.

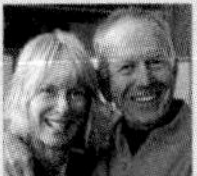

DIVERSE PERSPECTIVES: Being an Older Parent
Our names are Madeline and Steve. We are both almost 60, and we have a son in high school and a daughter in junior high school. We met at work when we were both in our 30s and got married at almost age 40. Both of us wanted children earlier in life but had been committed to our careers; we also wanted to spend the first few years of our marriage traveling.
Having children in our mid-40s was difficult physically—we didn't have as much energy as
we'd once had. But we've both noticed that we don't seem to get as stressed out about parenting as younger parents do
Lesson 21.1
HEALTH TECHNOLOGY
An application, or app, is a computer program that allows you to perform tasks on a smartphone or other device. Some apps are designed to help you use skills for healthy living—for example, by self-assessing your food content, self-monitoring your physical activity, or planning healthy meals. If well designed, apps can help you change your health behaviors, but not all apps are based on good health information. Before using an app, determine whether the people who developed it are health experts; ask people you know and trust about the app, and test it out for yourself. For more information about health-related apps, see the student section of the Health Opportunities Through Physical Education website.
CONNECT
Do you currently use any apps to help you live a healthier life? If so, what features do you think make a good health application? If not, what type of app might appeal to you? Can you imagine using a health app in the future?

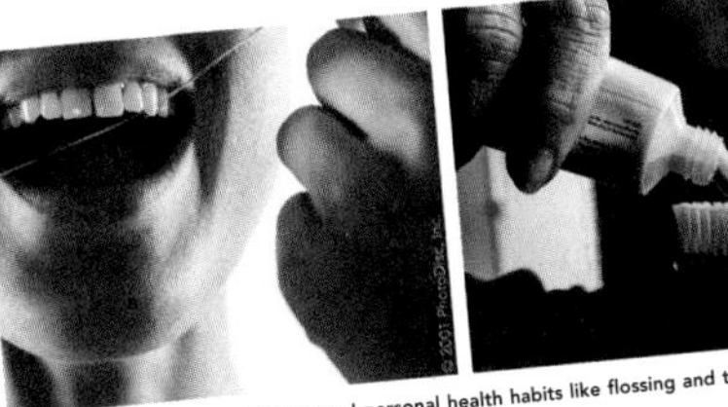

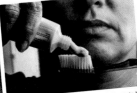

ADVOCACY IN ACTION: Provides you with personal, school, or community advocacy challenges.

SELF-ASSESSMENT: Helps you evaluate and reflect on your personal health habits related to a wide variety of behaviors, which can help you to prepare a plan for healthy living.

Lesson 35.1

ADVOCACY IN ACTION: Promoting Recycling

Not surprisingly, people are more likely to recycle when appropriate recycling bins are readily available. Evaluate your school to determine whether an *effective* recycling program is in place.

If your school doesn't provide recycling bins or lacks some needed options (e.g., paper, plastic, refuse, glass), determine what bins the school should add and what company or community organization will recycle the materials. You can even create a map showing where recycling bins should be located. Then write a one-page letter to the school board advocating for the purchase and appropriate placement of the needed recycling bins. Include information about the four Rs and explain why recycling is important for both environmental and personal health.

If your school already has adequate recycling bins, create posters to place above the bins that explain their importance and encourage students, teachers, and staff members to use them regularly.

SELF-ASSESSMENT: How Healthy Is My School Community?

Your school is an important community to which you belong. This assessment asks you to think about aspects of a healthy school community and consider your connection to your school. Answer each question by circling the proper response, then add up the total number of points as directed in the assessment. You may need to ask a teacher or school staff member for help in answering some of the questions in parts 1 and 2.

	Yes (2 points)	No (0 points)
Part 1: Health and safety		
My school . . .		
has a no tolerance policy for harassment or bullying.	2	0
has emergency plans, like evacuation routes, in place.	2	0
has active supervision in place to ensure safety and reduce violence.	2	0
is a safe physical environment.	2	0
does not allow smoking on campus.	2	0
is kept clean and bright.	2	0
provides help to those who want to quit smoking.	2	0
has at least one full-time nurse on campus.	2	0
provides counseling and mental health services.	2	0
Part 2: Nutrition and physical activity services		
My school . . .		
requires students to take physical education.	2	0
provides physical activities after school.	2	0
requires students to take health education.	2	0
promotes healthy food and beverage choices.	2	0
provides healthy and low-fat food.	2	0
has a clean and pleasant cafeteria.	2	0
Total points from parts 1 and 2: ______		
The higher the score, the healthier and safer the school community.		
Part 3: My school engagement		
As a member of my school, I . . .		
am involved in at least one club or organization at school.	2	0
... at my school.	2	0

Lesson 36.1

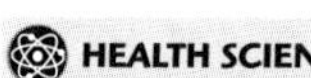

HEALTH SCIENCE

Malaria was eliminated in the United States by a concerted effort made from 1947 to 1951, yet somewhere in the world a child dies from malaria every 30 seconds. In Africa, one in every five childhood deaths is attributed to malaria. Poorer individuals are at highest risk because their homes and dwellings provide little protection from infected mosquitoes. They can't afford preventive medication or, if symptoms arise, medical care. The elimination of malaria in the United States was aided by spraying homes with mosquito-killing insecticides, spraying insecticides over large land areas, and removing mosquito nesting sites. In addition, U.S. residents have access to medicine that helps prevent and treat malaria.

The advances in chemical and medical science that contributed to effective insecticides and medications are certainly not new, yet malaria remains a global threat. This disparity illustrates the fact that even when science can solve a particular health problem, challenges may still exist in distributing the solution to those most in need. In addition, many developing countries have little in the way of organized public health services, and citizens often have no education or awareness of options that might exist. Therefore, humanitarians and scientists must often work together to make the greatest gains in global public health.

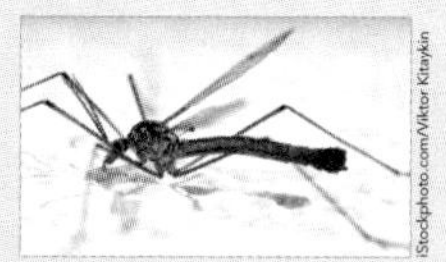
iStockphoto.com/Viktor Kitaykin

HEALTH SCIENCE: Focuses on the role of science in health and allows for cross-disciplinary learning and exploration.

of exercise, much of the world faces very different public health issues, and the biggest challenge in global public health is poverty.

Countries with a poor economy and low standards of living are sometimes referred to as **developing nations**, and these are the places where the majority of the world's people live. These countries often face particularly intense public health problems, including malnutrition and widespread disease (e.g., malaria, AIDS). As a result, major global health initiatives are focused on bringing vaccinations, antibiotics, safe water, and sustainable farming techniques to developing countries.

Another key effort focuses on creating educational opportunities for more children around the world. Access to education is considered a primary way to end the cycle of poverty and improve global public health. It opens doors for employment, which can bring individual freedom as well as opportunities for acquiring healthier food, safer living conditions, and higher-quality health care.

HEALTHY COMMUNICATION

If you had US$1,000 to donate to a group addressing a serious health problem, what would it be? Why? Would you choose to support a cause in the United States or donate to a group addressing a global health issue? Why? Share your response with a group of classmates or peers.

"Of all the forms of inequality, injustice in health care is the most shocking and inhumane."

—Martin Luther King, Jr.

HEALTHY COMMUNICATION: Uses your interpersonal communication skills in order to share your health knowledge, debate controversial topics, or promote healthy living among your peers.

HEALTH QUOTES: Provide quotes from famous people about health and wellness.

Comprehension Check

1. What types of organization serve the public health in the United States? Provide three specific examples.
2. What are the three levels of prevention addressed by public health services? Which are the most effective in improving public health?
3. What is the difference between the prevalence and the incidence of a disease?

767

MAKING HEALTHY DECISIONS: Time Management

Alexis was one of those people who was always going from one commitment to the next. Her friends rarely saw her sitting still, and she often complained about having too much to do. Alexis played on the softball team and volunteered at her church on the weekends. She also helped out around the house with cleaning and cooking. When her friend Deborah asked her to go to yoga class together as a way to manage stress, she said, "I totally want to—it would be really great—but I just don't have any free time." Later in the conversation, Deborah noticed Alexis talking about TV shows she'd been watching and showing off a new video game she'd been playing. Deborah wondered if Alexis was as busy as she seemed to be. Deborah herself worked two jobs, was an honor student, ran cross country, and played in the school orchestra.

For Discussion

What could Deborah suggest that Alexis do to make time for yoga class? What could Deborah say to Alexis that might help her better understand her time management needs? To help you answer these questions, review this chapter's Skills for Healthy Living feature.

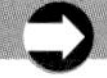

SKILLS FOR HEALTHY LIVING: Time Management

How you manage your time is an important part of your overall health. If you struggle with time management, you may have higher levels of stress and you may end up coping with your stress by engaging in destructive habits that seem to provide quick fixes, such as smoking or drinking alcohol. Poor time management can also interfere with your ability to create time for healthy pursuits, such as exercise.

Young people, like adults, often tend to book their schedules solid with work, school, errands, and other tasks they deem important. For example, you may be involved in a community organization, spend time tending to a school garden, play a sport, or care for an aging relative. The time you spend doing all of these activities is referred to as your committed time. What's left over is your free time. Learning to manage your free time can help you manage stress, avoid destructive habits, and make time for healthy habits. The following tips can help you with your time management:

- **Monitor your time.** Write down what you do during the course of each day. Record when you sleep, when you eat, when you're at school, when you're at work, and when you do all of the other things you do. Most people who track their use of time are surprised by the findings.
- **Evaluate your use of time.** Once you've tracked your time for several days, review your records to see how many hours you spend in various types of activities. For example, you can arrange all your activities into three categories: school and work, committed time, and free time. Then you can evaluate whether there is a good balance between the categories. Alternatively, you can think of all of your activities as fitting into three drawers: the lower drawer (not important or urgent), the middle drawer (important but not urgent), and the top drawer (urgent and important). If any drawer is overflowing, you may need to re-evaluate your commitments and priorities. Evaluating your time can help you decide whether you're using your time the way you want and need to use it. Having a lot of important and urgent things to do can add to your stress levels significantly.
- **Plan a schedule.** After you determine how much time you spend on various activities, work on creating a time management plan for yourself. Efficient time management means you get to do all the things you think are important so that you don't feel rushed or anxious, and it also allows you to make time for those things that you value, such as relaxation and recreational activities. Begin by blocking out your committed time (school, work, practice time). Then, make decisions about your free time.

need along the way. Most important, follow through with your plan so that you don't end up in a bind.

- Third, schedule in and plan time for yourself to do the things that you value (even when they don't seem important or urgent), such as exercising, reading a novel, or playing a musical instrument. Ensuring you are balanced and have the opportunities to relax and recover from the demands of life is critical to overall health. Often people do not take the time for these important activities unless they plan for them. It is also important to ensure that these activities do not interfere with obligations such as schoolwork.
- Finally, schedule some time every day for the unexpected. Meetings, appointments, and practices can run late, unexpected opportunities can arise, or other scheduled tasks can take longer than expected. Allowing some flexibility in each day can help you adjust your schedule to adapt to changing demands.

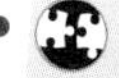

ACADEMIC CONNECTION: College and Career Skills

Being able to respond to precise instructions is an important skill for college and career readiness. For example, if you were asked to *analyze* how physical activity contributes to overall health, would you know how to respond? Would you be confident in your ability to *compare* carbohydrate and protein? What about your ability to *contrast* them? Each of these is different, and you must first understand what is being asked before you can accurately respond. The following are some of the most valuable skills for successful college admissions (performance on standardized tests like the SAT or ACT as well as for writing college admissions essays) and job performance.

- *Analyze:* Explain how each part functions or fits into the whole. For example, how does each type of physical activity (see the Physical Activity Pyramid) affect each component of health?
- *Persuade:* Take a stand on one side of an issue and convince others of the validity of that stance. Use facts, statistics, beliefs, opinions, and your personal view. Showing passion for your point of view can help you be persuasive.
- *Compare:* Find the common characteristics between two things. For example, carbohydrate and protein are both energy-yielding nutrients, and both contain 4 calories per gram.
- *Contrast:* Identify how people, events, or objects are different from one another. For example, carbohydrate is primarily used as fuel for the body, whereas protein is primarily used to build and repair tissues in the body.
- *Describe:* Present a clear picture of a person, place, thing, or idea. Try to write or speak so that the reader or listener could accurately visualize what you are saying.
- *Summarize:* State the meaning in a concise way (e.g., describe each of the factors that lead to teen stress and explain the relative importance of each).

MAKING HEALTHY DECISIONS: Asks you to apply the identified skill to evaluate potential solutions to the problems posed in the scenario.

SKILLS FOR HEALTHY LIVING: Provides guidelines for learning skills for healthy living that help you adopt healthy behaviors.

ACADEMIC CONNECTION: Relates concepts from other academic subject areas to health and wellness.

LIVING WELL NEWS: Provides an article to test your health-literacy skills.

LIVING WELL NEWS, ISSUE 30

Does a High-Carbohydrate Diet Contribute to Mild Cognitive Impairment?

Most adults have considered the possibility of dying from heart disease or cancer. We're all familiar with the fact that these diseases are among the most common causes of death. At the same time, Alzheimer's disease is contributing to more deaths each year (see figure 30.6). In fact, Alzheimer's affects 5.2 million adults in the United States, and that number is expected to triple by 2050. While we know that eating a diet lower in saturated fat may help us hold off heart disease or cancer, what do we know about how diet affects the risk of Alzheimer's?

Seeking to answer this question, Mayo Clinic researchers tracked the eating habits of 1,230 people between the ages of 70 and 89 for one year. Next, the 940 people who showed no sign of cognitive impairment were asked to return for a 15-month follow-up. By the study's fourth year, 200 of those 940 people were beginning to show mild cognitive impairment (MCI), which can include problems with memory, language, thinking, and judgment.

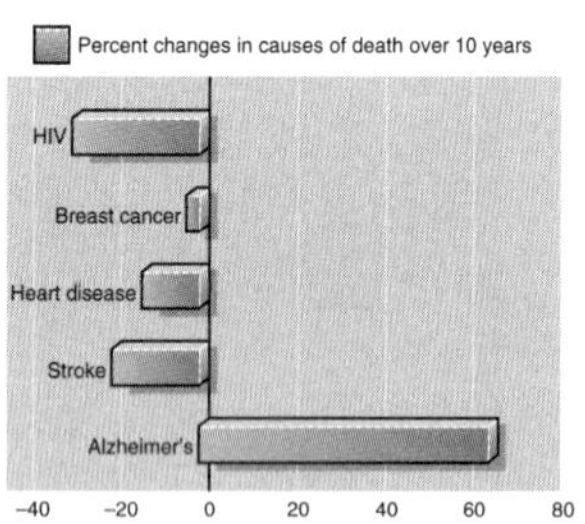

Figure 30.6 Recent changes in death rates. Alzheimer's has greatly increased while the others have decreased.

People with the highest carbohydrate intake were nearly twice as likely to develop MCI as people who ate a balanced diet.

"Not everyone with MCI goes on to develop Alzheimer's disease, but many do," says Professor Rosebud Roberts, a researcher in Mayo's epidemiology division in Rochester, Minnesota. "A high-carbohydrate intake could be bad for you because carbohydrates impact your glucose and insulin metabolism."

Since sugar fuels the brain, a moderate amount is essential. However, high levels of sugar may actually interfere with the brain's ability to use the sugar for fuel. Roberts says high glucose levels might affect the brain's blood vessels and also play a role in the development of plaques in the brain that interfere with normal neural functioning. "Those proteins are toxic to brain health and are found in the brains of people with Alzheimer's," states Roberts.

The study found that people whose diets had the highest intake of protein (e.g., from chicken, meat, or fish) reduced their risk of cognitive impairment by 21 percent. Those whose ... highest in fat (e.g., from nuts or hea... have ... DeMa... Cance... show... preve... diet ... heart...

Do ... dise... red... incr... dis...

CHAPTER REVIEW: Helps you reinforce what you've learned in the chapter's two lessons.

CHAPTER REVIEW

Reviewing Concepts and Vocabulary

As directed by your teacher, answer items 1 through 5 by correctly completing each sentence with a word or phrase.

1. Changes in motor skills, perception, and hearing are a normal part of ________ development.
2. The acquisition and development of skills such as language, problem solving, and reasoning are part of ________ development.
3. Periods of relatively rapid growth called ________ ________ can cause aches and pains as well as muscle cramps.
4. Bathing, preparing food, eating, and dressing are examples of ________ ________ ________.
5. Regular exercise has been shown to play a role in reducing the risk of ________, which is the leading cause of disability among people over the age of 80.

For items 6 through 10, as directed by your teacher, match each term in column 1 with the appropriate phrase in column 2.

6. abstract thinking	a. the way you solve problems and make decisions
7. reasoning skills	b. the number of years you have been alive
8. socioemotional development	c. includes self-esteem, empathy, and friendships
9. chronological age	d. how well your body systems are aging
10. physiological age	e. the ability to consider things that are not visible, immediate, or concrete

For items 11 through 15, as directed by your teacher, respond to each statement or question.

11. What is socioemotional development?
12. What are two things you should never do when caring for an infant?
13. Describe two health careers that might interest you.
14. Why might young adulthood be a stressful time? Provide two reasons.
15. Define *intrinsic motivation* and give an example.

THINKING CRITICALLY: Requires the use of critical-thinking skills to apply chapter information.

Thinking Critically

Write a response to the following prompt.

List and discuss the major physical and mental changes that occur with aging. Which ones can you affect through your own choices? What changes can you begin to make now to help you age well? Write a letter to yourself as you are now, and another letter to yourself at age 65, to remind yourself of these changes and motivate yourself to make healthy choices.

TAKE IT HOME: Provides an enrichment activity for use outside the classroom.

Take It Home

Think of a person you know and respect who is older than 65—for example, a parent, grandparent, neighbor, or family friend. Interview the person about his or her life. Find out what challenges the person faces and what steps he or she takes to try to overcome them. Ask the person what advice he or she has for you about staying healthy as you age. Write a brief report about what you learn.

Joggie Botma/fotolia.com

662

UNIT VII

Understanding Health and Wellness

Healthy People 2020 Goals

- Help people live high-quality, longer lives.
- Reduce preventable disease, injury, and early death.
- Increase awareness and understanding of what determines good health.
- Help people adopt a healthy lifestyle in order to achieve lifetime health, fitness, and wellness.
- Create environments that promote health, fitness, and wellness for all.
- Increase health literacy.
- Live high-quality, longer lives free of preventable diseases, injury, and early death.
- Increase the percentage of people who receive risk factor information.

Self-Assessment Features in This Unit

- The Wellness Questionnaire
- Stages of Health Behavior
- Healthy Living Skills

Making Healthy Decisions and Skills for Healthy Living Features in This Unit

- Self-Assessment
- Goal Setting
- Self-Planning

Special Features in This Unit

- Diverse Perspectives: Living With a Disability
- Consumer Corner: Don't Be Outsmarted! Finding High-Quality Health Information
- Advocacy in Action: Positive Attitudes

Living Well News Features in This Unit

- The State of Youth Health
- Do the Rich Get to Be Healthier?
- Can You Make a Contract for Good Health?

19

Introduction to Health and Wellness

In This Chapter

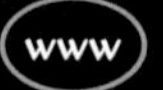

www **Student Web Resources**
www.HOPEtextbook.org/student

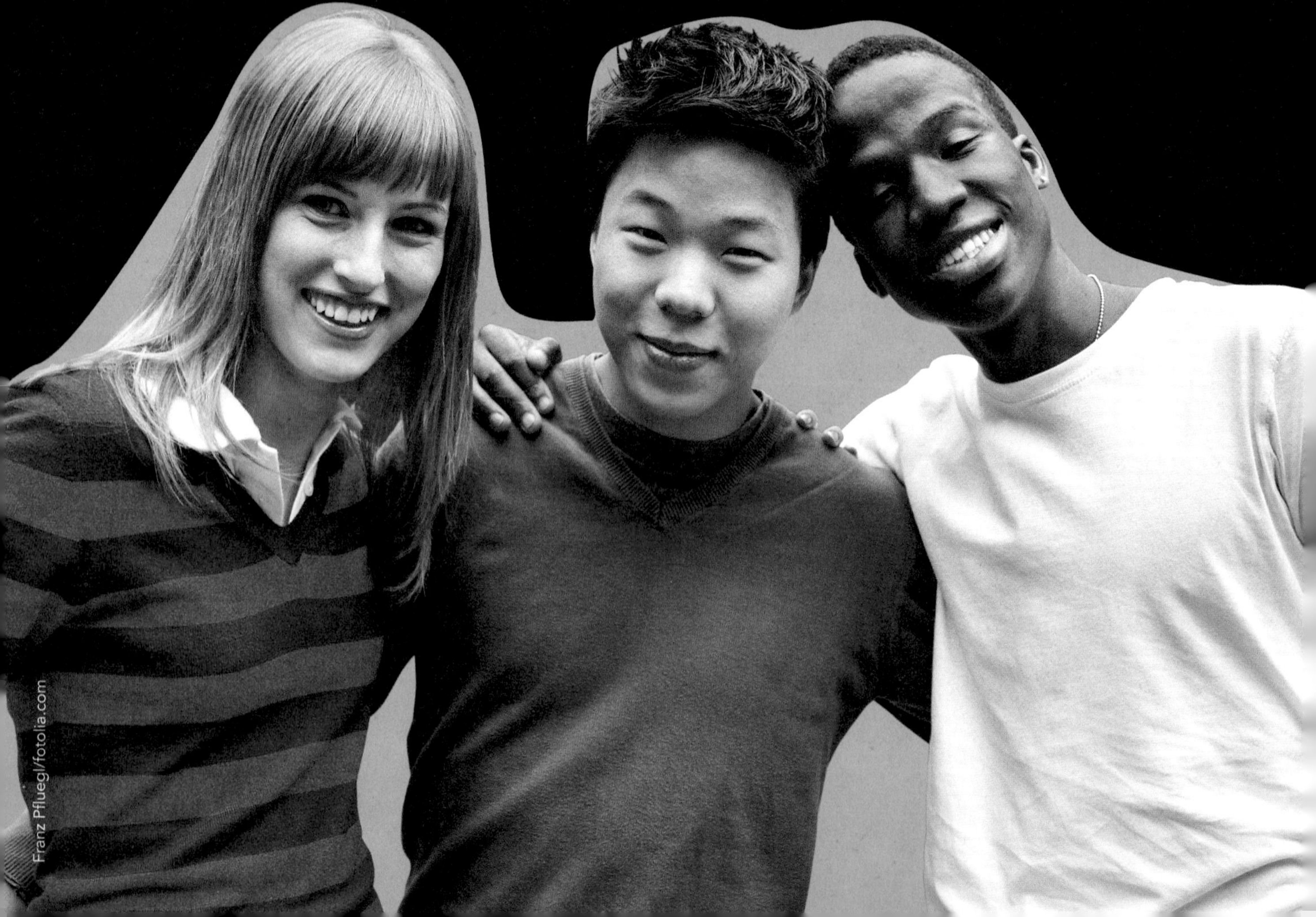

Franz Pfluegl/fotolia.com

Lesson 19.1

Health and Wellness

Lesson Objectives

After reading this lesson, you should be able to

1. define health and wellness and explain how they are related,
2. describe the five components of health and wellness and how they are related, and
3. answer common questions about health and wellness.

WWW 1 **Lesson Vocabulary**

health, *Healthy People 2020*, public health scientist, wellness, World Health Organization (WHO)

A large crowd was assembled to hear Dr. Lazarus, a **public health scientist**, discuss national health objectives. The title of her talk was "Health Is More Than Not Being Sick." She indicated that one major health objective "is to help all people live high-quality, longer lives." As the title of her talk suggests, Dr. Lazarus pointed out that **health** is more than freedom from disease; it also includes being *well* and enjoying a high quality of life. She emphasized that how you live your life can help you achieve both longer life and a higher quality of life.

Maggie, a first-year high school student, attended the talk with some of her friends because her mother was one of the organizers. Her grandfather and some of his friends also attended. After the talk, one of Maggie's friends said, "That was interesting, but why tell me about it? I don't have any health problems!" At the same time, Maggie's grandfather was saying half-jokingly to some of his friends, "That's good information, but why tell it to us old-timers? They need to talk to those kids while they still have a chance to prevent health problems!"

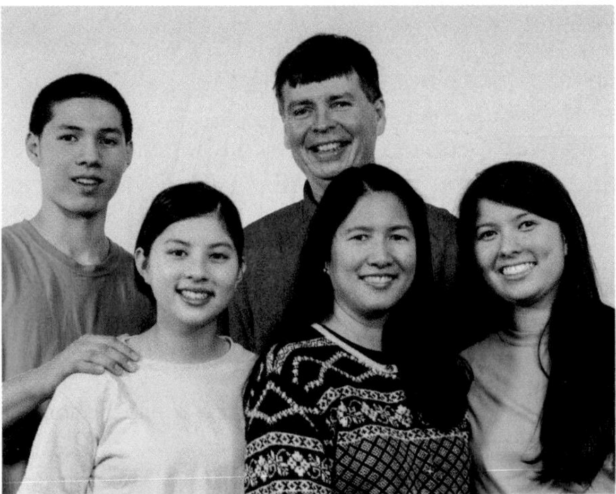

Health and wellness are important to people of all ages.

In part 2 of this book, you'll study all aspects of health, including **wellness**. You'll see that, although your health and wellness are not totally under your control, the choices you make and the way you live can make a big difference in both your health and your wellness—no matter what your age. In fact, it's never too soon or too late to learn more. This particular lesson defines health and wellness and describes their various components.

Moving From Illness to Wellness

On the way home from Dr. Lazarus' talk, Maggie, her mother, and her grandfather talked about health and wellness. "When I was a kid," said her grandfather, "we worried about polio and measles. We were more concerned about not getting sick than being well. But I can see that things have changed since then."

He's right. Prior to the 1940s, the leading causes of death in the U.S. were infectious diseases such as pneumonia, smallpox, and, as Maggie's grandfather recalled, polio. People also often died at younger ages than they do today. For example, a person born in 1900 had an average life expectancy of 47 years. Since the 1940s, however, life expectancy has been greatly increased by advancements in medical science (such as antibiotics, vaccines, and improved surgical techniques), improved public health practices

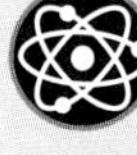

HEALTH SCIENCE

Every 10 years, scientists from more than 400 organizations work together to develop national health objectives for the United States. The most recent goals are included in a document called ***Healthy People 2020***, which, as its name suggests, identifies health goals to be accomplished by the year 2020. Public health scientists and other experts from all U.S. states, federal agencies such as the Centers for Disease Control and Prevention (CDC), and other public and private agencies developed the goals. They identify health objectives for all age groups, including teens.

The *Healthy People 2020* goals help health agencies and organizations prioritize their work. They also help teachers and schools plan what is taught in health classes and what types of health-related services to provide. In this book, key *Healthy People 2020* objectives are included on the opening page of each unit. Review these objectives to help you understand how the material you learn in this class relates to U.S. health goals. You can find more information about *Healthy People 2020* and various health organizations in the student section of the Health Opportunities Through Physical Education website.

(such as improved water and disposal of waste), and lifestyle changes (such as reduced tobacco use). As a result, a baby born today has an average life expectancy of about 80 years.

In 1947, the **World Health Organization (WHO)** issued a statement proclaiming that good health is not merely the absence of disease or illness; rather, it is a more complete state of being that includes wellness. Wellness is the *positive* aspect of health that includes having a good quality of life and a good sense of well-being as exhibited by a positive outlook on life.

The fact that good health includes wellness is illustrated in figure 19.1. The blue in the circle represents freedom from disease and illness, and the green in the circle represents wellness (quality of life). Illness is the negative aspect of health that we want to treat or prevent, and wellness is the positive aspect of health that we want to promote.

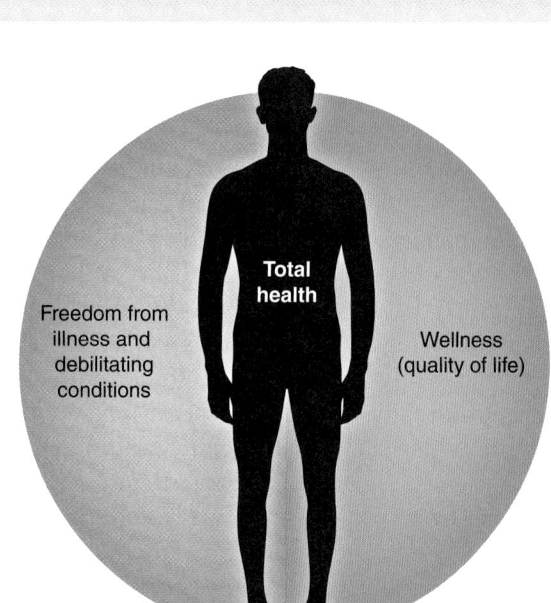

FIGURE 19.1 Being healthy means having wellness in addition to not being ill.

The Components of Health and Wellness

There are five components of health and wellness: intellectual, social, physical, emotional, and spiritual. The goal for each component of good health and wellness is to promote the positive while avoiding the negative (see figure 19.2). Look at the positive aspects at the top of the figure and negative aspects at the bottom. If you're informed, involved, fit, happy, and fulfilled, you've incorporated the positive aspects of the health components into your life. Thus you possess wellness, and your risk of illness is decreased.

The part can never be well unless the whole is well.

—Plato, Greek philosopher

Each of the five components of health and wellness is associated with all of the others. This interrelationship is often illustrated in the form of a chain (see figure 19.2). The chain can be no stronger than its weakest link. In addition, each link, or component, interacts with the others; in other words, if you change one component in a positive way, it strengthens all of the others. On the other hand, if one deteriorates, it weakens all of the others. Therefore, for your health and wellness chain to be strong, you must focus not just on one component but on all of them.

HEALTHY COMMUNICATION

Do you think any of the wellness components is more important than the others? Why or why not? Debate your perspective with several peers or classmates. Support your position with facts and be respectful of others' opinions.

Answering Health and Wellness Questions

During Dr. Lazarus' talk, she defined health and wellness as described in the preceding pages. Still, after the talk, many people had questions. Each question is included here, along with Dr. Lazarus' answers.

Question: Are there degrees of health and wellness?
Answer: Yes. There are different levels of health and wellness. A person who has a serious illness is different from a person who has a minor illness or who has risks for illness such as high blood pressure or high blood fat. In the same way, a person who has a high level of wellness has more positive components than a person who possesses less wellness.

Question: Can you be sick and still have wellness?
Answer: Yes. A person who has wellness is happy, fit, fulfilled, informed, and involved. A person can have a treatable disease, such as diabetes or cancer, and possess all of the components of wellness. In fact, research has shown that healthy lifestyle choices—such as eating well and doing regular physical activity—can help you reduce disease symptoms and risks while also contributing to a high quality of life.

Question: Can you be free of illness and not have good wellness?
Answer: Yes. Some people are not sick, meaning that they do not have a specific disease or illness, but also are not happy, fit, fulfilled, involved, and informed. Thus they are not well. Of course, optimal health includes wellness, so people who do not have good wellness do not have optimal health.

Question: Can you have good health and wellness if you have a disability?
Answer: Yes. Having a disability is an impairment that affects one's ability to perform certain typical functions. Most experts are quick to point out that having a disability does not necessarily mean that a person is handicapped. A disability can be associated with any health or wellness component. It may limit a person's ability to perform some of life's tasks, but good health—including wellness—can be present in people with a disability who also have a positive outlook on life.

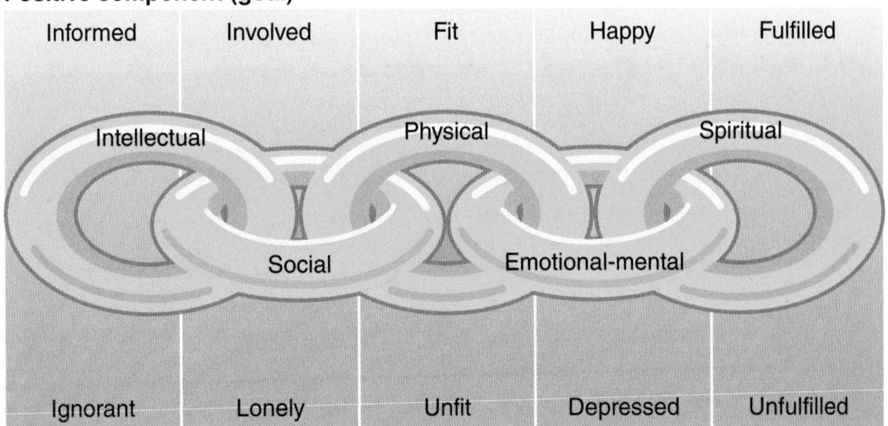

FIGURE 19.2 The total health and wellness chain.

Question: How do personal health and wellness goals differ from the national health goals described in *Healthy People 2020*?

Answer: The *Healthy People 2020* objectives are commonly referred to as goals for the community or for society. Personal health and wellness objectives are goals that each person sets to help his or her own health and wellness. National objectives help individuals set personal goals and are achieved when many individuals improve their health and wellness. For example, over the years, one national objective in the United States has been to reduce tobacco use. This national priority led to changes in public policy that encouraged people to change their personal behavior. Changes by many people over the past 20 years have resulted in better health for many individuals and improved national health.

Question: What about vocational (job-related) and environmental health and wellness? Why are they not included as components of health and wellness?

Answer: Health and wellness are personal states of being. Vocational and environment factors are very important to health and wellness, but they are not personal characteristics. Your job (vocation) and the environment (your surroundings) affect your health and wellness, so they are considered to be *determinants* of personal health and wellness rather than personal *characteristics* (health and wellness components).

In this lesson, you've learned about health and wellness and how they are defined. In the next lesson, you'll learn more about factors that determine health and wellness.

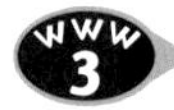

DIVERSE PERSPECTIVES: Living With a Disability

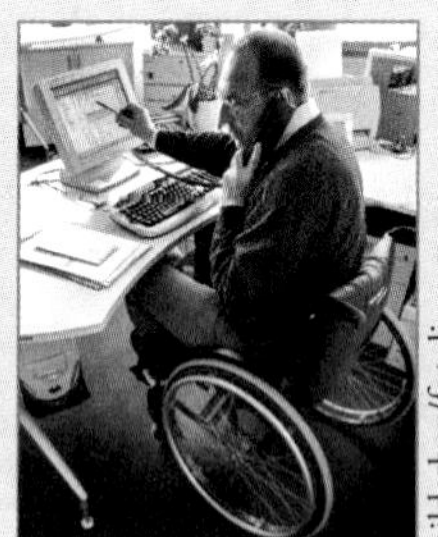

bilderbox/fotolia.com

Hi, my name is Travis. When I was 18, I was severely injured playing competitive ice hockey. My injury was to my spine. I have no sensation below my waist. I depend a lot on the care of others when it comes to meeting my basic daily needs. Sometimes I feel like I am a real burden on others. I think that is one of the hardest parts about having a disability like mine. But I am grateful that I still have my mind, that I'm not on a ventilator, that I have family around to support me. Sometimes I wish I could drive, that my level of injury was lower and that I had more physical movement, but I rarely ever think of those things. As the saying goes, my glass is always half-full . . . and I mostly try to think my glass is full. I know this sounds funny, but my life is full and busy. I started a foundation that raises money for spinal cord research and provides help to others in need. It isn't the life I imagined for myself when I was young, but I am proud of who I am now and what I've become.

Comprehension Check

1. Describe a hypothetical person who has good health, including good wellness.
2. List and describe the five components of health and wellness.
3. Identify and answer some often-asked questions about health and wellness.

SELF-ASSESSMENT: The Wellness Questionnaire

You've now learned about wellness and its several components. The Wellness Questionnaire will help you self-assess *your* current wellness. Use the following instructions.

1. Read each statement about wellness. Select one response for each statement. You can strongly agree, agree, disagree, or strongly disagree with each statement.
2. Record your responses as directed by your teacher. A worksheet may be provided.
3. Calculate your score for each of the five wellness components by adding the numbers associated with your responses to the three questions related to that component.
4. Add all five of your wellness component scores to get your overall wellness score.
5. Use table 19.1 to get your wellness rating for each wellness component and for your overall wellness. Record your ratings.

WELLNESS QUESTIONNAIRE

Wellness statement	Strongly agree	Agree	Disagree	Strongly disagree	Item score
1. I am physically fit.	4	3	2	1	
2. I can do the physical tasks needed in my work.	4	3	2	1	
3. I have the energy to be active in my free time.	4	3	2	1	
Physical wellness score (sum of the scores for items 1–3) =					
4. I am happy most of the time.	4	3	2	1	
5. I do not get stressed often.	4	3	2	1	
6. I like myself the way I am.	4	3	2	1	
Emotional wellness score (sum of the scores for items 4–6) =					
7. I have many friends.	4	3	2	1	
8. I am confident in social situations.	4	3	2	1	
9. I am close to my family.	4	3	2	1	
Social wellness score (sum of the scores for items 7–9) =					
10. I am an informed consumer.	4	3	2	1	
11. I check facts before making health decisions.	4	3	2	1	
12. I consult experts when I'm unsure of health facts.	4	3	2	1	
Intellectual wellness score (sum of the scores for items 10–12) =					
13. I feel a sense of purpose in my life.	4	3	2	1	
14. I feel spiritually fulfilled.	4	3	2	1	
15. I feel strong connections to the world around me.	4	3	2	1	
Spiritual wellness score (sum of the scores for items 13–15) =					
Total wellness score (sum of the five wellness scores) =					

TABLE 19.1 Rating Wellness

Wellness rating	Three-item score	Total wellness score
Good	10–12	>50
Marginal	8–9	40–49
Low	<7	<39

Lesson 19.2

Determinants of Health and Wellness

Lesson Objectives

After reading this lesson, you should be able to

1. describe the five types of determinants that influence health and wellness,
2. explain how each type of determinant is either in or out of your control, and
3. describe the five benefits of a healthy lifestyle.

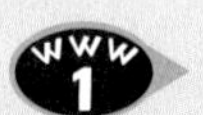

Lesson Vocabulary

determinant, medical scientist, priority healthy lifestyle choice, self-assessment, self-management skill, state of being

In this chapter's first lesson, you learned about health and wellness, each of which is a **state of being**—something that an individual person possesses. Your health and wellness are affected by many factors, which are referred to by public health and **medical scientists** as **determinants**. As the *Healthy People 2020* report indicates, you need to learn about these determinants in order to stay fit, healthy, and well.

> “One who has health has hope; and one who has hope has everything.”
>
> 
>
> —Ancient proverb

Determinants of Health and Wellness

In her talk about health, Dr. Lazarus described determinants of good health and wellness. She also noted that some determinants are more in your control than others. As shown in figure 19.3, five types of determinants affect your health and wellness (including two on the left of figure 19.3); lighter shades of orange indicate determinants over which you have less control, and darker shades indicate those over which you have more control.

Personal Determinants

Personal factors are determinants over which you have little or no control—for example, your heredity, your age, your sex, or a disability. They are shaded in a very light shade of orange. Even though you have little control over personal factors, they still affect your health and wellness. For example, some people inherit genes that put them at risk for certain diseases. As you grow older, risk increases for such diseases. Sex is also a factor. For example, males are more prone to storing abdominal fat than females, which places them at a higher risk for some diseases. We also know that women have a longer life expectancy than men. Of course, a personal disability can also affect your health and quality of life.

You'll learn more in other chapters about personal factors and their effect on your fitness, health, and wellness. Although you cannot control personal factors, you can be aware of them and prevent them from having an undue effect on your health and wellness. Being aware can also help you alter other determinants over which you do have control. For example, if you have a family history of heart disease, you can take special care to attend to risk factors for heart disease that you can control.

Environmental and Health Care Determinants

Your health and wellness are also affected by environmental factors. They are shown in a darker shade of orange than the personal factors because you do have some control over them. For example, as an adult, you can choose to live or work in a healthy environment, and you can recycle to help protect the environment. But you cannot personally control the quality of the air in your neighborhood, and you are limited in your control of other environmental factors (e.g., pollution in local rivers and streams).

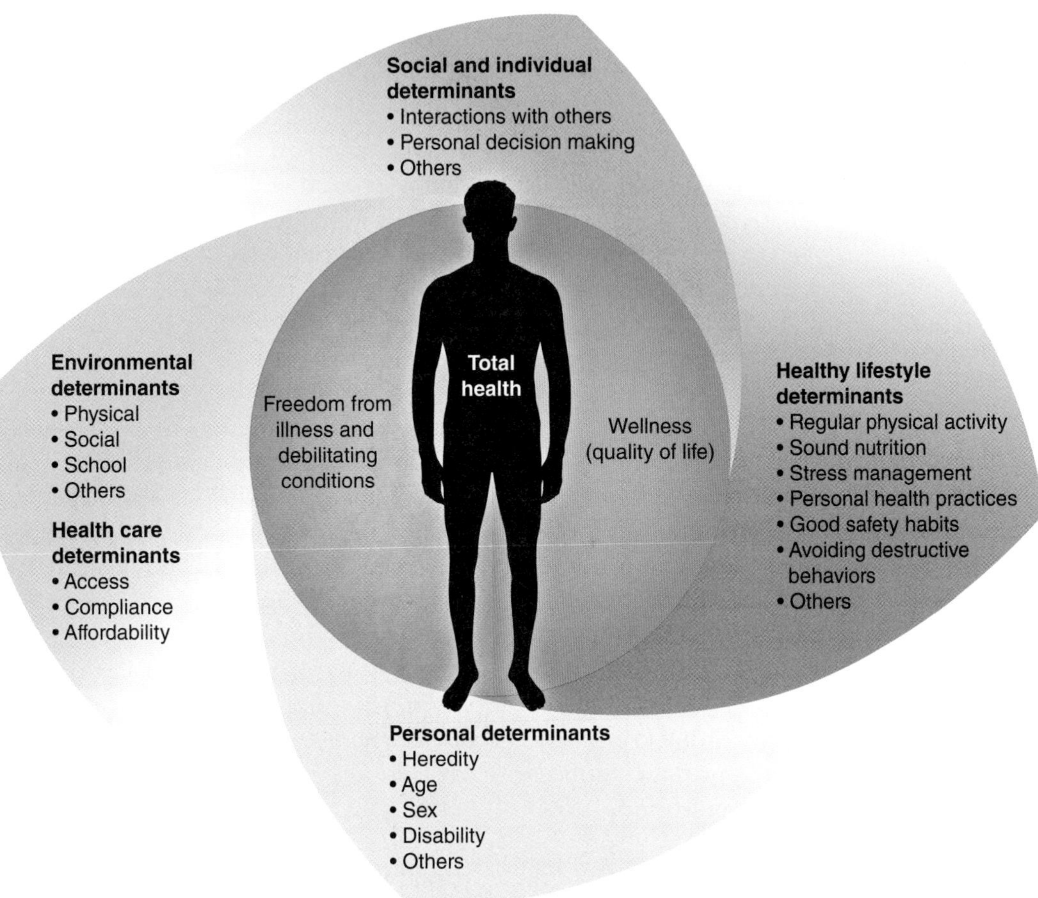

FIGURE 19.3 The five types of determinants of health and wellness (in bold).

Adapted, by permission, from C.B. Corbin et al., 2013, *Concepts of fitness and wellness*, 10th ed. (St. Louis, MO: McGraw-Hill Education). © The McGraw-Hill Companies.

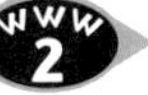

Environmental determinants can be subdivided into several groups. Physical environmental factors include, for example, air quality, water quality, and physical characteristics of your home, your school, and other human-made spaces you use. Social factors include the quality of the social environment in your home and community. To some extent, you cannot control your social environment because you may have to go to the school you are assigned to and live where your family lives. But you do have some control over your relationships and interactions with others. More information about these aspects is included in the next section of this lesson.

Health care refers to being able to see a doctor or other health care professional as needed and having access to health care facilities and medicine. Health care also includes opportunities to learn about prevention of illness and promotion of wellness. People who receive good health care live longer and have higher-quality lives compared to those who don't. This factor is shown in a darker shade of orange because you have some control over it. But health care is not equal for all people. For some, access is limited due to lack of money or insurance. Others simply do not take advantage of health care that is available to them. Still others seek care but do not comply with the recommendations given by their physicians or other health care providers. All three of these aspects—having access to good health care, seeking it when needed, and complying with health care recommendations—are important to your health and wellness.

Social and Individual Determinants

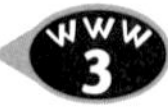

The people around you are part of your social environment. And of course the friends you choose, and the people you spend the most time with, affect

CONNECT

On a scale of 1 to 10, with 1 being the least and 10 being the most, how much does your closest friend (or group of friends) influence your health choices and behaviors? Is this influence more positive or more negative overall? How do you think *you* influence *their* behaviors and choices? Provide at least one example.

you more than people who play smaller roles in your social environment. The people closest to you and your interactions with them, including the decisions that you make with them, affect your health and wellness. Teens who hang out with friends who avoid destructive habits and practice healthy habits are more likely to be healthy and well than those who don't.

Individual factors are also important—for example, being a wise consumer by getting informed and making good decisions. In figure 19.3, social and individual factors are colored in a relatively dark shade of orange because you have considerable control over the choices that you make, both individually and with your family and friends.

Lifestyle Determinants

By far the most important determinants of personal health and wellness are your lifestyle choices—personal behaviors that you can adopt to improve your health and wellness. In most cases, they are factors over which you have a lot of control; therefore, they're shown in dark orange in figure 19.3.

Adopting a healthy lifestyle offers you many benefits. First, it reduces your risk of disease and early death. Nearly 60 percent of early deaths in the U.S. result from unhealthy lifestyle choices. In contrast, healthy lifestyle choices—such as getting regular physical activity, eating a well-balanced diet, avoiding smoking, and managing stress—are effective in preventing and treating various illnesses. For example, eating well and being active can help you prevent diseases such as heart disease and help manage conditions such as diabetes.

Like Maggie's grandfather in this chapter's first lesson, you might assume that because illness and disease are most common later in life, older people can't do anything about them. Or, like Maggie herself, you might share a common attitude among many teenagers: "I'm young and healthy. Why should I change what I do?" But evidence indicates that the disease process begins early in life. Therefore, making healthy lifestyle choices early in your life

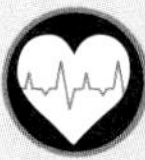

HEALTH TECHNOLOGY

The World Wide Web allows many people to get immediate access to all kinds of health and fitness information. Some of this information is good, but much of it is inaccurate. In each chapter of part 2, you'll find a web address that leads you to sound information about health and wellness. Look for special web symbols included throughout part 2; just type in the appropriate address from the first page of the chapter, and you'll find good, reliable information. For more information about health-related websites, see the student section of the Health Opportunities Through Physical Education website.

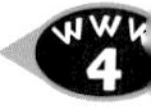

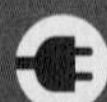

CONNECT

Visit the student section of the Health Opportunities Through Physical Education website. Select one or two of the web topics at this site and spend some time exploring them. How do you think accessing reliable health information online can affect a person's health behaviors? Briefly describe what you found at the websites and discuss your assessment of the information.

can do much to prevent disease and illness later on. The evidence also indicates that no matter how old you are, improving your lifestyle enhances your health and wellness.

As you work your way through part 2 of this book, you'll learn about each of the lifestyle choices listed in figure 19.3. Three of the most important ones are being active, eating well, and managing stress. As a result, they're sometimes called **priority healthy lifestyle choices** because, if adopted, they can make a huge difference in your personal health and wellness. However, many other lifestyle choices also influence your health and wellness—for example, simple personal health practices learned in elementary school (such as washing your hands, brushing your teeth, and getting adequate sleep), practicing good safety habits (such as wearing a seat belt and driving safely without being preoccupied), and avoiding destructive habits (such as tobacco and alcohol use).

Benefits of a Healthy Lifestyle for Teens

Living a healthy lifestyle helps you not only later in life—you can also enjoy many benefits now. They include looking and feeling good, learning better, enjoying daily life activities, and handling emergencies.

Looking Good

Do you care about how you look? Most people do. In fact, one study showed that 94 percent of all men and 99 percent of all women would change some part of their appearance if they could. People are most often concerned with their weight (weighing too much or too little), the size of their waist or thighs, their muscles, and their teeth and hair. Experts agree that regular physical activity and eating well are healthy lifestyle choices that help you look your best. You don't have to take drastic measures to feel good about your appearance.

Feeling Good

Besides looking better, people who practice a healthy lifestyle feel better. If you're active, and therefore more physically fit, you can resist fatigue, you're less likely to be injured, and you're capable of working more efficiently. National surveys indicate that active people who eat well also sleep well and are less likely to be depressed.

Learning Better

In recent years, health scientists have found that being active and eating well help you learn better. Studies show that teens who are active and fit score better on tests and are less likely to be absent from school; thus they learn more. In addition, teens who are active and eat regular healthy meals, especially breakfast, are less tired and more alert at school. Recent studies also show that regular exercise and good fitness are associated with high function in the parts of the brain that promote learning. Your learning is also helped by getting enough sleep and learning to manage stress.

Enjoying Life

Enjoying life is important for your personal wellness. But what if you're too tired on most days to

Healthy lifestyles can help you feel good and enjoy life.

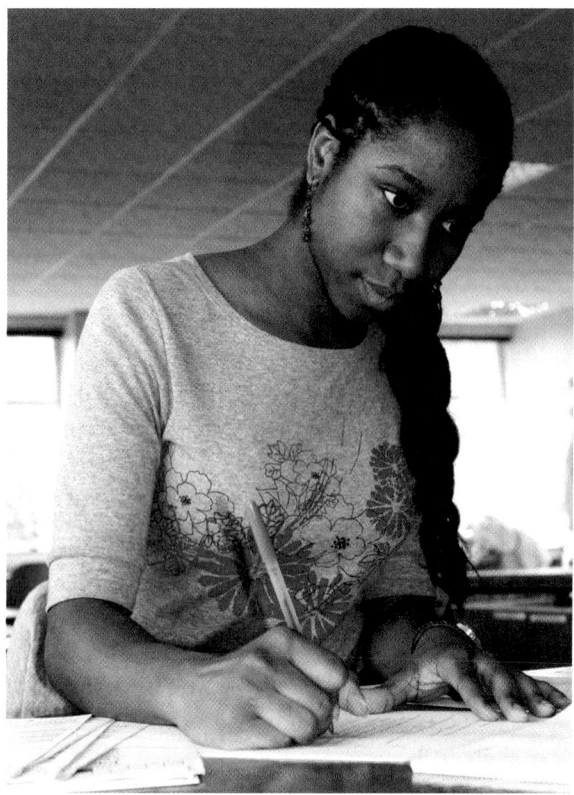

Teens who are active and eat regular healthy meals, especially breakfast, are more alert at school.

Laurence Gough - Fotolia

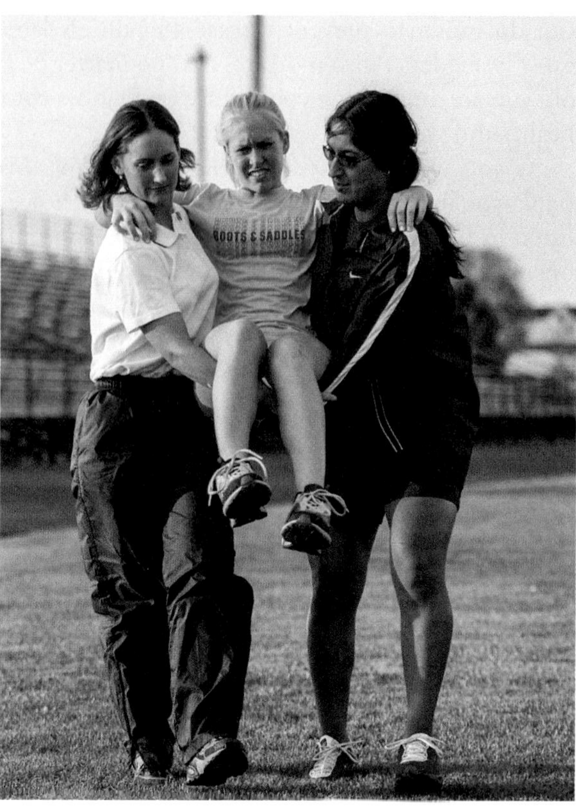

Good health helps you respond effectively in day-to-day demanding situations.

participate in the activities you really enjoy? Regular physical activity results in physical fitness, which is the key to being able to do more of the things you want to do. In addition, people who eat a good breakfast do not experience low energy during the day and are therefore better able to enjoy life to the fullest.

Meeting Emergencies

People who are fit, healthy, and well have the ability to handle emergencies and day-to-day demanding situations. For example, they are able to run for help, change a flat tire, and offer needed assistance to others.

Comprehension Check

1. Explain how each of the five types of determinants affects health and wellness.
2. Describe the amount of control you have over each of the five types of determinants.
3. Describe the five health benefits of a healthy lifestyle. How are they important both to teens and adults?

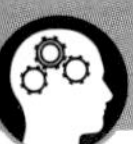

MAKING HEALTHY DECISIONS: Self-Assessment

When you take a trip, you typically plan ahead. After you choose a destination, you use a map to help you get where you want to go. Like a map, a **self-assessment** (or self-test) helps you know where you are (your current health status) and decide where you want to go (set goals for good health). Self-assessment is one type of healthy living skill (also called **self-management skill**), and many kinds of self-assessments exist. For example, you can assess your eating patterns, your stress level, your health risks, your knowledge, your current personal health habits, your physical fitness, and, as you did earlier in this chapter, your wellness status. You'll do self-assessments throughout this book.

After attending Dr. Lazarus' lecture about health, Maggie and her grandfather talked about what they had heard. They recalled Dr. Lazarus mentioning that most Americans do not have a realistic view of their own health. For example, as many as seven million people have type 2 diabetes but don't know it, and one in three adults has high blood pressure but doesn't know it.

For this reason, Dr. Lazarus urged her audience to get periodic medical checkups. But she also pointed out that people can use self-assessments to help track their health status. For example, she noted that many people use a home scale to self-assess their weight and that some count calories to assess their energy intake. Maggie's grandfather mentioned a friend with diabetes who did self-assessments of his blood sugar. And Maggie realized that she did self-assessments in physical education class to determine her cardiorespiratory endurance.

For Discussion

Dr. Lazarus suggested that people can learn to do self-assessments to help them plan for healthy living and set good health goals. But she also urged people to get regular medical exams to make sure that they are healthy and well. Discuss some ways in which Maggie's family could use self-assessments related to health. What kinds of self-assessment might different family members use? Might the self-assessments that Maggie and her younger brother perform be different from those done by her grandfather or her mother and father? What steps can Maggie and her family members take to make sure that their self-assessments are reliable and accurate? When answering these discussion questions, consider the guidelines in this chapter's Skills for Healthy Living feature.

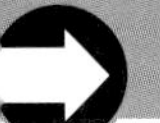

SKILLS FOR HEALTHY LIVING: Self-Assessment

As mentioned earlier, assessing your health and wellness is much like using a map; it helps you know where to go from here. You can assess your current health status to help you learn where you need to improve and make plans for doing so. Use the following guidelines as you learn to do personal health and wellness self-assessments.

- **Consider self-assessments of both health and wellness.** Tests of health and wellness assess your state of being. Examples include blood pressure tests, skin cancer screenings, dental exams for cavities, and wellness questionnaires.
- **Consider self-assessments of health and wellness determinants.** Examples include assessments of your dietary intake, activity level, use of time, personal health habits, social interactions, and personal actions, as well as environmental factors that affect your health and wellness.
- **Use a variety of self-assessments.** Using a variety of self-assessments helps you get a comprehensive profile of your health and wellness and the factors that determine them.
- **Use self-assessments for personal improvement.** Once you've learned to use

self-assessments, repeat them from time to time to monitor your progress. Avoid doing assessments too often, but check yourself periodically to see how you're doing. Change takes time, so assessing before changes have time to take place may cause you to be discouraged in meeting your goals.

- **Use recommended health standards rather than comparing yourself with others.** Sometimes people feel discouraged by their self-assessment results—often because they are comparing themselves with others. Doing so can lead to unrealistic expectations or self-criticism. A better approach is to use health standards, and you'll learn more about them throughout part 2 of this book.
- **Keep self-assessment results confidential.** Self-assessments are personal and confidential. The decision to share—or not share—health information is up to each person. In some cases, you're asked to share information with your teacher so that you can get feedback and advice. This is done with the understanding that the information is not to be shared with others. In other cases, you may work with a partner to perform a self-assessment. Prior to the self-assessment, you should reach an agreement about confidentiality with your partner, and you should both take the agreement seriously.
- **Learn from and periodically check with an expert.** Some self-assessments require more skill than others. For example, weighing yourself on a scale is easy, but checking your blood pressure is more difficult. Before performing a self-assessment, learn from an expert whenever possible. Your health or physical education teacher can help you with many self-assessments related to health and fitness.

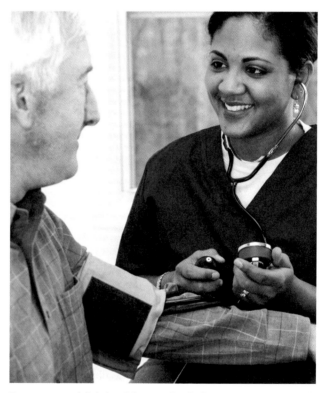

Doctors establish health standards for assessments such as blood pressure. Avoid comparisons to others and focus on standards for good health.

Rob/fotolia.com

- **Take advantage of health screenings.** Health agencies frequently offer free health screenings to help people detect problems. When performed by health experts, these screenings can provide you with good information and help you evaluate the accuracy of your self-assessments.
- **If you have concerns, seek advice from a professional, a parent or guardian, or a teacher.** Self-assessments are useful in assessing your current status and helping you plan programs to improve your health and wellness. They help you set goals and monitor your progress in meeting your goals. But even the people most skilled in self-assessment do not have the professional skills to interpret some health information. And incorrect interpretations of information gained from self-assessments can lead to anxiety and unnecessary concerns. If you have questions about self-assessment results, seek help from a qualified person.

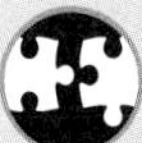

ACADEMIC CONNECTION: Percent and Percentages

Statistics is a branch of mathematics that helps us learn from data and make comparisons of measurements. In the health sciences, percentages are used to help us determine health behavior changes over time. A percentage is a portion, or share, of the whole. The whole (total) is expressed as 100 or 100 percent. Half of the whole is 50 percent of the whole. For example, a dollar is 100 cents, so a dime (10 cents) is 10 percent of a whole dollar. A quarter (25 cents) is 25 percent of a dollar. The Living Well News feature uses percents and percentages to help us understand tobacco use in the United States. In 2011, 45 percent of teens (45 of every 100) tried smoking. As shown in table 19.2, the percentage of teens who smoke has decreased in recent years.

The State of Youth Health

The Centers for Disease Control and Prevention (CDC), a U.S. government agency, has been keeping tabs on the health of the nation's youth for years. Specifically, the Youth Risk Behavior Surveillance System (YRBSS) tracks six categories of health-risk behavior among youth and young adults: (1) behaviors that contribute to violence and unintentional injury; (2) sexual behaviors that contribute to unintended pregnancy and sexually transmitted disease; (3) alcohol and other drug use; (4) tobacco use; (5) unhealthy dietary behaviors; and (6) inadequate physical activity. In addition, the YRBSS monitors the rates of obesity and asthma in the youth population. The most recent survey gathered data from 15,000 youth in grades 9 through 12.

All YRBSS data is reported and compared by sex, age, ethnicity, and state. For example, one item addresses the percentage of youth who have ever smoked a cigarette. Nationwide, 45 percent of students reported having tried a cigarette. White (44 percent) and Hispanic (49 percent) teens were more likely to have tried a cigarette than black (39 percent) teens. Males (46 percent) were more likely to have tried a cigarette than females (43 percent). Youth were most likely to smoke regularly in Kentucky (12 percent) and Wyoming (10 percent) and least likely to do so in Utah (2 percent) and Hawaii (4 percent). Smoking has declined significantly in teens over the last two decades. See table 19.2 for a sample of student smoking data that demonstrates this trend.

Information from the YRBSS helps health professionals and educators better understand youths' health behaviors and track those behaviors over time. "We are encouraged that more of today's high school students are choosing healthier, safer behaviors, such as wearing seat belts, and are avoiding behaviors that we know can cause them harm, such as binge drinking or riding with impaired drivers," said Howell Wechsler, director of CDC's Division of Adolescent and School Health. "However, these findings also show that despite improvements, there is a continued need for government agencies, community organizations, schools, parents, and other community members to work together to address the range of risk behaviors prevalent among our youth."

For Discussion

How honest do you think teens are when they fill out a survey about their health behaviors? Do you think they're more likely to be honest if the survey is anonymous (no name attached) and confidential (used only for the research study)? Why or why not? Why is it important for people to be honest when reporting their health information on a self-assessment? What about when reporting their information on a medical history form that will only be seen by a medical professional?

TABLE 19.2 Percentage of Students Who Have Ever Tried a Cigarette

2001	2003	2005	2007	2009	2011
64	58	54	50	46	45

From Youth Risk Behavior Surveillance System (YRBSS) 2011.

Reviewing Concepts and Vocabulary

As directed by your teacher, answer items 1 through 5 by correctly completing each sentence with a word or phrase.

1. _______ is more than just freedom from disease; it also involves optimal well-being.
2. __________ is the positive component of good health and is exemplified by a positive sense of well-being and a good quality of life.
3. Factors such as your heredity, your age, your sex, and a disability are examples of ____________ determinants over which you have little or no control.
4. Air quality is an example of a(n) ____________ determinant.
5. The friends you choose are all part of your ___________ environment.

For items 6 through 10, as directed by your teacher, match each term in column 1 with the appropriate phrase in column 2.

6. physical component	a. a sharp and engaged mind
7. emotional component	b. having healthy interactions with others
8. spiritual component	c. happiness
9. intellectual component	d. a sense of connection to the world and others and having a strong purpose in life
10. social component	e. being physically fit

For items 11 through 15, as directed by your teacher, respond to each statement or question.

11. What are the components of wellness?
12. How do health and wellness differ?
13. Why are environmental factors not listed as components of personal wellness?
14. Why is it important to learn how to conduct self-assessments?
15. What are the priority healthy lifestyle choices?

Thinking Critically

Write a paragraph in response to the following prompt.

A person with a physical disability or disease may still have wellness. Use a specific example to explain how this is possible.

Take It Home

Research some of the self-assessments related to health that are available online. Select one that you think would be of interest to a family member. Encourage that person to complete the self-assessment. You can find links to self-assessments in the student section of the Health Opportunities Through Physical Education website.

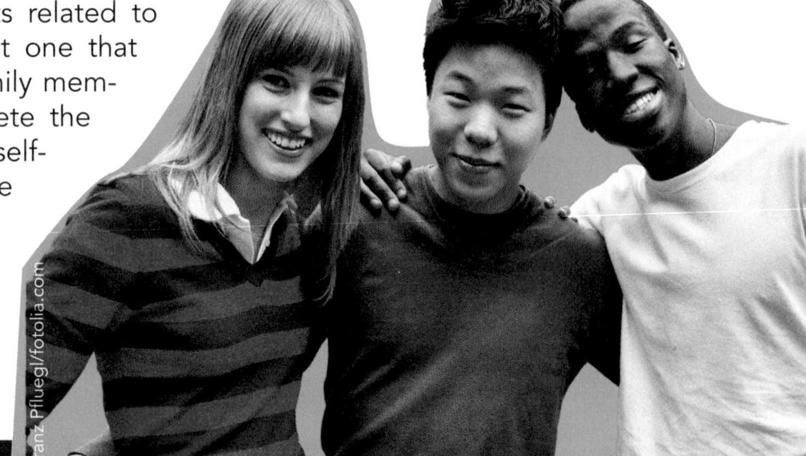

Franz Pfluegl/fotolia.com

20

Health Behavior Change and Personal Health

In This Chapter

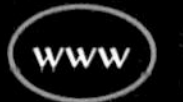

Student Web Resources
www.HOPEtextbook.org/student

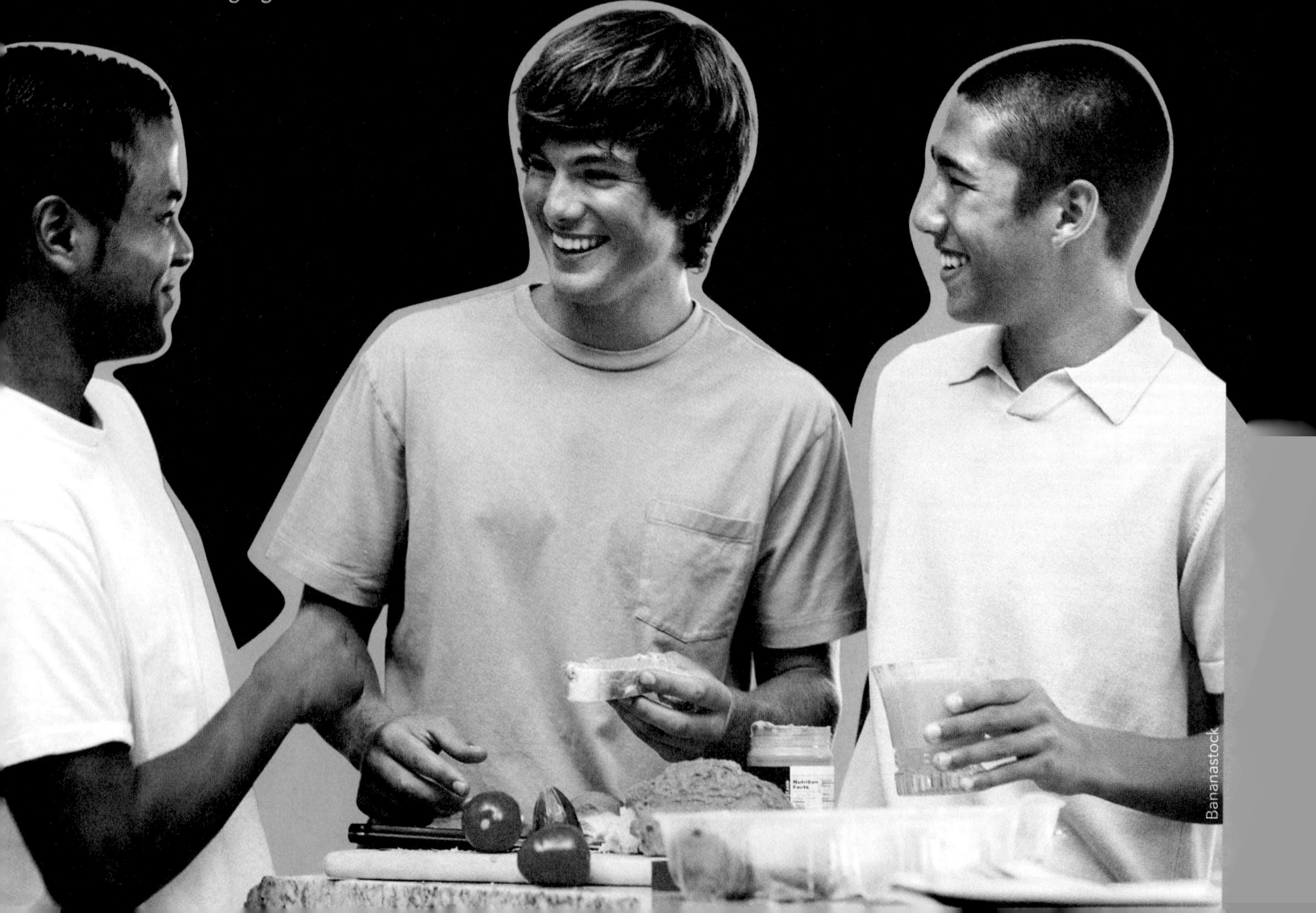

Bananastock

Lesson 20.1

Personal Health and Wellness

Lesson Objectives

After reading this lesson, you should be able to

1. explain the difference between controllable and uncontrollable risk factors,
2. describe several healthy lifestyle choices, and
3. identify and explain some environmental and social factors that affect health and wellness.

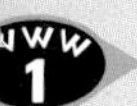

Lesson Vocabulary

accelerometer, controllable risk factor, healthy lifestyle, risk factor, sleep apnea, uncontrollable risk factor

If you asked every person you know, you'd probably find that most of them want to have good personal health and wellness. But how many are aware of all the things they can do to achieve those goals? In this lesson, you'll learn about healthy lifestyle choices and how they can help you achieve good personal health and wellness. You'll also learn about other factors that can influence your health and wellness.

Teens	Adults
1. Accidents (unintentional injuries)	1. Heart disease
2. Homicide	2. Cancers
3. Suicide	3. Chronic lower respiratory disease
4. Cancers	4. Stroke
5. Heart disease	5. Accidents (unintentional injuries)

FIGURE 20.1 The top five causes of death in teens versus adults.

Determinants and Other Risk Factors

A **risk factor**, as it relates to disease, is anything that increases your chance of getting sick (having a disease). Some determinants of health and wellness are associated with disease risk and are therefore considered to be risk factors; examples include age, sex, and heredity. These particular factors are called **uncontrollable risk factors**. For example, older people are more at risk of diseases that are the leading causes of death (such as heart disease, cancer, and diabetes) than are younger people (see figure 20.1). Similarly, men have a greater risk of heart disease than women. And people with a family history of a certain disease are typically more at risk for it than people who do not have such a history.

Determinants such as health care and environment are also related to risk. For example, people have lower risk if they have health insurance, regularly see medical professionals for health screening and treatment, and follow the advice given by medical professionals. These factors may be somewhat controllable by teens, but they are often controlled by other people in your life. Still, as you'll see later in this lesson, there are things that you can do as a teen to reduce your risks related to health care.

Your disease risk is also affected by where you live and work. For example, if you live or work in a highly polluted area, your risk is greater. Nor are environmental risk factors totally in your control. Teens usually cannot, for example, control where they live or go to school, though working teens may have some control over their working environment.

Factors where you can exert more control include the friends you associate with and the decisions you make. The factors over which you have the most control are your lifestyle choices. They are also among the most important factors in reducing your risk of disease.

> "It is health that is real wealth and not pieces of gold and silver."
>
> —Mahatma Gandhi, human rights leader

Health and Wellness Promotion

The focus of early health professionals was on diagnosis and treatment of illness. Treating disease is still a high-priority health goal in the United States, but it is equally important to help people prevent illness and improve their quality of life and sense of well-being throughout their lives (health promotion). As illustrated in figure 20.2, all three factors (treatment, prevention, and promotion) are important. Treatment helps you to avoid illness. Prevention involves taking steps to avoid future illness including minimizing your controllable risk factors. Promotion involves taking action to build good health and wellness for yourself and other members of society. The remainder of this lesson describes steps that you can take to reduce your risk of disease and promote your personal wellness. The focus here is on changing personal behaviors (making good lifestyle choices), but other determinants are also discussed—especially when they relate to risk factors that are in your personal control.

Healthy Lifestyle Choices

A **healthy lifestyle** is a way of living that helps you prevent illness and enhance your wellness. Healthy lifestyle choices make up one kind of determinant of your health and wellness; more specifically, they are often considered to be **controllable risk factors**. As you can see in figure 20.3, four major factors contribute to early death. The largest number of early deaths results from unhealthy lifestyle choices. These deaths could be prevented if people changed the way they live. Remember, too, that healthy lifestyle choices not only reduce your risk of disease and disease-related death but also enhance your wellness. For example, not smoking greatly reduces your risk of heart disease and cancer; it also increases the quality of your life, because you can breathe better, have a keener sense of smell, and spend less money on tobacco and medical care.

The following lifestyle choices are ones that you can adopt to promote good fitness, health, and wellness. Of course, these options benefit you only if you choose to do them. The choices you make have much to do with your personal fitness, health, and wellness. Each choice is discussed only briefly here, but most are discussed in greater detail in other sections of part 2 of this book.

Many aspects of a person's lifestyle can be changed to improve his or her health and wellness. Ten are discussed here. Three of these—being physically active, eating well, and managing stress—are sometimes called priority healthy lifestyle choices because they can help so many people. Statistics

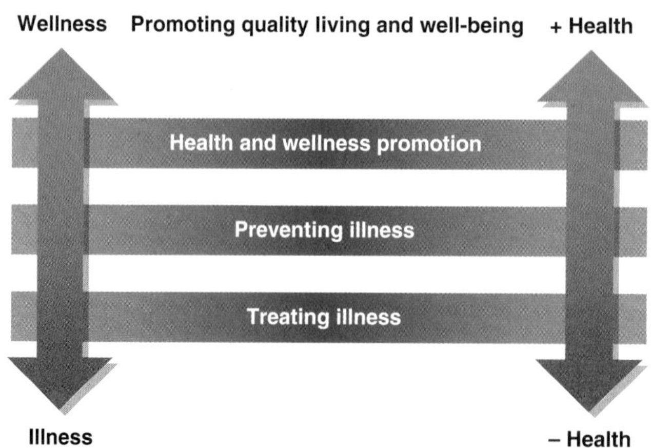

FIGURE 20.2 Health and wellness: from treatment to promotion.

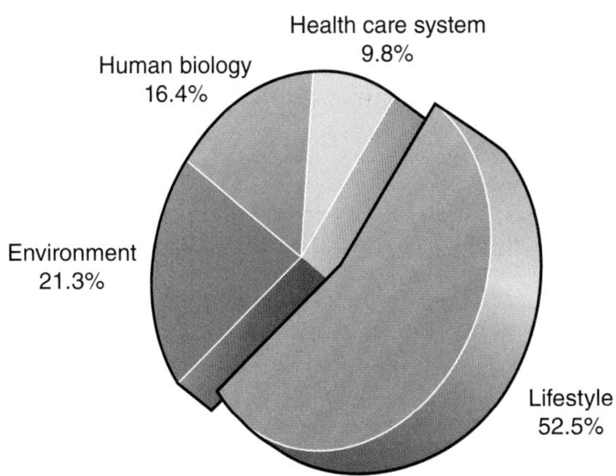

FIGURE 20.3 Four main factors contribute to early death.

Reprinted, by permission, from C. Corbin, G. Le Masurier, and K. McConnell, 2014, *Fitness for life*, 6th ed. (Champaign, IL: Human Kinetics), 407.

indicate that the majority of teens do *not* do regular physical activity, do *not* follow important dietary guidelines, and *do* report being stressed on a regular basis.

Be Physically Active

Among the health goals set forth in the U.S. government's *Healthy People 2020* report, being physically active is one of the most important. Changing your lifestyle from inactive to active can do more for your health and wellness than most other changes. In fact, being physically active can also help you manage stress, so its benefits are doubled. In addition, physical activity helps you reduce many risk factors, such as high blood pressure and high blood fat. Physical activity also builds good health-related physical fitness, including cardiorespiratory endurance, strength, muscular endurance, power, flexibility, and healthy body composition. Fitness is associated with reduced disease risk and with wellness factors such as having the energy to enjoy leisure activities without fatigue, being able to work without fatigue, and looking and feeling good.

Eat Properly

What kinds of food do you typically eat? Are your meals generally high in fat? Do you eat plenty of fruits, vegetables, and grains? Do you limit unhealthy fats and get adequate protein in your diet? Many children, teens, and adults do not eat a balanced diet—a diet that includes healthy amounts of important food groups. Some also don't eat breakfast—a very important meal. Skipping breakfast

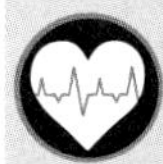

HEALTH TECHNOLOGY

Considerable evidence shows that getting too little sleep can lead to health problems. Teens need about nine hours of sleep per night, but 90 percent of teens report getting less than that, and 25 percent report getting less than 6.5 hours per night. However, your number of sleep hours per night isn't the only thing that's important. Your sleep patterns also matter. People who wake up numerous times, or toss and turn frequently during the night, are not getting restful sleep. In fact, for years, scientists have used sophisticated machines to detect **sleep apnea** and other serious sleep disturbances. Now, an **accelerometer**, such as one worn to count steps, can also be used to determine movement patterns during the night.

Experts do caution against overgeneralizing conclusions based on sleep reports from sleep-tracking devices. They point out that a person can sleep well most of the time but still have periodic restless nights. In addition, sleep trackers do not sense levels of sleep (e.g., light versus deep sleep) and cannot directly determine the amount of sleep you get. As a result, experts acknowledge that use of a sleep tracker could result in the cost of an unnecessary medical visit if the tracker suggests a problem where none exists. Even so, sleep trackers can be useful in screening for sleep problems in people who frequently feel tired or suspect that they have a sleep problem. If a sleep tracker indicates that your sleep is interrupted frequently, consult an expert for more analysis. For more information about sleep-tracking devices, see the student section of the Health Opportunities Through Physical Education website.

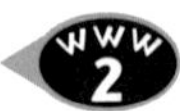

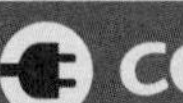

CONNECT

Investigate sleep-tracking devices. Evaluate the pros and cons of using such a device. Check to see if activity-tracking devices cost more when they also include sleep-tracking capability.

(and other meals) can burden you with fatigue, lack of attention, and poor school performance.

With all this in mind, one major U.S. health goal is to improve the nutrition of all citizens. The goals set forth in *Healthy People 2020* outline ways to improve your health and wellness by changing your eating habits. Together, regular physical activity and sound nutrition do more to reduce your disease risk than all other factors except tobacco avoidance. Eating well gives you the energy for work and play, whereas overeating contributes to overweight and obesity—problems that are all too common among Americans today.

Manage Stress

You've probably had periods of stress and know how it can affect you in the short term. But did you know that stress can also cause health problems and detract from your personal well-being and quality of life? Most people are well aware of the stress experienced by business people, elected officials, and other people in high-stress jobs, but many of us sometimes forget that stress affects everyone—including teens. You can help yourself by learning stress management techniques to use before tests and in other times of high stress. You can also reduce stress by learning to manage your time effectively. See the book's chapter on stress management.

Adopt Good Personal Health Habits

In kindergarten or first grade, you most likely learned about personal health habits, such as regularly brushing and flossing your teeth, washing your hands before meals and after using the bathroom, and getting enough sleep. Because these habits are often taught in elementary school, many teens feel that they're not still important—but they are! Table 20.1 summarizes key personal health habits and provides some related information you may not know.

Avoid Destructive Habits

Just as adopting healthy habits contributes to good health, practicing destructive habits detracts from your health and wellness. Examples include smoking, other tobacco use, legal or illegal drug abuse, and alcohol abuse. These destructive habits can impair your fitness, detract from your performance of physical activities, and result in various diseases, lowered feelings of well-being, and reduced quality of life. Another destructive practice is risky sexual behavior.

Young people sometimes claim, "I can do these things and they don't hurt me." This attitude results in part from the fact that, although many destructive behaviors do cause immediate harmful effects, other negative effects can take years to develop. As a result, it's not uncommon for older people to say, "I wish I'd listened when I was younger." If you really want to see the effects of a destructive behavior, interview a person who has done the behavior for years. If you select a person you know and care about, you may even be able to help that person.

Adopt Safety Practices

Daily news reports are filled with accounts of injury and death caused by motor vehicle crashes. Other common causes of death and injury include falling, poisoning, drowning, fire, bicycle accidents, and accidents in and around the home. Many of these outcomes could have been prevented if simple safety rules had been followed. As a result, one U.S. health goal is to reduce the number of deaths and injuries caused by accidents.

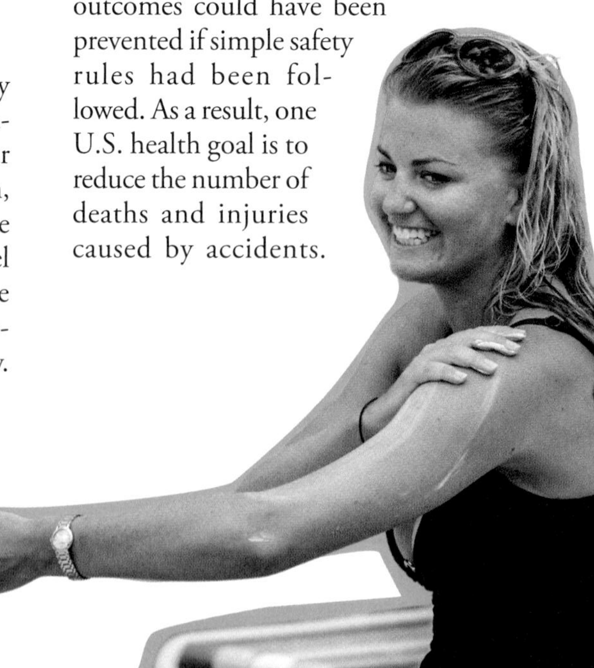

Adopting good personal health habits like applying sunscreen before sun exposure is part of a healthy lifestyle.

TABLE 20.1 Personal Health Habits

Health habit	Healthy action	Health information
Oral care	• Regular brushing • Regular flossing • Regular cleaning and screening	It's well known that oral care helps you look your best and prevents erosion of teeth, bones, and mouth tissues (periodontitis). You may not know that the bacteria that cause periodontitis have also been found in plaque in the arteries, which can lead to heart disease.
Sleep	• Getting nine hours of sleep each night • Avoiding sleep during the day	Many people think that the need for sleep dramatically decreases during the teen years. However, studies show that teens need nine hours of sleep per night. Unfortunately, teens get an average of only 7.5 hours, and one in four teens gets 6.5 hours or less. Why does this matter? Lack of adequate sleep is associated with poor grades, depression, and sleepiness during school. It's also important to get good-quality sleep. Teens who snooze during the day often do not sleep well at night.
Hand washing	• Washing your hands regularly, especially before eating and after using the bathroom, working, playing sports, or coming into contact with a sick person • Washing properly with soap • Using hand sanitizer when hand washing is not possible	Hand washing is a basic practice learned in elementary school, but it's no less important at any other age, including your teen years. Washing your hands regularly—and well—is your first line of defense against the spread of many illnesses, including flu, colds, gastrointestinal infections (e.g., diarrhea), skin infections, and some more serious diseases, such as bronchitis, hepatitis A, and meningitis. Students lose millions of days of school attendance each year due to illnesses that might have been prevented by hand washing.
Careful coughing and sneezing	• Covering your mouth and nose with a tissue • Disposing of tissues in a wastebasket • Coughing or sneezing into your upper sleeve (not your hands) when you don't have a tissue	The healthy actions listed here are part of what the U.S. Centers for Disease Control and Prevention has described as proper etiquette for coughing and sneezing. Etiquette refers to social rules that benefit people. Using good etiquette when coughing or sneezing reduces the risk of infectious illness in all settings. It's especially important in crowded places and in medical settings such as hospitals and doctors' offices.
Posture	• Sitting with good posture • Standing with good posture • Lifting with good posture • Using good body mechanics during daily activities • Using backpacks safely and with good posture	Poor posture is associated with many health problems and is also important to wellness. For example, it is associated with back and neck pain (and 80 percent of people in the U.S. experience back pain at some point). Poor posture can also lead to unnecessary fatigue. In addition, many school-age people carry backpacks, and you should learn how to use your backpack properly—with good posture. Here are some guidelines provided by the National Safety Council (a U.S. nonprofit group): • Limit the weight of your backpack to no more than 15 to 20 percent of your body weight. • Use both straps (not just one on one shoulder). • Wear your pack over your midback, where your muscles are the strongest. • If you have to lean forward to carry the pack, it's too heavy—lighten the load. • Don't bend at the waist when carrying a backpack (instead, bend your legs to squat with your back straight). Other guidelines are available at the safety council's website (www.nsc.org).

> continued

TABLE 20.1 > continued

Health habit	Healthy action	Health information
Skin care	• Using sunscreen that blocks UVA and UVB light • Avoiding lengthy exposure to the sun, especially at high altitude and in the late spring, summer, and early fall • Avoiding sun lamps, tanning beds, and tanning salons • Getting screened for abnormal skin growths and seeking medical help if in doubt	Tanning is a common practice among teens—but one that has resulted in an ever-increasing rate of skin cancer. The most dangerous kind of skin cancer is melanoma because it can spread to other parts of the body. Use the ABCDE rule when checking for skin cancer symptoms. A = Is one half of the skin growth (mole or other skin irregularity) different from the other half (**asymmetry**)? B = Are the **borders** of the growth irregular? C = Does the **color** of the growth vary (e.g., tan, brown, black, or another color)? D = Is the **diameter** of the spot larger than 6 mm (larger than a standard pencil eraser)? E = Has the mole or spot changed in appearance (**evolution**)? Research indicates that the use of tanning booths increases a person's risk of skin cancer. Some states prohibit their use by teens without a parent's permission.
Other	• Learning first aid so that you can help yourself and others if an accident occurs • Working with others to improve school and community environments so that they are safe and promote health	Health problems can be associated with the availability of health care (or lack thereof). You may not be in control of all aspects of the health care system, but there are some things you can do, such as those listed here, to help prevent disease and promote wellness.

You can do your part by making healthy lifestyle choices such as the following: wearing a seat belt, wearing a helmet when cycling or in-line skating, making sure that poisonous substances are properly labeled, installing and maintaining smoke detectors, practicing water safety, and keeping your home in good repair. And don't forget—being physically fit can help prevent accidents, too.

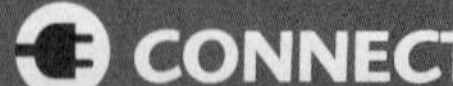

In what ways does your family influence your adoption of healthy behaviors? In what ways do your peers influence your adoption of healthy behaviors? Provide specific examples. Which has a greater influence on your behaviors—family or peers? Explain your answer.

Learn About First Aid and CPR

Even people who make healthy lifestyle choices and adopt good safety practices can have accidents. Because accidents can happen to anyone, everyone should have a first aid kit handy and know how to administer first aid. Other important first aid skills include bleeding control, the Heimlich maneuver to relieve choking, cardiopulmonary resuscitation (CPR), and use of an automated external defibrillator (AED) to restore effective cardiac rhythm. The National Heart, Lung, and Blood Institute defines an AED as a portable device that checks the heart rhythm. If needed, it can send an electric shock to the heart to try to restore a normal heart rhythm. AEDs are used to treat heart attacks.

Medical and health scientists have been doing research for many years to find the best ways of giving first aid to people whose heart or breathing has stopped. As a result, over the past 50 years, new methods of CPR have been developed, thus saving thousands of lives. Mouth-to-mouth resuscitation was first used in France in the 1700s, and medical doctors in the late 1800s used chest compression to revive people. Doctors used these procedures for a long time before they were finally recommended to the general public in the 1960s. Since then, the

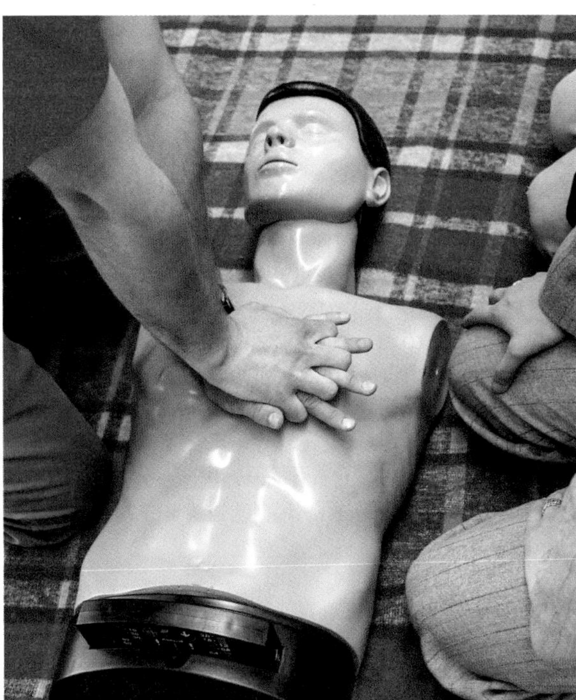

Knowing how to perform CPR is an important first aid skill.

Roman Milert/fotolia.com

guidelines for using mouth-to-mouth breathing and chest compressions have changed dramatically. In addition, the proper use of AEDs by the general public has become an essential part of CPR training and implementation. Training and certification are now offered by many schools and several national organizations. See the book's chapter on safety and first aid.

Seek and Follow Appropriate Medical Advice

Even if you make healthy lifestyle choices and stick with them, you may occasionally become ill. In those cases, seek and follow appropriate medical advice. In fact, for best results, get regular medical and dental checkups to help prevent problems before they start. Consult your own physician and dentist to determine how often you should have a checkup. Some people avoid seeking medical help because they fear they may be ill. However, this practice is dangerous, because early detection can be crucial to an ultimate cure. As noted earlier, getting the best medical help is not always under your control. If this is the case for you, seek help through your school nurse or guidance counselor.

During your school years, many decisions about your health care are made for you by others. For example, you may receive inoculations (vaccinations) for various diseases, such as polio, flu, measles, and mumps. The U.S. Centers for Disease Control and Prevention (CDC) provides a vaccination schedule for children and teens (for details, see the student section of the Health Opportunities Through Physical Education website). After your school years, you become responsible for your own inoculation schedule—and for various health checks, such as annual health screenings with a physician and screenings for heart disease, diabetes, various forms of cancer, and other conditions. Many diseases can be prevented or minimized by early detection through screening. See the book's chapter on health care consumerism.

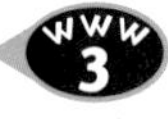

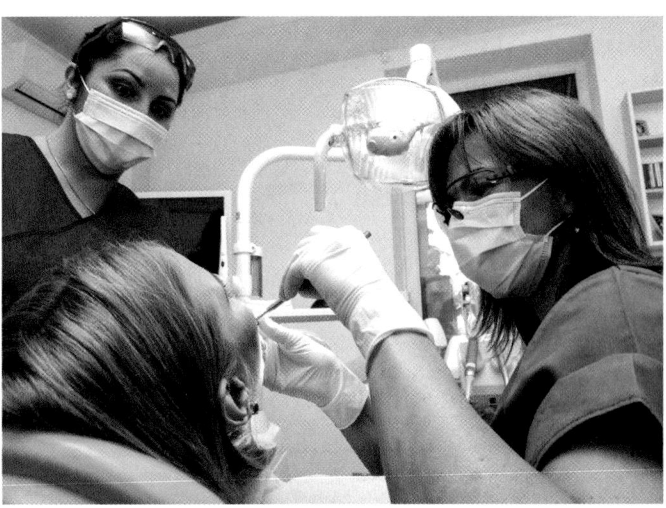

Getting regular dental checkups will help prevent problems before they start.

© Grecu Mihail Alin/Dreamstime

Make Efforts to Improve the Environment

As noted earlier, the environment is something over which you have limited control. Still, there are things you can do to change your immediate environment; in other words, even here your behavior can make a difference. Your physical environment includes the air, land, water, plants, and other physical things that exist around you. We know that certain physical environments can be very harmful to a person's health. You may be unable to change some aspects of your physical environment, such as where you live. You can, however, take action to improve your environment by, for example, not exposing yourself unnecessarily to smoke-filled places, avoiding excessive exposure to the sun, and being careful about using pollutants, such as weed killers. You can also reduce your exposure to air pollution by exercising away from heavily traveled streets.

Other steps that you can take include recycling many items (such as cans, plastic bottles, and plastic bags) and conserving water and electricity. You can also help people in your community who are working to improve the "built environment," which refers to the physical characteristics of your neighborhood. Doing so—for example, by adding sidewalks and bike paths and improving street lighting and crossings—increases residents' participation in physical activity, such as walking and biking in neighborhoods. See the book's chapter on a healthy environment.

CONSUMER CORNER: Don't Be Outsmarted! Finding High-Quality Health Information

Living a healthy lifestyle requires you to seek out and use appropriate health information. Not all information about health is truthful or reliable. In fact, many health-related websites are really trying to sell you products or services, and they may not be committed to accuracy. Medline, an online database compiled by the U.S. National Library of Medicine, recommends that you take the following steps when seeking health information online.

- **Consider the source.** Know who is responsible for the site. Use sites created by recognized authorities and organizations.
- **Focus on quality.** Rely on sites with a clear and qualified editorial board and expert contributors.
- **Be a cyberskeptic.** Avoid claims that seem too good to be true—they usually are. Also, confirm information by using more than one source.
- **Look for the evidence.** Rely on medical research, not opinion.
- **Check for currency.** Look for the latest information.
- **Beware of bias.** Check to see if the site is supported by public funds, private donations, or commercial advertising. Nonprofit and government websites are less likely to include bias information compared to commercial sites that use advertisements.
- **Protect your privacy.** Health information should be confidential. Check to see if the site has a privacy policy and be careful with any information you share.
- **Consult with your health professional.** Good websites can help you become informed, but health care professionals provide the best medical information.

Consumer Challenge

Visit a government website (typically with the web extension .gov) to review a health topic (e.g., www.cdc.gov or www.fitness.gov). Compare information from this website with a commercial website that contains information on the same topic.

Seek Friends Who Support You and Who Practice Healthy Behaviors

Talking to others is a form of social interaction. So is doing things with others. Research shows that your social interactions (behaviors) have much to do with your health and wellness. For example, studies show that people with a large number of friends throughout life live longer. Regular interactions with friends can promote better brain function, thus leading to a better quality of life. Positive social interactions also contribute to happiness, which is one indicator of wellness. A recent study indicates that friends can even help each other prevent weight gain. More generally, having friends who make healthy decisions helps you make good decisions. On the other hand, having friends who practice destructive habits and make negative health decisions can lead you to make unhealthy decisions. Which scenario do you choose?

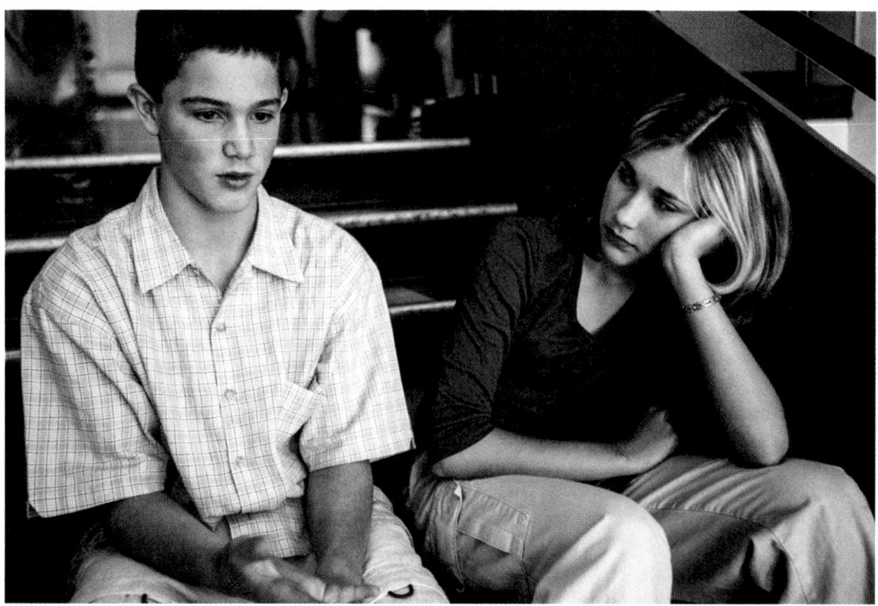

Supportive friends are important to good health and wellness.
Photodisc

Comprehension Check

1. Explain the difference between controllable and uncontrollable risk factors.
2. Describe the three priority healthy lifestyle choices, as well as four or more additional healthy lifestyle choices.
3. Explain how environmental and social factors affect health and wellness.

SELF-ASSESSMENT: Stages of Health Behavior

The questionnaire presented here will help you self-assess your current health behaviors. It does not include all health behaviors but is designed to provide useful information about selected health habits. Record your results as directed by your teacher. A worksheet containing the questionnaire may be provided. Follow these directions.

1. Read the three statements related to each health behavior. Record the number (1 to 5) that best represents your current stage.
2. Add the scores for the three statements for each behavior (e.g., physical activity, nutrition) to get a score for that behavior.
3. Add the first five health behavior scores to get your overall health behavior score. *Note:* Because of the personal nature of the destructive habits section of the questionnaire, the three-item score for that section is not included in your total score. You should determine your destructive habits score, but you are not required to note your responses on your worksheet.
4. Use table 20.2 to get ratings for each health behavior and for your overall health behavior.

Stages of Health Behavior Questionnaire

Health behavior	Stage 1: Change needed	Stage 2: Thinking about change	Stage 3: Planning for change	Stage 4: Some change made	Stage 5: Regular healthy behavior	Item score
1. Do 60 minutes of activity per day.	1	2	3	4	5	
2. Do vigorous activity three days a week.	1	2	3	4	5	
3. Do muscle fitness and flexibility exercise three days a week.	1	2	3	4	5	
Physical activity score (sum of the scores for items 1–3) =						
4. Eat three well-balanced meals per day.	1	2	3	4	5	
5. Choose fruits and vegetables for half of daily food consumption.	1	2	3	4	5	
6. Balance calories taken in with calories expended.	1	2	3	4	5	
Nutrition score (sum of the scores for items 4–6) =						
7. Have learned stress management skills.	1	2	3	4	5	
8. Manage time effectively.	1	2	3	4	5	
9. Do physical activity or stress reduction exercises to manage stress.	1	2	3	4	5	
Stress management score (sum of the scores for items 7–9) =						

Health behavior	Stage 1: Change needed	Stage 2: Thinking about change	Stage 3: Planning for change	Stage 4: Some change made	Stage 5: Regular healthy behavior	Item score
10. Get nine hours of good sleep each night.	1	2	3	4	5	
11. Floss and brush teeth at least twice a day.	1	2	3	4	5	
12. Wash hands regularly.	1	2	3	4	5	
Personal health habits score (sum of the scores for items 10–12) =						
13. Get regular medical and dental exams and follow the advice of health professionals.	1	2	3	4	5	
14. Wear appropriate safety equipment when biking or participating in a sport and wear a seat belt when driving.	1	2	3	4	5	
15. Drive safely and do not use phone while driving.	1	2	3	4	5	
Safety and medical practices score (sum of the scores for items 13–15) =						
16. Avoid use of tobacco.*	1	2	3	4	5	
17. Do not abuse drugs or alcohol.*	1	2	3	4	5	
18. Avoid risky sexual behavior.*	1	2	3	4	5	
Destructive habits score (sum of the scores for items 16–18) =						
Total health behavior score (sum of the five wellness scores)** =						

*Answer these questions for your own use, but responses are not required on your worksheet.

**Your total score does *not* include your destructive habits score (see the note accompanying those questions in the table).

TABLE 20.2 Rating Health Behaviors

Health behavior rating	Three-item score	Total health behavior score
Good	13–15	>65
Marginal	10–12	50–64
Low	<9	<49

Lesson 20.2

Changing Health Behaviors

Lesson Objectives

After reading this lesson, you should be able to

1. describe the four types of groups that, along with personal actions, influence your health;
2. describe the five stages of health behavior and how they relate to change; and
3. describe the theories used to study health behavior change.

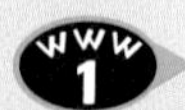

Lesson Vocabulary

cognitive theory, community health, global health, health behavior, health psychology, personal health, SMART goal, stages of health behavior change

Health and wellness are important to looking good, feeling good, enjoying life, and preventing disease and illness. Many factors determine your state of health and wellness. For this reason, a person is somewhat—but not totally—in control of day-to-day health and wellness. At the personal level, you can't control your age and your heredity, but you are in control of your personal behaviors that influence your health. This lesson explains the process of behavior change and introduces you to several theories used to help understand **health behaviors**.

Groups and Health

Personal health refers to your own health and wellness. It involves the choices and actions you take as an individual that affect your health. It includes everything from your exercise habits to how often you floss your teeth. Personal health and group health influence each other. As the arrow at the top of figure 20.4 indicates, the personal health of each group member influences the health of the total group. At the same time, as indicated by the arrow at the bottom of the figure, behaviors and interactions within a group affect each member's personal health. For example, if your friends and family practice good health behaviors, you're more likely to adopt good personal health practices as well.

A collection of groups makes up a community—for example, a school, a worksite, a neighborhood, or a town. The health and wellness of a community (**community health**) depend on the personal health

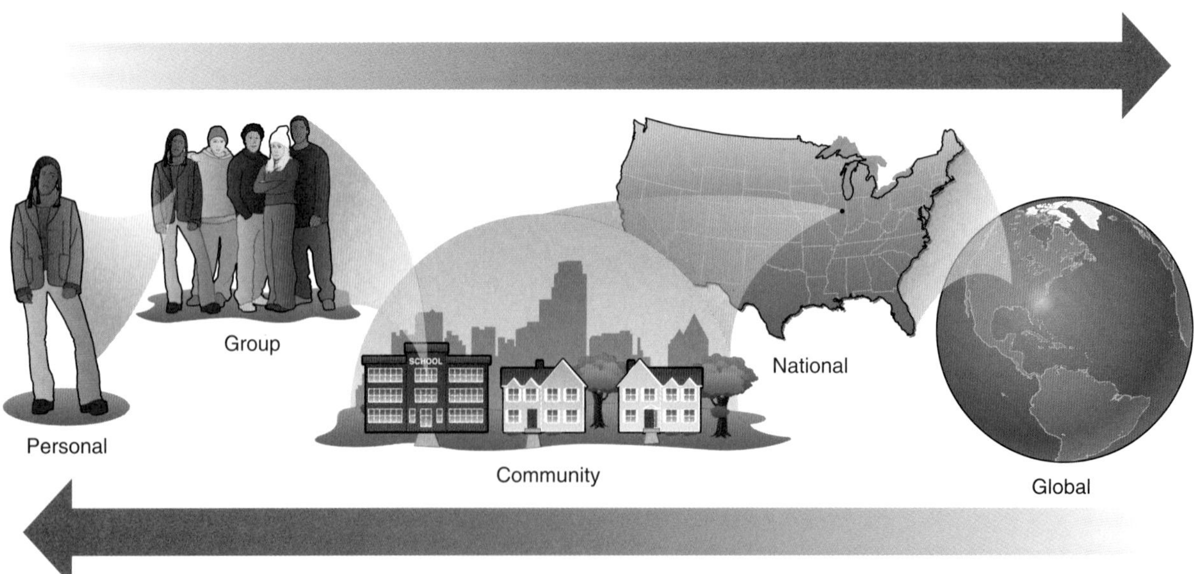

FIGURE 20.4 The relationship between personal health and group health.

of individuals in the community. At the same time, the community's rules, laws, and common practices affect the health of the groups and individuals that make up the community. For example, if a school or workplace limits smoking, the risk of disease is reduced for everyone in that environment. Similarly, if the available food includes healthy options, such as fresh fruits and vegetables, it is easier for people in the community to be healthy.

> "The first wealth is health."
>
> —Ralph Waldo Emerson, poet

The United States is made up of the communities in towns, cities, and counties that are located in various states. Like communities, nations have health policies and practices that influence the health of their individuals and groups. For example, the CDC works to promote good health and control diseases, and other agencies work to protect food and regulate drugs. Health laws and policies, such as public smoking bans, vary from county to county. As indicated by the top arrow in figure 20.4, the health and wellness of individuals, groups, and communities influence the health and wellness of the nation. As indicated by the arrow at the bottom of figure 20.4, the reverse is also true; that is, national policies and health practices influence the health of individuals, groups, and communities within the nation.

Global health refers to the health of everyone on our planet. In the United States, we are fortunate to live in a nation and in communities that provide treated water, safe waste disposal, and high-quality health care for most (though not all) citizens. But these things do not hold true globally. Many nations still face illness and epidemics not common in the United States. In addition, health practices in one country can influence the health of another nation and its citizens. For example, air pollution created in one nation can affect the entire planet, and an epidemic in one nation can put the health of people in other nations at risk.

Each of us can most influence health and wellness at the personal level. What we do individually also affects the health of people in both smaller and larger groups. Likewise, the health practices and policies in force in our groups, communities, nation, and global population affect us as individuals. Part 2 of this book focuses on enhancing your personal health and wellness. However, you'll also study the effects of social interactions in all types of groups and environments on your personal health and wellness.

Stages of Health Behavior

Researchers know that health behaviors can be changed. They also know that changes occur not all at once but in stages. Dr. James Prochaska and his colleagues developed the "stages of change" idea beginning in the 1970s as a result of research related to smoking behavior; therefore, the example given in figure 20.5 relates to smoking. There are five **stages of health behavior change**, ranging from precontemplation to maintenance. The goal is to move from lower stages to higher stages; the ultimate goal, of course, is stage five.

In the first stage, a person refuses to recognize that change is necessary. For example, a smoker may deny the need to stop smoking. The person might say, "I have no intention to stop." A person at stage 2 is thinking about making a change but has not

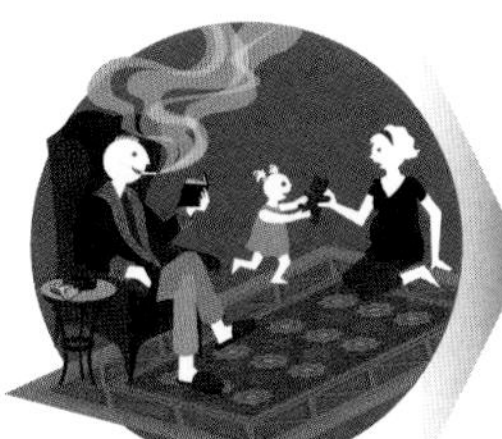

Stage 1: Precontemplation
You have no intention to change the behavior.

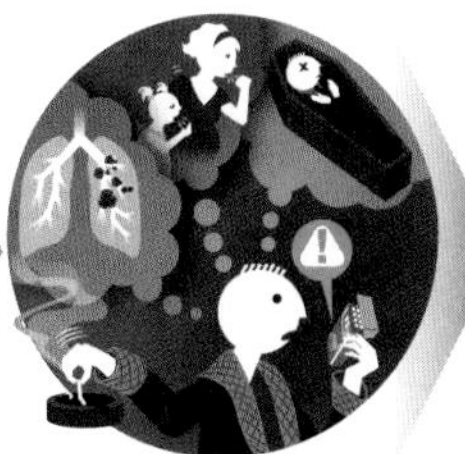

Stage 2: Contemplation
You acknowledge an intention to change the behavior.

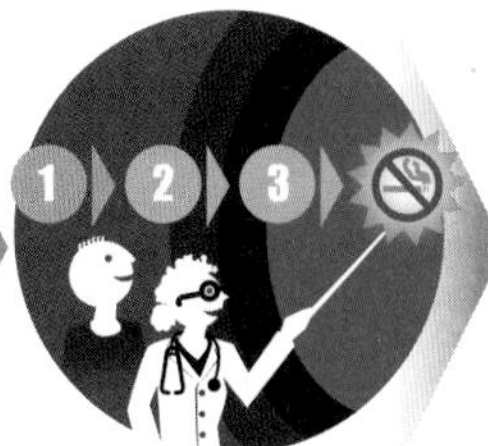

Stage 3: Preparation
You actively plan to change the behavior.

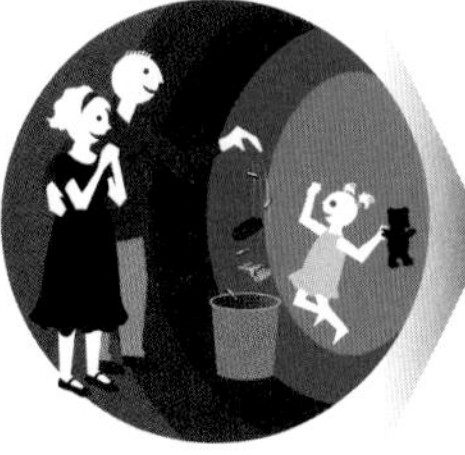

Stage 4: Action
You change the behavior.

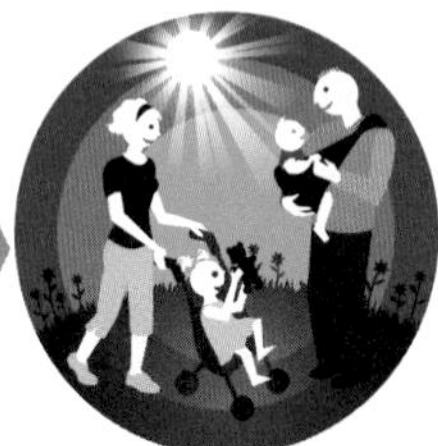

Stage 5: Maintenance
You sustain the behavior change for at least six months.

FIGURE 20.5 Stages of health behavior.

HEALTH SCIENCE

One particular area of the general field of health science is called **health psychology**. Psychology is the study of human behavior, and health psychologists study health behaviors. They are especially interested in finding ways to help people change their behaviors to promote good health. The health psychologists who developed our understanding of the stages of health behavior used information gained from several theories, which are often called **cognitive theories**. The terms *cognitive* and *cognition* refer to thinking and reasoning. Thus cognitive theories address a person's ability to use information to make reasonable decisions and create reasonable solutions to problems. Several theories that are used to explain health behaviors are described in the following discussion.

Transtheoretical Model

The stages of health behavior (stages of change) described in this chapter are based on research that uses a framework called the transtheoretical model. The stages represent levels of motivation for change, ranging from low motivation to high motivation and regular behavior change. Two concepts especially important to this model are self-confidence (also called self-efficacy) and decisional balance. Self-confidence helps you dare to change. Decisional balance involves balancing the positives and negatives of making a change; if there are more positives than negatives, you're motivated to make the change.

Social Learning Theory

According to this theory, also called social cognitive theory, people learn from their interactions with other people. We watch and listen to others, and we shape our attitudes and behaviors based on role models (e.g., parents, friends, teachers). Modeling means imitating or trying out behaviors displayed by those around us. To model a behavior, a person must be motivated—he or she must want to try. So motivation is important to this theory. Self-confidence (self-efficacy) is also important because it helps you be motivated to try a new behavior and stick with it.

Self-Determination Theory

Human motivation is central to self-determination theory. To be motivated, people have to feel competent, which is similar to feeling self-confident. Also important is autonomy (self-determination)—the freedom to make your own decisions. Autonomy helps people feel internally motivated. A third important feature of this theory is relatedness. People are more likely to be motivated if they feel that they are related to or involved in the world around them.

Theory of Planned Behavior

This theory holds that positive attitudes and personal beliefs motivate people to behave in a certain way. According to the theory, positive attitudes and beliefs help you want to change. People who *state* an intention to change (e.g., make a New Year's resolution) are more likely to actually make changes than people who do not state such an intention. As in social learning theory, feelings of confidence are important here. Having self-confidence helps people both state their intention to change and actually make the change. The theory of planned behavior originated from an earlier theory called the theory of reasoned action. Both theories emphasize the fact that you can use cognitions (thinking) to help motivate your behavior and make good decisions.

Health Belief Model

This model states that people will take action to change their health if they have an interest in health matters, feel susceptible to a particular illness, believe that the benefits of treatment or action outweigh the barriers, or think a potential illness could be serious. The health belief model is often used to determine the likelihood that someone will follow the health recommendations they are given by a health professional.

HEALTHY COMMUNICATION

Many businesses and schools are smoke-free environments. Some towns, cities, and states now ban smoking in all public places, including outdoor spaces. Do you think such policies designed to protect public health are fair and justified? Why or why not? Share your opinion with a peer or classmate. Support your opinion with facts and respect each other's opinions.

taken steps to implement it. This person might say, "I'm thinking about stopping." At stage 3, a person has not only thought about changing but also taken steps toward making the change. In the example shown in the figure, the person might have accessed a website for advice about how to stop smoking or investigated joining a smoking cessation group.

By the time a person reaches stage 4, he or she has already made some changes but still needs to make more. The person in figure 20.5 might have cut down the number of cigarettes per day or even stopped smoking for a few days. At stage 5, a person has made a definitive change and is sticking with it. For example, he or she might have stopped smoking for six months or more. This stage is often referred to as maintenance, because the person is adopting the healthy behavior on a regular basis.

It would be nice if people who want to change health behaviors could always move quickly from stage 1 to stage 5. But this is not always the case. For example, smokers who quit (reach maintenance) often do not find success right away. For some smokers, it takes several tries over a period of many months. Others move through the stages more quickly. Regardless of how long it takes, people often move from a low stage to a higher stage and then fall back to a lower stage. Then they try again, each time moving to a higher stage. Of course, there are exceptions, but gradual change is most common. Since the original research, the stages have been used to help people improve all sorts of health behaviors, including eating patterns, physical activity, adoption of personal health habits, and avoidance of destructive habits other than smoking.

You can find more information about theories of health behavior change in the student section of the Health Opportunities Through Physical Education website.

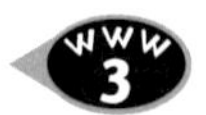

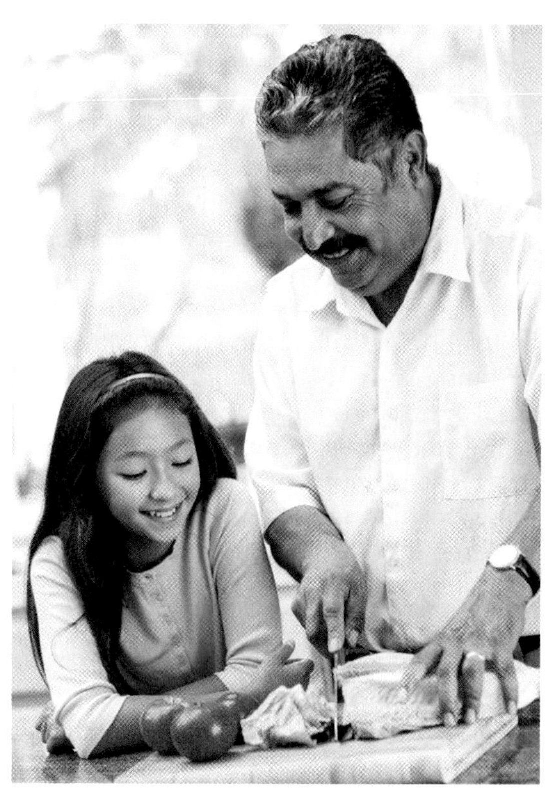

Learning from interactions with other people is part of the social learning theory.

Monkey Business/fotolia.com

Comprehension Check

1. Identify the four types of groups that, along with personal actions, influence your health; also explain how personal health is related to group health.
2. List and describe the five stages of health behavior change; explain how they relate to behavior change.
3. Describe one of the theories used to study health behavior change.

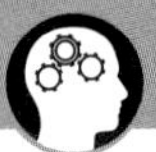

MAKING HEALTHY DECISIONS: Goal Setting

We all know people who have tried to change a health behavior but have not been successful in making permanent change. They are in stage 2 for behavior change. They may have tried to make lifestyle changes but may have fallen short because they failed to set good goals. This feature highlights what are called **SMART goals** for one personal health behavior: sleep.

Ms. Gonzales, the health education teacher, noticed that Emma was not turning in her assignments on time. Emma had always been a good student, but was falling behind and risked getting a poor grade. After class, Ms. Gonzales asked Emma, "Are you okay? You seem a bit tired." Emma said, "I am sorry for getting my homework in late. I have had so much to do lately and I haven't gotten enough sleep. I fell asleep while I was trying to do my homework last night. I'm sorry."

Ms. Gonzales asked Emma if she could stop by after school for a visit. When they met, Ms. Gonzales said, "Maybe you need to make a plan to improve your sleep habits. Maybe setting some SMART goals would help." With Ms. Gonzales' help, they used the acronym SMART to set some goals. Emma prepared several goals to help improve her sleep habits. She made sure that her goals corresponded with each letter in the acronym.

- **S**pecific means identifying very specific things you want to accomplish.
- **M**easurable means being sure you can easily evaluate the goal to see if you have accomplished it.
- **A**ttainable means that they challenge you and are not too hard or too easy.
- **R**ealistic means that they are reasonable for you and that you can expect to accomplish them if you put in the effort.
- **T**imely means the goal can be achieved in the time allotted and the goal is right for you at this time.

Emma wrote down her goals and put them into action.

For Discussion

Why is it important for Emma to use the SMART formula in setting her goals? What are some examples of SMART goals that Emma might write to improve her sleep habits? What are some things that Emma can do to help her implement her goals? In answering these questions, consider the guidelines presented in this chapter's Skills for Healthy Living feature.

SKILLS FOR HEALTHY LIVING: Goal Setting

Now that you know about SMART goals, you can begin developing goals of your own. As you work through this course, you'll have the opportunity to set goals for a variety of health behaviors using the Healthy Living Plan worksheet presented in later chapters. The following guidelines will help you as you identify and develop your personal goals.

- **Use the SMART formula.** Use the formula and goals described by Ms. Gonzales in the Making Healthy Decisions sidebar.
- **Choose a few goals at a time.** Part 2 of this book prompts you to establish goals for adopting a variety of healthy behaviors, but at any given time you should choose a few goals to focus on rather than working on all of your goals at once. Trying to do too much often leads to failure. Narrowing down to a few goals at a time can help you succeed.
- **Focus on modifying behavior when setting short-term goals.** Short-term goals are goals that can be accomplished in days or weeks. When setting short-term goals, focus on changing your behaviors (e.g., getting in bed by a specific time, eating five servings of fruits and vegetables every day for two weeks or walking 30 minutes every day for two weeks). If you change your behavior, then fitness, health, and wellness will follow.

- **Over the long term you can focus on the process and the product.** As noted, short-term goals focus on behavior change (changing the process). Product goals are outcomes that result from changing the process (behavior). For example, if you do strength training (the process), you will increase the number of push-ups you can do (product). It takes time to change strength (the product), so product goals—such as increasing the number of push-ups you can do—are not especially good as short-term goals.
- **Put your goals in writing.** Writing down a goal represents a personal commitment and increases your chance of meeting that goal. You'll get the chance to write down your goals as you do the activities in this book.
- **Know your reasons for setting your goals.** Those who set goals for reasons other than their own personal improvement often fail. Ask yourself *why* you are setting each goal. Make sure you're setting goals for yourself based on your own needs and interests.
- **Self-assess periodically and keep logs.** Doing self-assessments helps you set appropriate goals and determine whether you've met them. Keeping logs helps you determine whether you're meeting your goals. Focus on improvement by working toward goals that are slightly higher than your current self-assessment results.
- **Reward yourself.** Achieving a personal goal is rewarding. It feels good. Congratulate yourself for your accomplishment.
- **Revise if necessary.** If you find that a goal is too difficult to accomplish, don't be afraid to revise it. Revising a goal is better than quitting because you didn't reach an unrealistic goal.
- **Consider maintenance goals.** Improvement is not always necessary. Once you reach the highest level of change, consider setting a goal of maintenance. For example, if your weight is healthy, then it is a healthy behavior for you to eat food containing enough calories to balance the calories you expend. In this case, it would not be healthy to restrict your calories so that you lose weight. Maintaining a healthy energy balance and a healthy weight are good goals.

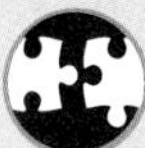

ACADEMIC CONNECTION: Domain-Specific Language

Part of meeting standards in English language arts is demonstrating the acquisition of domain-specific words and phrases. This means that you are expected to learn vocabulary words that are particular to different subject areas, or disciplines. In each lesson of this text, you are provided a list of vocabulary words that are specific to fitness, health, and wellness. Take the time to study the definition of each vocabulary word (see the glossary or the study section of the website for definitions) and observe how the word is used in its appropriate context (where it appears in the text and how it is used). Try to use each vocabulary word in a new sentence after you have become familiar with it.

Do the Rich Get to Be Healthier?

Having less than a high school education and earning less than US$12,000 annually may increase your risk of heart disease, according to the journal *BMC Cardiovascular Disorders*. Additional published studies also suggest a relationship between heart disease and socioeconomic factors such as income, education, and ethnicity. Other conditions that have been associated with lower income include obesity, sleep quality, and diabetes risk (see figure 20.6).

When people can't afford to buy fresh fruits and vegetables, they often opt for cheaper "fast food" that is not optimal for good health. Lower-income workers and blue-collar laborers also often experience impaired sleep quality when they get stuck with night shifts or "swing shifts." In addition, people with more money are more likely to regularly see a doctor and dentist for proper preventive care, more likely belong to a health club, and more likely to get medicine they need.

As health advocate Dennis Carlson has said, "A solid health foundation is built on awareness, information, and then action." But all of these things are harder for people who are poor to sustain, as policy expert Beth Trout points out: "Education and awareness are great, but they do you less good if you live in a dangerous, unwalkable neighborhood with lots of fast food and no supermarkets; if you have little control in your work life; and if you are constantly worried about money, housing, and safety."

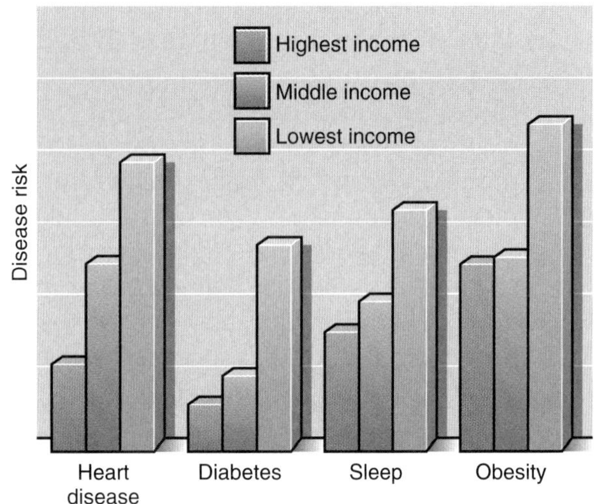

Figure 20.6 The relationship between income level and common health concerns.

For Discussion

Brainstorm a list of ways that society could help all people be healthier regardless of economic status. Think of as many realistic examples as you can, then share your ideas with those of a peer or classmate. Compare your ideas and work together to create a list of your top three ideas. Negotiate and compromise as needed to build consensus (agreement).

CHAPTER REVIEW

Reviewing Concepts and Vocabulary

As directed by your teacher, answer items 1 through 5 by correctly completing each sentence with a word or phrase.

1. A collection of groups makes up a ________________.
2. ________ ________ refers to the health of everyone on our planet.
3. Short-term goals should focus on changing behavior or goals referred to as ________________ goals.
4. Tobacco, alcohol, and drug use are all forms of ______________ habits.
5. A ______ factor is anything that increases the chances that you will get sick.

For items 6 through 10, as directed by your teacher, match each term in column 1 with the appropriate phrase in column 2.

6. precontemplation	a. making a change such as engaging in physical activity
7. contemplation	b. maintaining a behavior change for six months
8. preparation	c. thinking about making a behavior change
9. action	d. taking steps toward making a behavior change
10. commitment	e. stage where a person has not yet considered a health change

For items 11 through 15, as directed by your teacher, respond to each statement or question.

11. What does self-determination theory say about behavior change?
12. What are two examples of personal health habits?
13. What is a controllable risk factor? Provide an example.
14. What characterizes a SMART goal?
15. Describe the relationship between process and product goals.

Thinking Critically

Write a paragraph to answer the following questions.

Sheldon is thinking about cutting back on his consumption of sugary drinks. Last weekend, at the grocery store with his dad, he spent some time looking at alternatives, such as naturally flavored water. What stage of change best describes Sheldon's current status? What is one thing you could do to help him move to the next stage?

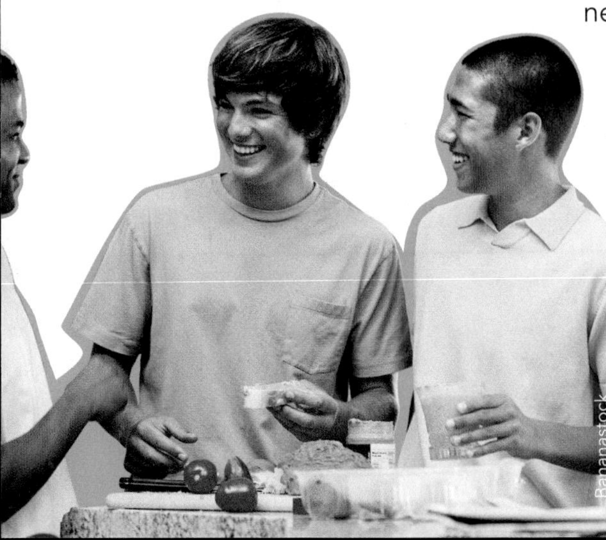
Bananastock

Take It Home

Teach a parent or guardian what you've learned about the stages of behavior change. Work together with a partner to create an illustration or diagram that explains the stages. Use the illustration or diagram when having the discussion with your parent or guardian. You may want to use an example of a specific behavior (e.g., being more active, eating better).

21

Choosing Healthy Lifestyles

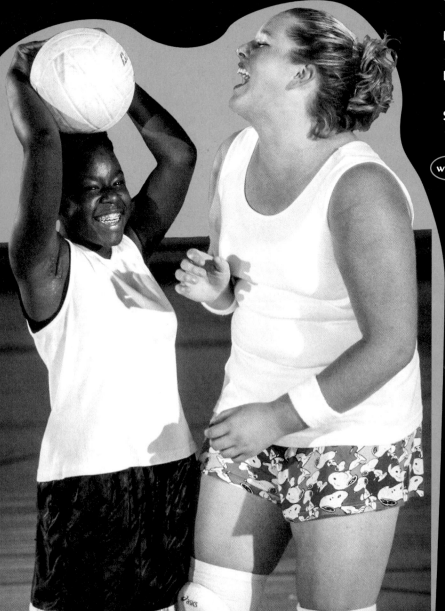

In This Chapter

Student Web Resources
www.HOPEtextbook.org/student

Lesson 21.1

Skills for Healthy Living

Lesson Objectives

After reading this lesson, you should be able to

1. explain the meaning of the term skills for healthy living,
2. explain each of the skills for healthy living, and
3. describe how the skills help you be healthy and well.

WWW 1 **Lesson Vocabulary**

self-regulation skills, skills for healthy living

Alex went to a lecture about health by Dr. Lazarus. He listened carefully and decided that he wanted to make some changes in his life—and try to help his parents make some changes. Alex felt stressed about his schoolwork. He knew that he had to reduce his stress level and that he needed to establish a more regular routine. He was also concerned because his dad smoked cigarettes and neither of his parents exercised regularly. Alex wasn't sure how to go about making changes in his own life, much less how to help his parents make changes. By consulting with his health teacher, he found out that using **skills for healthy living** would help him.

Experts in health behavior have proven that people who learn skills for healthy living (also known as self-management skills or **self-regulation skills**)—and use them regularly—can make changes in their health behaviors and stick with those changes. A skill is the ability to perform a task well, and a person's skills improve with regular practice.

There are many kinds of skills. For example, typing is a physical skill that helps you use a computer. Playing a musical instrument is a physical skill that helps you create sound. Being able to squat down and back up safely is a physical skill that helps you with gardening or performing various household tasks. Throwing is a physical skill that helps you participate in various sports. The more you practice a physical skill, the better you get at it. But not all skills are physical. For example, calculation skills are necessary in math, writing skills are important in language arts, and critical thinking skills are necessary in almost all areas of study.

Skills for healthy living are similar to the skills just described. They can help you accomplish a desired goal or keep doing a good thing that you already do. For example, building good time management skills can help you make time to engage in a new activity, such as learning to cook healthy foods. You might also use good time management to help you maintain a workout schedule that you already have in place even when new time demands emerge. Like other skills, skills for healthy living can be learned and improved with practice.

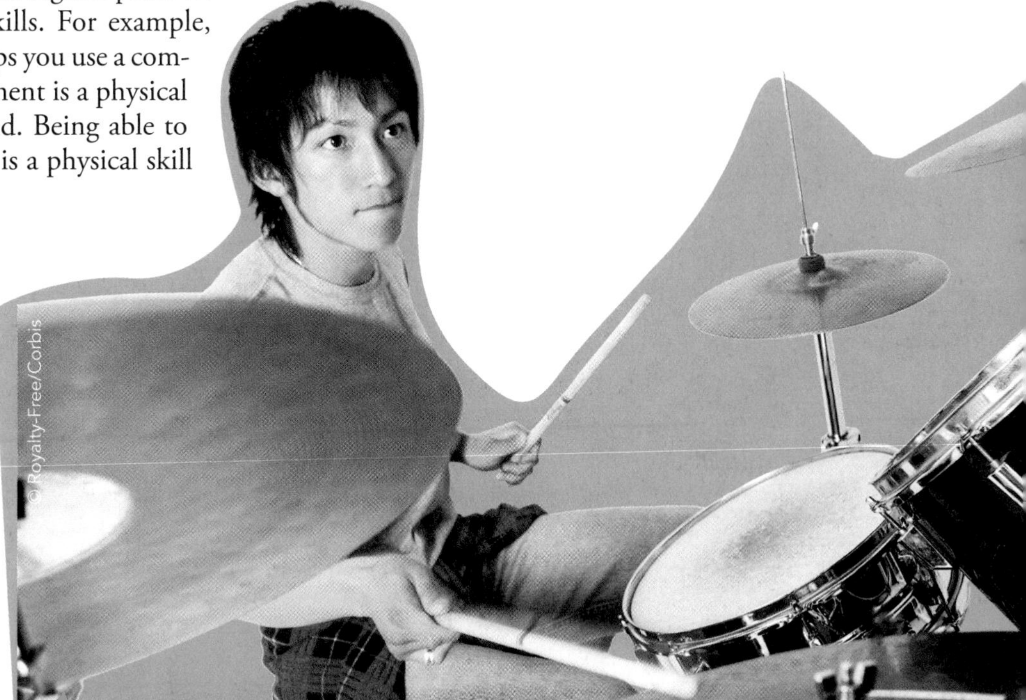

A skill is the ability to perform a task well, and a person's skills improve with regular practice.

Skills for Healthy Living

In this lesson, you'll learn about 14 skills for healthy living, as well as 6 personal characteristics that are similar to skills and that help you make behavior changes. These skills are similar to self-management skills taught in physical education. In health education, they apply to a variety of health behaviors and are called skills for healthy living. The 14 skills for healthy living are described in detail in table 21.1.

TABLE 21.1 Skills for Healthy Living

Skill	Description	Benefits
Self-assessment	A person with self-assessment skill can evaluate his or her current status for markers of health and wellness or particular health behaviors. Examples include assessing your personal fitness, dietary nutrition, and stress level.	• Helps you objectively determine your current status. • Helps you set goals and plan a program to change your health behavior.
Goal setting	A person with goal-setting skill can set goals that are SMART (specific, measurable, attainable, realistic, and timely) for changing his or her health behaviors.	• Provides a road map for change. • Helps you prepare a plan for changing your health behavior.
Self-planning	This skill has five steps (discussed in this chapter's lesson titled Self-Planning) that serve as an outline for planning your personal program for health behavior change.	• Helps you commit in writing to goals and changing your behavior. • Provides a measuring stick for evaluating whether you've accomplished your goals.
Self-monitoring	This skill helps you keep records (logs or a journal) to see whether you're actually doing what you think you're doing—whether you're meeting personal goals and complying with your planned program for changing your health behavior.	• Helps you evaluate your progress in meeting goals and adhering to your program. • Helps you stay motivated to stick with your program. • Helps you keep useful records.
Overcoming barriers	This skill helps you find ways to stick with a behavior change despite obstacles such as lack of time, lack of safe places to be active, and difficulty selecting healthy foods.	• Helps you begin making changes. • Helps you stick with your changes. • Helps you eliminate excuses and succeed.
Time management	This skill helps you schedule time efficiently so that you have more time for the important things in your life.	• Helps you see how you use your time. • Helps you take care of priorities. • Helps you reduce stress.
Relapse prevention	This skill helps you stick with healthy behaviors even when you have problems getting motivated or when other people or situations tempt you to make unhealthy decisions.	• Helps you adhere to healthy behaviors. • Helps you persist and meet your goals.
Finding social support	This skill helps you stick with healthy behaviors by getting support from friends and family members.	• Helps you adhere to healthy behaviors. • Helps you prevent relapse.

Skill	Description	Benefits
Providing social support	Being a healthy citizen includes being able to help others when they are at risk for injury, illness, or death. This skill involves identifying risks, communicating effectively, and finding appropriate resources.	• Helps you build self-confidence and social wellness. • Helps you develop social responsibility.
Saying no	This skill helps you avoid doing things you don't want to do, especially when you're under pressure from friends or other people.	• Helps you adhere to healthy behaviors. • Helps you stay on track to meet your goals.
Conflict resolution	This skill helps you resolve problems that arise at school, at home, or in other circumstances.	• Helps you reduce stress. • Helps you maintain friendships and other good relationships.
Critical thinking	This skill enables you to find and interpret information that helps you make good decisions and solve problems related to your health. For example, one critical thinking skill that you will address in part 2 of this book is evaluating nutrition information.	• Helps you set goals. • Helps you plan your program. • Helps you be a wise health consumer.
Performance	This type of skill involves performing tasks of daily living (e.g., typing, cooking) and tasks that make your leisure time enjoyable (e.g., playing a sport).	• Helps you enjoy life. • Contributes to healthy living.
Self-help	This type of skill helps you be safe and healthy and able to help others as well. Examples include knowing first aid and CPR, using safety equipment (e.g., helmet and pads for roller blading), and practicing good personal health habits (e.g., tooth brushing and flossing).	• Helps you be healthy and well. • Helps you be safe and avoid injury. • Allows you to contribute to the health and safety of others.

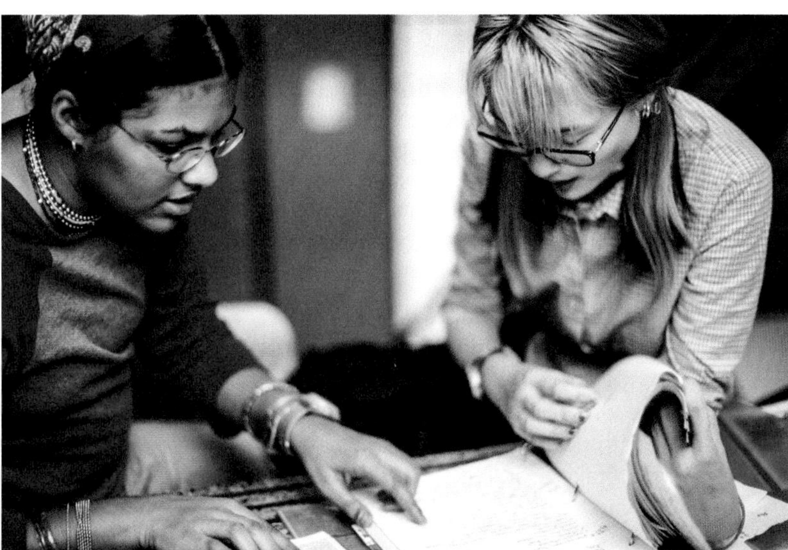

Knowledge is a personal characteristic that functions as a skill for healthy living and it will help you set goals and plan for healthy living.

Photodisc

Personal Characteristics That Function as Skills for Healthy Living

Health scientists have demonstrated that acquiring certain personal characteristics can also help you adopt healthy behaviors. These six characteristics are not exactly skills, but you can improve them with practice, and they do help you adopt healthy behaviors. Therefore, they function as skills for healthy living (self-management) and are considered as such in part 2 of this book. These six characteristics are described in table 21.2. You can self-assess the six characteristics and the 14 skills for healthy living (20 in all) using the questionnaire in the self-assessment in this chapter.

Time and health are two precious assets that we don't recognize and appreciate until they have been depleted. ”

—Denis Waitley, motivational speaker and writer

HEALTHY COMMUNICATION

Which personal characteristic discussed in this chapter do you think is most important in helping you to be healthy? Force yourself to select only one of the characteristics. Share your selection and the reasons for your selection with a classmate. Engage in active listening and determine where you both agree and disagree. Did listening to your classmate change your perspective?

Though it's important to know about the skills described in tables 21.1 and 21.2, being aware of them doesn't mean that you can automatically use them effectively. You also need to know how and when to use them, and you need to *practice* using them. Throughout part 2 of this book, you'll learn more about these skills and get the opportunity to practice using them. For best results, practice them on your own as well as in class. For example, the best athletes practice their skills outside of practice sessions—that's part of why they're the best. If you want to be good at using the skills of healthy living, practice them at every opportunity.

TABLE 21.2 Personal Characteristics That Function as Skills for Healthy Living

Skill	Description	Benefits
Knowledge	Knowledge involves more than just knowing and remembering facts. Higher-order forms of knowledge include understanding (ability to interpret, summarize, and explain ideas), application (ability to use ideas), analysis (ability to examine parts of an idea), evaluation (ability to assess an idea), and synthesis (ability to put ideas together). You're developing your knowledge of health throughout this course.	• Helps you make good decisions about health and wellness. • Provides a basis for critical thinking. • Helps you set goals and plan for healthy living. • Helps you be a wise health consumer.
Positive attitude	An attitude is a personal feeling or set of feelings about something. Health scientists know that people with positive attitudes are more likely to adopt healthy behaviors than people with negative attitudes. It's important to learn to take a positive attitude and to change your attitude when needed.	• Helps you enjoy life. • Motivates you to make healthy lifestyle choices. • Helps you stick with your pursuit of your goals.
Ability to identify risk factors	Risk factors are characteristics that make you more likely to have a disease or health condition. You can maximize good health by identifying your risk factors and getting screening to see if you have certain conditions.	• Helps you resist disease and other health problems. • Helps you make changes to reduce them.

Skill	Description	Benefits
Intrinsic motivation	Motivation involves having an incentive or reason for doing a certain behavior. There are two types. *Intrinsic* motivation spurs you to do a behavior because you enjoy it or want to do it. *Extrinsic* motivation encourages you to do a behavior because of a reward or incentive provided by someone else (e.g., being paid for earning a high grade). Over the long haul, intrinsic motivation is more effective in helping you change your health behaviors. Though motivation is not technically a skill, it can be classified as a skill for healthy living because it can help you adopt healthy behaviors.	• Helps you stick with your goals. • Helps you give good effort and enjoy your efforts. • Helps you adopt new behaviors and try new things (e.g., new foods or activities).
Self-confidence (self-efficacy)	Self-confidence is the belief that you can perform a task successfully. People with self-confidence (also called self-efficacy) believe that they will be successful in performing a specific task. It's possible to be confident in one area while not so confident in another. Self-confidence is not exactly a skill, but building your self-confidence can help you adopt healthy behaviors. Practice using positive self-talk and setting SMART goals. Using positive role models can help you build confidence.	• Helps you succeed in your endeavors. • Helps you stick with your pursuit of your goals. • Helps you give good effort and enjoy your efforts. • Helps you adopt new behaviors and try new things (e.g., new foods or activities). • Helps you react positively to criticism.
Positive self-perception	A self-perception is a way of seeing yourself. Types of self-perception include social, scholastic, physical, and global.	• Helps you succeed in your endeavors. • Helps you stick with your pursuit of your goals. • Helps you give good effort and enjoy your efforts. • Helps you adopt new behaviors and try new things (e.g., new foods or activities). • Helps you react positively to criticism.

ADVOCACY IN ACTION: Positive Attitudes

To advocate for something is to publicly recommend or support it. Throughout part 2 of this book, you're given opportunities to advocate on behalf of a variety of health issues in a variety of ways. We know that positive attitudes can help you make healthy decisions and achieve overall good health. Begin your advocacy work by initiating a positive attitudes campaign. Design posters of inspirational sayings and quotes to place around campus. Include information that helps others understand the link between positive attitudes and making healthy decisions.

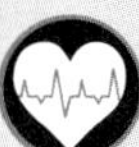

HEALTH TECHNOLOGY

An application, or app, is a computer program that allows you to perform tasks on a smartphone or other device. Some apps are designed to help you use skills for healthy living—for example, by self-assessing your food content, self-monitoring your physical activity, or planning healthy meals. If well designed, apps can help you change your health behaviors, but not all apps are based on good health information. Before using an app, determine whether the people who developed it are health experts; ask people you know and trust about the app, and test it out for yourself. For more information about health-related apps, see the student section of the Health Opportunities Through Physical Education website.

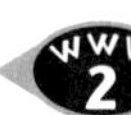

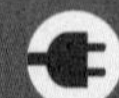

CONNECT

Do you currently use any apps to help you live a healthier life? If so, what features do you think make a good health application? If not, what type of app might appeal to you? Can you imagine using a health app in the future?

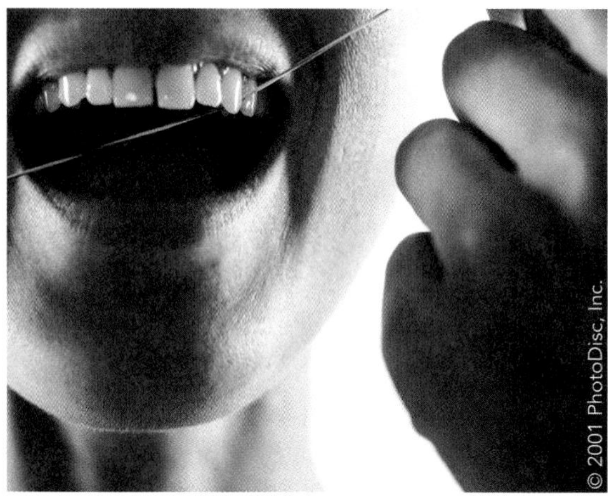

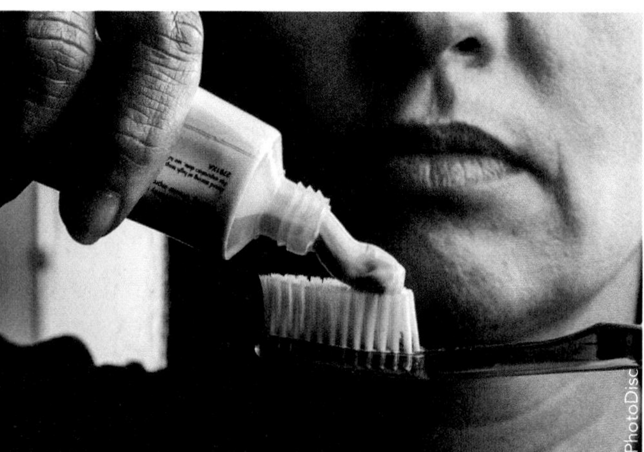

Self-help skills such as practicing good personal health habits like flossing and tooth brushing help you to be healthy and well.

Comprehension Check

1. What is the meaning of the term skills for healthy living?
2. List each of the skills for healthy living and explain one of them in more detail.
3. Explain how the skills for healthy living can help you be healthy and well.

SELF-ASSESSMENT: Healthy Living Skills

The following questionnaire will help you see which of the skills (and characteristics) for healthy living you already possess and which ones you need to develop or improve. As directed by your teacher, record your results. A worksheet may be provided. Follow these instructions.

1. Read each of the 20 skills and characteristics. Circle the number (1 to 4) that best represents your response (use regularly, use rarely, developing this skill, and do not have this skill).
2. Add the scores for the 20 skills and characteristics to get a total score.
3. Use table 21.3 to get your rating for each healthy living skill and for your total score.

Healthy Living Skills Questionnaire

Healthy living skills and characteristics	I have this skill or characteristic and use it regularly.	I have this skill or characteristic but rarely use it.	I am developing this type of skill or characteristic.	I do not have this type of skill or characteristic.	Score
1. Self-assessment	4	3	2	1	
2. Goal setting	4	3	2	1	
3. Self-planning	4	3	2	1	
4. Self-monitoring	4	3	2	1	
5. Overcoming barriers	4	3	2	1	
6. Time management	4	3	2	1	
7. Relapse prevention	4	3	2	1	
8. Finding social support	4	3	2	1	
9. Providing social support	4	3	2	1	
10. Saying no	4	3	2	1	
11. Conflict resolution	4	3	2	1	
12. Critical thinking	4	3	2	1	
13. Performance	4	3	2	1	
14. Self-help	4	3	2	1	
15. Knowledge	4	3	2	1	
16. Positive attitude	4	3	2	1	
17. Ability to identify risk factors	4	3	2	1	
18. Intrinsic motivation	4	3	2	1	
19. Self-confidence (self-efficacy)	4	3	2	1	
20. Positive self-perceptions	4	3	2	1	
Total score and total rating =					

TABLE 21.3 Rating Chart

Wellness rating	One-item score	Total score*
Good	4	>80
Marginal	2–3	64–79
Low	<1	<63

*It is desirable to be skilled in all areas; therefore, even if you have a good total rating, you should work to improve your skills in any area for which you have a score below 4.

Lesson 21.2

Planning for Healthy Living

Lesson Objectives

After reading this lesson, you should be able to

1. describe the five steps in program planning,
2. describe the SMART formula for goal setting, and
3. explain how you can be accountable for carrying out your plan.

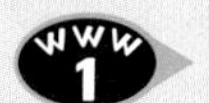

Lesson Vocabulary

accountability, action steps, enabler, health behavior contract

Living a healthy life isn't always easy. Some healthy behaviors may come naturally to you, and others may be more challenging. For example, you might find it easy to refuse cigarettes if you come from a nonsmoking family and the smell of cigarette smoke is unappealing to you. Other healthy behaviors might be more difficult for you to start doing or to maintain. You might dislike the taste of vegetables and thus struggle to eat enough of them. Or you might feel you don't have the ability to say no to friends who try to convince you to try risky behaviors, such as experimenting with abuse of drugs.

In addition, many healthy decisions are hard to maintain throughout life. You can help yourself maintain healthy behaviors over the long term by learning how to make decisions thoughtfully and plan carefully.

The Five Steps in Making a Healthy Living Plan

Planning for healthy living (program planning) is a skill that takes time to develop and must be intentionally practiced. You'll have opportunities throughout part 2 of this book to make healthy living plans for various areas of life. All of them will use the five-step process explained here. For an example of a complete plan, see the Sample Healthy Living Plan.

Step 1: Determining Your Personal Needs—Self-Assessment

The first step toward preparing a healthy living plan and making healthy decisions is to collect information about your personal needs. Throughout this book, you'll do many self-assessments that help you understand your current health status so that you can plan where you want to go. Some self-assessments may show you that you're already healthy, and others may draw your attention to areas where you could improve. Even when the results of a self-assessment show you that you're healthy in that area, you can always use the planning process to sustain or enhance your healthy behavior.

Step 2: Considering Your Healthy Behavior Options

After determining your personal needs, the next step is to consider your options for healthy behavior—for example, what types of physical activity are available to you, what changes you can make in your diet, or what approaches are available for ending an unhealthy habit (e.g., nicotine aids, smoking cessation groups). Regardless of the behavior you want to change, explore your options and reflect on which ones might be best for you based on your personal strengths and weaknesses, as well as the barriers you might face in trying to change the behavior.

Step 3: Setting Your Goals

Effective planning involves setting both short-term and long-term goals. Short-term goals are those that you can reasonably achieve in several weeks, whereas long-term goals require months and sometimes even years. Identify both short- and long-term goals for any health behavior you try to change. Remember that all goals should be SMART goals (see figure 21.1).

Sample Healthy Living Plan

STEP 1: Determining Your Personal Needs

The behavior I want to change is: I want to be better prepared for emergencies.

Starting date: April 2

The self-assessment I conducted relating to this behavior is: My Emergency Preparedness.

The results of the self-assessment are: I am not well prepared to meet emergencies.

STEP 2: Determining Your Options

The options available to me for changing this behavior are:

1. Take a first aid and CPR class.
2. Get a first aid kit for my house and car.

One personal strength I possess to help me change this behavior is:

I have good self-motivation and follow through on commitments.

One personal weakness I have that might make changing this behavior difficult is:

I am a little shy and might not be comfortable in a community first aid class.

The barriers I may face in trying to change my behavior are:

1. I live in a small town and there may not be classes available to me.
2. I don't have much extra money for buying supplies.

STEP 3: Setting Goals

Short-term goals (1 day to 1 month):	Target date:
1. Sign up for a first aid or CPR class.	May 10
2. Make a list of items for my home first aid kit.	May 6

> continued

Sample Healthy Living Plan > continued

Long-term goal (more than a month): Target date:

I will get certified in both CPR and first aid and will have at least one first aid kit made. July 10

STEP 4: Structuring Your Healthy Living Plan and Establishing Accountability

The action steps I need to take first to help me achieve my goals are:

1. Look up options for CPR or first aid classes in the community.
2. Research whether or not there are online CPR or first aid classes I can take.
3. Go to the store and make a list of available items and their prices.

To help me be successful in making this change, I will use the following accountability strategy or strategies:

- ☑ Behavioral contract
- ☐ Social support
- ☐ Behavioral journal or log
- ☐ Other: ______

Step 5: Implementing Your Plan and Evaluating Your Progress

Short-term goal 1	☑ Met	☐ Not met	Date: April 21
Short-term goal 2	☐ Met	☑ Not met	Date: July 15
Long-term goal	☑ Met	☐ Not met	Date: July 15

If you met your goal, what contributed most to your success?

I was persistent, and my school counselor helped me find a free CPR class in the community.

If you did not meet your goal, what contributed most to your lack of success?

I met all of my goals, but I was late in meeting my second short-term goal because I had a problem with my car.

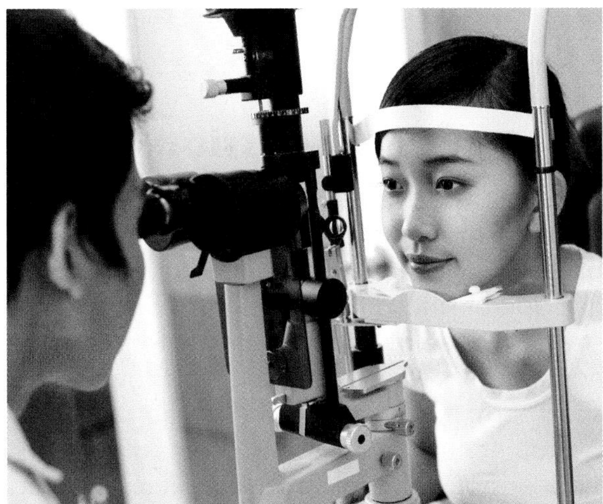

Getting regular check-ups may be one of the healthy options available to you.

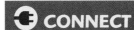

SMART Goal Reminder

S = Specific

M = Measurable

A = Attainable

R = Realistic

T = Timely

FIGURE 21.1 SMART goal reminder.

Step 4: Structuring Your Healthy Living Plan and Establishing Accountability

In step 4 of the planning process, you use the information that you developed in steps 1, 2, and 3. For each goal, write down **action steps**.

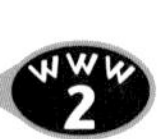

In addition to establishing your action plan, identify the strategy that you'll use for **accountability**. Being accountable means that you follow through with the goals and commitments you make to yourself and others. Two ways to hold yourself accountable are to develop family and peer support and to use self-monitoring strategies. Each of these strategies is discussed in this chapter's Skills for Healthy Living feature.

Step 5: Implementing Your Plan and Evaluating Your Progress

After you've been implementing your action steps for a while, make time to evaluate your progress. Ask yourself whether your goals still seem reasonable. Review your action steps and decide whether they're helping you achieve your goal.

> "Good health and good sense are two of life's greatest blessings."
>
> —Publilius Syrus, Roman philosopher

Using Self-Planning Skills

The five steps in planning for healthy living are presented here to help you learn how to plan your own behavior change (self-planning). You'll begin to learn to do self-planning for many kinds of healthy behavior.

CONNECT

You will benefit from your healthy living plan only if you follow it. How might a person's family help him or her carry out a healthy living plan?

Comprehension Check

1. What are the five steps in planning for healthy living?
2. What does each letter in the SMART (goal setting) formula represent?
3. What is accountability and why is it important in planning?

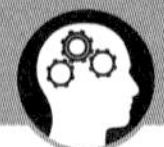

MAKING HEALTHY DECISIONS: Self-Planning

Josefita wanted to change a specific health behavior—her eating. During her annual physical exam, she had been told that her blood sugar level was higher than it should be. It was not high enough for her to be considered diabetic, but the doctor had said that she was prediabetic. High blood sugar is sometimes associated with being overweight, but Josefita was not overweight. However, her doctor and dietitian did advise her to make some dietary changes. Specifically, they recommended that Josefita eat fewer high-fat foods, reduce her consumption of foods high in simple sugar (e.g., candy, doughnuts, pastries), and eat more foods high in fiber (e.g., fruits, vegetables). They also advised her to eat regular, well-balanced meals (rather than skipping meals) and to eat meals rich in nutrients.

For Discussion

How might Josefita be able to use the five steps in program planning to change her eating patterns? How could she use the advice of her doctor and dietitian to carry out the five steps? If Josefita follows her doctor's advice, how might her health improve? Provide one short-term and one long-term example. What is another healthy behavior Josefita might consider adopting? Explain your choice. To guide your thinking about these questions, use the Skills for Healthy Living feature.

SKILLS FOR HEALTHY LIVING: Self-Planning

Now that you know about the five self-planning steps, you can use the following guidelines to help you create plans that work for you over the long term. You can also use the guidelines to help family members and friends who want to change their health behavior.

- **Use the five steps in sequence.** Start with step 1 (determining your needs), then work your way through all five steps.
- **Don't try to do too much.** Plan a program that reasonably challenges you but isn't overly difficult. If you try to accomplish too much all at once, you may not be effective in carrying out your plan. Setting SMART goals is critical to success.
- **Be specific.** Just as SMART goals are specific, your program should be specific. It should clearly lay out (in writing) the actions that you will take to meet your goals.
- **Revise if necessary.** The fifth step in program planning is to try your program and evaluate it. However, you don't have to wait until you've finished your program to revise it. If you find that it isn't working, revise it when you discover the problem.
- **Seek family support.** Tell family members about your plan and ask for their support. Family members may want to help by making health behavior changes themselves to support the changes you're making. This will help you to be accountable.
- **Seek peer support.** Identify a trusted friend or group of people who will help you stay on track as your implement your plan. Choose a buddy or group of friends who will be supportive. Avoid negative "**enablers**"—people who make it easier (enable you) to engage in a destructive habit or make it harder to stay on track with your positive behavior changes. This will help you to be accountable.
- **Self-monitor for progress.** Keep a behavior journal or log. Keeping records not only lets you know if you're successful in your plan; it can also provide reinforcement to help you stick with your plan. Choose a specific time each day to record your progress. Some experts recommend making daily entries in your log just before bedtime. Some plans may require more frequent entries (e.g., recording after lunch, after dinner, and at bedtime). This will help you to be accountable.

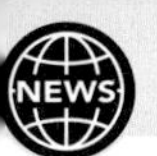

LIVING WELL NEWS, ISSUE 21

Can You Make a Contract for Good Health?

A **health behavior contract** is an agreement you make with yourself to change a specific health behavior. Research shows that behavioral contracts can help you stick with your plan for changing your health behavior. Behavioral contracts have been used in school classes to help students both meet academic goals and adopt healthy behaviors. In many ways, a personal plan based on the five steps for program planning *is* a health behavior contract. It is a written statement of what you plan to do to change your behavior.

Still, some experts recommend supplementing your plan with a health behavior contract to give you another incentive for sticking with your plan. You can do a contract alone or with someone else, such as a parent or teacher. The contract is typically signed and witnessed to give it a prominent place in your life. Here's a sample contract:

Based on awareness of my personal health, I ____________________ (name) have decided to set the following health-related goal: ______________________________

My health behavior goal is ____ (long-term SMART goal).

My intrinsic (internal) motivation for wanting to achieve this goal is

____

____

____.

The difficulties I anticipate facing in making this change are

____

____

____.

The specific actions or behaviors I will take to reach my goal are (short-term SMART goals)

____

____

____.

I will reward achievement of my goal by ______________________________ (extrinsic motivation). If I fail to achieve my goal I will forfeit this reward.

I will review this contract on (date) ____________________.

Signature: ________________________________

Signature of witness: ________________________________

For Discussion

What do you think of the idea of a behavioral contract? How might it be helpful? Some contracts include a punishment if the contract is not fulfilled. What do you think of that idea?

Reviewing Concepts and Vocabulary

As directed by your teacher, answer items 1 through 5 by correctly completing each sentence with a word or phrase.

1. Skills for healthy living are also called ________________________ skills.
2. Skills for healthy living can be ________________ with practice.
3. Self-__________________ helps you identify your current health status.
4. The skill that helps you solve problems with others is ______________ resolution.
5. ____________ steps are things that you can do immediately to progress toward a behavior change.

For items 6 through 10, as directed by your teacher, match each term in column 1 with the appropriate phrase in column 2.

6. step 1	a. structuring your healthy living plan and establishing accountability
7. step 2	b. setting your goals
8. step 3	c. determining your personal needs (self-assessing)
9. step 4	d. implementing your plan and evaluating your progress
10. step 5	e. considering your healthy behavior options

For items 11 through 15, as directed by your teacher, respond to each statement or question.

11. Describe three skills for healthy living and explain why they are important.
12. Describe two characteristics that are similar to skills for healthy living and explain why they are important.
13. Describe the five steps in program planning.
14. Describe at least three guidelines for planning for healthy living (self-planning).
15. What is a health behavior contract? Explain.

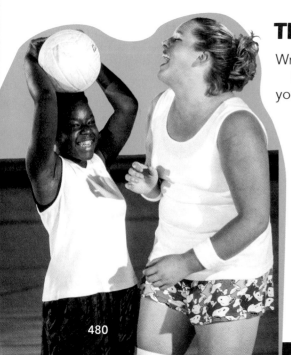

Thinking Critically

Write a paragraph to answer the following questions.

How is knowledge important to your health? How can it help you achieve positive behavior change?

Take It Home

Share the self-assessment from this chapter with at least one family member. Ask the person(s) to complete the self-assessment, then share information with the person(s) about each of the healthy living skills. Consider setting a family goal that focuses on improving one healthy living skill each week or month.

UNIT VIII

Preventing Disease and Seeking Care

Healthy People 2020 Goals

- Help people live high-quality, longer lives.
- Reduce disease, injury, and early death.
- Increase awareness and understanding of what determines good health.
- Help people adopt healthy lifestyles for lifetime health, fitness, and wellness.
- Create environments that promote health, fitness, and wellness for all.
- Improve emotional wellness.
- Decrease suicide, and suicide attempts, among teens.
- Increase availability of treatment for depression and anxiety.
- Increase counseling and wellness checkups.
- Increase school health education.
- Reduce the rate of HIV transmission among adolescents and adults.
- Increase annual flu and other vaccinations.
- Reduce the proportion of adolescents who are considered obese.
- Prevent inappropriate weight gain among adolescents and young adults.
- Reduce the overall cancer death rate.
- Reduce the percentage of teens who use artificial tanning.
- Increase the proportion of teens who take measures to protect against skin cancer.
- Improve the health literacy of the population.
- Increase the number of teens who have had a wellness checkup in the past year.

Self-Assessment Features in This Unit

- Body Mass Index
- My Disease Prevention IQ
- My Self-Esteem

Making Healthy Decisions and Skills for Healthy Living Features in This Unit

- Self-Confidence
- Identifying Risk Factors
- Providing Social Support

Special Features in This Unit

- Diverse Perspectives: Being Overweight
- Consumer Corner: Choosing Hand Sanitizers
- Advocacy in Action: Mental Health Awareness

Living Well News Features in This Unit

- Yo-Yo Dieting Is Up and Down
- Can Hot Temperatures Make Us Vulnerable to Disease?
- Teens Under the Knife

22

Understanding Your Body

In This Chapter

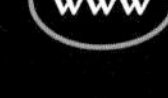

Student Web Resources

www.HOPEtextbook.org/student

BananaStock

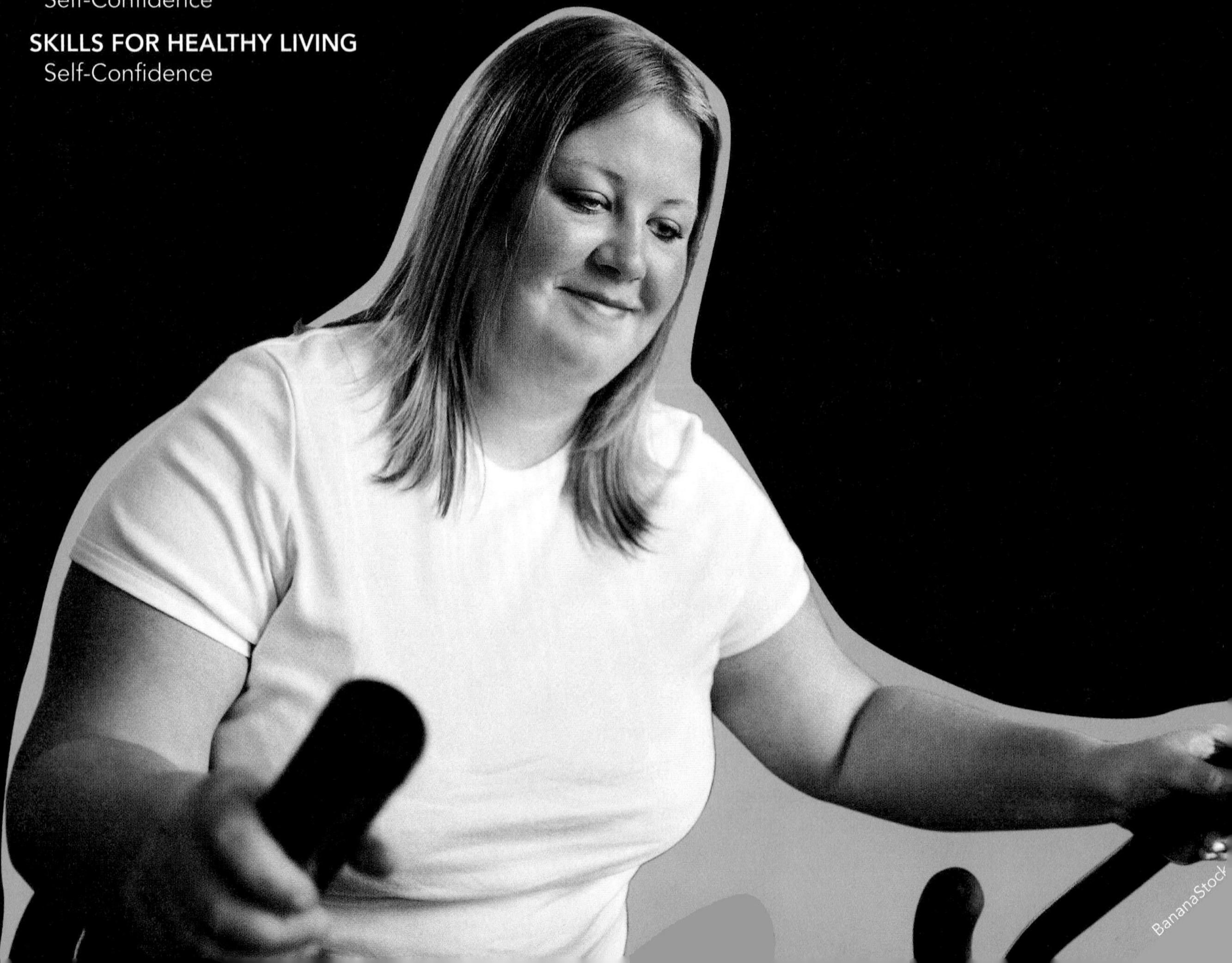

Lesson 22.1

Body Systems

Lesson Objectives

After reading this lesson, you should be able to

1. identify all of the major body systems,
2. identify the major components of each body system, and
3. explain the primary function of each body system.

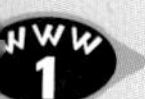

Lesson Vocabulary

alveoli, cardiac muscle, coronary circulation, cystic fibrosis, gene, hormones, kidney dialysis, nephrons, phenotype, pulmonary circulation, skeletal muscle, smooth muscle, systemic circulation

The human body is an amazing thing. Every second of the day, it sets off electrical impulses and chemical messengers, satisfies its need for oxygen, circulates blood and filters waste products, and regulates its acid–base balance and temperature. All the while, it allows you to think, dream, laugh, cry, jump, play, listen, learn, grow, and do everything else you do.

The intricacy and complexity of the body take years of study to understand, and science is still uncovering the body's many secrets. This lesson introduces you to the 11 major body systems and how they work together to maintain health and functioning. It also introduces the concept of genetics and the role that genes play in regulating major body systems.

Body Systems

The human body's 11 major body systems include the following: respiratory, circulatory, skeletal, muscular, integumentary, endocrine, nervous, digestive, excretory, reproductive, and immune. Each system performs its own specific functions, but all of the systems must also work together and support each other for the body to maintain optimal health and well-being.

For example, in order for you to play soccer on a hot day, your nervous, muscular, skeletal, respiratory, and circulatory systems must work together to create movement and supply your body with needed oxygen; in addition, your integumentary system must function optimally to allow heat to escape through your skin in the form of sweat. In fact, almost every system in your body affects all of the others; some of these interrelationships are summarized in table 22.1.

Circulatory System

Your circulatory system moves blood and oxygen through your body (see figure 22.1). Its operations include three kinds of circulation: pulmonary, coronary, and systemic. **Pulmonary circulation** moves blood from your heart to your lungs and back to your heart; **coronary circulation** provides your heart tissue itself with necessary blood and nutrients; and **systemic circulation** involves all of the arteries and veins that feed the rest of your body. During systemic circulation, your blood also passes through your kidneys and liver, where it is cleaned of toxins and waste products.

Respiratory System

Your respiratory system includes your mouth, nose, trachea, lungs, and diaphragm. Its primary functions are to supply your blood with oxygen and expel carbon dioxide. Oxygen enters your nose and mouth, then passes down through your trachea and into your lungs. More specifically, your trachea divides into two smaller tubes called bronchi, which then divide into smaller tubes. These tubes lead directly to your lungs, where they continue to divide and connect to tiny air sacs called **alveoli**. At this level, oxygen exchange takes place through a network of capillary beds (very small blood vessels). Once fully developed, your lungs contain about 600

TABLE 22.1 Interrelationship of Body Systems

System	Examples of interaction with other body systems
Circulatory	Circulates oxygen from the lungs to muscles to support movement; moves nutrients from the digestive system to all cells in the body; moves hormones through the body for the endocrine system.
Respiratory	Provides oxygen to all systems and removes carbon dioxide from all systems so that cells can survive and function.
Muscular	Moves bones to produce movement and exert force; necessary to produce bone growth for the skeletal system; contracts the heart to provide circulation for the circulatory system.
Skeletal	Bones act as levers to facilitate movement in concert with muscular systems; gives structure to the body; protects the brain for the nervous system; produces blood cells for the immune system.
Nervous	Sends messages to muscles to support movement; controls organs (e.g., stomach, intestines) for the digestive and excretory systems.
Digestive	Breaks down food into nutrients needed by all systems; sustains healthy bacteria in the colon for the immune system.
Excretory	Removes wastes from the body for the digestive system; helps remove water from food and deliver it to the blood for the circulatory system.
Endocrine	Provides hormones needed for the reproductive system; provides chemical messengers needed to regulate the brain and nervous system.
Immune	Protects all systems of the body from disease.
Integumentary	Includes skin, hair, and nails; protects the muscles and bones of the muscular and skeletal systems; protects the organs of the digestive system; protects the body from germs for the immune system.
Reproductive	Secretes (via the testes and ovaries) hormones essential for the maturation of the skeletal and muscular systems during adolescent growth spurts; is intensely interconnected with and mutually supportive of the endocrine system.

million alveoli. The respiratory system is presented in figure 22.2.

Muscular System

Your muscular system is responsible for all movements in your body and consists of more than 650 muscles (see figure 22.3). Muscular tissue falls into one of three categories: cardiac, smooth, and skeletal. **Cardiac muscle** refers to the muscle of your heart, which is distinctive in that it contracts automatically and regularly. On average, the heart contracts 70 times per minute and pumps five quarts (liters) of blood each minute.

Smooth muscle is found in the walls of other hollow organs, such as your esophagus, stomach,

Genetics and Cystic Fibrosis

Cystic fibrosis is a genetic disorder caused by inheriting a particular defective gene from each parent. The genes interfere with the acid balance in the lungs, making it more likely that bacteria will grow. The resulting inflammation leads to the accumulation of mucus, which plugs the airways and causes damage that interferes with breathing and leads to a persistent cough. Cystic fibrosis can affect individuals of all races, but it is five times more common in whites than Hispanics or blacks.

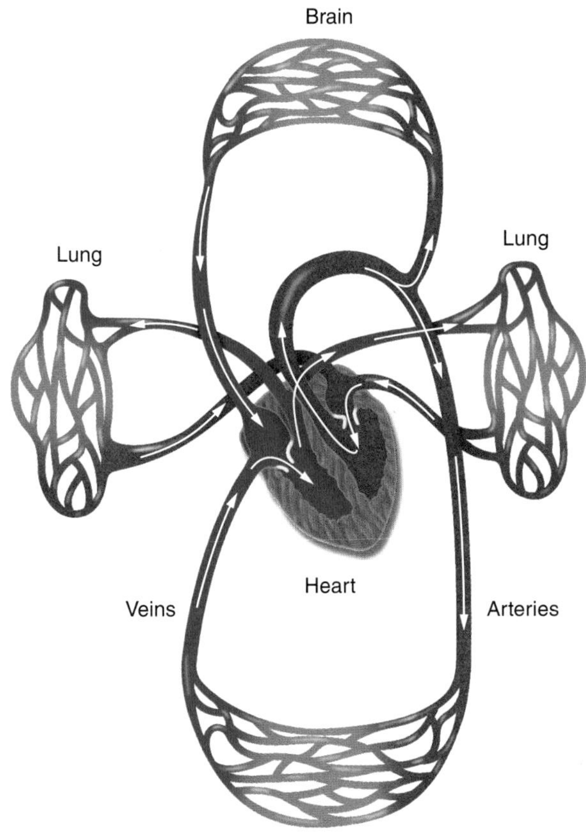

FIGURE 22.1 The circulatory system.

intestines, and (for females) uterus. Its primary role is to contract in order to reduce the size of the organ and create force or movement. As a result, smooth muscle plays a critical role in most body functions. For example, it contracts your esophagus, stomach, and digestive organs in order to push food through your digestive system. It also contracts the uterus to deliver a baby. Smooth muscle function is involuntary, meaning that it contracts automatically in response to stimulation from the nervous system.

Skeletal muscle controls all motor activities and is under your voluntary control. As the name implies, skeletal muscles are attached to your bones in order to give them stability and leverage.

The Skeletal System

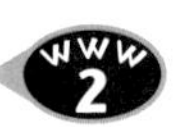

Your skeletal system is made up of your bones and the network of tendons, ligaments, and cartilage that connects them. Bones also act as levers. Human infants are born with 300 to 350 bones, some of which fuse together as the body develops. By the time most children reach the age of nine, they have 206 bones. The skeletal system performs vital functions, including support, movement, protection, blood cell production, calcium storage, and hormone regulation.

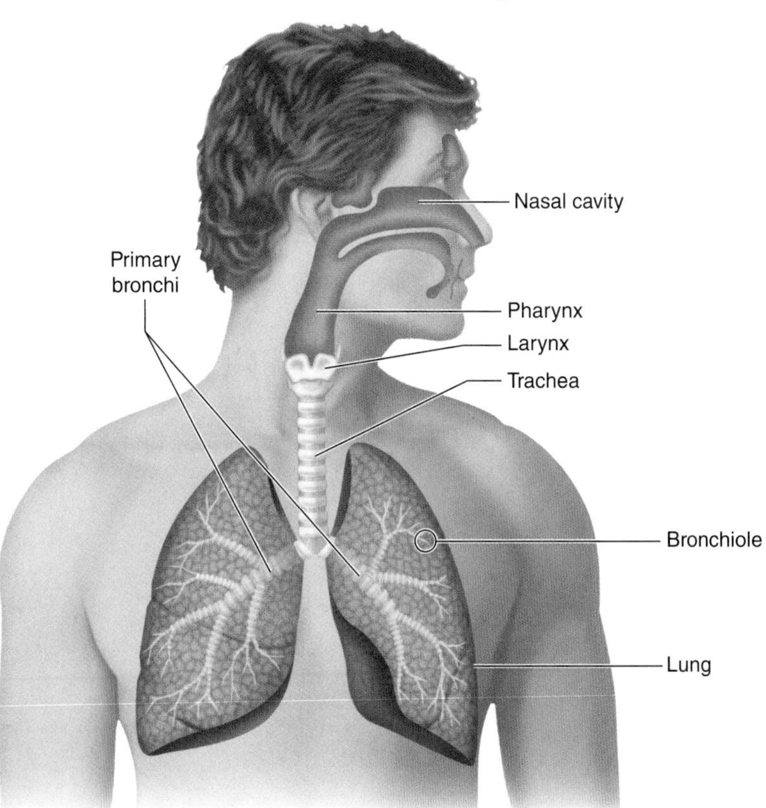

FIGURE 22.2 The respiratory system.

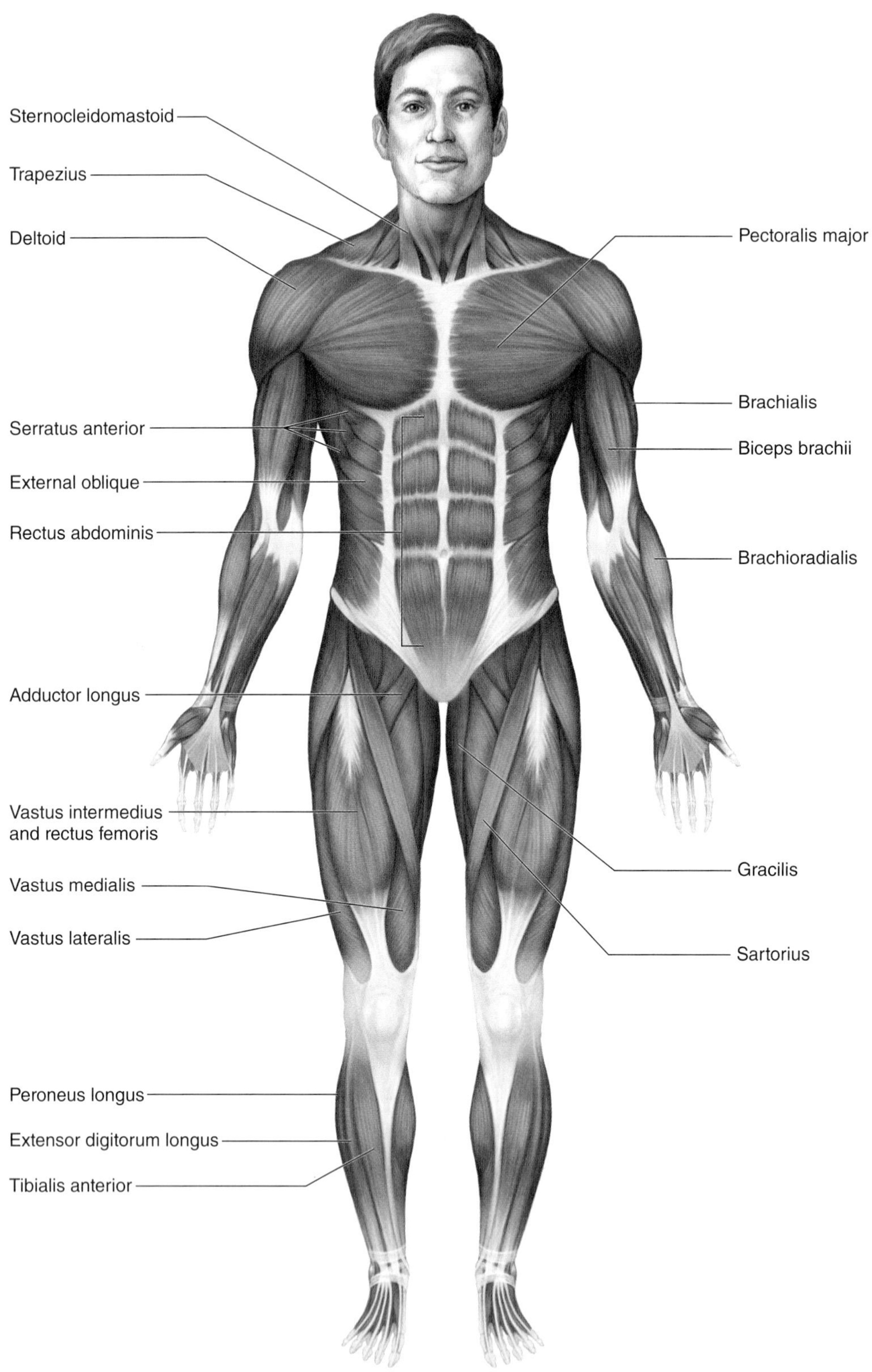
Sternocleidomastoid
Trapezius
Deltoid
Serratus anterior
External oblique
Rectus abdominis
Adductor longus
Vastus intermedius and rectus femoris
Vastus medialis
Vastus lateralis
Peroneus longus
Extensor digitorum longus
Tibialis anterior
Pectoralis major
Brachialis
Biceps brachii
Brachioradialis
Gracilis
Sartorius

FIGURE 22.3 The muscular system.

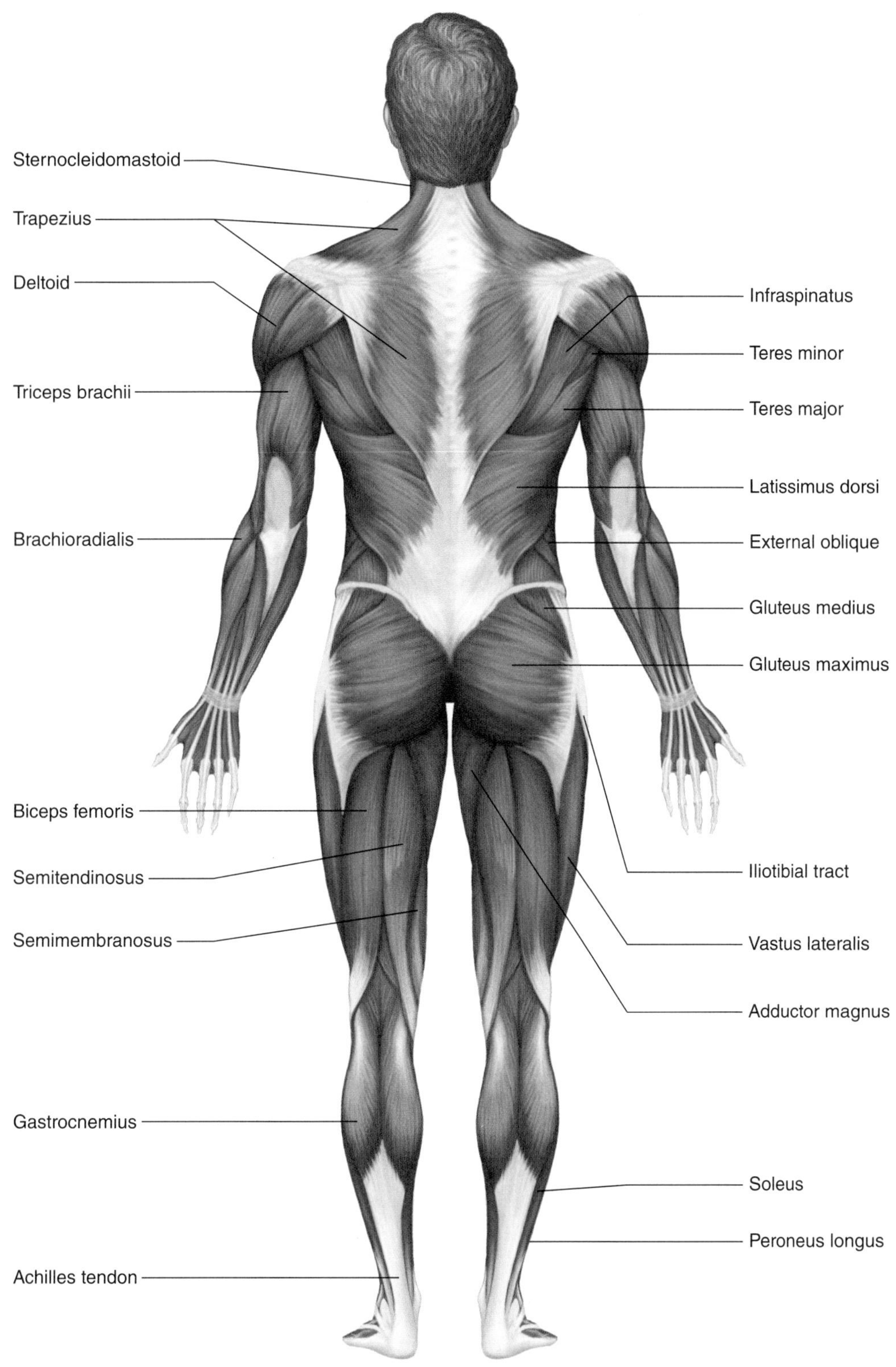
Sternocleidomastoid
Trapezius
Deltoid
Triceps brachii
Brachioradialis
Biceps femoris
Semitendinosus
Semimembranosus
Gastrocnemius
Achilles tendon
Infraspinatus
Teres minor
Teres major
Latissimus dorsi
External oblique
Gluteus medius
Gluteus maximus
Iliotibial tract
Vastus lateralis
Adductor magnus
Soleus
Peroneus longus

A typical bone has a dense and tough outer layer as well as an inner spongy layer that is lighter and slightly flexible (see figure 22.4). In the middle of some bones is the jelly-like bone marrow, where new cells are constantly being produced for blood. Teeth are considered part of the skeletal system, but they are not counted as bones. They are made of dentin and enamel, which is the strongest substance in your body. Teeth also play a key role in your digestive system because they help break down food so that it can be swallowed safely and then transported into the stomach.

Your skeletal system consists of two distinctive parts: your axial skeleton and your appendicular skeleton (see figure 22.4). Your axial skeleton totals 80 bones and consists of your vertebral column, rib cage, and skull. It transmits the weight from your head, trunk, and upper extremities down to your lower extremities at your hip joints. It is responsible for the upright posture of humans. Your appen-

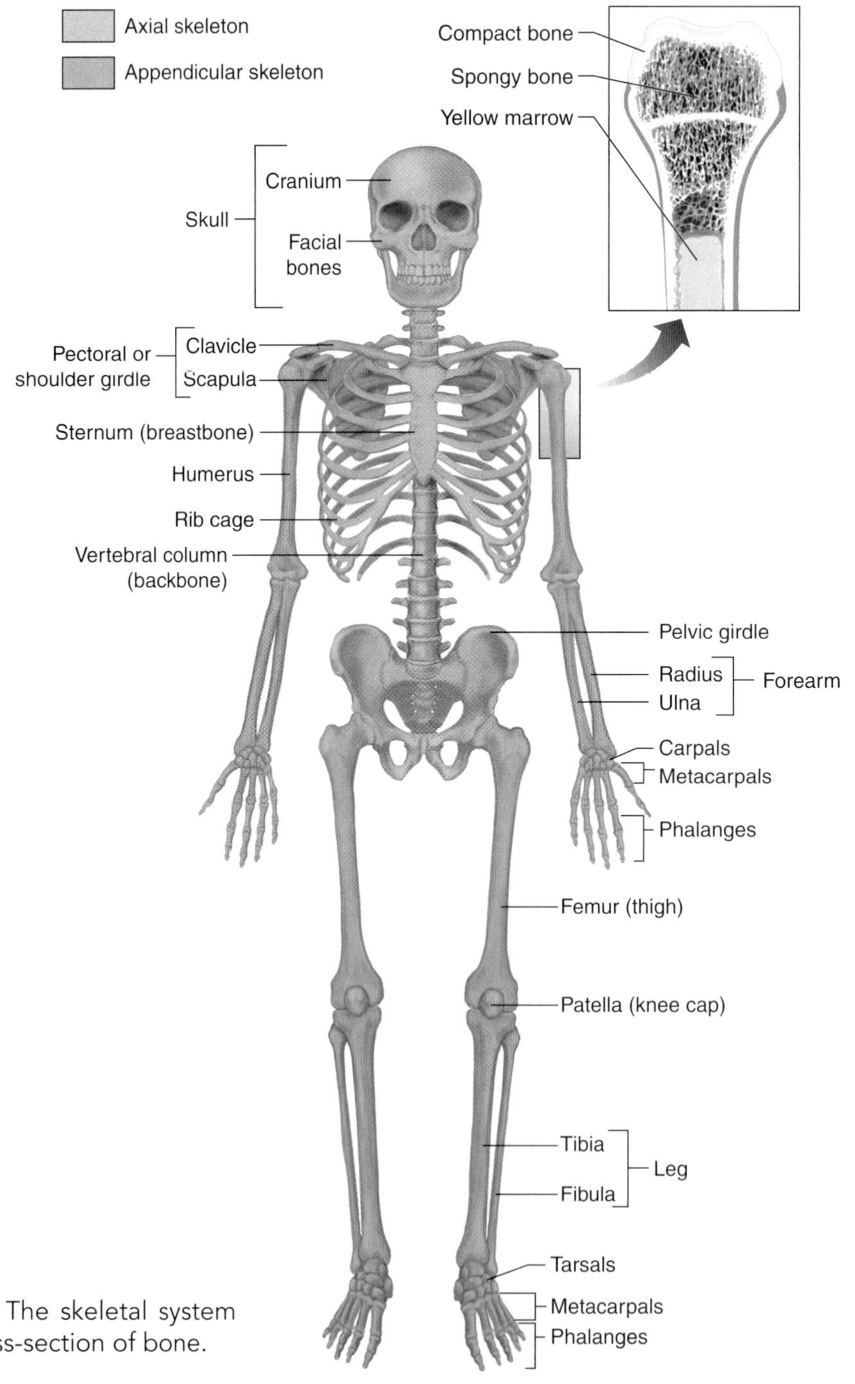

FIGURE 22.4 The skeletal system including a cross-section of bone.

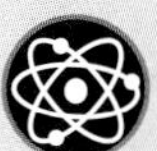

HEALTH SCIENCE

Your muscular system has strong genetic influences, and the types of muscle tissue that you have can influence your athletic abilities. For example, certain genes are associated with particular muscle proteins that can affect muscle contraction. In fact, one team of Australian researchers discovered the "gene for speed." They studied more than 400 Australian Olympic athletes and another 400 individuals who were not competitive athletes. The gene for speed was missing in 20 percent of the general population but was present in all of the Olympic athletes who competed in power sports (e.g., sprinting, high jumping, long jumping).

dicular skeleton totals 126 bones and is formed by your pectoral girdle (shoulder and shoulder blades), upper limbs, pelvic girdle (hips), and lower limbs. It makes walking, running, and other movements possible and protects the major organs responsible for your digestion, excretion, and reproduction.

Nervous System

Your nervous system provides all of the electrical signals that control your movements. It is made up of two main parts: your central nervous system (CNS) and your peripheral nervous system. Your CNS includes your brain and spinal cord (see figure 22.5). Your peripheral nervous system consists of a network of nerves that link your brain and spinal cord to the rest of your body.

Some of these nerves transmit sensory information from your eyes, ears, skin, and other sensory organs to your CNS. Others communicate with your muscles and glands. You're not aware of all of these actions because many of them (e.g., digestion, breathing) are autonomic, meaning that they happen automatically. Other nerves carry signals that you produce in your brain and control more consciously in order to perform actions such as chewing, walking, picking up a pen, and raising your arm in class.

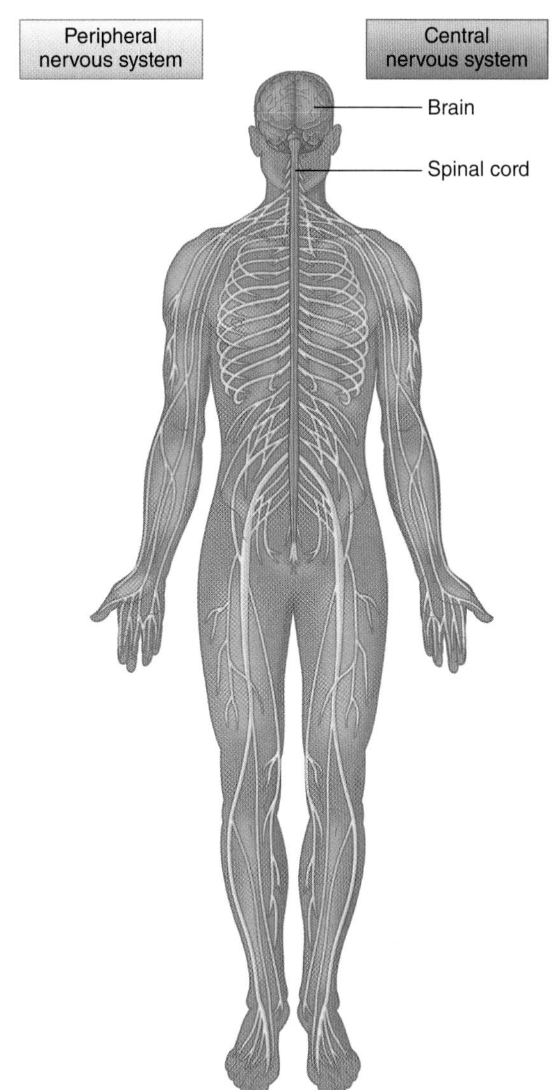

FIGURE 22.5 The nervous system.

Digestive System

Your digestive system gets the nutrients you eat into your body, where they are broken down into usable parts and absorbed. Digestion begins in your mouth with chewing and the secretion of saliva, which begins to break down some carbohydrates. It continues in your stomach, where your food is churned and broken down, and in your small intestine, where most nutrients are absorbed by your body. Your large intestine helps extract water

Crohn's Disease

Crohn's disease is an inflammatory bowel disease that extends into the deeper layers of the intestinal wall. It is a chronic condition that may recur throughout life and causes bloating, discomfort, pain, diarrhea, and other symptoms. About 20 percent of Crohn's cases appear to run in families. Scientists have identified several genes that contribute to the development of this disease.

from your food and moves waste products out of your body (see figure 22.6). Like other major body systems, digestion depends on the work of the circulatory, endocrine, and nervous systems in order to function properly.

Excretory System

Your excretory system eliminates metabolic wastes from your body and helps maintain proper fluid balance. This system involves the work of your kidneys, bladder, urethra, and skin. Your kidneys play a critical function in this system, since all blood

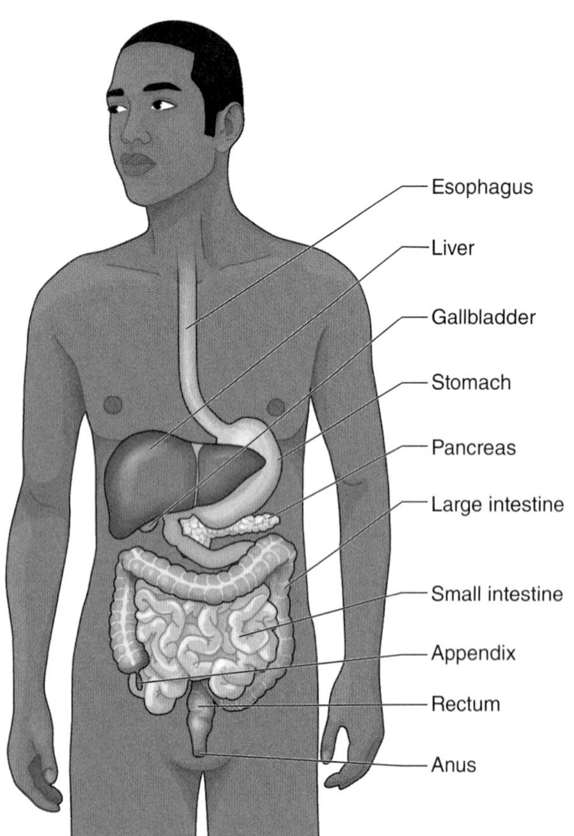

FIGURE 22.6 The digestive system.

passes through them to be cleaned of toxins. Each kidney weighs about 0.25 pound (0.1 kilogram) and contains one million filtering units known as **nephrons**. The glands associated with the kidneys (adrenal glands) also monitor and regulate the fluid balance in your body. Your kidneys deliver unneeded fluid, vitamins, and minerals, as well as toxins, to your bladder for elimination as urine.

Kidney damage can result from chronic high blood pressure, diabetes, and overuse of certain medications (e.g., the painkillers acetaminophen and ibuprofen). Once the kidneys are damaged beyond normal functioning, a person requires kidney dialysis or a transplant in order to survive. **Kidney dialysis** involves running all of the blood in the body through an external filtering system multiple times each week.

Endocrine System

Your endocrine system consists of glands that produce and secrete a variety of hormones throughout your body. **Hormones**, or chemical messengers, communicate information from one cell to another and coordinate functions throughout your body and between body systems. Major endocrine glands include your hypothalamus, pituitary, thyroid, parathyroid, adrenal, pineal, and reproductive organs (see figure 22.7). Disruptions to the endocrine system can affect growth and development, metabolism, and reproductive functions (e.g., ovulation in females, sperm production in males).

Immune System

Your immune system protects you from infection. It is a complex network consisting of your tonsils, lymph nodes, lymphatic vessels, spleen, thymus, and bone marrow. This system fights disease by attacking each threat it faces with a specialized

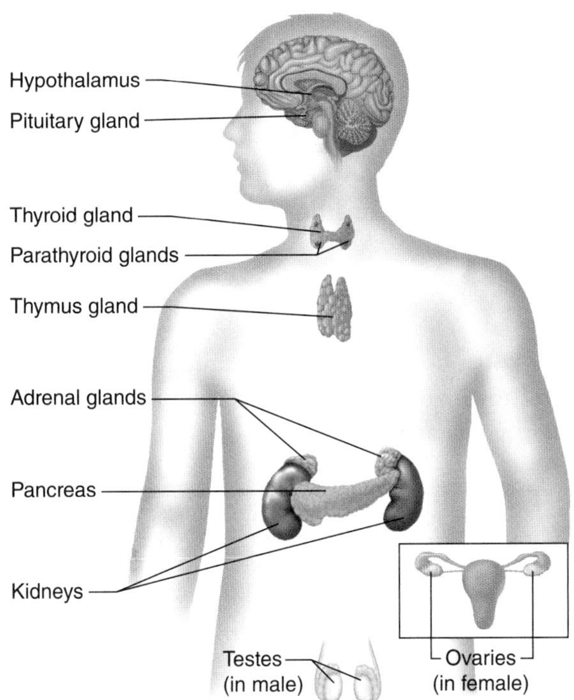

FIGURE 22.7 The major endocrine glands. Two of the most important glands in the body, the hypothalamus and pituitary glands, are located in the brain.

response. As you go through life and are exposed to more threats, your body builds its immunity. When you're exposed to a particular threat, such as chicken pox (not as common anymore because of vaccine), your immune system creates a memory of the threat that enables it to launch a very specific, quick, and aggressive response if the threat returns. Your immune system also plays a role in many disease processes and is discussed further in the chapter titled Diseases and Disability.

Integumentary System

Your integumentary system consists of your skin, hair, and nails. Most important of these is your skin, which is the largest single organ of your body. Your skin protects and cushions your body's organs and provides a physical barrier to keep out foreign materials. It consists of three layers: epidermis, dermis, and subcutis. The epidermis is the outermost layer of your skin. It consists of dead cells on top and live, reproducing cells toward the bottom. Your dermis is your middle layer of skin; it contains its own blood supply and is home to your sweat glands and hair roots. It also contains collagen, which gives your skin strength and elasticity. Your deepest layer of the skin is the subcutis, where adipose (fat) tissue provides cushioning for your organs and insulation to help your body maintain a stable temperature.

HEALTHY COMMUNICATION

Select one of the major body systems presented in this chapter. Write one or two verses of a rap song or poem to explain the body system to an elementary or middle school student. Include the system's functions and major organs and give advice for keeping it healthy.

Reproductive System

The human reproductive system allows for the conception, development, and delivery of offspring. It differs, of course, between males and females but ultimately serves the overall purpose of reproduction. In the male reproductive system, sperm is produced in the testicles for release through the penis during sexual activity. The female reproductive system includes the uterus, ovaries, fallopian tubes, vagina, and external genitalia. The female

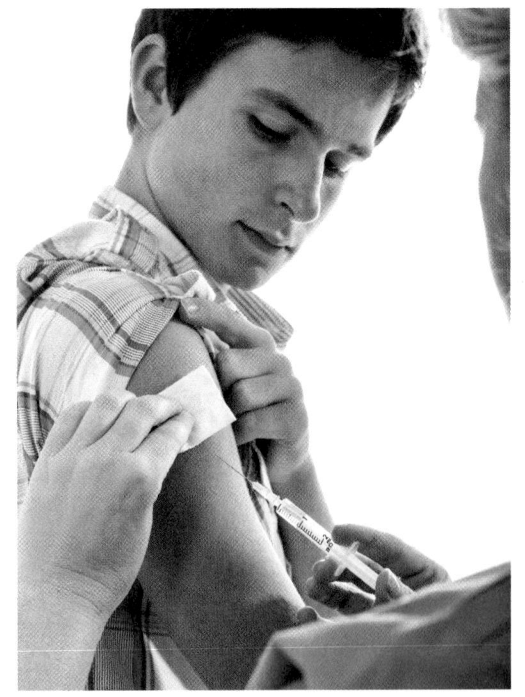

Vaccinations help your body build its immunity.

© Alexander Raths/Dreamstime

Genes and Skin Color

One of the most obvious phenotype characteristics that distinguishes members of our species is skin color. Human skin color covers a tremendous range, and variations can be correlated with factors such as climate, continent, and culture. Still, scientists know very little about the underlying genetics of skin color, and even the number of genes involved in the expression of skin color remains unknown.

menstrual cycle is a monthly cycle that results in the release of a mature egg and prepares the walls of the uterus to implant the egg if it is fertilized by sperm. If fertilization does not occur, the lining of the uterus is shed through menstruation, and the cycle begins again.

Genetics and the Body

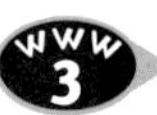

Genetics plays a large role in determining how well each of your body systems functions on its own and how well your systems work together. Almost every cell in your body carries a complete set of **genes** (genotype) and all of the information necessary to make you. These instructions are unique to you and are encoded in your DNA—long, twisting, ladder-shaped molecules that store a particular pattern, or code, based on how they are organized. Strands of DNA form your chromosomes, which combine to create your genes, which in turn create the proteins that ultimately affect every aspect of who you are. Thus your genes influence everything about you—for example, what type of muscle cells you have, how well you see and smell, how efficiently your body uses energy, and how you think and solve problems.

We are often most aware of genetic influences when we look at a person's physical characteristics. The way in which your genes are visibly expressed is known as your **phenotype**, which includes, for example, your height, eye and hair color, and skin color. A phenotype has both a genetic and an environmental influence. Height, for instance, is mostly a genetic trait, but it is also affected by the quality of your diet during times of critical bone development, which can also influence how strong your bones become. So genetics and lifestyle choices work together to influence who you are and how healthy you are.

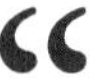

> Yet this is health: To have a body functioning so perfectly that when its few simple needs are met it never calls attention to its own existence. ”
>
> —Bertha Stuart Dyment, author

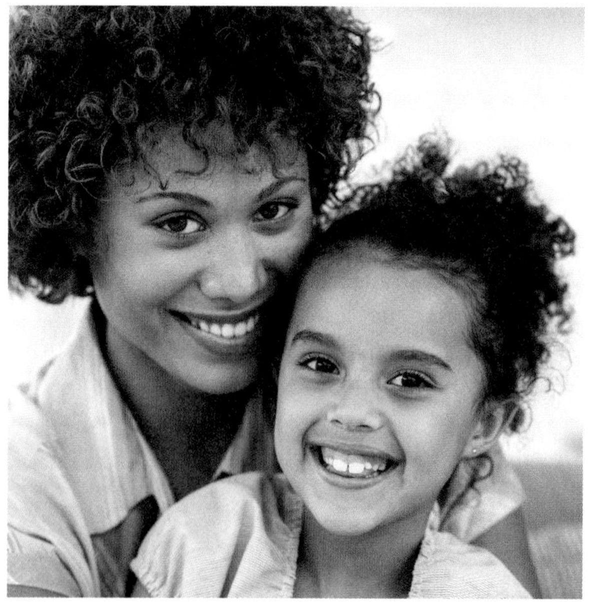

Genes play a role in determining how well our body systems work together and are visibly expressed through eye, hair, and skin color.

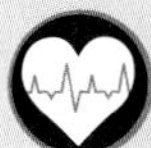

HEALTH TECHNOLOGY

Scientists have been working to develop artificial organs since the late 1800s. Many people have benefited from artificial joint replacements, and progress on other organs has been rapid over the last 30 years. For example, the first temporary artificial heart was used in 2007, and a permanent artificial heart was recently approved for use, though its size and life span need improvement before it can be widely applied. Scientists are also developing artificial bladders, skin, blood vessels, and even blood itself. These advances provide hope for people suffering from a fatal or debilitating illness and for those waiting for an organ donation or transplant.

Some research on artificial organs remains controversial, such as the development of artificial wombs and the creation of implantable computer chips that might directly affect brain function. Some biomedical ethicists also question whether the goal of prolonging life through the development of an artificial human body is a good thing, either for individuals or for society.

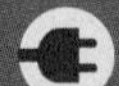

CONNECT

How do you think your cultural background and personal values influence your thoughts about using artificial organs to prolong life? How do your background and personal values influence your thinking about becoming an organ donor when you die? What other factors go into making the decision of whether or not to become an organ donor?

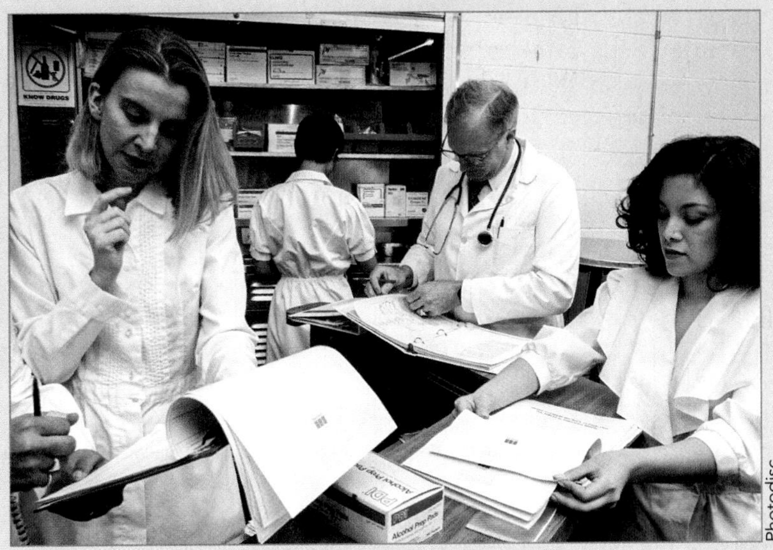

Photodisc

Comprehension Check

1. Identify the 11 different body systems.
2. Identify and describe key components of each system.
3. Briefly describe the function of each system.

SELF-ASSESSMENT: Body Mass Index

1. Measure your height in inches (or meters) without shoes.
2. Measure your weight in pounds (or kilograms) without shoes. If you're wearing street clothes (as opposed to lightweight gym clothing), subtract 2 pounds (0.9 kilogram) from your weight.
3. Determine your BMI using the BMI calculation chart or either of the following formulas.

$$\frac{\text{weight (lb)}}{\text{height (in.)} \times \text{height (in.)}} \times 703 = \text{BMI}$$

$$\frac{\text{weight (kg)}}{\text{height (m)} \times \text{height (m)}} = \text{BMI}$$

4. Use table 22.2 to find your BMI rating, and record your BMI score and rating.

Height																																	
4' 6"	25	25	26	26	27	28	29	30	31	32	34	35	36	37	39	40	41	42	43	45	46	47	48	49	51	52	53	54	56	57	58	59	60
4' 7"	24	24	25	25	26	27	28	29	30	31	32	34	35	36	37	38	39	40	41	43	45	46	47	48	49	50	51	52	54	55	56	57	58
4' 8"	23	23	24	24	25	26	27	28	29	30	31	32	34	35	36	37	38	39	40	42	43	44	45	46	47	48	49	50	52	53	54	55	56
4' 9"	22	22	23	23	24	25	26	27	28	29	30	31	32	34	35	36	37	38	39	40	42	42	43	44	45	47	48	49	50	51	52	53	54
4' 10"	21	22	22	23	23	24	25	26	27	28	29	30	31	32	34	35	36	37	38	39	40	41	42	43	44	45	46	47	48	49	50	51	52
4' 11"	20	21	21	22	22	23	24	25	26	27	28	29	30	31	32	33	34	35	36	37	38	39	40	41	42	43	45	46	46	47	48	49	50
5' 0"	19	20	20	21	21	22	23	24	25	26	27	28	29	30	31	32	33	34	35	36	37	38	39	40	41	42	43	44	45	46	47	48	49
5' 1"	18	19	19	20	21	22	23	24	25	26	26	27	28	29	30	31	32	33	34	35	36	37	38	39	40	41	42	43	43	44	45	46	47
5' 2"	18	18	18	19	20	21	22	23	24	25	26	27	27	28	29	30	31	32	33	34	35	36	37	37	38	39	40	41	42	43	44	45	46
5' 3"	17	18	18	19	19	20	21	22	23	24	25	26	27	27	28	29	30	31	32	33	34	35	35	36	37	38	39	40	41	42	43	43	44
5' 4"	17	17	17	18	19	20	21	21	22	23	24	25	26	27	27	28	29	30	31	32	33	33	34	35	36	37	38	39	39	40	41	42	43
5' 5"	16	17	17	17	18	19	20	21	22	22	23	24	25	26	27	27	28	29	30	31	32	32	33	34	35	36	37	37	38	39	40	41	42
5' 6"	15	16	16	17	18	19	19	20	21	22	23	23	24	25	26	27	27	28	29	30	31	31	32	33	34	35	36	36	37	38	39	40	40
5' 7"	15	15	16	16	17	18	19	20	20	21	22	23	23	24	25	26	27	27	28	29	30	31	31	32	33	34	34	35	36	37	38	38	39
5' 8"	14	15	15	16	17	17	18	19	20	21	21	22	23	24	24	25	26	27	27	28	29	30	30	31	32	33	33	34	35	36	36	37	38
5' 9"	14	15	15	15	16	17	18	18	19	20	21	21	22	23	24	24	25	26	27	27	28	29	30	30	31	32	32	33	34	35	35	36	37
5' 10"	13	14	14	15	16	17	17	18	19	19	20	21	22	22	23	24	24	25	26	27	27	28	29	29	30	31	32	32	33	34	34	35	36
5' 11"	13	14	14	15	15	16	17	17	18	19	20	20	21	22	22	23	24	24	25	26	26	27	28	29	29	30	31	31	32	33	33	34	35
6' 0"	13	13	14	14	15	16	16	17	18	18	19	20	20	21	22	22	23	24	24	25	26	26	27	28	28	29	30	31	31	32	33	33	34
6' 1"	12	13	13	14	15	15	16	16	17	18	18	19	20	20	21	22	22	23	24	24	25	26	26	27	28	28	29	30	30	31	32	32	33
6' 2"	12	12	13	13	14	15	15	16	17	17	18	19	19	20	21	21	22	22	23	24	24	25	26	26	27	28	28	29	30	30	31	31	32
6' 3"	11	12	12	13	14	14	15	15	16	17	17	18	19	19	20	21	21	22	22	23	24	24	25	26	26	27	27	28	29	29	30	31	31
6' 4"	11	12	12	13	13	14	15	15	16	16	17	18	18	19	20	20	21	21	22	23	23	24	24	25	26	26	27	27	28	29	29	30	30
Weight	90	95	100	105	110	115	120	125	130	135	140	145	150	155	160	165	170	175	180	185	190	195	200	205	210	215	220	225	230	235	240	245	250

BMI calculation chart. Locate your height in the left column and your weight in pounds in the bottom row. The box where the selected row and column intersect is your BMI score.

TABLE 22.2 Rating Chart: Body Mass Index

	13 years old		14 years old		15 years old		16 years old		17 years old		18 years old	
	Male	Female	Male	Female	Male	Female	Male	Female	Male	Female	Male	Female
Very lean	≤15.4	≤15.3	≤16.0	≤15.8	≤16.5	≤16.3	≤17.1	≤16.8	≤17.7	≤17.2	≤18.2	≤17.5
Good fitness	15.5–21.3	15.4–22.0	16.1–22.1	15.9–22.8	16.6–22.9	16.4–23.5	17.2–23.7	16.9–24.1	17.8–24.4	17.3–24.6	18.3–25.1	17.6–25.1
Marginal fitness	21.4–23.5	22.1–23.7	22.2–24.4	22.9–24.5	23.0–25.2	23.6–25.3	23.8–25.9	24.2–26.0	24.5–26.6	24.7–27.6	25.2–27.4	25.2–27.1
Low fitness	≥23.6	≥23.8	≥24.5	≥24.6	≥25.3	≥25.4	≥26.0	≥26.1	≥26.7	≥27.7	≥27.5	≥27.2

Data based on *Fitnessgram*.

Waist-to-Hip Ratio (Male and Female)

1. Measure your hips at the largest point (the largest circumference of your buttocks). Make sure that the tape is at the same level (horizontal to the ground) in the front, in the back, and on your sides. The tape should be snug but not so tight as to cause indentations in your skin (do not use an elastic tape). Stand with your feet together when making the measurement.
2. Measure your waist at the smallest circumference (called the natural waist). If there is no natural waist, measure at the level of the umbilicus. Measure at the end of a normal inspiration (just after a normal in-breath). Do not suck in to make your waist smaller. This measurement is slightly different from the one used to measure waist girth by itself.
3. To calculate your waist-to-hip ratio, divide your waist girth by your hip girth.
4. Find your ratio in table 22.3 to determine your rating.
5. Record your hip and waist measurements and rating.

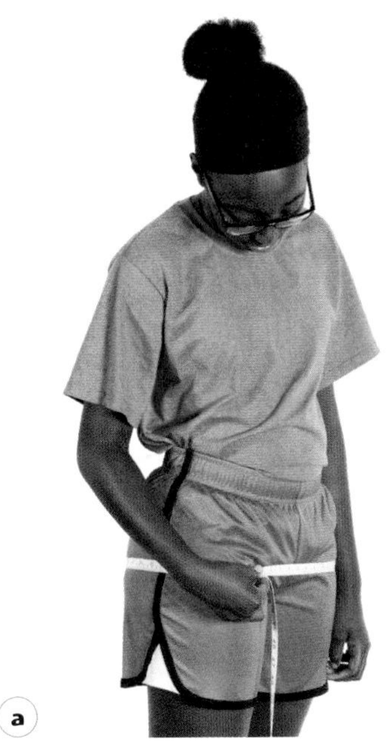

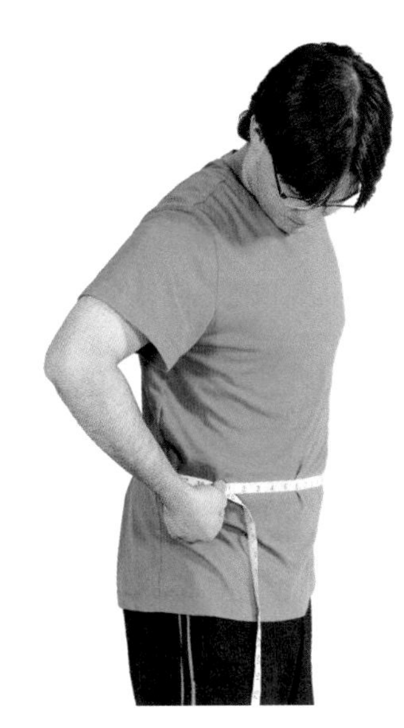

To determine your waist-to-hip ratio, measure *(a)* your hips and *(b)* your waist.

TABLE 22.3 Rating Chart: Waist-to-Hip Ratio

	Male	Female
Good fitness zone	≤0.90	≤0.79
Marginal	0.91–1.0	0.80–0.85
Low fitness zone	≥1.1	≥0.86

Planning for Healthy Living

Use the Healthy Living Plan worksheet to make a plan to improve or maintain your weight or body composition. Monitor the steps you take toward meeting your goals and repeat this self-assessment in one to three months to help determine the success of your plan.

Lesson 22.2

Healthy Body Weight

Lesson Objectives

After reading this lesson, you should be able to

1. define *body mass index (BMI)*, *overweight*, and *obesity*;
2. understand the health risks associated with overweight and obesity; and
3. understand the relationship between physical activity, weight, and health.

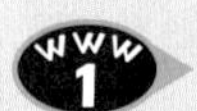

Lesson Vocabulary

body composition, body mass index (BMI), essential body fat, lower body fat, obesity, overweight, storage fat, toxic food environment, upper body fat, weight cycling

Have you seen news stories about obesity and disease risk? How about advertisements for weight loss? Do you ever think about your weight or feel pressured to change your weight? Obesity and overweight have increased dramatically in the United States since 1990, and this trend has led to growing concerns about related health risks, such as heart disease and diabetes. This lesson defines overweight and obesity and explores their relationship to health and disease. It also considers the relationships between weight, physical activity, genetics, and society.

The Obesity Epidemic

Obesity is common in American society today. Approximately one-third of all adults are overweight or obese, and 17 percent of children aged 2 to 19 are considered obese. Experts have named this current crisis the "obesity epidemic" because obesity has increased rapidly over the past 20 years. This crisis has many causes, and of the biggest is the rise in physical inactivity; indeed, sedentary living has become the norm. In addition, foods that are high in fat and low in nutrients are more readily available and less expensive than ever before. As a result, it has become easier and easier for people to put on unwanted weight. Reversing this trend is a major public health goal, and experts agree that it is a complex effort requiring many societal changes and individual commitments. For example, in 2013 the American Medical Association formally classified obesity as a disease. The change aids in the fight against obesity-related diseases such as type 2 diabetes and heart disease, and might also improve funding for obesity drugs, surgery, and counseling.

Weight and Body Mass Index

A person's body weight is simply the number of pounds or kilograms he or she weighs, and weight by itself is often of little value in determining health risk. A more useful measure is **body mass index (BMI)**, which is the standard way to measure a person's weight in relation to height. BMI provides a better reflection of health status because it considers the body's overall mass. By definition, the mass of an object is its weight divided by its total volume (the amount of space the body takes up). Body mass index can be calculated by dividing a person's weight (in kilograms) by his or her height (in meters squared); it can also be figured by means of a formula in inches and pounds. BMI can be used to determine whether a person is **overweight**—that is, whether he or she has too much weight per unit of body height or mass. For more information, refer to the BMI chart presented in this chapter's Self-Assessment feature.

Body mass index is a relatively easy and inexpensive way to determine weight status in large populations. As a result, it is often used in large studies that seek to determine the relationship between body weight and health. This type of research has shown that excessive body weight as measured by BMI may be associated with diseases such as diabetes, heart disease, cancer, and arthritis. Very low body weight may also be a sign of disease—or of malnutrition.

These risk assessments are based on the averages of large populations, and individual differences do exist in healthy body weight. For example, BMI does not directly measure body composition (amount of muscle versus amount of fat), nor does it reflect the location of weight on the body, and both of these factors are known to affect health. BMI also does not register a person's lifestyle, in particular diet and physical activity. As a result, it's possible to be overweight as defined by BMI while also being very active and healthy. It's also possible to have a normal weight as defined by BMI and be very unfit and unhealthy. Genetics also plays a large role in size and weight, and individual differences need to be considered when interpreting BMI results.

In spite of the limitations of BMI, there is an established relationship between a high BMI and health risk. As you learned in the self-assessment, the health standards for BMI for teens vary by age and gender. For adults, the CDC uses 25 as the standard for overweight and 30 as the standard for obesity. If you have a high BMI but are very active and eat well, you may want to do follow-up self-assessments to determine your percentage of body fat.

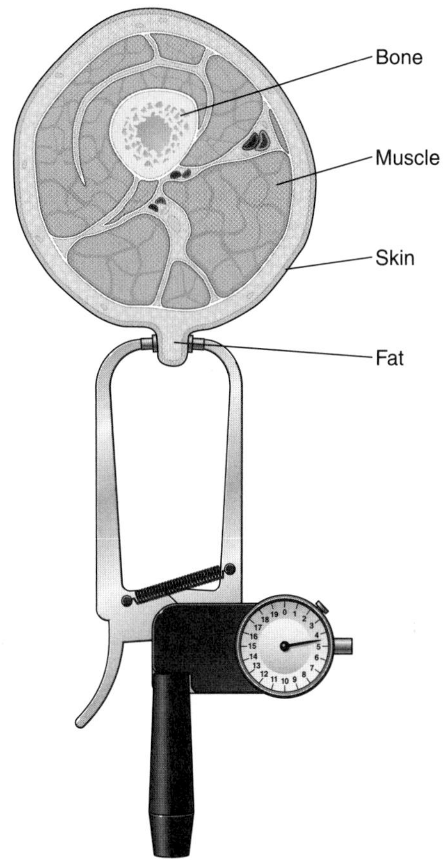

FIGURE 22.8 Using a skinfold measurement caliper.

Body Composition

Body composition refers to the ratio of fat to lean tissue in a person's total body mass. A high level of fat, regardless of overall weight, is associated with heart disease, diabetes, and certain cancers. Human beings do need a certain amount of body fat to survive, and this amount is called **essential body fat.** It cushions and insulates organs and aids in nervous system functions. It also plays a role in hormone regulation and reproductive health, particularly in women. Additional body fat (beyond essential fat) is called **storage fat**, and up to a certain point it does not appear to be harmful for health. Healthy body fat levels range from 13 to 31 percent for women and 6 to 25 percent for men. Genetics, physical activity level, and age are examples of factors that can influence total body fat levels.

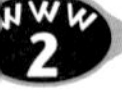

If a person has too much body fat per unit of body mass, he or she is considered obese. Measuring body fat is more challenging than measuring BMI, and several common methods are used, each of which involves potential error. The most commonly used technique is skinfold measurement, wherein calipers are used to measure subcutaneous fat, which is fat located directly under the skin (see figure 22.8). This technique assumes that about half of a person's total fat is subcutaneous and that the remainder is found in and around the organs.

In addition to special equipment, taking skinfold measurements requires special training. Measurements should be performed by a person who has learned proper technique and practiced this technique to ensure consistency and accuracy.

Another commonly used technique for measuring body fat is bioelectrical impedance analysis. You can read about it in the Health Technology feature presented in this lesson. Getting an accurate assessment of your body fat level can help you determine if other assessments such as BMI are effective for you. If you have a high BMI but a low level of body fat, this indicates that the BMI is not an effective technique for you.

Body Fat Distribution

As you've seen, total body fat provides information about an individual's health risks. However, even greater insight can be gained by noting the location of the fat, which is known as a person's fat distribution pattern. Research shows that fat tissue acts differently depending on where it is located and that different fat distribution patterns come with different degrees of health risk.

When fat is found in the upper body, particularly around the stomach area, it is called an **upper body fat** distribution pattern or apple shape (see figure 22.9). Fat found in this area and around the abdominal organs is very active and responsive to hormones, particularly testosterone. Fat located in the abdominal cavity can enter the bloodstream more easily, which makes it easier to lose, but it also means that the fat can enter the liver and be converted into dangerous cholesterol. As a result, abdominal fat has been associated with high cholesterol and risk for heart disease.

Fat located in the lower body, particularly around the hips and thighs, is called a **lower body fat** distribution pattern or pear shape (refer to figure 22.9). Fat in this location is much less active than abdominal fat. Generally speaking, lower body fat is considered much less harmful than abdominal fat to overall health. As a result, it can often be more resistant to weight loss efforts. The waist-to-hip ratio is a simple measure that can help determine a person's disease risks based on fat distribution (see this chapter's Self-Assessment feature).

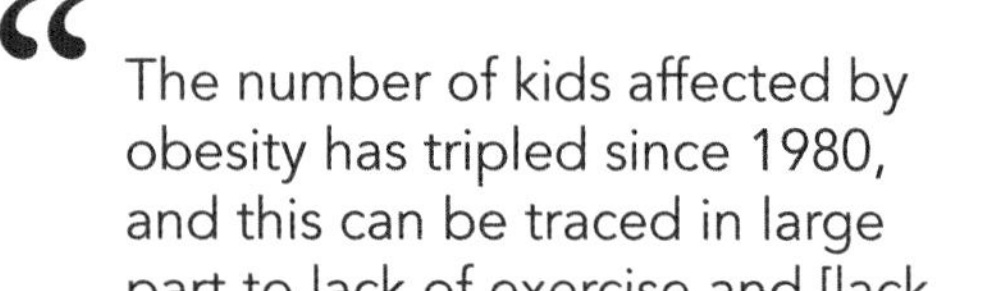

"The number of kids affected by obesity has tripled since 1980, and this can be traced in large part to lack of exercise and [lack of] a healthy diet."

—Virginia Foxx, U.S. congresswoman

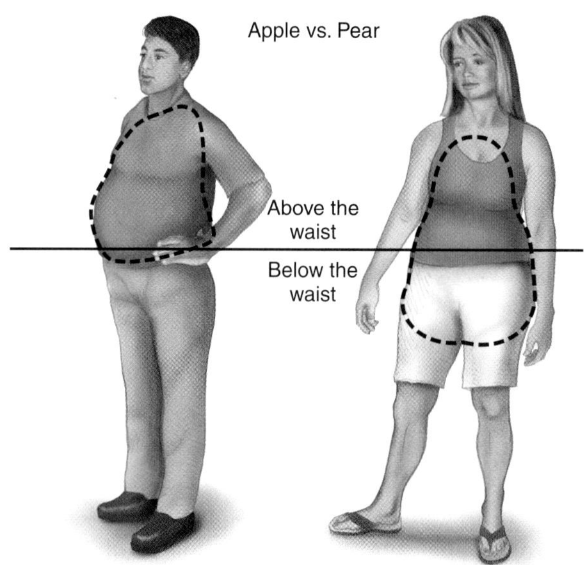

FIGURE 22.9 Apple versus pear body shape.

Health at Every Size

Because weight, body composition, and fat distribution pattern can be associated with disease risk, you need to understand them and evaluate your personal status. Regardless of the results, you also need to understand that none of these factors alone defines a person's total health status. American culture often assumes that fat always means unhealthy and that skinny always means healthy. We also tend to believe that a person's weight is a direct reflection of his or her lifestyle.

These assumptions are simplistic, and believing them can lead a person to make poor health decisions. Research has clearly demonstrated, for example, that individuals of normal weight who are unfit and sedentary face a higher risk for many diseases than those who are slightly overweight but

DIVERSE PERSPECTIVES: Being Overweight

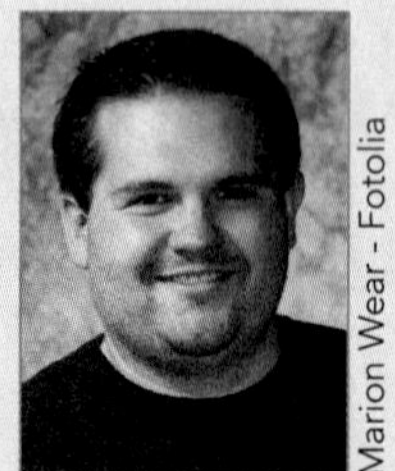

Marion Wear - Fotolia

My name is Christian, and I'm overweight. I have struggled with my weight most of my life. I remember being in elementary school and being teased and bullied by other kids. Both of my parents are obese. They're hard on me because they don't want me to be like them. My mom is always on my case to diet and exercise. I try not to be hard on myself, but it's a challenge because I feel like a failure sometimes. Not everyone looks at me like I must be lazy or stupid, but enough people do that it makes me self-conscious. Even when I look happy and okay on the outside, I'm often feeling insecure deep down. I wish people would get to know me before they judge me. I'm a pretty good student and a good musician. I don't really understand why being overweight makes me a bad person in some people's eyes.

physically fit and exercising regularly. In addition, being slightly overweight but having a stable weight may be healthier than engaging in a series of fad diets that result in cycles of weight loss and weight gain. In fact, **weight cycling**—the repeated gaining and losing of weight—may increase weight, fat, and disease risk over time.

Genetic influences on weight, body composition, and body fat are also very powerful. We are not all made to be the same general size. Genetic research has demonstrated that people respond differently to changes in physical activity patterns and diet. Some individuals lose weight or maintain a healthy weight more easily, while others find it more challenging to do so.

In addition, it is generally easier for individuals with higher incomes to take steps such as buying healthy foods, joining a health club, hiring a personal trainer, and purchasing exercise gear. People in better socioeconomic conditions also enjoy greater safety in their parks and greater access to social programs, such as athletic clubs, sport leagues, and parks and recreation programs. Socioeconomic status also makes a difference in how an individual is affected by **toxic food environments**—that is, environments in which food is plentiful and inexpensive but also higher than necessary in calories and fat.

We should encourage all people to seek out their healthiest weight by eating a healthy diet and engaging in regular physical activity and exercise. We should also be compassionate and encouraging to all people and not assume that someone who carries a few extra pounds is simply not trying hard. Reducing obesity over the long term depends on providing both a physically and an emotionally safe place for individuals to pursue a healthy lifestyle.

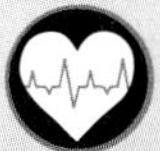

HEALTH TECHNOLOGY

Body fat scales have become popular in recent years. These scales use bioelectrical impedance analysis to give you an estimate of your body fat level. They estimate your fat level based on how a small amount of electricity moves through your body. In order to use this technology accurately, you need to understand how it works.

When you step onto the electrical sensors on the scale, a small electrical current is sent up one leg and down the other. The scale measures how quickly the current covers the distance and how much of the current is returned. This is relevant because water conducts electrical currents, and your muscle tissue is about 70 percent water when normally hydrated. The scale's programming assumes that you're properly hydrated and that the current is traveling through muscle tissue that contains a known amount of water.

However, if you step on the scale after exercising very hard and sweating heavily, your body may be dehydrated. As a result, the current will not move as quickly as it normally would, and the scale will assume that you have less muscle tissue than you actually do. As a result, it will report a higher level of body fat than you really have.

Many consumers fail to understand this basic science and then become perplexed when they measure their body fat after a hard workout only to see that it has apparently gone up! Therefore, being well hydrated is critical for using this technology effectively at home.

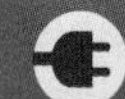

CONNECT

How might using a body fat scale at home affect your feelings about your health? Do you think it would affect your health behaviors? Why or why not?

Comprehension Check

1. What is BMI, and what can it tell you about your health?
2. Why is the location of fat on the body an important factor to consider in determining a person's health risks?
3. Describe the relationship between physical activity, weight, and health.

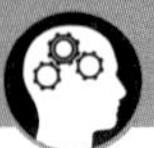

MAKING HEALTHY DECISIONS: Self-Confidence

Olivia has always hated speaking in front of the class and has always doubted her own ideas. As a kid, she would purposefully misspell words in the spelling bee just so she could sit down. Now that she's in high school, it seems like she's expected to speak in front of the class more often.

Group projects and reports also cause Olivia a lot of stress because she feels nervous about sharing her ideas with her group. She's also very self-conscious about her appearance and size: "I don't want to look like an idiot if I'm wrong. I don't want to be blamed for failing, and I don't want people to call me fat or stupid." As a result, she usually doesn't contribute much. Sometimes, she gets angry with herself because she knows that the group is making mistakes or is not doing the task as carefully as she would if she worked alone. Still, she stays quiet.

Will seems just the opposite of Olivia, and she often envies him for how easy it seems for him to be in front of the class. Indeed, Will is a bit of a class clown, always cracking jokes about other people or doing silly stunts. The truth, however, is that Will wishes he wasn't always trying to be funny: "I try to make people laugh because I'm afraid they'll be laughing *at* me if they aren't laughing *with* me." Will is tall and lanky and wears glasses. He feels like a "nerd" and has noticed that no one seems to comment on how he looks because they think of him as "the funny kid" in class. Will does like being popular, but he hates his own appearance, and most of the time he doesn't feel very confident at all.

For Discussion

Despite their differences, both Olivia and Will lack self-confidence. What should Olivia do in order to build her self-confidence? How could others help her? What should Will do to build his self-confidence? Do you think that covering up his insecurity with humor will help him become more confident? When answering these questions, refer to this chapter's Skills for Healthy Living feature for more information.

SKILLS FOR HEALTHY LIVING: Self-Confidence

Everyone suffers from a lack of confidence now and then. Self-doubt can be triggered by uncertainty, competition, or change. For some people, however, a more general lack of self-confidence interferes with daily life and can even lead to social isolation. Building your self-confidence is important to your mental health. It also makes you more likely to be physically active and to resist peer pressure to engage in risky behaviors.

During the teenage years, self-confidence is disproportionately connected to how a person perceives his or her appearance and social status. As a result, teens with body weight issues are more likely to suffer from low self-confidence. A lack of self-confidence is also closely associated with fear of failure.

The good news is that self-confidence is a matter of perception, and building self-confidence is a skill that can be learned. To build your self-confidence, use the following suggestions.

- **Keep a success journal.** Keep track of everything you do well each day. We often focus too much on a few things, such as appearance, and don't pay attention to all of the ways in which we succeed on a daily basis. Focusing on your strengths helps you feel more confident about your abilities.
- **Be your best self.** One quick way to create self-doubt is to compare yourself negatively with others and pass judgment on yourself. No one is good at everything, yet we often compare ourselves with lots of different people—each one very good at something—and assume that we should be better at everything than we are. Stop negatively comparing yourself with others; instead, focus on being the best *you* that you can be.

- **Set small goals that you're sure to reach with effort.** If you set goals that are out of your reach, you won't be able to achieve them, and failing to reach a goal often contributes to low self-confidence. On the other hand, reaching a goal that is well thought out can boost your self-confidence.
- **Work on self-improvements.** We all have weaknesses in our skills and abilities that can contribute to self-doubt. Seek out ways to improve your skills and abilities. If you lack confidence because you aren't good at, say, math or reading, take steps to get help and improve your ability in that area. For example, if you don't feel confident in physical education, practice some of the skills you're learning in class when you're outside of class. You're likely to see improvement in most skills with practice, and when you do your self-confidence will improve.
- **Walk the walk.** If you lack self-confidence, this fact is probably visible to others in the way you carry yourself. Practice holding your head up and using good posture. Standing up straight and walking with a sense of purpose can do wonders for your self-confidence, and it shows others that you're a confident individual.
- **Avoid negative talk.** Try not to think or say negative things about yourself or others. Negative self-talk only serves to reduce your self-confidence, and when you communicate with others in a negative way they often do the same. Positive attitudes are contagious, and surrounding yourself with positive people helps you feel more self-confident.

ACADEMIC CONNECTION: The Scientific Method

The scientific method is a way to ask and answer scientific questions by making observations and doing experiments. The advancement of science and human understanding relies on the use of an unbiased and fair method of scientific discovery. Sometimes the scientific method yields conflicting results, such as in this chapter's Living Well News feature. When this happens, scientists will seek to replicate (or duplicate) other researchers' findings and add to their discoveries until a more definitive answer is found.

Following are the steps of the scientific method:

1. Ask a question. Every scientific discovery begins with a specific question.
2. Do background research. Sound science depends on knowing and understanding what others before you have learned. Knowing this information helps you to add to the body of knowledge on a topic in a meaningful way.
3. Construct a hypothesis. A hypothesis is an educated guess about the answer to the question as well as the reason for that guess.
4. Test the hypothesis by doing an experiment. Here, a scientist does the experiment in pursuit of the truth.
5. Analyze the data and draw a conclusion. Once the experiment is concluded, the scientist determines the findings based on careful analysis.
6. Communicate the results. Advancing knowledge depends on sharing what is learned. Scientists communicate their results in academic and scientific journals.

Yo-Yo Dieting Is Up and Down

Yo-yo dieting, also called "weight cycling," can be a frustrating experience for people with weight problems. The term refers to a decrease of 10 pounds (4.5 kilograms) or more of body weight, followed by weight regain after the regimen ends (see figure 22.10). This process can lead to emotional upheaval and health problems.

When a diet includes very low calorie intake, the body first adapts to conserve energy by slowing down its metabolism. When the near-starvation period is then followed by a return to former eating habits, the body reacts by storing fat faster. This is why many dieters end up heavier than they were before their initial weight loss efforts.

Dr. Tracy Bale and her colleagues at the University of Pennsylvania found that dieting itself can change how the brain responds to the process. Based on experiments with mice, the researchers observed that switching from near starvation to overeating can lead to changes in the brain. In other words, the experience of near starvation (severe dieting) effectively taught the rodents to overindulge in high-calorie foods as soon as they had access to them, just in case there would be another period of starvation in the future.

However, not everyone agrees that yo-yo dieting is always unhealthy. At least one study suggests that losing weight, even if it's gained right back, is better than remaining obese all the time. Based on experiments with mice, researchers found that yo-yo dieters may be healthier and live longer than those who do nothing about their weight. Dr. Edward List, a scientist at Ohio University's Edison Biotechnology Institute and lead author of the study report, concludes that gaining and losing weight by itself does not seem detrimental to one's life expectancy. Still, significant weight changes can result in some damage that is hard to reverse, such as muscle being lost during rapid weight loss and then replaced by fat gain. Another potential problem is the emotional toll of repeated bouts of success followed by failure.

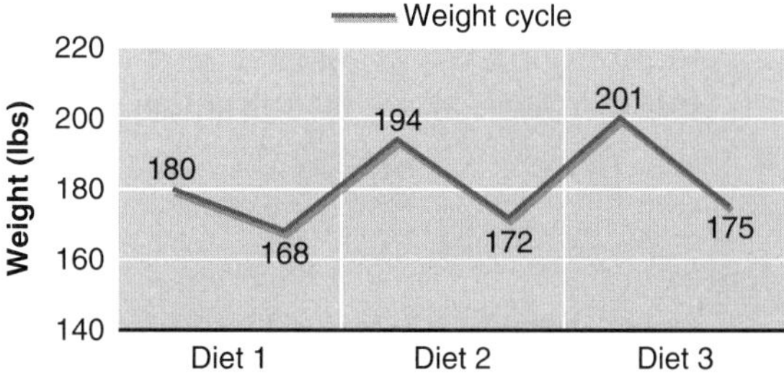

Figure 22.10 Cycle of weight loss and regain.

For Discussion

Given the conflicting research results, do you think it is better for an overweight person's overall health to try to lose weight, even if he or she regains the weight each time? Why or why not?

CHAPTER REVIEW

Reviewing Concepts and Vocabulary

As directed by your teacher, answer items 1 through 5 by correctly completing each sentence with a word or phrase.

1. Your respiratory system includes your mouth, nose, trachea, ________, and ________.
2. Nervous system functions that happen automatically, such as breathing, are called ____________.
3. Most nutrients are absorbed through the ___________ intestine.
4. Fat tissue is located in the _____________ layer of the skin.
5. Repeatedly gaining and losing weight is called _________ _________.

For items 6 through 10, as directed by your teacher, match each term in column 1 with the appropriate phrase in column 2.

6. skinfold	a. weight per unit of height
7. bioelectrical impedance	b. measuring subcutaneous fat
8. body mass index	c. normal hydration required for accuracy
9. upper body fat	d. body fat required for normal physiological function
10. essential body fat	e. fat located around the internal organs

For items 11 through 15, as directed by your teacher, respond to each statement or question.

11. Name the two branches of the nervous system.
12. What is one difference between skeletal and cardiac muscle?
13. Give two examples of how a phenotype may be expressed.
14. Which body fat distribution pattern is more dangerous to health? Why?
15. What is a toxic food environment?

Thinking Critically

Write a paragraph in response to the following questions.

Jenna struggles with her weight. She walks her dog for almost an hour every day after school and goes to aerobics classes at the local gym at least three times a week. Still, most people consider Jenna fat, and sometimes she gets teased at school. She is 5 feet 4 inches (1.6 meters) tall, weighs 170 pounds (77 kilograms), and has a classic pear shape.

What would you tell Jenna about her weight and health? Do you think she is at great risk for disease?

Take It Home

Ask a friend or family member if you can conduct a body weight assessment for him or her. Use the self-assessment presented in this chapter to determine the person's body mass index and waist-to-hip ratio. Once you've gathered and evaluated the information, give the person an interpretation of what the results may mean for his or her health. Write a report presenting your interpretation. If you don't have a scale and tape measure at home, use your own results from this chapter to write your report. If you are comfortable doing so, share your report with a friend or family member and tell him or her what you've learned from doing the self-assessments.

23

Diseases and Disability

In This Chapter

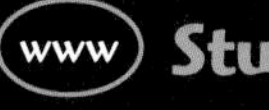

www **Student Web Resources**
www.HOPEtextbook.org/student

Alexander Raths/fotolia.com

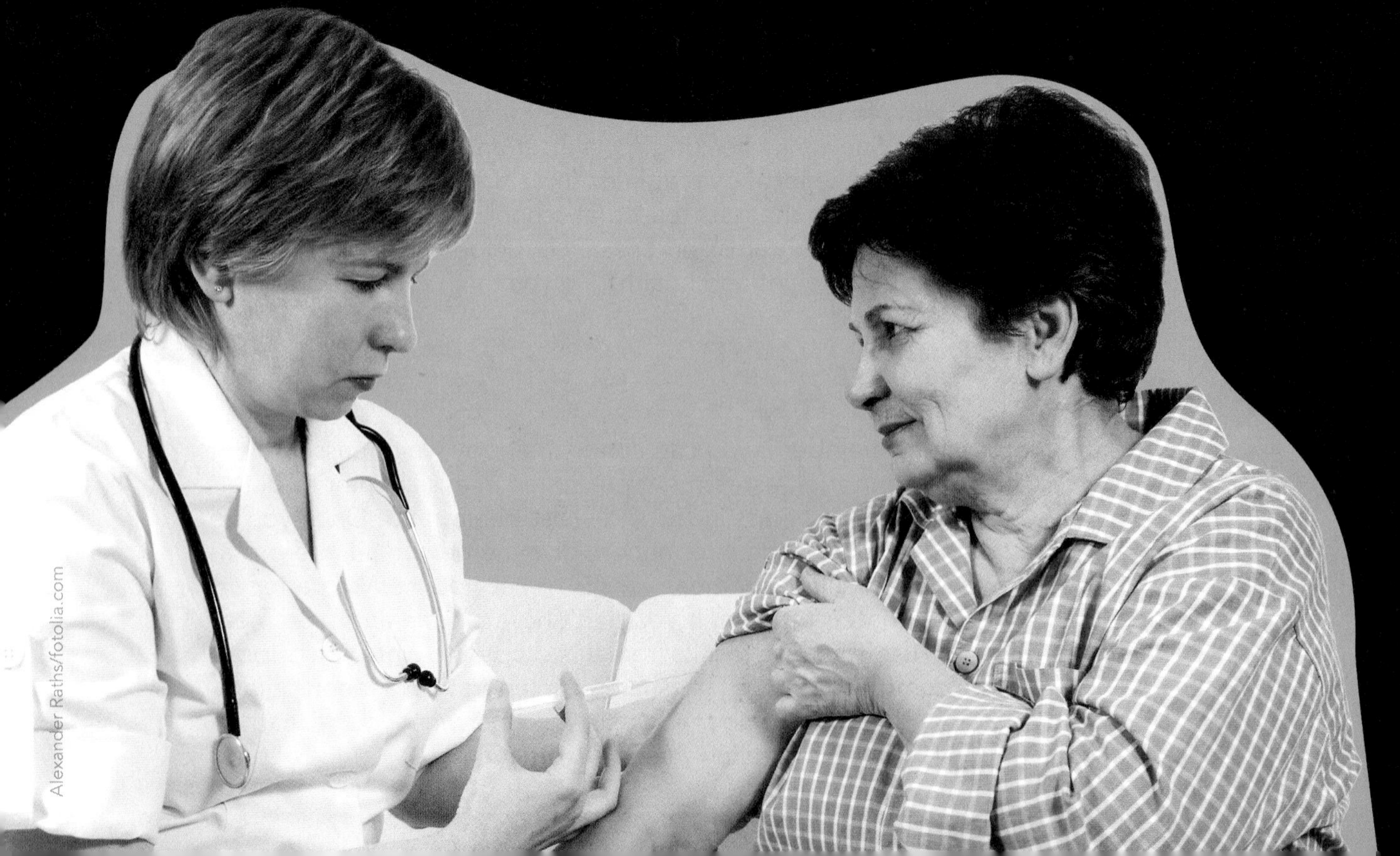

Lesson 23.1

Infectious Diseases

Lesson Objectives

After reading this lesson, you should be able to

1. understand what infectious diseases are and what causes them,
2. give examples of infectious diseases, and
3. understand how to protect yourself from common infectious diseases.

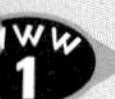

Lesson Vocabulary

acquired immune deficiency syndrome (AIDS), antibiotic, athlete's foot, bacteria, fungi, human immunodeficiency virus (HIV), immune system, influenza, localized infections, pathogen, protozoan, systemic infections, viruses

Have you ever had a cold or the flu? Did you have chicken pox when you were a kid? Have you ever had a bout of food poisoning that caused you to vomit or have diarrhea? If you answered yes to any of these questions, then you've had an infectious disease. These diseases are all around us, and learning about how they are spread and how your body works to fight them can help you reduce your risk of getting sick.

What Are Infectious Diseases?

Living organisms are in the air, on you, and in you all of the time. These small organisms are known as microorganisms. They are not visible to the naked eye and often require powerful magnification in order to be seen. Your mouth, skin, and digestive tract host millions of these microorganisms, which are part of a normal, healthy system. However, some dangerous microorganisms can enter the body, multiply, and cause serious illness. These microorganisms are known as **pathogens**, and the diseases they cause are known as infectious diseases.

Infections can be systemic or localized. **Systemic infections** affect the entire body, not just a single organ or body part; examples include the flu and the common cold. **Localized infections** affect only one body part or organ; examples include athlete's foot and infected wounds.

Methods of Transmission

Pathogens are spread in a number of ways, such as contact with infected people, animals, or objects. Direct contact occurs, for example, from kissing, sharing straws, sexual contact, or even a blood transfusion from an infected donor. Indirect contact

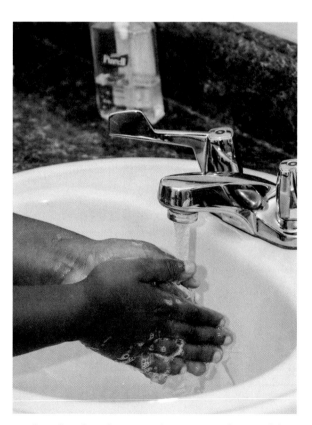

Washing hands with soap and water is one key guideline in preventing infectious diseases.

occurs when you touch an object (e.g., cell phone, computer keyboard, doorknob) where a pathogen is found. One of the most effective ways to reduce your risk of acquiring an infection is to wash your hands regularly.

Pathogens can also spread through airborne transmission. This occurs when a pathogen is in small droplets of water in the air, such as when an infected person sneezes. Germs can also travel through the air as small particles that can be inhaled. Finally, pathogens can travel in hosts, such as insects, animals, and food. As a result, you can be exposed to an infectious disease by coming into contact with an infected animal, being bitten by a pathogen-carrying insect, or eating contaminated food.

CONNECT

Identify three ways in which your friends' and family members' habits can affect your likelihood of getting an infectious disease. How do your own habits influence your susceptibility, or vulnerability, to infectious disease?

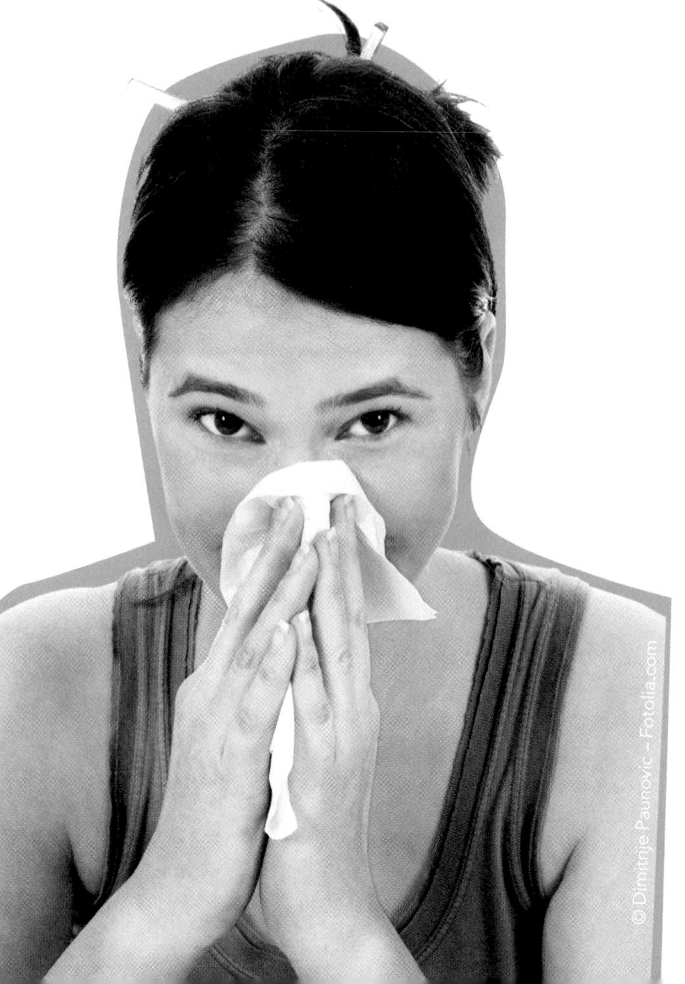

You can help prevent airborne transmission of pathogens by covering your mouth and nose with a tissue or handkerchief when you sneeze or cough. If you don't have a tissue or handkerchief, sneeze or cough into your upper sleeve rather than into your hands or directly into the air.

Your Body's Defenses

Because pathogens are always in the environment, your body has defenses to protect you against pathogens and the infections they can cause. First, you have physical and chemical defenses that can prevent a pathogen from entering your body. These defenses include your skin, mucous membranes, saliva and tears, and digestive system. Your skin acts as a barrier and contains acids that can kill some pathogens. The skin also sheds regularly, which allows you to shed pathogens as well. Your body's mucous membranes, such as those in your nasal passages, secrete mucus that captures or kills many pathogens, which can then be washed away or expelled from your body. Your tears and saliva work in a similar manner. Your digestive system, including stomach acid, can kill and move some pathogens through your body and eliminate them before they cause severe damage.

The Immune System

If a pathogen gets through your other defenses and enters your body, your **immune system** is designed to attack and kill it. It fights infection and disease by attacking each type of threat it faces with a specialized response that either disables or destroys the pathogen. The organs of the immune system are positioned throughout the body (see figure 23.1). They are called lymphoid organs because they are home to lymphocytes, which are small white blood cells that are the key players in the immune response. Bone marrow—the soft tissue in the hollow center of bones—is the source of all blood cells, including lymphocytes. The thymus is a lymphoid organ that lies behind the breastbone, and the lymph nodes are small bean-shaped glands

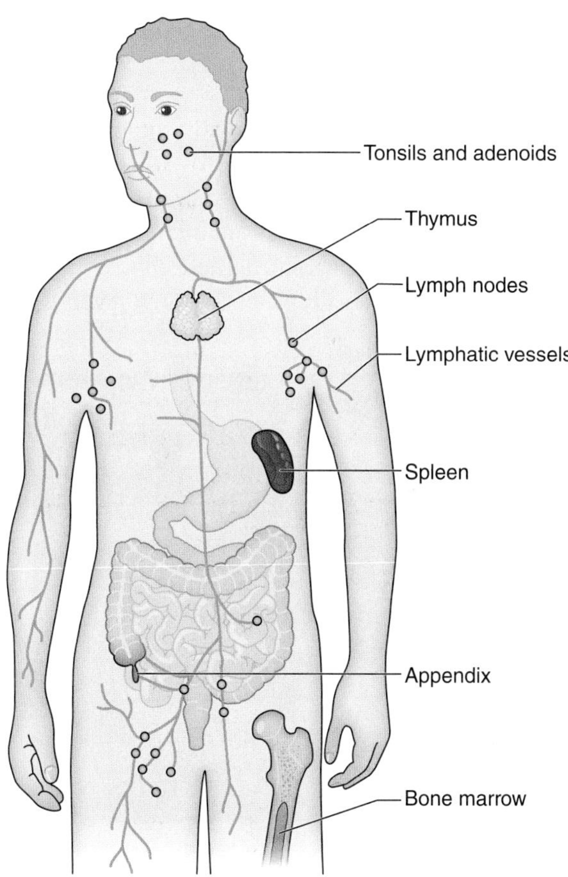

FIGURE 23.1 Your immune system, which consists of numerous components, fights infection and disease.

located throughout the body. Clusters of lymph nodes are in the neck, armpits, abdomen, and groin. The spleen is a flattened organ at the upper left of the abdomen. Like the lymph nodes, the spleen contains compartments where immune cells gather and work. The spleen serves as a meeting ground where immune defenses confront antigens (invaders). Other lymphoid tissues are throughout the body, especially in areas that serve as gateways for the body such as the linings of the digestive tract, airways, and lungs. These tissues include the tonsils, adenoids, and appendix. The lymphatic system mirrors the major blood vessels of the body, which allows cells and fluids to be exchanged between the blood and lymphatic vessels. This enables the lymphatic system to monitor the body for threats. Pathogens that pass through this system are attacked by specialized cells and killed. Together, these systems form your immune response.

Common Causes of Infectious Disease

The dangerous microorganisms called pathogens come in various forms, including bacteria, viruses, and fungi. The following discussion provides more detail, along with some examples.

Bacterial Infections

Bacteria are simple, single-cell organisms found in the air and soil, in food, and on plants and animals. Most bacteria are harmless to your health and some are helpful in digesting your food. Some can be dangerous because they give off poisonous substances known as toxins. About 100 known bacteria are dangerous to people.

One of the most common bacterial diseases that affects teens is strep throat. Strep, or streptococcus, bacteria typically invade the nose and throat and are transferred by contact with the mucus of an infected person. The infection is diagnosed by means of a throat swab performed by a physician. Common symptoms include sore throat, headache, fever, and swollen lymph nodes on the sides of the neck. Other common bacterial infections are lyme disease, bacterial meningitis, and tuberculosis. Most bacterial diseases are treated with an **antibiotic**—a kind of prescription drug that kills or inhibits the bacteria.

Viruses and Viral Infections

Viruses can multiply only once they have entered a living cell. Once inside, they take over the cell's reproductive cycle and ultimately cause cell damage or cell death. Viruses can be airborne, and they can also be found in body fluids, as in the case of **acquired immune deficiency syndrome (AIDS)**. A virus also does not respond to antibiotics. Some of the most common viral infections are described in the following sections.

Influenza and the Common Cold

Influenza, or flu, is a common viral infection that attacks the upper respiratory system. You can catch the flu by breathing in airborne droplets containing the virus or by coming into contact with a contaminated surface and touching the eyes, mouth, or nose. Symptoms include high fever, sore throat, headache, and cough.

HEALTH SCIENCE

Smallpox is an infectious disease that in earlier times killed millions of people worldwide. In 1796, physician Edward Jenner noticed that people who had contracted a related but less serious disease called cowpox seemed to develop a resistance to smallpox. To test his theory, he exposed a healthy boy to the cowpox disease. Once the boy recovered from that disease, Jenner injected him with the live smallpox virus. The boy did not get sick because he had developed immune defenses from cowpox that destroyed the smallpox virus.

Today, of course, vaccines are common, and they are given in one of two basic forms. Live vaccines are weakened versions of a pathogen, whereas inactivated vaccines consist of dead or incomplete forms of the pathogen. Both forms stimulate the body's immune system to develop antibodies that are associated with the disease in question. If the body is later exposed to the same pathogen, or disease-causing agent, it will recognize it and destroy it.

Vaccination is one of the greatest health science advancements in the modern era; it has helped reduce or eliminate illness and death due to various diseases worldwide. In fact, the U.S. Centers for Disease Control and Prevention (CDC) has identified 28 diseases that are preventable through vaccination, including hepatitis A and B, influenza, human papillomavirus, smallpox, measles, mumps, and yellow fever.

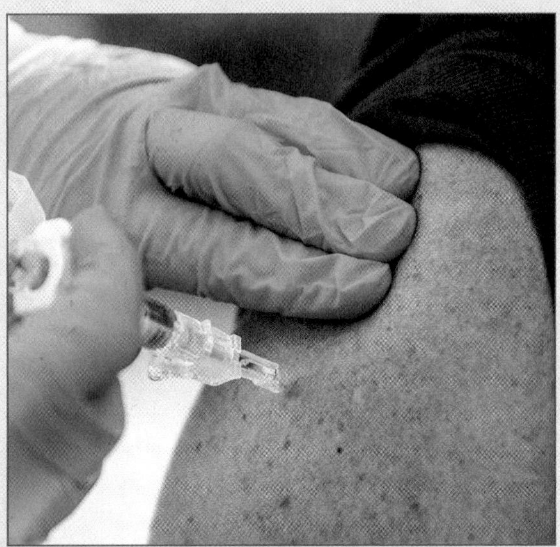

Immunization helps prevent many infectious diseases.

A serious case of the flu can be dangerous, and flu poses a significant threat to infants and elderly people. In the United States, as many as 30,000 people die from influenza each year. In recent years, flu vaccinations have become more common, and their use can help prevent large-scale outbreaks (see this chapter's Health Science feature for more on vaccination).

Many people mistake a common cold for influenza because it can produce similar symptoms; colds, however, are caused by different viruses. In addition, most colds last only 3 to 7 days, whereas the flu can last 10 days or more. Despite the large number of over-the-counter (OTC) cold remedies, there is no cure for the common cold. In fact, viral infections of all types have no known cure. The best-known remedies for overcoming a virus are rest, a balanced diet, and plenty of fluids. Over-the-counter and prescription medications may help you treat the symptoms of a cold or other virus. This can help your body in its own recovery process.

HEALTHY COMMUNICATION

Influenza is especially dangerous for older adults and young children. Thus it is important for members of both groups to understand how influenza is transmitted and what steps they can take to reduce their chance of getting the disease. If you were given 60 seconds to educate and influence members of each group, what would you say? How would your messages differ between the two groups?

Acquired Immune Deficiency Syndrome

Acquired immune deficiency syndrome (AIDS) is a sexually transmitted infection (STI) caused by the **human immunodeficiency virus (HIV)**. HIV is found in bodily fluids of infected people and can be transmitted to others through sexual contact and in blood (e.g., by sharing a needle). Pregnant women can also transmit the virus to a fetus through shared blood or to an infant through breast milk. HIV gradually attacks the immune system, making the infected person susceptible to many other infections and diseases. In almost all people, HIV progresses to AIDS over time. Remaining abstinent from both sexual activity and drug use is the only way for an adult to eliminate the risk of acquiring HIV and AIDS.

According to the U.S. government's National Institutes of Health (NIH), AIDS is the sixth leading cause of death among people aged 25 to 44 in the United States. Youth aged 13 to 24 account for about 5 percent of all U.S. AIDS cases. You can learn more about HIV and AIDS, other sexually transmitted infections, and their prevention and treatment in the student section of the Health Opportunities Through Physical Education website.

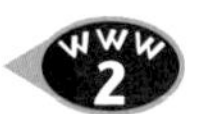

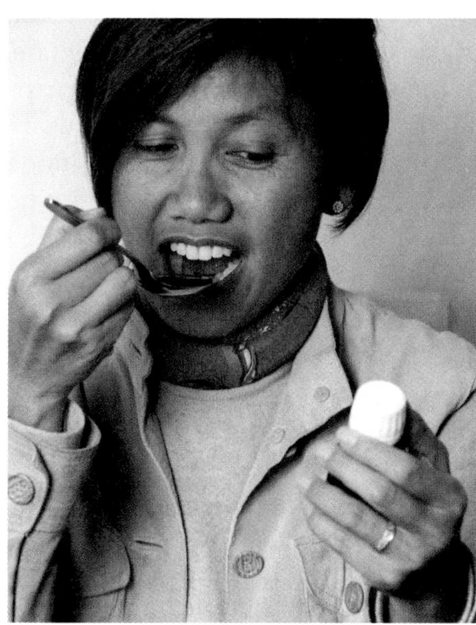

Over-the-counter medications may help relieve symptoms but they do not cure the common cold.

Hepatitis

Hepatitis is an infection of the liver that results in serious inflammation of that organ. There are five types, the most common of which are hepatitis A, B, and C. The main symptoms of these three types are fever, nausea, abdominal pain, and jaundice (yellowing of the skin).

Hepatitis A is most commonly transmitted in drinking water or food contaminated with the virus. Since the virus is found in feces, it spreads easily in settings marked by poor sanitation or poor personal hygiene. Hepatitis A can also be contracted by eating fruit, vegetables, or other foods contaminated during handling or by eating raw shellfish harvested from contaminated water.

Hepatitis B is spread through contact with blood or body fluid from an infected person; thus common causes of transmission include sharing needles and having unprotected sex. Most cases of hepatitis B are short term, and many infected people are not aware of being sick because the symptoms are generally mild and resemble those of the flu.

Hepatitis C, however, can lead to permanent liver damage as well as cirrhosis (scarring of the liver), liver cancer, and liver failure. Like hepatitis B, hepatitis C is spread through contact with an infected person's blood and produces mild symptoms. Unlike hepatitis B, it is usually chronic (long term), and an infected person typically has it for 15 years before being diagnosed.

Vaccines exist for hepatitis A and B. They are typically required for anyone working in the health care industry. Anyone with hepatitis should seek medical care from a physician.

Fungi and Fungal Infections

Fungi are single-cell and multicell organisms that thrive in warm, humid environments; examples are yeast, mold, and mushrooms. About half of all known fungi are dangerous to humans. Infection is typically caused by a fungus landing on the skin or being inhaled into the lungs, which can result in an internal infection. A fungus can also be ingested in spoiled food. A fungus attacks the body by releasing

Travel-Related Viruses

Severe acute respiratory syndrome (SARS) is a viral disease caused by a coronavirus. It was discovered in Asia in 2003; it then spread to two dozen countries on four continents within a few months. SARS typically begins with a high fever, headache, and body aches. It may result in a dry cough. Most people who contract SARS develop pneumonia or other respiratory infections, and it is considered more dangerous and deadly than common influenza. In fact, SARS is one of several viral diseases that threaten global health. Fortunately, SARS is relatively rare, but it does prove that infectious diseases can spread unexpectedly.

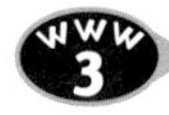

You should also be aware of some other globally active viral diseases when traveling overseas, including avian influenza, yellow fever, and dengue fever. The CDC maintains a database of travel-related health concerns and provides up-to-date recommendations about inoculations and medications needed for safe travel.

enzymes that digest or dissolve cells that it contacts. Fungal infections are treated with antifungal medications and creams.

One common fungal infection is **athlete's foot.** It begins like other fungal infections when a small amount of the fungus lands on the skin. It then multiplies in the warm, moist environment of the sock and shoe. You're more likely to get athlete's foot if you wear closed-toed shoes lacking good ventilation, sweat often, have wet feet for long periods, or get a toenail or skin infection on a foot. To prevent athlete's foot, change shoes often, allow shoes to air out, change socks frequently, and wash your feet thoroughly every day.

Protozoan Infections

A **protozoan** is a single-cell organism that can move through the body in search of food. It attacks the body by releasing enzymes or toxins that can destroy or damage cells. Malaria is a protozoan-based disease that attacks the red blood cells and is common in parts of Africa and many tropical locations. Malaria is transmitted by 50 of the 480 known mosquito species around the globe. In the United States, malaria-carrying mosquitoes were eliminated in the late 1940s and early 1950s. Today, malaria is rare in the United States and is typically seen only in people who have traveled to a malaria-infected country.

Other Types of Pathogens

Infectious diseases can also be caused by larger pathogens, such as lice, mites, and some worms. For example, the trichina worm can live in the muscle tissue of various animals, including bears, foxes, and pigs. If an infected animal is consumed, the worm can invade the person who ate the contaminated meat. It can then cause a foodborne illness known as trichinosis. The best prevention against trichinosis and other pathogens transferred in food and meat products is to ensure that all food is properly handled (cleaned, separated, and stored safely) and that meat is fully cooked at an appropriate temperature.

Preventing Infectious Disease

We're all exposed to potential sources of infection every day. To reduce your chance of becoming ill with an infectious disease, follow these guidelines.

- **Wash your hands with soap and water.** This is especially important before and after preparing food, before eating, and after using the toilet. Use sanitizers when soap and water are not available.
- **Cover your nose and mouth when coughing or sneezing.** Use a tissue or handkerchief to cover your nose and mouth fully, or sneeze or cough into a sleeve. Try to keep your hands clean, or wash them immediately if you must use them to cover your cough or sneeze. Covering properly helps reduce the spread of infection to others.
- **Get vaccinated.** Immunization drastically reduces your chances of contracting many diseases.

CONSUMER CORNER: Choosing Hand Sanitizers

The popularity of alcohol-based hand sanitizers has skyrocketed in recent years. They are readily available in most convenience stores, grocery stores, and pharmacies and can often be found in public restrooms, cruise ship lobbies, schools, hospitals, and even outdoor play areas. Most alcohol-based hand sanitizers offer good protection against a host of germs, including bacteria, fungi, and other pathogens. They typically contain isopropanol, ethanol, n-propanol, or a combination of these ingredients. When selecting and using a hand sanitizer, consider the following points.

- Purchase a sanitizer with an alcohol content of 60 to 95 percent. Anything less makes the product ineffective.
- Sanitizers come in the form of foam, liquid, and gel. Foam sanitizers are excellent but often more expensive. Select a thicker gel sanitizer, since research shows that more of it makes it onto your hands.
- Use an adequate amount of the product to completely wet all surfaces of your hands and fingers. Rub your hands together for 10 to 15 seconds. If your hands dry before then, you haven't used enough.
- If your hands are visibly soiled, don't rely on hand sanitizers to do the job. Research shows that sanitizers are not effective when excess dirt and debris are on the hands.
- When possible, wash your hands with warm soapy water before using an alcohol-based hand sanitizer. This combination is your best bet for killing a wide range of germs.

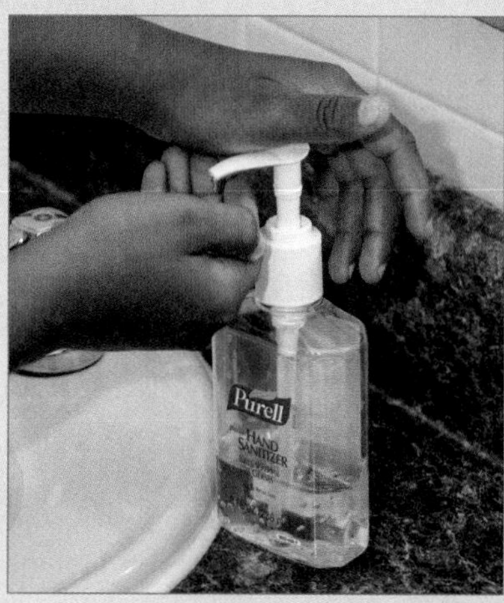

Use an adequate amount of hand sanitizer to completely wet all surfaces of the hands and fingers.

Consumer Challenge

How should hands be washed in order to provide the best protection against disease? For the answer, visit the CDC website (www.cdc.gov).

- **Stay home.** Don't go to school if you're vomiting, have diarrhea, are coughing and sneezing, or have a fever.
- **Prepare food safely.** Keep counters and other kitchen surfaces clean when preparing meals. Promptly refrigerate leftovers—don't let cooked foods remain at room temperature for extended periods.
- **Remain abstinent or, if sexually active, practice safe sex.** The best method of avoiding any STI is to practice abstinence. If you are sexually active, always use a condom and remain sexually monogamous. You can learn more about the role contraceptives play in disease prevention by visiting the student section of the Health Opportunities Through Physical Education website. WWW 4
- **Don't share personal items.** Use your own toothbrush, comb, and razor. Avoid sharing drinking glasses or dining utensils.
- **Travel wisely.** Don't travel in confined spaces like trains and planes when you're ill.

Comprehension Check

1. What is an infectious disease? List three types of pathogens that cause infectious disease.
2. Briefly describe two specific examples of infectious disease.
3. Identify four ways to protect yourself from infectious disease.

SELF-ASSESSMENT: My Disease Prevention IQ

Indicate your level of agreement with each statement in the questionnaire. Record the number of points associated with each response and add them together for your total. Interpret your disease prevention IQ score using the scale provided at the end of the questionnaire. *Note:* This is for your personal information and is not intended to be turned in to your teacher.

	Always 3	Sometimes 2	Never 1
Behaviors related to chronic disease			
1. I balance calories (calories in equal calories out) to maintain a healthy weight.	3	2	1
2. I participate in moderate to vigorous physical activity for 60 minutes every day.	3	2	1
3. I do muscle-fitness exercises (e.g., push-ups, sit-ups) at least two to three times per week.	3	2	1
4. I don't smoke or use any tobacco products.	3	2	1
5. I eat at least five servings of fruits and vegetables every day.	3	2	1
6. I avoid foods and drinks high in sugar and caffeine.	3	2	1
7. I avoid foods high in fat.	3	2	1
8. I regularly protect myself from the sun by wearing sunscreen, a hat, and long sleeves and long pants.	3	2	1
9. I go to the doctor regularly for checkups.	3	2	1

	Always 3	Sometimes 2	Never 1
Behaviors related to infectious disease			
10. I wash my hands every time I use the restroom and when I prepare or eat food.	3	2	1
11. I get appropriate vaccinations, including a yearly flu shot.	3	2	1
12. I stay home when I am sick and may be contagious.	3	2	1
13. I use only clean surfaces and utensils when preparing or eating food.	3	2	1
14. I avoid sharing personal items (e.g., razors, utensils, drinking cups, bottles).	3	2	1
15. I help keep a clean house, especially the kitchen and bathroom.	3	2	1
16. I cover my mouth with a tissue or handkerchief when I cough or sneeze or use my sleeve or forearm.	3	2	1
17. I protect myself from sexually transmitted infections.	3	2	1

Add up your points.
My disease prevention IQ score is: ___________

A score of 40 to 51 indicates lower risk, meaning that your habits and behaviors lower your risk for chronic and infectious diseases. Work to maintain or even strengthen your healthy habits.

A score of 30 to 39 indicates moderate risk, meaning that you have some good habits, but others might be putting you at risk. Try to be more consistent in your habits and adopt more healthy habits.

A score of 29 or lower indicates higher risk, meaning that your habits and behaviors may be putting you at higher risk for chronic and infectious diseases. It's time to make some changes.

✓ Planning for Healthy Living

Use the Healthy Living Plan worksheet to improve one or more of your disease prevention habits.

Lesson 23.2

Chronic Diseases and Disabilities

Lesson Objectives

After reading this lesson, you should be able to

1. identify and describe the most common chronic diseases in our society;
2. describe the consequences of chronic diseases; and
3. define disability and identify common types of disabilities, and differentiate between a disability and a handicap.

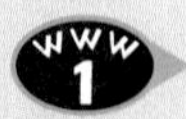

Lesson Vocabulary

Americans With Disabilities Act, arteriosclerosis, atherosclerosis, cancer, cardiovascular disease (CVD), chronic disease, coronary heart disease, dementia, diabetes, disability, hypertension, stroke

Most infectious diseases go away once the infection is attacked by your immune system or is properly treated. **Chronic diseases** last a long time, sometimes a lifetime. Most people who live into old age develop at least one chronic disease. If a friend or family member has had cancer or high blood pressure, or if you know someone with diabetes or arthritis, then you know someone whose health has been affected by a chronic disease. In fact, chronic diseases are the most common causes of death in the United States.

Although it's the most serious, death isn't the only consequence of a chronic disease. Chronic disease can progress into disability with time, lack of treatment, or an aggressive form of the illness. But disabilities don't always develop as a result of a chronic disease. Some disabilities may be present from birth. Examples are vision, hearing, mobility, or cognitive impairments. In this lesson you'll learn about common chronic diseases and how to interact respectfully with people who have disabilities.

Chronic Diseases

In the previous lesson you learned about infectious diseases such as the flu and cold. When you get the flu or catch a cold, you have an acute illness, or one that you get over within a relatively short time. Imagine, though, if those cold or flu symptoms never went away, and if the limitations they put on your activities never let up. In the following sections you'll learn about common chronic diseases and what you can do now to avoid them.

Cardiovascular Disease

Cardiovascular disease (CVD) refers to chronic diseases that affect the circulatory system. One in four Americans has one or more cardiovascular diseases, and these diseases contribute to 60 percent of all deaths in the nation. The most common cardiovascular diseases are discussed here; many other forms also exist.

Coronary Heart Disease

The most common form of CVD is **coronary heart disease**, in which the arteries in the heart become clogged or hardened. This is the leading cause of death in the United States. Clogged arteries, a condition called **atherosclerosis** (figure 23.2), can result from eating a high-fat diet, getting too little exercise, smoking, or being very overweight.

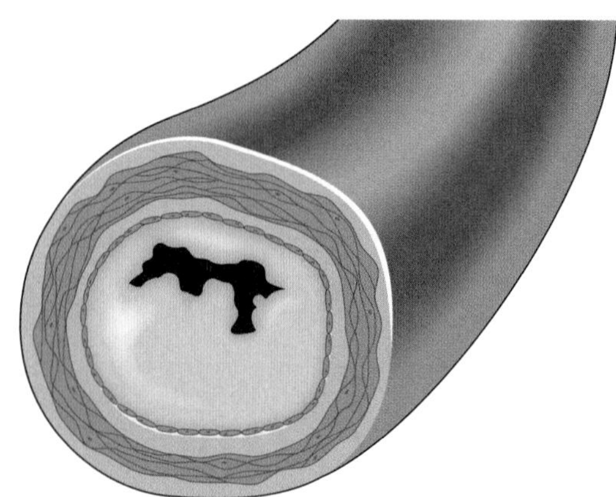

FIGURE 23.2 Plaque buildup in coronary heart disease.

Hardened (inflexible) arteries, a condition called **arteriosclerosis**, tend to occur as we age, but we can limit its effects by living a healthy lifestyle. Both of these cardiovascular diseases can decrease blood flow to the heart muscle, which can lead to chest pain known as angina and heart attacks. A heart attack is a cutting off of blood flow to a portion of the heart, which causes the cells in that area to die. Figure 23.3 shows how a blood clot or piece of plaque can break loose and block blood flow to the heart.

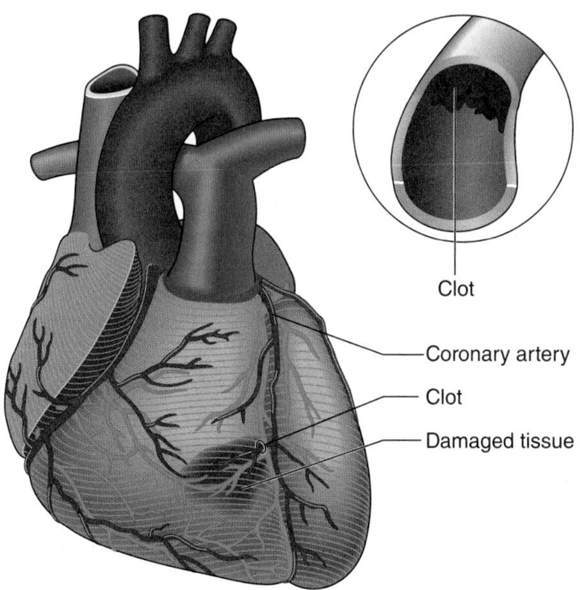

FIGURE 23.3 A blood clot can cause a heart attack by preventing the heart from getting enough oxygenated blood.

Stroke

Inadequate blood supply can also damage the brain. For example, atherosclerosis or a blood clot can block an artery that supplies the brain with blood and cause a **stroke**. This is the most common type of stroke, and it is called an ischemic stroke (inadequate blood supply). A stroke can also occur if a blood vessel in the brain bursts, causing severe bleeding; this type is known as a hemorrhagic stroke. Some strokes are severe enough to cause death, and many others result in disability. This is the fourth leading cause of death in the United States. A person has a **disability** when he or she is unable to perform activities or actions in the way they would normally be performed due to a restriction or impairment (see the Disability section later in this lesson for more information). After a stroke, many people have speech or movement disability due to the damage caused in the brain.

Peripheral Artery Disease

Atherosclerosis can also occur in arteries that take blood to parts of the body other than the heart, and this condition is called peripheral artery disease (PAD). It can compromise circulation to organs and limbs, resulting in symptoms that include leg pain, muscle aches, poor nail or hair growth, decreased temperature in one leg or arm, or sores and wounds on the toes that don't heal properly. About eight million Americans have PAD. The risk of developing it increases with age, and it is more common among people who smoke or have diabetes, high blood pressure, or high cholesterol.

High Blood Pressure

Another form of CVD is high blood pressure, also known as **hypertension**. Each time your heart beats, it moves blood through your arteries at high speed and with a certain amount of force. The amount, or measure, of that force is your blood pressure. People with high blood pressure have higher than normal amounts of force in their arteries, which can damage artery walls as it pushes blood against them. High blood pressure is a risk factor for both coronary heart disease and stroke.

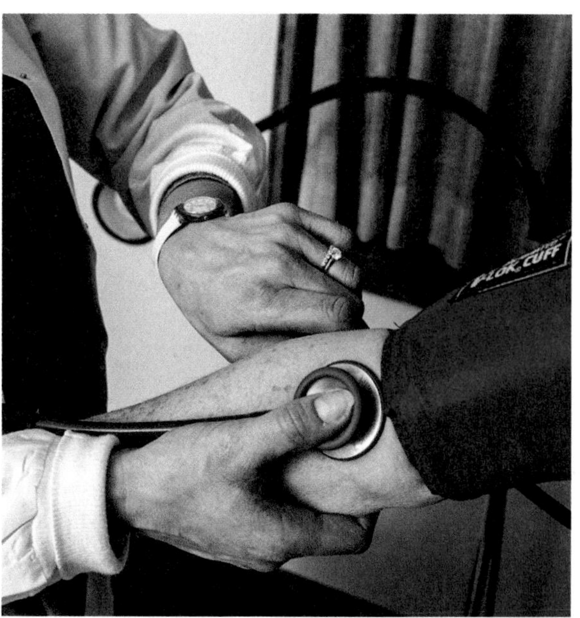

Monitoring blood pressure is a tool for reducing the risk of coronary heart disease and stroke.

PhotoDisc

HEALTH TECHNOLOGY

Scanning and imaging technologies can help determine whether a person has a chronic disease. The common X ray is still useful in assessing damage to bones and other structures. Technological advances have also produced methods for seeing three-dimensional and color images of internal parts of the body. For example, computed tomography (CT) scans provide a series of images stacked together to form a three-dimensional image of an organ or other body area (like slices of bread stacked together to form a loaf). Another technique is magnetic resonance imaging (MRI), which uses a magnetic field and pulses of radio wave energy to form pictures of organs and other structures inside the body. MRI images can show more detail than either conventional X rays or CT scans.

Such technologies have many uses. For example, they can help find cancers and detect blockages in arteries and veins that occur with cardiovascular disease. Ongoing technological advances in scanning and imaging are continuing to make the machines increasingly sophisticated and the resulting images sharper and more useful.

CONNECT

What if you could have a free medical scan of all your body systems that would locate any infections or diseases and tell you of any physical abnormalities or early signs of disease? Would you want to do it? Could there be any negative aspects to the scan? Do you think medical insurance should pay for this type of preventive screening? Why or why not?

Cancer

The term **cancer** refers to uncontrolled growth of abnormal cells in the body. There are dozens of types of cancer; see table 23.1 for information about some of the more common types. In the United States, the most common types among men are prostate, lung, and colon cancer, and the most common types among women are breast, lung, and colon cancer. Cancer is the second leading cause of death in the United States, accounting for more than half a million deaths per year.

Symptoms, treatment, and survival rate for cancer depend on the type and location of the cancer and how advanced it is at the time of the diagnosis. Though all cancers are different, common symptoms of cancer are fatigue, fever, chills, loss of appetite, weight loss, and night sweats. Regular physical exams and cancer screenings are important for catching cancers in developing stages, when they can often be effectively removed or stopped. Great advances have been made in cancer screenings and treatments, and many common cancers, such as prostate and breast cancer, have increasing survival rates. If left untreated or if treatment is ineffective, cancer can spread to multiple organs. Known risks

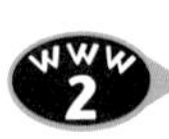

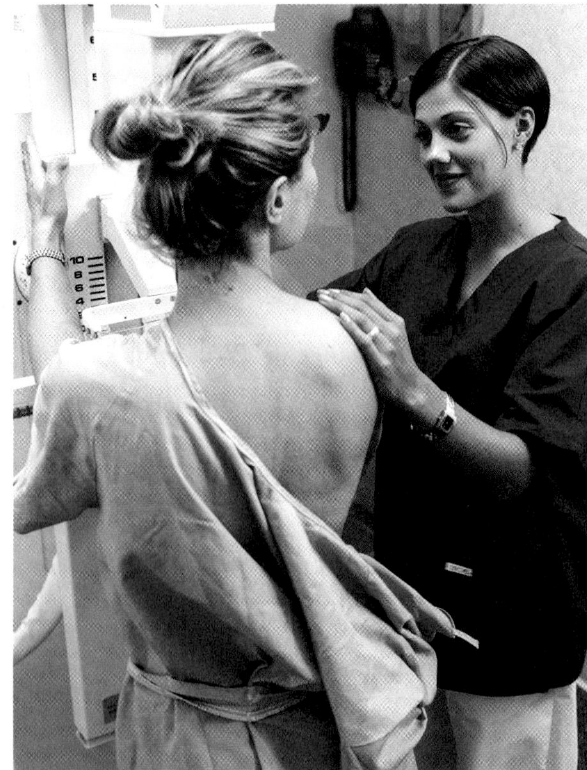

Cancer screenings are important for catching cancers in developing stages.

ImageState Photos

TABLE 23.1 Common Types of Cancer

Type of cancer	Description	Risk factors
Bladder	Most commonly attacks the cells lining the inside of the bladder.	Smoking, family history of bladder cancer, exposure to arsenic and other workplace chemicals
Breast	Multiple types exist. This is the most commonly diagnosed cancer among women; men may also get it.	Increasing age, early first menstrual period, family history of breast or uterine cancer, being overweight, physical inactivity, high alcohol consumption, genetics
Colon	Attacks the colon or rectum. It is the third most common type of cancer among women and the second most common among men.	Family history of colon cancer, history of polyps, being over the age of 50, smoking, high-fat diet
Leukemia	Cancer of the bone marrow and blood cells. Multiple types exist, including some that are most common among children.	Genetics, exposure to radiation, smoking, certain related disorders and diseases
Lung	This is the leading cause of cancer deaths among both men and women.	Tobacco smoke, pollution, family history, asbestos and radon exposure, being over age 65
Melanoma	This is a skin cancer caused by excessive sun exposure.	Accumulated sun exposure or tanning bed, severe sunburns that blister (especially before age 18)
Prostate	Attacks the male prostate gland and is the leading cause of cancer among men.	Being over age 65, family history of prostate cancer, being African American, genetics

Preventing Skin Cancer

Only half of all teens report using sunscreen on a regular basis, and 80 percent believe that tan skin makes people look healthier. Although those with light skin are more susceptible to skin cancer, it does not mean that people with dark skin are immune to skin cancer. Unfortunately, sun exposure is especially risky for teens because the teenage years are a time of rapid cell division. Over the long term, tanning reduces skin elasticity, which leads to more wrinkles and can cause uneven skin tones as seen with sun spots and age spots. Tanning also significantly increases the chances of developing skin cancer. To help prevent skin cancer, follow these recommendations from the CDC.

- Seek shade, especially during midday hours.
- Wear clothing that protects your skin, such as long pants, long-sleeve shirts, and hats. You can also wear clothing made with sun-protective fabric (i.e., fabric treated specifically to protect from the sun's rays).
- Wear a hat with a wide brim to shade your face, head, ears, and neck.
- Wear sunglasses that wrap around and block both UVA (long wave) and UVB (short wave) rays. Ultraviolet (UV) rays penetrate the earth's atmosphere and are responsible for damage to the skin.
- Use sunscreen with a sun protection factor (SPF) of 15 or higher and with both UVA and UVB protection.
- Avoid indoor tanning.

for cancer include lifestyle factors such as smoking, physical inactivity, high-fat diet, and exposure to ultraviolet radiation from the sun (e.g., through sunbathing, tanning, or spending time outdoors without using sunscreen and other proper precautions).

Lung Disease

The term *lung disease* refers to a number of conditions that affect the lungs and the ability to take in and use an adequate amount of oxygen. It is the third leading cause of death in the United States. One common lung disease is inflammation of the lungs, or asthma, which can result in spasms of the lung tissue that cause wheezing and breathing difficulty. Asthma can be managed with proper medication, and individuals with this condition can lead normal lives.

Another common lung disease is chronic obstructive pulmonary disease, or COPD. It involves difficulty in exhaling air from the lungs, and the trapped air can cause coughing and tissue damage. Two forms of COPD are emphysema and bronchitis (see figure 23.4). Emphysema occurs when air sacs in the lungs are gradually destroyed, making the person progressively short of breath. In bronchitis, the lung's mucous membrane becomes inflamed, and the swelling causes coughing spells. Both emphysema and bronchitis can be caused by and made worse by smoking.

Lung disease can also result from bacterial infections, such as pneumonia and tuberculosis. Lung cancer, commonly associated with smoking, is one of the most common cancers in the United States. Many other forms of lung disease also exist, and lung disease is the third most common cause of death in the United States.

Dementia and Alzheimer's Disease

Dementia involves loss of brain function over time (see figure 23.5). It can affect memory, thinking, language use, judgment, and behavior. Most causes of dementia are irreversible, meaning that the damage caused to the brain cannot be repaired. The most common cause of dementia symptoms is Alzheimer's disease, which has a genetic component and tends to run in families. It is the sixth leading cause of death in the United States. It is also more common among females, people over age 65, and people with a history of high blood pressure or head trauma. Alzheimer's affects more than five million people in the United States.

Since people with the disease are unable to fully care for themselves, many families are left to provide unpaid and unskilled care for family members with Alzheimer's or another cause of dementia. Caregivers have physical, emotional, and financial strain, which can put their own health at risk. To learn more, visit the student section of the Health Opportunities Through Physical Education website.

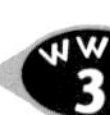

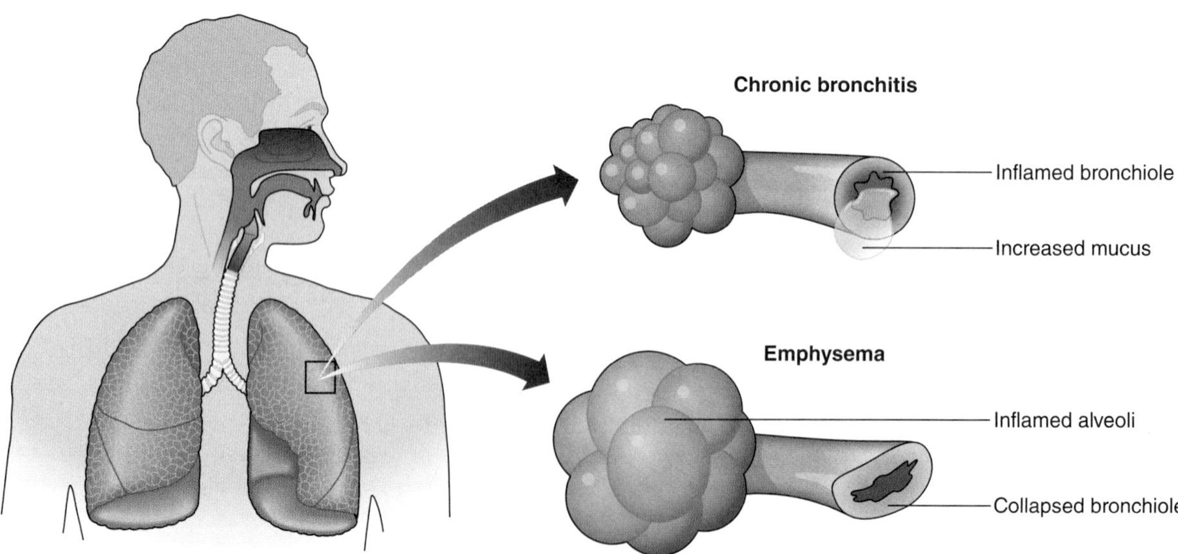

FIGURE 23.4 In emphysema, the airways collapse and damaged air sacs enlarge, causing shortness of breath and wheezing. In chronic bronchitis, the airways become inflamed and filled with mucus.

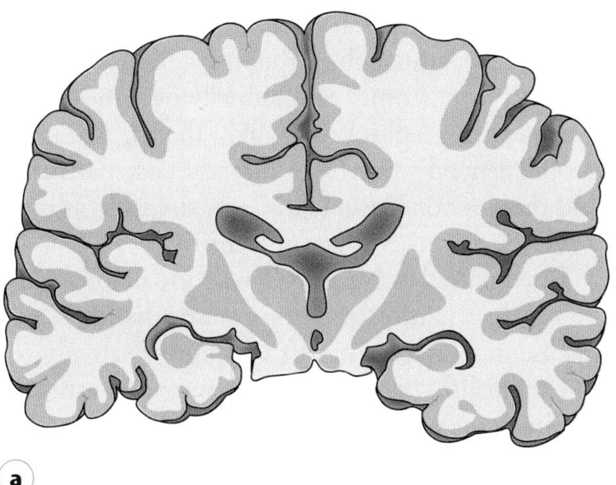

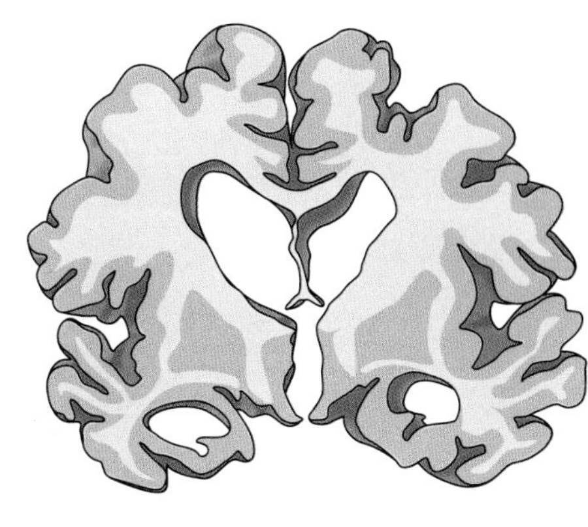

a b

FIGURE 23.5 When compared with (*a*) a normal brain, (*b*) a cross-section of brain with Alzheimer's disease is smaller and shriveled.

Diabetes

Diabetes is a chronic disease related to having too much sugar (glucose) in the blood. It is the seventh leading cause of death in the United States. The body is normally able to use blood sugar or store it in muscle and liver cells with help from the hormone insulin. Produced by the pancreas, insulin acts like a key that opens the way for sugar to enter the cells. This process is critical because the human body cannot function properly if cells cannot access needed fuel from blood sugar. Diabetes results from either a lack of insulin (type 1 diabetes) or improperly functioning insulin (type 2 diabetes).

Type 1 diabetes has a strong genetic component and is most likely to develop in childhood, adolescence, or early adulthood. Symptoms include excessive thirst, hunger, weight loss, and frequent urination. Those with type 1 diabetes must monitor blood sugar and take insulin before eating in order to properly use the sugar in their blood.

Type 2 diabetes is strongly related to obesity and can develop at any age. In recent years, type 2 diabetes (formerly referred to as adult-onset diabetes) has become more common in the United States among children, teenagers, and young adults as obesity rates in these populations have increased. It typically requires a combination of medication, exercise, and a healthy diet for management. Many may not exhibit symptoms until the disease is relatively severe. Symptoms can include any of those for type 1 as well as blurred vision and frequent infections. The symptoms of diabetes may not be present in the early stages of the disease. Because many people with type 2 diabetes are often overweight or obese, weight loss is often effective in treatment. However, diabetes can occur in people who are not obese or overweight.

Pregnant women can also develop a form of diabetes, called gestational diabetes, which can put both mother and infant at risk for immediate and long-term complications. Altogether, according to the American Diabetes Association, about 8 percent of Americans, including 1 in every 400 children, have diabetes.

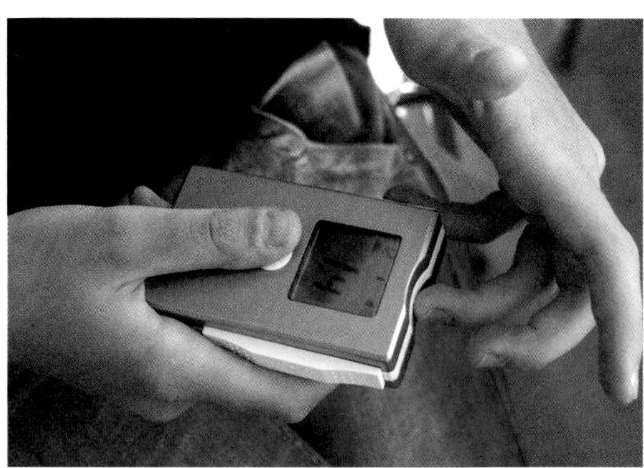

Monitoring blood sugar is a regular part of managing diabetes.

Phototom/fotolia.com

Osteoporosis

Osteoporosis is a chronic disease in which the bones lose density and become weaker (see figure 23.6). It can result from the body either being unable to

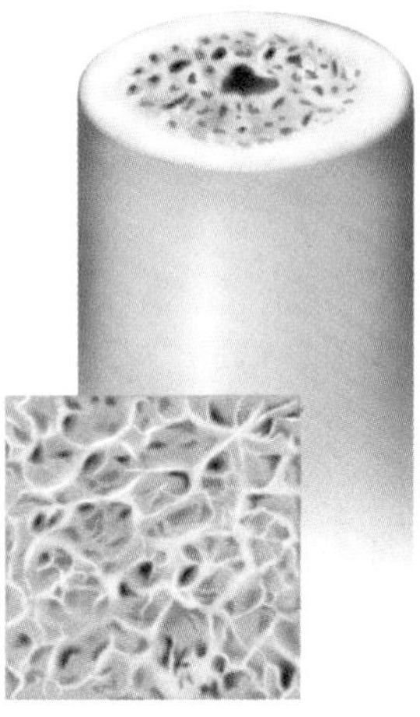

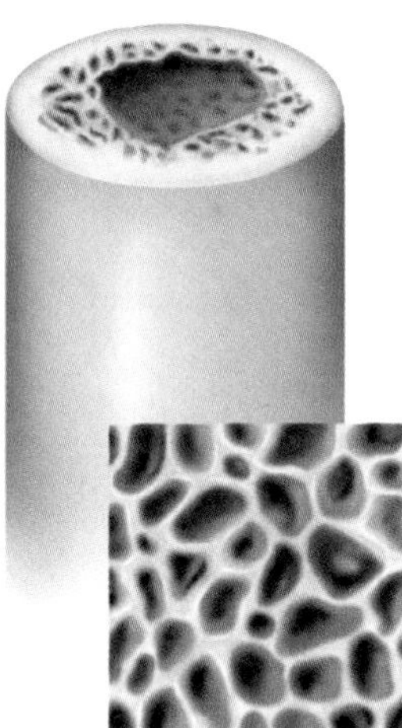

FIGURE 23.6 Osteoporosis involves a decrease in bone density.

make new bone or absorbing calcium and phosphate from the bones. The disease affects one of every five women and one of every four men in the United States over the age of 50. Its primary cause involves normal changes in the levels of estrogen and testosterone associated with aging. Risk is increased for people who smoke, are underweight, have vitamin D deficiency, or are bedridden. Risk is also higher for women of European heritage.

Some young people can develop osteoporosis if they have an eating disorder for an extended time. This situation is particularly dangerous because their bones are still developing (peak bone density generally occurs between the ages of 25 and 30). You can help your bones develop properly—and reduce your risk of osteoporosis—by engaging in weight-bearing physical activity and eating a balanced diet during your adolescent and early adult years.

Arthritis

Arthritis (Greek word meaning joint and *itis* meaning inflammation) involves inflammation and damage in the joints (see figure 23.7). There are more than a hundred types of arthritis and related joint conditions. Two of the most common forms of arthritis are osteoarthritis and rheumatoid arthritis. Osteoarthritis is also called degenerative joint disease or degenerative arthritis. It affects about 33 million Americans and is the most common chronic joint condition. Osteoarthritis results from joint overuse. It is most common in joints that bear weight such as the knees, hips, feet, and spine. It often comes on gradually over months or even years. Except for the pain in the affected joint, people generally don't feel sick from osteoarthritis, and there is no unusual fatigue or tiredness as there is with some other types of arthritis.

Rheumatoid arthritis (RA) is a form of inflammatory arthritis and is an autoimmune disease (i.e., a disease in which the body's immune system attacks its own healthy tissues). With rheumatoid arthritis, the immune system attacks the synovium, a thin membrane that lines the joints. The attack causes fluid to build up in the joints resulting in pain and inflammation. Rheumatoid arthritis is a chronic disease that is systemic, meaning it can also attack other parts of the body. Most people with RA have intermittent bouts of intense disease activity called flares. For others, the disease is continuously active and gets worse over time. Some people with RA enjoy long periods of remission where no disease activity or symptoms are present.

Though arthritis is commonly thought of as a disease of older adulthood, some variation of it also affects about 1 in every 250 people under the age of 18. Common symptoms of many types of arthritis are stiffness, swelling, joint pain, and loss of joint mobility. Methods for managing the disease's effects on daily living vary by type and often include exercise, proper diet, physical therapy, medication, and, in some cases, joint replacement surgery. Maintaining

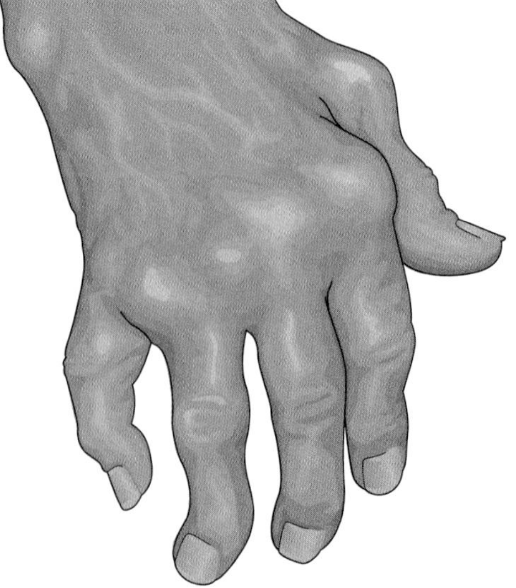

FIGURE 23.7 Severe arthritis can result in deformities and pain that dramatically affect mobility.

a healthy weight, participating in low-impact exercise and physical activity, using good posture and body mechanics when doing active jobs and chores, and appropriately treating joint injuries like sprains and strains can help reduce likelihood of getting arthritis later in life.

Preventing Chronic Disease

Many chapters in part 2 of this book address ways of preventing chronic disease. For now, review the following suggestions for reducing your risk of chronic diseases such as coronary heart disease, diabetes, cancer, and lung disease. You can find more detailed information about smoking, body weight, exercise, and diet in the chapters dedicated to those topics.

Avoid Tobacco Use

- Avoiding tobacco, especially in the form of cigarettes, is the single most important way to prevent all forms of cardiovascular disease as well as lung disease and cancer.

Get Daily Physical Activity and Limit Screen Time

- Do aerobic exercise: Most of the 60 or more minutes of daily recommended physical activity should be of either moderate or vigorous intensity. Do vigorous physical activity at least three days per week.
- Do muscle-strengthening exercise: As part of the 60 or more minutes of daily recommended physical activity, do muscle-strengthening activity at least three days per week.
- Engage in bone-strengthening exercise: As part of the 60 or more minutes of daily physical activity, do bone-strengthening physical activity (weight-bearing exercise) at least three days per week.
- Limit screen time use (e.g., television, computer and tablet, video game, app) to no more than two hours a day.

Eat a Healthy Diet

- Limit your consumption of saturated fat (e.g., in meat products).
- Eat a generous amount of fruits and vegetables.
- Eat cereal and grain products in their whole-grain, high-fiber form.
- Limit your consumption of sugar and sugar-based beverages.
- Avoid excessive calorie intake from any source.
- Limit your sodium intake.

Disability

Disabilities are reported by about 21 percent of the U.S. population each year. Disabilities can include physical, cognitive or intellectual, emotional, and mobility impairments (see table 23.2). People with a disability share the same hopes and dreams for their lives as people who do not have a disability. One part of our social responsibility to each other is to make efforts to ensure that people with disabilities have the same opportunities available to individuals without a disability.

Some people confuse being handicapped with having a disability. You can have a disability or impairment without being handicapped. Being handicapped limits or prevents the fulfillment of a role.

In the legal arena, the **Americans With Disabilities Act** ensures the civil rights of all Americans who have a mental or physical disability. The law protects individuals with all forms of disability, including those that emerge as part of a chronic disease, such as cancer or AIDS. The law guarantees equal opportunity in employment, public services, public transportation, public accommodations, and communication. A similar law, the Individuals With Disabilities Education Act, ensures equal opportunity in education.

In your own interactions, treat individuals with a disability respectfully. Don't refer to a person in terms of his or her disability. For example, avoid saying, "This is my blind friend Sarah." If it is necessary or helpful to alert others of a person's disability, then introduce the person first. For example, say "This is my friend Sarah; she is visually impaired." Use the person's name first and remember that a person with a disability is a human being, just as you are.

> "All interest in disease and death is only another expression of interest in life."
>
> —Thomas Mann, author

TABLE 23.2 Common Forms of Disability

Disability	Things to know	Things to consider
Vision impairments	• Visual impairment, including blindness, affects 2 percent of the population. • The chance of vision impairment increases with age. • Common causes of visual impairment include diabetes, cataracts (cloudiness in the eye), glaucoma (pressure in the eye), and macular degeneration (related to aging).	• Avoid startling the person. • Speak up right away. • Speak clearly and pay attention to your use of nonverbal gestures. • Use clear descriptions of where things are located and who is nearby. • Do not touch the person or a guide dog without permission. • If the person asks to be guided, extend your arm and allow him or her to hold on to it.
Hearing impairments	• Hearing impairment affects 3.5 percent of the population. • The chance of hearing impairment increases with age (it affects one-third of adults over age 60). • Listening to loud music through earbuds or headphones might increase your risk of hearing impairment over time.	• Touch the person gently on the arm or shoulder to get his or her attention. • Stand directly in front of the person when speaking so that he or she can see your mouth when you speak. • Do not shout. • Speak slowly and clearly. • Use sign language if you and the person both know it.
Mobility impairments	• Impaired mobility affects about 7 percent of the population. • Mobility impairment can result from disease, injury, or a birth defect. • Mobility aids and prosthetics can help many individuals maintain their independence.	• Be patient and move only as quickly as the individual does. • Give assistance only if asked. • If a person uses a wheelchair or is seated, squat down or sit. When possible, avoid "talking down" to the person. • Be positive and encouraging if the person wants to try an activity, sport, or physical task.
Cognitive impairments	• There are a wide range of cognitive impairments. • Cognitive impairments include conditions such as Down syndrome, traumatic brain injury, autism, and dementia. • Aging contributes to cognitive impairments like dementia.	• Move to a quiet place free of noise and distractions. • Be willing to repeat yourself without becoming frustrated. • Be patient and allow more time for the person to respond to questions or demands.
Emotional impairments	• Emotional impairments can include a wide range of emotional disorders (see chapter on emotional health and wellness). • Emotional impairments can also involve serious sensory impairments such as hearing voices or hallucinating.	• Be patient and empathetic. • If a person seems to suffer from hearing voices or hallucinations, a calm, controlled, and careful approach to interactions is recommended. In these instances avoid physical contact or sudden movements.

Comprehension Check

1. Identify and describe the most common chronic diseases.
2. Describe the consequences of chronic diseases.
3. What is the difference between a handicap and a disability?

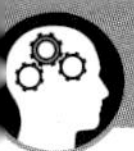

MAKING HEALTHY DECISIONS: Identifying Risk Factors

Yesenia noticed that her older sister, Selena, had recently gained a little weight and seemed to be sick a lot. In addition, in the last few months, Selena had often complained of being cold and thirsty. Most nights, the sisters were home alone because their mom worked two jobs and their dad had passed away three years earlier due to heart disease. The girls tended to eat fast food or frozen meals for dinner and spent a lot of time in front of the computer. Yesenia did play softball at school, but Selena preferred fashion and art and spent most of her time designing clothes or following the latest trends online.

The girls' older brother, Marcos, weighed 250 pounds (113 kilograms) and had been diagnosed with type 2 diabetes at age 17. His doctor had told him that he needed to lose weight, exercise daily, and go on a special diet if he wanted to improve his health and reduce his own chance of developing heart disease. Since then, Marcos had been pretty good about taking walks and lifting weights at the community center, and sometimes he cooked for himself and his sisters at home.

For Discussion

What chronic diseases and disorders seem to run in this family? What behaviors contribute to their risk for developing chronic disease? Which sister is at increased risk based on her behavior? What healthy behaviors do members of the family practice? What should Yesenia say to Selena about her behavior and health risks? To help you answer these questions, read this chapter's Skills for Healthy Living feature.

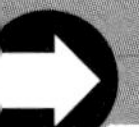

SKILLS FOR HEALTHY LIVING: Identifying Risk Factors

To prevent infectious and chronic diseases, you need to recognize and monitor risk factors and take effective action. Take the time to get familiar with common diseases and their risk factors and monitor your decisions and behaviors. Here are some helpful tips.

- **Know your family history.** Spend some time learning about your family history of disease. For relatives who have passed away, find out if any chronic disease contributed to their deaths. For relatives who are still alive, learn about what diseases they have been diagnosed with and at what ages they were diagnosed. Consider your grandparents, parents, and siblings first, but also ask about aunts, uncles, and first cousins. If you're adopted and don't know your family's genetic history, pay extra attention to lifestyle factors and take all of the preventive measures you can in relation to the most common chronic diseases.
- **Learn the risks.** Get familiar with the risks for the most common diseases. Many chronic diseases share common risks, such as physical inactivity, poor diet, and smoking. Some diseases, however, have very specific risk factors. The CDC and the (U.S.) National Institutes of Health are good sources of accurate information about diseases and risk factors.
- **Monitor your behaviors.** We often fail to pay careful attention to our lifestyle behaviors. When you're trying to determine your disease risk, however, you need to assess your behaviors. You can find quizzes on the web or even in smartphone or tablet apps to help you evaluate your behaviors and their associated risks for disease. You can also track your healthy and unhealthy choices in a log or journal in order to see patterns over time—especially in your physical (in)activity and dietary habits.
- **Make healthy decisions.** Once you know which diseases run in your family, the risk factors for common chronic diseases, and the habits and behaviors you already have, you can begin to make informed decisions to improve your health and reduce your risks. It's also useful to consult with experts, such as physicians, dietitians, and trainers.

Can Hot Temperatures Make Us Vulnerable to Disease?

Changing weather patterns are bringing hotter weather to many parts of the United States. According to the National Climatic Data Center, this trend has been most pronounced in the past two decades. More generally, since 1895 the lower 48 states have seen temperature increases of about 0.12°F (0.07°C) per decade, and six of the nation's warmest years on record have occurred since 1998.

How does this warming trend relate to health? For one thing, the adult Culex mosquito that carries West Nile virus does best in hot, dry weather, but water is necessary for the larval stage. As a result, spikes in West Nile cases, such as one that occurred in the summer of 2012, are likely to become more regular occurrences (table 23.3 shows the top four U.S. states for West Nile).

Hot weather creates more warm, damp places in which mosquitoes can lay eggs. The warmth also allows the eggs to hatch faster and the larvae to mature faster. As a result, the mosquitoes spend more of their life span in a flying state, says Janet de la Rossi, and published expert on West Nile virus transmission. Warmer weather also promotes the growth of the virus within the mosquito itself. "Taken together, we see a greater risk for overall transmission to humans," says Michael Smith of the Centers for Disease Control and Prevention.

What can be done about these trends? "Killing mosquitoes that carry disease has been proven to cut down disease rates," said de la Rossi. Most eradication programs spray for mosquitoes at least six times per season, at a cost of US$60,000 to US$100,000 per treatment. Unfortunately, local budget cuts across the country are reducing funds available for mosquito control (abatement) projects. More than 1,100 localities throughout the country currently use mosquito control programs, but most are seriously threatened by budget issues.

In California, the problem is compounded by the large number of foreclosed and abandoned houses, some of which have stagnant swimming pools filled with mosquitoes. These mosquitoes can be pumped out along with the stagnant water—when there is money to pay the cost. "When funds aren't provided, the pumps aren't in the field, and the mosquito population thrives," said Dave White, former mosquito control expert, who was laid off two months ago.

At the same time, Lilly Doppler, a biologist states that "a warm winter, early spring, and hot summer have been so much a factor in a surge in the mosquito population that I honestly don't believe that (cuts have) played a factor with respect to this outbreak." Others in government who are making the budget cuts argue that individuals can take their own precautions against getting bitten by mosquitoes (e.g., applying mosquito repellent, wearing long sleeves and pants, staying in screened areas) and that the government does not need to pay for control programs when other issues are more pressing.

TABLE 23.3 Top Four U.S. States for West Nile Virus

State	Cases of West Nile	Deaths from West Nile
Texas	1,868	89
Louisiana	335	16
South Dakota	203	3
Oklahoma	191	17

Centers for Disease Control and Prevention 2012.

For Discussion

How does the weather affect mosquito outbreaks? Name two things you could do to help reduce the presence of mosquitos in your yard, school, or neighborhood. What steps could you take individually to help prevent yourself from being bit by an infected mosquito?

CHAPTER REVIEW

Reviewing Concepts and Vocabulary

As directed by your teacher, answer items 1 through 5 by correctly completing each sentence with a word or phrase.

1. A dangerous microorganism that causes a disease is known as a ___________.
2. When a disease is transmitted by sharing a straw or by kissing, it is being spread through __________ transmission.
3. Yeast, mold, and mushrooms are examples of ____________.
4. High blood pressure, also known as __________, is a form of cardiovascular disease.
5. ____________ is a chronic disease in which the bones lose density and become weaker.

For items 6 through 10, as directed by your teacher, match each term in column 1 with the appropriate phrase in column 2.

6. lymphocytes	a. uncontrolled, abnormal cell growth
7. arthritis	b. hard, rigid arteries
8. arteriosclerosis	c. white blood cells that attack pathogens
9. atherosclerosis	d. clogged arteries
10. cancer	e. inflammation or damage to the joints

For items 11 through 15, as directed by your teacher, respond to each statement or question.

11. What is an infectious disease?
12. Describe two differences between influenza and the common cold.
13. What is the name of the virus that causes AIDS, and what does AIDS stand for?
14. List four types of cancer.
15. What is a disability? Describe one type of disability.

Thinking Critically

Write a paragraph in response to the following question.

During lunch you overhear your classmate Sarah making fun of another classmate, Martin, who has a mild form of Down syndrome. The things Sarah said about Martin are untrue and cruel. You know Martin to be a kind, funny, and smart person with a really big heart. What would you say to Sarah about the fact that she made fun of someone with a disability?

Take It Home

Share with your family members what you've learned about preventing chronic illnesses. Discuss with them what steps should be taken as a family to help reduce risks for cardiovascular disease, cancer, and diabetes. If a particular disease runs in your family, pay extra attention to the prevention of that disease. Identify three to five action steps that your family can take together to improve overall health and reduce the risk of chronic disease.

24

Emotional Health and Wellness

In This Chapter

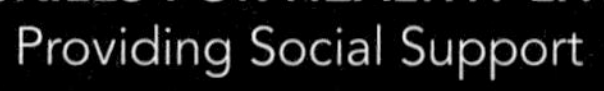

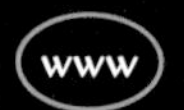

Student Web Resources

www.HOPEtextbook.org/student

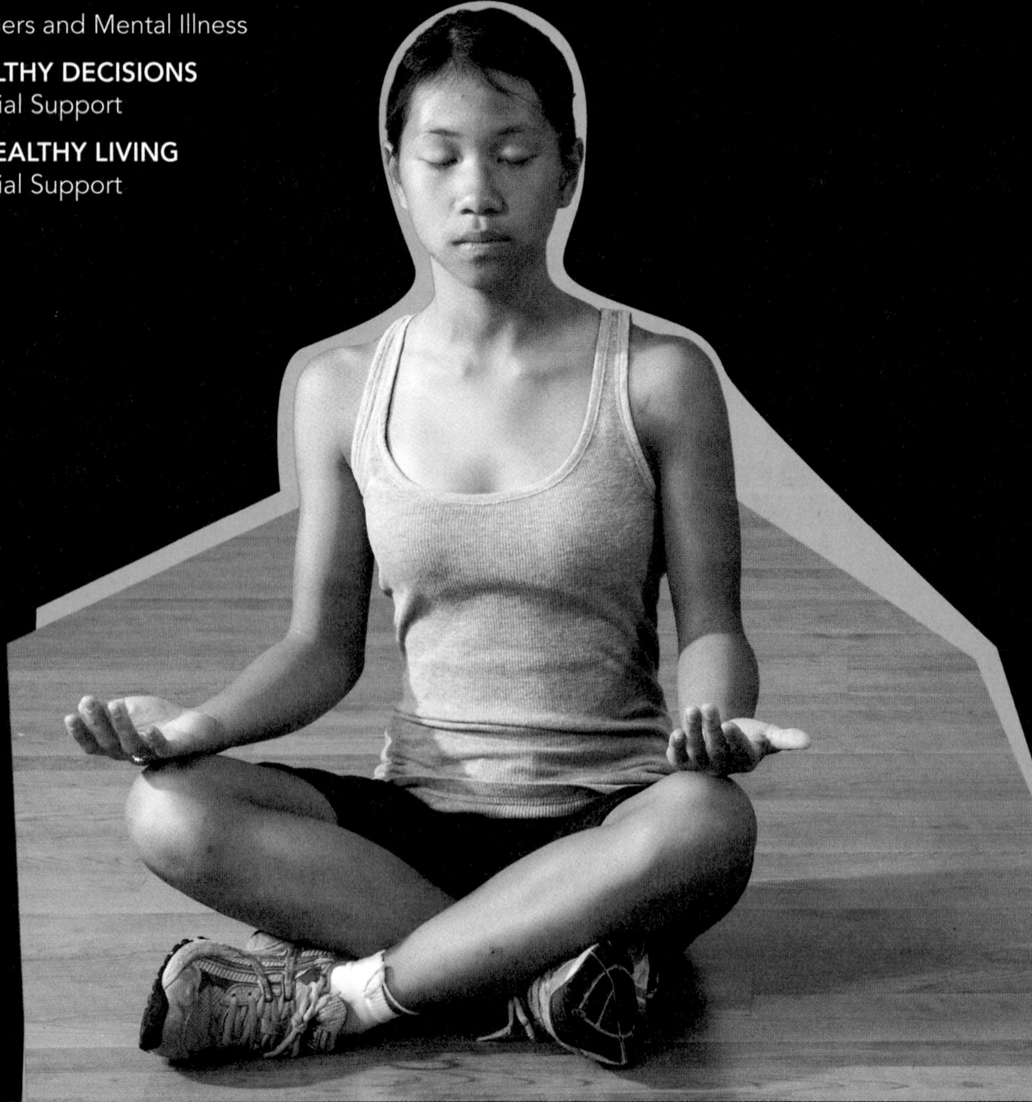

Lesson 24.1

Mental and Emotional Wellness

Lesson Objectives

After reading this lesson, you should be able to

1. identify factors that contribute to emotional wellness;
2. define *personality*, *self-esteem*, and *body image*, and explain their importance to emotional health and wellness; and
3. explain how spiritual health and wellness relate to emotional health and wellness.

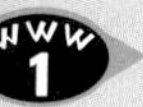

Lesson Vocabulary

body image, emotional wellness, personality, self-esteem, spirituality

How would you describe your personality to others? Can you identify your strengths and weaknesses? How do you feel about who you are and how you look? How do you respond when you feel sad or angry? Your answers to such questions can give you insight into your emotional health. This lesson introduces the most important aspects of good emotional health and wellness.

Emotional Health and Wellness

You learned earlier that health and wellness have five components. Emotional health and wellness is one of them. Like health in general, emotional health requires freedom from illness (in this case mental illness) and possession of emotional wellness (emotional well-being). This lesson will focus on emotional (mental) well-being and the next lesson will focus on mental illness. People with emotional wellness have a realistic understanding of their life circumstances and are able to understand and effectively use the options available to them. They can also assess situations accurately and make decisions that are in the best interest of both themselves and others. As a result, an emotionally healthy person can engage fully in life and cope with day-to-day challenges. Some indicators of good emotional health are identified in figure 24.1.

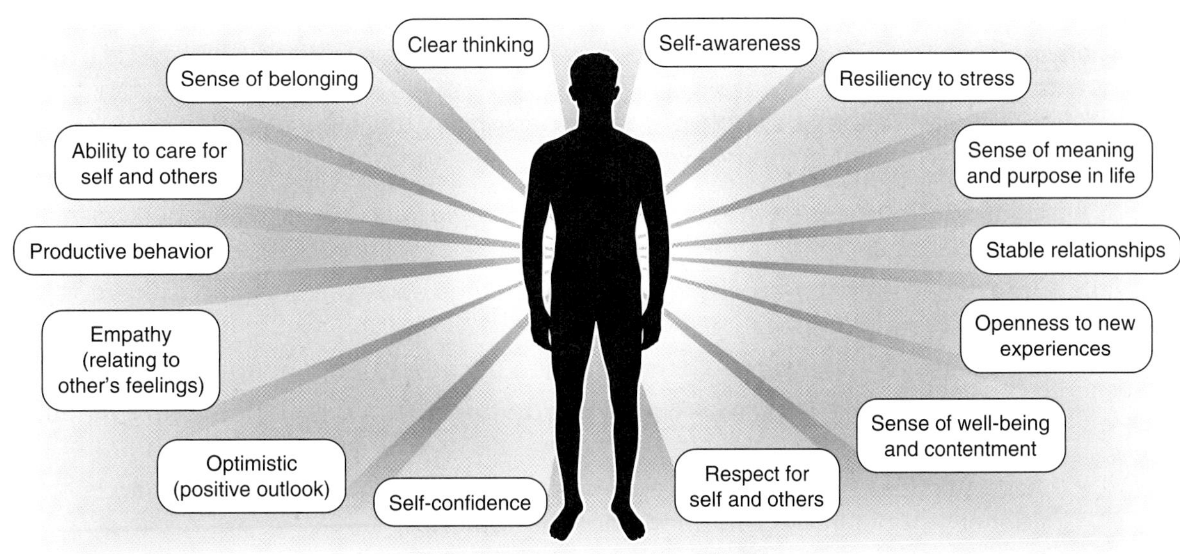

FIGURE 24.1 An emotionally healthy person displays some or all of these indicators.

Everyone experiences some challenges in life that might compromise emotional health and wellness. For example, a girl who is emotionally healthy during high school might experience some reduction in health status when she starts college if new academic challenges affect her self-confidence and she feels disconnected from her new community. As a result, she might not feel content, might find herself lacking motivation, and might become easily discouraged. This wouldn't mean that she had a mental illness, but it would mean that her emotional health wasn't as good as it could be. In your own life, you can use many of the skills for healthy living presented in part 2 of this book to help you develop strong mental health.

Emotional Wellness

Emotion is a normal part of living, and an emotionally healthy person isn't someone who never experiences sadness or fear or who is always happy. What good **emotional wellness** does mean is that you're able to use your thoughts to understand and control the effects that your emotions have on your behavior. It means that you can recognize your own and others' emotional reactions and determine whether a given reaction is helpful—or not. Good health is more than freedom from illness (i.e., mental and emotional illnesses); it includes emotional wellness as shown by being happy and not depressed or sad.

You can also be supportive of your friends and family members and be happy when they exhibit healthy emotional responses. For example, it's okay for you and others to cry in sad situations or feel frustrated when something doesn't go as planned. We all need to allow ourselves and others the time and space to experience healthy emotional responses. However, when an emotional response, such as anger, is expressed in a destructive way—for example, in a violent outburst—it is not emotionally healthy. You can help yourself attain and maintain good emotional health by learning to understand your emotions and control your behavioral responses.

Personality

Think about your close friends and family members. Some are energetic and talkative, some are quieter and more reflective, others are neat and well organized, and still others are spontaneous and messy. Each person you know has a different **personality**—the unique mixture of qualities and traits that distinguishes him or her from others. Personality traits influence how we react to the challenges of life, interpret and express our feelings, and resolve conflicts with others.

Healthy Personality Traits

Many personality traits contribute to your overall emotional wellness. Some traits (such as carefulness) may help you avoid danger, whereas others (such as resilience) may help you resist disease. Here's a sample of healthy personality traits that are often considered to be characteristics of emotional wellness.

- **Conscientiousness**—tendency to conduct yourself according to an inner sense of what is right and wrong; having a strong sense of self-awareness and knowledge
- **Emotional stability**—ability to manage feelings and reactions and behave in a reasoned and consistent manner
- **Openness to experience**—demonstration of curiosity and independence
- **Optimism**—positive outlook on life and tendency to find the positive in various situations
- **Assertiveness**—ability to express emotions, needs, and desires clearly and confidently without impinging on the rights of others
- **Resilience**—ability to adapt to change and stressful events in healthy and flexible ways

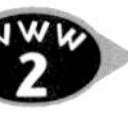

As a result, your personality plays a role in your emotional health and wellness. Many personality traits exist, but individuals with certain traits seem to have better overall health (see the list titled Healthy Personality Traits). Personality traits are often established early in life, and they are influenced by genetics and by relationships with parents, siblings, friends, teachers, and others. It is possible to influence your personality traits, or to manage a trait (e.g., being disorganized), by working throughout your life to develop healthy life skills—for example, time management.

CONNECT

Do you think you were born with your personality type, or do you think your family environment has created your personality? What personality traits do you share with your family members?

Self-Esteem

Positive self-esteem is foundational to good emotional wellness. **Self-esteem** refers to the way in which a person perceives himself or herself. It is a combination of self-confidence and self-respect. A person exhibits positive self-esteem in feeling that he or she can cope with daily challenges and is worthy of happiness. People with positive self-esteem have confidence in themselves, solve problems effectively without excessive worry, confront or eliminate things that cause them fear or anxiety, take appropriate risks, and nurture themselves and their relationships with others. High self-esteem is not, however, the same thing as arrogance—a sense of superiority over others that results in an overbearing or dominating personality. You can be self-confident and self-accepting without being arrogant.

Research shows that people with positive (or high) self-esteem are more likely to engage in healthy behaviors, such as exercise and healthy

Tips for Healthy Self-Esteem

- **Accept who you are.** Make a list of your good qualities and skills and post it in a location where you will see it every day. Don't be too hard on yourself.
- **Keep track of your accomplishments.** Write them down every day and share them with a supportive friend, teacher, or family member.
- **Develop your own values.** Don't try to be someone else. Know who you are and take healthy pride in your identity.
- **Accept your strengths and weaknesses and set goals for yourself.** No one is perfect. Don't focus on things you can't change about yourself. Instead, think of constructive things you can do to improve in areas that you do control.
- **Don't be afraid to take healthy risks.** It's impossible to make it through life without failure. The important thing is to learn from your failures.
- **Find friends who support you.** Don't allow yourself to be mistreated or constantly put down. Anyone who repeatedly treats you with disrespect does not deserve to be in your life. Similarly, support the people in your life.
- **Respect yourself and others.** People who respect themselves and others are more likely to be respected by others. Don't be judgmental toward yourself or other people. Instead, be encouraging and supportive. You'll feel better about yourself, and others will respond in kind.
- **Join groups that promote your self-esteem.** Participate in clubs and organizations that you enjoy and that use and appreciate your strengths. Accept praise and compliments for the contributions you make.
- **Be careful not to behave arrogantly.** Take pride in your work and who you are without acting as if you're better than others.

eating, and are better able to avoid unhealthy behaviors, such as smoking and excessive drinking. People with low self-esteem, on the other hand, don't have much respect for themselves. They tend to judge themselves harshly and think negatively about their own abilities. Research has shown that low self-esteem is associated with risky and unhealthy behaviors among teenagers, such as drug and alcohol use, dropping out of school, and developing eating disorders.

Body Image

Many people of all ages struggle with body image. Your **body image** includes your thoughts, feelings, and behaviors related to your body size, shape, and appearance. Body image is strongly related to overall self-esteem, especially among teenagers. Many experts believe that young people often struggle with body image due to the pressure they feel when they compare themselves with unrealistic media representations of attractiveness. Other influences on body image include parents, friends, teachers, coaches, and health care workers.

In some cases, a single negative or critical comment about a person's body or appearance can be devastating, especially when it comes from a trusted friend, family member, or role model. When we make negative comments about someone's appearance, or tease someone because of how he or she looks, we contribute to negative body image. Instead, we should celebrate individual differences in appearance and focus on the positive personality characteristics and abilities that each person possesses. You can learn more about body image by visiting the student section of the Health Opportunities Through Physical Education website.

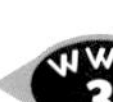

CONNECT

How do you think the media influences your body image? Explain what you see as the three most significant media influences on your body image. Debate your perspective with your peers. Support your position with facts and be respectful of others' opinions.

> "Optimism is the faith that leads to achievement. Nothing can be done without hope and confidence."
>
> —Helen Keller

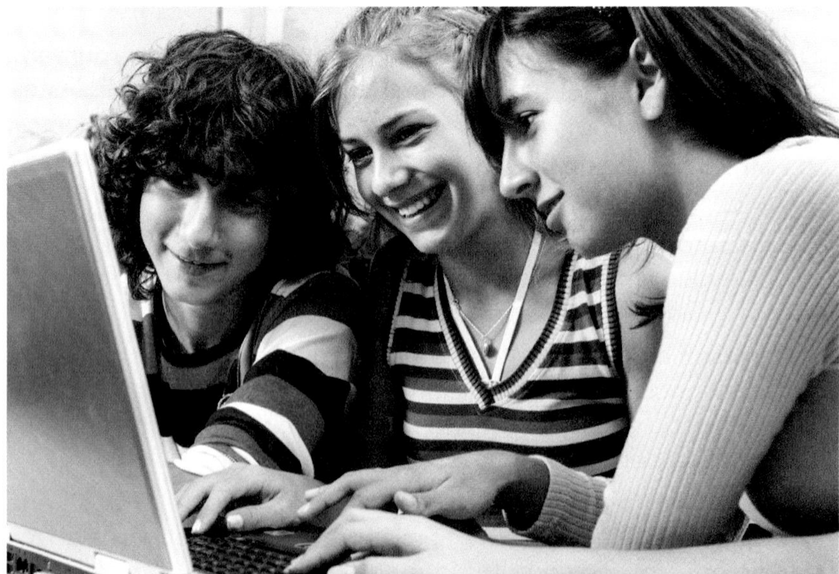

Friends, as well as parents, teachers, coaches, health care workers, and the media, can influence body image.

gajatz - Fotolia.com

Spiritual Wellness

In modern society, we often seek to boost our self-esteem or validate our worth by acquiring material possessions. Many people believe that getting more or better stuff will make them happier. Sooner or later, however, most people come to understand that inner happiness is not achieved by simply having more, and they seek out other ways to find or create meaning and purpose in their lives. There's a name for this process. **Spirituality** is defined by the National Center for Complementary and Alternative Medicine as "an individual's sense of purpose and meaning in life, beyond material values." Spirituality is one component of health and wellness and all are interrelated. Spiritual fulfillment specifically relates to emotional health and wellness. It is generally understood to include three facets: relationships, values, and meaningful purpose in life. See the chapter on the introduction to health and wellness for the total health and wellness chain.

- **Relationships.** When we seek to connect with other people, we contemplate who we are in relation to others and what we truly value. When we treat others with respect and dignity, we manifest our own spirituality.
- **Values.** Our personal values are the principles that guide our decisions and actions. Your values are reflected in the rules by which you conduct your own life and the positions you stand for. When we pursue spiritual well-being, we look deeply into our own values and beliefs and seek to align our life choices and actions with them.
- **Meaningful purpose in life.** Why are you here on earth? What is it you're here to do? Spiritual wellness is associated with articulating your individual purpose in life and making choices that align with and develop that purpose. People begin to question their purpose as children and adolescents; they revisit this inner seeking throughout life.

Spirituality is different from religion. A religion is a system of beliefs, practices, rituals, and symbols designed to connect one to a sacred or divine being. Not all human beings participate in organized religion, but all have spiritual needs and longings, and research shows that spiritual well-being is important to physical health. For example, the National Cancer Institute suggests that spirituality contributes to physical health by decreasing anxiety and depression, reducing alcohol and drug use, reducing blood pressure and risk of heart disease, and increasing a person's coping ability and overall feelings of hope, optimism, satisfaction, and inner peace.

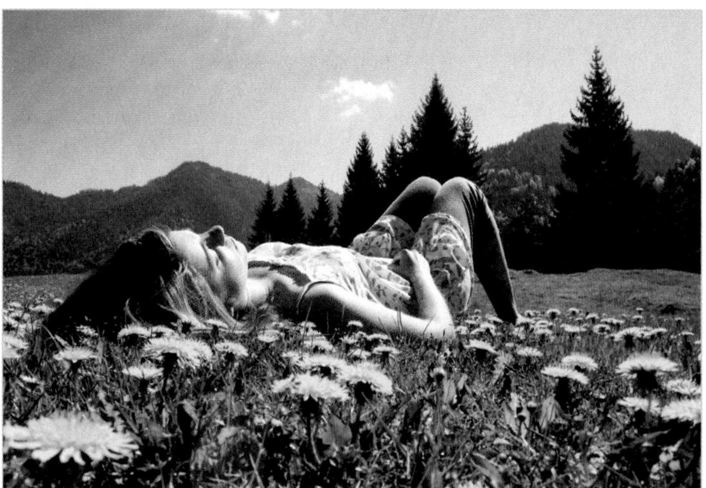

Practicing spirituality can be done through physical pursuits, religious practices, and contemplation or mediation.

pixhunter.com - Fotolia

> continued

> continued

People practice spiritual wellness in a variety of ways. There is no single right way to seek spiritual wellness because spirituality itself is tied to individual values. Here are some common contemporary spiritual practices.

- **Physical pursuits.** Yoga, intentional relaxation, hiking, and other nature activities are common ways that people connect to their own sense of spirituality.
- **Religious practices.** Religious practices, church attendance, retreats, and other religious activities are central to many people's sense of spirituality. Keep in mind that these are often practiced together. Many religious practices also include contemplation and altruism.
- **Contemplation or meditation.** These practices concentrate the mind on a subject, question, object, or "nothingness" (blankness or openness). Often, people keep track of their contemplations and meditations in a journal. Another common spiritual practice is to contemplate gratitude or specific things for which you're grateful.
- **Mindfulness.** This practice involves being fully present in the moment in a nonjudgmental state of observation. One way of practicing mindfulness is to awaken fully into an experience such as painting, drawing, music, or sculpting. In fact, anything can be a mindful activity if one is fully immersed in the moment and in touch with his or her innermost feelings.
- **Prayer.** This practice involves focusing oneself in communication with a sacred or divine being. Prayer takes many forms and may include words of praise, sharing of concerns, and petitions for guidance.
- **Altruism.** This is the act of giving yourself or your time due to genuine concern for others. Many people find that practicing altruism connects them to their own spirituality; in practicing selflessness, they get in touch with their deepest personal values.

Comprehension Check

1. Identify factors that contribute to emotional wellness.
2. What is one reason why it's important to have good self-esteem and why is it important to emotional health and wellness?
3. How does spiritual health and wellness relate to emotional health and wellness?

SELF-ASSESSMENT: My Self-Esteem

Your level of self-esteem is a good indicator of both your overall emotional health and wellness and your risk for becoming depressed or engaging in unhealthy behaviors. Self-esteem is a complicated thing to measure accurately, and no single test gets at all of its elements. Still, questionnaires like this one can help you get a sense of your overall self-esteem. More important, answering these questions can help you identify any qualities in yourself that could make you vulnerable to low self-esteem.

This questionnaire includes a list of statements addressing your general feelings about yourself. For each statement, circle the response that most accurately reflects how you feel. Try to be honest.

1. I feel like I am a person of worth on an equal plane with others.	Strongly agree	Agree	Disagree	Strongly disagree
2. I feel that I have a number of good qualities.	Strongly agree	Agree	Disagree	Strongly disagree
3. All in all, I am inclined to feel that I am a failure.	Strongly agree	Agree	Disagree	Strongly disagree
4. I am able to do things as well as most other people.	Strongly agree	Agree	Disagree	Strongly disagree
5. I feel I do not have much to be proud of.	Strongly agree	Agree	Disagree	Strongly disagree
6. I take a positive attitude toward myself.	Strongly agree	Agree	Disagree	Strongly disagree
7. On the whole, I am satisfied with myself.	Strongly agree	Agree	Disagree	Strongly disagree
8. I wish I could have more respect for myself.	Strongly agree	Agree	Disagree	Strongly disagree
9. I certainly feel useless at times.	Strongly agree	Agree	Disagree	Strongly disagree
10. At times I think I am no good at all.	Strongly agree	Agree	Disagree	Strongly disagree

To determine your score, complete the following calculations.

For items 1, 2, 4, 6, and 7, give yourself the following points for each response: strongly agree = 3, agree = 2, disagree = 1, strongly disagree = 0.

Item 1:_____ Item 2:_____ Item 4:_____ Item 6:_____ Item 7:_____

For items 3, 5, 8, 9, and 10, give yourself the following points for each response: strongly agree = 0, agree = 1, disagree = 2, strongly disagree = 3.

Item 3:_____ Item 5:_____ Item 8:_____ Item 9:_____ Item 10:_____

Total the points for all 10 items and write your score below.

My Self-Esteem score is: __________.

Higher scores are suggestive of a higher self-esteem. If your score is below 15, consider setting goals to improve your self-esteem. If your score is 15 or higher, consider ways to maintain your self-esteem (see lesson 24.1 of this chapter).

Planning for Healthy Living

Use the Healthy Living Plan worksheet to improve your self-esteem.

Lesson 24.2

Mental Disorders and Mental Illness

Lesson Objectives

After reading this lesson, you should be able to

1. identify and describe common mental disorders,
2. recognize the stages of coping with death and dying and know what to do if someone exhibits them, and
3. explain three treatment options for mental disorders.

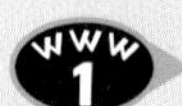

Lesson Vocabulary

anorexia nervosa, anxiety disorder, attention-deficit/hyperactivity disorder (ADHD), bulimia, compulsive behavior, depression, generalized anxiety disorder, manic-depressive disorder, mental disorder, muscle dysmorphia, obsession, phobias, post-traumatic stress disorder, psychotherapy, suicide

Do you know anyone who suffers from a mental disorder? Mental disorders affect one in four adults and one in ten adolescents each year and are often left untreated. This lesson introduces some of the most common mental disorders and their treatments.

Mental Disorders

In the previous lesson, you learned about emotional health and wellness. The focus was on the positive and having good emotional wellness. This lesson describes a variety of disorders associated with emotional (mental) health and wellness. Because the term *mental* is commonly used as medical descriptor for these disorders, the terms **mental disorder** or mental illness will be used (rather than emotional disorders).

A mental disorder is an illness that affects a person's mind and reduces his or her ability to function. Mental disorders, or mental illnesses, involve behaviors, thoughts, or emotions (e.g., anger, fear, sadness, envy) that are unusual or inappropriate to a given situation. Many factors can contribute to the development of a mental disorder, and in some cases there is no clear reason why a person develops a disorder. Possible contributing factors include heredity, traumatic experience, and brain damage resulting from injury, accident, heavy alcohol or drug use, or illness. Even today, societies sometimes stigmatize individuals with mental illness; however, many people will experience some degree of mental illness at some point in life.

Anxiety Disorders

Are you afraid of heights or of flying? What about public speaking? Have you ever experienced sudden anxiety (perhaps a feeling of nervousness or a rapid heart rate or breath rate) for a reason you didn't understand? When such feelings occur regularly or interfere with a person's ability to function normally, they are considered signs of an **anxiety disorder**. **Generalized anxiety disorder** involves feelings of intense worry, fear, or anxiety that do not stem from a specific source or cause. In contrast, intense fear and anxiety that do relate to a specific situation or object (e.g., heights, crowds, spiders) are called **phobias**.

Anxiety disorder can also appear as an unwanted thought or image that takes control of the mind. Such thoughts or images are called **obsessions**, and they can lead to **compulsive behaviors**, which are unreasonable behaviors done in an attempt to prevent a feared outcome. For example, individuals obsessed with germs and a fear of disease may feel compelled to wash their hands many times a day, even when they are already very clean.

Another type of anxiety disorder is called **post-traumatic stress disorder**. In this condition, an individual who has experienced or witnessed a traumatic event, such as a war or terrorist attack,

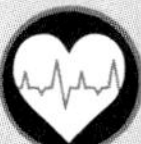

HEALTH TECHNOLOGY

Treating phobias has traditionally involved repeated exposure to a fearful situation so that the person can gradually adjust and overcome his or her fears. For example, people with a fear of heights (acrophobia) might begin treatment by standing on a platform positioned only slightly off the ground while applying techniques such as deep breathing to reduce their anxiety response, then progressively move higher until they are able to stand on top of a multistory building. This type of therapy can involve tremendous amounts of time and many unpredictable elements.

Advances in computer technology allow a similar process to be performed in a more controlled and safe environment. In virtual reality exposure therapy, the patient wears a head-mounted display and headphones so that both sight and sound are controlled. The virtual world can be precisely adjusted by the therapist to produce the desired exposure and the resulting anxiety, and the patient can revisit the setting or situation as often as needed to successfully conquer his or her fear.

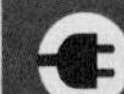

CONNECT

When you immerse yourself in a virtual world by becoming a character in a video game or taking on an avatar, you enter a type of virtual reality. When you are engaged in a virtual reality, do you think it helps or hurts your ability to focus and concentrate? Can you imagine using virtual technology to help you overcome a phobia?

experiences intense flashbacks or nightmares that produce high anxiety and may interfere with his or her sleep, concentration, and relationships.

Eating Disorders

Eating disorders are mental disorders in which anxiety and other emotions are expressed through behaviors related to food and eating. Eating disorders are not simply about appetite and hunger; rather, they are complex psychological disorders. Two eating disorders you may have heard of are anorexia nervosa and bulimia. Individuals with **anorexia nervosa** believe they're fat even when they're dangerously thin; as a result, they may restrict their eating to the point of starvation. Symptoms

What Is a Panic Attack?

Anyone can suffer a panic attack in a life-threatening or otherwise very stressful situation. However, a person with panic disorder (a type of anxiety disorder) experiences regular panic attacks that can come at any time and for no apparent reason. A panic attack can produce the following symptoms.

- Rapid heart rate and breathing
- Pain or discomfort in the chest
- Fear of choking or suffocating
- Uncontrolled trembling or shaking
- Nausea, dizziness, or lightheadedness
- Fear of losing control or dying

Panic disorder often begins during adolescence, and it can be treated with medication and therapy. Left untreated, it can lead to depression, phobia, or substance abuse.

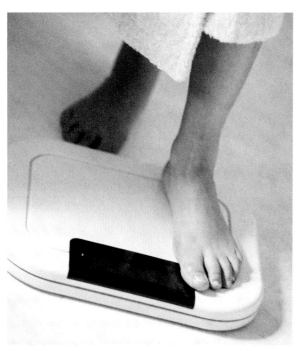

Eating disorders trigger anxiety and other emotions such as body image issues.

Eyewire

include extreme weight loss, dry skin, poor temperature regulation (feeling cold), and body image issues (e.g., feeling fat despite being very thin). Anorexia is a very serious disease that can lead to death if not treated properly. Treatment can be a long process involving multiple health care professionals; to be successful, it must address the underlying anxiety and emotional problems.

Bulimia involves uncontrolled episodes of bingeing (eating a large amount of food) and purging (trying to get rid of the food). Purging sometimes involves forcing the body to vomit but might also include using laxatives, weight loss pills, or even exercise (if it is done for the purpose of getting rid of calories and if the individual has an uncontrollable compulsion to exercise). Individuals with bulimia often eat in order to deal with an unwanted emotion or thought but then feel that they must get rid of the calories in order to remain attractive and in control.

Teenage females are more likely than males to suffer from eating disorders; in fact, about 90 percent of teens with eating disorders in the U.S. are female. Males who experience anxiety about their bodies may engage in different types of unhealthy behavior—for example, consuming excessive protein, obsessively engaging in weightlifting or prolonged training to build muscle, or taking hormones or unnecessary supplements in order to build muscle or change their body shape. Males who take such actions may have a disorder known as **muscle dysmorphia**, which is not considered an eating disorder per se but is a similar form of mental illness that can have serious consequences for long-term health. This is especially true when people use steroids or other drugs to increase muscle size or enhance performance.

Eating disorders are complex conditions that can be very difficult to understand. If you suspect a friend or family member might have an eating disorder, it is important to recognize that you cannot "fix" or help that person on your own. According to the National Eating Disorders Association, when sharing your concerns with a person who might have an eating disorder, you should avoid placing any blame, shame, or guilt on the other person and avoid being stubborn or forceful with your opinions. Set aside time to talk openly, provide support, express your specific concerns, and be committed to listening to the other person even if they don't seem to understand or agree with what you are saying. If the person is open to the conversation, encourage them to see a doctor or mental health professional. If you try talking to the person and are still concerned, share your concerns with a trusted adult or health professional. For more information about eating disorders and similar conditions, see the student section of the Health Opportunities Through Physical Education website.

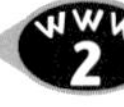

Mood Disorders

When a person experiences extreme emotions that prevent him or her from functioning normally, the person may be experiencing a mood disorder. About 10 percent of Americans experience a mood disorder

HEALTHY COMMUNICATION

You suspect that a friend may have bulimia. She has always struggled with her appearance, and she talks many times a day about being fat. She also makes regular trips to the bathroom after meals and seems very emotional. Lately, she has been excessively hyper and always wants to go work out to "burn off calories." How should you handle this situation? If you chose to confront her with your concerns, what would you say?

each year, and women are 50 percent more likely than men to experience such a disorder at some point in life. A mood disorder can increase a person's risk for heart disease, diabetes, and other diseases. Fortunately, good treatment enables most people with a mood disorder to lead a productive life.

Depression is a mood disorder in which a person feels extreme sadness and hopelessness. The risk of developing depression increases throughout childhood and into adolescence. By the age of 18, about 10 percent of teenagers have experienced an episode of depression. Girls report depression at a higher rate than boys do, and depression is the leading cause of disability among all Americans between the ages of 15 and 44. Depression puts an individual at risk for **suicide** (the taking of one's own life) (see figure 24.2).

In some cases, episodes of depression alternate with periods of extreme excitability and restlessness in a condition known as **manic-depressive**

Grief, Death, and Dying

When a loved one dies, those left behind often feel extreme grief and sadness. Grief can be intense and last a long time, but it is a normal emotion that differs from depression. The typical stages that people go through when coping with the death of a loved one are illustrated in figure 24.3. Some people go through these stages in a different order than others, and some do not experience all of the stages. The person who died may also have experienced the stages if he or she knew that death was imminent and came to terms with that reality.

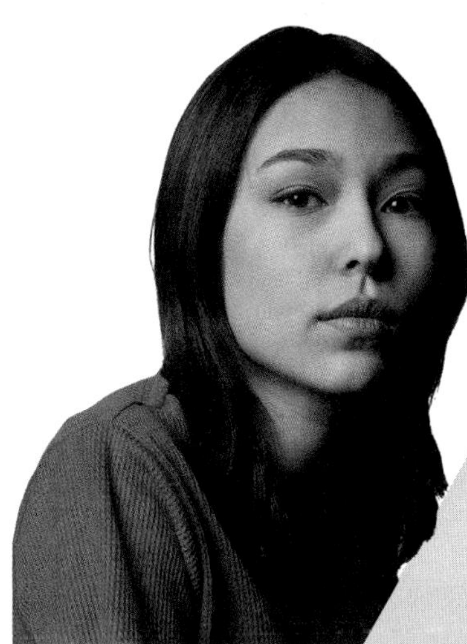

Warning signs of depression in teens

- Irritability or anger
- Extreme sensitivity to criticism
- Withdrawing from parents or some friends
- Change in appetite, significant weight loss or weight gain
- Change in sleep patterns (difficulty sleeping or sleeping too much, especially during the day time)
- Changes in activity patterns (becoming sluggish or frantic)
- Loss of energy
- Feelings of worthlessness or guilt
- Difficulty thinking or concentrating
- Loss of interest in usual activities
- Repeated thoughts or statements about death or suicide

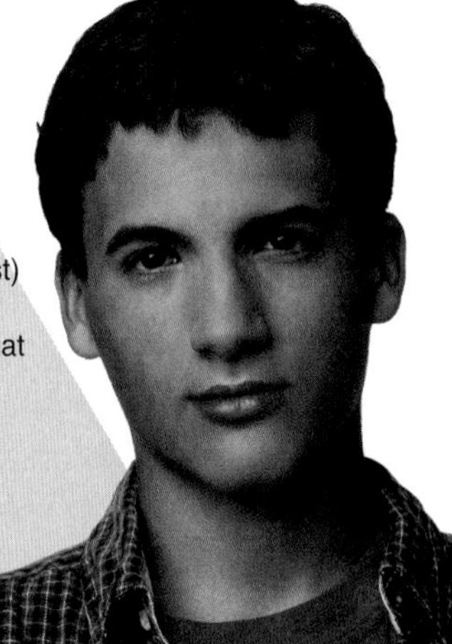

Warning signs of suicide

- A history of depression or the existence of the signs of depression (see previous list)
- Expressions of self-hatred
- Excessive risk-taking behaviors along with a careless attitude ("It doesn't matter what happens to me anyway.")
- A direct statement about committing suicide ("I'm going to end it all.")
- An indirect statement about suicide ("You won't have to worry about me being here by then.")
- Final preparations such as giving away possessions, writing revealing letters, or repairing damaged relationships (before planning to say good-bye)
- A preoccupation with themes of death
- Significant changes to personal appearance

FIGURE 24.2 Depression is a serious illness that can lead someone to commit suicide. Recognizing signs of depression and suicide can help you to help others.

disorder or bipolar disorder. When a person is overly excited and restless, he or she may be experiencing a manic episode. People in a manic state may speak so quickly and move around so rapidly that it is difficult to understand them or keep up with their actions. In manic-depressive disorder, manic episodes may last days or weeks and alternate with periods of serious depression. Manic-depressive disorder affects about 2 percent of teens each year.

Self-Injury

Sometimes people cope with emotion, stress, or trauma by injuring themselves through actions such as cutting or burning their skin. This type of behavior is called self-injury. It is a serious problem that can become a compulsive behavior and can be associated with mental disorders such as depression and eating disorders. People who engage in cutting often wear concealing clothing and if confronted may tell lies to cover up the truth. If you or someone you know engages in cutting or other self-injury, tell a trusted adult so that the person can get help in coping with emotions in a healthier way.

Attention-Deficit/ Hyperactivity Disorder

Attention-deficit/hyperactivity disorder (ADHD) is the most common mental disorder diagnosed in children and young adults. Specifically, about 9 percent of teens between the ages of 13 and 18 are diagnosed with ADHD. The disorder can involve a combination of factors, including hyperactivity (excessive energy), inattention (being unable to stay focused), and problems with impulse control (lacking patience and self-control). When ADHD is not properly diagnosed and treated, it can lead to problem behaviors such as drug or alcohol abuse, problems with the law, dropping out of school, and inability to hold down a job. Medications and therapy are used to treat ADHD. Having clear and consistent rules and routines is also helpful to managing the condition.

> "If I feel depressed I will sing. If I feel sad I will laugh. . . . Today I will be the master of my emotions."
>
> —Og Mandino, author

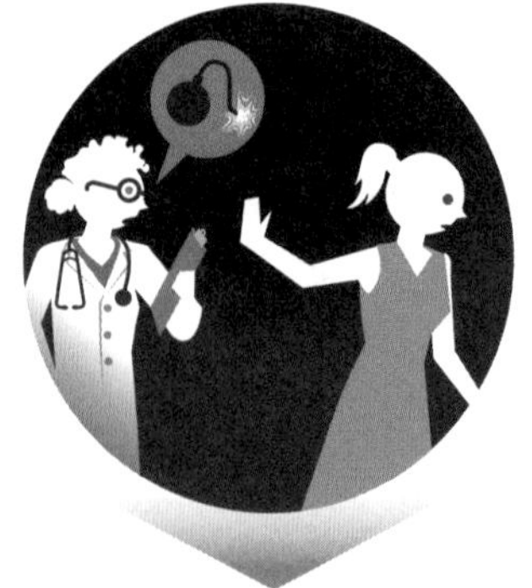
Denial
This isn't happening to me!

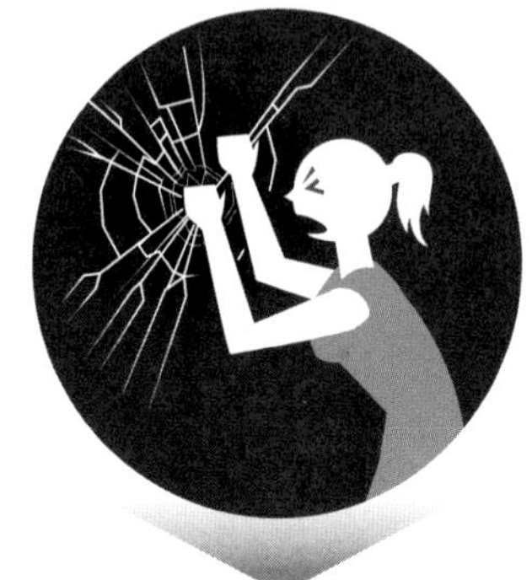
Anger
Why is this happening to me?

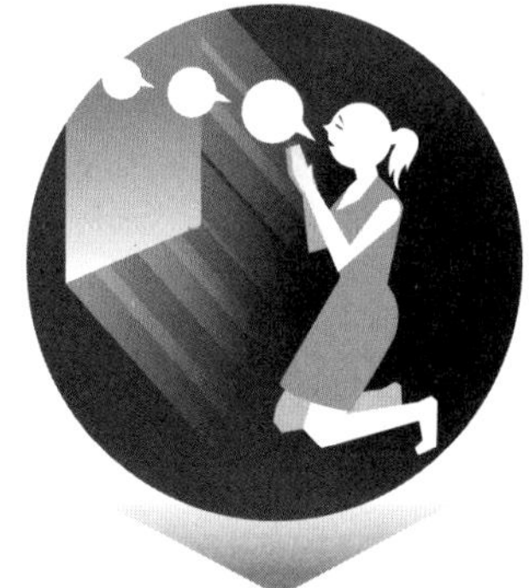
Bargaining
I promise I'll be a better person if...

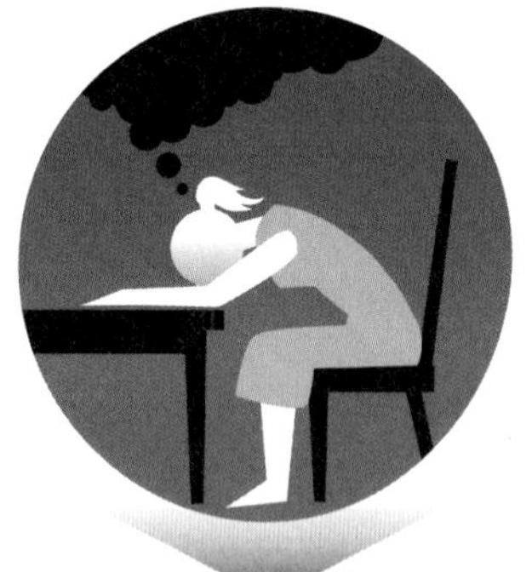
Depression
I don't care anymore.

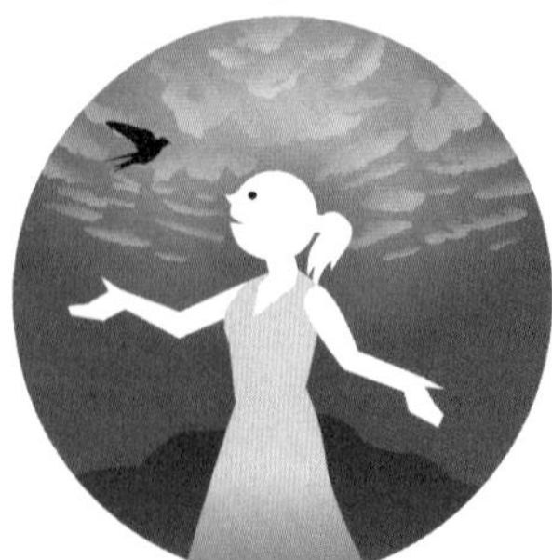
Acceptance
I'm ready for whatever comes.

FIGURE 24.3 Stages of coping with death and dying.

ADVOCACY IN ACTION: Mental Health Awareness

Working in a small group, research one of the mental disorders discussed in this chapter. Gather information about the disorder's causes, risk factors, major symptoms, and treatment options. Next, speak to your school's leaders and health providers to gather information about relevant mental health services available on site. Then create a poster or other presentation about the disorder to share the information you've put together. Finally, as a class, share your collective work by organizing a mental health awareness advocacy campaign.

Treating Mental Disorders

Many treatment options are available for mental disorders. The exact treatment or combination of treatments depends on the disorder and the person. Treatment may be provided by a health care team, which can include a physician, a pharmacist, and a mental health professional (e.g., psychologist, psychiatrist, or social worker). Common treatment options include psychotherapy, counseling, medication, and substance abuse counseling. Additional treatments, such as hospitalization, may be used in more severe situations. In some cases, a mental disorder is so severe that a doctor, loved one, or guardian oversees the care until the affected individual is well enough to participate in decision making.

Counseling and Psychotherapy

Psychotherapy and counseling are methods of treating mental disorders that involve talking about the condition and related issues with a mental health care provider. During psychotherapy or counseling sessions, a person learns about his or her condition and his or her moods, feelings, thoughts, and behaviors. The person uses insights and knowledge gained from the treatment to learn coping and stress management skills.

There are many types of psychotherapy, each with its own approach to improving a person's emotional wellness. Psychotherapy can often be successfully completed in a few months, but in some cases long-term treatment is helpful. It can be done one-on-one, in a group, or with family members.

Medication

Medication does not cure a mental disorder, but it can provide significant relief from symptoms and help the individual function more fully. Psychiatric medication can also help other treatments, such as psychotherapy, to be more effective. The selection of medication depends on the particular situation and how the person's body responds. Here are some of the most commonly used classes of prescription psychiatric medication.

- **Antidepressant medications.** Antidepressants are used to treat various types of depression and sometimes other conditions. They can help improve such symptoms as sadness, hopelessness, lack of energy, difficulty concentrating, and lack of interest in activities. Antidepressants are grouped into more specific categories determined by how they affect brain chemistry.

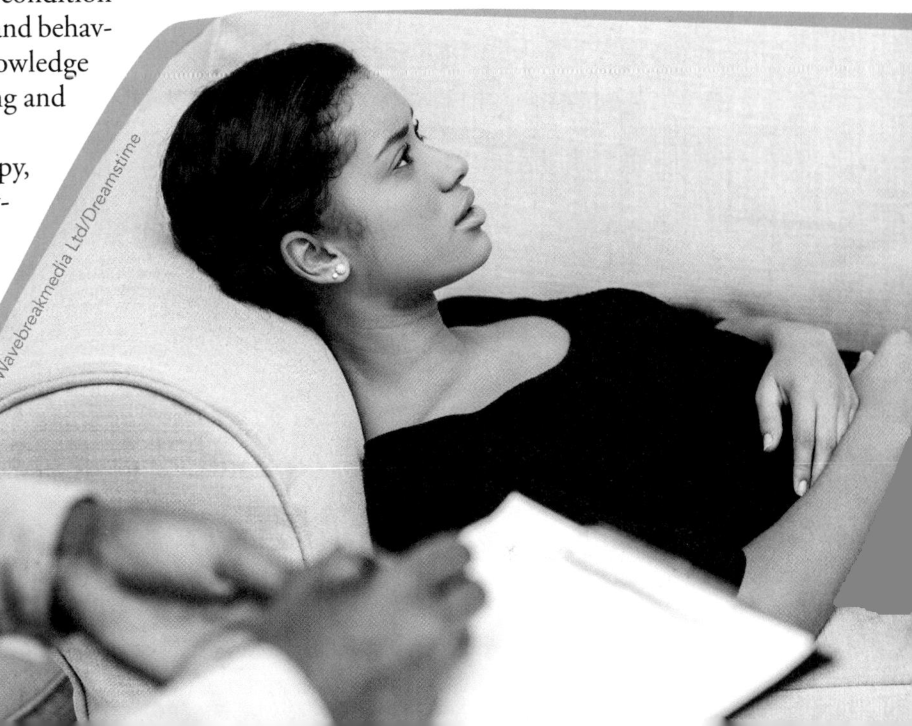

Psychotherapy helps to treat mental disorders and can be done in a group setting.

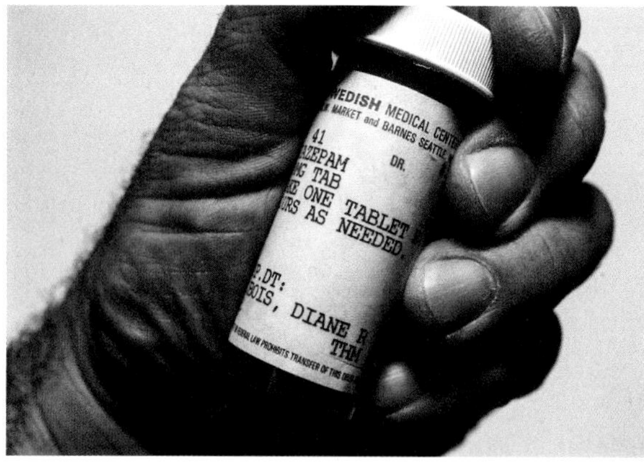

Medication can be used to treat some of the symptoms associated with mental illness.
PhotoDisc

- **Mood-stabilizing medications.** Mood stabilizers are most commonly used to treat bipolar disorder, which is characterized by alternating episodes of mania and depression. Sometimes they are used with antidepressants to treat depression.
- **Anti-anxiety medications.** These medications are used to treat anxiety disorders, such as generalized anxiety disorder and panic disorder. They may also help reduce agitation and insomnia. They are typically fast acting, helping relieve symptoms in as little as 30 to 60 minutes. One major drawback, however, is their potential for addiction.
- **Antipsychotic medications.** Also called neuroleptics, these medications are typically used to treat psychotic disorders such as schizophrenia. Psychotic disorders involve a loss of contact with reality.

Substance Abuse Counseling

Substance abuse commonly occurs along with mental illness; in such cases, it often interferes with treatment and worsens the problem. If an individual cannot stop using drugs or alcohol on his or her own, specialized treatment is needed. For children and adolescents, treatment for substance abuse and mental health issues should include parental and physician involvement. All types of treatment are proven to be more effective when parents or guardians are informed and are actively involved. Substance abuse treatments are discussed in later chapters and include the following:

- Psychotherapy
- Medication
- Hospitalization to address withdrawal (detox)
- Support groups, such as 12-step programs

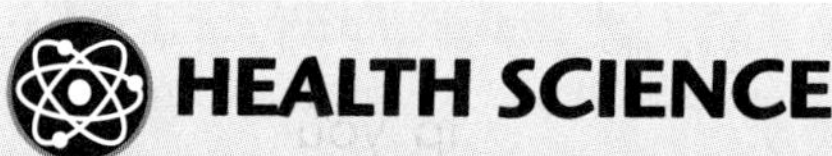

HEALTH SCIENCE

Brain cells are called neurons, and they communicate with each other by using electrical signals to release chemical messengers from one cell to another. These messengers, called neurotransmitters or neurochemicals, carry out specific jobs and help regulate your body functions and emotions. Some of the most common neurochemicals are serotonin, dopamine, and norepinephrine.

When we are in a state of good emotional health and wellness, this complex communication system works well and without interruption. However, the effectiveness of neurochemicals can be limited by various conditions in the brain. When this happens, normal brain communication breaks down, and mental health may suffer. To learn more about the science of mental health, visit the student section of the Health Opportunities Through Physical Education website.

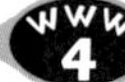

Comprehension Check

1. Explain three types of anxiety disorder.
2. List the stages of coping with death and dying.
3. List three treatment options for mental disorders and describe one in more detail.

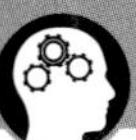

MAKING HEALTHY DECISIONS: Providing Social Support

Anton is a high school senior and star baseball player. You've been Anton's friend since elementary school and have always liked his positive outlook, outgoing nature, and generous spirit. Anton lives with his grandmother and doesn't have any other family nearby. He's always helping his grandma around the house and telling stories about her. He also spends a lot of time with his girlfriend, Zelia.

Lately, however, you've noticed that Anton doesn't talk much about his grandmother and that he seems to be more reserved than usual. In addition, Zelia has mentioned that Anton seems distant with her lately even though they haven't been fighting or having any problems. Last week, you saw Anton hanging out by himself after school even though he was supposed to be at baseball practice. When you asked him about it, he said he was tired and he acted irritated that you were bothering him. When you asked him to go grab a bite to eat, he shrugged his shoulders and said, "I'm not hungry. What's the point anyway?" And just yesterday, Anton drifted off in class, and when the teacher called on him he didn't know the answer to the question. After class, he said that he was "worthless and stupid" and that he was going home.

For Discussion

What do you think might be wrong with Anton? Is there reason to be concerned for his health? What might you do to help him and provide him with social support? In answering these questions, consider the information presented in figure 24.2 and in this chapter's Skills for Healthy Living feature.

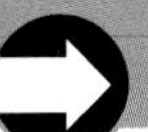

SKILLS FOR HEALTHY LIVING: Providing Social Support

Most people who attempt suicide do not really want to die but see suicide as the only way out of a painful or intolerable situation. Sometimes a person who attempts suicide lacks the support that he or she needs in order to overcome painful circumstances; such a person's suicide attempt is a call for help. With these realities in mind, you can see the value of being able to provide support to someone in need. In order to do so, it is essential to know how to communicate effectively and who to talk to for help. If someone you know displays signs of depression or suicidal thinking, get involved and seek help. Here are some guidelines.

- **Tell a trusted adult about your concerns.** Do not keep your concerns or your knowledge a secret, even if the other person is asking you to. When it comes to depression and suicide, secrets can be deadly, and keeping a friend's secret is not the right or healthy thing to do.
- **Take threats seriously.** If someone you know displays warning signs, don't excuse them or brush them off.
- **Listen and care.** If a person confides suicidal intentions to you, listen for the reasons that the person feels that way. Understanding where the person is coming from can help you convey the situation more effectively to others and may ultimately help the person get the support that he or she needs.
- **Don't belittle or challenge.** If you dismiss a person's threats about suicide, he or she may take that dismissal as a challenge.
- **Monitor the warning signs.** If the person seems to be getting worse, let others know, such as the person's parents, siblings, spouse, or counselor.

If you have serious concerns about a friend and don't know where to turn, call the National Suicide Prevention Lifeline at 1-800-273-TALK(8255).

Teens Under the Knife

If you think plastic surgery is something that only adults do, think again. According to the American Society of Plastic Surgeons, patients aged 18 and younger undergo well over 100,000 plastic surgery procedures each year. Some of the most common types of plastic surgery chosen by teens include nose jobs, breast reduction surgery, and correction of protruding ears, asymmetrical breasts, and scarring caused by acne or injury.

Teens seek such surgeries for many reasons. One often-cited reason is the desire to put an end to cruel comments made by other kids or teens—years of cruel remarks can drive a teen to take surgical action. For example, Jenna, a teenager from Texas, had surgery because she was often on the receiving end of Dumbo jokes about her protruding ears. Such reasons are also given by many adults, but teens often feel even greater pressure to fit in with others in terms of their appearance. For this reason, teens often report that their self-image and self-confidence improve when their perceived physical shortcomings are addressed.

Even so, many psychologists and physicians express concern about teenagers getting elective plastic surgery for any reason. These experts state that peer pressure and peer acceptance are viewed as particularly important among teens. They also note that teens pay a lot of attention to social messaging, social norms, and social expectations that will ultimately fade as they move into adulthood.

It's certainly true that body image plays a particularly prominent role in perceptions of overall health and well-being among teens. Most teens compare themselves and others with media images—often unfavorably, since popular culture tends to promote images and standards of physical attractiveness that are difficult, if not impossible, to attain. These days, computer manipulations, air brushing, and specialty makeup have established flawless skin, eyes, and noses as the norm. In addition, some common media images, such as the bodies of runway models, contradict what can be reasonably attained by most people even if they practice healthy behaviors. For example, fashion models weigh an average of 23 percent less than other U.S. females, but their images are perceived by many people as being normal.

In this environment, going under the knife for a permanent change in appearance may not be wise. "Often, individuals regret their decisions once they've grown into adulthood and found greater self-esteem through their professional and personal accomplishments," said Dr. Priyah Punjab, director of the Adolescent Self-Esteem Center of Los Angeles. Meanwhile, plastic surgeon Dr. Mark Macintosh not only supports plastic surgery for teens—he promotes it. "It's a cruel, competitive world out there, and we should feel obligated to do anything we can to help our kids thrive," said Macintosh. However, the National Institutes of Health (NIH) in the United States raises concerns about the medical risks associated with plastic surgery and also notes that both boys and girls continue to develop and change into their early twenties.

For Discussion

At what age do you think it's okay for a person to have elective plastic surgery? Why? Debate your perspective with a peer whose views differ from yours. Listen to each other's opinions and determine where you agree and disagree.

Reviewing Concepts and Vocabulary

As directed by your teacher, answer items 1 through 5 by correctly completing each sentence with a word or phrase.

1. ____________ health is your ability to use your thoughts in order to understand and control the effect your emotions have on your behavior.
2. The ability to adapt to change and stressful events in healthy and flexible ways is known as ______________.
3. People with positive _________________ are more likely to engage in healthy behaviors such as exercise and healthy eating.
4. ________________ is a mood disorder in which a person feels extreme sadness and hopelessness.
5. _________ _________ is an eating disorder that occurs when an individual does not eat enough food to stay healthy.

For items 6 through 10, as directed by your teacher, match each term in column 1 with the appropriate phrase in column 2.

6. conscientiousness
7. body image
8. phobia
9. muscle dysmorphia
10. post-traumatic stress disorder

a. intense fear and anxiety caused by a specific situation or object
b. your thoughts, feelings, and actions about your body shape or size
c. disorder typically seen in males that involves intense desire to become more muscular
d. anxiety disorder in which an individual has intense flashbacks or nightmares related to a traumatic event
e. conducting oneself according to an inner sense of right and wrong

For items 11 through 15, as directed by your teacher, respond to each statement or question.

11. Describe three healthy personality characteristics.
12. What is body image?
13. List two symptoms of a panic attack.
14. Identify and briefly explain one treatment for mental disorders.
15. What are three characteristics of attention-deficit/hyperactivity disorder?

Thinking Critically

Write a paragraph in response to the following statement.

Identify a positive personality characteristic you possess and use an example to explain how that characteristic helped you make a healthy choice.

Take It Home

Keep an accomplishment journal for one week and ask a family member to do the same. Write down your successes and the things you do well—no matter how big or how small. Each night, share your accomplishments with your family member and ask that person to share his or her accomplishments for the day.

UNIT IX

Embracing Priority Lifestyles

Healthy People 2020 Goals

- Increase the number of people at a healthy weight.
- Reduce the number of people, including teens, who are overweight or obese.
- Prevent inappropriate weight gain among teens.
- Reduce disordered eating among adolescents.
- Reduce the percentage of teens who do no leisure-time activity.
- Increase trips made by walking and biking.
- Improve health literacy.
- Increase fruit, vegetable, and whole-grain consumption.
- Reduce the consumption of calories from saturated fats and added sugars.
- Increase the number of people who get adequate calcium in their daily diet.
- Increase availability of healthy snacks.
- Achieve high-quality, longer lives. Reduce preventable disease, injury, and early deaths.
- Create environments that promote health, fitness, and wellness for all.
- Adopt healthy lifestyles for health and wellness.
- Increase comprehensive school health education.
- Increase the number of teens who do regular muscle fitness exercises.
- Increase out-of-school activities for teens.
- Increase overall cardiovascular health.
- Reduce heart disease, stroke, cancer, diabetes, high blood pressure, and osteoporosis.
- Improve teens' comprehension of health promotion and disease prevention concepts.
- Increase education to promote health-enhancing behaviors and reduce health risks.
- Increase availability of stress reduction programs.

Self-Assessment Features in This Unit

- Energy Balance
- What Motivates Your Eating?
- Stress Management

Making Healthy Decisions and Skills for Healthy Living Features in This Unit

- Self-Monitoring
- Nutrition Information
- Time Management

Special Features in This Unit

- Diverse Perspectives: Being Vegan
- Consumer Corner: Selecting Diet Products and Services
- Consumer Corner: Can Vitamins Really Reduce Stress?

Living Well News Features in This Unit

- Can a Trip to Your Local Drug Store Help You Lose Weight?
- Eating Out May Be Both Deceiving and Unhealthy
- Stress at Work: Can Worksite Health Promotion Help?

25

Nutrition: Foundations for Healthy Eating

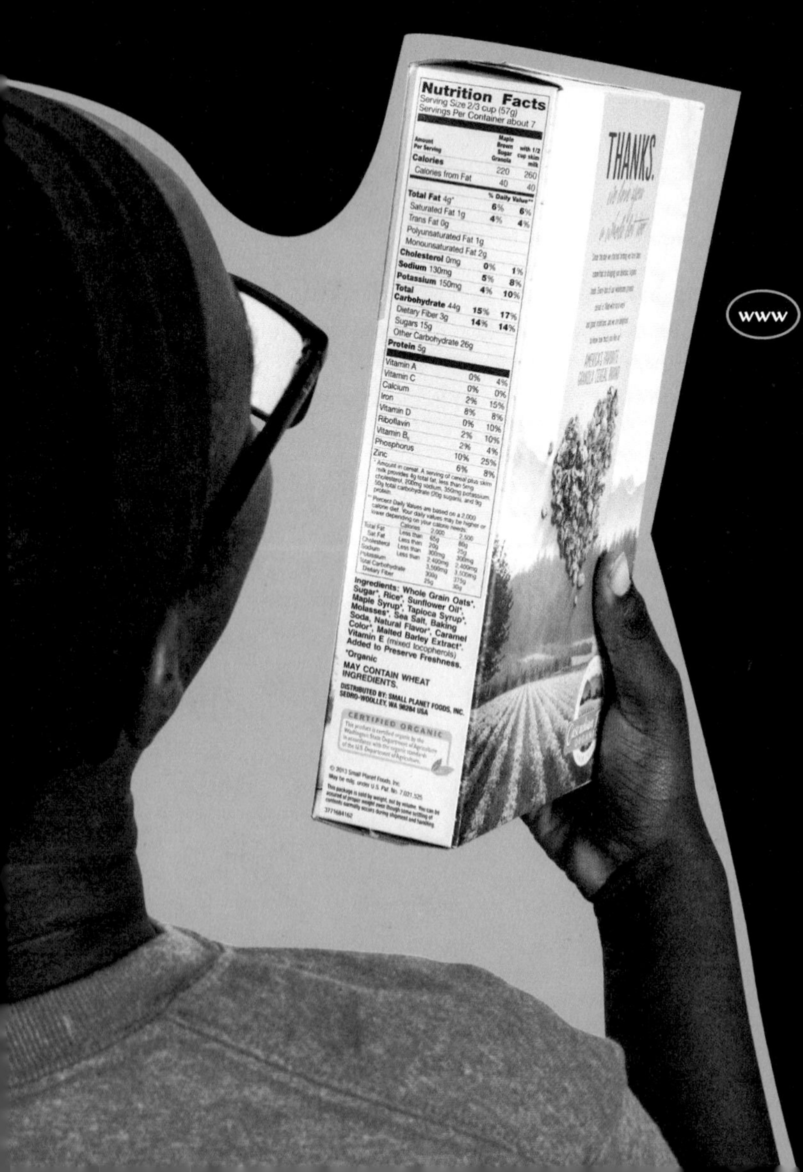

In This Chapter

www Student Web Resources

www.HOPEtextbook.org/student

Lesson 25.1

Basic Nutrients

Lesson Objectives

After reading this lesson, you should be able to

1. list and describe the three macronutrients,
2. list and describe the two major types of micronutrients, and
3. explain the functions of major macronutrients and micronutrients.

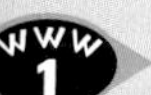

Lesson Vocabulary

calorie, carbohydrate, cholesterol, essential amino acid, insoluble fiber, macronutrients, micronutrients, mineral, nutrient-dense food, protein, saturated fat, soluble fiber, unsaturated fat, vitamins

Sitting down to a meal with delicious food can be a wonderful experience. However, experts tell us that Americans live in a toxic food environment. They mean that large quantities of food are available and that much of it contains added salt, fat, and sugar. As a result, Americans often consume too many daily calories while getting too few of the essential (and other important) nutrients. Perhaps it is not surprising, then, that nutrition has become a national focus in the United States due to rising rates of obesity and illness, such as heart disease and diabetes.

Fortunately, nutrition information is easy to find; unfortunately, the information is not always accurate. This lesson introduces you to the basics of good nutrition and provides you with the foundation necessary for making sense of nutrition information.

Basic Nutrients

Everything you consume can be classified into six major nutrient categories: carbohydrate, protein, fat, vitamin, mineral, and water. Items in the first three categories provide your body with calories and thus are known as energy-yielding nutrients. They are also called **macronutrients** because they are needed in large quantities (macro means large). Items in the remaining three categories—vitamin, mineral, and water—provide no direct energy or calories but are critical to chemical reactions in your body. They are known as non-energy-yielding nutrients and also as **micronutrients** because they are needed in smaller quantities.

Energy-Yielding Nutrients

Carbohydrate, protein, and fat provide your body with energy. Energy is often measured using **calories**. The term *calorie* is short for the proper scientific term *kilocalorie* (abbreviated as kcal), which represents the amount of energy required to raise the temperature of a liter of water one degree centigrade (Celsius) at sea level. The U.S. Department of Agriculture (USDA) recommends that most of the calories in your diet come from carbohydrates and that fewer of your calories come from protein and fat. Figure 25.1 shows the portion of your daily diet that should come from each of these nutrients. Table 25.1 shows recommended daily caloric intake varied by age and gender.

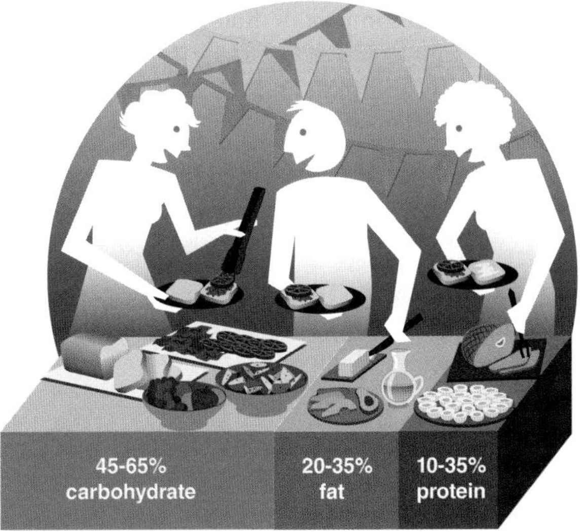

FIGURE 25.1 Percentage of calories recommended by the USDA for carbohydrate, protein, and fat.

TABLE 25.1 Recommended Daily Caloric Intake by Age and Gender

Gender and age	Estimated daily calories needed by those who are not physically active*
All children 2–3 yrs.	1,000
All children 4–8 yrs.	1,200–1,400
Girls 9–13 yrs.	1,600
Boys 9–13 yrs.	1,800
Girls 14–18 yrs.	1,800
Boys 14–18 yrs.	2,200
Females 19–30 yrs.	2,000
Males 19–30 yrs.	2,400
Females 31–50 yrs.	1,800
Males 31–50 yrs.	2,200
Females 51+ yrs.	1,600
Males 51+ yrs.	2,000

*These amounts are appropriate for individuals who get less than 30 minutes of moderate physical activity on most days. Those who are more active need more total calories and have a higher limit for empty calories. To find your personal total calorie needs and empty calories limit, enter your information into http://MyPlate.gov.

USDA's Center for Nutrition Policy and Promotion.

Carbohydrate

Carbohydrate is your body's main source of energy, and it provides the foundation for a healthy diet. Most of the cells in your body rely on carbohydrate for energy; even the metabolism of fat requires carbohydrate energy. Dietary carbohydrate comes in multiple forms, and not all carbohydrate-rich foods are healthy food choices.

The two main classifications of carbohydrates are simple and complex. Simple carbohydrate, also called simple sugar, is naturally found in foods such as fruits and milk and can also be refined to create products such as table sugar and corn syrup. Complex carbohydrate is found in the starch and fiber contained in foods such as whole-grain breads and vegetables. Most of the sugar in a healthy diet should come in the form of complex carbohydrate. Both simple and complex carbohydrates provide four calories per gram of weight.

The healthiest complex carbohydrate choices are high in fiber. These choices are typically known as **nutrient-dense foods** because they contain high levels of vitamins, minerals, and other important nutrients while remaining relatively low in calories.

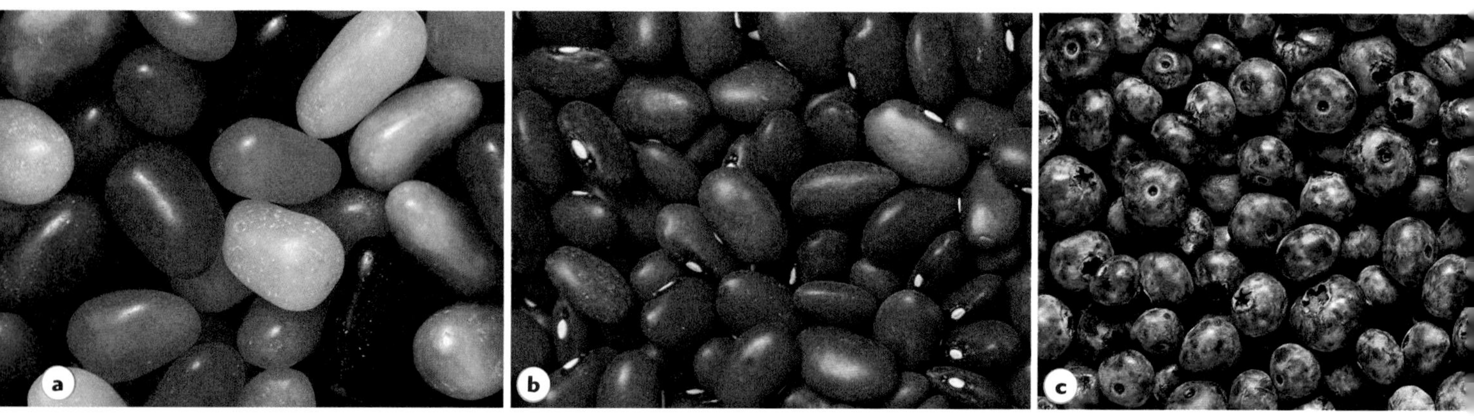

Examples of carbohydrate: *(a)* simple sugar (candy); *(b)* complex carbohydrate (beans); *(c)* fiber (fruit).

Apples, whole-grain bread, broiled salmon, steamed vegetables, and black beans are examples of nutrient-dense foods.

Dietary fiber can be soluble or insoluble. **Soluble fiber** is partially digestible and absorbs water as it passes through your digestive system. **Insoluble fiber** is not digestible; it passes through your digestive tract without being broken down or used. Insoluble fiber is often found on the outer layer of fruits, grains, and vegetables. Both types of fiber are important for good health because they help absorb damaging substances in your body and maintain normal digestive function. Both types are contained in most fruits, vegetables, and grains in their natural form.

As a general rule, the more unprocessed a food is, the more likely it is to provide nutrient-dense, fiber-rich, complex carbohydrate. For example, eating a whole apple, including the skin, provides more nutrients, more fiber, and less sugar than eating processed apple sauce. Similarly, bread made from whole-grain flour rather than white flour provides more fiber and more nutrients. White flour is made by removing much of the insoluble fiber from the original grain before grinding it and bleaching it.

Protein

Protein refers to a group of nutrients that build, repair, and maintain your body cells. Protein is easily found in animal products, such as meat, eggs, cheese, and milk; some of these may be high in fat. Some protein can also be found in plants, including grains, beans, and vegetables. Like carbohydrate, protein contains four calories per gram of weight. However, protein is not as easily used by the body for fuel as carbohydrate. As a result, only 12 percent to 15 percent of the calories you eat in the form of protein will be used directly for energy.

Carbohydrate is also used to generate and repair tissue. During digestion, your body breaks down protein into smaller building blocks known as amino acids. Twenty known amino acids are required by the human body for normal functioning, and nine of them must be obtained in the diet because the body cannot make them. If you consume these nine, your body will manufacture the remaining eleven. For this reason, the nine are known as **essential amino acids**.

A food that provides all nine essential amino acids in proper proportion is referred to as a complete protein. Examples include all animal products (e.g., meat, eggs, cheese, milk). A food that provides some of the essential amino acids is referred to as an incomplete protein. Examples include most grains, beans, and vegetables. It is possible to combine incomplete protein sources to make a complete protein; such foods are referred to as complementary protein sources. One example is black beans served with brown rice, which also has the virtue of being high in fiber and low in fat. A vegetarian (a person who doesn't eat meat) must be careful to eat a good variety of incomplete protein sources so that all of the essential amino acids are available for his or her body to use.

Fat

Fat is found in animal products and some plant products (e.g., nuts, vegetable oils). Unlike carbohydrate and protein, fat contains nine calories per gram of weight. As a result, foods higher in fat provide more calories and can be a significant contributor to weight gain if they are not monitored in your diet. However, fat is essential for normal physiological functioning. Specifically, it helps dissolve and carry certain vitamins, aids in the growth and repair of your tissues, and is critical for normal functioning in your nervous system, including brain functioning. As a result, your diet must contain an adequate amount of appropriate fat.

Fat is classified as either saturated or unsaturated. **Saturated fat** is found in animal products and is generally solid at room temperature. Examples include lard, butter, milk fat, and meat fat. **Unsaturated fat** is more typically found in vegetable products (e.g., oils) and tends to be liquid at room temperature. Examples include sunflower, corn, soybean, peanut, almond, and olive oils. Fish also produce unsaturated fat in their cells. Though a healthy diet includes both types of fat, unsaturated fat is considered healthier for the human body. In fact, according to the USDA, less than 30 percent (or up to 35 percent according to the Institute of Medicine) of the total calories you consume should come from fat in general, and no more than 10 percent of your total calories should come from saturated fat.

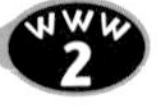

Sometimes unsaturated fat (e.g., sunflower oil) is chemically altered to look and act like saturated fat; in this case, it is called trans-fatty acid or hydrogenated fat. Trans-fatty acid has been found

DIVERSE PERSPECTIVES: Being Vegan

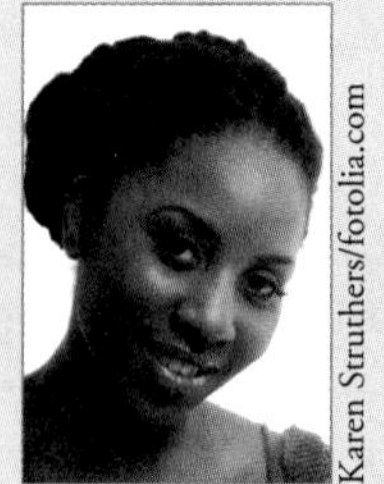
Karen Struthers/fotolia.com

My name is Erin, and I started eating a vegan diet in college after I took a course on the ethical treatment of animals. As a vegan, I don't consume any animal or animal-derived products, including eggs, milk, cheese, and cereal and bread products that use these ingredients. Some people choose to eat a vegan diet because of a health condition they have, like heart or kidney disease. I'm still young, and I live a healthy lifestyle, so eating vegan is a health choice for me too, but it is also an ethical decision. I am an animal lover and believe that all animals deserve humane treatment. I struggle with the idea of chickens or other animals being raised just to be used for human consumption. I know that my individual decision to be vegan won't change the world, but it's important to me and my personal sense of values.

Sometimes it's really difficult. A lot of restaurants don't have very many creative or good vegan options, so I prefer to eat a snack before I leave home so that I won't go hungry if that happens. Parties, barbeques, and other celebrations can also be a challenge if there aren't enough options for me. I do have to be careful to get all of the nutrients I need. I see a dietitian once a year to evaluate my diet, and I am also good about getting regular medical checkups. Learning to cook vegan foods has opened my eyes to a wider range of grains, beans, vegetables, and fruits, and I am happy with my decision. I have a lot of energy, my weight is never an issue for me, and I am at peace knowing I am living according to my personal sense of values.

in processed bakery foods (e.g., cakes) and has often been used to prolong a food's shelf life. You can be sure that a food contains trans-fatty acid if you see a term such as "hydrogenated" or "partially hydrogenated" in the ingredient list. The Food and Drug Administration (FDA) has now banned trans fat, but it has been left on the sample food label later in this chapter.

You should also pay attention to your intake of **cholesterol**, which is different from but related to fat. Cholesterol is a waxy, fatlike substance found in the cells of all mammals, including humans. A small amount of cholesterol is needed to make hormones and provide structure to your cell membranes. You consume cholesterol whenever you eat animal products, and even if you don't eat animal products, your body is able to use other fat to make cholesterol in your liver. People who eat a lot of saturated fat or trans-fatty acid are more likely to produce more cholesterol in their liver and thus have more cholesterol in their blood. High blood cholesterol puts you at risk for atherosclerosis and other cardiovascular diseases. To help prevent high cholesterol, and thus reduce your risk for cardiovascular disease, experts recommend consuming a diet that is low in saturated fat, trans-fatty acid, and cholesterol.

Non-Energy-Yielding Nutrients

Vitamins, minerals, and water provide no direct calories, or energy, for your body to use. Vitamins and minerals are also needed in smaller quantities than carbohydrate, fat, and protein. As a result, they are called non-energy-yielding nutrients, or micronutrients. Still, they are essential for normal functioning of your body. They are used in the chemical reactions that break down and release energy from the other nutrients, and they are necessary for the normal growth, development, and maintenance of your body.

Vitamins

Vitamins are organic compounds that are essential to your body's normal growth, functioning, and maintenance. Vitamins support chemical reactions in your body that are necessary for effectively using carbohydrate, protein, and fat. Your body needs many vitamins for healthy functioning, and the actions of vitamins are often interrelated. As a result, a deficiency in just one vitamin can affect the actions of other vitamins and cause profound health problems.

Vitamins are needed, for example, for your body's growth and repair. Vitamin C and the B vitamins are water soluble, meaning that they dissolve in water and are carried to your cells in your bloodstream. Because your body cannot store B and C vitamins, you must eat foods containing them every day. In contrast, vitamins A, D, E, and K dissolve in fat and are stored in fat cells in your liver and fat tissues. They can be dangerous, however, if they build up to excessive levels. For example, consuming vitamin A at a level that exceeds the recommended limit can cause liver scarring and damage. The best way to get the vitamins you need is to eat a well-balanced diet that is rich in nutrient-dense foods. Vitamin functions and food sources are presented in table 25.2.

Minerals

Minerals are essential nutrients that help regulate the activities of your cells. Twenty-five minerals have been identified as important for the human body. Minerals are present in all plants and animals, and a well-balanced diet is likely to provide you with an adequate amount of all necessary minerals. Table 25.3 shows some major functions and food sources of the most important minerals.

Some minerals are especially important for young people—for example, calcium and iron. Calcium helps build and maintain your bones. Sometime between the ages of 20 and 25, your body is still developing its bone structure and has yet to reach its peak bone mass. The body then gradually loses its ability to take calcium from food and store it in the bones. Eventually, the body begins to take calcium out of the bones to help with normal functions. Therefore, it is critical for your bones to reach their maximum possible density during your teenage years. This is particularly important for females, who are at greater risk of losing bone mass later in life. In fact, though osteoporosis (loss of bone mass) is a disease associated with older ages, the framework for prevention is set during your teenage years. You need to get enough calcium and do weight-bearing exercises (e.g., walking, jogging,

TABLE 25.2 Vitamin Functions and Food Sources

Vitamin	Function	Food sources
B_1 (thiamine)	Helps release energy from carbohydrate	Pork, organ meat, legumes, greens
B_2 (riboflavin)	Helps break down carbohydrate and protein	Meat, milk products, eggs, green and yellow vegetables
B_6 (pyridoxine)	Helps break down protein and glucose	Yeast, nuts, beans, liver, fish, rice
B_{12} (cobalamin)	Aids formation of nucleic and amino acids	Meat, milk products, eggs, fish
Biotin	Aids formation of amino, nucleic, and fatty acids and glycogen	Eggs, liver, yeast
Folacin (folic acid)	Helps build DNA and protein	Yeast, wheat germ, liver, greens
Pantothenic acid	Involved in reactions with carbohydrate and protein	Most unprocessed foods
Niacin	Helps release energy from carbohydrate and protein	Milk, meat, whole-grain or enriched cereals, legumes
C (ascorbic acid)	Aids formation of hormones, bone tissue, and collagen	Fruits, tomatoes, potatoes, green leafy vegetables
A (retinol)	Helps produce normal mucus and is part of a chemical necessary for vision	Butter, margarine, liver, eggs, green or yellow vegetables
D	Aids absorption of calcium and phosphorous	Liver, fortified milk, fatty fish
E (tocopherol)	Prevents damage to cell membranes and vitamin A	Vegetable oils
K	Aids blood clotting	Leafy vegetables

TABLE 25.3 Mineral Functions and Food Sources

Mineral	Function	Food sources
Calcium	Builds and maintains teeth and bones; helps blood clot; helps nerves and muscles function	Cheese, milk, dark green vegetables, sardines, legumes
Iron	Helps transfer oxygen in red blood cells and other cells	Liver, red meat, dark green vegetables, shellfish, whole-grain cereals
Magnesium	Aids breakdown of glucose and protein; regulates body fluids	Green vegetables, grains, nuts, beans, yeast
Phosphorus	Builds and maintains teeth and bones; helps release energy from nutrients	Meat, poultry, fish, eggs, legumes, milk products
Potassium	Regulates fluid balance in cells; helps nerves function	Oranges, bananas, meat, bran, potatoes, dried beans
Sodium	Regulates internal water balance; helps nerves function	Most foods, table salt
Zinc	Helps transport carbon dioxide; helps wounds heal	Meat, shellfish, whole grains, milk, legumes

weightlifting)—now and throughout your life—to stimulate your bone development and help prevent osteoporosis later.

Your body needs iron for proper formation and functioning of your red blood cells, which carry oxygen to your muscles and other tissues. Insufficient iron in the blood causes iron-deficiency anemia, which can leave you feeling tired all the time and interfere with your ability to do daily activities. The best dietary source of easily absorbed iron is meat. Some iron can also be obtained from beans, seeds, dark leafy greens, and grains. People who don't eat meat or animal products should make sure to consume other foods high in iron.

Another important mineral is sodium; however, in contrast with calcium and iron, the concern here is getting too much of it. Sodium is naturally present in many foods. Because it is a preservative and also enhances flavor, it is also commonly added to many foods, and it is especially high in some—for example, chips, lunch meat, fast food, processed food, and canned food. As a result, much of the sodium that Americans consume is hidden, and most consume far more than they need. This poses a problem because excess sodium is directly associated with high blood pressure; therefore, people with high blood pressure must take extra precautions to limit sodium in their diet. The best way to reduce your sodium intake is to eat a diet that is high in whole foods—especially fruits, vegetables, and whole grains—and low in processed foods. For more ideas, see table 25.4.

Vitamin and Mineral Supplements

If you're considering a vitamin or mineral supplement, talk to your parent or guardian, physician, or a registered dietitian (RD) first. The American Medical Association does recommend that most Americans take a general vitamin and mineral supplement, but this recommendation exists because most Americans do not eat proper, well-balanced meals. The best approach is to establish a healthy diet first, then consider possible supplements. If you decide to take a supplement, the Academy of Nutrition and Dietetics recommends avoiding any supplement that provides more than 100 percent of the Recommended Dietary Allowance (RDA) for each vitamin or mineral unless prescribed by a physician.

HEALTHY COMMUNICATION

Do you believe that taking vitamin and mineral supplements is an important part of being healthy? Share your perspective with a friend or classmate in a concise but thoughtful way. Support your position with facts and respect each other's opinions.

TABLE 25.6 Resting Metabolism (Calories) for Males Aged 16 or Older

	Weight (lb)					
Height (in.)	100	120	150	180	200	≥220
60–64	1,360	1,480	1,670	1,860	1,980	2,110
65–68	1,410	1,540	1,720	1,910	2,035	2,160
69–72	1,460	1,590	1,770	1,960	2,085	2,210
≥73	1,490	1,610	1,800	1,985	2,110	2,235

To convert inches to centimeters, multiply by 2.54. To convert pounds to kilograms, multiply by 0.45.

TABLE 25.7 Resting Metabolism (Calories) for Females Aged 12 to 15

	Weight (lb)					
Height (in.)	90	100	120	150	180	≥200
60–64	1,275	1,320	1,410	1,540	1,670	1,755
65–68	1,295	1,340	1,425	1,560	1,690	1,775
69–72	1,315	1,360	1,445	1,575	1,705	1,795
≥73	1,325	1,370	1,455	1,585	1,715	1,800

To convert inches to centimeters, multiply by 2.54. To convert pounds to kilograms, multiply by 0.45.

TABLE 25.8 Resting Metabolism (Calories) for Females Aged 16 or Older

	Weight (lb)					
Height (in.)	90	100	120	150	180	≥200
60–64	1,260	1,300	1,390	1,520	1,650	1,740
65–68	1,275	1,320	1,405	1,540	1,670	1,755
69–72	1,295	1,340	1,425	1,555	1,685	1,775
≥73	1,305	1,350	1,440	1,565	1,700	1,785

To convert inches to centimeters, multiply by 2.54. To convert pounds to kilograms, multiply by 0.45.

- Mowing the lawn expends 316 calories per hour for a person of Sandy's size, or about 5.25 calories per minute (316 ÷ 60 = about 5.25). Thus in mowing the lawn for 15 minutes, he expended about 79 calories (5.25 × 15 = 79).

Sandy recorded his calories expended in his activity log (see figure 25.3). His calories expended in physical activity totaled 355. He added this number to his resting metabolism of 1,800 to determine that his total energy expenditure for the day was 2,155 calories (355 + 1,800 = 2,155).

Prepare an activity log similar to the one that Sandy prepared. Record each activity you performed on the day of your log. Use the compendium for physical activity or a physical activity calculator to determine the number of calories you expended in each activity that you performed. Total the calories expended in these activities. Then add this calorie total to your resting metabolism calories to determine your total calories expended for the day.

Activity	Minutes	Calories per hour	Calories
	Morning		
Physical education: Burn It Up workout	30	340	170
Walk to and from classes	10	318	53
	Afternoon		
Walk to and from classes	10	318	53
	Evening		
Mow lawn	15	316	79
Daily activity total	65		355
Resting metabolism			1,800
Total daily calories expended			2,155

Figure 25.3 Sandy's activities for Wednesday.

Step 3: Evaluate Your Calorie Balance

Compare your calorie expenditure to your calorie intake to see if your calories balance for the day. Sandy expended 2,155 calories for the day but consumed 2,551, so he consumed 396 calories more than he expended (2,551 – 2,155 = 396). It's not unusual to consume more calories than expended on one day, then consume less than expended on another. However, if Sandy regularly consumed 396 calories a day more than he expended, he would gain body fat over time.

Determine if you have energy balance (calorie intake equals calorie expenditure) or if you have imbalance. Subtract the smaller number (whether calorie intake or calorie expenditure) from the larger number.

✔ Planning for Healthy Living

Use the Healthy Living Plan worksheet to set goals and develop a plan to maintain or improve your energy balance. Monitor the steps you take toward meeting your goals and repeat this self-assessment in one to three months to help determine the success of your plan.

Lesson 25.2

Healthy Eating: My Plate

Lesson Objectives

After reading this lesson, you should be able to

1. read and understand a food label,
2. indicate each food group and its recommended intake based on established dietary guidelines, and
3. identify examples of healthy food choices from each food group.

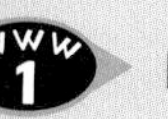

Lesson Vocabulary

empty calories, health claim, nutrient claim, structure/function claim

Eating well day after day can be a challenge. Fortunately, several great resources are available to help you make healthy food choices on a daily basis. Food labels are found on most food products and can be used to help you make informed decisions about which ones to buy and eat. In addition, the USDA and the U.S. Department of Health and Human Services (HHS) work together to develop and issue the Dietary Guidelines for Americans, which are updated every five years. These guidelines help American consumers make informed food choices in order to eat healthier calories, maintain or reduce weight as appropriate, and prevent diseases such as heart disease and diabetes. The guidelines also form the basis for the recommended intake associated with each of the major food groups. The recommended intakes are illustrated in the MyPlate guidelines. Each of these tools and resources is introduced in this chapter.

Selecting Healthy Foods: Using Food Labels

One of the most important tools available to help you select healthy foods is the nutrition facts label found on most food packages. The nutrition label gives you information about the food's serving size and content, including carbohydrate, protein, fat, and selected vitamins and minerals. It also tells you how much carbohydrate, protein, and fat the food has as a percentage of daily intake based on a 2,000-calorie diet. Your individual needs may differ from the label depending on whether you need more or less than 2,000 calories per day. Each aspect of the food label is explained in figure 25.4.

When reading a food label, consider the suggested serving size and how many servings are contained in the package. Many people make the mistake of assuming that the numbers listed on a food label apply to the entire package. For example, look at the label shown in figure 25.4. It indicates 60 calories per serving, but two and a half servings are contained in the can. As a result, if you ate the whole can, you would be eating 150 calories. In addition, eating the entire can would give you more than a whole day's worth of recommended sodium—just from that one food! As you can see, a food label gives you specific information related to essential nutrients that can be very useful in making dietary decisions. The FDA requires labels such as the one shown in figure 25.4. These labels are different from labels on the front or back of the box provided by manufacturers. Also, trans fat has been banned by the FDA, but it must be included on the label until the trans fat ban is fully implemented.

Nutrient Claims on Food Packages

In addition to the labels required by the FDA, some foods contain additional claim provided by the manufacturer. For example, you may have noticed markings about "fat free" cookies, "lean beef," or "low sodium" canned foods. In the United States, such **nutrient claims** are regulated by the Food and Drug Administration (FDA) and can appear only if the food meets certain standards. Nutrient claims can help you make informed choices, but you need

First look at the serving size and the number of servings in the package. To determine the calories for the entire package, multiply the servings per package by the calories per serving (i.e., 2.5 x 60). *Note:* The serving size and your idea of a serving size may be different.

Here you can see how many grams of carbohydrate, protein, and fat are in a serving. You can estimate the number of calories for each by using basic math. Multiply the fat grams by 9 calories, the carbohydrate grams by 4 calories, and the protein grams by 4 calories. These calculations are not exact, but they are a reasonable guide.

Chicken Noodle Soup

Nutrition Facts

Serving Size 1/2 cup (120 ml) condensed soup

Servings Per Container about 2.5

Amount Per Serving

Calories 60 **Calories from Fat** 15

	% Daily Value*
Total Fat 1.5g	2%
Saturated Fat 0.5g	3%
Trans Fat 0g	
Cholesterol 15mg	
Sodium 890mg	37%
Total Carbohydrate 8g	3%
Dietary Fiber 1g	4%
Sugars 1g	
Protein 3g	

Vitamin A	4%	Calcium	0%
Vitamin C	2%	Iron	2%

*Percent Daily Values are based on a 2,000 calorie diet. Your Daily Values may be higher or lower depending on your calorie needs:

	Calories	2,000	2,500
Total Fat	Less than	65g	80g
Saturated Fat	Less than	20g	25g
Cholesterol	Less than	300mg	300mg
Sodium	Less than	2,400mg	2,400mg
Total Carbohydrate		300g	375g
Dietary Fiber		25g	30g

Use this as a quick reference to determine how much fat is in the food.

Notice that you can quickly determine if trans-fatty acids, cholesterol, or sodium, are present in the food. In this case, one serving of soup is giving you 37% of the sodium you need all day. If you ate the entire can of soup, you would exceed your recommended sodium intake. *Note:* The FDA has banned trans fat, but it is included on food labels until the ban is fully implemented.

Here you can see the percentages of the daily serving recommendations for 4 of the most important vitamins and minerals.

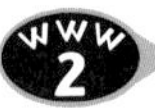

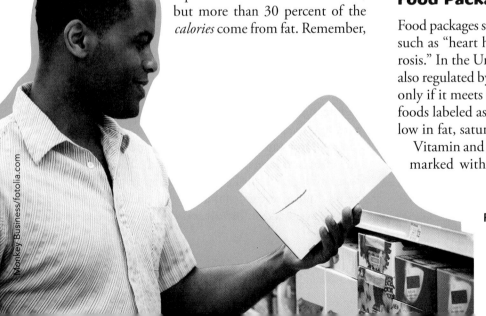

FIGURE 25.4 Sample food label.

to know their specific meanings and remember that they apply to a single serving (not necessarily the whole packaged amount).

Table 25.9 presents a few sample claims and their real meanings. Notice, for example, that a food may be labeled "fat free" even if it contains a small amount of fat (less than half a gram per serving). Some foods, such as milk and packaged meat, are advertised as being 2 percent fat (or 98 percent fat free). This is true when the calculations are based on weight. For example, 2 percent of the *weight* of a glass of 2 percent milk comes from fat, but more than 30 percent of the *calories* come from fat. Remember, every gram of fat contains 9 calories—more than twice as much as contained in the same weight of carbohydrate or protein. To determine the true percentage of fat calories in a given food, divide the total calories from fat per serving by the overall calorie total per serving, then multiply the result by 100. For the food label shown in figure 25.4, one serving contains 15 calories from fat, and the overall calories per serving is 60 ($15 \div 60 = 0.25 \times 100 = 25$), so the fat content is 25 percent.

Disease and Structure Claims on Food Packages

Food packages sometimes also contain health claims such as "heart healthy" or "helps prevent osteoporosis." In the United States, such **health claims** are also regulated by the FDA and can appear on a food only if it meets certain requirements. For example, foods labeled as being good for your heart must be low in fat, saturated fat, and cholesterol.

Vitamin and mineral supplements are sometimes marked with similar claims related to a body

Monkey Business/fotolia.com

Reviewing nutrient claims on food packages can help you make informed choices.

TABLE 25.9 Examples of Nutrient Claims on Food Packages

Nutrient claim	What it means
Fat free	Less than 0.5 g of fat per serving
Low fat	3 g or less of fat per serving
Lean	Less than 10 g of fat, 4 g of saturated fat, and 95 mg of cholesterol per serving
Light (lite)	1/3 fewer calories or no more than 1/2 the fat of the higher-calorie, higher-fat version; or no more than 1/2 the sodium of the higher-sodium version
Cholesterol free	Less than 2 mg of cholesterol and 2 g or less of saturated fat per serving

structure or function, such as "improves eye sight" or "builds strong bones." However, these **structure/function claims** are *not* regulated; therefore, supplement marketers who use these claims must also include a statement indicating that the claim is not endorsed by the Food and Drug Administration. This statement is often in fine print and is difficult to locate on the package.

Dietary Guidelines for Americans

Dietary Guidelines for Americans is a U.S. government document based on extensive research about foods, their effects on health, and the current strengths and weaknesses of the typical American diet. The guidelines state that a healthy diet should

- emphasize fruits, vegetables, whole grains, and fat-free or low-fat dairy products;
- include lean meat, poultry, fish, beans, eggs, and nuts; and
- be low in saturated fat, trans fat, cholesterol, salt (sodium), and added sugar.

The guidelines are reflected in specific recommendations made for each food group. The 2010 Dietary Guidelines for Americans also have guidelines for vegetarians, vegans, and other special diets. Dietary guidelines also exist that address the different needs of other cultures and countries. To learn more about the Dietary Guidelines for Americans and other dietary guidelines, visit the student section of the Health Opportunities Through Physical Education website.

MyPlate

To help you meet the dietary guidelines, the USDA suggests following the MyPlate recommendations for each major food group (see figure 25.5). Note that half of the plate is made up of fruits and vegetables. Yet studies show that fewer than 5 percent of teenagers eat the recommended amount of fruits and vegetables on a daily basis. Teenage girls should consume 1 1/2 cups of fruit each day, and teenage boys should consume 2 cups daily. All fresh fruits count toward meeting the requirement, though measurements may vary. For example, half a cup of dried fruit (e.g., raisins, dried apples) counts as a full cup of fruit.

Similarly, teenage girls should eat 2 1/2 cups of vegetables per day, and teenage boys should eat 3 cups daily. You should also vary the vegetables you eat. Your diet should include servings of dark green vegetables, red and orange vegetables, beans and peas, and starchy vegetables. All have a role to play in your overall nutrition.

Grains and protein sources make up the other half of the plate. Both of these sources are recommended in amounts referred to as "ounce equivalents" (see tables 25.10 and 25.11 for examples). For grains, teenage girls should eat three to six ounce equivalents per day, and teenage boys should eat four to eight. You should also eat at least half of your grains in the form of whole grain. You can improve your whole-grain intake by choosing whole-grain bread, brown rice, and whole wheat pasta while limiting your consumption of bakery products, white bread, and white rice. For protein sources, teenage girls should consume five ounce equivalents daily, and teenage boys should consume six and a half per day.

The dairy group completes the MyPlate illustration. Both teenage girls and teenage boys need three cups of dairy food each day. Choose low-fat or fat-free options and limit your intake of dairy products containing added sugar (e.g., sweetened milk or yogurt). Vegans should consult the guidelines to determine how they can get the amount of calcium they need.

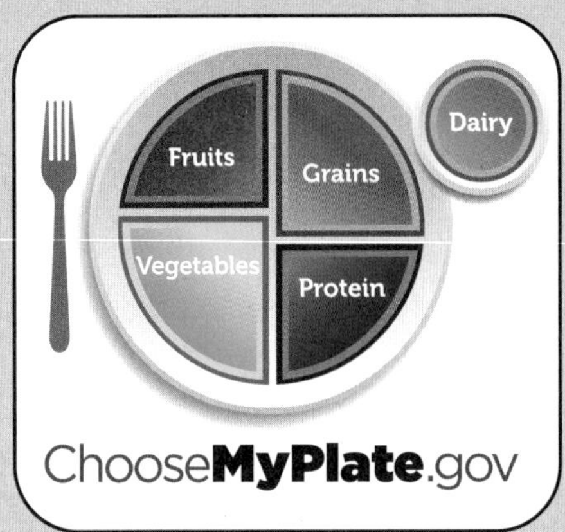

1. **Balance calories.**
   Find out how many calories you need for a day as a first step in managing your weight.
   Go to *www.ChooseMyPlate.gov* to find your calorie level. Being physically active also helps you balance calories.

2. **Enjoy your food, but eat less.**
   Take the time to fully enjoy your food as you eat it. Eating too fast or when your attention is elsewhere may lead to eating too many calories. Pay attention to hunger and fullness cues before, during, and after meals. Use them to recognize when to eat and when you've had enough.

3. **Avoid oversized portions.**
   Use a smaller plate, bowl, and glass. Portion out foods before you eat. When eating out, choose a smaller size option, share a dish, or take home part of your meal.

4. **Eat these foods more often.**
   Eat more vegetables, fruits, whole grains, and fat-free or 1% milk and dairy products. These foods have the nutrients you need for health including potassium, calcium, vitamin D, and fiber. Make them the basis for meals and snacks.

5. **Make half your plate fruits and vegetables.**
   Choose red, orange, and dark green vegetables like tomatoes, sweet potatoes, and broccoli, along with other vegetables for your meals. Add fruit to meals as part of main or side dishes or as dessert.

6. **Switch to fat-free or low-fat (1%) milk.**
   They have the same amount of calcium and other essential nutrients as whole milk, but fewer calories and less saturated fat.

7. **Make half your grains whole grains.**
   To eat more whole grains, substitute a whole-grain product for a refined product such as eating whole wheat bread instead of white bread or brown rice instead of white rice.

8. **Eat these foods less often.**
   Cut back on foods high in solid fats, added sugars, and salt. They include cakes, cookies, ice cream, candies, sweetened drinks, pizza, and fatty meats like ribs, sausages, bacon, and hot dogs. Use these foods as occasional treats, not everyday foods.

9. **Compare sodium in foods.**
   Use the nutrition facts label to choose lower sodium versions of foods like soup, bread, and frozen meals. Select canned foods labeled *low sodium*, *reduced sodium*, or *no salt added*.

10. **Drink water instead of sugary drinks.**
    Cut calories by drinking water or unsweetened beverages. Soda, energy drinks, and sports drinks are a major source of added sugar, and calories, in American diets.

FIGURE 25.5 Follow these 10 tips for creating a great plate.
USDA's Center for Nutrition Policy and Promotion.

TABLE 25.10 Ounce Equivalents for Grains

Food	1 oz. (28 g) equivalent	Common portion and number of oz. (28 g) equivalents
Bagel	1 mini bagel	1 large bagel = 4 oz. equivalents
Bread	1 regular slice	2 regular slices = 2 oz. equivalents
Muffin	1 small (2 1/2 in. or 6 1/2 cm in diameter), plain or wheat	1 large (3 1/2 in. or 9 cm) = 3 oz. equivalents
Pancake	1 small (4 1/2 in. or 11 1/2 cm) pancake	3 pancakes = 3 oz. equivalents
Pasta	1/2 cup cooked	1 cup cooked = 2 oz. equivalents
Popcorn	3 cups popped	1 mini microwave bag or 100 cal. bag = 2 oz. equivalents
Rice	1/2 cup cooked	1 cup cooked = 2 oz. equivalents
Tortilla	1 small (6 in. or 15 cm), flour	1 large (12 in. or 30 cm) = 4 oz. equivalents

From U.S. Department of Agriculture 2011.

TABLE 25.11 Ounce Equivalents for Protein Sources

Food	1 oz. (28 g) equivalent	Common portion and number of oz. (28 g) equivalents
Meat	1 oz. cooked meat	1 small steak = 3–4 oz. equivalents
Poultry	1 oz. cooked turkey or chicken without skin	1 small chicken breast = 3 oz. equivalents
Seafood	1 oz. cooked fish or shellfish	1 can tuna = 3–4 oz. equivalents 1 salmon steak = 4–6 oz. equivalents
Eggs	1 egg	1 whole egg = 1 oz. equivalent 3 egg whites = 2 oz. equivalents
Nuts and seeds	1/2 oz. (14 g) nuts or seeds or 1 tbsp peanut butter	1 oz. nuts or seeds = 2 oz. equivalents
Beans and peas	1/4 cup cooked peas or beans	1 cup bean soup = 2 oz. equivalents

From U.S. Department of Agriculture 2011.

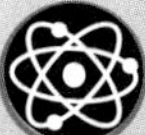

HEALTH SCIENCE

Have you ever wondered how scientists figure out how many calories the human body uses for various functions and activities? The answer is calorimetry, which is the measurement of heat released or stored within a closed system. Calorimetry can be used to determine how much heat the human body releases during a given activity. Doing so requires a metabolic chamber large enough for a person to live in during the study. The chamber allows scientists to measure exactly how much heat an individual gives off while eating, sleeping, or engaging in a physical activity.

Since this type of measurement is expensive and not very practical, scientists also estimate calorie expenditure by measuring how much oxygen a person uses. This approach works because every liter of oxygen the body uses requires five kilocalories of energy. As a result, scientists can have people breathe into a special analyzer that compares how much oxygen is inhaled versus how much is exhaled. The difference tells them how much oxygen a person used and therefore how many kilocalories were required. This form of calorimetry allows scientists to measure energy expenditure (calorie use) in a wide variety of settings and activities.

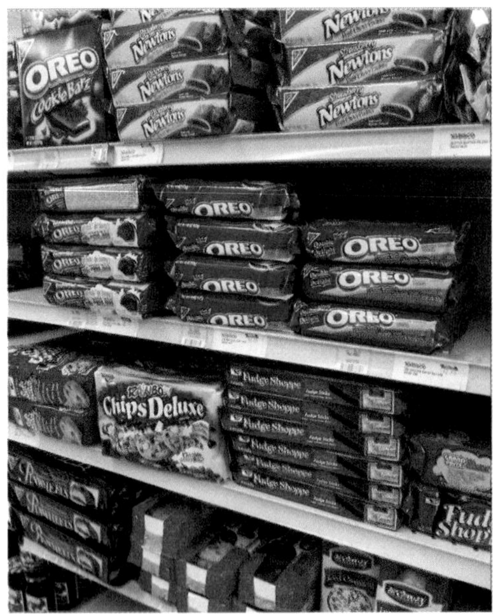

Packaged snack foods are often high in empty calories.
Human Kinetics/Kelly Huff

Recommendations also exist for oils in the diet. Teenage girls should not consume more than five teaspoons of oil each day, and teenage boys should not consume more than six teaspoons daily. Oils are most commonly found in nuts, fish, cooking oil, and salad dressing. The best way to limit your oil intake is to avoid fried food and limit your use of oily dressings and sauces.

Understanding Empty Calories

As you may recall, foods that are high in vitamins and minerals and low in calories are known as nutrient-dense foods. But some foods are just the opposite; they contain **empty calories**—calories that come from solid fat or added sugar. Examples of solid fat include trans-fatty acid, butter, beef fat, and shortening. Examples of added sugar include table sugar and corn syrup. These ingredients can be found in many foods, especially processed foods such as cakes, cookies, ice cream, hot dogs, sausages, chips, and soft drinks. Even some fancy coffee drinks (e.g., caramel latte) can be very high in empty calories. Other examples are presented in table 25.12.

You should strictly limit your consumption of empty calories. This doesn't mean that you must avoid the food completely, but a healthier option is often available, such as low-fat hot dogs, fat-free cheese and milk, sugar-free drinks, and baked crackers and chips. Be aware, however, that some of these better options still contain a lot of empty calories or may pose other health risks. If you are considering a food with a lot of empty calories, know that it contributes to overeating and weight gain and provides you with little nourishment.

TABLE 25.12 Examples of Foods High in Empty Calories

Food and portion	Estimated total calories	Estimated empty calories
1 cup whole milk	149	63
1 cup frozen yogurt	224	119
3 fried chicken wings with skin and batter	478	382
1 medium glazed doughnut	255	170
1 medium order of French fries	431	185
1 slice pepperoni pizza	340	139
1 bottle of regular soda	192	192

From U.S. Department of Agriculture 2011.

Comprehension Check

1. Describe three things you can learn about a food by reading its nutrition label.
2. What do the Dietary Guidelines for Americans say that we should eat less of?
3. What are empty calories? Provide three examples of foods high in empty calories.

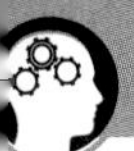

MAKING HEALTHY DECISIONS: Self-Monitoring

Over the past two years, Chloe had gained more pounds than she should have, and she felt more tired and sluggish than she used to. Lately, she'd been trying to eat a healthier diet. However, even though she'd been working on changing her eating habits, she didn't notice any changes in her weight or her energy level. When she wrote about her struggles in an essay for English class, her teacher noted that she had seen Chloe snacking on chips and candy during breaks and afterschool events. She wondered if Chloe was aware of these habits. After considering her teacher's comments, Chloe started keeping track of her food intake. When she reviewed her food log, she noticed that her main meals were pretty healthy but that she was snacking on food with empty calories between meals. This surprised her because she had thought she was just having "a few chips or a couple of pieces of candy" at a time and hadn't thought it was that important.

For Discussion

What did self-monitoring teach Chloe about her habits? What are some other situations where self-monitoring might help someone better understand his or her behavior? Is there a behavior that you might benefit from tracking? Use the guidelines presented in this chapter's Skills for Healthy Living feature to help you begin self-monitoring a health behavior of your own.

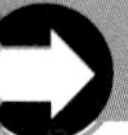

SKILLS FOR HEALTHY LIVING: Self-Monitoring

Self-monitoring means keeping track of your own behaviors. For example, many people wish to lose weight, but few people keep a detailed log of the calories they eat. Effective self-monitoring involves writing down what you eat, what you're doing while eating, and how you feel before and after eating. Tracking these factors for even a short time allows you to clearly see your own choices and patterns. It also focuses your attention and increases your self-awareness. In short, it brings clarity to exactly what behaviors you're doing and which ones need changing.

You can self-monitor any health behavior or habit for which you have a goal or desired outcome—for example, your diet, physical activity, smoking, drinking, or even time spent watching TV or playing video games. To be effective, you must self-monitor with honesty and without cheating. Done right, self-monitoring is like holding up a mirror to yourself and allowing yourself to see what is really happening and what you need to do to change it. If you decide to self-monitor a health behavior, use the following guidelines as a starting point.

- **Write things down.** Don't assume you can simply remember what you did.
- **Record information as frequently as possible.** Your log will be more accurate if you record your behavior as it happens, or at least several times a day. If you record your behaviors only at night, you might forget something or feel too tired and miss the day entirely.
- **Be honest and record your current behaviors.** Self-monitoring works only if you record what you're actually doing. This is one of the biggest challenges for most people. Sometimes people write down what they wish they had done or what they know they should have done, rather than what they did do. Self-monitoring is useful only if you're willing to look openly and honestly at your choices and actions.
- **Reflect on your behaviors and set goals.** Look over your journal or log after a week or two. What patterns do you see? Can you accurately understand

your own behaviors? You may need to continue self-monitoring a while longer, or you may be ready to set goals and begin changing your behavior.

- **As you begin to change, write down your goals and continue to monitor your actions.** Once you see what your behaviors look like, you can set reasonable goals for change. If monitoring your TV watching reveals that you watch an average of five hours each day, you might set a goal of watching no more than three and a half hours daily. Keep monitoring your actions to see if you meet your goal; if so, consider whether or not to change it again. In this case, your final goal might be to watch TV for no more than two hours each day.
- **Take advantage of relevant technology and social support.** Depending on the health behavior you're tracking, you might find that a social support group exists in your community that could help you stay honest and be accountable for your actions. Apps for electronic devices also offer ways to monitor and track a wide range of behaviors. Using one of these options might help you be consistent in your efforts.

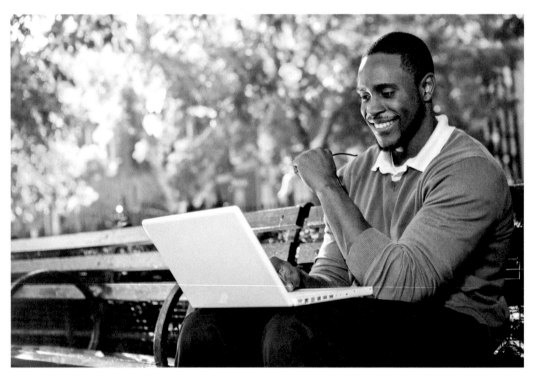

Monitoring and tracking health behaviors can be made easier with the use of technology.
Joselito Briones

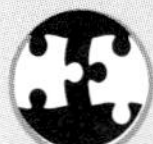

ACADEMIC CONNECTION: Mathematical Literacy

Developing literacy is an important part of being a good critical thinker. There are various types of literacy. Traditionally, a literate person was considered to be a person who could read and write with reasonable proficiency (ability). Today we speak of literacy in a number of ways. For example, in the chapter on health care consumerism, you will read about what it means to have health literacy. Mathematical literacy (also called qualitative literacy) refers to the knowledge of and confidence with basic mathematical and analytical concepts and operations that are required for problem solving, decision making, economic productivity, and real-world applications. The ability to read information in graphic form is a part of mathematical literacy. This chapter's Living Well News feature uses a bar graph to represent the percentages of obesity in various populations.

A bar graph is especially useful in making comparisons of group information. Each bar illustrates the percentage of a group that has a given characteristic. The height of the bar represents the percentage of a group that has that characteristic. For example, in figure 25.6 the bar for people 60 years of age and older is higher than the bar for other age groups, indicating that a higher percentage of older people (39.7) are obese compared to younger people (32.6 to 36.6).

The ability to interpret the data available in a graph and to decipher trends and patterns that emerge from the graphical representation is a part of mathematical literacy. Developing mathematical literacy requires practice. Whenever you are presented with data in graphs, take the time to read and understand the information.

Can a Trip to Your Local Drug Store Help You Lose Weight?

One in three adults in the U.S. is considered overweight or obese (see figure 25.6). Thus it is not surprising that, according to the U.S. Centers for Disease Control and Prevention, the use of weight loss supplements is on the rise. An article published in the *American Journal of Clinical Nutrition* stated that about 15 percent of Americans have used weight loss supplements (20 percent of women and 10 percent of men). In fact, weight loss supplements are big business. The Nutrition Business Journal, a market research firm, reported that about US$1.7 billion was spent on weight loss pills in 2007. Unlike prescription drugs, however, these products do not require a doctor's prescription; nor are they subject to the same rigorous standards applied to prescription drugs. More alarming, the U.S. Food and Drug Administration (FDA) warns that most over-the-counter (OTC) weight loss drugs are ineffective and that many can carry dangerous side effects.

"I used to think weight loss pills were just harmless pills of hope," said Dr. Anthony Smart, a general physician in the Seattle area. Over the last five years, however, he has seen an increasing number of patients taking weight loss supplements who complain of heart palpitations and chest pain.

Amy Fredlund, CEO of a leading dietary supplement company, states that the majority of weight loss supplements are safe and that the majority of problems that do exist involve obscure imported brands. However, other experts—including physicians, pharmacists, and government scientists—state that even mainstream weight loss supplements could be risky.

Consider ephedra, an herbal stimulant that gained popularity as a weight loss supplement in the 1990s. Ephedra-related problems included heart attacks, seizures, and deaths, leading the FDA to ban the supplement in 2004. As more Americans continue to be obese and the supplement industry continues to grow, the conflict between safety and hopelessness will undoubtedly continue.

For Discussion

What are some alternatives to weight loss supplements that a person could consider if they wanted to lose weight? What individuals or sources of information might a person consult when trying to decide whether or not to use a weight loss supplement? Why do you think some people choose to take these types of supplements?

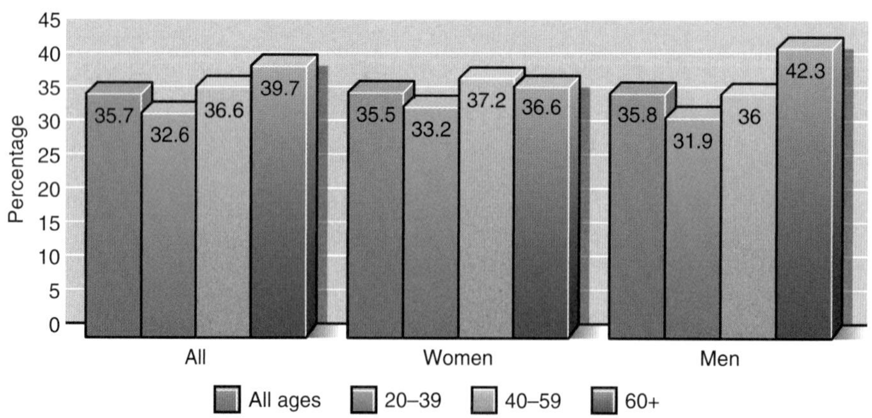

Figure 25.6 Obesity in the United States.
From CDC, NHNES 2009-2010.

Reviewing Concepts and Vocabulary

As directed by your teacher, answer items 1 through 5 by correctly completing each sentence with a word or phrase.

1. Carbohydrate, ____________________, and fat provide energy to the human body.
2. __________ __________ is unsaturated fat (e.g., sunflower oil) that is chemically altered to look and act like saturated fat.
3. Fat that comes primarily from plant sources and is liquid at room temperature is called ________________________ fat.
4. Your body needs ___________ essential amino acids from the foods you eat.
5. __________________ is a mineral necessary for optimal bone growth.

For items 6 through 10, as directed by your teacher, match each term in column 1 with the appropriate phrase in column 2.

6. saturated fat	a. carbohydrate, fat, protein
7. unsaturated fat	b. solid at room temperature
8. macronutrient	c. vitamin and minerals
9. micronutrient	d. chemically altered fat
10. trans-fatty acid	e. most vegetable oils

For items 11 through 15, as directed by your teacher, respond to each statement or question.

11. Explain the difference between soluble and insoluble fiber.
12. What is an incomplete protein?
13. What is cholesterol?
14. Why is calcium an important mineral for teens?
15. What is a nutrient claim? Give one example.

Thinking Critically

Write a paragraph in response to the following questions.

Scott likes to eat hamburgers, fries, and chocolate shakes. For lunch, he often eats pepperoni pizza with extra cheese dipped in ranch dressing. He doesn't like to eat fruits and vegetables. Scott is 17, is not overweight, and has no current health problems. What changes would you advise Scott to make in his diet? Why?

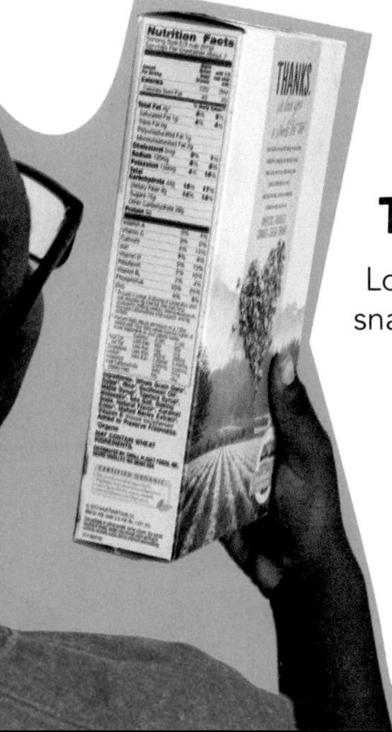

Take It Home

Look through the foods in your house and select five that you might normally snack on. Study each label and complete the following steps.

1. Write down the name of each food, the serving size, and the number of servings in the package.
2. Rank the foods in writing according to the amount of fat per serving (least fat = 1 and most fat = 5). Repeat this process for fat and fiber content.
3. Determine which snack is the healthiest and which is the least healthy. Explain your selections to a family member.

26

Nutrition: Energy Balance and Consumer Nutrition

In This Chapter

Student Web Resources
www.HOPEtextbook.org/student

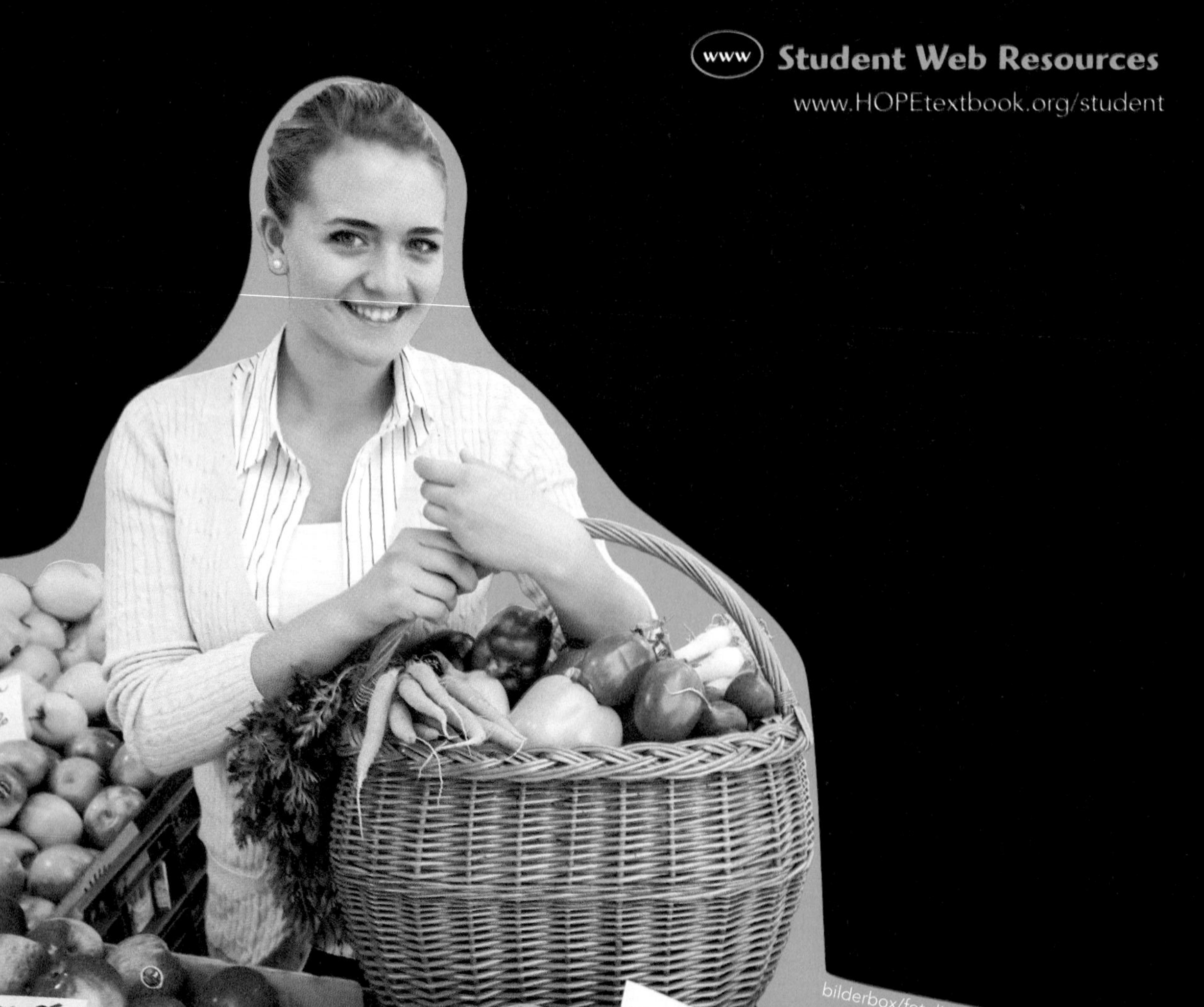

bilderbox/fotolia.com

Lesson 26.1

Energy Balance

Lesson Objectives

After reading this lesson, you should be able to

1. explain energy balance in relation to nutrition and health,
2. describe the difference between hunger and appetite and how each can affect healthy eating, and
3. explain why diets tend to fail and describe weight gain and maintenance.

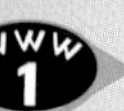

Lesson Vocabulary

appetite, hunger, negative energy balance, positive energy balance, resting metabolic rate, satiety

A newborn baby has an innate ability to know when it is hungry and needs food and when it is full. This natural ability to maintain energy balance is the result of a complex set of monitoring and feedback systems in the body. As we grow, we interact with our environment—which includes various societal influences on our diet—and we begin to respond to other types of cues that can influence our eating behaviors. This lesson introduces you to energy balance, hunger, and appetite, as well as the factors that influence them. It also discusses weight loss and dieting.

What Is Energy Balance?

Energy balance is the relationship between energy intake (what you eat) and energy output (what you do). Your energy intake is the total number of calories you consume in the form of carbohydrate, protein, and fat. Your energy output is the total energy you use for digestion, basic body functions, and physical activity. When your energy intake and output are the same, you're in a state of energy balance or equilibrium.

If you take in more calories than you use, you're in a state of **positive energy balance**. This means that you have more energy than you need, and the extra energy gets stored in your body. It's like a bank account balance. If you put more money into the account than you take out, you have a positive balance. However, maintaining a positive energy balance over a period of time causes weight gain and can negatively affect your health. Conversely, if you use more calories than you take in, you're in a state of **negative energy balance**. Over time, this state results in weight loss; it can also be a sign of starvation, illness, or disease. Energy balance is illustrated in figure 26.1.

Energy Expenditure

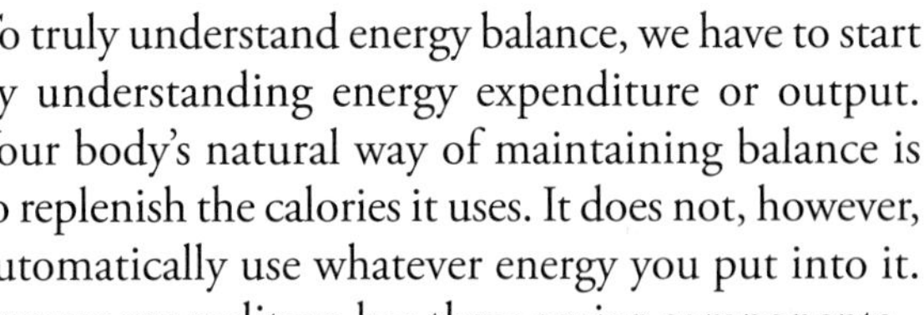

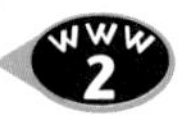

To truly understand energy balance, we have to start by understanding energy expenditure or output. Your body's natural way of maintaining balance is to replenish the calories it uses. It does not, however, automatically use whatever energy you put into it. Energy expenditure has three major components.

1. *The energy you need in order to maintain normal functions, such as breathing, circulating blood, and maintaining tissues (e.g., liver,*

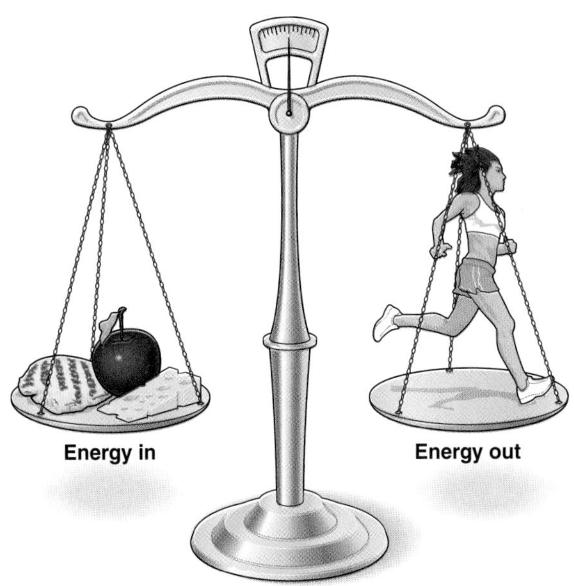

FIGURE 26.1 Energy balance.

brain, muscles). The number of calories you use for these functions is called your **resting metabolic rate**, which is influenced by a variety of factors (see figure 26.2).

2. *The energy you need to ingest and digest food.* This process starts with chewing, continues through swallowing, and ends with moving food through your intestines.
3. *The energy you use in movement and physical activity.*

Your body uses most of its energy (60 percent to 70 percent) to maintain normal functions of survival, about 10 percent for ingestion and digestion of food, and the remainder for movement and physical activity (see figure 26.3).

Some stimulants (e.g., caffeine) are marketed as tools for increasing your metabolism—thus helping you burn (use) more calories—but their effect is minimal, and they can cause damaging side effects. A better solution is exercise. The more movement and activity you do, the more your energy expenditure increases. In addition, movement is the source of energy expenditure that you can control directly through your own actions. In fact, an extremely active person might double his or her energy expenditure through activity. In addition, active bodies often consist of more muscle tissue, which naturally raises the metabolic rate, thus using more calories.

Energy Intake

Your energy intake, or the number of calories you consume each day, makes up the other half of the energy balance equation. You need to balance the number of calories you eat with the number you use in order to remain in energy balance. Recall that calories come from the carbohydrate, fat, and protein you eat. Teenage girls from ages 14 to 18 who are not active need to eat about 1,800 calories each day. Teenage boys from ages 14 to 18 who are not active need to eat about 2,200 calories each day. As just explained, your energy needs will rise as physical activity and exercise levels increase. How much you choose to eat can also be influenced by our hunger, satiety, and appetite. Each of these factors is explained in this lesson.

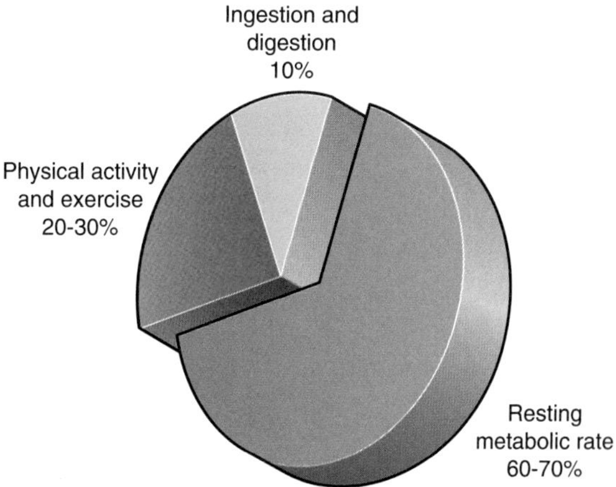

FIGURE 26.3 Contributors to daily energy expenditure.

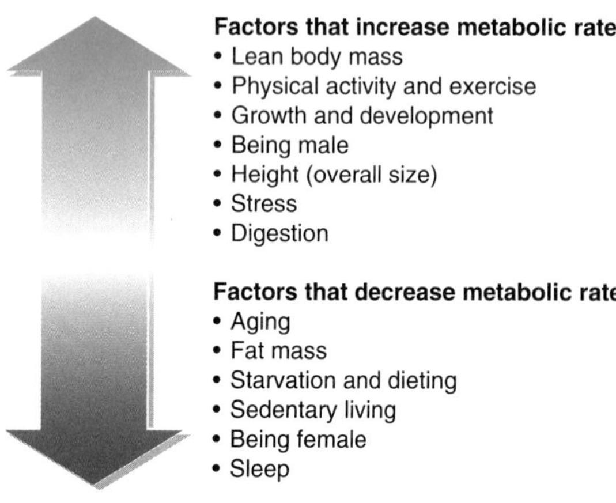

Factors that increase metabolic rate
• Lean body mass
• Physical activity and exercise
• Growth and development
• Being male
• Height (overall size)
• Stress
• Digestion
Factors that decrease metabolic rate
• Aging
• Fat mass
• Starvation and dieting
• Sedentary living
• Being female
• Sleep

FIGURE 26.2 Influences on resting metabolic rate.

Hunger and Satiety

Your body regulates your food consumption through a series of internal and external cues and stimuli. **Hunger** is your physiological drive to eat. When it's time to eat, your body tells you so through a set of internal changes, including a drop in blood sugar and the onset of stomach contractions. Other parts of your body also play a role in establishing your hunger—specifically, your brain, central nervous system (CNS), endocrine system, and digestive system. When you eat, your blood sugar and nutrient levels rise, and your hormone and neurotransmitter levels change, all of which eventually tells your brain and your body that you're full and therefore that it's time to stop eating.

When your body is well balanced and you're comfortable between meals, you're in a state of **satiety**, or fullness. The systems that contribute to hunger and satiety are complicated and very intricate. Studies have shown that certain conditions—for example, imbalances in hormones and neurotransmitters—can make it more difficult for some individuals to feel full. Figure 26.4 shows the relationship between hunger, satiation, and satiety.

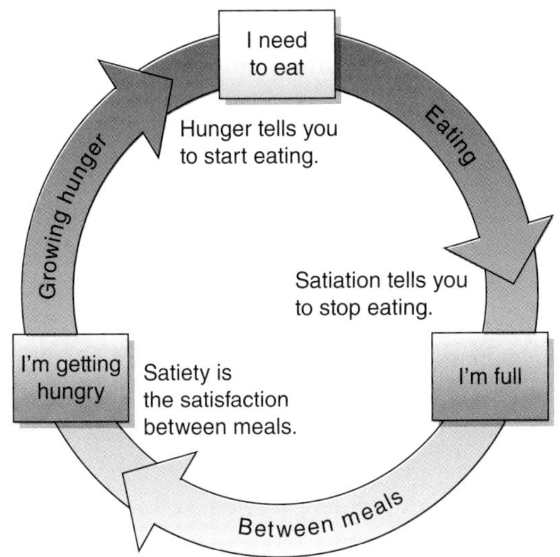

FIGURE 26.4 Hunger, satiation, and satiety are cues that tell you when to start and stop eating.

Appetite

Physiological hunger isn't the only thing that affects your food intake. Have you ever eaten popcorn at a movie or a hot dog at a ball game even though you didn't feel hungry? As these examples illustrate, our choices about what—and when—to eat can be influenced by our psychological needs. Whereas your hunger is your *physiological* drive to eat, your **appetite** is your *psychological* drive to eat. Thus it's different from your hunger. Appetite has to do with the pleasure you derive from food. It can be triggered by the sight and smell of food or even the sound of food cooking. On the other hand, if you're sick with a cold or the flu, the sight or smell of food can make you feel nauseated.

Appetite is influenced by many factors, including traditions. For example, people often associate eating with celebrations, holidays, particular family gatherings, and religious traditions. We may also associate eating with particular circumstances. Some people snack when they watch TV or when they get home from work or school—even if they aren't hungry. Others eat dessert after dinner even if they just ate a very large and satisfying meal.

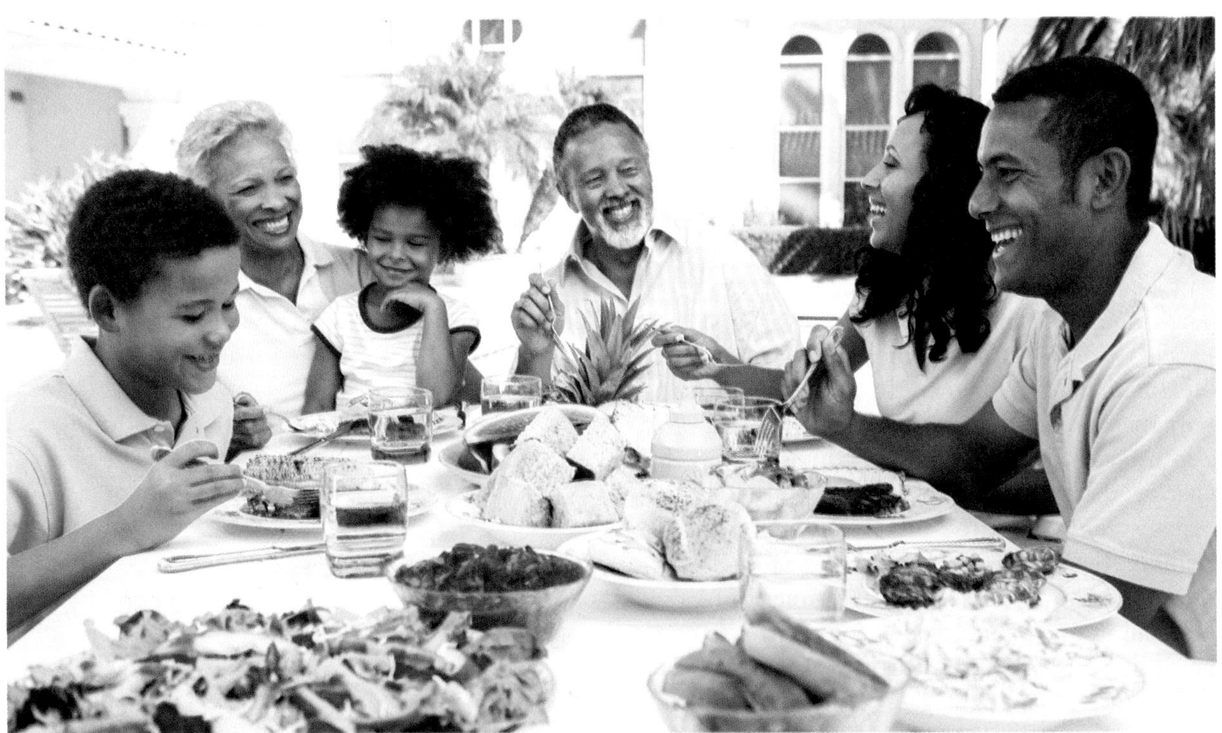

Appetite is influenced by many factors. We often associate eating with family gatherings for example.

Monkey Business/fotolia.com

Emotions also play a particularly important role in appetite. Is there a food you tend to eat when you feel sad or lonely? How about when you feel happy? Do you eat a lot, or nothing at all, when you feel stressed about a major exam? Most people let emotions affect their eating habits in consistent ways; therefore, understanding what circumstances and emotions trigger you to eat can prevent you from taking in unnecessary calories. Getting control of your appetite is a critical part of establishing and maintaining healthy eating habits.

> "If hunger is not the problem, then eating is not the solution."
>
> —Anonymous

Consequences of Energy Imbalance

When energy balance is not maintained, weight loss or weight gain may occur. In American society, many individuals seem to have a chronic (long-term) positive energy balance that results in gradual weight gain during the adult years. This weight gain may result in obesity and may bring many health risks. As a result, many people take various measures to try and lose weight. Other individuals struggle with trying to gain weight even when they maintain a positive energy balance.

Energy Needs Throughout Life

The amount of energy, or the number of calories, a person needs will change as the person goes through life. Infants and children need a lot of energy to support their growing bodies. Teenage girls and boys also use energy to support growth, as well as the changes that occur during puberty. Once a person reaches adult maturity, his or her energy needs stabilize, then gradually decrease (see table 26.1).

Studies show that the average American gains one-half to one pound (about one-quarter to one-half kilogram) per year after the age of 25. The reason for adult weight gain is not fully known, but likely contributors include lack of physical activity combined with poor eating habits, slower metabolism, and gradual loss of muscle mass. The best way we know of to reduce adult-onset weight gain is to remain physically active throughout life. It also helps to practice healthy eating and engage in regular self-monitoring.

Weight Loss Diets

It's very likely that either you or someone you know has tried to lose weight by going on a diet. In fact, dieting for weight loss is so common in the United States that it almost seems normal, and many people chase after the latest dieting trends year after year. At any given time, as many as 50 percent of American women and 25 percent of American men are reported to be on a weight loss diet. The average age of a first diet among American females is eight years.

Despite these trends, a third of Americans remain obese. How can it be that so many Americans diet while obesity rates remain so high? The fact is, most diets that people try don't work over the long term. Almost any diet, when followed, can result in some weight loss over the first few weeks or months. However, most diets are hard to follow (and many

TABLE 26.1 Energy Needs Across the Life Span

Age (years)	Calories per day (sedentary → active*)
Children 2–3	1,000 → 1,400
Females	
4–8	1,200 → 1,800
9–13	1,600 → 2,200
14–18	1,800 → 2,400
19–30	2,000 → 2,400
31–50	1,800 → 2,200
51+	1,600 → 2,200
Males	
4–8	1,400 → 2,000
9–13	1,800 → 2,600
14–18	2,200 → 3,200
19–30	2,400 → 3,000
31–50	2,200 → 3,000
51+	2,000 → 2,800

*Active means doing daily activity equivalent to walking 3 miles at 3 to 5 miles per hour (4.8 kilometers at 4.8 to 8 kilometers per hour).

From U.S. Department of Agriculture 2005.

are even unhealthy or outright dangerous). As a result, many people "go off" of their diet after a short time and end up returning to the same poor eating habits they practiced before trying the diet. Only about 5 percent of those who do lose weight maintain the weight loss for a year or longer.

The National Weight Control Registry (NWCR) tracks and studies people who have successfully lost weight and kept it off. Though people can be successful using a wide range of diets, the most common behaviors associated with long-term weight loss include reducing overall caloric intake and fat intake, increasing energy expenditure through regular exercise, and having strong social support during the process. We also know that healthy weight reduction should occur slowly—at a rate of one-half to two pounds (about one-quarter to one kilogram) per week. To achieve this reduction, a person needs to expend about 500 more calories per day than he or she eats.

When you consider these findings together, the truth is that the most successful weight loss efforts focus on eating a well-balanced diet and getting enough regular physical activity. This approach

Are Energy Drinks a Good Thing?

Energy drinks are the fastest-growing beverage market in the United States; in 2011, for example, energy drink sales exceeded US$9 billion. Much of the energy drink market is directed at teenagers, and one in three teenagers reports regularly consuming energy drinks. Many young people believe that energy drinks can help them perform better in school, sports, and other activities. Others use energy drinks for the "buzz" or sensation they feel shortly after drinking them. This effect results from a stimulant, usually caffeine, and many energy drinks contain two to seven times more caffeine than a typical can of soda (see table 26.2).

TABLE 26.2 Caffeine Levels of Common Beverages

Beverage	Caffeine (mg)
Coffee—1 cup	115–175
Coca-Cola—12 oz. (355 ml)	47
Energy drink—1 serving	80–360
Hot cocoa—1 cup	10–17
Tea, black—1 cup	32–176
Tea, green—1 cup	25

Even so, because energy drinks are classified as supplements rather than beverages, they fall outside of U.S. regulations governing caffeine. This is no small matter. In 2007, half of all reported cases of caffeine overdose occurred in people under the age of 19, and this risk is increasing with the rise in consumption of energy drinks by teens. Most energy drinks also add herbal stimulants, such as ginseng, ginkgo biloba, and guarana.

While the United States has been slow to study the effect of energy drinks on teenagers, research from several other countries has demonstrated that the side effects of consuming energy drinks can include liver damage, kidney failure, respiratory disorders, agitation, confusion, seizures, psychotic conditions, nausea, vomiting, abdominal pain, abnormal heart rhythms, hypertension, heart attack, heart failure, and even death. High levels of caffeine consumption may also interfere with normal growth and development, particularly of the bones.

In addition, despite their name, energy drinks provide little usable energy for the body. If you're feeling sluggish or tired—or if you want to maximize your performance—the healthiest, safest, and most effective approach is to eat nutrient-dense foods, drink adequate water, do regular physical activity, and get a full eight to nine hours of rest each night. If you consume caffeine on a daily basis and decide to stop, reduce your intake gradually (over a period of one to two weeks) in order to limit withdrawal effects, such as headache and irritability.

HEALTHY COMMUNICATION

How often do you and your friends use energy drinks? What are the main reasons that you do or don't use them? Do you worry about the short- or long-term health risks associated with drinking these beverages? Share your opinions with your classmates. Support your perspective with facts and be respectful of others' opinions.

is not the same as "going on a diet." Instead, it means adopting long-term health behaviors in line with the prevailing recommendations for diet and physical activity.

Weight Loss Surgery

Many people struggle with issues of weight and associated diseases. Surgery is an extreme approach to weight loss that may be needed by some individuals who are unable to engage in normal activities of daily living and who have related health conditions (e.g., diabetes). Multiple types of weight loss surgery are available. Some use staples or bands to reduce stomach size; others redirect food to enter the intestinal system further along than usual, which reduces the amount of food absorbed by the body. These procedures, known as bariatric surgeries, carry significant risks and should be considered only in extreme cases after noninvasive approaches have been exhausted. Successful weight loss surgery can enable a person to lose as much as half of his or her body weight over a two-year period. However, long-term success still depends on making permanent changes in diet and physical activity.

Gaining Weight

Weight gain (especially as muscle mass) is often desired by certain people such as young males. For those who wish to gain weight, combining proper physical activity with adequate nutrition is the best method. Strength and muscular endurance exercises can help with weight gain. Resistance exercises like weightlifting are especially effective because they help the body build lean tissue (muscle). It is important to remember that physical activity burns calories and that muscle burns more calories than fat. Therefore, if you are trying to gain weight, it is very important to increase your intake of calories as you train and build muscle. A special diet (i.e., one with high protein) is not needed for weight gain and can be dangerous. It is also important to remember that genetic influences play a powerful role in body size and shape. Not everyone is meant to be heavily muscular and not everyone will respond to training or dietary changes in exactly the same way.

CONNECT

What does growing up in contemporary society teach you about dieting, weight, and health? Which type of media do you think has the biggest effect on people's perceptions of dieting, weight loss, weight gain, and health? Are men and women affected differently by these media narratives? How does the media affect *your* decisions about dieting, weight loss, or weight gain?

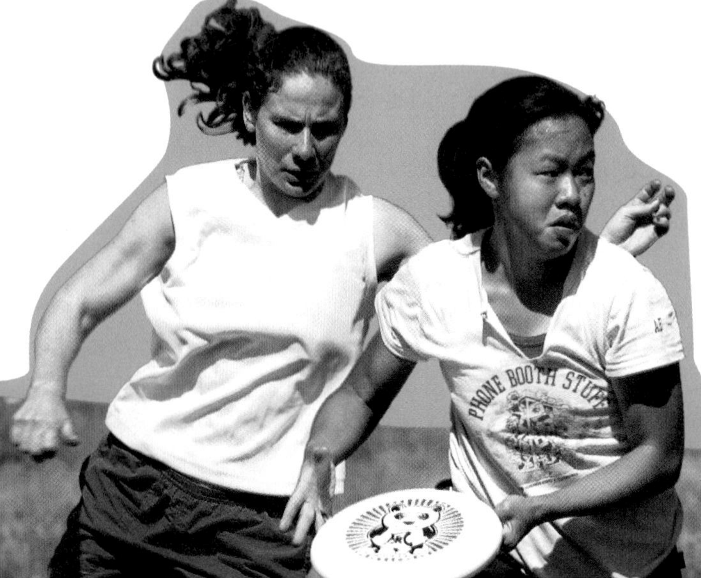

Unlike fad diets, regular physical activity can help you lose weight and keep it off.

CONSUMER CORNER: Selecting Diet Products and Services

There is no shortage of diet products and services in U.S. society. The problem is that many of them are not safe or effective, and even among those that are, it can be challenging to know which is the best choice. The following guidelines can help you make an informed decision if you ever need to lose weight.

- **Put safety and effectiveness first.** A safe and effective diet usually results in a loss of one or two pounds (about one-half to one kilogram) per week. Diets that promise rapid weight loss are more likely to be dangerous and less likely to produce long-term benefits.
- **Choose a plan that is flexible.** Not everyone likes the same foods. Any good diet plan allows for personal choice and options.
- **Choose a plan that is balanced.** We all need a balanced diet. No product or service is safe or effective in the long run if it doesn't offer a balance of foods and food groups. Diets that limit choices or focus on only one food group are not likely to provide balance.
- **Choose a plan that is comfortable.** A good diet should be comfortable and even enjoyable. Programs that provide recipes and allow for eating out and attending special functions are more realistic and more likely to help you succeed in the long term.
- **Choose a plan that advocates activity.** Every good weight loss product or service should advocate regular physical activity and provide some basic guidelines to follow.
- **Choose a plan that is educational.** Good weight loss products and services provide information about issues such as how to shop and cook in ways that are sustainable in the long term. Plans that provide you with food or limit you to prepackaged food may be easy, but they don't help you develop the healthy eating skills you need throughout life.
- **Involve your doctor.** Be careful about any plan that includes supplements or limits your food choices. Talk to your doctor before starting any weight loss diet.
- **Consider your needs.** Choose a program or plan that fits your level of commitment, your food preferences, and your budget. You're bound to fail if the program requires too much of your time or includes mostly foods that you don't enjoy.

Consumer Challenge

What diet programs and services are you familiar with? To learn more about some of the best-known options, visit the student section of the Health Opportunities Through Physical Education website.

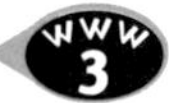

Comprehension Check

1. What is the difference between positive and negative energy balance?
2. How does hunger differ from appetite?
3. What are some reasons that most diets fail in the long term? Describe weight gain and maintenance.

SELF-ASSESSMENT: What Motivates Your Eating?

What motivates you to eat or not to eat? Do certain situations, emotions, or traditions affect what you choose to eat? This self-assessment will help you better understand what motivates your eating behaviors so that you can better manage them. Indicate your level of agreement with each statement, then total your score from each section and consider your findings. Record your results as directed by your teacher.

Situational factors

When your favorite foods are around the house, do you eat them even if you aren't hungry?					
Never 1	Rarely 2	Occasionally 3	Frequently 4	Always 5	
When you're eating out, do you try to get the most food you can for the money you're spending?					
Never 1	Rarely 2	Occasionally 3	Frequently 4	Always 5	
If you see an advertisement for a specific food or restaurant—or if you're passing a bakery, candy shop, or other appealing display—do you stop and get that food?					
Never 1	Rarely 2	Occasionally 3	Frequently 4	Always 5	

Total your score: _____
3–6: You may occasionally eat when you shouldn't, but overall you're in pretty good control in tempting situations.
7–9: You might want to pay attention to which situations tempt you to eat when you aren't hungry and ask yourself why you eat in these situations.
10–15: Your eating may be too determined by situations. Try to focus on your own hunger cues rather than on what the situation suggests.

Emotional factors

Do you eat when you're bored even if you're not hungry?				
Never 1	Rarely 2	Occasionally 3	Frequently 4	Always 5
Do you eat to cope with feelings of sadness, hopelessness, or loneliness?				
Never 1	Rarely 2	Occasionally 3	Frequently 4	Always 5
Do you eat when you're happy or excited, even if you're not hungry?				
Never 1	Rarely 2	Occasionally 3	Frequently 4	Always 5
Do you eat when you're feeling anxious or stressed?				
Never 1	Rarely 2	Occasionally 3	Frequently 4	Always 5

Total your score: _____
4–8: Your emotions don't seem to affect your eating habits very often.
9–12: Your emotions sometimes get the best of you when it comes to eating. Pay attention to how you feel and what you eat and try not to let emotions dictate when or what you eat.
13–20: You're often or always eating in response to your emotions rather than your own hunger. Work on finding healthy ways to cope with your emotions and pay careful attention to your feelings of hunger and fullness.

Social factors

<table>
<tr><td colspan="5">Do you eat when you're at a party or celebration in order to fit in and be social?</td><td rowspan="6">Total your score: _____
3–6: You seem not to let social situations control your eating very often.
7–9: Some social situations may be causing you to eat even when you're not hungry. Try not to give in to social pressures to eat if you're not feeling hungry.
10–15: Social situations may be getting the best of you when it comes to eating. Explain to your friends and family members that you're working on improving your eating habits and ask for their support.</td></tr>
<tr><td>Never
1</td><td>Rarely
2</td><td>Occasionally
3</td><td>Frequently
4</td><td>Always
5</td></tr>
<tr><td colspan="5">Do you eat when your friends are eating, even if you're not hungry?</td></tr>
<tr><td>Never
1</td><td>Rarely
2</td><td>Occasionally
3</td><td>Frequently
4</td><td>Always
5</td></tr>
<tr><td colspan="5">Do you feel like you're being rude or disrespectful if you don't eat everything on your plate?</td></tr>
<tr><td>Never
1</td><td>Rarely
2</td><td>Occasionally
3</td><td>Frequently
4</td><td>Always
5</td></tr>
</table>

✓ Planning for Healthy Living

Use the Healthy Living Plan worksheet to change any negative eating motivation or habit you may have.

Lesson 26.2

Healthy Eating Habits

Lesson Objectives

After reading this lesson, you should be able to

1. identify several ways to plan and shop for healthy foods,
2. make healthy food choices when eating in a cafeteria or restaurant, and
3. identify specific steps to reduce or eliminate the risk of food poisoning.

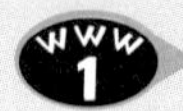

Lesson Vocabulary

nutritionist, registered dietitian (RD)

Many people know something about basic nutrition and understand some general facts about carbohydrate, fat, and protein. It can be challenging, however, to use that knowledge to make changes in your eating habits. People often struggle with selecting or preparing healthy food options, and some people think they can't make healthy choices when eating out. The challenge is heightened by the fact that much of the information available about nutrition and diet is misleading or inaccurate. As a result, many people don't know who to trust for advice. This lesson provides some practical solutions.

Making Healthy Choices: Planning Ahead

You eat in a variety of places, including your home, school, and car. Since high-fat and high-calorie foods are all around us, it's important to plan ahead to ensure that you have healthy options available. More generally, healthy living requires learning to plan meals, shop for and cook healthy foods, and, when necessary, select the healthiest prepared foods.

When you eat at home, begin by planning your meals. In fact, it's best to both plan meals and do your food shopping *after* eating a good, healthy meal so that you're not hungry—and thus more vulnerable to temptation—while you plan and shop. To plan, think about what you might want to eat for breakfast, lunch, and dinner over the next several days (or week). Write down the meals and add all of the necessary ingredients to your grocery list; include some healthy snack options as well.

At the grocery store, choose the particular ingredients and foods that are tasty and provide the healthiest options for your planned meals. Use food labels to help you select lower-fat and lower-calorie options, consider fresh or fresh-frozen vegetables instead of canned to reduce salt intake, and select leaner cuts of meat or substitute poultry or fish. Lean meats—those with less than 5 grams of fat per 3.5-ounce (100-gram) serving—include eye of round roast and steak, sirloin tip side steak,

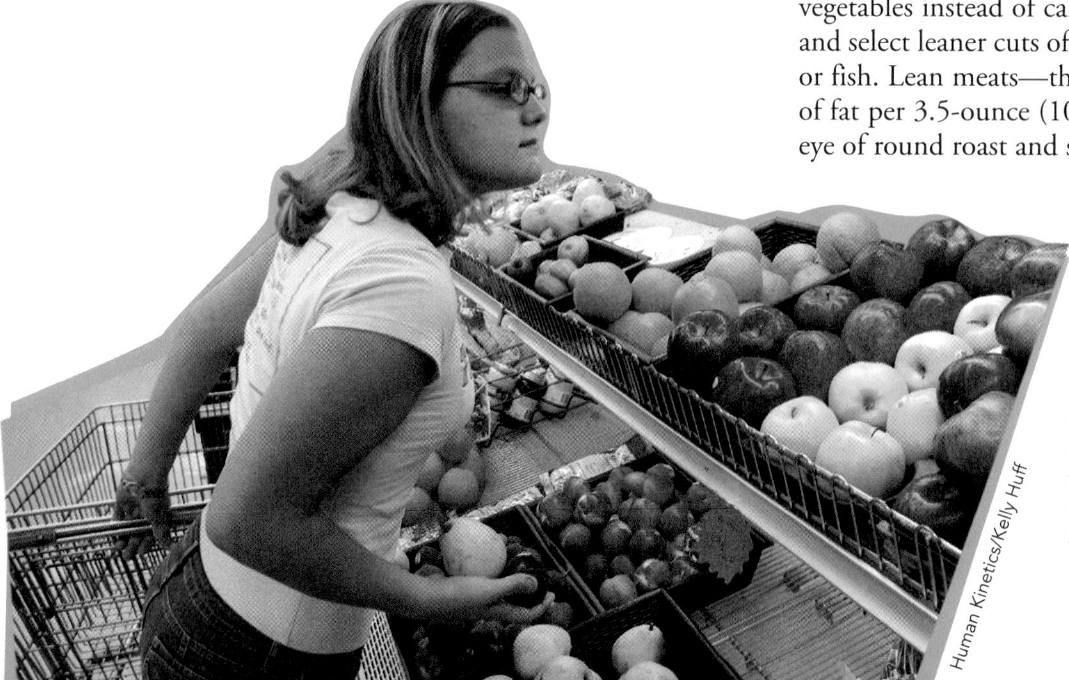
Human Kinetics/Kelly Huff

It can be a challenge to make healthy food choices when shopping; the fruits and vegetables available in the colorful produce section are a good place to start.

top round roast and steak, bottom round roast and steak, and top sirloin. Additional suggestions for choosing healthier groceries are found in table 26.3.

While shopping, think also about how you'll cook your meals. If you'd planned to make fried chicken, consider using a baked crust instead. If your planned menu called for frozen fish sticks, consider baked or fresh fish options instead of fried or battered ones. The key to successful meal planning is not to deny yourself particular foods or meals that you enjoy but rather to be intentional in selecting the healthiest ingredients available and choosing the healthiest and tastiest cooking methods you can. Stir frying and sautéing are better options than deep frying; other healthy choices include baking, grilling, steaming, and broiling. When serving food, put cream-based sauces on the side, avoid adding butter to vegetables and breads before they're served, and use salt-free seasonings instead of table salt.

Eating Healthily in a Cafeteria or Restaurant

It can be even more challenging to eat well when you're not in control of the shopping or food preparation. However, if you pay attention to your choices, you can almost always find a healthy food option. You can also reduce the chance of giving in to the temptation of less healthy foods if you observe a few general precautions.

WWW 2

- **Don't skip breakfast.** Eating a healthy breakfast every day can ensure that you're not overly hungry during midmorning breaks and at lunch.
- **Start with a glass of water.** Even if you're having another beverage with your meal, ask for a glass of water and drink it first. We often mistake thirst for hunger. Making sure you're adequately hydrated will help you avoid eating too much.
- **Put vegetables on your plate first.** A fresh salad or fresh steamed vegetables will take up space on your plate and discourage you from filling it up with less healthy choices.
- **Select fresh fruit.** Eating a piece of fruit with your meal can reduce sugar cravings and help you limit sugary drinks or desserts.
- **Carry your own snacks.** Having healthy snacks available can keep you from selecting unhealthy vending machine options and prevent you from getting too hungry. If the cafeteria or restaurant doesn't have as many healthy food options as you'd like, having a healthy snack with your meal might also keep you from making poor choices to satisfy your hunger.
- **Don't start with dessert.** Not only should you not start with dessert; you should also avoid selecting your dessert until you've completely finished your meal and beverage. Once the dessert is on your plate, you're more likely to eat it even if you're not hungry.

TABLE 26.3 Shopping for Healthier Foods

Traditional option	Healthier option
Whole or 2% milk	Fat-free milk or low-fat soy milk
Regular cheese	Low-fat, part-skim, or fat-free cheese
Yogurt	Fat-free yogurt without added fruit (add your own at home to reduce unnecessary sugar)
Meat	Leaner cuts of meat (or removing excess fat at home before cooking), pinto or black beans as substitute in dishes (e.g., chili, tacos)
Salad dressing	Fat-free or low-fat dressing
Canned vegetables	Fresh or fresh-frozen vegetables without added sauce or cheese
Canned fruit in heavy syrup	Fresh fruits or canned fruits in their own juice
Cooking oil, shortening, butter	Olive oil cooking spray for stir-frying or sautéing
Soup	Low-sodium, fat-free (or low-fat) soup; broth-based instead of cream-based when possible
Ice cream	Fat-free yogurt, sorbet, or low-fat ice cream
Potato or tortilla chips	Pretzels, whole-grain crackers, low-fat popcorn, baked chips

Healthy Snacks

Most teenagers snack throughout the day, particularly when they get home from a day at school. The calories you eat in an afterschool snack can add up quickly and contribute to unnecessary weight gain. Try to keep healthy snack options available at home and make an effort to eat them. It might even help to post a reminder in the kitchen about the healthy snack options available to you. Consider simple snacks such as the following items:

- Pretzels
- Carrot or celery sticks dipped lightly in fat-free ranch dressing or teriyaki sauce
- Apples with a small amount of fat-free cheese
- Bananas, oranges, raisins, grapes, and other "grab and go" fruits
- Low-fat or fat-free yogurt without added sugar
- Whole-grain crackers and breads
- Low-fat turkey slices
- A small handful of almonds, other nuts, or seeds
- Air-popped popcorn

Choose your beverage wisely as well. Avoid sugary drinks (e.g., sodas, energy drinks, other non-nutritious drinks). Start with a glass of water to satisfy your thirst. If you still want something more to drink, consider fat-free milk, fat-free soy milk, or fruit juice without added sugar.

- **Don't skimp.** This may run contrary to what you think, but the key to healthy eating is to select healthy foods—not simply to eat less. In fact, eating too little can make you develop cravings and eat worse foods later in the day. Eat a well-balanced meal that includes low-fat, high-fiber foods so that you'll be satisfied without overeating.
- **Stop when you're full.** You don't have to finish everything you ordered. Ask for a takeout box for the portion you don't need. In restaurants that serve large portions, ask for the box at the beginning of the meal and put half of the food in the box before you start eating.
- **Make requests.** When possible, request changes in your food to make it healthier. For example, when ordering a hamburger, eliminate the mayonnaise and cheese (substitute mustard or ketchup). If a fish or meat dish is served with a heavy sauce on top, request that the sauce be served on the side or left off. You can also ask for salad dressings to be served on the side and for vegetables to be steamed and served without butter.

Most states require restaurants to provide nutrition information about their foods. In some cases, this information appears on the menu; in others, you have to ask for it. Don't be shy about requesting the information or using it to help you make good

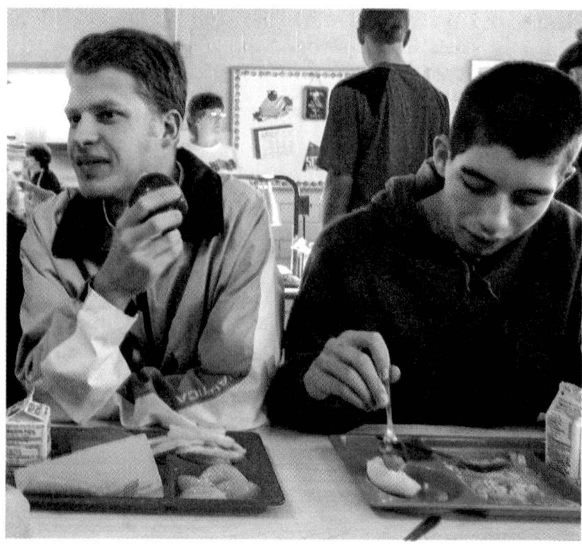

Make careful choices when eating out or at school.

choices. More and more traditional restaurants, and even some fast food outlets, are providing healthy food options. Eating out today doesn't have to be an unhealthy experience; nor should you take it as a license to ignore nutrition recommendations or common sense.

Although there are many healthy food options when eating out, there is considerable research on the benefits of family dining (i.e., eating together as a family at home). People tend to eat more nutritious foods and they are more likely to share in the food preparation. Also, people are more likely to eat slowly and less likely to watch TV or text while they are eating.

Changing Bad Eating Habits

Changing your eating habits can be hard even if you've moved past the state of contemplation and are ready for action. Don't try to make every desired change at once. Set a reasonable plan that includes weekly short-term goals and celebrate your achievements along the way. Try to avoid using weight loss as a measure of success when making dietary changes; focus instead on your behaviors. For example, if you're trying to reduce overall calories, begin with one or two changes, such as switching from regular to diet soda or from regular cheese to fat-free cheese.

Once you've demonstrated success at those changes, add a few more; for example, consider eliminating a late night snack or switching from a vending machine snack to a healthier one that you bring from home. Such changes add up over time, and you're more likely to be successful over the long term if you avoid taking on too much at once. The idea is not to think of the changes as short-term fixes but to make them last.

Preparing Food Safely

Have you ever had a stomachache or felt nauseous after eating? If so, you may have experienced food poisoning, also known as foodborne illness. This can last from one hour to two days. Each year, one in every six individuals suffers a case of food poisoning and 3,000 people die from it. Preventing foodborne illness at home begins with proper food handling, preparation, and cooking. The U.S.

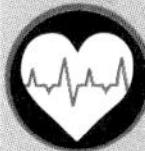

HEALTH TECHNOLOGY

Modern research has led to the discovery and isolation of phytochemicals—chemical compounds that occur naturally in plants and perform important functions in the human body. Phytochemicals are not considered to be essential nutrients because we do not develop deficiency diseases if we consume too little of them. However, consuming them can reduce the risks of developing various illnesses, including heart disease, cancer, type 2 diabetes, infections, eye diseases, and other conditions related to premature aging. Today, scientists study the thousands of known phytochemicals and their effects on health while also continuing to discover new phytochemicals.

Phytochemicals tend to be associated with the colors and pigments of fruits and vegetables, and they tend to hold up well when heated (cooked) and stored. Most phytochemicals work in groups, and though it's possible to buy supplements containing phytochemicals, our still-limited understanding of their properties and functions makes eating them in foods a better alternative. Some of the best-known phytochemicals are carotenoids (e.g., lycopene), phytoestrogens (e.g., isoflavones), and flavonoids (e.g., phenols). The best way to benefit from phytochemicals is to eat a good assortment of fruits and vegetables every day.

CONNECT

Identify two phytochemicals and the specific roles they might play in disease prevention. To help you research your answer, visit the student section of the Health Opportunities Through Physical Education website.

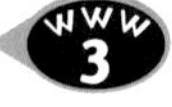

Centers for Disease Control and Prevention (CDC) recommends the following rules.

- **Clean.** Always begin by washing your hands in warm soapy water for at least 20 seconds. Wash all utensils and cutting boards with soapy water and clean all surfaces with a bleach solution after using them. Wash all fruits and vegetables—even those that you peel, to prevent bacteria from spreading to the inside during peeling or cutting.
- **Separate.** When shopping for food and when storing food in your refrigerator, separate produce from meats, eggs, and poultry. When preparing foods, use separate utensils and cutting boards for produce and meats. Using the same cutting utensils and surfaces can result in cross-contamination with bacteria and other pathogens.
- **Cook.** Cook foods to their proper temperatures (see table 26.4); where necessary, use a food thermometer to check the food's internal temperature. Serve foods immediately, making sure to keep them warm—above 140°F (60°C). Cold and uncooked foods (e.g., coleslaw, dips, and salads) should be kept chilled and should not be left out at room temperature for more than two hours.
- **Chill.** When a meal is finished, place leftovers in the refrigerator immediately. When cooling hot foods, use shallow dishes to allow the food to cool thoroughly, quickly, and evenly. When marinating foods, place them in the refrigerator and dispose of unused marinade. Respect expiration dates and inspect foods for mold and foul odors before eating them, since foods can spoil even when properly chilled.

TABLE 26.4 Proper Cooking Temperatures

Food	Temperature
Ground beef	165°F (74°C)
Fresh meat, lamb, poultry	135° F (58°C) for steak, 165°F (74°C) for all others
Pork	145°F (63°C)
Eggs and egg dishes	Until yoke and white are firm for eggs; 140°F (60°C) for egg dishes
Seafood	145°F (63°C) or until flesh is opaque and separates easily with a fork
Leftovers	165°F (74°C)

Trustworthy Sources of Nutrition Information

Anyone can *claim* to have nutrition knowledge, and in many states anyone can use the term **nutritionist** without having to meet specific educational standards. In contrast, a person who has studied nutrition at a recognized college or university, holds a certification in the field, and possesses full knowledge of nutrition is either a **registered dietitian (RD)** or a dietetic technician, registered (DTR). Other health professionals may possess nutrition knowledge, but be careful about assuming that their education has been formal or that they are as knowledgeable about all aspects of nutrition as they could be.

Comprehension Check

1. List five healthy choices a person can make when shopping for groceries.
2. What are three things a person can do to eat healthily in a cafeteria or restaurant?
3. What are the four steps to prevent food poisoning when preparing, cooking, and serving food?

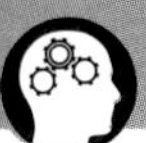

MAKING HEALTHY DECISIONS: Nutrition Information

Sarah is a high school sophomore who is interested in nutrition and tries to eat healthily. Lately, however, you've noticed that Sarah has stopped eating certain foods and that she makes all sorts of strange claims that she never used to make. For example, she won't eat any fish because she heard that fish is contaminated with mercury, she eats only raw vegetables because she heard that cooked ones lose their nutritional value, and she stopped eating citrus fruits because she heard from her mom that they cause diabetes.

Sarah has also started taking various vitamins in her drinks a few times a day. When you ask Sarah why she believes all these things are beneficial, she said "because my mom told me." When you ask her about her new vitamin supplements, she says that her mom has been buying them from a neighbor who says he is a nutritionist. It seems, however, that Sarah's habits are getting worse—not better—and that she thinks her vitamins are more important than the food she eats.

For Discussion

What concerns do you have about Sarah's choices? Do you think she should question the information she's hearing? Why or why not? Where would you recommend that Sarah go to get better information? How should she decide whether nutrition information is accurate? When answering these questions, consider the guidelines in this chapter's Skills for Healthy Living feature.

SKILLS FOR HEALTHY LIVING: Nutrition Information

It's not hard to find nutrition information. If you search the web for information about most any health topic, you're likely to get thousands of hits. Sometimes it seems that everyone has an opinion or perspective about what to eat, how to eat, when to eat, and so on. Unfortunately, much of the information out there is not rooted in good science; instead, it's often profit driven or based on individual experiences that don't apply to other people. Use available resources such as food labels, food charts in restaurants, and MyPlate resources. When you look for nutrition information, use the following guidelines.

- **Consider the URL address.** Sites with the suffix *.gov* (governmental), *.edu* (education), or *.org* (organization) are often the most reliable sources of nutrition information. Sites with the suffix *.com* (commercial) may or may not be reliable and are more likely to use biased information to sell a product or service.
- **Consider the author or publisher.** Is the website written or published by a reputable organization, such as the CDC, the Academy of Nutrition and Dietetics, or the U.S. National Institutes of Health? What are the author's or organization's credentials? Remember—anyone can claim to know about nutrition, but registered dietitians are the most qualified to present information about nutrition.
- **Consider the date.** Is the website current? Has the site been updated lately? Nutrition information changes, and U.S. guidelines are updated every five years. Make sure the information you're reading is as current as possible.
- **Consider the motivation.** Is the website aimed at selling a supplement, program, or other product? If so, compare the information you find there with information from more neutral sites. Sites designed to sell a product often use only the research they have sponsored or other findings that support their interests—even if that information is not well supported by other studies. There are no quick fixes or miracles in dieting and nutrition. Such claims should be a warning to scrutinize the information carefully. Also be very cautious about sites featuring extensive testimonials without research to support them.

Eating Out May Be Both Deceiving and Unhealthy

When you sit down at a family restaurant or place an order at your favorite fast food spot, chances are that your food will *not* meet federal nutrition recommendations. In fact, researchers from Tufts University in Boston tested 157 meals from 33 individual or small-chain restaurants and found the average meal contains two to three times the calories a person needs at a single sitting, and more than half of what is needed for an entire day (see table 26.5 for examples).

An 'On the Menu' report issued by the National Restaurant Association states that the industry is "employing a wide range" of healthy living strategies, including putting nutrition information on menus and order boards. It references Kids LiveWell, the first voluntary national program to encourage restaurants to offer healthful children's menu items. The report says, "We launched with 19 restaurant companies two years ago and now have more than 140 companies representing more than 40,000 locations."

Medical professionals, however, say that restaurant industry standards are out of line. For example, the industry-favored "Healthy Dining" seal of approval allows up to 2,000 milligrams of sodium per entrée, even though the standard recommended *daily* allowance for adults is only 2,300 milligrams.

A related study showed that kids and teens who eat in a restaurant on any given day consume more fat and sugar than they do when they eat at home. Of the 9,000 teens studied, 24 percent had eaten at a takeout or fast food restaurant on each day they were questioned. The study showed that adolescents ate an additional 310 calories on days when they ate at a takeout or fast food restaurant. Drinks proved to be a major culprit; regular menu drinks (e.g., sodas, shakes) had an average of 310 calories. In some regards, full-service restaurants proved to be even worse than takeout and fast food spots; in particular, entrées at family style restaurants averaged more calories, fat, and sodium than fast food options.

For Discussion

What is your favorite restaurant? What is your favorite meal there? Have you evaluated the fat and sodium content of the meal? If it were high in fat and sodium, would that influence your choice? Why or why not? Nutrition information for fast food restaurants can be found online.

TABLE 26.5 Nutritional Content of Sample Restaurant Dishes

Dish	Calories	Fat (% RDA)	Sodium (% RDA)
Domino's Ultimate Pepperoni Pizza—1 slice	280	13 g (20)	650 mg (27)
Famous Dave's Sampler Platter with Boneless Wings	2,880	181 g (278)	7,580 mg (316)
McDonald's Sausage Biscuit With Egg	560	33 g (51)	1,170 mg (49)
Ruby Tuesday Parmesan Chicken Pasta Without Biscuit	1,345	74 g (114)	3,481 mg (145)
Subway 6" Spicy Italian on Wheat Bread	480	24 g (37)	1,520 mg (63)
Taco Bell XXL Grilled Stuft Burrito	880	42 g (65)	2,020 mg (84)

Reviewing Concepts and Vocabulary

As directed by your teacher, answer items 1 through 5 by correctly completing each sentence with a word or phrase.

1. Your _____________ can be influenced by circumstances, emotions, and traditions.
2. Most people who go on a diet do not keep the weight off for longer than ___________.
3. A __________ ____________ is a licensed professional and a good source of nutrition information.
4. Substances found in plants, called ___________, perform important functions in the human body.
5. The sensation of fullness is known as _________.

For items 6 through 10, as directed by your teacher, match each term in column 1 with the appropriate phrase in column 2.

6. positive energy balance
7. negative energy balance
8. hunger
9. appetite
10. resting metabolic rate

a. the calories you burn each day just to survive
b. the physiological need to eat
c. taking in more calories than you use
d. the psychological drive to eat
e. using more calories than you take in

For items 11 through 15, as directed by your teacher, respond to each statement or question.

11. How is age related to a person's energy needs?
12. What does the National Weight Control Registry teach us about effective long-term weight loss?
13. Describe two ways to make healthy choices when shopping for groceries. Give specific examples.
14. How long can you safely leave cooked food out at room temperature?
15. Describe two guidelines for evaluating nutrition information online.

Thinking Critically

Write a response to the following prompt.

You and some friends are planning a birthday party and want it to be a fun and healthy event. Make a list of eight healthy snacks you could serve at the party. For each snack, identify all of the ingredients and explain how to prepare it. Include tips for making sure the food preparation is safe.

Take It Home

Pick a meal that you and your family eat on a regular basis. Ask a parent or guardian for the recipe or look it up in a cookbook. Write down all of the ingredients, then identify at least two ways to make the meal healthier. Write down the changes and explain why they would be healthier. Share your modified meal idea with a family member and encourage your family to try the healthier option.

27

Stress Management

In This Chapter

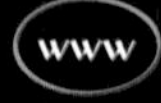

Student Web Resources

www.HOPEtextbook.org/student

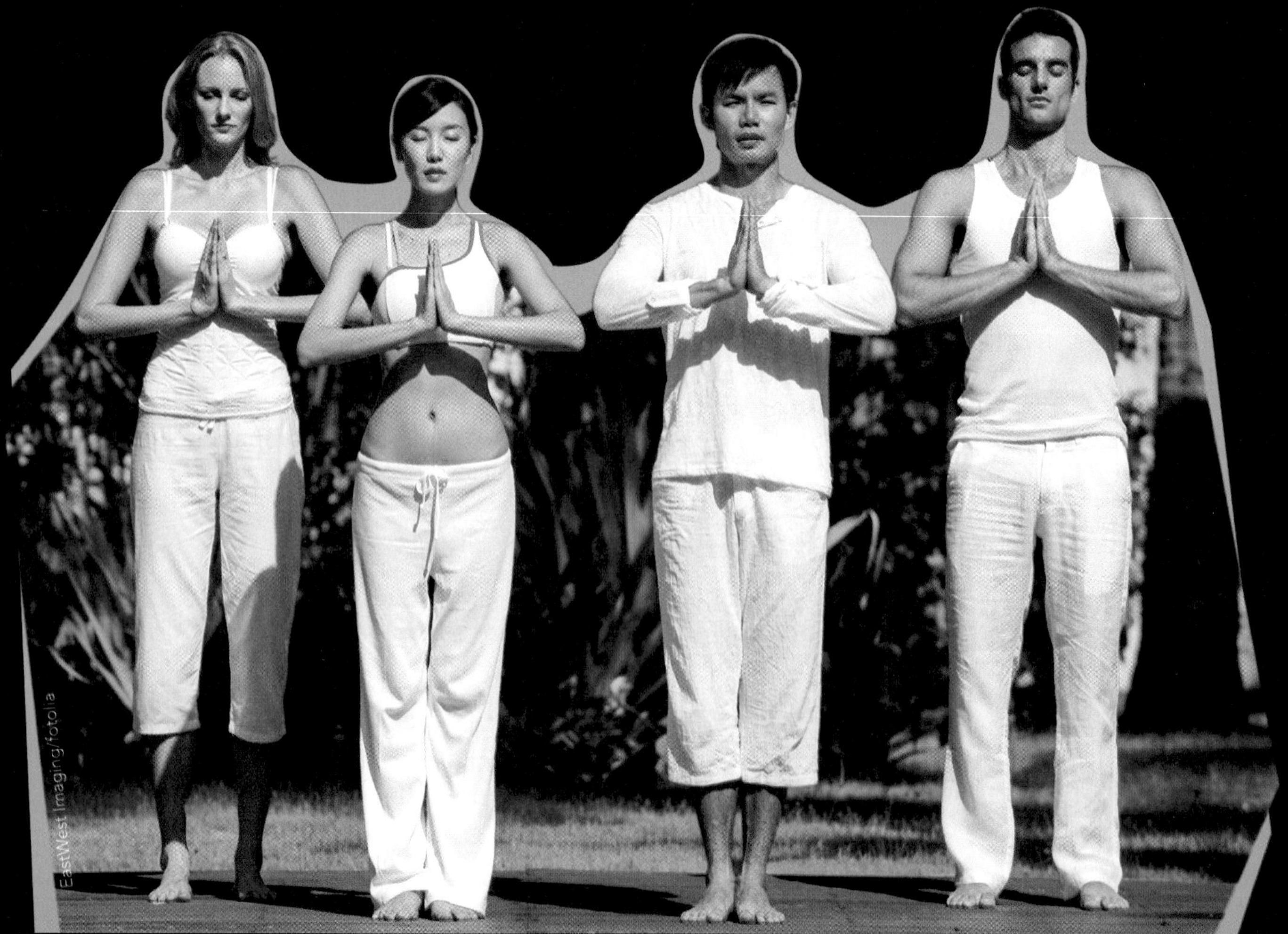

EastWest Imaging/fotolia

Lesson 27.1

Understanding and Avoiding Stress

Lesson Objectives

After reading this lesson, you should be able to

1. explain how the body responds to stress,
2. identify the positive and negative aspects of stress, and
3. understand how different people can react differently to the same stressor.

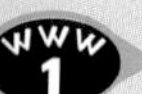

WWW
1

Lesson Vocabulary

assertiveness, distress, eustress, fight-or-flight response, stressor

When someone asks how you're feeling, do you ever answer by saying that you're stressed or "stressed out"? Do you ever feel like there are too many demands on your time? Do you worry about your performance on tests and homework? Everyone experiences stress, and the teenage years can be particularly stressful. This lesson introduces you to the concept of stress and discusses how the body reacts to stress. Understanding stress, its causes, and its symptoms can help you learn to manage it more effectively.

Understanding Stress

Stress is the body's reaction to a difficult or demanding situation. Renowned stress researcher Hans Selye defined stress as the "nonspecific response of the body to any demand or change." Selye named this response the general adaptation syndrome. His theory (see figure 27.1) described the general way in which all people respond when they experience a **stressor**—something that causes or contributes to stress. Stressors can be physical (e.g., pain, thirst, hunger, illness), emotional (e.g., worry, fear, anger, love), or social (e.g., relationships). Some stressors—for example, flying, taking a test, speaking in public, and facing schedule or financial demands—are common among most people. Others vary by the individual. People tend to be stressed whenever a situation feels out of their control—when they feel that they don't have the ability to cope with or manage the situation effectively. Regardless of the particular stressor, the general adaptation syndrome is the set of physiological reactions we all experience in response to stress.

The first stage of the general adaptation syndrome is the alarm reaction. Any stressor that you experience starts your body's alarm response (see figure 27.2), also known as the stress response or the **fight-or-flight response**. The term *fight-or-flight* reflects the fact that these physiological changes prepare the body to either engage in a physical fight

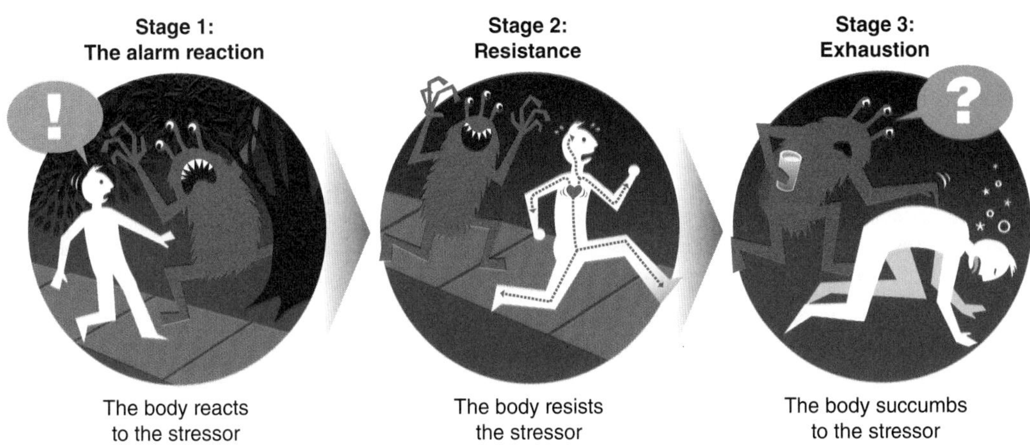

Stage 1:
The alarm reaction
Stage 2:
Resistance
Stage 3:
Exhaustion
!
?
The body reacts to the stressor
The body resists the stressor
The body succumbs to the stressor

FIGURE 27.1 The general adaptation syndrome.

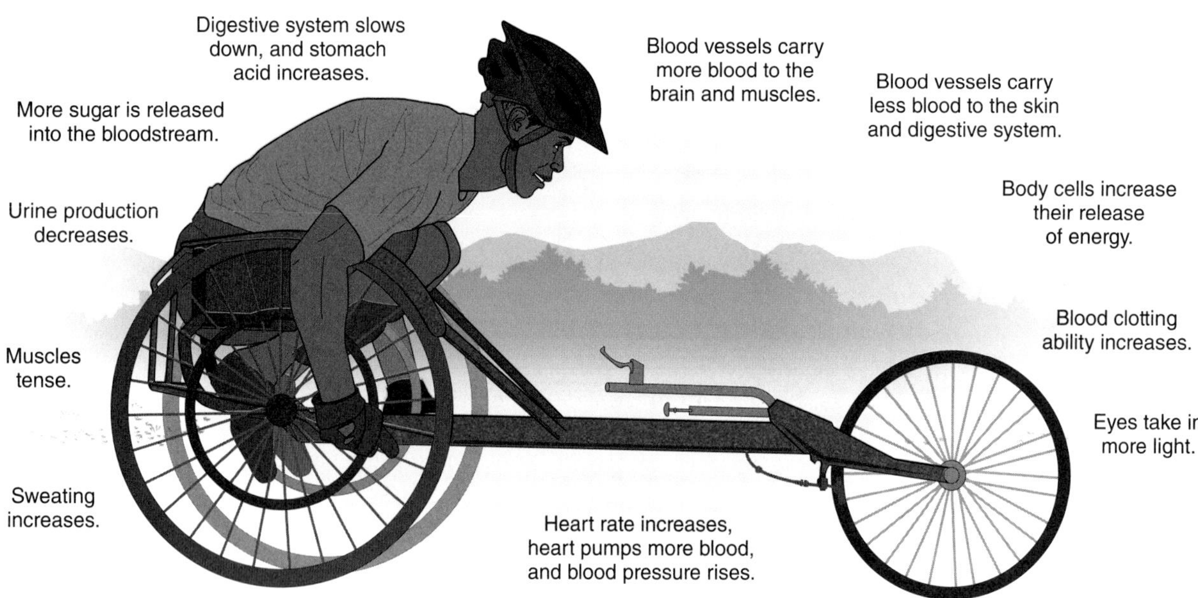

Digestive system slows down, and stomach acid increases.
More sugar is released into the bloodstream.
Urine production decreases.
Muscles tense.
Sweating increases.
Blood vessels carry more blood to the brain and muscles.
Blood vessels carry less blood to the skin and digestive system.
Body cells increase their release of energy.
Blood clotting ability increases.
Eyes take in more light.
Heart rate increases, heart pumps more blood, and blood pressure rises.

FIGURE 27.2 The stress response.

or flee (run) from a stressful situation. Fighting and fleeing can be appropriate in some life-and-death situations. If a car is racing toward you, you need to flee—to get out of the way. If a big dog backs you into a corner, you may have no choice but to fight. In such circumstances, fleeing or fighting can save your life.

In modern society, most of our stressors are not immediately life threatening. Even so, your body acts as if you're preparing for a physical response: blood flows to your muscles, your pupils get bigger, your blood pressure increases, your heart beats faster, and your breathing rate goes up.

The second stage of the general adaptation syndrome is resistance. In this stage, your body works to resist or minimize the potential long-term effect of the stress response on your systems. If stress is not effectively managed, it can cause a wide range of negative symptoms (see table 27.1).

Extreme cases—in which the body is not able to effectively manage stress over a long time, or in which the stressor itself is ongoing or chronic—can lead to the exhaustion stage of the general adaptation syndrome. In this stage, illness and disease can occur. In fact, chronic stress can play a role in the development or progression of several diseases and disorders, including coronary heart disease, diabetes, depression, and Alzheimer's disease.

WWW 2

Stress and Performance

Though we often categorize all stress as negative stress, or **distress**, not all stress is bad. Stress can be a challenge that helps us learn, grow, and develop. Indeed, a certain amount of stress is desirable because it helps us be alert and prepares our bodies for optimal performance. This type of stress is called **eustress**, or positive stress.

TABLE 27.1 Effects of Stress on the Body

Type of impact	Symptoms
Cognitive	Headaches, insomnia, difficulty remembering things, inability to concentrate
Physiological	Increased heart rate, hypertension, gastrointestinal problems, frequent illness, increased respiratory rate, disruption of metabolism
Behavioral	Disrupted eating habits, grinding of teeth, hostility, increased use of substances, difficulty communicating with others, social isolation
Emotional	Crying, fatigue, anxiety, depression, hypervigilance, impulsiveness, irritability

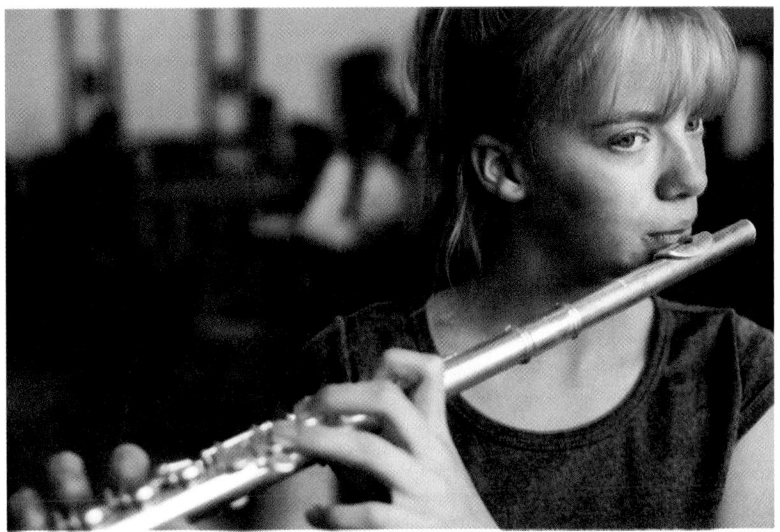

Feeling some stress will motivate you to practice before your concert performance.

Photodisc

For example, if you're preparing for a big exam and you experience no stress at all, you might be lazy and lack the motivation to study. As a result, you might perform poorly. On the other hand, if you feel overly stressed—if you experience distress—you might have too much nervous energy to concentrate while studying or you might be unable to remember the things you did manage to study. In this situation, as in many others, an ideal amount of stress will optimize your performance. Feeling some stress will motivate you to study and heighten your brain function and your senses during the exam, thus allowing you to perform at your best. Figure 27.3 illustrates the relationship between stress and performance.

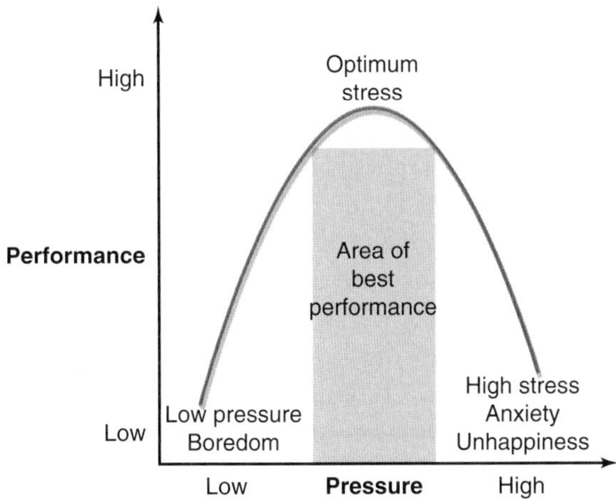

FIGURE 27.3 The relationship between stress and performance.

> "Stress is the spice of life; the absence of stress is death."
>
> —Hans Selye, stress researcher

Sources of Stress

As you probably already know, you'll face many stressors during high school in particular and during your teenage years overall. The number one stress reported by middle and high school students is academic pressure (e.g., getting good grades, preparing for college). The second-leading source of stress reported among these groups involves relationships—with parents, romantic partners, and friends. Other commonly reported sources include financial concerns, responsibilities at home, body image struggles, peer pressure, popularity concerns, bullying (including cyberbullying), and criticism and disapproval. Though you can't always control the daily stressors you face as a teenager, you can learn to manage your emotional reactions in stressful situations, build your coping skills, and learn relaxation techniques that can help you minimize the effect of stress. In some ways stress is similar to pain. You are the one who experiences it and despite the saying "I feel your pain," you really don't. You can feel your own pain, but not the pain of others. Likewise, you perceive a stressor, but others may view the same situation in a very different manner. One person may see a snake and immediately run

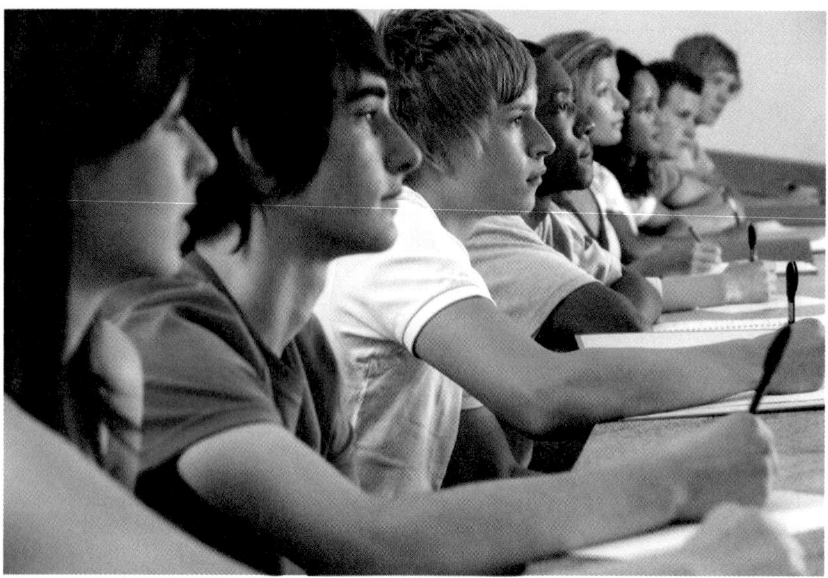

Academic pressure is the number one stressor reported by middle and high school students.

Monkey Business - Fotolia.com

away; another person may see the same snake and want to pick it up and learn more about it. Previous knowledge and experience and coping skills will determine why two people react so differently to the same stimulus. The remainder of this lesson and all of the next lesson provide you with important information and help you learn skills that can help you better manage stressors in your life.

> **CONNECT**
>
> How much do you think peer pressure influences your individual stress level? What are the most common stressors you feel as a result of peer pressure? Explain each stressor and analyze how it affects your stress level.

Avoiding Stressful Situations

The next lesson addresses stress management techniques that can help you handle stressful situations—something we all need to be able to do. But sometimes the best thing you can do is avoid a stressor altogether. Skills that you can use to stay out of stressful situations include assertiveness, avoidance decision making, and time management.

Assertiveness

Has anyone ever sabotaged your studying by coaxing you to play video games or go to the mall instead? If so, you can benefit from learning to say no or offer a better alternative, such as "I'll meet up with you later after my homework is done." Doing so requires **assertiveness**—standing up for your own needs, interests, and desires. Assertiveness is not the same as aggressiveness. Both are direct forms of communication, but aggressive behavior is direct communication without regard for the rights and feelings of others, whereas assertive behavior is direct while respecting others. Passive behavior, in contrast, involves not standing up for your rights—for example, not doing or saying anything even when you believe someone is taking advantage of you.

Most people have to practice becoming assertive. People often mistakenly believe that being assertive means being rude. In reality, assertive behavior means simply and directly stating your feelings. For example, if a classmate asks you to lend him or her your homework, you can answer by saying, "That makes me feel uncomfortable. I can't do it." This is a direct and honest response. An aggressive response, on the other hand, would involve saying something like, "You're stupid. Do your own homework." And a passive person would likely give the homework to the classmate because he or she doesn't want to "cause trouble" or thinks something like, "If I don't give him my homework, he won't like me."

Remember—your feelings are your feelings, and you have a right to express them. This doesn't mean that you'll always get what you want, but at least it lets others know where you stand. Most people admire someone who can be honest and forthright in a respectful manner.

Like most things in life, being assertive gets easier with practice. It may seem uncomfortable at first, but you can practice assertive responses in front of a mirror when no one else is around. If you can't be assertive in a practice situation, it's unlikely that you'll be assertive in life situations. You might want to start with some easier scenarios, such as how you would respond if you ordered food and received the wrong order. A passive response would be to say nothing and accept the order as it is. An aggressive response would be to say something like, "Can't you get anything right? This is not what I ordered!" An assertive response would be something like, "This is not what I ordered. Would you please take it back and bring me my order?"

Developing assertiveness skills is one way you can avoid some of the potential stressors in your life. Being assertive helps you stand up for yourself and effectively defuse potential conflicts. As a result, it allows you to avoid getting yourself into situations that you don't want to be in.

Avoidance Decision Making

You can also avoid some situations simply by making smart choices. For example, if getting caught in heavy traffic causes you to feel stressed, you can try to run errands at less busy times of the day. If your home environment is stressful and studying at home causes you stress, you might choose to study in the library before or after school. If you're at a park and see someone who makes you feel uncomfortable, you can choose to leave the park and go home. The key is to avoid getting yourself into situations that you know will be stressful and to remove yourself from situations that might become uncomfortable or stressful.

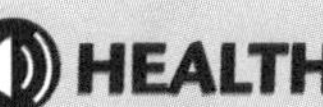

HEALTHY COMMUNICATION

What are some situations in which it's important to be assertive? What are some things that make a person assertive and not aggressive? Do you think assertive behavior is interpreted differently in males than in females? Support your opinions with facts and be respectful of others' opinions.

Time Management

Many stressors are related to time constraints—for example, being overscheduled, running late to an important meeting, and forgetting to study for an exam. All three are examples of how poor time management skills can create stressful situations that you might otherwise avoid. Teach yourself to take on the most important or pressing tasks first. For example, first do your homework that is due tomorrow, then tackle the big paper due in two weeks. If you're faced with a large or tedious task, break it down into smaller parts or spread the project over

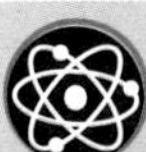

HEALTH SCIENCE

Neuroscientists (scientists who study the brain) have documented the effects of stressful events on brain circuits and brain development. Stressful events experienced early in life can affect the brain's networks in ways that help or hurt how a person might react to stressful events later in life. Stressful or traumatic events can also inhibit the brain's reward system. This system normally makes us feel pleasure when, for example, we eat a nice meal or spend time with good friends. But individuals who undergo extreme stress, such as war veterans, often report a lack of pleasure from normal activities. Scientists are working to develop medications that can repair or mimic the reward system in order to more effectively treat mental health conditions that might result from stress.

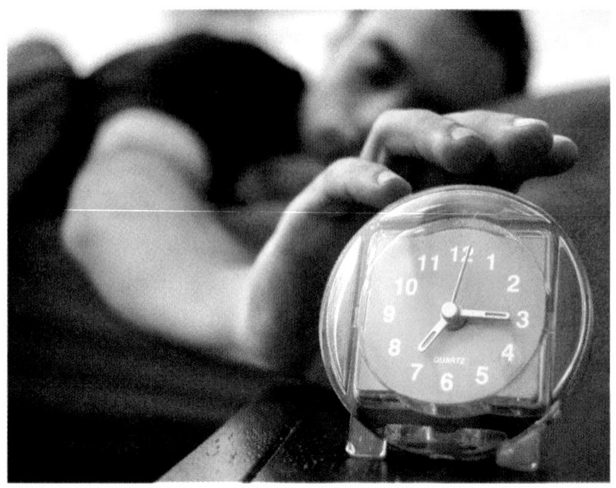

Time management is a key to avoiding stressful situations.

diego cervo/fotolia.com

a longer period of time. If you have to memorize twenty new vocabulary words by next week, learn three words per day rather than trying to learn them all at once.

Other ways to decrease stress by managing your time effectively including making a list of things to do and keeping a schedule to organize your daily life. Even if you're the type of person who thrives on pressure and likes to press right up to a deadline, you'll find it beneficial to allow for the unexpected—the computer glitch, the traffic jam, the unexpected homework assignment. In this way, good time management can help you avoid stress and maximize your performance. For more information about time management, see this chapter's Skills for Healthy Living feature.

CONSUMER CORNER: Can Vitamins Really Reduce Stress?

Many vitamin and supplement products are marketed as helping people reduce or manage stress and its symptoms. Unfortunately, most of these claims are supported by little or no scientific evidence that they hold true in healthy individuals. The stress response can reduce some vitamin levels in the blood, and it is important to restore them to normal levels through either a healthy diet or a modest vitamin or multivitamin supplement. But no vitamin can keep stress out of your life, and the best way to reduce stress is to learn how to recognize its symptoms and causes and how to manage it through a variety of strategies like those presented later in this chapter.

If you're thinking of taking a vitamin to reduce stress (or for some other reason), are you assertive enough to discuss it with your personal health care professional or school nurse? When considering taking a vitamin, ask yourself the following questions.

- Does this vitamin offer a proven health benefit?
- Does the research support the use of this vitamin for people with my health status?
- Is this vitamin known to treat a medical condition or help prevent disease?
- What is the recommended dose for this vitamin?
- When and for how long should I take this vitamin?

Comprehension Check

1. How does the body respond to stress?
2. What are the positive and negative aspects of stress?
3. Explain how the same situation might be a stressor to one person but not to another.

SELF-ASSESSMENT: Stress Management

Indicate how frequently each of the following statements applies to you. Total the points associated with your responses to get your stress management score. Then use the descriptions accompanying the table to interpret your score.

SELF-ASSESSMENT QUESTIONNAIRE

	Rarely	Sometimes	Frequently	Always
I feel pressure to do things I don't really want to do.	1	2	3	4
I am anxious about doing well in my classes.	1	2	3	4
I feel like there's no one I can turn to who will understand how I feel.	1	2	3	4
I'm so busy, I rarely have time for myself.	1	2	3	4
I drink lots of caffeine to maintain my energy throughout the day.	1	2	3	4
I eat fast food that's not good for me because I don't have the time for anything else.	1	2	3	4
I cannot find the time or energy to enjoy the activities that are important to me.	1	2	3	4
I get less than six hours of sleep at night.	1	2	3	4
It is necessary to multitask to accomplish everything I need to do.	1	2	3	4
I feel guilty if I relax and do nothing.	1	2	3	4
My stress management score is ___________.				

A score of 10 to 19 = lower risk. You have a low risk for stress-related health problems. Keep up the good work, but consider learning and practicing a stress management technique or two in case things change.

A score of 20 to 29 = moderate risk. You have a moderate risk for stress-related health problems. You should practice a stress management technique two or three days per week.

A score of 30 to 40 = higher risk. You are at high risk for stress-related health problems. It's time to make some changes. It would be great if you could practice a stress management technique on a daily basis.

Planning for Healthy Living

Use the Healthy Living Plan worksheet to set goals and develop a plan to help you control and manage your stress through stress management techniques. Monitor the steps you take toward meeting your goals and repeat this self-assessment in one to three months to help determine the success of your plan.

Lesson 27.2

Stress Management Techniques

Lesson Objectives

After reading this lesson, you should be able to

1. describe a variety of stress management techniques,
2. explain how physical activity and exercise can help you manage stress, and
3. describe a method of practicing mindfulness.

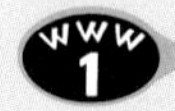

Lesson Vocabulary

asanas, biofeedback, mindfulness, reframing

Many methods are available to help you successfully manage stress. Some are mainly physical, and some are mostly mental, but the fact is that your mind and body are connected. What affects your mind affects your body, and what affects your body affects your mind. We tend to talk about mind and body as if they are totally separate, perhaps because we have separated them through our language—different words describe different parts, functions, and concepts. The reality, however, is that these parts, functions, and concepts often overlap or coordinate with each other. Therefore, learning stress management techniques helps your whole human system operate more efficiently. Stress management is a type of fine tuning that helps us better cope with the stressors of daily living.

Reframing

Because stress involves perception, one way to deal with it is to change your perception or reframe the situation. For example, if you think a teacher is being too hard on you, you might consider the possibility that the teacher is not picking on you but is devoting time to you because he or she thinks you can do better. Or, if you believe you have to dress like people in a certain group at school, you might consider the fact that it's more important to be who you are than what others might like you to be.

Of course, **reframing** doesn't always solve a problem. There are times when people are just plain mean spirited and you can't reframe them into being nicer. You can, however, reframe your response to mean people. You can practice not letting anger, vengefulness, or jealousy get the best of you. As the saying goes, when life gives you lemons, you can choose to make lemonade. For example, when you have to wait in a long line, instead of complaining about the wait, you can find a productive way to use your time—perhaps listening to your favorite song, reading a book, or practicing deep breathing.

Mindfulness

Mindfulness means being in the moment. Too often, our thoughts dwell on the past or on the future. Of course, we should learn from the past, and we should plan for the future, but many people seem to ignore the here and now. When is the last time you were lost in the moment, or when time seemed to stand still? These are examples of being mindful—times when you are fully present and immersed in a particular moment.

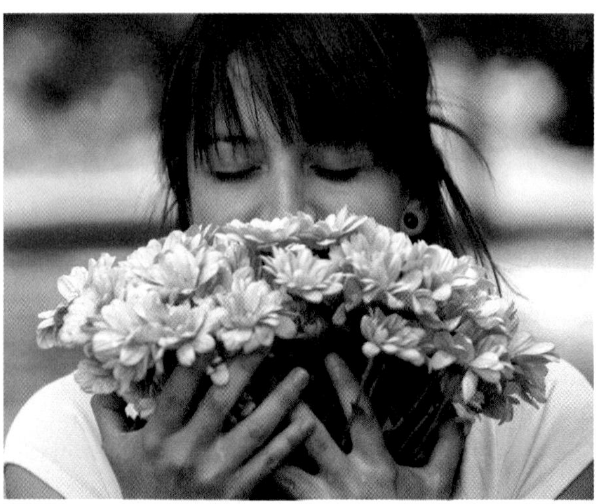

Mindfulness means being fully present and immersed in a particular moment.

Andres Rodriguez - Fotolia

One way to practice being mindful is to put a single raisin, grape, or sunflower seed in your mouth. Take a few minutes to explore the texture, the aroma, the feel, and the taste. More than likely, you will find this experience far different from your usual eating. In fact, in daily life, it's not unusual for people to eat without even noticing it, because they may be multitasking—watching TV, playing a video game, or texting while eating.

Although multitasking is common, we all need at least a little time each day when we can be more aware of what is going on in our bodies. Ask yourself, "Are my muscles tense? Am I breathing rapidly? Is my heart rate fast?" If so, you can consciously let go of the tension, slow down your breathing and lower your heart rate. They are all under your control, and the more you practice, the better you get at being in control and being in the moment. Sometimes we just need time to be, not do. As some popular motivational speakers like to say, "We are human beings, not human doings." Since we spend plenty of time doing, it's important to devote some time to just being.

Breathing

To a large extent, if you can control your breathing, you can control your stress. It may seem strange to pay attention to breathing; after all, you've been doing it all your life. But there are special kinds of breathing that can help you better handle stress. Practices that use breathing to manage stress include yoga, tai chi, and some types of meditation.

A good way to start using breathing as a stress management technique is to simply observe your breathing. Find a quiet place, sit in a comfortable position, and close your eyes. Now, just pay attention to five to ten cycles of your breathing. What did you notice? Did anything surprise you—for example, noticing a space between your inhalation and your exhalation? Did you feel silly? Did your thoughts wander? Did you notice whether or not you were breathing through your mouth or your nose? Was your breathing faster or slower than you expected?

Simply becoming aware of your breathing can help you focus. In addition, once you know how you normally breathe, you can experiment with a special kind of breathing called "so hum" breathing. To use this technique, say the word "soooo" (to yourself, not out loud) as you inhale (for the length of the inhalation) and say to yourself the word "hummmm" for the length of your exhalation. Even though it may seem strange to do this, after repeating the so hum breathing for several cycles, you will become more relaxed. And as with most things that are new, you'll find that the more you practice this type of breathing, the better you get at it—and the more in control of your stress you become.

Some people prefer to do this type of breathing by simply saying the "so" and the "hum" as just described. Others like to fill in the space between the inhalation and the exhalation with the word "and." Thus they say "soooo" internally on the inhalation, then "and" in the space between inhalation and exhalation, then "hummmm" on the exhalation, then "and" again, and so on. Try each method to see which you prefer. If you don't have allergies, asthma, or a cold, inhale through your nose and exhale through your mouth.

Another breathing technique used for stress reduction is called breath counting. It involves simply counting your exhalations, up to ten, then starting over. If your thoughts wander or you forget which breath you were on, just start over at one. It's very common to lose track or to find your thoughts wandering—and it's perfectly okay. Some people do this practice for as long as twenty minutes, but if you have less time, try five minutes. Like so hum breathing, it may seem a bit strange at first, but it is very relaxing to most people who give it a chance.

Practices that use breathing to manage stress include yoga, tai chi, and some types of meditation.

Guided Imagery

This practice involves allowing someone to guide you to a relaxing place in your mind. It is similar to controlled daydreaming. Using a prompt—whether it be a computer application, video game, podcast, digital audio recording, or skilled teacher—you can allow yourself to be led to a safe and relaxing place in your mind, no matter where you are. You can find many guided imagery programs and activities by doing a web search for the phrase "guided imagery." Although the word *imagery* suggests something visual to many people, guided imagery can also involve your other senses, as in the smell of a rose, the taste of chocolate, the feel of sand on your toes, or the sound of a gentle rain.

Body Scanning

Most people can manage their stress simply by scanning their body for any unwanted or unneeded tension. To try this technique, start from your head and end at your toes. Focus on the muscles of your forehead. Check for any unwanted or unneeded tension. You can wrinkle your forehead to see what your tension feels like, then consciously let go of it. You can follow this same pattern for other muscle groups. Next, for example, check the muscles around your closed eyes. When you find any unwanted or unneeded tension, let it go. Release it. Progress through your jaw muscles; your tongue muscles; your shoulder muscles; the muscles of your arms, hands, and fingers; your back muscles; the muscles of your chest and stomach; the muscles of your hip girdle (hips and buttocks); and, finally, the muscles of your legs, feet, and toes.

Physical Activity

Physical activity and exercise are natural mechanisms for managing stress. Taking a brisk walk or a jog, or doing some resistance or stretching exercises, or yoga or tai chi, can help your body balance the naturally occurring changes that result from the fight-or-flight response (see figure 27.2). Noncompetitive physical activity, especially when done slowly (e.g., yoga), allows your body to return to its normal physiological state more quickly following stress.

For stress management purposes, deemphasize competition when engaging in physical activity. Competition causes stress in most people. This doesn't mean that you should always avoid competition, which actually meets other human needs. It just means that if you're exercising to relieve stress, it's better to stick to noncompetitive activities. Moderate physical activity performed a few hours before bedtime also helps you get to sleep.

Yoga

Yoga has been around for thousands of years, and in recent years it has become very popular in the United States. Yoga positions (**asanas**) use sustained stretching to help people become more flexible; as a result, many people use yoga as a type of exercise. However, yoga is much more than a stretching exercise; some types of yoga also involve breathing and body awareness. Therefore, if you like to combine physical and mental types of stress management, you'll probably be attracted to yoga. Yoga classes are now available in many settings across the United States, including preschools; elementary, middle, and high schools; and colleges and universities. In addition, many businesses offer yoga classes or encourage their employees who work at desks or work stations to practice "desktop yoga" (i.e., yoga-like exercises that can be done while sitting at a desk) in order to reduce muscular tension.

Tai Chi

Tai chi chuan, usually referred to in the United States simply as tai chi, has been around for hundreds of years. It involves a series of movements performed in a slow, focused manner accompanied by deep breathing. It is a noncompetitive and self-paced system of gentle physical exercise and stretching. Each posture flows into the next without pause, ensuring that the body is in constant motion.

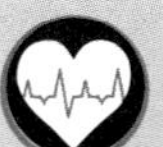

HEALTH TECHNOLOGY

Many technological applications are now available to help people control stress. **Biofeedback** machines, for example, are very popular and range from very expensive to very inexpensive. These machines allow you to monitor body systems and functions such as muscular tension, heart rate, blood pressure, electrical conductance on the skin, skin temperature, and brain waves. The *bio* part of the name means life, and *feedback* means information—in this case, about your performance. So biofeedback machines measure your physiological (life) functions and give you information about them that can help you gain better control over your body in order to reduce stress. Some biofeedback devices look very much like medical devices, whereas others look more like video games. Biofeedback devices can be purchased through major online retailers.

CONNECT

Are you interested in trying biofeedback as a way to learn how to control your stress? What about this technology do you think would (or would not) help you?

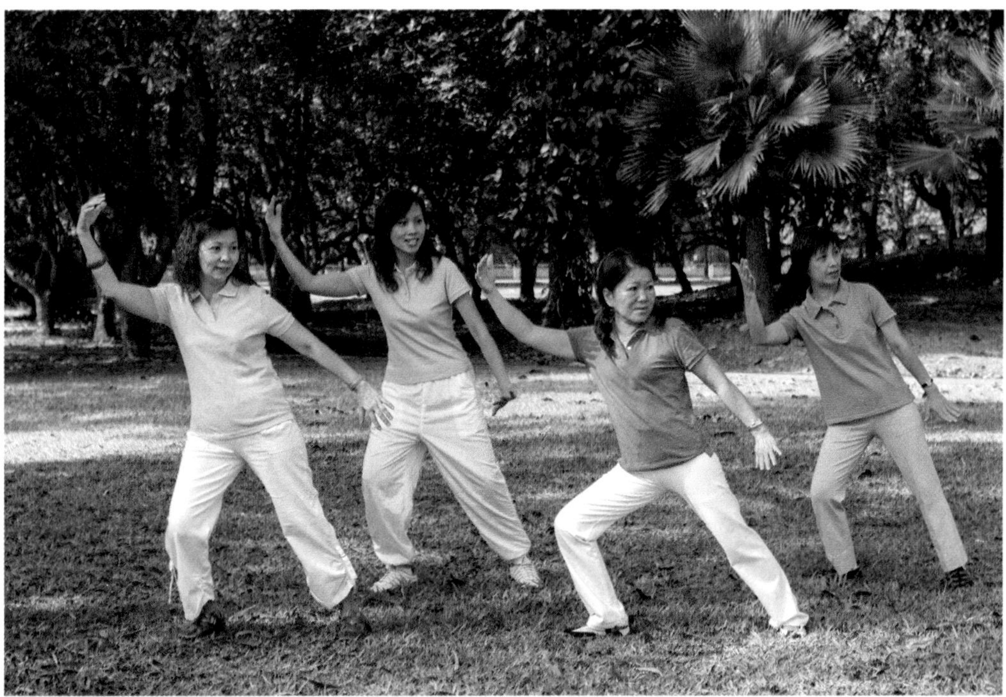

Tai chi is a self-paced system of gentle physical exercise and stretching that keeps the body in constant motion.

EastWest Imaging

Comprehension Check

1. Describe two stress management techniques that do not involve physical activity.
2. Explain how physical activity and exercise can help you manage stress.
3. Describe a method of practicing mindfulness.

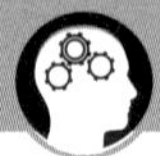

MAKING HEALTHY DECISIONS: Time Management

Alexis was one of those people who was always going from one commitment to the next. Her friends rarely saw her sitting still, and she often complained about having too much to do. Alexis played on the softball team and volunteered at her church on the weekends. She also helped out around the house with cleaning and cooking. When her friend Deborah asked her to go to yoga class together as a way to manage stress, she said, "I totally want to—it would be really great—but I just don't have any free time." Later in the conversation, Deborah noticed Alexis talking about TV shows she'd been watching and showing off a new video game she'd been playing. Deborah wondered if Alexis was as busy as she seemed to be. Deborah herself worked two jobs, was an honor student, ran cross country, and played in the school orchestra.

For Discussion

What could Deborah suggest that Alexis do to make time for yoga class? What could Deborah say to Alexis that might help her better understand her time management needs? To help you answer these questions, review this chapter's Skills for Healthy Living feature.

SKILLS FOR HEALTHY LIVING: Time Management

How you manage your time is an important part of your overall health. If you struggle with time management, you may have higher levels of stress and you may end up coping with your stress by engaging in destructive habits that seem to provide quick fixes, such as smoking or drinking alcohol. Poor time management can also interfere with your ability to create time for healthy pursuits, such as exercise.

Young people, like adults, often tend to book their schedules solid with work, school, errands, and other tasks they deem important. For example, you may be involved in a community organization, spend time tending to a school garden, play a sport, or care for an aging relative. The time you spend doing all of these activities is referred to as your committed time. What's left over is your free time. Learning to manage your free time can help you manage stress, avoid destructive habits, and make time for healthy habits. The following tips can help you with your time management:

- **Monitor your time.** Write down what you do during the course of each day. Record when you sleep, when you eat, when you're at school, when you're at work, and when you do all of the other things you do. Most people who track their use of time are surprised by the findings.
- **Evaluate your use of time.** Once you've tracked your time for several days, review your records to see how many hours you spend in various types of activities. For example, you can arrange all your activities into three categories: school and work, committed time, and free time. Then you can evaluate whether there is a good balance between the categories. Alternatively, you can think of all of your activities as fitting into three drawers: the lower drawer (not important or urgent), the middle drawer (important but not urgent), and the top drawer (urgent and important). If any drawer is overflowing, you may need to re-evaluate your commitments and priorities. Evaluating your time can help you decide whether you're using your time the way you want and need to use it. Having a lot of important and urgent things to do can add to your stress levels significantly.
- **Plan a schedule.** After you determine how much time you spend on various activities, work on creating a time management plan for yourself. Efficient time management means you get to do all the things you think are important so that you don't feel rushed or anxious, and it also allows you to make time for those things that you value, such as relaxation and recreational activities. Begin by blocking out your committed time (school, work, practice time). Then, make decisions about your free time.

When making decisions about your time, consider some of the following tips:

- First, schedule time for those things that are most important and most urgent (for example, an assignment worth a lot of points that is due tomorrow is important to your academic success and has a clear, time-sensitive deadline). It is typically better to allot more time than you think you might need to get these tasks done.
- Second, make a plan to complete those items that are important to you but may not be as urgent. Plan ahead and schedule in the time you need along the way. Most important, follow through with your plan so that you don't end up in a bind.
- Third, schedule in and plan time for yourself to do the things that you value (even when they don't seem important or urgent), such as exercising, reading a novel, or playing a musical instrument. Ensuring you are balanced and have the opportunities to relax and recover from the demands of life is critical to overall health. Often people do not take the time for these important activities unless they plan for them. It is also important to ensure that these activities do not interfere with obligations such as schoolwork.
- Finally, schedule some time every day for the unexpected. Meetings, appointments, and practices can run late, unexpected opportunities can arise, or other scheduled tasks can take longer than expected. Allowing some flexibility in each day can help you adjust your schedule to adapt to changing demands.

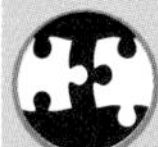

ACADEMIC CONNECTION: College and Career Skills

Being able to respond to precise instructions is an important skill for college and career readiness. For example, if you were asked to *analyze* how physical activity contributes to overall health, would you know how to respond? Would you be confident in your ability to *compare* carbohydrate and protein? What about your ability to *contrast* them? Each of these is different, and you must first understand what is being asked before you can accurately respond. The following are some of the most valuable skills for successful college admissions (performance on standardized tests like the SAT or ACT as well as for writing college admissions essays) and job performance.

- *Analyze:* Explain how each part functions or fits into the whole. For example, how does each type of physical activity (see the Physical Activity Pyramid) affect each component of health?
- *Persuade:* Take a stand on one side of an issue and convince others of the validity of that stance. Use facts, statistics, beliefs, opinions, and your personal view. Showing passion for your point of view can help you be persuasive.
- *Compare:* Find the common characteristics between two things. For example, carbohydrate and protein are both energy-yielding nutrients, and both contain 4 calories per gram.
- *Contrast:* Identify how people, events, or objects are different from one another. For example, carbohydrate is primarily used as fuel for the body, whereas protein is primarily used to build and repair tissues in the body.
- *Describe:* Present a clear picture of a person, place, thing, or idea. Try to write or speak so that the reader or listener could accurately visualize what you are saying.
- *Summarize:* State the meaning in a concise way (e.g., describe each of the factors that lead to teen stress and explain the relative importance of each).

Stress at Work: Can Worksite Health Promotion Help?

According to the American Psychological Association, 69 percent of people report that their work is a significant source of stress, 41 percent report feeling stressed at work on a regular basis, and 51 percent report that stress reduces their work productivity. According to the U.S. Bureau of Labor Statistics, people suffering from stress, anxiety, and related disorders miss an average of 25 work days each year. In contrast, the average number of days missed due to physical illness or injury is only 6. And according to health economist Dr. Roesch, job stress is estimated to cost the U.S. industry more than US$300 billion a year in absenteeism; turnover; diminished productivity; and medical, legal, and insurance costs.

What can be done about these costs? According to the U.S. Centers for Disease Control and Prevention, health care spending can be reduced by implementing and expanding evidence-based programs to promote workplace health, which would also improve the health of many Americans. Evidence shows, for example, that workplace health programs can positively influence social norms; help establish effective health policies; promote healthy behaviors such as practicing stress management techniques; improve people's health knowledge and skills; provide needed health screenings, immunizations, and follow-up care; and reduce on-the-job exposure to substances and hazards that can cause disease or injury. And when done well—using evidence-based best practices—comprehensive worksite health programs can yield an average $3 return on every $1 spent over a two- to five-year period (see figure 27.4).

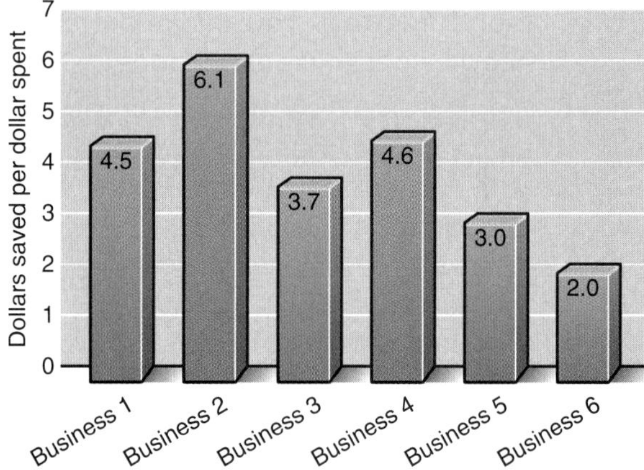

FIGURE 27.4 Return on investments for worksite health promotion programs.

For Discussion

How important do you think it is for employers to provide health promotion programs at work? What services and benefits do you think should be part of a good worksite health promotion program?

CHAPTER REVIEW

Reviewing Concepts and Vocabulary

As directed by your teacher, answer items 1 through 5 by correctly completing each sentence with a word or phrase.

1. The practice of using your imagination, or an actual visual or sound presentation, to help you relax is known as __________ __________.
2. If you're often late or tend to wait until the last minute to complete your homework, the best stress management technique for you would be __________ __________.
3. Identify two types of stress management breathing discussed in this chapter: ____________ ____________ and ____________ ____________.
4. Identify two physiological changes that happen in people who are under stress: __________ __________ __________ and ____________ ____________.
5. ________________ involves paying close attention to what you're doing at the moment.

For items 6 through 10, as directed by your teacher, match each term in column 1 with the appropriate phrase in column 2.

6. yoga
7. tai chi
8. body scanning
9. reframing
10. guided imagery

a. changing the way you view a situation
b. uses asanas or postures
c. slow, flowing movements done in sequence
d. focusing step by step on different body parts
e. using soothing words or images to help manage stress

For items 11 through 15, as directed by your teacher, respond to each statement or question.

11. Explain the relationship between performance and stress.
12. Briefly describe the fight-or-flight response.
13. How does assertiveness differ from aggression?
14. What is mindfulness?
15. Describe one breathing exercise for stress management.

Thinking Critically

Write a paragraph in response to the following questions.

Stress is something that most people think of as a negative aspect of life. However, it would be dangerous or even deadly if people did not have a stress response. Why?

Take It Home

Select a relaxation technique from this chapter and explain it to at least one of your family members. Then work together to try out the technique. Rate your stress before and after the session. Make a family relaxation plan that will help you build relaxation into your daily lives.

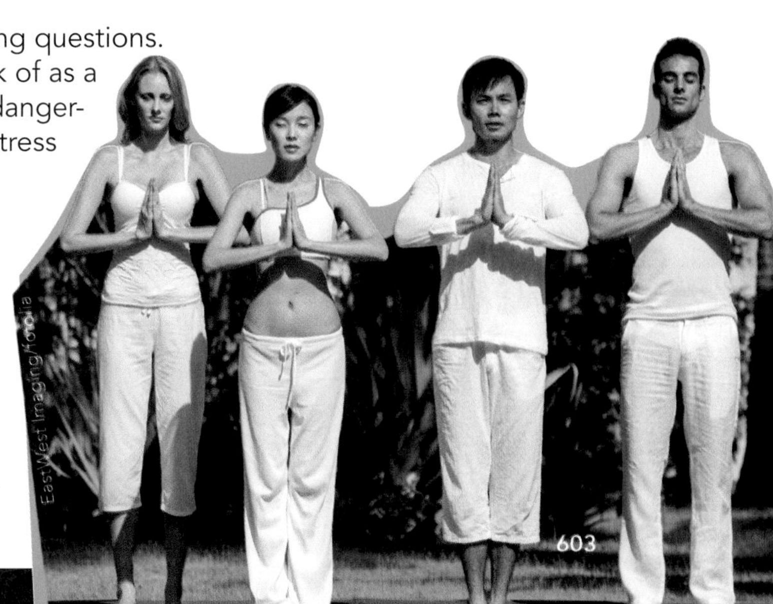
EastWest Imaging/fotolia

UNIT X

Building Relationships and Lifelong Health

Healthy People 2020 Goals

- Increase the proportion of pregnant women who receive early and adequate prenatal care.
- Reduce sexual violence.
- Reduce the rate of all infant deaths and death among children.
- Reduce the rate of adolescent and young adult deaths.
- Increase the proportion of adolescents who are connected to a parent or other positive adult caregiver.
- Reduce adolescent and young adult perpetration of and victimization by crimes.
- Increase the proportion of adults who report having someone with whom they can talk about their health.
- Increase the proportion of teens that prohibit harassment based on a student's sexual orientation or gender identity.
- Reduce bullying and fighting among adolescents.
- Increase the proportion of older adults with reduced cognitive functioning who engage in light, moderate, or vigorous leisure-time activities.
- Improve health literacy.

Self-Assessment Features in This Unit

- My Health Care Consumer Skills
- Rate Your Relationships
- My Spiritual Wellness

Making Healthy Decisions and Skills for Healthy Living Features in This Unit

- Critical Thinking
- Conflict Resolution
- Intrinsic Motivation

Special Features in This Unit

- Advocacy in Action: Know Your Medical History
- Diverse Perspectives: Sexual Orientation
- Diverse Perspectives: Being an Older Parent

Living Well News Features in This Unit

- What Are the Most Common Types of Health Insurance?
- Changing Marriage Patterns
- Does a High-Carbohydrate Diet Contribute to Mild Cognitive Impairment?

28

Health Care Consumerism

In This Chapter

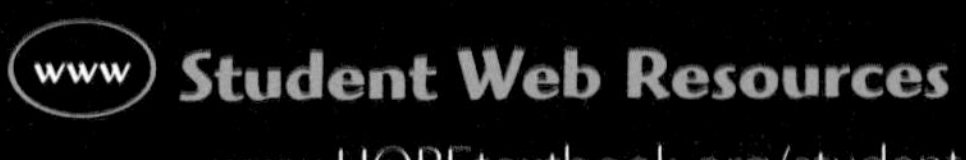

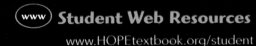

Student Web Resources

www.HOPEtextbook.org/student

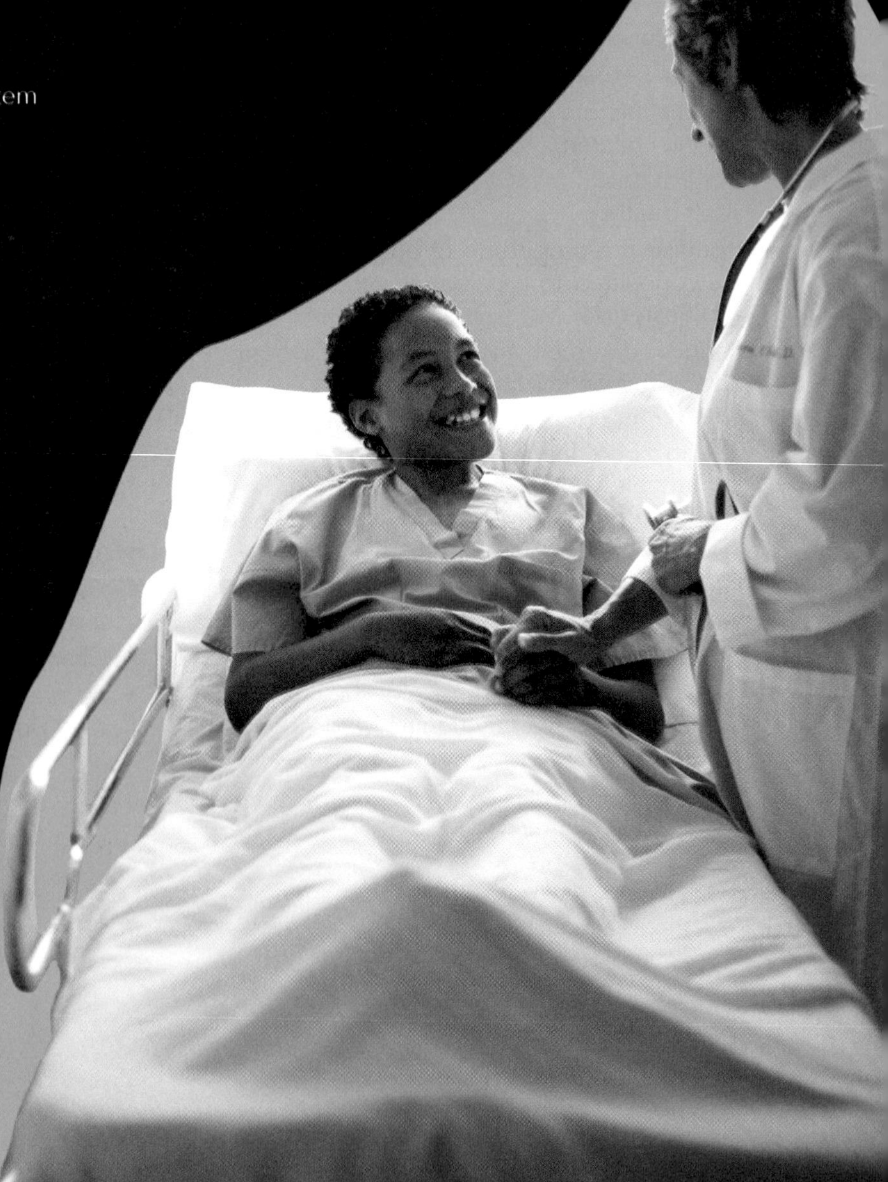

Photodisc

Lesson 28.1

Health Literacy and Consumer Skills

Lesson Objectives

After reading this lesson, you should be able to

1. explain the importance of knowing your medical history and what should be included,
2. describe your consumer rights in terms of health care, and
3. explain the value of health literacy.

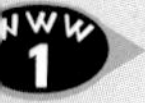

Lesson Vocabulary

culturally and linguistically appropriate services (CLAS), electronic medical records, health literacy, medical history, telemedicine

Chances are good that you've not had to make many choices about your medical or dental care without help from a parent or guardian. Even so, it's not too early to get more involved in your own care. Of course, your parents or guardians have a deep interest in your health. But you, the patient, are the person who actually feels the pain of an illness or injury. Only you know how your condition makes you feel. In addition, the earlier people become actively involved in their own health care, the more likely it is that any necessary intervention will be successful.

This lesson focuses on what it means to have health literacy and explores key issues to help you be an effective consumer of health care. The discussion uses the general term *health care provider* because, depending on the reason you seek treatment, you may visit a doctor, dentist, mental health professional, nurse, dental hygienist, nurse practitioner, pharmacist, physician assistant, physical therapist, occupational therapist, athletic trainer, chiropractor, public health official, or any of many other types of health professionals.

> "I am interested in getting people to use the health care system at the right time, getting them to see the doctor early enough, before a small health problem turns serious."
>
> —Donna Shalala, former U.S. Secretary of Health and Human Services

How Is a Health Care Consumer Different From Other Types of Consumers?

When you're looking for health care, you have choices to make and questions to answer: what health care professional to see, how much the health care will cost, how to pay for it, where to go if your usual health care provider is not available, and how to get to your health care provider. It's a lot different from buying a video game online or going to a few stores to compare prices and return policies. Here are some more major differences between being a health care consumer and buying other products.

1. *If you have something seriously wrong, you can't afford to put it off like you can if you're buying a new phone or new shoes.* If you're really sick or injured, you need help right away.
2. *You likely don't have the time or the information to comparison-shop.* For many products, it's easy these days to go online, find out what different companies charge for the same product, and choose the least expensive offer. But it's not easy to find out the costs of medical services and determine which health care professional is the best match for your needs—medically or financially.
3. *Unlike shopping for a product online, you generally have to go to wherever the health care professional is located, which can be difficult due to factors such as time, money, and distance.* Of course, some medications and medical equipment can be ordered

online and delivered to your home. However, even with the advent of **telemedicine** and **electronic medical records**—which allow patients to talk with doctors from a distance and access their records online—there will always be a need to see health care providers in person on some occasions.

4. *In medical care your options for bargaining are very limited.* In many commercial transactions, people can bargain for a good deal. For example, when people buy a house or car, or even when they shop at a flea market or garage sale, they can make an offer that the seller will either accept or turn down. One situation in which bargaining might be possible is that of a health care professional not included on an insurance company's list of preferred providers. In this case, the patient could ask (bargain) with the health care professional to accept the same fee that he or she would be paid if included as a preferred provider. Most of the time, however, you do not get to negotiate the price of health care services and products.

5. *In health care, you generally don't have options such as getting two for one, getting a refund, or returning a product you aren't satisfied with.*

For these reasons and others, health care consumer groups and health literacy organizations have developed guidelines and materials to help people navigate the health care system and learn how to stay healthy.

CONNECT

How do you think the web has influenced health care consumerism? How might it influence the doctor–patient relationship? Think of as many realistic examples as you can, then share your ideas with those of a peer or classmate. Compare your ideas and work collaboratively to come up with a response you agree on. Negotiate and compromise as needed to build consensus (agreement).

Health Literacy

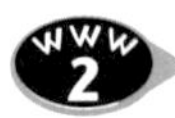

The U.S. government's *Healthy People 2020* report defines **health literacy** as "the degree to which individuals have the capacity to obtain, process, and understand basic health information and services needed to make appropriate health decisions." The U.S. Department of Health and Human Services (HHS) further explains that health literacy depends on having good knowledge of health topics, effectively engaging cultural factors (e.g., language differences), knowing how to fill out complex forms and locate health providers and services, engaging in self-care and chronic-disease management (e.g., asthma control), understanding mathematical concepts (e.g., probability, risk), and being able to perform key tasks (e.g., calculating cholesterol and blood sugar levels, measuring medications, understanding nutrition labels).

Health literacy is closely tied to the skill of critical thinking (for more on this connection, see the Skills for Healthy Living feature). It is not something that people just have; it must be acquired and developed. Although health literacy does involve some degree of common sense, many aspects of health care require special—and sometimes technical—knowledge. Generally speaking, the more knowledgeable you are, the more likely you are to have positive health outcomes. On the other hand, if you give vague information to your health care professional, you may get unspecific treatment.

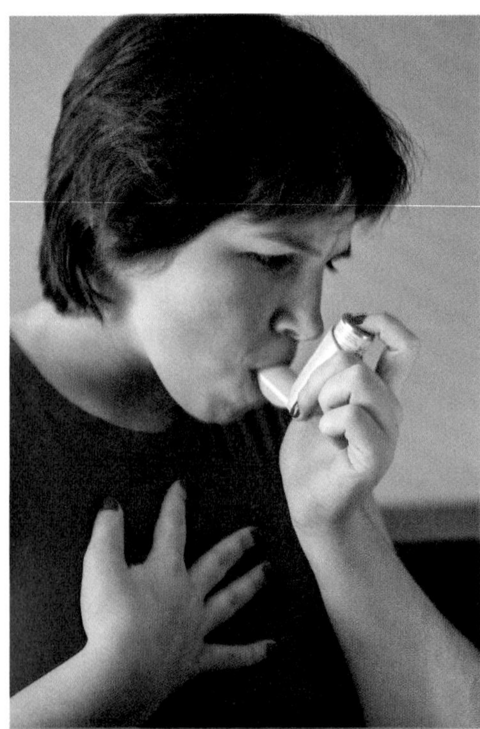

Understanding chronic-disease management such as asthma control is just one aspect of health literacy.

Linguistic and Cultural Barriers to Health Literacy

A patient who speaks a different language from the health care provider often has the right to an interpreter (for spoken language) or translator (for written language). Many health care providers and hospitals employ interpreters and translators or subscribe to a service that provides them via telecommunication. Even if a patient speaks the same language as the health care provider, the patient may not always understand the medical or technical language that the health care provider uses. All patients have the right to an explanation that they understand.

In addition, the practice of providing **culturally and linguistically appropriate services (CLAS)** sets standards to ensure that a patient's treatment is not only understandable but also appropriate, whenever possible, within the patient's culture. For example, in some cultures people don't eat certain kinds of food. If a person is put on a special diet for medical reasons, that diet should not include foods prohibited by the person's religion or other cultural tradition.

Knowing Your Consumer Rights and Responsibilities

To participate effectively in your own health care and develop your health literacy, you must know your responsibilities and rights as a health care consumer. For example, you have the responsibility to be honest and forthcoming with your health care providers. You are expected to answer their questions honestly and provide an accurate **medical history**. This history should include all information that can help your medical professional give you the best possible treatment for your specific situation. Information that may be included in a medical history is identified in the accompanying text box. You are also expected to ask questions of your health care provider whenever you need clarification or have a concern.

In addition to these responsibilities, you have certain rights as a health care consumer. In the United States, the Patient's Bill of Rights, created by the government in 1998, affirms the following rights that you hold as a health care consumer.

- **Information.** You have the right to accurate and easily understood information.
- **Choice.** You have the right to a choice of health care providers and to high-quality health care.
- **Access.** If you have severe pain, an injury, or a sudden illness that may put your health in serious danger, you have the right to emergency care whenever and wherever needed.
- **Participation.** You have the right to know your treatment options and to participate in decisions about your care.

Keeping Track of Your Medical History

To ensure that you receive the best possible medical treatment, keep track of your medical history. Specifically, record the following types of information:

- Any prescription medications used during the past six months, including name, dose taken, and reason for taking
- Any over-the-counter (OTC) medications, vitamins, and supplements used during the past six months, including product name, dose taken, and reason for taking
- Any known allergies to medication
- All previous vaccinations and the date of each
- Past major medical events (e.g., surgeries, hospitalizations, tests, treatments, medical problems)
- Known family history of heart disease, cancer, or other disease or disorder (including parents, grandparents, siblings, aunts and uncles, and cousins)

ADVOCACY IN ACTION: Know Your Medical History

Everyone needs to understand his or her health history. As a classroom, design a Know Your Medical History campaign to help your peers gather information about their own health histories. Design a form that can be used to collect critical health information (use the text box titled Keeping Track of Your Medical History as a guide). Set up a table on campus to help fellow students learn why it's important to know their medical history. Provide them with the form you developed and invite them to sign a pledge stating that they will learn their own medical history. Consider providing ribbons, stickers, or pins to all of your peers who sign the pledge. Because of confidentiality issues, however, do not ask anyone to give their medical history to you.

- **Respect.** You have the right to considerate, respectful, and nondiscriminatory care.
- **Confidentiality.** You have the right to talk in confidence with your health care providers.
- **Complaints.** You have the right to a fair, fast, and objective review of any complaints you have against your health care provider or facility.

Trust and Confidentiality

It's crucial that you tell your health care providers the truth, even if it includes something about which you feel embarrassed or the topic is a sensitive one. For example, your providers need to know about medications you are taking, previous illnesses, sexual behavior, and any use of alcohol or other drugs. If you don't tell the truth, you're unlikely to get the treatment you need.

Most state laws provide for special relationships that allow confidentiality between doctors and patients, attorneys and clients, priests and those who confess to them, and guardians and their wards. In health care, such laws mean that your doctor will keep your medical information confidential. This fact can be controversial because some parents and guardians believe that if they are paying the medical bills, the health care professional should not hold back any information about their children. Open communication is encouraged with parents (guardians). Of course, a child is always free to communicate any medical information to his or her parents or guardians. But, for a variety of reasons, they sometimes choose not to.

HEALTHY COMMUNICATION

Do you think it is fair for a minor to be able to keep medical information private from parents or guardians? Why or why not? What personal values influence your perspective? How do you think cultural influences affect your perspective? Share your perspectives with a peer and show respect for each other's opinions.

Comprehension Check

1. Why is it important to know your medical history and what should be included?
2. Describe three rights that you have as a health care consumer.
3. Explain the value of health literacy.

SELF-ASSESSMENT: My Health Care Consumer Skills

For each question, select the answer (yes or no) that best describes you or your situation. Record your results as directed by your teacher.

1. I have access to (or know where to find) my medical history, including my immunization records.
   a. yes
   b. no
2. I have a medical home (a place where I can see the same health care provider) when I need medical care.
   a. yes
   b. no
3. I know what health care services are available at my school.
   a. yes
   b. no
4. If I don't understand my health care professional, I am not afraid to ask for clarification.
   a. yes
   b. no
5. I always tell the truth when my health care professional asks me about my behavior or my medical history, even if it might be embarrassing (e.g., sexual behavior, drug or alcohol use).
   a. yes
   b. no
6. If I am having a problem with my health, I try to learn as much as I can about my condition.
   a. yes
   b. no
7. I feel comfortable talking to my parents or guardian when I am not feeling well.
   a. yes
   b. no
8. When I am told by my health care professional what I should do to get better, I follow all the directions that I am given.
   a. yes
   b. no
9. If my condition gets worse, despite following my health care provider's advice, I have no problem calling for additional help.
   a. yes
   b. no
10. I know where to get medical care if my health care provider is not available.
    a. yes
    b. no
11. I know how to determine whether a website is a reliable source of medical information.
    a. yes
    b. no

12. I understand what patient–doctor confidentiality means.
    a. yes
    b. no
13. I am willing to ask for a medical translator (if needed for me or a friend or family member).
    a. yes
    b. no
14. I believe that it is my responsibility to do what it takes to help myself get well.
    a. yes
    b. no
15. I know where my local public health department is located.
    a. yes
    b. no

To score this self-assessment, count the number of yes answers that you circled. If the total is 12 to 15, you're a very good health care consumer; keep up the good work. If the total is 9 to 11, you can become a very good health care consumer with a little help (e.g., talking to your parents or your school nurse, learning more about your medical history, and so on). If the total is 8 or below, review this chapter to build your skills as a health care consumer.

✓ Planning for Healthy Living

Use the Healthy Living Plan worksheet to improve your skills as a health consumer.

Lesson 28.2

Self-Care and the Health Care System

Lesson Objectives

After reading this lesson, you should be able to

1. explain the importance of personal responsibility when seeking medical care and using the health care system,
2. identify two ways in which a person might get medical insurance, and
3. explain three things you should look for when selecting a physician.

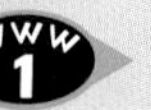

Lesson Vocabulary

medical home, patient education, public health, self-care, support group

In many ways, this entire book addresses self-care. More specifically, the things you learn by reading the book, doing the self-assessments, performing online research, taking quizzes, and making behavior changes all help you take better care of your health.

Self-care does not replace medical care; it complements it. Your self-care is affected in part by the choices you make. It is also influenced by whether or not you have health insurance and whom you select as your health care providers—for example, family physician, specialist, dentist, physician assistant, or nurse practitioner. Your school probably has a school nurse and may even have its own health clinic. Your community may also have a free health clinic or a clinic that charges on a sliding scale according to ability to pay.

You must make many decisions when selecting health care professionals and deciding what type of health care is best suited to you. In this lesson, you'll learn about self-care and health care options.

Self-Care

Self-care involves all of the decisions you make and the actions you take to maintain your health. It includes knowing when you are at risk for a health problem (e.g., asthma increases the risk of complications from the flu). Self-care and medical care work hand in hand. Your health care professional may tell you what to do to get better, but you're responsible for actually doing the things you should do. For example, if you're an athlete with an injury, a physical therapist may assign you exercises, but you're responsible for doing them as directed. That is one type of self-care. Similarly, although vaccination (which helps prevent disease) is not something you give to yourself, self-care is required in order for you to make and keep an appointment to get vaccinated.

Self-care is often tied to **patient education**. For example, if you have diabetes, you have likely been given education to help you learn to monitor your glucose level, know what your diet and exercise programs should be, and know when and how to take injections or other medications. In this case,

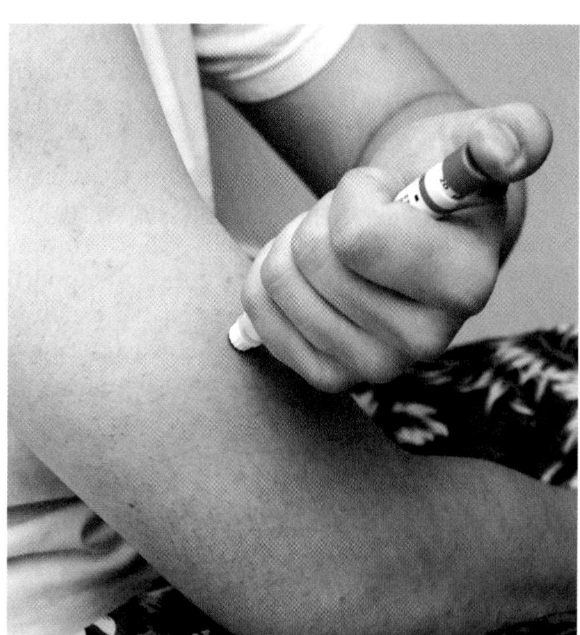

Effective self-care is often based on patient education such as a person who is allergic to bee stings learning how to use an epipen (an epinephrine shot to prevent severe reactions).

Nebojsa Bobic/fotolia.com

self-care involves doing the things you need to do to control your disease, and patient education includes the information, coaching, counseling, and behavior modification techniques provided by your health care provider. Many years ago, the life expectancy for people with type 1 (early-onset) diabetes was not very high. Now, however, when people with diabetes receive patient education and practice self-care, they are able to live as long as people who don't have diabetes.

Support Groups

Support groups, which bring together people who have similar problems, can play an important role in maintaining good health. As discussed in this book's chapters on alcohol and drugs, support groups can help people quit addictive and destructive behaviors. They can also help people meet other goals, such as losing weight, maintaining an exercise program, and learning how to eat well. In fact, just about every health condition or concern you can think of has a support group. For rare conditions, where few people with the condition live near each other, support groups can operate through social media.

As with self-care, support groups do not take the place of medical care but complement it. Most support groups are led not by professionals but by people who have the same problem or concern shared by other members of the group. Some hybrid groups combine medical care with support. For example, a doctor might give a presentation, after which members take the floor and share their problems and successes. In all support groups, members share information, emotional support, moral support, and tactics that enable them to become healthier. We all know that when we have a supportive environment, we are much more likely to succeed in facing difficult situations.

Specialty Camps and Workshops

Many camps and workshops are available for young people who want to learn more about their own health concern in a fun and supportive environment. Thousands of young people have participated in such experiences to learn how to lose weight, control asthma and diabetes, overcome addiction, and deal with a host of other specific conditions. Some programs incorporate sports, crafts, ropes courses, horseback riding, and other activities. The camps and workshops are typically sponsored by an organization associated with a specific health condition, such as the American Diabetes Association, the American Lung Association, or the American Cancer Society. They may be free or inexpensive for people who qualify.

The Health Care System

The health care system includes all available medical services, the ways in which medical care is paid for, and the programs and services aimed at preventing disease and disability. In the health care system, physicians work with nurses and other health care providers to care for patients.

Medical Home

Patient-centered medicine is a term used to describe a form of medical practice that focuses on the patient's needs and concerns rather than the doctor's. One important part of this approach is to facilitate communication between medical specialists to optimize each person's treatment.

In order for this approach to be successful, each patient needs a primary point of contact in the health care system through which he or she receives medical attention. This point of contact is termed your **medical home**. A patient-centered medical home is a health care delivery system in which patients have an ongoing relationship with a personal physician who provides comprehensive and culturally and linguistically appropriate care. This physician also takes responsibility for coordinating care with other providers.

For many people, their medical home is their primary care physician—a medical doctor who takes care of most routine medical needs. Most primary care physicians have training in family practice, internal medicine, or pediatrics. Your medical home as a student could be your primary care physician, but it could also be your school nurse, and some schools even have their own doctors. Some also have their own school psychologist or psychiatrist. In addition, most high schools have school counselors. All of these professionals can be part of your medical home, depending on your particular needs.

The advantage of having a medical home is that you get to see someone who knows you and your background. Seeing a different person each time you need health care can be more time consuming, and you are more likely to have gaps in the services you receive. Many **public health** departments provide free or inexpensive medical services such as vaccines and testing for sexually transmitted infection (STI). Check to see what medical service your local public health department offers.

Think about it this way: Many people like to get their hair cut by the same person because that person knows what they want. As a result, loyalty often develops between a stylist and a customer. The same kind of relationship—on a deeper level—can develop between a patient and a health care provider who establish a level of trust that enhances their communication. Thus establishing your medical home is one way to enhance your health care experience.

School-Based Health Clinics

Many health care professionals believe that school-based health clinics make sense because children and young adults spend so much of their time at school. In fact, a school-based clinic can be a person's medical home. However, not everyone likes school-based clinics. Some parents and guardians feel that these clinics assume responsibilities that should be their own. Other parents and guardians like school-based clinics because if their child gets sick at school, they don't have to leave work to pick up the child. They know that the child is being taken care of by a health care professional. In addition, medical checkups can be performed at school without making an appointment and an extra trip to another health care provider. And, of course, people can still choose—the presence of a school-based clinic doesn't mean that everyone has to use it.

Emergency Rooms

For a variety of reasons, many people use emergency rooms as their only access to the medical care system. In emergencies, of course, this is exactly what people should do. But many people go to the emergency room for other reasons—for example, because it's always open, they don't have a medical home, their usual health care provider is not open, they don't want to wait for an appointment, an emergency room attends to everyone who shows up regardless of ability to pay, or the person doesn't know of any other options.

Emergency care is much more expensive than care from a primary health care professional, but it is essential in certain circumstances. Examples include when experiencing chest pain, difficulty breathing, severe injury, or poisoning. In many cases, if patients attended to medical problems in their early stages, there would be less need to go to an emergency room.

Selecting a Physician

The relationship you have with your primary care physician can affect the quality of the advice and care you receive. Most people in the United States have a choice when it comes to a selecting a primary care physician. Whether you are part of a health maintenance organization (HMO)—in

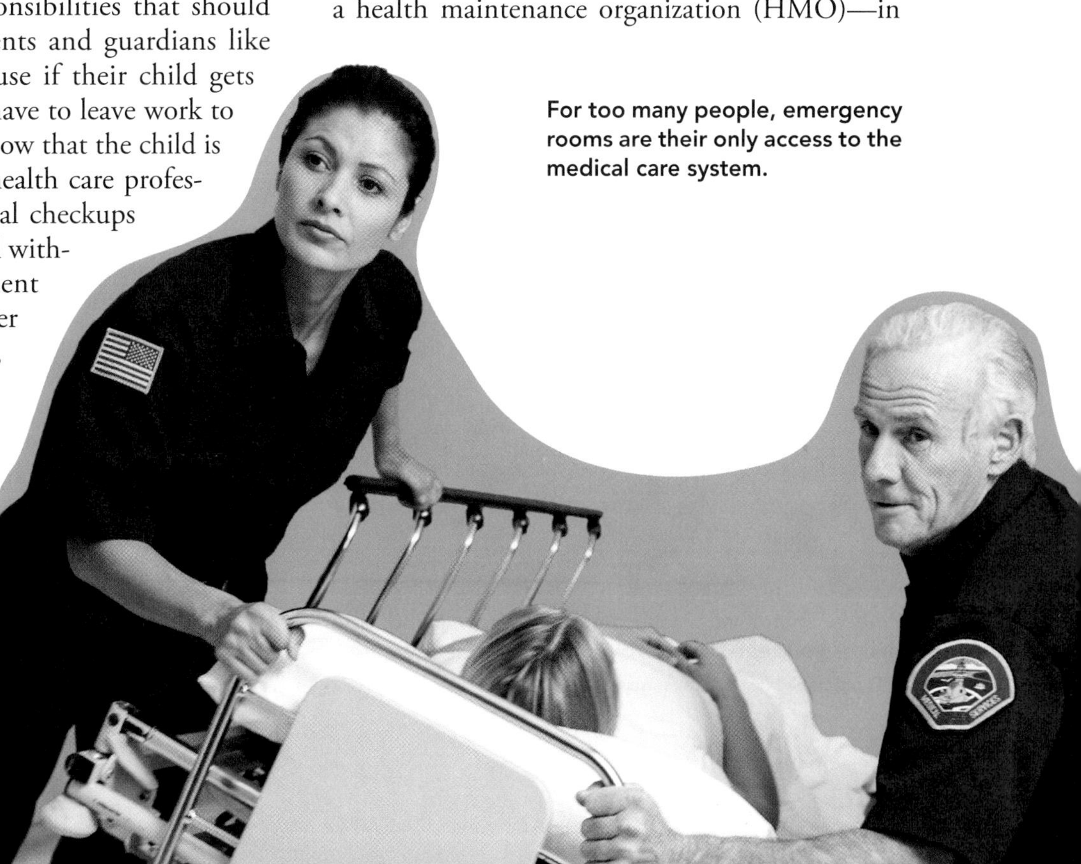

For too many people, emergency rooms are their only access to the medical care system.

which all medical services are connected within a network—or are free to choose any doctor in your area, you generally get to pick which doctor is best for you. (See this chapter's Living Well News feature.) Sometimes the choice is a hard one. When selecting a doctor, consider the following factors.

- **Professional ability.** The first and foremost concern on anyone's mind when choosing a doctor should be the physician's credentials. Remember to consider specialties and board certifications.
- **Male or female.** Ask yourself whether you're more comfortable seeing a male or female doctor. Your answer may vary according to the particular medical service.
- **Connection.** Pay attention to how well you connect with your doctor. Do you feel that you are heard? Do you feel respected? Would you recommend this doctor to others?
- **Bedside manner.** Does the doctor have a professional but empathetic tone? Your doctor should listen to what you have to say and respond in ways that show he or she not only hears but also takes seriously what you have to say.
- **Availability.** Is the doctor always booked? Is it hard to schedule appointments? It's important to be able to get care when you need it.
- **Insurance.** Know your insurance and select a doctor who will be covered.
- **Reputation.** It's no longer difficult to find out how others feel about particular doctors. It is easy to get online and do some checking. If doctors are unpopular or have made serious mistakes, they are likely listed with concerns expressed online. However, the Internet can also be misleading on issues like this. A small incident may be overstated or a disgruntled patient may simply lie. For this reason, don't rely solely on online comments when selecting a health care provider. Cross reference them with the other factors.

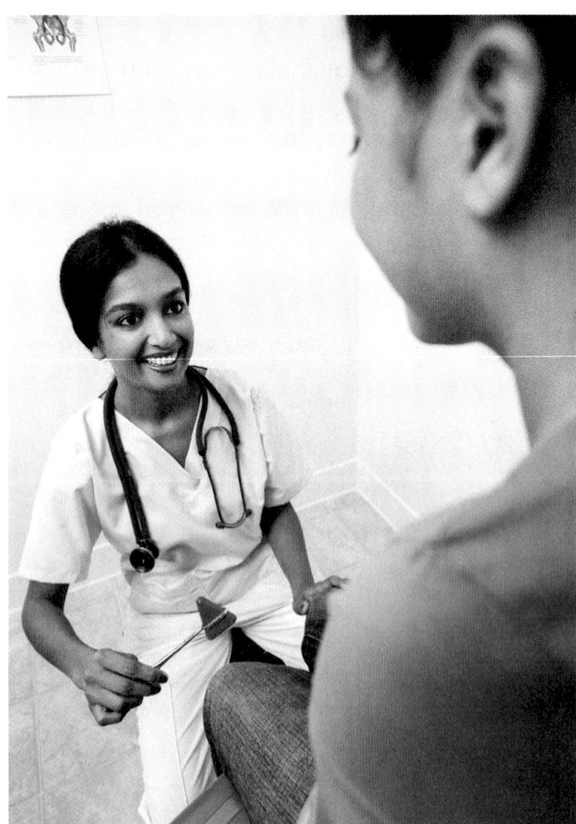

Find a doctor who can communicate well and who makes you feel comfortable about your health care.

© Photographerlondon | Dreamstime.com

Medical Coverage

Part of accessing health care involves making sure you can afford to pay for medical treatment when you need it. One way to meet medical expenses is to purchase medical insurance. According to the U.S. Census Bureau, 84 percent of Americans have some type of health insurance, and those who do are more likely to access the health care system and to have better health. As a teenager, if you have health insurance, you're most likely covered through a parent's or guardian's plan.

Most insured Americans have private group insurance that is provided by an employer, who negotiates the cost of the insurance with the insurance provider and usually helps pay the premium. An insurance premium is a set amount of money paid into the plan up front so that members of the group can have access to financial help and services when they need them. If you're covered on a parent's or guardian's insurance plan, that person is contributing a set amount from each paycheck to cover your premium. As a result, a good health insurance plan is an important benefit to look for when you're considering potential employers.

Other forms of insurance are also available. Plans such as Medicaid and Medicare are subsidized (partially or fully paid) by the U.S. government to help

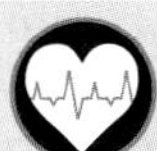

HEALTH TECHNOLOGY

About two out of three people with Internet access look up medical information online. Two out of five people, for example, use physician rating websites to learn more about their doctor. Unfortunately, only a small number of people rate their doctors online, so the results you find may be based on just a handful of ratings. In addition, since people may be more likely to rate a doctor when they've had a bad experience, you should be careful in judging how accurate online ratings really are. If anyone has ever written bad things about you online, you know that what they say can be wrong or unfair. That's a major problem with online ratings. Some people just like to post negative comments about others, whether or not they're true.

Some health care organizations are rated by groups such as Healthgrades, a health care quality reporting group. Before you use an online ratings site, find out more about the group doing the rating. Is it an independent group, or is it funded by one of the health organizations being rated? Does it have a good system for determining its ratings?

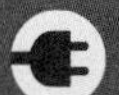

CONNECT

Have you used a physician rating system when deciding which health care provider to see? Do you think you would do so in the future? Why or why not?

low-income and elderly people obtain affordable medical care. Young, healthy people can also elect to pay for individual insurance plans. Those who don't have access to group care and cannot afford comprehensive individual insurance may choose to purchase catastrophic insurance. This type of plan costs less each month but can be used only if you suffer a very serious health condition.

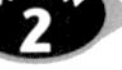

The Affordable Care Act (ACA) allows people who don't have insurance from other sources to be able to purchase their own health insurance. The costs vary from state to state and according to income (i.e., people with low incomes may qualify for a subsidy). If people refuse to buy insurance, they must pay a penalty. Insurance companies cannot refuse to insure people because of a preexisting condition, as many companies did before the ACA. Immigrants who are lawfully in the United States can buy health insurance, but immigrants who are undocumented cannot purchase it.

Comprehension Check

1. What role does personal responsibility play in seeking medical care and using the health care system?
2. Identify two ways in which a person can get medical insurance.
3. What are three things to look for when selecting a physician?

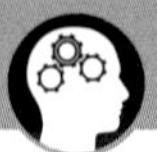

MAKING HEALTHY DECISIONS: Critical Thinking

Renny was recently diagnosed with a stomach ulcer. Her doctor prescribed medication for her and told her to try to reduce her stress. After the appointment, Renny noticed that her stomach hurt even worse. She stopped taking her medication because she assumed it was causing her increase in pain. Things got so bad that she stopped wanting to eat any solid food. She was able to eat in small amounts over the course of the day and drank mostly fruit juices and soda for the calories.

Renny's aunt told her that she should take a multivitamin and eat licorice because it has an ingredient that helps with digestion. Renny tried that for a while, then started drinking milk after her sister said that it might coat her stomach. The whole situation was making her feel even more stressed out, and the idea of managing her stress was overwhelming. The only thing she found helpful was sleeping, so she was often just lying around and resting.

For Discussion

What weaknesses do you see in Renny's critical thinking about her health problem? Name at least two. What are two specific steps Renny could take to improve her thinking about this issue? To help you answer these questions, refer to the Skills for Healthy Living feature.

SKILLS FOR HEALTHY LIVING: Critical Thinking

Critical thinking is the process of actively and skillfully conceptualizing (generating or creating), applying, analyzing, synthesizing, and evaluating information. Critical thinking is influenced by observation, experience, reflection, reasoning, and communication. Ultimately, it serves as a guide to belief and action. More specifically, it enables you to find and interpret information that helps you make decisions and solve problems in order to live a healthy lifestyle.

Your critical thinking is affected by the work you do as part of your formal education, as well as the way in which you process other life experiences and learn from them. To develop and use critical thinking skills in relation to your health and wellness, consider the following tips.

- **Readily admit a lack of understanding or information and ask questions.** No one knows everything about all aspects of health, wellness, and medicine. Smart people know when to ask others.
- **Be curious.** Health information changes, and you need to stay curious enough to seek updated information on issues related to your health.
- **Be interested in finding new solutions.** Many health issues have more than one solution. Sometimes the ability to try a new approach or solution makes the difference.
- **Be willing to examine beliefs, assumptions, and opinions and weigh them against facts.** The more you learn, the more you're likely to have your previous beliefs and opinions challenged. Accept the challenge and don't be afraid to grow.
- **Listen carefully to others.** Listening to others is essential for your health care. Learn to listen and to follow medical advice.
- **Make critical thinking a lifelong process and self-assess your ability to think critically.** Continually train yourself to think better. Like most skills, developing strong critical thinking takes effort.
- **Suspend judgment until all facts have been gathered and considered.** Jumping to conclusions and making swift judgments shuts off your ability to gather more information and learn. Keep an open mind.
- **Look for evidence to support assumptions and beliefs.** Don't just look at evidence to prove a different point of view wrong. Make a practice of looking

for evidence that supports your health beliefs and assumptions. If you can't find any, consider alternative perspectives.

- **Don't be afraid to update your thinking as you learn more.** It's okay to change your mind on an issue in light of new information.
- **Examine problems closely.** Be sure of what it is you really want to know before you seek solutions.
- **Reject information that is incorrect or irrelevant.** Don't be influenced by scams and quackery.

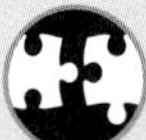

ACADEMIC CONNECTION: Sources of Information

When reading and analyzing writing and research, you need to recognize the difference between primary and secondary sources of information and use each appropriately. Each is described as follows.

Primary Sources

A primary source is an original object or document—the raw material or firsthand information. Primary sources include historical and legal documents, eyewitness accounts, results of experiments, statistical data, pieces of creative writing, and art objects. Here are some primary sources used in health and fitness:

- Journals or periodicals are the main type of publications in which scientific research is reported. *Exercise and Science in Sports and Medicine* and the *Journal of Health, Physical Education, Recreation and Dance (JOPERD)* are examples of periodicals used in health and fitness.
- These are detailed accounts of research conducted in pursuit of higher academic degrees such as a master of science (MS) degree.
- Conference papers are an important avenue for reporting new research or developments.
- Reports are individual publications containing research. These include many governmental reports. For example, the CDC often reports on data from the Youth Risk Behavior Surveillance System.

Secondary Sources

A secondary source is something written about a primary source. Secondary sources include comments on, interpretations of, and discussions about the original material. You can think of secondary sources as secondhand information. Examples of secondary sources of health and fitness information are articles in newspapers or popular magazines, textbooks, book or movie reviews, and articles in scholarly journals that discuss or evaluate someone else's original research.

What Are the Most Common Types of Health Insurance?

Most people who have a health care policy through their employer (and many who are self-insured) are enrolled in some type of managed care plan—either a health maintenance organizations (HMO) or a preferred provider organization (PPO). A less common alternative is a point-of-service (POS) plan, which combines the features of an HMO and a PPO (see figure 28.1). All managed care plans contract with doctors, hospitals, clinics, and other health care providers such as pharmacies, labs, X ray centers, and medical equipment vendors. This group of contracted health care providers is known as the health plan's network.

In some types of managed care plans, you may be required to receive all of your health care services from providers in the insurer's network. This is the case with HMOs, which require you to select a primary care physician (PCP), who is responsible for managing and coordinating your health care. When you need to see a specialist or receive a diagnostic service (e.g., a lab test or X ray), you must get a referral from your PCP. If you don't have a referral or you choose to see a provider outside of your HMO's network, you will most likely pay most or all of the cost. Even when you see a doctor within your HMO's network, you'll likely make a co-payment (due at the time of service), and you may also have to meet a deductible (a set amount that you pay yourself before your insurance benefits take over).

In other managed care plans, you may be able to receive care from providers who are not part of the network, but you will pay a larger share of the cost to receive those services. A preferred provider organization contracts with a network of preferred providers from whom you can choose. You do not need to select a PCP or get a referral to see other providers in the network. As with an HMO, you will have a co-payment and a deductible to meet.

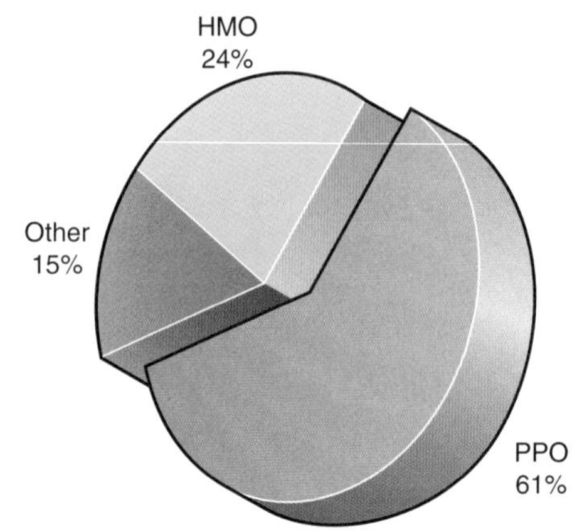

Figure 28.1 Health insurance plans.

For Discussion

Are you covered by any health care insurance that you know of? What would be the advantages and disadvantages of getting your medical care from a plan like an HMO? How much of every dollar earned would you be willing to pay in order to have quality medical insurance? Explain your response.

CHAPTER REVIEW

Reviewing Concepts and Vocabulary

As directed by your teacher, answer items 1 through 5 by correctly completing the sentence with a word or phrase.

1. A regular health care provider is referred to as a medical __________.
2. A group of people who get together to discuss health concerns or conditions that they have in common is called a(n) ____________ ____________.
3. A health care professional who teaches a patient how to take care of his or her condition or disease is providing ________________________.
4. A person with asthma or diabetes who learns how to manage his or her symptoms is practicing ____________ ____________.
5. One type of managed care plan is an HMO, which stands for ____________ ____________ ____________.

For items 6 through 10, as directed by your teacher, match each term in column 1 with the appropriate phrase in column 2.

6. CLAS	a. related to the skill of critical thinking
7. specialty camp	b. views health from a collective, group, or population perspective
8. public health	c. more expensive than care from a primary health care provider
9. health literacy	d. culturally and linguistically appropriate services (CLAS)
10. emergency care	e. for young people who want to learn more about their own health concerns

For items 11 through 15, as directed by your teacher, respond to each statement or question.

11. Describe two things you should look for when selecting a physician.
12. List two reasons that a person might choose to get help at an emergency room rather than seeing a regular physician.
13. Why is patient education important?
14. What is critical thinking?
15. What are two steps you could take to improve your critical thinking skills?

Thinking Critically

Write a paragraph in response to the following question.

When José arrived at his doctor's office, the receptionist spoke to him in English, but José's first language was Spanish and he had a hard time figuring out what he was supposed to do. What would be the best solution to José's problem?

Take It Home

Talk with your parents or guardians about your health care insurance. Find out if you have HMO, PPO, or another form of insurance. Learn about your medical co-payments and deductibles and find out what will happen to your insurance if you leave home or go to college.

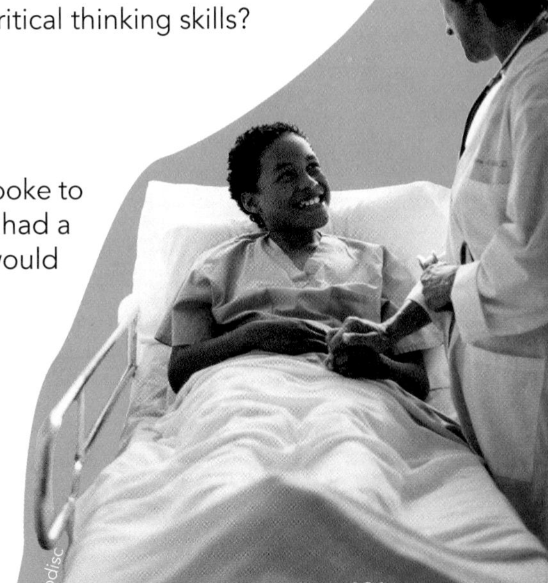

Photodisc

29

Family Living and Healthy Relationships

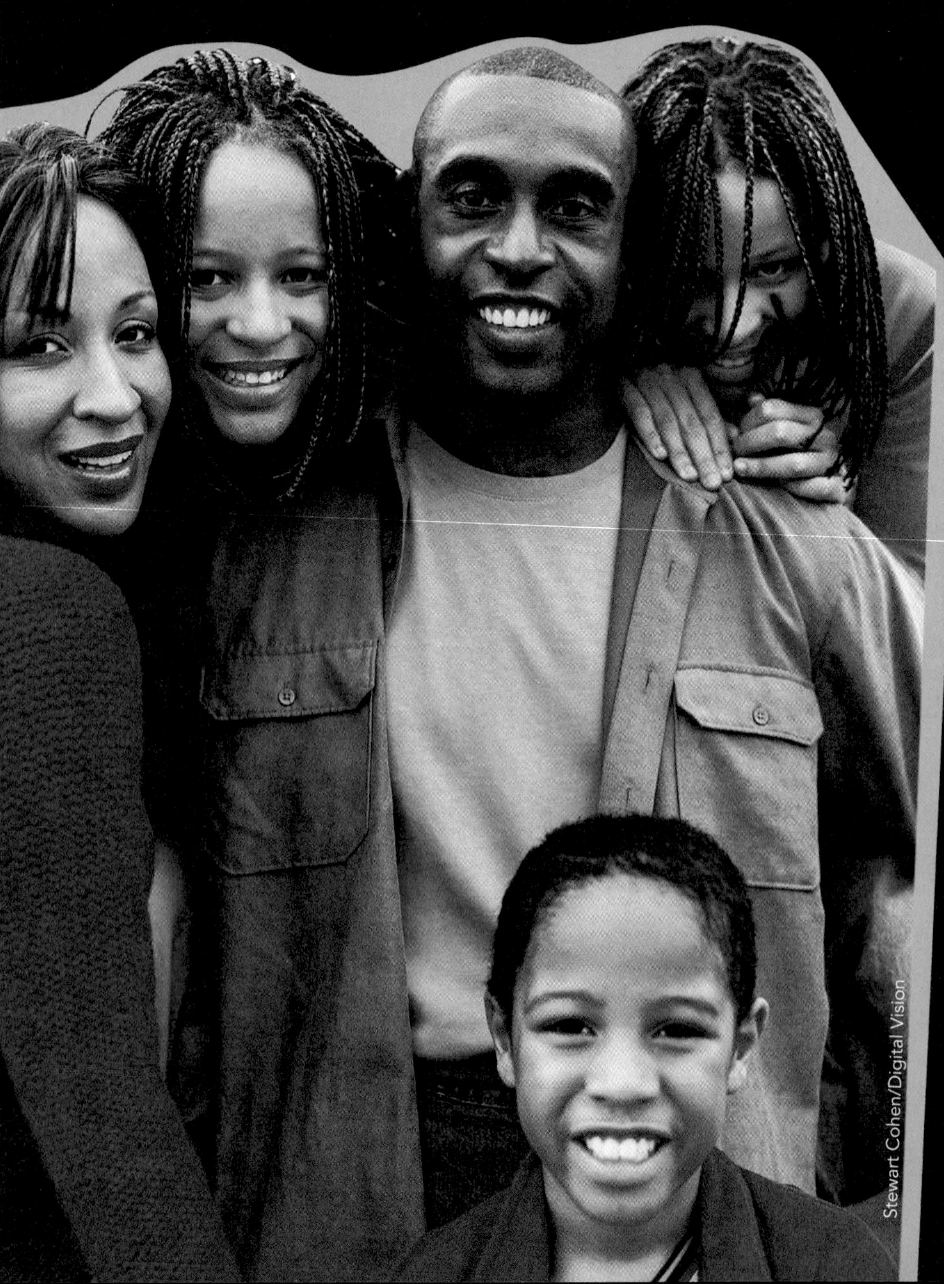
Stewart Cohen/Digital Vision

In This Chapter

Student Web Resources

www.HOPEtextbook.org/student

Lesson 29.1

Family Life and Family Structure

Lesson Objectives

After reading this lesson, you should be able to

1. describe types of family in contemporary society,
2. define gender roles and explain how they have changed over time,
3. explain three factors that contribute to marriage success, and
4. describe the difference between divorce and separation.

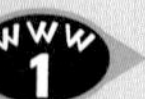

Lesson Vocabulary

blended family, culture, divorce, empty nest, extended family, family role, gender, nuclear family, role model, separation, sex, traditional family

The family has historically been viewed as the most important force in shaping human development. Family offers a place of security and stability for people, each with his or her own roles. In this lesson, various types of families and the roles fulfilled by family members will be described. Marriage, parenting, and family dynamics will be discussed as well.

Family and Family Types

Family is defined in many different ways. One definition is a group of people who are related to each other. Another refers to a group of people living under one roof. Many definitions exist and we'll explore some of them.

The term **nuclear family**, sometimes referred to as a **traditional family**, is commonly defined as a father and mother with children. In this family unit, the mother was often seen as the primary caretaker of the children who stayed at home to care for the household while the father went to work each day. The most recent census indicates that less than half of all households now have both a husband and wife, and not all households have children. Roles have changed over the years for many reasons, one of which is the fact that in many families both parents now work full time outside of the home. This arrangement means that the caretaking of children is often a shared responsibility between parents and others, such as **extended family** members (e.g., grandparents, aunts, uncles), as well as babysitters, day care providers, neighbors, friends, and after-school program providers.

Today more than a quarter of all households have only one person. Also, many households have only two people under the same roof (without children), but those in the household consider themselves to be a family. People in one- or two-person family households are typically part of an extended family, but those other family members do not live under the same roof. These people may include those older in age with grown children, those who have no children, or those who have children who do not live with them.

Families with children now have a variety of different forms, including single-parent, adoptive (i.e., with at least one adopted child), divorced, blended (formed when a parent remarries), and gay and lesbian families. Thus the term *family* has broadened and now refers not only to bloodlines but also to an individual's living and social arrangements, which often consist of more than those people who are related by blood.

Families with children, regardless of type, tend to cycle through four stages of development: beginning, parenting, **empty nest**, and retirement (see figure 29.1). The beginning stage is the time when the newly united couple, or the individual, creates the home and adjusts to the new personal and social status. In this stage, people plan their future and move forward to realize their dreams. The parenting stage begins, of course, with the birth or adoption of the first child and lasts until the youngest child leaves the family home. Today many parents stay in this stage for a longer time than was traditionally the case, since adult children are more often living at home longer or returning home after college.

It is now fairly common for sons and daughters to live at home with parents into their young adulthood.

When the last child leaves home, parents find themselves in the empty nest stage. Traditionally, parents have been middle aged when they arrive at this point. Some parents have difficulty adjusting to this period of their lives, whereas others enjoy their new freedom. In the retirement stage, adults are typically ending their careers and enjoying the freedom of no longer having to be responsible for a job. However, in today's society, more people are continuing to work at an older age, and some even launch second careers. During this stage, a new role as a grandparent is common. Many indicate that being a grandparent has the benefits of a loving bond with grandchildren without the day-to-day responsibilities of parenting.

Whatever family type you find yourself in, a healthy family provides you with love and support. Generally, our first lessons about relating to others come from our family members. Young people tend to model their behavior on the examples they see most often—those of their parents, siblings, and extended family members, who fill similar functions and roles across family types. That is, individuals fulfill child-rearing roles whether they are part of a two-parent family, a single-parent family, a **blended family**, a divorced family, or a gay or lesbian family.

CONNECT

In what ways do you model the behaviors and relationships you see in your family? Do you treat your friends or your dating partner in ways that mirror what you see in your home? Overall, are these influences more positive or more negative?

Family Roles

Most families share similar roles in that they teach family members about love, respect, responsibility, social interaction, communication, and other life skills necessary for living apart from the family, coping with change, and being financially independent. However, roles for each family member vary from family to family. In today's society **family roles** aren't as clear-cut as they may have been for previous generations. There was a time when society expected only the adult male in the household to work each day while the adult female stayed home to take care of the house and children.

Today both adults (in two-parent and blended families) in the household often work outside of the home and share the financial duties, household chores, and child rearing. In single-parent families, of course, one individual is primarily responsible for all aspects of breadwinning, finances, chores,

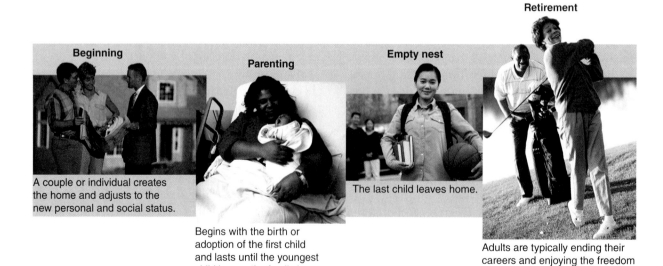

FIGURE 29.1 Four stages of development of families.

and child rearing. Most gay and lesbian families consist of two adults and function in much the same manner as heterosexual two-parent and blended families. Familial roles and responsibilities will continue to evolve in response to changes in economic conditions, in the definition of family roles, and in society more generally.

Role Models

Parents serve as **role models** who impart values and information to their children. Parenting also requires a set of skills that are learned on the job—for example, patience, emotion management, health promotion, disease prevention, time management, and communication. The lessons that a child needs to learn often come through trial and error; therefore, a parent must have plenty of patience to allow the process to happen. Children can be very trying, and parents must know how to keep their frustration and other emotions in check while disciplining with love.

Parents also need to know how to handle various kinds of hurt—whether it be first aid situations, colds, the flu, bruised feelings, or emotional distress—in their children. They must model a healthy lifestyle for their children to emulate. Many of the diseases and illnesses experienced by average Americans result directly from poor lifestyle habits (e.g., poor eating, sleeping, and exercise patterns). Parents are called on to provide their children with the best environment possible and to help them develop the necessary tools for meeting the ever-changing world around them. One of the most important tools parents can give their children is the ability to communicate effectively. Good communication—both within and outside of the family—can go a long way toward preparing family members for a lifetime of success and happiness.

Parents are not the only role models for children. The learning that takes place outside of the home and the classroom is often the most influential in the lives of young people. This is the case due to the constant flow of information received from teachers, friends, peers, and the media. Such sources provide young people with a continuous stream of information that sometimes includes questionable information. This misinformation is often not discussed fully with parents or educators. As a result, the misinformation is often regarded as accurate when it really is not. The importance of good role models outside the family cannot be underestimated.

Gender Roles

Our ideas of what it means to be male or female are structured by the messages—both direct and indirect—that we receive from family, friends, and the media. In considering these messages, it is useful to understand the distinction between sex and gender. **Sex** refers to the biological factors (male or female) that influence your fitness, health, and wellness. The word **gender** has a similar but slightly different meaning. It refers to social and cultural roles of people (masculine or feminine). For example, in the past, some roles were identified as gender appropriate for males only (masculine) or females only (feminine). Generally speaking, males were (traditionally) expected to be independent and physically active, whereas females were traditionally expected to be more social and cooperative. For example, young boys may be encouraged to play sports while young girls may be encouraged to play with dolls. Society

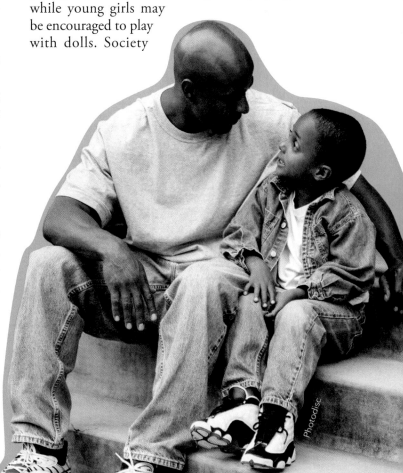

Parents serve as role models who impart values and information to their children.

asserts and reinforces such expectations even before children are born (e.g., blue for baby boys and pink for baby girls). This type of socialization continues for a lifetime. It is, among other things, the basis for the stereotypes that we see in our **culture**.

> "What can you do to promote world peace? Go home and love your family."
>
> —Mother Teresa

Over time, stereotypes have diminished, especially in Western culture. For example, girls and women who often did not have opportunities to participate in sports prior to the 1970s now are regular participants. Activities previously considered appropriate only for males are now considered to be appropriate for both sexes (male and female).

Roles in a family or social group are influenced by gender stereotype. As noted earlier, some roles have traditionally been considered to be masculine (to be fulfilled by males) or feminine (to be fulfilled by females). Some families adhere to strict role expectations, whereas others do not. For example, in some families the man works and the woman stays home. Over time, role expectations have changed, as is the case when parents both work outside the home or the father stays home as the primary care giver. In today's society, men and women can both pursue most any desired career, educational path, or role (whether in a relationship or in society more generally). In other words, we are much less bound by traditional roles than people were in previous generations.

Family Dynamics and Stability

Marriage plays an important role in most cultures around the world. In the United States, it is a legal bond that typically involves permanence and sexual and emotional exclusivity. Marriage provides stability and fulfills many social, emotional, financial, and sexual expectations and needs. According to a study done by the Pew Research Center to determine why people get married, the top three factors are being in love, making a lifelong commitment, and companionship. Ninety-three percent of the people interviewed felt being in love was the number one reason for marriage; 87 percent felt making a lifelong commitment was important while 81 percent felt having a companion was significant. Couples who get married are also more likely to live longer compared to their single counterparts.

HEALTHY COMMUNICATION

How do you feel about traditional gender roles for males and females? Do you seek relationships where traditional gender-specific behaviors are expected? Why or why not? Share your perspective with a friend or classmate. Support your perspective with reasons and facts and be respectful of other opinions.

The term *marriage* was traditionally used to describe only a legal union between a man and a woman, but that is no longer the case. In June 2013, the U.S. Supreme Court declared part of the Defense of Marriage Act (DOMA) unconstitutional, which had defined marriage solely as a legal union between a man and a woman. The Supreme Court ruling declared that same-sex couples who are legally married deserve the same legal rights enjoyed by other married couples under federal law. There are a number of states that are legalizing gay marriage. States that may not yet recognize gay marriage may recognize civil unions or domestic partnerships. Civil unions provide legal recognition to a couple's relationship and provide some legal rights similar to those given to spouses in marriages. Domestic partnerships are broadly defined as a committed relationship between two adults of the same sex.

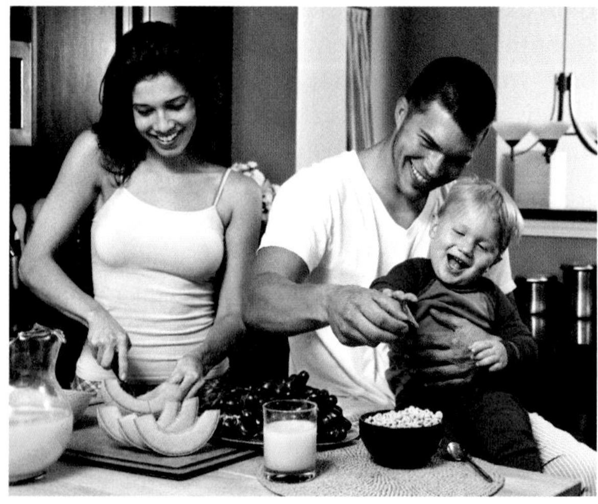

Marriage is a legal bond that provides stability.
iofoto/fotolia.com

HEALTH SCIENCE

According to researchers at Harvard University, individuals who have strong relationships with family, friends, and their community experience happier and healthier lives. Such people live longer and experience fewer health problems. For example, connecting with others reduces the effects of stress and improves the functioning of the coronary artery, digestive, and immune systems. Research also shows that exhibiting caring behavior triggers hormones that reduce stress. This means that when people take action to promote social support and express affection, they bring about life-enhancing effects. This is encouraging news for families, because every day provides an opportunity to engage with other human beings and practice this proven strategy for improving the health of both the caregiver and the receiver.

Marriage success can be attributed to a variety of factors including the age of the individuals; the length of the relationship and the engagement; the presence or absence of shared interests, values, and goals; the attitudes of each individual's parents or guardians toward the marriage partner; and the individuals' views about having and raising children. For more information related to marriage, 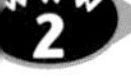 see the student section of the Health Opportunities Through Physical Education website.

Although marriage is a lifetime commitment for some, the expectations associated with marriage may be difficult to maintain, and married couples may go through periods where their happiness alternately diminishes and increases. The highest degrees of happiness are typically found in the beginning stages of the relationship and upon the birth of the first child. Happiness tends to level off as the couple raises adolescents. It increases again as children reach young adulthood and move out, and as the retirement years get closer.

Some couples who experience trouble in their relationship try separation rather than divorce. The most common type of **separation** is a test period that is not legally recognized. In this approach, any shared property or possessions are still co-owned by the couple. Couples may use a separation to assess their relationship and decide whether they want to work at staying together.

Though many marriages last, others end in **divorce**, which is a legal termination of the marriage, wherein the property, the custody and support of any children, and possibly spousal support are negotiated by the divorcing individuals or decided by a judge or court. According to the American Psychological Association, approximately 40 to 50 percent of married U.S. couples divorce, and for people who marry again the divorce rate is even higher. Divorce rates also tend to be higher for younger individuals.

Most people marry with the intention of having a permanent relationship. When divorce happens, it often results from multiple causes, and it differs for each couple. Divorce also goes beyond the termination of the marriage itself; it often has a ripple effect and influences every aspect of a person's life. Divorced individuals often have to establish their individual identity all over again, since changes take place in their financial status, living arrangements, friendships, family relationships, and possibly even work situations. Children are also affected by divorce and may not understand why their parents are divorcing. While children may initially feel fearful of the changes associated with divorce, they can overcome the anxiety and grow up having very positive relationships with both their mother and their father, as well as with a spouse of their own.

Comprehension Check

1. Describe the types of family in contemporary society.
2. Define gender roles and explain how they have changed over time.
3. Explain three factors that contribute to marriage success.
4. Describe the difference between divorce and separation.

SELF-ASSESSMENT: Rate Your Relationships

Think about a family member, friend, or boyfriend or girlfriend you are close to. Select the answer (yes or no) to the following questions. Record your results as directed by your teacher.

1. This person encourages me to try new things.
   a. yes
   b. no
2. This person is supportive of the things I do.
   a. yes
   b. no
3. We have similar common interests and values.
   a. yes
   b. no
4. It is easy to share my feelings (e.g., happy, sad, frustrated, and so on) with this person.
   a. yes
   b. no
5. This person respects me and our relationship.
   a. yes
   b. no
6. This person is not liked very well by my other friends.
   a. yes
   b. no
7. This person gets jealous when I talk with or hang out with other people.
   a. yes
   b. no
8. This person thinks I'm too involved in different activities.
   a. yes
   b. no
9. This person puts me down or criticizes me.
   a. yes
   b. no
10. This person pressures me to do things I don't want to do.
    a. yes
    b. no

Planning for Healthy Living

Use the Healthy Living Plan worksheet to improve your relationship skills.

Lesson 29.2

Relationships

Lesson Objectives

After reading this lesson, you should be able to

1. describe the three main qualities that most people value in their friendships,
2. explain how peer pressure can be both positive and negative,
3. describe the four roles that people may play in a bullying situation, and
4. list at least four healthy dating expectations that you have for yourself.

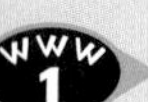

Lesson Vocabulary

assertive behavior, bullying, casual friendship, close friendship, cyberbullying, date rape, dating violence, harassment, manipulation, online dating, peer pressure, platonic friendship, refusal skills, sexual coercion

Humans are social beings; we have an innate desire to belong, feel accepted, and be wanted. In fact, your ability to relate with others often determines how happy and successful you will be throughout your life. More specifically, your ability to give and receive love and support is related to your attainment of a healthy and productive life. Relationships can bring much sorrow—and much joy—to your life. Entering into any relationship demands that we take risks. These risks frequently put us outside of our comfort zone, but without them our growth and development would be stunted. In this lesson, you'll learn about different types of relationships and some of the characteristics that define them.

What Is a Relationship?

Relationships are connections between people. They can be strong and last a lifetime (e.g., a parent–child relationship) or short and superficial (e.g., a relationship with a short-term employer). Relationships can involve romance or be based on friendship. A friendship is likely to be based on shared interests and values. Friends play an important role in helping us grow and mature.

Different people look for different qualities in friends. The most valued qualities are honesty, confidentiality, empathy, and tolerance. Trustworthiness is valued and expected because we want our friends to be fair, sincere, and straightforward. We want to know that we can confide in our friends and not worry that they will disclose information (confidentiality). Empathy is the ability to understand how another person feels; without this trait, it would be difficult for friends to understand one another. Tolerance allows friends to remain friends through adversity. Friends do not always get along, but good friends find a way to work through the rough patches.

Long-standing mature relationships provide an opportunity for mutual caring, openness, disclosure, commitment, trust, and tenderness. As people mature, they have more opportunity and capacity for relationships on many levels.

Safe and Healthy Peer Relationships

As you mature, your peer relationships will take on different aspects. Many young people maintain friendships initiated during their school years, while others focus on new relationships as they enter college or the work force. Friendships also vary in commitment and level of significance, and they are dynamic and may continue to evolve over time. Many people enjoy friends that include both males and females, and interacting with a range of peers can enrich your life and encourage your growth and development beyond young adulthood.

Three basic types of friendship are casual, platonic, and close. **Casual friendship** occurs between individuals who share some commonalities (e.g., classmates or co-workers); it is not characterized by the formation of a deep bond. **Platonic friendship** often involves a member of the opposite sex and is characterized by affection but not romantic involvement. **Close friendship** is punctuated by emotional ties and the sharing of intimate personal information. When problems arise, it is generally to these close friends that we turn for support and guidance.

Regardless of the type, positive friendships are built on shared morals and values and common interests. They are characterized by trust, dependability, predictability, and accountability. Maintaining such a friendship requires work and loyalty. Loyal friends are respectful of each other. They encourage and support one another in both easy and difficult times.

Peer pressure can affect one's decisions and actions including relationships with friends. On the positive side, peer pressure can encourage us to try new things and be better in some way. Our peers can also serve as role models for us to emulate, thus helping us grow. Negative peer pressure, on the other hand, encourages us to make poor decisions and behave badly and thus ultimately leads to negative consequences. People of all ages can be influenced by negative peer pressure, which is often exerted through **manipulation**—indirect pressure to get you to do something inappropriate or harassing. **Harassment** often includes name calling, teasing, or **bullying**.

Resisting Negative Peer Pressure

One way to address negative peer pressure is to try to avoid it. For example, we know that teens with friends that have destructive health habits (e.g., smoking, use of drugs) are more likely to adopt these habits than people with friends who do not have destructive habits. Finding friends with similar values reduces chances for negative peer pressure. Whenever possible, try to develop and maintain friendships with people that you know share your values and interests. Be true to yourself and your beliefs by asserting your goals and values; this may reduce your risk of potentially harmful consequences.

Being assertive and practicing refusal skills can be very helpful in standing up for yourself if needed. **Assertive behavior** involves making a firm verbal statement that lets another person know how you feel. **Refusal skills** are techniques for saying no and sticking with it. The following three steps help you to be assertive and use refusal skills.

1. **State your position.** Demonstrate that you mean no. You can do this both verbally and through nonverbal cues. For example, you might say no and state a reason, or you might say no and raise your hand to signify clearly that you are not interested.

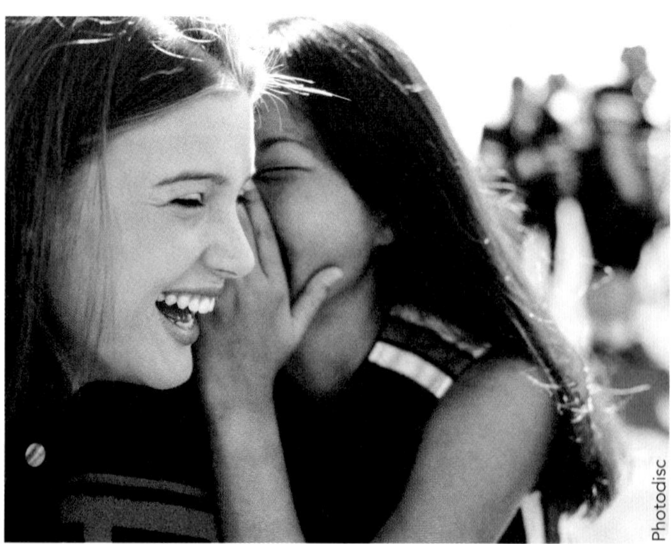

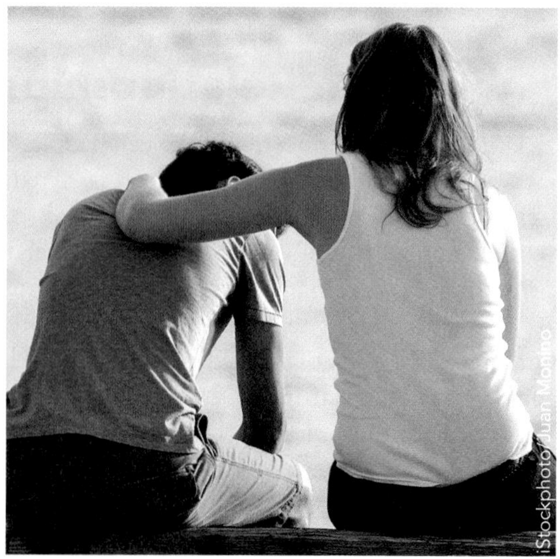

Close friendships are punctuated by emotional ties and the sharing of intimate personal information allowing friends to turn to each other for support and guidance.

2. **Suggest an alternative activity.** If you are being pressured to take part in an activity you are not comfortable with, suggest an alternative. You might also provide reasons for doing so.

3. **Stick with your position.** Stay positive and firm while you make clear that you are not interested in the suggested activity or behavior. Use strong words and body language and look your friend in the eye. If this does not work, remove yourself immediately from the situation. In the best case scenario, your friends will honor your requests. Occasionally, you may have friends who are aggressive and who continue to apply pressure and make you uncomfortable. If your personality tends toward being passive, you may find it difficult to refuse your friends. Assertive behavior takes practice. With practice, you get better at it and it will serve you well throughout your life.

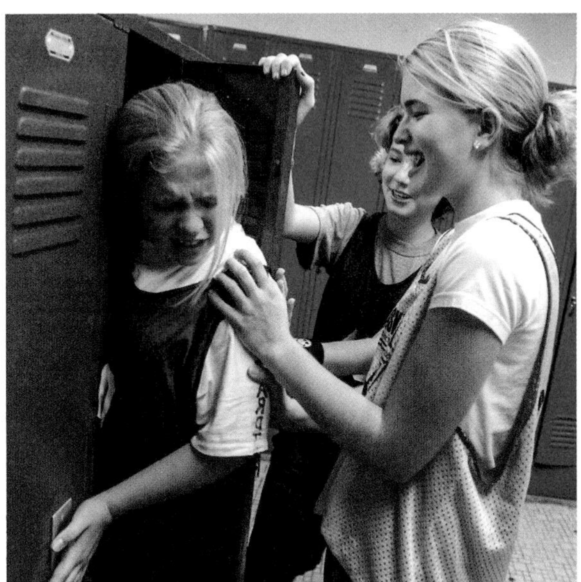

Bullying can take three main forms: verbal, social, or physical.

Bullying

Bullying involves an imbalance of power between a bully and his or her victim. It is the act of repeatedly doing or saying something to intimidate or dominate another person. It might involve making threats, spreading rumors, physically or verbally attacking someone, or purposefully excluding someone from a group. Bullying takes three main forms: (1) verbal, in which someone says or writes mean things; (2) social, which involves hurting someone's reputation or relationships; and (3) physical, which includes hurting a person's body or damaging his or her possessions. Bullying is covered under the federal civil rights laws enforced by the U.S. Department of Education and the U.S. Department of Justice. Punishment varies from a fine or imprisonment of up to one year (or both). If bodily injury results or if an act includes the use, attempted use, or threatened use of a dangerous weapon, punishment can be a fine or imprisonment up to ten years (or both).

Bullying may involve only the bully and the person being bullied, or other people. Other people can play a variety of roles in bullying, including assistant, reinforcer, outsider, and defender. An individual who assists the bully (assistant) does so by encouraging him or her and perhaps even joining in the act of bullying. A person who reinforces the bully's behavior (reinforcer) does so by being part of the audience; this person doesn't participate in the bullying itself but does encourage the bully to continue. An outsider neither encourages the bully's behavior nor defends the individual being bullied. In contrast, a defender helps the person *being* bullied by comforting him or her and perhaps by coming to his or her defense during the bullying incident itself.

Stopping bullying can be a difficult task, since much of it happens subtly and often isn't noticed. Aside from witnessing an incident of bullying, how can you know when there is a problem? Here are some signs that a person may be getting bullied: unexplainable injuries; lost or destroyed clothing, electronics, or other personal items; changes in eating habits, such as coming home from school hungry (because a bully took his or her lunch or lunch money); difficulty with sleeping; decline in grades or desire to go to school; participation in fewer school activities than usual; and self-destructive behaviors (e.g., cutting). There are also signs that a person may be acting as a bully. They include getting into physical or verbal fights; having friends who are bullies; being more aggressive than normal; being sent to the principal's office for being verbally or physically aggressive; having unexplained money or belongings; and blaming others for their actions. The following are some statistics about bullying.

- Approximately one in seven students in grades kindergarten through 12 is either a bully or has been bullied.

- About 56 percent of students have witnessed a bullying crime at school.
- Approximately 71 percent of students report that bullying is an ongoing problem.
- One out of every 10 students drops out or changes schools because of repeated bullying.
- Revenge for bullying is one of the strongest motivations for school shootings.

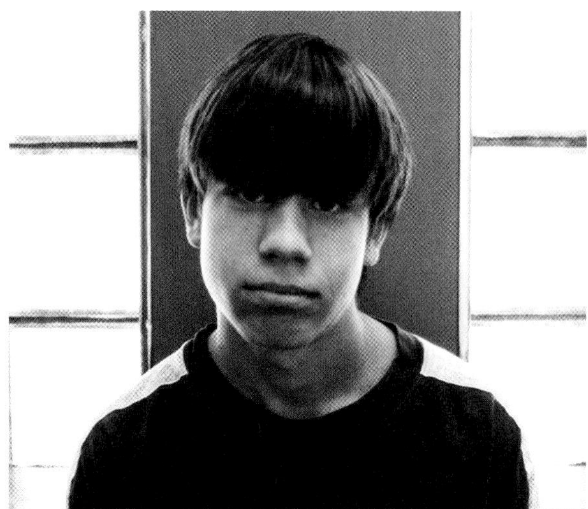

A person who is bullied may not want to go to school—just one of several signs of bullying.
Photodisc

If you are being bullied, try the following tips.

- If you feel safe, talk to the bullying student and tell them in a strong, calm voice to leave you alone.
- Walk away from the bully.
- Tell an adult right away about the incident. While this may feel like you are tattling, adults can't help unless they know it is happening.
- If possible, try to avoid the bully and make sure you have a friend with you. Many bullies are less likely to bully multiple people.

Cyberbullying

Cyberbullying involves electronic technology, such as cell phones, computers, tablets, and social media sites. It can happen 24-7, since messages and images can be posted anonymously and distributed quickly to a large audience at any time. In addition, once a message or image is posted, it can be difficult or impossible to fully remove.

The signs of cyberbullying are much the same as those for bullying in general. The main difference involves the consistency and amount of bullying that can be done via technology. It isn't done just on the school playground, in the lunchroom, or between classes. Rather, it can happen all day and all night long, and many more people can see the bullying when it is posted to a social media website or distributed electronically. Cyberbullying can lead to anxiety, depression, and even suicide due to the ongoing bullying. Students must also realize that what they post online can have lasting consequences when they apply for college or a job. Recruiters will search for people to see the kinds of posts they make as well as the posts that are made about them. Cyberbullies and their parents may also face legal charges for cyberbullying. For more information about cyberbullying, see the student section of the Health Opportunities Through Physical Education website.

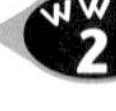

Dating Relationships

Dating can be described as an extension of a friendship. Dating allows students an opportunity to strengthen self-esteem; being liked by a friend encourages people to gain confidence in how they feel about themselves. Dating also helps to improve social skills and assists in students understanding personal needs.

The dynamics of dating relationships are similar to those of a friendship-based relationship, except for the level of intimacy that is shared. In fact, a dating relationship often begins as a friendship, then develops into a relationship that includes another level of intimacy when two people share a physical attraction. Dating relationships are nonmarital—usually exclusive—relationships between two people that may or may not include a sexual relationship.

As a dating relationship becomes more serious, trust becomes more and more important. Trust is established over time and is earned as a result of proven commitment. When this kind of trust is experienced by two individuals who are capable of an emotionally mature and physically satisfying relationship, it can be one of the most gratifying experiences in life. When you enter into any type of relationship, your personal values will be questioned, affirmed, and challenged. You must

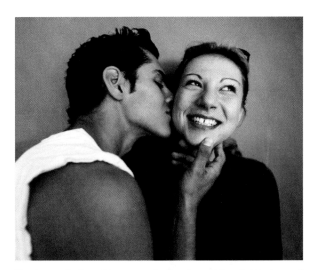

Dating relationships are similar to a friendship-based relationship, except for the level of intimacy that is shared.

Photodisc

consider your own values when making decisions about relationships. If you decide to behave in ways that conflict with your values, you will cause yourself distress and feelings of guilt, shame, and loss of self-respect.

Setting Limits

Dating can be an enjoyable experience; it can give you opportunities to develop your social skills and learn more about yourself. Some people, for example, discover new interests and ways of expressing themselves through dating. At the same time, dating can put you at risk for unwanted peer pressure—for example, pressure to participate in sexual activity or other high-risk activities such as using drugs. It is important to remember that abstinence in both sexual activity and drug use is the only prevention method for not getting pregnant, not getting sexually transmitted infections, and not using and abusing drugs. It is also the only prevention method that works 100 percent of the time. Therefore, before you go on a date, you should determine who else will be present, what time you and your date need to be home, and how you will get from one place to another. Plan for your safety and self-control. First and foremost, avoid places where there will be alcohol or other drugs. Also avoid being alone with a date or in an isolated place.

Parents and other caregivers often set limits on where you can go, who you can go with, and how late you can stay out. In most cases, however, it is ultimately up to you and your date to make the final decisions because your parents or caregivers aren't around. As a responsible individual, you will set your own limits about where you will go and what you will do on dates. Communicating these limits to your date before going out helps you avoid risky and sometimes embarrassing situations.

DIVERSE PERSPECTIVES: Sexual Orientation

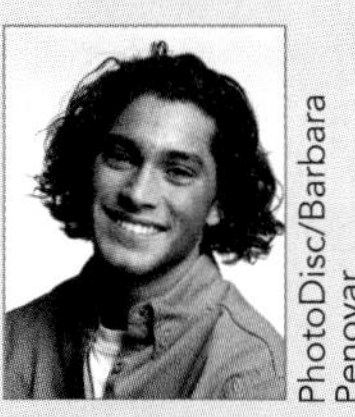

PhotoDisc/Barbara Penoyar

My name is James, and I am gay. I knew I was different from most of my friends early in my life. I remember having a crush on another boy when I was in middle school, and I remember not knowing what to do, what to think, or who to talk to. My family is very traditional and conservative. I was raised in a faith tradition that isn't always very accepting of gays and lesbians, and I am from a small town where everyone seems to know everyone else's business. This made it really difficult.

I came out in high school, and at first most of my family members and friends weren't accepting. I moved out and lived with a friend whose parents were more tolerant. I went through a time of depression and even had a failed suicide attempt after that. Even though society has changed some of its views and I can see role models on popular television shows or among great athletes, I still felt like I didn't belong, or like I wasn't valued. The family I lived with saved my life and gave me a sense of inner strength and self-confidence. They also helped build bridges for me with my own family. I was lucky to have them when I did.

I realized later on that being a gay teenager is harder than being a gay adult. The pressures are greater, and the challenges to fit in and be accepted are just worse at that time in life for everyone. I want my story to be a sign of hope for other teens who may struggle like I did. It gets better.

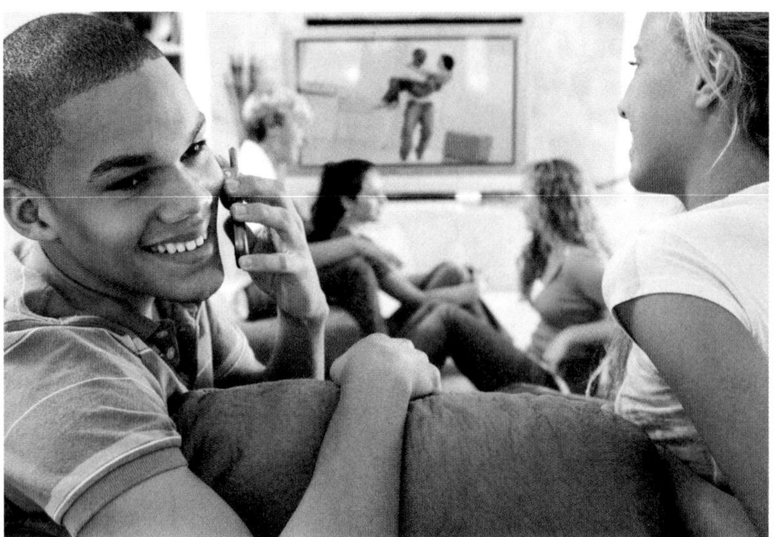

Avoiding being alone with a date is just one limit you could set when dating.

Monkey Business/fotolia.com

Healthy dating begins with your own expectations. Expect to be treated with consideration and respect. Expect that your partner respect your values. Expect that you have the courage—and remember that you have the right—to say no to any activity or behavior for which you are not ready. Remember: no one has the right to force unwanted advances on you. These expectations may seem obvious, but dating can sometimes obscure the obvious.

Satisfying and secure relationships take skill and effort and often share certain identifiable traits. Key traits include trust, predictability, and faith. In fact, trust is punctuated by a sense of predictability, meaning that you can predict your partner's behavior based on the fact that you have witnessed consistent positive behavior from him or her in the past. When your partner demonstrates consistent dependability, you know that you can rely on him or her, particularly when you need support the most. Having faith in your partner allows you to feel that you are certain about his or her intentions and principles. These characteristics—trust, predictability, and faith—are crucial to a satisfying relationship, and can be used as a measuring stick for deciding whether a given relationship is a healthy one.

Teens should also consider dating a variety of people as they begin to date. Too often, teens think that they will be with the first person they date for the rest of their life, which is usually not the case. Dating is one part of the high school experience, whether it is for a one-time trip to the movies or a school dance or lasts for an extended period of time. It should not be an all-consuming experience. The person you date should be supportive of you and the activities you are involved with; should encourage you to be the best person you can; and should hold values and goals similar to yours. Too many teens "fall in love" only to find that the person they are dating does not share their values and goals for their future. Teens need to understand that while breaking up is difficult to do, many of the dating and friendship relationships they have in high school will change, and the qualities they are drawn to in a partner may also change dramatically as they continue to mature.

Breaking Up

When ending a relationship, break up with the person face to face rather than through texting, social media, or e-mail. While breaking up in person may be more difficult to do, it is also more respectful and less hurtful. It may feel easier to hide behind a phone or computer, but it is also much easier to be hurtful through media than it is in person.

In addition, break up with the person sooner rather than later. You cannot change the other person, and thinking that you can will lead only to arguments and hurt feelings. Breaking up is not the time to pick a fight or blame each other; in fact, it is often just time to move on. Finally, before breaking up, make sure of what both you and the other person need—is it time to talk with each other, or is it time for a clean break to get away from each other?

Also, if someone breaks up with you, it is important to respect their decision. While it may be painful, moving on and giving the person the space they request is part of being a mature and responsible person.

Valuing Your Social Health

Dating relationships during the teen years can support healthy growth and development and lead to life-changing experiences. People who enter into such relationships with strong values and morals often fondly remember their first dating relationships. If you can resist the hormone-influenced urges and social pressures that tend to lead people toward high-risk behaviors—including sexual activity and drug and alcohol use—your dating relationships are likely to generate positive feelings of self-respect and self-esteem.

On the other hand, overcoming a bad reputation (whether it is based on real or assumed behaviors) is a difficult task. Teens are often judged not only by their peers but also by their teachers and other adults in the community. Family relationships can also become strained and difficult when parents learn that their children have stepped past the limits they set to protect them. When faced with the question of whether or not to become sexually active or partake in other risky behaviors, think critically, evaluate the risks, and ask yourself, "How will this activity affect my goals for my future?" It is important to remember that remaining abstinent when dating is the only way to ensure that there won't be unintended consequences such as pregnancy and sexually transmitted infections. Your teacher may provide you with more information on this topic.

Dating Violence

Dating violence occurs in the form of various kinds of physical, emotional or psychological, and sexual abuse within a dating relationship, and unfortunately it occurs more often than was once assumed. In fact, adolescents and young adults sometimes misinterpret abusive behavior by a dating partner as a sign of caring. In reality, a dating partner should never disrespect, dominate, or exert force or excessive control over you. Here are some sobering statistics about dating violence from the U.S. Centers for Disease Control and Prevention.

- One-fourth of high school girls have been abused physically or sexually.
- Young women between the ages of 16 and 24 are roughly three times more likely than the rest of the population to be abused by an intimate partner.
- Half of males and females who experience rape or physical or sexual abuse attempt to commit suicide. Rape is any kind of penetration of another person regardless of gender without the victim's consent. **Date rape** is the same as rape except it is committed by a person known to the victim in a dating situation.
- About 1.5 million high school boys and girls report being intentionally hit or physically harmed in the last year by someone with whom they were romantically involved.
- At least half of all violent crimes occur after the offender, the victim, or both have been drinking alcohol.
- In one in three sexual assaults, the offender was intoxicated. Sexual assault is any type of sexual contact or behavior that occurs without the clear consent of the receiver.

Basic signs that a relationship may be headed for trouble include manipulation, put-downs, excessive control over the dating partner's behavior, control over the partner's outside friendships, jealousy and possessiveness, scaring or threatening the partner, and general lack of respect. A healthy relationship should never involve **sexual coercion** (i.e., the unwanted sexual penetration that occurs after a person is pressured in a nonphysical way) or sexual violence (i.e., any sexual act that is committed against someone's will). If you find yourself in a situation characterized by one or more of these factors, seek outside help from parents, teachers, or school counselors. Like all forms of violence, dating violence traumatizes victims and leaves emotional scars. It can also result in unintentional pregnancy and sexually transmitted infections such as HIV. Your teacher may provide you with more information on this topic.

It is also critical to take measures that reduce your risk of experiencing dating violence. Make sure that your dates take place in well-lit public areas. Encourage your date to invite others. Date as part of a group until you know him or her better. Avoid using alcohol and other drugs on dates and immediately remove yourself from any situation involving alcohol or drugs—they increase your risk for violence and trouble. Always tell a parent or guardian who you are with and where you intend to go on your date. Bring a cell phone and some extra money in case you need to get home on your own.

HEALTH TECHNOLOGY

While traditional dating is the best option for many, online dating is an increasingly popular alternative. **Online dating**, also called Internet dating, involves searching for a romantic partner on the Internet. This practice has grown in popularity due to social media sites, including some teen dating sites. As always, you need to be very careful about any information you consider providing and you should talk with a parent or guardian before using an online dating site. Online dating can be very risky. Here are some tips to help keep you safe.

1. **Protect your personal information.** Never give out your real name, address, or phone number online to a person you don't know. Also do not give out other personal information, such as where you go to school or the names of teams or organizations of which you are a part. Choose an online dating name that cannot be linked to your real name.
2. **Read all information available.** Start out slowly by reading all of the profile information about other members along with carefully evaluating the information. Then trust your instincts about what you find. Remember that not everything put on the Internet is the truth. People will exaggerate the truth about themselves as well as lie about who they really are.
3. **Protect your privacy.** Create a new e-mail account that you use only for online dating. Make sure that you sign your e-mail only with your dating name.
4. **Don't be afraid to stop.** If a conversation ever becomes uncomfortable, terminate it and contact the dating site's administrators about it.
5. **Share photo with care.** Use extreme caution if you are asked to share a photo with someone you don't know. Always ask to see a current photo of that person as well and be aware that he or she may send a fake photo.
6. **Use alternate forms of communication.** If you are going to talk on the phone with someone you met online, protect yourself. Do not give out your phone number. Enter *67 before dialing so that the other person won't be able to see your number. Consider using a communication app (e.g., Skype) as a way to avoid using your phone number.
7. **Meet in public.** If you get to the point in your relationship where you want to meet face to face, never allow the person to pick you up at home, school, or work. Schedule a meeting during the day at a public place where there are a lot of people around who could help you if needed; in addition, consider bringing a friend with you to the date. Make sure to tell a friend or family member about your date and give them a phone number, information about the meeting time and place, and a picture of the person you are meeting.

As with any relationship, you need to get to know the person you're talking with before telling too much about yourself. Be cautious about online dating. You never know who may really be at the other end of the computer connection.

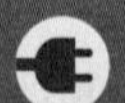

CONNECT

What could be some benefits of online dating? What are some risks of online dating? If you haven't already, do you think you will participate in online dating? Why or why not?

Overcoming Abuse

For those who have suffered abuse or dating violence, it is important to remember that they have not done anything to justify being treated in an abusive way. All forms of abuse are illegal and should be reported to the authorities. Reporting such an incident can be instrumental in preventing further abuse. All U.S. states have laws and policies to facilitate the reporting of abuse, often anonymously. In addition, help for victims of abuse is also offered by health care facilities, educational institutions, and places of worship. Victims should seek out this assistance in order to protect themselves and others from future abuse and to receive emotional and spiritual support. According to the Centers for Disease Control and Prevention, approximately one in five women and one in seven men who experienced rape or physical violence by an intimate partner first experienced some form of partner violence between the ages of 11 and 17.

Abusers also need help; in fact, they are likely to have been victimized in their own past. According to a research study, 35 percent of abusers had also been victims of abuse. Abusers often see violence as a way of life and view it as normal behavior. Support and counseling provided by mental health professionals can help both the abuse victim and the abuser. To prevent and overcome abuse, all individuals need to learn skills for developing and maintaining healthy and safe relationships.

> "You don't develop courage by being happy in your relationships every day. You develop it by surviving difficult times and challenging adversity."
>
> —Epicurus, ancient Greek philosopher

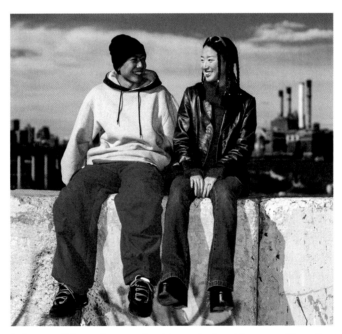

It is possible to have a healthy relationship even if you've been abused.

Photodisc

Comprehension Check

1. Describe the three main qualities that most people tend to value in their friendships.
2. Explain how peer pressure can be both positive and negative.
3. Describe the four roles (other than the bully) that people may play in a bullying situation.
4. List at least four healthy dating expectations that you have for yourself.

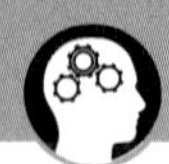

MAKING HEALTHY DECISIONS: Conflict Resolution

Sofia and Ariana have been best friends since third grade. When they began their first year of high school, Sofia began dating Mateo, a senior, and spending less time with Ariana. Mateo convinced Sofia that she should stop playing soccer in order to spend more time with him. He has a reputation for being a partier and getting in trouble at school. Sofia now seems to be spending more and more of her time with Mateo, and when Ariana tries to talk to Sofia at school or on the phone, Mateo pressures Sofia to stop talking. He also seems to dictate to her who she can and cannot talk to, as well as what she can and cannot do.

Ariana decided she would stop by Sofia's house one day after soccer practice to talk with her about Mateo's controlling behavior. As soon as Ariana told Sofia that she didn't think Mateo was good for her and that he was controlling her life, Sofia started yelling at Ariana, and they ended up in a big fight. It has now been over a week since Ariana tried to talk with Sofia about Mateo, and they haven't spoken to each other. In fact, Sofia has begun telling their friends that Ariana is the one trying to control her life.

For Discussion

Using the seven skills for conflict resolution (see the Skills for Healthy Living feature), explain how Ariana could have approached Sofia about her relationship with Mateo in a principled manner rather than being confrontational. How would you rewrite the scenario between Sofia and Ariana using the seven steps of conflict resolution?

SKILLS FOR HEALTHY LIVING: Conflict Resolution

Conflict is a part of life. It happens between friends and family members, as well as with individuals we don't like and may not even know. Although most people don't like conflict and tend to ignore it, others are confrontational. Thus it's important to know how to resolve conflict through constructive engagement, which can produce better outcomes and relationships. You can use conflict resolution skills to settle a disagreement in a responsible way. Conflicts should be resolved through conversation—not violence.

Conflict resolution approaches can be classified into three primary groups: soft, hard, and principled. Soft and hard responses tend to lead to winners and losers rather than resolution. People who approach conflicts with a soft response tend to withdraw or avoid conflict and may even deny that a conflict exists. On the other hand, people who approach conflicts with a hard response tend to be confrontational and aggressive. These individuals have the goal of winning the conflict rather than resolving it through a cooperative resolution. In contrast, people who approach conflicts with a principled response seek a resolution that preserves the relationship and addresses the needs of both parties. Ideally, a person who falls into the soft or hard group will use the following seven skills to become more of a principled responder when handling a conflict.

- **Remain calm.** Be patient and stay in control of your emotions. If you are calm, you are less likely to harm yourself or others.
- **Set a positive tone.** Avoid blaming and shaming, using put-downs, and making threats. Instead, show that you want to be fair as you work together to resolve the conflict.
- **Define the conflict.** Have each person describe the conflict, either in conversation or in writing. Be brief and to the point.
- **Take responsibility for personal actions.** Do not cover up any of your behavior. Apologize if any of your actions were wrong or may have contributed to the conflict.
- **Listen to the needs and feelings of others.** Do not interrupt when another person is speaking. When it is your turn,

use "I" messages (i.e., state your needs and feelings and do not focus on the traits or behaviors of someone else). Show respect.

- **List and evaluate possible solutions.** Identify as many solutions as possible. Then examine each solution to determine whether it is healthful, safe, legal, in accordance with family guidelines and good character, and nonviolent.
- **Agree on a solution.** Select a responsible solution. State what each party will do. Make a written agreement, if necessary. Restate and summarize the agreement to help each person honor it.

These steps give you a healthy way to help resolve conflicts. Realize that not every conflict will require using all seven steps; nor will you always use them in exactly the order in which they are listed here. Each conflict, each situation, is different, as is each individual. The goal is to use conflict resolution skills appropriately in order to contribute to a cooperative resolution for all.

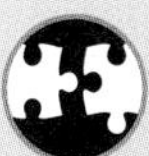

ACADEMIC CONNECTION: Relationships Between Concepts and Terms

Part of meeting the standards for English language arts is the ability to understand the relationships between concepts and terms. In part 2 of this book you have worked with groups of different but related concepts and terms such as bullying, cyberbullying, sexting, sexual coercion, and sexual assault as well as drug addiction, drug dependence, and drug tolerance. Do you understand the differences between these related sets of terms? Are you able to appreciate why they are similar and how they are different? Use the glossary or the study section of the website to look up each term to help you distinguish between them. Can you identify another set of related terms you have learned in this book?

Changing Marriage Patterns

In 1960, 72 percent of U.S. adults aged 18 or older were married. Today that figure is just 51 percent. According to U.S. Census data, the age at which people elect to get married for the first time is also increasing. In 1960, the median age at first marriage was 20.3 for females and 22.8 for males. By 2012, these ages had risen to 26.6 for females and 28.6 for males.

Age at first marriage varies greatly between countries. Compared with other regions of the world, the United States and northwestern Europe are characterized by relatively later ages of first marriage, as well as a larger proportion of the population who remain single and more emphasis on nuclear family rather than extended family.

Traditionally, marriage has served to mark the transition to adulthood and the beginning of a new family. Over the last half century, however, family dynamics have changed, as more young adults have cohabited and delayed marriage. Many young people are now comfortable with delaying marriage until their late 20s or early 30s (see figure 29.2). Today, in fact, only 20 percent of those aged 18 to 29 are married, compared with 59 percent of that same group in 1960.

"There may be some wisdom in waiting," says sociologist Rebecca Johhanson. "The likelihood that a first marriage will break up within 10 years is highest among those individuals who get married under the age of 18 and lowest among those who are married after the age of 25."

On the other hand, "delayed marriage increases the number of years when a nonmarital pregnancy might occur and decreases the likelihood of starting a family," states marriage and family therapist Bill O'Reilly.

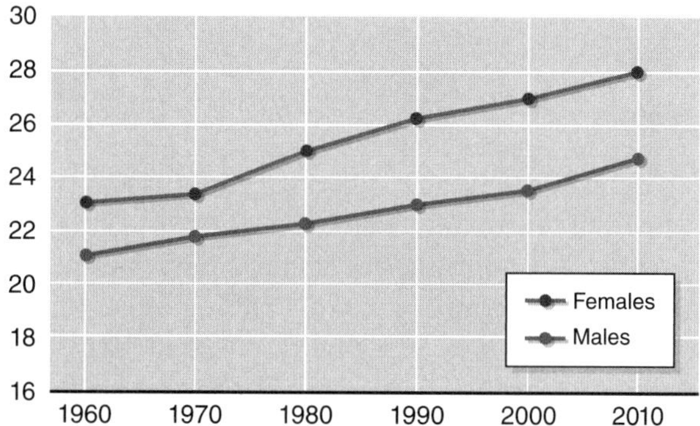

Figure 29.2 Increasing marital age.

For Discussion

Why do you think more young people are waiting longer to get married than in previous generations? What benefits do you see in marrying later? What disadvantages?

Reviewing Concepts and Vocabulary

As directed by your teacher, answer items 1 through 5 by correctly completing each sentence with a word or phrase.

1. A _______ family—consisting of a mother, a father, and at least one child—has been the typical depiction of the American family.
2. ________ refers to the biological factors (male or female) that influence your fitness, health, and wellness.
3. ________ is a set of rules governing behavior in a society. It is influenced by morals, values, and religious beliefs.
4. _________ is a characteristic valued by most people that involves the ability to understand how another person feels.
5. Techniques used to help an individual say no and stick with it are referred to as _______________ skills.

For items 6 through 10, as directed by your teacher, match each term in column 1 with the appropriate phrase in column 2.

Column 1	Column 2
6. manipulation	a. relationship, often with a member of the opposite sex, in which there is no romantic involvement
7. separation	b. social and cultural roles of people
8. gender	c. searching for a romantic partner on the Internet
9. online dating	d. indirect pressure to get you to do something inappropriate
10. platonic friendship	e. test period for couples that is not legally recognized

For items 11 through 15, as directed by your teacher, respond to each statement or question.

11. List and briefly explain the four stages of development that all families tend to cycle through.
12. What is the primary difference between bullying and cyberbullying?
13. Why do you think the divorce rate is higher among people who get married at a younger age?
14. List the factors that predict marriage success.
15. Explain the three steps for using refusal skills.

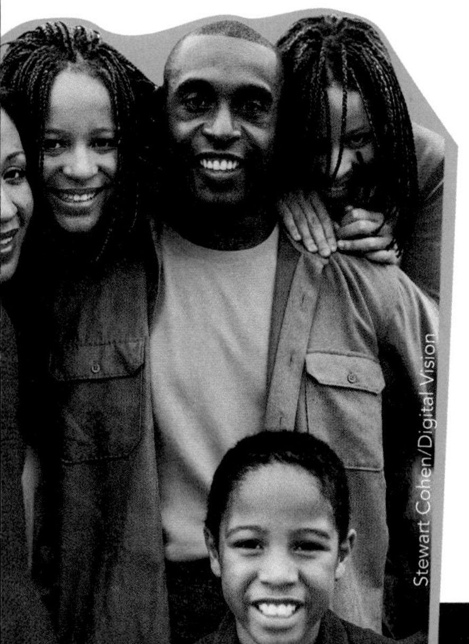
Stewart Cohen/Digital Vision

Thinking Critically

Write a paragraph in response to the following question.

Have you ever really thought about the characteristics that your perfect partner might have? What characteristics do you value the most? List four characteristics and indicate why they are so important to you.

Take It Home

Talk to a parent, guardian, or other trusted adult about online dating. Make a list of the pros and cons of online dating as compared with traditional dating. Discuss any differences in rules or parameters (e.g., appropriate age to start dating) between the two types.

30

Health and Wellness Throughout Life

In This Chapter

LESSON 30.1
Healthy Children and Adolescents

SELF-ASSESSMENT
My Spiritual Wellness

LESSON 30.2
Aging Well

MAKING HEALTHY DECISIONS
Intrinsic Motivation

SKILLS FOR HEALTHY LIVING
Intrinsic Motivation

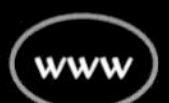

Student Web Resources

www.HOPEtextbook.org/student

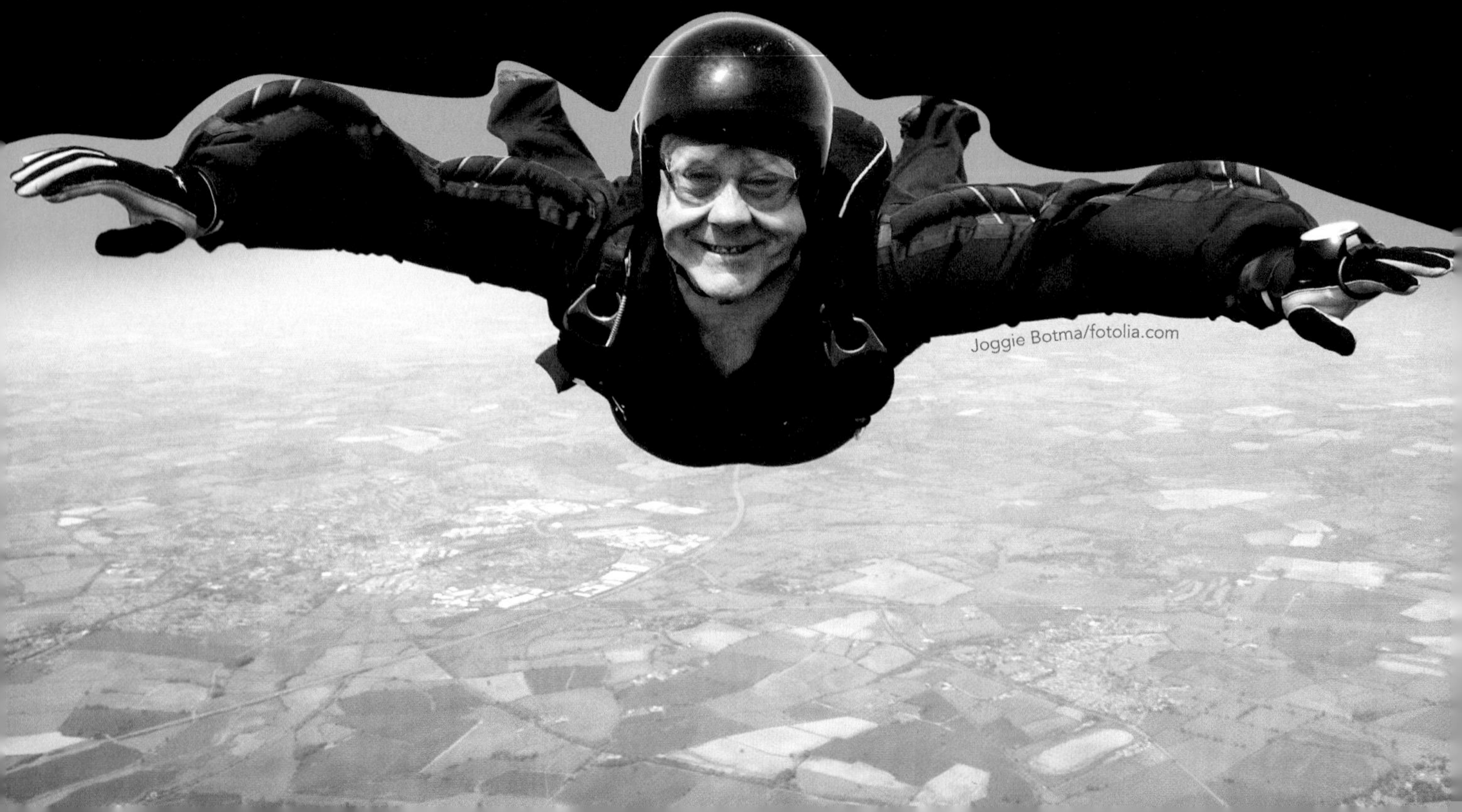

Joggie Botma/fotolia.com

Lesson 30.1

Healthy Children and Adolescents

Lesson Objectives

After reading this lesson, you should be able to

1. identify major developmental milestones in infants and young children,
2. describe puberty and list the secondary sex characteristics of males and females, and
3. identify career options in health and wellness.

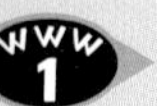

Lesson Vocabulary

abstract thinking, adolescents, cognitive development, developmental milestones, growth spurts, impulse control, physical development, puberty, reasoning skills, secondary sex characteristics, socioemotional development

What do you remember about yourself as a young child? How have you changed over the years? Childhood and adolescence are times of tremendous change. Infants, children, preadolescents, and adolescents all experience rapid—and normal—changes in physical, cognitive, social, and emotional development. Developing fully in each of these areas helps us achieve wellness in all stages of life.

The Life Span

The average adult life span in the United States is 82 years for females and 76 years for males. Over the course of an average life span, a person passes through six developmental phases (see figure 30.1). Each phase is marked by unique factors related to well-being. In infants, children, and adolescents, growth and developmental factors are most prominent as the body and brain reach maturity. During young adulthood and middle adulthood, factors related to maintaining emotional and physical health and managing stress become prominent. The older adult years are often marked by declining physical, emotional, and mental health; challenges to social well-being; and the stress associated with these changes.

Infants and Children

The first two stages of the life span are infancy and childhood. Two of the most obvious markers of **physical development** in infants and children are weight and height. Parents and physicians track changes in weight and height to make sure that the child is properly nourished and healthy. Physical development also involves changes in motor skills (movement abilities) and sensory perceptions. It is particularly rapid during the first two years of life.

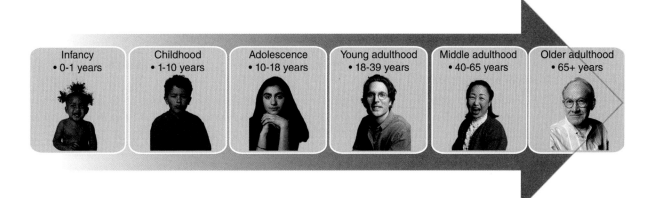

FIGURE 30.1 Stages of the life span.

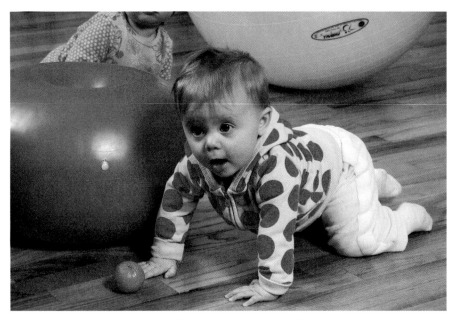

Learning to crawl is just one of many developmental milestones expected in a typically developing infant.

Each physical change brings new abilities and new learning.

Cognitive development is the acquisition and development of skills such as language use, problem solving, and reasoning. Emotional and social development involves expressing feelings about self, others, and things. It also involves relating well to others. Because emotional development and social development are closely related, they are often referred to as **socioemotional development**. Markers of socioemotional growth are self-esteem, empathy, and friendship.

Developmental milestones are the physical and behavioral signs one expects to see in a typically developing infant or child during a period or at a particular age. Table 30.1 presents some of the major physical, cognitive, and socioemotional milestones for infants and young children.

TABLE 30.1 Developmental Milestones for Infants and Young Children

Age	Milestones
0–6 months	Grows rapidly (doubles birth weight), follows objects with eyes, reaches with both hands, places objects in mouth, turns over unassisted, recognizes parents with smile at 2 to 3 months, responds to adult interaction by 6 months.
7–12 months	Triples birth weight, doubles birth length, begins to grow teeth, stands up, crawls and begins to walk unassisted, begins to distinguish strangers, experiments with sounds, develops sense of self, distinguishes between good and bad, begins to attract attention with giggles and shouting, has sense of humor, demonstrates separation anxiety from parents.
1–3 years	Continues to grow and gain weight (at a slower rate), has emerging teeth, runs, climbs, pushes and pulls, can learn taught skills, has fully developed range of emotions, moves from playing alone to having a set of friends, understands friendship, uses short sentences such as "me want cookie."
4–6 years	Continues to grow 2 to 3 inches (5 to 7.5 centimeters) per year; legs lengthen; eats and drinks independently; hops, skips, and throws; has emerging molars and some permanent teeth; generally wants to please others; can follow rules and play in groups; selects own friends; uses a vocabulary of 2,100 words.

Caring for Infants

If you're caring for an infant, talk with his or her parents or guardians for guidance. Make sure you know what to do and what not to do.

Be sure to know

- what to do when the baby cries,
- what to do if you suspect that the baby is sick,
- how to properly put on a diaper,
- how to bathe the baby safely,
- how to give the baby a bottle and burp the baby safely, and
- how to properly pick up and hold the baby.

Do not

- leave the baby alone,
- hit or shake the baby,
- yell or scream at the baby, or
- give the baby any toys or objects that could be swallowed.

Adolescence

The third stage of the life span is called adolescence. **Adolescents** are individuals between the ages of 10 and 19. The period in which the body undergoes sexual development is known as **puberty**. Puberty begins sometime between the ages of 10 and the late teens. Physical changes that occur during puberty include the development of **secondary sex characteristics** (see figure 30.2), and the start of ovulation in girls and sperm production in boys. At this time, the body can undergo rapid **growth spurts**. During this time, bone length increases; this growth can cause aches and pains as well as muscle cramps.

Physical changes can also alter how the body moves and reacts. As a result, it can sometimes feel awkward to do activities and sports that are normally easy or familiar. Both girls and boys may also feel self-conscious about their appearance during this time. Rest assured that it's normal for adolescents to feel self-conscious about changes in body size, shape, and appearance. The physical changes that accompany puberty are normal. They can occur at different times and rates in different people.

Girls are particularly at risk of dropping out of physical activity as they progress through adolescence. At this time they typically have an increase in overall body fat, develop breasts, start menstruating, and undergo changes in body shape. These developments can cause self-consciousness and a perceived drop in skill or ability. Don't let this stop you from being active. While boys are more likely than girls to remain active during the teenage years, activity rates among boys also decline during adolescence. Continuing to be physically active throughout your teenage years helps you practice healthy habits in adulthood. Being physically active also helps prevent weight gain and can improve self-esteem. Be supportive of friends and encourage each other to stay active.

Because growth takes a great deal of energy, both boys and girls experiencing puberty often notice an increase in appetite. Though it's normal to eat more during this time, you should select healthy and nutrient-dense foods that give your body the nourishment it needs.

You also experience cognitive changes during adolescence as parts of your brain change and grow. For one thing, you improve considerably at **abstract thinking**—the ability to consider things that are not visible, immediate, or concrete. You also improve your **reasoning skills**—your ability

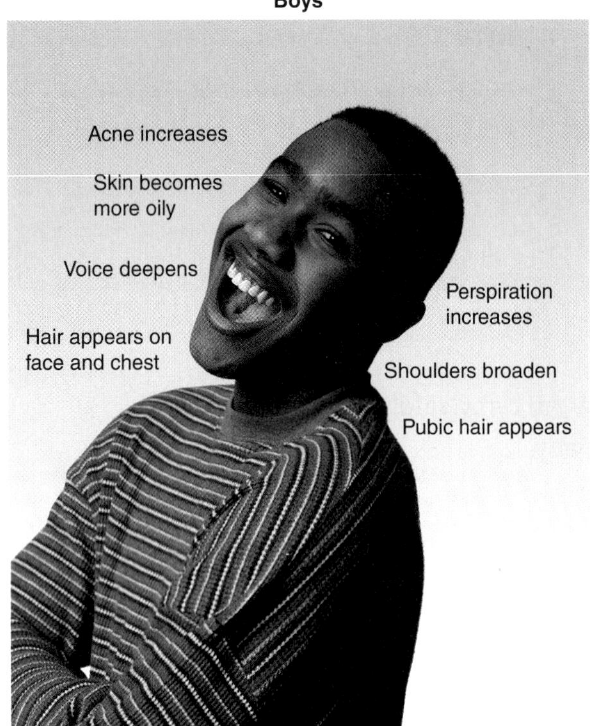

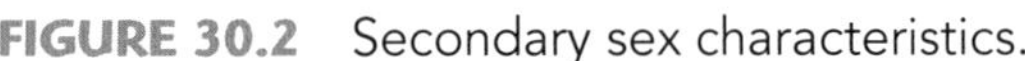

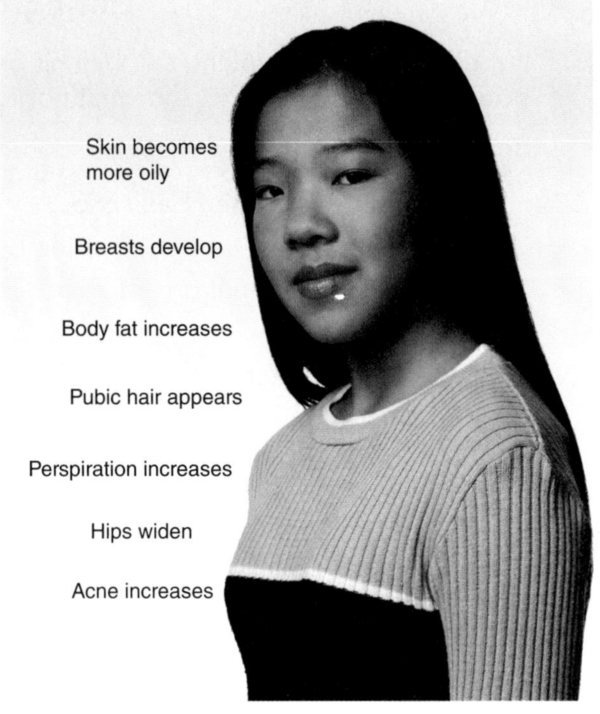

FIGURE 30.2 Secondary sex characteristics.

to solve problems and make decisions. Together, these changes allow you to think more critically and evaluate ideas more carefully. As your brain matures and develops, you may notice improvements in your ability to do math, solve scientific questions, and express complex ideas.

Adolescence can also bring uncertain and changing emotions. Many preteens and teenagers have emotions that at times seem uncontrollable. This emotional uncertainty results in part from an increase in hormones, such as estrogen and testosterone. As a result, despite adolescents' maturing cognitive abilities, they may also have challenges with **impulse control**—the ability to resist making rapid decisions without fully considering the consequences. It's important to think twice about any sudden or rash decisions you are tempted to make. You also need to consider the possible effects on your health and wellness. Examples include driving aggressively, drinking, using drugs, and being violent.

In addition, adolescence is a time of intense self-discovery and searching. This search for identity and self-expression is a normal part of the adolescent experience. You may find yourself seeking meaning and purpose in your life. You may question your values and beliefs as you work to define what's important to you. You may also feel like experimenting with your identity and personality. For example, you might try different clothing and hairstyle choices and other forms of expression. All of this emotional change—along with the physical changes your body is going through—can make your teenage years a turbulent yet exciting time.

CONNECT

What are some of the ways in which you express your individuality? How do your peers influence how you choose to express your individuality? Does peer pressure make it easier or harder to express your individuality as a teenager? Debate your perspective with your peers. Support your position with facts and be respectful of each other's opinions.

> Adolescence represents an inner emotional upheaval, a struggle between the eternal human wish to cling to the past and the equally powerful wish to get on with the future.
>
> —Louise J. Kaplan, psychologist and author

Adolescence is also a stage when you begin to define goals and plans. Deciding on a potential job path or career can be overwhelming and stressful. As you explore your interests, consider the following tips and suggestions:

- **Explore career clusters.** Explore clusters or groups of occupations with common features first. Once you see which clusters appeal to your interests, you can explore specific options in more detail.
- **Take skills and interest assessments.** Taking assessments will help you discover your interests, skills, values, or other traits. You can complete self-assessments in each chapter.
- **Understand needed skills.** Knowing about specific skills that are needed for jobs and careers will help you to make informed decisions when choosing college and job training options.
- **Set goals and stay positive.** Use the skills you have learned in this book to help you set career goals and to stay positive as you work to achieve them.
- **Study career and labor market information.** Spend some time getting to know labor market information. This includes data about occupations, industries, skills, salaries, job openings, and job satisfaction. Updated, local labor market information is a critical part of the puzzle when planning for a career.
- **Don't overlook unique or nontraditional career paths.** Make sure you consider all the options before deciding on a career path. Nontraditional careers, military options, and self-employment are often overlooked.

One example of a career cluster includes jobs related to health and wellness (see table 30.2). Many of these involve working directly with a variety of people in health care settings. Other options (e.g., medical research, laboratory work) are more removed from the general public. You can learn about more career options in health and fitness, as well as in other areas, by visiting the student section of the Health Opportunities Through Physical Education website.

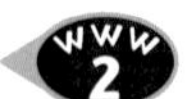

Young Adulthood

The fourth stage of the life span is young adulthood. This is marked by major milestones including beginning a career, college graduation, marriage, and the birth of children. During this time, self-identity is more firmly set. People begin to establish themselves as contributing members of society. You're likely to enjoy good physical health during these years if you follow recommendations for physical activity and nutrition.

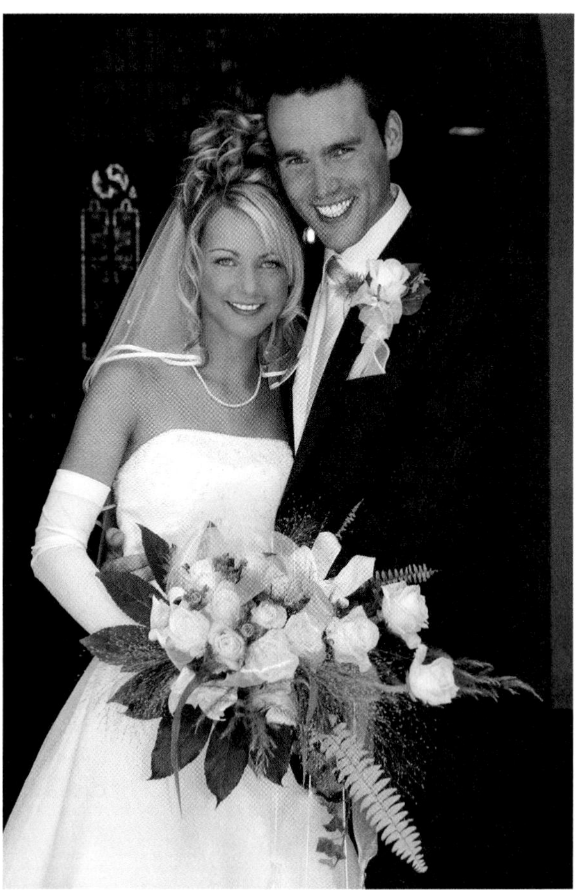

Defining moments for many people during young adulthood include beginning a career, college graduation, marriage, and the birth of children.

Christoph Hohnel - Fotolia

TABLE 30.2 Careers in Health and Wellness

Career	What do they do?	Who do they serve?
Chiropractor	Preserves and restores health through structural manipulation.	The general public and those with chronic pain or illness, typically in a private practice
Dentist	Preserves and restores oral health.	The general public, typically in a private practice
Dietitian PhotoDisc	Uses nutrition to maximize health and aid recovery from illness.	Variable by interest and specialty (e.g., the general public, children, athletes, people in hospital and rehabilitation settings)
Exercise physiologist	Specializes in the role of exercise for prevention and treatment of disease or enhancement of athletic performance.	Variable by interest and specialty (e.g., people with illness or injury, the general public, elite athletes)
Forensic scientist	Applies scientific methods to the investigation of legal problems; may be a doctor, dentist, pathologist, or other health care specialist.	Law enforcement officials, attorneys, crime victims and their families
Health education specialist Monika Adamczyk/fotolia.com	Encourages healthy behaviors through education and health promotion.	Variable by interest and specialty (e.g., schoolchildren, underserved populations, older people, other subgroups); typically in schools, public health offices, or private settings
Laboratory technician	Conducts laboratory tests to aid in the diagnosis and treatment of disease.	The general public at hospitals and medical clinics (e.g., conducting tests); other technicians and professionals in laboratory settings (e.g., analyzing blood work)
Medical researcher	Uses science and experimentation to advance the field of medicine and health care.	Other researchers in a lab; the general public when conducting clinical trials

Career	What do they do?	Who do they serve?
Naturopathic doctor	Focuses on whole-patient wellness through a practice of medicine that blends ancient natural therapies with current medical advances.	The general public (may specialize in children, pregnant women, aging people, other subgroups)
Nurse michaeljung - Fotolia	Provides focused, hands-on, highly personalized care to promote health, prevent disease, and help patients cope with illness.	The general public in hospitals and clinics (may specialize in children, pregnant women, aging people, other subgroups)
Personal trainer iofoto/fotolia.com	Designs and oversees personalized fitness and exercise programs; motivates and monitors improvements in health and fitness.	The general public (may specialize in strength and conditioning for athletes)
Pharmacist	Specializes in medications; dispenses prescription medications and works with doctors to determine proper medications and dosages for patients.	The general public through pharmacies located in a variety of settings
Physical or occupational therapist	Diagnoses and treats injuries and pain; oversees rehabilitation efforts.	The general public (may specialize in children, aging people, athletes, other subgroups) in a variety of settings (e.g., hospitals, private practices)
Physical education teacher	Uses scientific and education programming knowledge to teach physical activity, sport, and exercise and to promote healthy living.	School-aged children, families, and communities

> continued

TABLE 30.2 > continued

Career	What do they do?	Who do they serve?
Physician Photodisc	Diagnoses disease and prescribes treatments; may practice in a specialty (e.g., general medicine, surgery, dermatology).	The general public in settings ranging from private practices to hospitals and clinics
Psychologist or psychiatrist	Provides counseling and sometimes medical care to promote positive mental health; may be a medical doctor.	The general public or those who have mental illness in private practice, hospitals, and clinics
Public health professional	Works with populations of people; conducts research; plans, implements, and evaluates prevention and other health-related programs; oversees health promotion initiatives.	The general public in settings ranging from schools, public health departments, neighborhoods, communities, and even national and international programs
Social worker	Counsels individuals, families, and communities in need and provides a range of assistance and support.	The general public (often people with particular needs, such as children, poor people, and elderly people)
Wellness coach	Provides guidance, motivation, and support for positive behavior changes related to wellness; often holds certain health credentials.	The general public through private practice

However, since major life transitions during these years can be stressful, young adults are more susceptible to sadness and depression than younger or older people. Common sources of stress are financial strain and relationship challenges. If you develop a strong sense of identity and good coping skills now, you'll position yourself to make your early adulthood a positive and productive time.

Comprehension Check

1. Identify three major developmental milestones that occur during the first year of life.
2. List the secondary sex characteristics that develop during puberty for boys and girls.
3. Compare two careers related to health and wellness.

SELF-ASSESSMENT: My Spiritual Wellness

Spiritual wellness plays a significant role in many of life's developmental stages. Whether you are coming to terms with your sense of identity as an adolescent, negotiating with a spouse on how to raise a child as a young adult, or grappling with death and dying in older adulthood, your spirituality will impact your decisions and your overall wellness.

Spiritual wellness depends on many qualities, traits, and actions. Some experts in spiritual health refer to these elements as your "spiritual muscles" because they provide the foundation necessary for developing a strong sense of spiritual wellness. This self-assessment will help you examine your spiritual muscles. Respond to each statement honestly and openly, then calculate your score and evaluate it according to the guidelines at the end of the assessment.

I have a good sense of humor and giggle or laugh often. (humor)

Never	Rarely	Occasionally	Frequently	Always
1	2	3	4	5

I am able to forgive others if they've hurt my feelings or wronged me in some way. (forgiveness)

Never	Rarely	Occasionally	Frequently	Always
1	2	3	4	5

I am a curious person—I ask questions, seek out options and ideas, and am generally interested in learning. (curiosity)

Never	Rarely	Occasionally	Frequently	Always
1	2	3	4	5

I stick to the things I start and am persistent in pursuing my goals. (persistence)

Never	Rarely	Occasionally	Frequently	Always
1	2	3	4	5

I can move forward and make progress even if I feel scared. (courage)

Never	Rarely	Occasionally	Frequently	Always
1	2	3	4	5

I am able to wait for the right time to move forward or to seek acknowledgement for the things I do. (patience)

Never	Rarely	Occasionally	Frequently	Always
1	2	3	4	5

I feel a sense of purpose in my life. (optimism)

Never	Rarely	Occasionally	Frequently	Always
1	2	3	4	5

I have a general belief that things end up well and that there is a purpose for all things. (faith)

Never	Rarely	Occasionally	Frequently	Always
1	2	3	4	5

> continued

> continued

I trust my intuition and listen to my gut. (intuition)

Never	Rarely	Occasionally	Frequently	Always
1	2	3	4	5

I am able to care for someone or something without expecting recognition or reward for my actions. (compassion)

Never	Rarely	Occasionally	Frequently	Always
1	2	3	4	5

I am honest in my daily life and live according to a personal code of conduct. (integrity)

Never	Rarely	Occasionally	Frequently	Always
1	2	3	4	5

I treat others as I would like to be treated and seek to be kind and serve others. (humility)

Never	Rarely	Occasionally	Frequently	Always
1	2	3	4	5

I am imaginative and creative. (creativity)

Never	Rarely	Occasionally	Frequently	Always
1	2	3	4	5

I can love others without conditions and accept them for who they are. (unconditional love)

Never	Rarely	Occasionally	Frequently	Always
1	2	3	4	5

Total your score: _____

If your total score is 56 to 70, your spiritual muscles are strong. Continue seeking ways to cultivate your spirituality. If your total score is 29 to 42, your spiritual muscles are fairly strong, but something is holding you back. Reflect on your responses and identify three areas where you can improve. Write down what you can do to exercise those spiritual muscles more often and set some short- and long-term goals for doing so. If your total score is 14 to 28, your spiritual muscles are not as strong as they could be. Reflect on the list and identify five or more areas where you can improve. Write down what you can do to exercise your spiritual muscles more often and set some short- and long-term goals for doing so.

Planning for Healthy Living

Use the Healthy Living Plan worksheet to focus on developing one or more aspects of your spiritual health.

Lesson 30.2

Aging Well

Lesson Objectives

After reading this lesson, you should be able to

1. identify the benefits of regular physical activity during the aging process,
2. understand how aging affects dietary needs and preferences, and
3. identify common sources of stress for aging individuals.

WWW 1 **Lesson Vocabulary**

activities of daily living, chronological age, physiological age

We're all growing older every day, but aging is a slow process that affects each of us differently. As a result, it is somewhat subjective. Most young people consider anyone who is 10 to 20 years older than themselves to be old, and many people over 60 still think of themselves as young and vital. In reality, decisions you make now can affect the aging process that you'll experience decades from now. For example, eating a balanced diet and doing weight-bearing exercises can help you develop strong bones that protect you from osteoporosis later in life and keep you safe if you fall or have a traumatic accident.

Conversely, if you choose, for example, to start smoking at a young age, you can accelerate the aging process of your skin and organs, making you look and feel older. You can also begin a slow process of damaging your lungs in a way that results in cancer 20 years down the road.

This lesson explores some of the ways in which aging is affected by healthy lifestyles choices and how the aging process affects healthy lifestyle recommendations.

Middle and Older Adulthood

The fifth and sixth stages of the life span are middle and older adulthood. At these stages, it is important to maintain emotional and physical health. Managing stress is also an important factor at this age, too. Adults have more care and support responsibilities for themselves, children not quite on their own, or parents in older generations. There can be changes in oneself with new career and personal goals or in a relationship with children moving out of the

DIVERSE PERSPECTIVES: Being an Older Parent

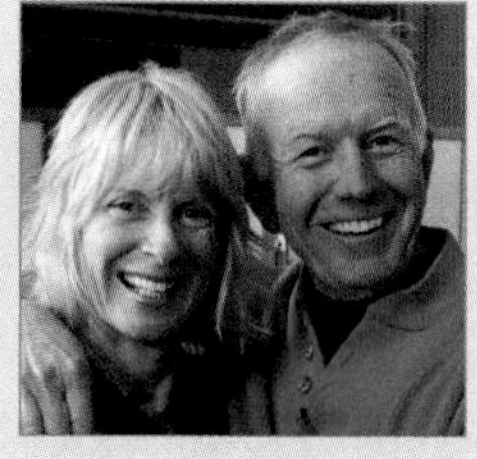

Our names are Madeline and Steve. We are both almost 60, and we have a son in high school and a daughter in junior high school. We met at work when we were both in our 30s and got married at almost age 40. Both of us wanted children earlier in life but had been committed to our careers; we also wanted to spend the first few years of our marriage traveling.

Having children in our mid-40s was difficult physically—we didn't have as much energy as we'd once had. But we've both noticed that we don't seem to get as stressed out about parenting as younger parents do, and we're financially more secure than a lot of younger parents. Our kids are great, but I know they think we aren't as cool as some of their friends' parents. When the kids were younger we often felt uncomfortable around much younger parents as well. We know it embarrasses our kids when strangers say, "Are these your grandparents?" That's probably one of the hardest parts.

house. As for physiological changes, some people start getting back or joint pain, wrinkles, or vision loss. Women experience menopause at this time, too. Although there can be many changes at these stages, people generally feel more established.

Physical Activity and Aging

Regular physical activity is beneficial to people of every age. A person is never too old to participate in some sort of physical activity. Still, as people move through the middle-age years and into the senior years, the habits they developed in their teens and young adulthood have a considerable effect. Regular physical activity has been shown to delay the onset of most chronic diseases, reduce adult weight gain, improve mood, and delay disease- and illness-related death (see figure 30.3). Regular exercise has also been shown to help reduce the risk of dementia—the leading cause of disability among people over 80.

Just as important, when older people engage in physical activity and exercise, they retain a higher level of fitness and are generally more mobile. As a result, they are better able to manage **activities of daily living**, such as bathing, preparing food, eating, and dressing. This ability allows them to remain independent, productive citizens for longer periods of time. Active older adults can also play more with their grandchildren and great-grandchildren, travel more often and more easily, participate in more leisure activities, and remain more socially engaged and connected to their communities. Physical activity and exercise recommendations for older adults are presented in figure 30.4. In short, being active throughout your life is one of the most important things you can do to ensure wellness as you age.

Nutrition and Aging

Eating well throughout your life also plays a critical role in how well you will remain as you age. Overall, people's nutritional needs are similar at all ages. All teens, adults, and older adults should eat a balanced diet of nutritionally dense foods. They should all minimize intake of saturated fat and sodium, eat plenty of fiber and foods rich in antioxidants, and limit their intake of alcohol.

Some differences, however, do exist. For example, most adults require fewer daily calories as they age because of decreased metabolic rate. After the age of 19, the recommended daily calories decrease by 10 per year for men and by 7 per year for women. As a result, by the time a person reaches age 70, daily need is about 350 to 500 calories lower than it was at age 20. But if a person remains physically active throughout life, and therefore loses less muscle, his caloric need will be a bit higher than that of a sedentary person.

Though caloric need may drop with age, some nutrient needs may increase—for example, calcium and vitamins B_6, B_{12}, C, and D. As a result, older people need to eat high-quality, nutrient-dense

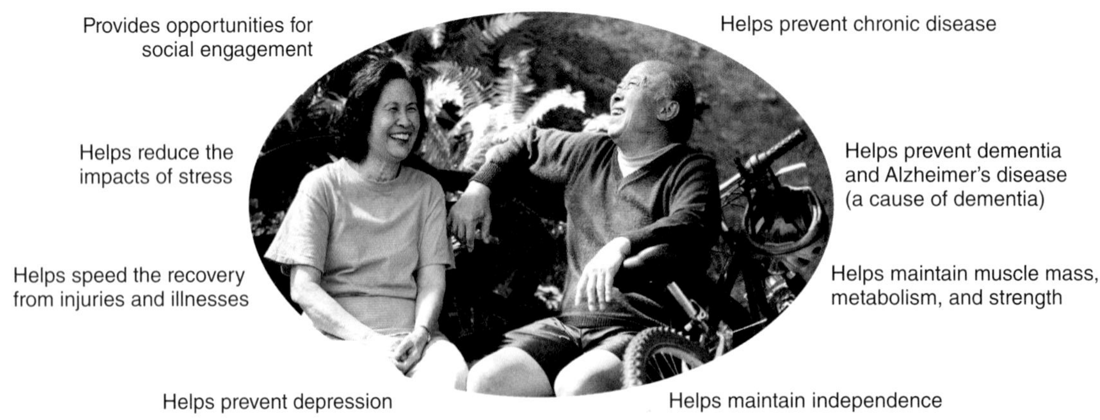
Provides opportunities for social engagement
Helps prevent chronic disease
Helps reduce the impacts of stress
Helps prevent dementia and Alzheimer's disease (a cause of dementia)
Helps speed the recovery from injuries and illnesses
Helps maintain muscle mass, metabolism, and strength
Helps prevent depression
Helps maintain independence

FIGURE 30.3 The benefits of physical activity for older adults. Some of these could apply to middle adulthood, too.

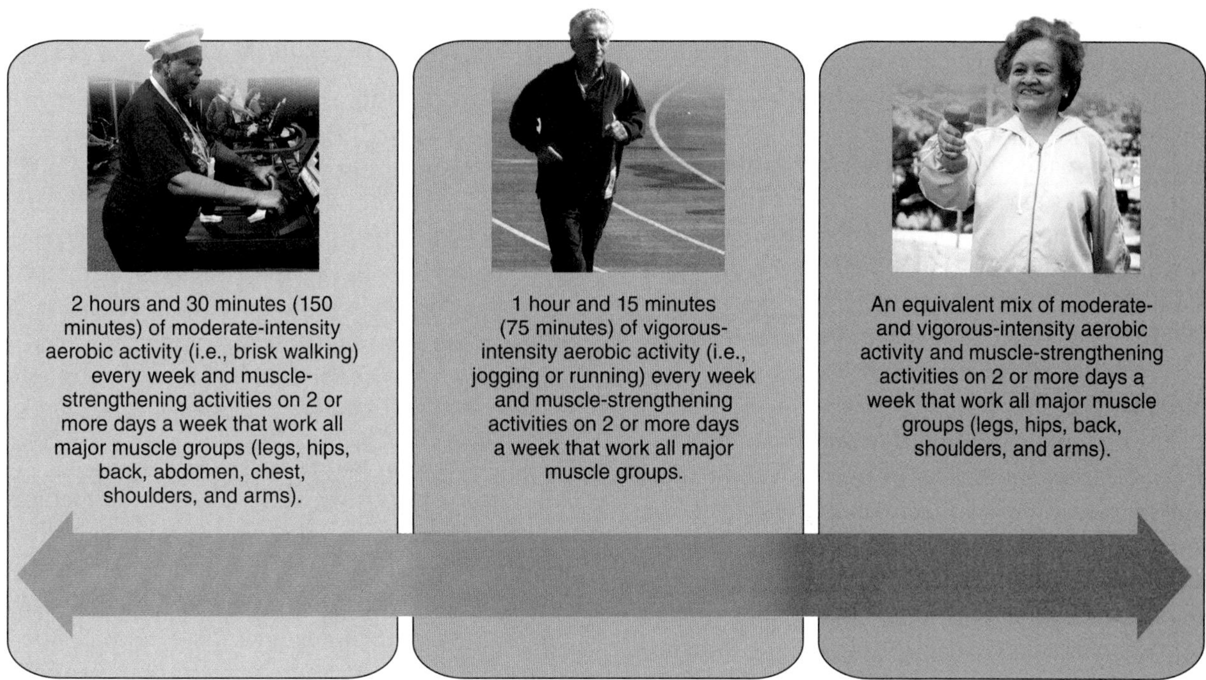

FIGURE 30.4 Physical activity and exercise recommendations for middle-aged and older adults: three options.

foods. Dietary needs and nutrition status can also be affected by many diseases and health conditions. In addition, an aging person's ability to get proper nutrition can be hindered by poverty or economic struggle, tooth loss, certain medications, lack of social support, and loss of independence.

What Does It Mean to Grow Old?

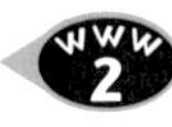

In 2011, a Londoner named Fauja Singh completed his seventh marathon at the age of 100; he had run his first at the age of 89. We often think of aging as

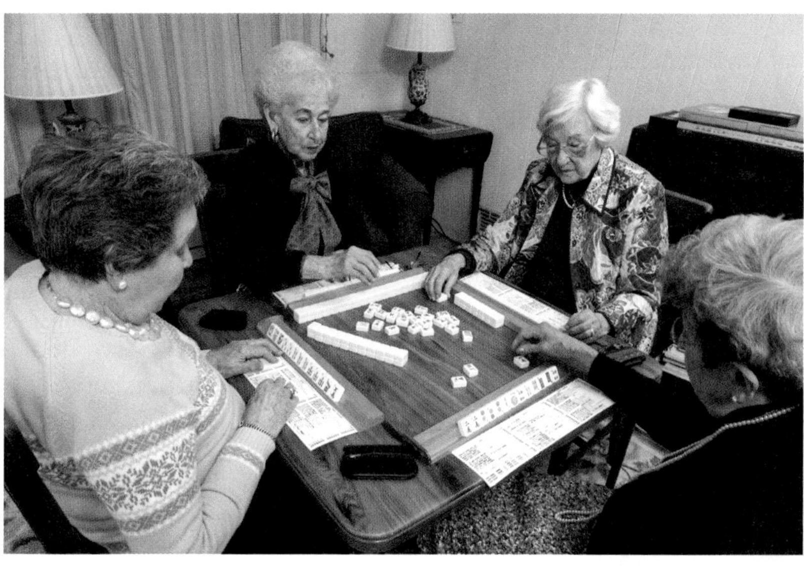

Most adults require fewer daily calories as they age because of decreased metabolic rate.

robert lerich/fotolia.com

a process of becoming weaker and frailer. However, people like Fauja Singh have demonstrated that the fact of aging itself is not nearly as important as how we choose to age. Research shows that the lifestyle choices we make throughout life affect our health and wellness more strongly than our **chronological age** (numeric age) does. This is particularly true as we move through midlife and into older ages. Maintaining a healthy lifestyle can keep your **physiological age**—the effective age of your body based on its ability to function well—lower than your chronological age.

Throughout part 2 of this book, you're reading about various aspects of health and wellness and considering what affects your health in all the components of wellness. As you continue through life and eventually enter old age, making healthy lifestyle choices is critical to your ability to stay healthy, maintain your independence, and enhance your quality of life.

Stresses of Aging

Albert is a retired military officer who lost his wife two years ago. He has no children and was an only child. Albert has arthritis and takes several medications for heart and blood pressure problems. When his wife, Patricia, was alive, she picked up his medications, helped with meal preparation, and managed some of the household tasks. As a result, Albert rarely felt uneasy or alone. Now, without her help, Albert now finds himself struggling. He doesn't have money to hire help and he has to ask neighbors to pick up his medications. He stresses for days about whom to ask and hates to inconvenience his busy, younger neighbors. His pain is sometimes so bad that he struggles to prepare his meals, and he feels he has no one to turn to. Figuring out what to eat and getting groceries are also sources of stress.

Stress is a part of all stages of life. In Albert's younger years, he might have felt stress mostly in relation to his military job. As an older adult, his stress relates largely to managing his pain and living in daily isolation. Understanding stressors and managing stress effectively are part of a lifelong process that can greatly affect how well we age.

Older adults do experience some common, and sometimes unfamiliar, stressors (see figure 30.5). However, many studies have shown that older adults report less stress overall. It's possible that older adults have the same degree of stressful situations but have learned to deal with stress better and become more resilient over time. The wisdom that comes with age can help a person put common stressors in perspective. An older adult who has managed difficult times in the past may not seem as bothered by stressful experiences in older age.

HEALTHY COMMUNICATION

How are older adults portrayed in the media? Do you think media stereotypes influence your perceptions of older adults? What experiences do you have with older adults? How do you think those experiences influence your views of aging? Share your perspectives with a friend or classmate. Use facts to support your position, and be respectful of each other's perspectives.

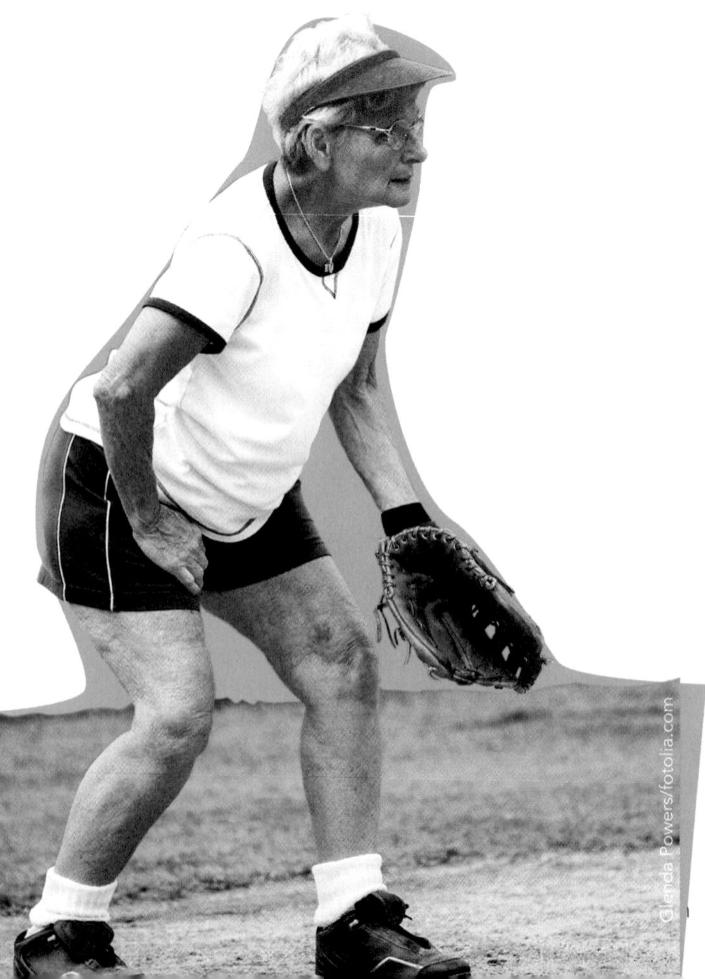

Lifestyle choices we make throughout life affect our health and wellness more strongly than our chronological age does.

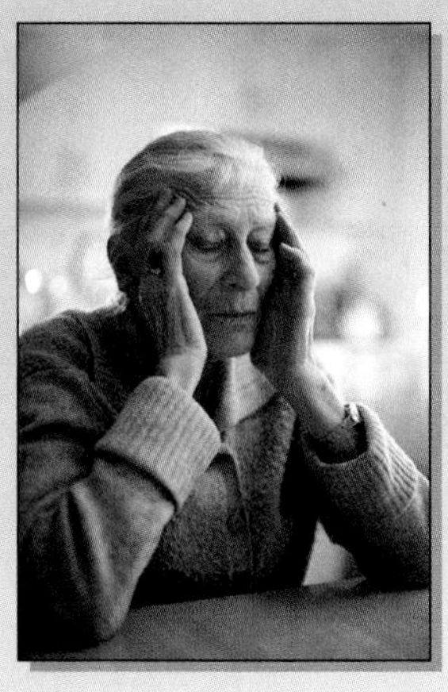

Death of spouse or lifelong friends

Financial strains

Health issues and problems

Depression and social isolation

Fear of loss of memories and concentration

Pain and discomfort from illness or treatments

Loss of independence

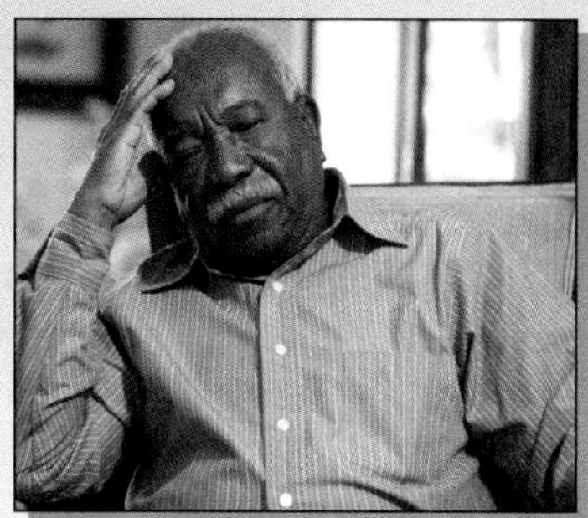

FIGURE 30.5 Common causes of stress in older adults.

Learning to cope with stress in the earlier stages of life—and doing so throughout life—not only helps you slow down the aging process and reduce your risk of disease, but it can also help you be more resilient later in life.

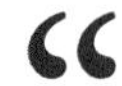

I think that age as a number is not nearly as important as health. You can be in poor health and be pretty miserable at 40 or 50. If you're in good health, you can enjoy things into your 80s. ”

—Bob Barker, entertainer

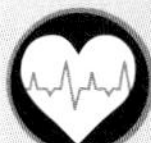

HEALTH TECHNOLOGY

Homes that can respond to the environment on their own used to be a futuristic idea, but that is changing. Now technologies make living at home possible for more people who are dealing with disability or age-related changes. For example, in-home monitoring systems help caregivers and health care workers see and talk with people even if they're not nearby. They can conduct basic physical exams, track medication use, and monitor vital signs from a distance.

In addition, computer technology now allows a person to control the home's temperature, lighting, security, and electronics using voice commands or applications without needing to get up. Devices such as lighting and temperature sensors and controls can even be programmed to make adjustments as a person moves around in the home. And voice commands or remote controls can fill a bathtub with water, raise a toilet seat, or turn on a faucet.

Soon, the integration of global positioning system (GPS) technology will create even more options. For example, smart home controls could notify someone when public transportation (e.g., a bus) is approaching the house. As new technologies are integrated into home living, the possibilities will continue to grow for people to remain independent and age comfortably and safely within their own homes.

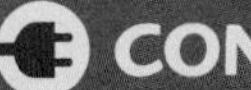

CONNECT

How do you think technology will affect the way you live in the future? Do you think technology will help you live a longer and better life? Why or why not?

HEALTH SCIENCE

Studies show that pet owners are more likely than other people to live longer and to recover from major health events, such as heart attacks. Research has also shown that interaction with animals can lower blood pressure and reduce feelings of anxiety and stress. Incorporating animals into the care of people with disease, disability, or aging-related impairment is referred to as animal-assisted intervention (AAI). A variety of populations have benefited, including elderly people, cancer and cardiac patients, those with autism, and people with anxiety or social disorders.

Some animals are used specifically for therapeutic purposes and can help patients relax and engage more fully in therapy. Animals can also provide direct assistance, as in the case of dogs that help people with vision impairments. Service dogs can also directly assist people by opening doors and cabinets or retrieving items such as phones or clothing. Many types of animals—including cats, fish, and birds—can provide companionship to aging people whose circumstances limit their interactions with people. Regardless of whether the animal is a beloved family pet or a working therapy dog, they provide unconditional love and a steady presence that can benefit the health of their human companions.

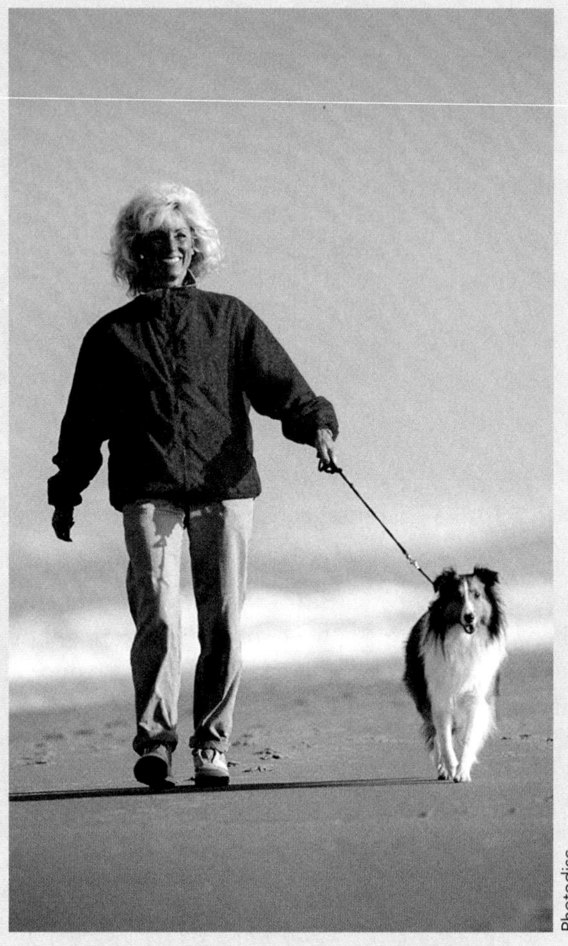

Photodisc

Comprehension Check

1. What are the benefits of physical activity in older adults?
2. What is one physical change that occurs with aging that might influence a person's diet or eating habits?
3. What are five common stressors that older adults may encounter?

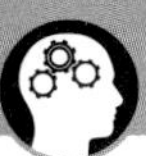

MAKING HEALTHY DECISIONS: Intrinsic Motivation

Damon is a high school senior who loves to win. Recently, his school sponsored a Walk the Globe challenge, and Damon was excited to participate. The walk raised money for Alzheimer's disease research. He thought it might help him get in shape, and he also had his heart set on winning the grand prize—a new iPad. The idea of the challenge, sponsored by the school's wellness club, was to see who could walk enough steps to make it "around the world" the fastest.

Damon was one of the first students to register and pick up his pedometer and walking chart. Every time you saw Damon, in school or around the neighborhood, he was walking and bragging about how he was going to win the prize. He seemed highly motivated, and he even lost a few pounds and gained a little more energy. As it turned out, he finished in second place and won a free water bottle. Despite his strong result, Damon stopped walking and actually seemed to sulk a little. Other students were surprised because he had seemed so motivated during the contest.

For Discussion

Does Damon seem to be intrinsically or extrinsically motivated? How can you tell? (To learn about these kinds of motivation, see the Skills for Healthy Living feature.) What are some things that Damon could do to become more intrinsically motivated? How might the campus wellness club help students build intrinsic motivation when they put together their next campus challenge?

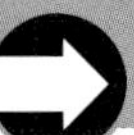

SKILLS FOR HEALTHY LIVING: Intrinsic Motivation

Intrinsic motivation involves doing something not because it brings recognition or reward but because you enjoy it or value it. For example, people who participate in healthy activities (e.g., exercise, healthy eating) for intrinsic reasons do so because they value the health benefits and enjoy the active lifestyle.

Extrinsic motivation, on the other hand, refers to doing something to get an external reward or avoid a punishment. Extrinsic motivation can sometimes motivate someone to begin a healthy behavior or avoid an unhealthy behavior, but it eventually fades away when the reward is achieved or is no longer valued.

As a result, change in health behaviors depends on intrinsic motivation. Here are some tips to help you develop your intrinsic motivation:

- **Learn and understand the benefits of healthy behaviors.** Knowledge can be a factor in developing internal reasons for choosing to live a healthy lifestyle.
- **Appreciate the effects of healthy living over your life span.** Talk to people who are older than you and are healthy and energetic. Compare them with others who are unhealthy. Think about how you would like to be in 5, 10, 20, or 30 years. Use that vision to motivate your choices now.
- **Give yourself credit for trying.** Sometimes the greatest reward comes from doing something challenging, even if you don't fully succeed. Commend yourself for having courage, persevering, and keeping a positive attitude. Believing that success is all or nothing is a quick way to undermine your own intrinsic motivation.
- **Set achievable goals, not just aspirations.** It's okay to dream big and hope for great things. Set small, realistic goals for yourself. Doing so can help you reach your dreams and build your intrinsic motivation in the process.
- **Find friends who share your value of healthy living.** When people share a value or appreciation for something, they find joy in the process of doing it together.
- **Stick with positive self-talk.** Avoid cutting yourself down or punishing yourself if you don't succeed at a goal. Remind yourself that you can and will do better the next time you try.

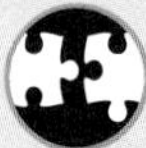

ACADEMIC CONNECTION: The Metric System

In the United States we typically express measurements in what are called U.S. customary units. However, most of the rest of the world and much of the scientific community use the metric system. Metric is a system of measurement that has three main units: the meter (m) for length, the gram (g) for weight, and the second (s) for time. Each of these main measures is then expressed as larger or smaller units based on a standard prefix (see table). For example, a kilogram is the same as 1,000 grams, and a centimeter is the same as one hundredth (1/100) of a meter. If a man's height is 200 centimeters, how many meters tall is he? If a woman's weight is 60,000 grams, how many kilograms does she weigh?

Common Big and Small Numbers

Name	Number	Prefix	Symbol
trillion	1,000,000,000,000	tera	T
billion	1,000,000,000	giga	G
million	1,000,000	mega	M
thousand	1,000	kilo	k
hundred	100	hecto	h
ten	10	deka	da
Unit	**1**		
tenth	0.1	deci	d
hundredth	0.01	centi	c
thousandth	0.001	milli	m
millionth	0.000 001	micro	μ
billionth	0.000 000 001	nano	n
trillionth	0.000 000 000 001	pico	p

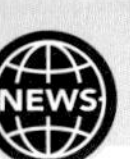

Does a High-Carbohydrate Diet Contribute to Mild Cognitive Impairment?

Most adults have considered the possibility of dying from heart disease or cancer. We're all familiar with the fact that these diseases are among the most common causes of death. At the same time, Alzheimer's disease is contributing to more deaths each year (see figure 30.6). In fact, Alzheimer's affects 5.2 million adults in the United States, and that number is expected to triple by 2050. While we know that eating a diet lower in saturated fat may help us hold off heart disease or cancer, what do we know about how diet affects the risk of Alzheimer's?

Seeking to answer this question, Mayo Clinic researchers tracked the eating habits of 1,230 people between the ages of 70 and 89 for one year. Next, the 940 people who showed no sign of cognitive impairment were asked to return for a 15-month follow-up. By the study's fourth year, 200 of those 940 people were beginning to show mild cognitive impairment (MCI), which can include problems with memory, language, thinking, and judgment.

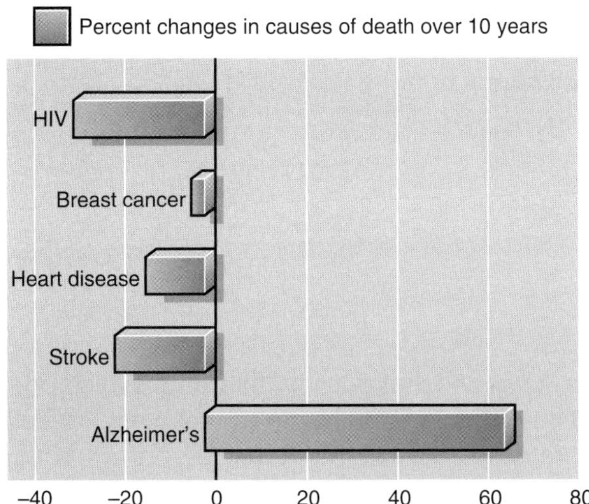

Figure 30.6 Recent changes in death rates. Alzheimer's has greatly increased while the others have decreased.

People with the highest carbohydrate intake were nearly twice as likely to develop MCI as people who ate a balanced diet.

"Not everyone with MCI goes on to develop Alzheimer's disease, but many do," says Professor Rosebud Roberts, a researcher in Mayo's epidemiology division in Rochester, Minnesota. "A high-carbohydrate intake could be bad for you because carbohydrates impact your glucose and insulin metabolism."

Since sugar fuels the brain, a moderate amount is essential. However, high levels of sugar may actually interfere with the brain's ability to use the sugar for fuel. Roberts says high glucose levels might affect the brain's blood vessels and also play a role in the development of plaques in the brain that interfere with normal neural functioning. "Those proteins are toxic to brain health and are found in the brains of people with Alzheimer's," states Roberts.

The study found that people whose diets had the highest intake of protein (e.g., from chicken, meat, or fish) reduced their risk of cognitive impairment by 21 percent. Those whose diets were highest in fat (e.g., from nuts or healthy oils) were 42 percent less likely to have cognitive impairment. However, Janet DeMarzo, a medical doctor with the American Cancer Society, warns that "while these results show the benefits of a high-fat diet for the prevention of cognitive impairment, the same diet proves to increase the risk of cancer and heart disease."

For Discussion

Do you think older adults at risk for Alzheimer's disease should eat a high-fat diet, which might reduce the chance of cognitive impairment but increase the risk of cancer and cardiovascular disease? Why or why not?

Reviewing Concepts and Vocabulary

As directed by your teacher, answer items 1 through 5 by correctly completing each sentence with a word or phrase.

1. Changes in motor skills, perception, and hearing are a normal part of ______________ development.
2. The acquisition and development of skills such as language, problem solving, and reasoning are part of __________________ development.
3. Periods of relatively rapid growth called _________ _________ can cause aches and pains as well as muscle cramps.
4. Bathing, preparing food, eating, and dressing are examples of __________________ __________________ __________________ __________________.
5. Regular exercise has been shown to play a role in reducing the risk of __________, which is the leading cause of disability among people over the age of 80.

For items 6 through 10, as directed by your teacher, match each term in column 1 with the appropriate phrase in column 2.

6. abstract thinking
7. reasoning skills
8. socioemotional development
9. chronological age
10. physiological age

a. the way you solve problems and make decisions
b. the number of years you have been alive
c. includes self-esteem, empathy, and friendships
d. how well your body systems are aging
e. the ability to consider things that are not visible, immediate, or concrete

For items 11 through 15, as directed by your teacher, respond to each statement or question.

11. What is socioemotional development?
12. What are two things you should never do when caring for an infant?
13. Describe two health careers that might interest you.
14. Why might young adulthood be a stressful time? Provide two reasons.
15. Define *intrinsic motivation* and give an example.

Thinking Critically

Write a response to the following prompt.

List and discuss the major physical and mental changes that occur with aging. Which ones can you affect through your own choices? What changes can you begin to make now to help you age well? Write a letter to yourself as you are now, and another letter to yourself at age 65, to remind yourself of these changes and motivate yourself to make healthy choices.

Take It Home

Think of a person you know and respect who is older than 65—for example, a parent, grandparent, neighbor, or family friend. Interview the person about his or her life. Find out what challenges the person faces and what steps he or she takes to try to overcome them. Ask the person what advice he or she has for you about staying healthy as you age. Write a brief report about what you learn.

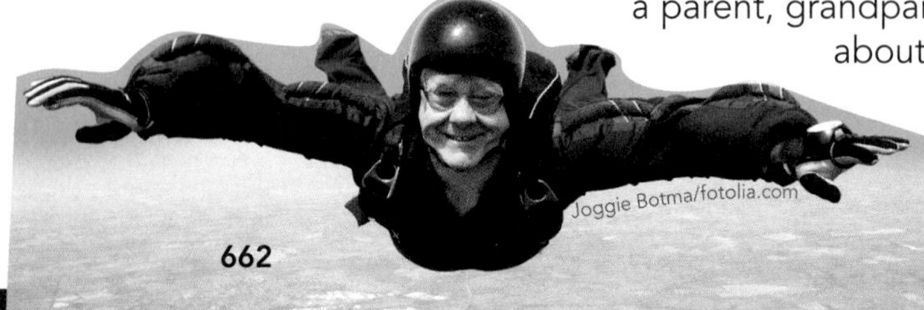
Joggie Botma/fotolia.com

UNIT XI

Avoiding Destructive Habits

Healthy People 2020 Goals

- Reduce tobacco use by adolescents.
- Reduce the initiation of tobacco use among children, adolescents, and young adults.
- Reduce exposure to secondhand smoke.
- Increase tobacco-free environments in schools.
- Reduce the proportion of adolescents and young adults (in grades 6 through 12) exposed to tobacco advertising and promotion.
- Reduce the sale of tobacco to minors.
- Reduce the proportion of adolescents who ride with a driver who has been drinking alcohol.
- Increase the number of states with ignition interlock laws for impaired driving offenders.
- Reduce binge drinking of alcohol.
- Reduce average annual alcohol consumption.
- Reduce fatalities related to alcohol-impaired driving (0.08 blood alcohol content or higher).
- Increase the proportion of adolescents who never engage in substance abuse.
- Increase the proportion of adolescents who disapprove of substance abuse.
- Increase the proportion of adolescents who perceive great risk associated with substance abuse.
- Reduce drug-induced deaths.
- Reduce steroid use among adolescents.
- Reduce nonmedical use of prescription drugs.
- Reduce the proportion of adolescents who use inhalants.
- Reduce the proportion of adolescents who have been offered, sold, or given an illegal drug on school property.

Self-Assessment Features in This Unit

- My Tobacco Knowledge
- My Alcohol Knowledge
- My Drug Knowledge

Making Healthy Decisions and Skills for Healthy Living Features in This Unit

- Preventing Relapse
- Finding Social Support
- Building Refusal Skills

Special Features in This Unit

- Advocacy in Action: Tackling Tobacco Ads
- Diverse Perspectives: Alcoholism
- Consumer Corner: Selecting and Using Over-the-Counter Drugs

Living Well News Features in This Unit

- What's in That Cigarette You're Smoking?
- Are Americans Set Up to Become Alcoholics?
- Is Aspirin a Miracle Drug?

31

Tobacco

In This Chapter

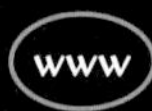

Student Web Resources

www.HOPEtextbook.org/student

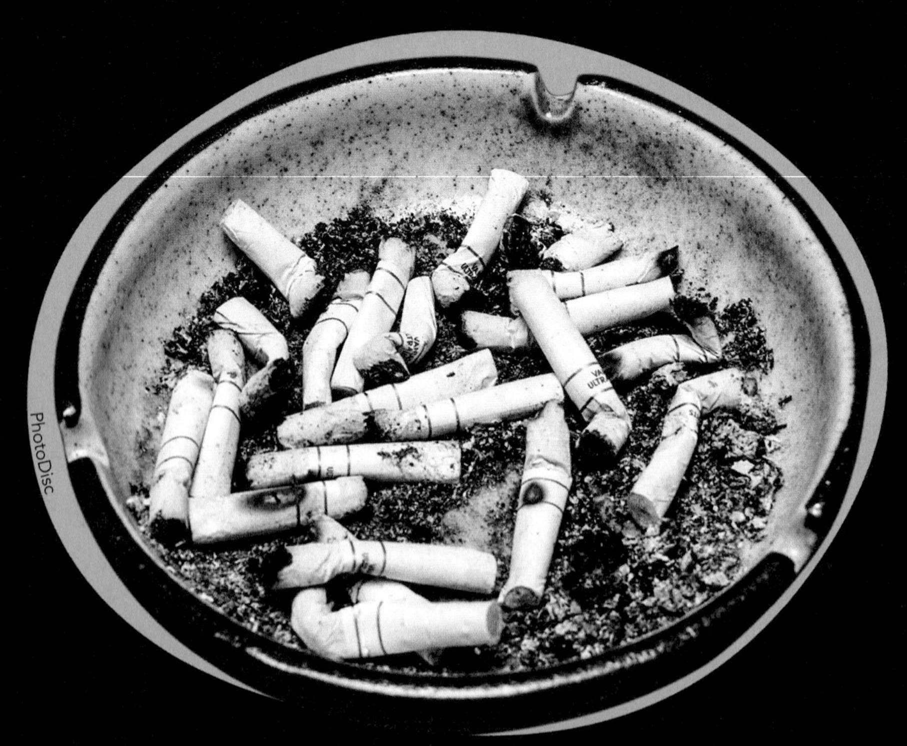

PhotoDisc

Lesson 31.1

Health Hazards of Tobacco Use

Lesson Objectives

After reading this lesson, you should be able to

1. explain how using tobacco or smoking began,
2. list at least three reasons that people use tobacco or smoke, and
3. list at least three diseases or disorders caused by tobacco.

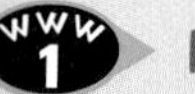

Lesson Vocabulary

neurotransmitter, secondhand smoke, smokeless tobacco, sudden infant death syndrome (SIDS)

What do the U.S. Centers for Disease Control and Prevention (CDC), the American Cancer Society, the American Heart Association, the American Lung Association, and the American Medical Association have in common? They all recognize that tobacco use is the number one cause of preventable disease in the United States.

Most Americans who smoke started doing so before the age of 18, and according to the CDC about 70 percent of current smokers want to quit. This chapter explores the reasons that people smoke, the health risks of using tobacco, trends of smoking and smokeless tobacco use in the United States, ways to stop smoking, U.S. laws affecting tobacco use, and how tobacco use in the United States compares with use in other countries.

History

Some experts trace the tobacco plant more than 8,000 years into the past. You may already know that Native Americans have historically used tobacco in religious ceremonies and as medicine. You may also know that tobacco was, and still is, a common and important crop in certain parts of the United States. Of course, people were not aware of the health risks associated with tobacco use until extensive research was conducted in relatively recent times. Even before science produced strong research, however, cigarettes were referred to as "coffin nails," thus linking them to premature death. Still, many people believed that tobacco had healing powers.

This was not the first (or the last) time that a product or procedure intended for healing caused more harm than good. For example, over a period of centuries, bloodletting (intentional bleeding using leeches) was the treatment of choice for many diseases and disorders; in this practice, blood was removed from the body in the belief that doing so would remove toxins or poisons. Neither bloodletting nor tobacco use are included in modern medical practice. To the contrary, tobacco use is responsible for about 400,000 to 450,000 premature deaths per year.

Perhaps someday there will be so few smokers that ash trays will be valued as collector's items. That's what happened in the case of spittoons, which were common when many more people used **smokeless tobacco**. These people needed to spit frequently, rather than swallow the tobacco juice that mixed with their saliva. As a result, spittoons were as common as trash cans in bars, restaurants, and even private homes. Over time, spitting came to be viewed as unsanitary and offensive; laws were passed against spitting, and spittoons became a thing of the past. Unfortunately, as smokeless tobacco became less popular, smoking became more popular.

Types of Tobacco

Tobacco is legally available to adults in the U.S. in many different forms. Manufactured cigarettes are the most commonly used forms followed by cigars (large cigars, cigarillos, and little cigars), smokeless tobacco (chewing tobacco and snuff), pipe smoking, and small pockets of hookahs (water pipes). Other forms include bidis cigarettes (hand rolled in special leaves) mostly from India and kreteks (cigarettes containing cloves and tobacco). These modes of tobacco use are not considered to be safe with long-term use.

The Health Risks of Tobacco Use

Tobacco use poses many health risks. Figure 31.1 provides a partial list of diseases and disorders associated with or made worse by smoking.

Figure 31.2 shows the number of deaths attributed to smoking and **secondhand smoke**, as well as the major causes of death. The two major killers are respiratory disease and heart disease. Many of the health problems associated with smoking, such as cancer and heart and lung disease, do not occur until a person has smoked regularly for many years. As a result, people in their teens sometimes find it hard to feel concerned about something that might happen to them in 20 or 30 years. Either they can't imagine being that much older, or they believe that they'll be able to stop smoking before it's too late. However, as discussed later in this chapter, it can be very difficult to quit smoking. In addition, some of the negative effects can arise much sooner than others—for example, bad breath, yellowing of the fingernails, and asthma. Thirdhand smoke is when the smoke clings to clothes, walls, furniture, and so on. It can remain even if smoking has ceased and it may be associated with some increased risk of cancers.

Cardiovascular diseases
- Heart attacks
- Stroke
- Heart disease
- Atherosclerosis
- High blood pressure
- Angina (chest pain)

Respiratory diseases
- Emphysema
- Chronic bronchitis
- Asthma

Other
- Diabetes
- Stomach ulcers
- Gum disease
- Bad breath
- Yellowing of fingernails
- Premature wrinkling
- Osteoporosis
- Reduced fertility
- Erectile dysfunction

Cancers
- Lung cancer
- Throat cancer
- Mouth cancer
- Other organ cancers

FIGURE 31.1 A partial list of diseases and disorders associated with or made worse by smoking.

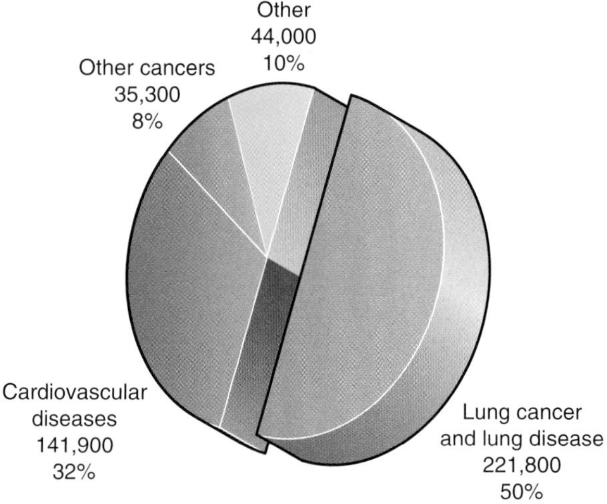

FIGURE 31.2 Deaths attributed to smoking.

Data is from www.cdc.gov/tobacco/data_statistics/tables/health/attrdeaths/.

HEALTHY COMMUNICATION

If teenage smokers could see 20 years into their future and knew for certain that smoking would cause them to develop cancer in their 40s, do you think this knowledge would be enough to make them kick the habit? Why or why not? Debate your perspectives with a peer who has different views from yours. Listen to each other's opinions and determine where you agree and disagree.

Smoking and Pregnancy

According to the March of Dimes (a U.S. nonprofit organization that advocates for infant health), exposure to tobacco during and after pregnancy (including secondhand smoke) puts embryos and babies at risk for developing many health problems including **sudden infant death syndrome (SIDS)** (see figure 31.3).

Why Do People Smoke?

People smoke for many reasons. Some people think smoking is necessary in order to fit in with their

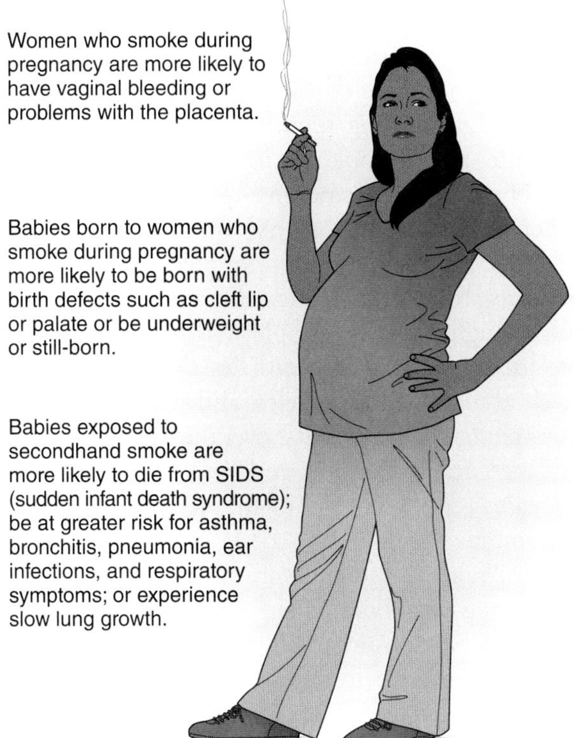

Women who smoke during pregnancy are more likely to have vaginal bleeding or problems with the placenta.
Babies born to women who smoke during pregnancy are more likely to be born with birth defects such as cleft lip or palate or be underweight or still-born.
Babies exposed to secondhand smoke are more likely to die from SIDS (sudden infant death syndrome); be at greater risk for asthma, bronchitis, pneumonia, ear infections, and respiratory symptoms; or experience slow lung growth.

FIGURE 31.3 Effects of smoking on infant health.

friends who smoke, although peer pressure is not the top reason that people smoke. Some people who smoke want to imitate their favorite actor or singer. In addition, if a parent smokes, you're more likely to smoke. Some people also try smoking out of simple curiosity, others smoke as an act of rebellion, and some think it will help them lose weight. And then of course there's advertising.

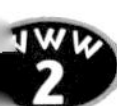

Overall, men use tobacco products more than women, but the gap between males and females has been narrowing. Most people think they're not very affected by advertising, but research tells a different story. And think about it: Tobacco manufacturers wouldn't spend hundreds of millions of dollars each year in advertising and promotion if it didn't work.

CONNECT

Do members of your immediate family smoke? Do you think their choices regarding smoking have influenced (or will influence) your likelihood of smoking? Why or why not?

When you ask people who've tried smoking if their first experience of it was pleasant, most say no. Some people get dizzy or light headed, some cough, some feel nauseous, and others simply don't like the taste or the overall experience. If most people's first impression of smoking is bad, why do some people try it again and again? Smoking is an acquired taste. As with food, you sometimes come to like something only after trying it many times. With smoking, this process is encouraged by the addictive element of nicotine and even chemicals or additives—such as menthol—that tobacco companies add to cigarettes. People may grow to like the taste and the feeling of smoking that is made more intense by their dependence on nicotine.

In fact, if you count each puff of a cigarette as a dose, or hit, no other drug is used as frequently as nicotine. According to the National Institute on Drug Abuse (NIDA) (a research group of the U.S. government), cigarettes and other forms of tobacco (including cigars, pipe tobacco, snuff, and chewing tobacco) contain not only nicotine but also hundreds of other chemicals and substances (see figure 31.4). Nicotine is the addictive ingredient, and it is readily absorbed into the bloodstream whenever a tobacco product is chewed or inhaled. In fact, nicotine reaches the brain within 10 seconds of inhalation. For each cigarette, a typical smoker takes 10 puffs over a period of five minutes. Thus, a person who smokes about 1 1/2 packs (30 cigarettes) daily gets 300 hits of nicotine in his or her brain every day.

Sometimes people can be tricked into believing that light cigarettes are safer than regular cigarettes. This is not true. In fact, there is no established safe level of tobacco smoking. Sidestream smoke, or secondhand smoke, can be more dangerous than smoke that is directly inhaled from a cigarette, cigar, or pipe because the particles in the secondhand smoke are smaller. Most people are not exposed to secondhand smoke as often as smokers are exposed to direct smoke, though. Of course, smokers breathe in both direct and secondhand smoke.

When nicotine enters a person's bloodstream, it immediately stimulates his or her adrenal glands to release the hormone epinephrine (adrenaline). Epinephrine, in turn, stimulates the person's central nervous system and increases his or her blood pressure, respiration, and heart rate. In addition,

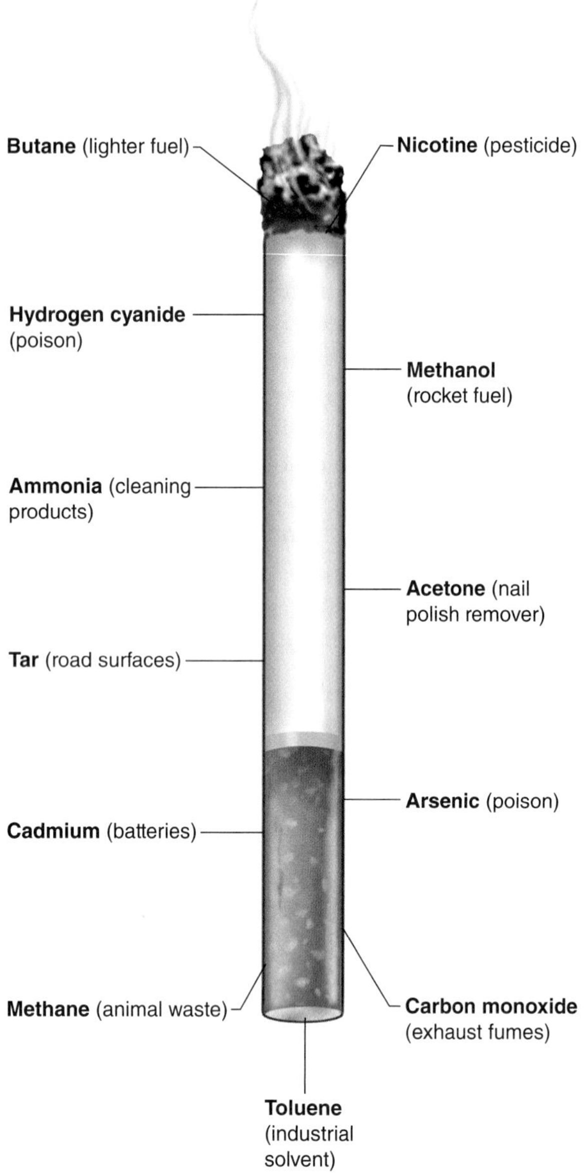

FIGURE 31.4 Cigarettes contain many harmful substances that are used in many other ways in addition to nicotine.

glucose is released into the person's blood, and insulin output from his or her pancreas is suppressed. These effects result in chronically higher blood sugar among nicotine users. Nicotine in cigarettes and in smokeless tobacco are both harmful. Nicotine from smoking may enter the body faster than nicotine absorbed through the mouth or gums. If the same amount of nicotine enters the body, regardless of the source, they are equally harmful, though. Because people tend to use tobacco products at a level that satisfies them, the blood levels of nicotine in smokeless and smoked tobacco users tend to be very similar over the period of a day.

Like cocaine, heroin, and marijuana, nicotine increases a person's level of the **neurotransmitter** dopamine, which affects the brain pathways that control reward and pleasure. For many tobacco users, long-term brain changes induced by continued nicotine exposure result in addiction—a condition of compulsive drug seeking and use, even in the face of negative consequences. Nicotine is actually more addictive than drugs like cocaine, but cocaine has a much greater potential for causing immediate harm than nicotine.

Comprehension Check

1. Give a historical reason why people used tobacco before there were tobacco companies.
2. What are two influences in society that increase the chance that a person will use tobacco?
3. How can using tobacco products during pregnancy be harmful to the embryo or fetus?

SELF-ASSESSMENT: My Tobacco Knowledge

Take the following quiz to see how much you know about the dangers of smoking and tobacco use.

1. Chemicals are added to tobacco when cigarettes are made.
   a. true
   b. false
2. Nicotine is classified as a drug.
   a. true
   b. false
3. The average smoker begins to smoke at age 22.
   a. true
   b. false
4. Peers influence teens to begin smoking more than any other influence.
   a. true
   b. false
5. Light cigarettes are healthier than regular cigarettes.
   a. true
   b. false
6. There are such things as safe cigarettes.
   a. true
   b. false
7. Nicotine is more addictive than cocaine.
   a. true
   b. false
8. The nicotine in chewing tobacco is less harmful than the nicotine in cigarettes.
   a. true
   b. false
9. Smoke inhaled directly from a cigarette is more dangerous than secondhand smoke.
   a. true
   b. false
10. Men are more likely to smoke than women.
    a. true
    b. false

Here are the correct answers: question 1 a, 2 a, 3 b, 4 b, 5 b, 6 b, 7 a, 8 b, 9 b, and 10 a. If you got nine or ten answers right, you really know your stuff. If you got seven or eight right, you're ahead of most people but still have some things to learn. If you got five or six right, you could stand to brush up on the facts. If you got four or fewer right, seek out more information.

Planning for Healthy Living

Use the Healthy Living Plan worksheet to help you quit smoking (if you smoke) or to continue being smoke free throughout your life. If relevant, consider whether you would use modern technology to help you.

Lesson 31.2

Marketing, Policies, Cessation, and Advocacy

Lesson Objectives

After reading this lesson, you should be able to

1. describe current trends in tobacco smoking among young people,
2. name two policies that discourage people from smoking, and
3. describe at least three methods of smoking cessation.

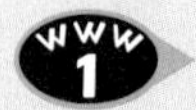

Lesson Vocabulary

countermarketing, media literacy, product placement, social marketing

In the United States, about 20 percent of people smoke, and a little more than 3 percent use smokeless tobacco. Turned around, these numbers mean that 80 percent of Americans do *not* smoke, and 97 percent don't use smokeless tobacco. Among U.S. high school students in 2010, according to the CDC, about 17 percent smoked, and 6 percent used smokeless tobacco. Clearly, the overwhelming majority of high school students do not use any kind of tobacco product.

The graph presented in figure 31.5 shows U.S. smoking trends from 1965 to 2009. As you can see, the rate of tobacco use has been going down among both adults and teens. A short-term rise did occur in teen smoking in the 1990s, due in part to a drop in cigarette prices at the time. In fact, it is estimated that every 10 percent reduction in the cost of cigarettes increases cigarette use among teenagers by 7 percent.

There are many reasons that fewer people in the United States smoke today than in years past. In a textbook such as this one, you might expect to be presented with only facts about how harmful tobacco is to your health, but years of experience show that facts alone are not enough to decrease the number of smokers or to stop people from starting to smoke. Fortunately, several tactics *have* helped decrease tobacco use in the U.S.—increased price, policy and law changes, **countermarketing**, **social marketing**, and education.

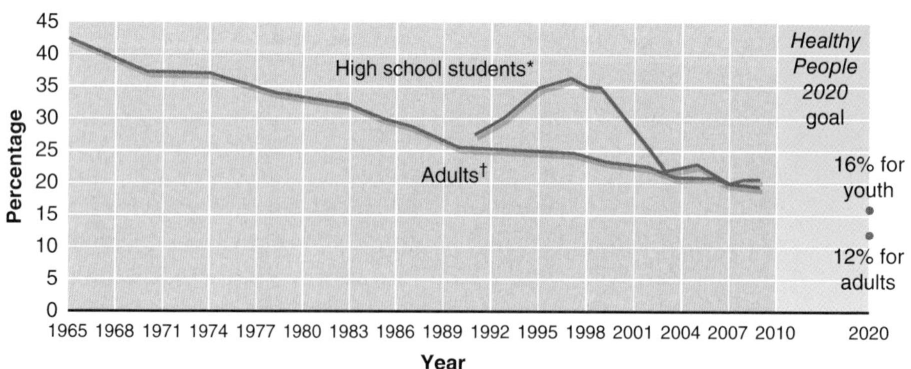

FIGURE 31.5 Trends in smoking among high school students and adults from 1965 to 2009.
From www.cdc.gov/chronicdisease/resources/publications/AAG/osh.htm.

Price

Price is important because the more expensive tobacco products are—whether due to price increases set by manufacturers or to increased taxes levied on tobacco products—the more likely it is that some smokers will either cut back or quit. Part of the reason is that people who earn less money tend to use tobacco products at a higher rate than people who earn more money. In addition, there comes a point with any product at which people feel that enough is enough and decide to cut back, stop, or switch to a cheaper alternative. For example, when the movie rental service Netflix raised its prices in 2011, it lost more than 800,000 customers; the company responded by lowering its prices. In the marketing of any product, price matters, and tobacco products are no exception.

With this in mind, many public health professionals have advocated for higher taxes on tobacco products, which would raise their overall price, thus meaning that fewer people would smoke. In addition, the money raised through the higher taxes could be used to help fund programs to help people quit using tobacco. Unfortunately, very few states have used tobacco taxes for tobacco prevention or cessation programs because these funds tend to go into general accounts and are spent on things like roads, bridges, and other needed products and services.

In another strategy, the state attorney generals of 46 U.S. states sued the largest four tobacco companies in 1998 for the medical costs of tobacco-related diseases and disorders that were paid by taxpayers. In the resulting Tobacco Master Settlement Agreement, the tobacco companies agreed to pay billions of dollars to the states in exchange for an agreement that the tobacco companies could not be held legally responsible for harm caused by tobacco products. Tobacco companies also agreed to cut back or eliminate advertising to youth.

Policies and Laws

In recent years, many policies and laws have dramatically changed how people view smoking in the United States. It is now hard to believe that at one time people could smoke on airplanes, in movie theaters, in school teachers' lounges, and even in hospitals. Smoke-free laws have been implemented in the majority of U.S. states, as well as the District of Columbia, Puerto Rico, the U.S. Virgin Islands, and hundreds of U.S. cities and counties that don't have statewide bans.

Many workplaces have created their own smoke-free policies—for example, banning smoking in company vehicles or even anywhere on the organization's property. Not surprisingly, more than 3,500 U.S. hospitals have also banned smoking on their property—inside or outside. In addition, nearly 800 college campuses have enacted total smoking bans.

Smoking bans have been passed for several reasons. Probably the most important one is to protect others from secondhand smoke. Just as construction companies require their workers to wear helmets to protect them from injury, policies and laws have been passed to protect workers from the dangers of secondhand smoke. The CDC estimates that exposure to secondhand smoke causes 46,000 deaths per year in the United States alone.

When children are exposed to secondhand smoke at home, they are more likely to suffer severe asthma attacks and other respiratory conditions, such as bronchitis, coughing, and sneezing. For these and

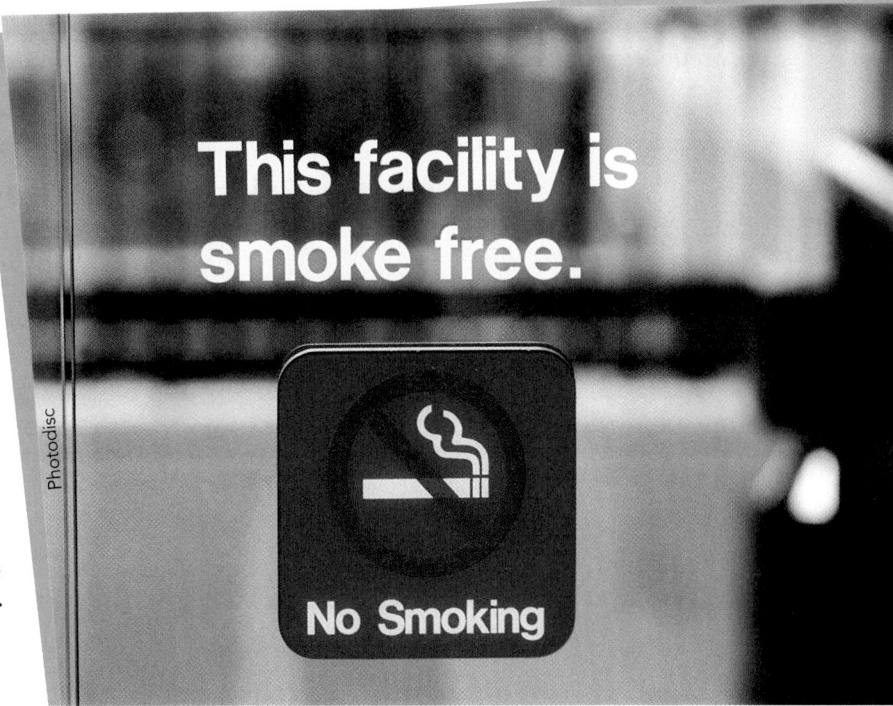
This facility is smoke free.
No Smoking
Photodisc

Where there are fewer places for people to smoke, more people quit smoking.

other reasons, 34 states have passed laws prohibiting smoking in commercial day care centers, and 33 prohibit smoking in home-based child care centers. Smoking bans reduce the risks of heart attack in both smokers and nonsmokers and thus are considered an effective mechanism for creating a healthier society.

Another reason for laws and policies against tobacco use is the fact that nonsmokers greatly outnumber smokers. The greater the gap grows between nonsmokers and smokers, the more likely communities are to enact policies and laws restricting smoking. Nonsmokers find it unfair to have to inhale secondhand smoke at work or in restaurants and other public places.

As you might expect, where there are fewer places for people to smoke, more people quit smoking. With the passage of more and more smoking bans—along with other factors such as the prohibition of cigarette lighters on airplanes—the habit of smoking is becoming increasingly difficult for people to maintain.

Legal Age for Buying Tobacco Products

In most U.S. states, it is illegal for a person under the age of 18 to purchase tobacco products (in a few states, the legal age is 19). New York City passed a law restricting the purchase of tobacco until the age of 21. Many communities conduct compliance checks by having people under the legal age try to buy tobacco in order to see if the business operator properly checks identification rather than selling the product to the minor. Businesses that sell to minors are often fined, and many times the employee who sold to the minor is fired. If a business repeatedly sells tobacco to minors, it may lose its license to sell tobacco products. It is also illegal for adults to purchase tobacco for minors.

Depending on state law, minors who try to purchase tobacco products could also be fined or assigned to perform community service. Purchasing tobacco (or alcohol) with a fake ID is a much more serious offense, and it is also illegal to make, manufacture, or sell fake IDs; doing so can result in a felony conviction and a large fine.

CONNECT

Oddly, although it's illegal for minors to purchase tobacco products, it's not always against the law for them to use these products depending on what state they live in. Do you think it should be illegal for minors to smoke at all? Debate your perspective with your peers. Support your position with facts and be respectful of each other's opinions.

Smoking, Fires, and Housing Policies

According to the U.S. Fire Administration, almost a thousand people are killed by smoking-related fires each year in the United States, and 25 percent of those who die are family members, friends, or neighbors of the smokers who cause the fires. One-third of those who die in these fires are the children of the smokers.

Why Are the Rules Different for Young People?

Laws are often enacted for the purpose of protecting young people. The belief is that youths have not fully matured and therefore may not be able to make effective decisions about certain issues that carry high stakes. That's part of the reason we have separate juvenile and adult courts.

Even the tobacco industry now takes an official stand against young people smoking. Industry representatives say that opting to smoke or not to smoke is an adult decision. Of course, this stance leads some young people to think that smoking makes them more grown up. The fact is that almost 80 percent of adult smokers started smoking before the age of 18—and the younger people are when they start smoking, the greater their health risks later in life.

These grim statistics have led some communities to make laws requiring landlords to disclose whether or not they prohibit smoking. Such laws do not require landlords to have smoke-free buildings, but they do require landlords to disclose their smoking policy to prospective tenants. Do they allow smoking anywhere? Do they allow smoking in designated areas? Do they have smoke-free units? Do they mandate how far away from windows and doors a smoker must be while smoking?

This information allows prospective tenants to evaluate whether they and their family will be exposed to secondhand smoke and whether the apartment complex may have a greater fire risk due to smoking. When landlords do offer nonsmoking rental complexes, they make all units safer for everyone.

Marketing and Countermarketing

As a result of the Tobacco Master Settlement Agreement's restrictions on tobacco advertising, billboard advertisements for tobacco products disappeared, as did tobacco advertising at sport events. Big tobacco companies hire clever marketers, however, and they have managed to keep their message in front of young people. One common strategy they use is **product placement**—arranging for a product to appear prominently in a television show, movie, or other media production. The idea is that if people see a famous actor, musician, or athlete using a product, they will be encouraged to use the product themselves. It is illegal for tobacco companies to pay to have their product displayed, but they can promote product placement.

This technique often works. For example, a tobacco company can encourage the makers of a movie to show an actor smoking its brand of cigarette, and audience members may not even think about the fact that they're seeing an advertisement. According to the nonprofit organization Breathe California of Sacramento-Emigrant Trails, there were far fewer incidences of smoking in movies in 2009 than in 2003—but still many. Of the films nominated for Academy Awards in 2013, 61 percent showed people smoking usually without mentioning any consequences.

Although athletes today are more likely to talk publicly about tobacco prevention than to advertise tobacco products, they can of course be seen *using*

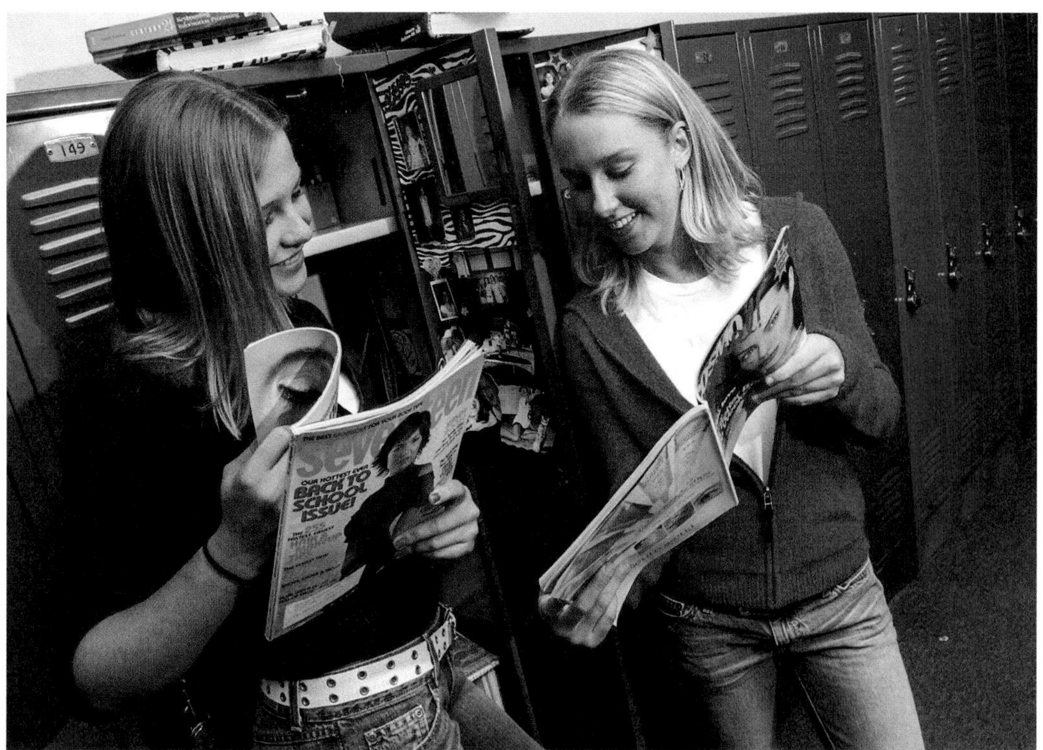

Be aware of marketing tactics in magazines and other media.

 ADVOCACY IN ACTION: Tackling Tobacco Ads

Analyze and write a summary of how tobacco products are portrayed in your preferred media source (e.g., favorite magazine, website, television show). For example, is tobacco openly advertised? Are images of people smoking shown in ways other than direct advertisements? Do you see product placements? Now, write a letter to the creators or publishers of the media source explaining your observations and the potential effect the tobacco ads or images might have on young people. Conclude your letter by advocating for a specific change.

tobacco products off the field if they do so. Mindful of athletes' status as role models, the Campaign for Tobacco-Free Kids launched a project called Knock Tobacco Out of the Park that succeeded in getting Major League Baseball to ban tobacco use by players, coaches, and managers at games (see figure 31.6). This was no small feat, given that smokeless tobacco had been part of the game of baseball for many years. In fact, the area where relief pitchers warm up is called the bullpen, which some think was named after ads for the Bull Durham brand of tobacco that used to appear near the area. The Campaign for Tobacco-Free Kids also gives awards every year to outstanding youth anti-tobacco advocates.

As a result of the Knock Tobacco Out of the Park campaign, major league players, managers, and coaches are no longer allowed to carry a tobacco tin or package in their uniforms at any time when fans are in the ballpark. They are also prohibited from using smokeless tobacco during televised interviews, autograph signings, team-sponsored appearances, and other events where they interact with fans.

Of course, the concern for smokeless or spit tobacco is because of the health hazards related to

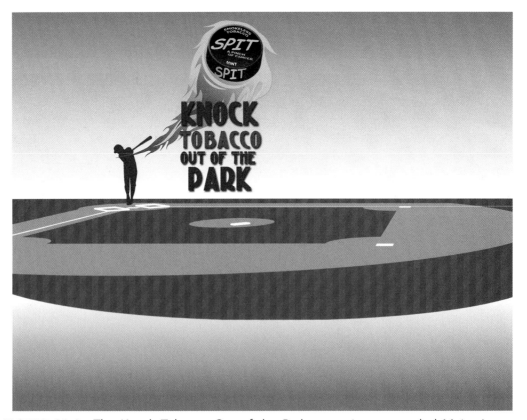

FIGURE 31.6 The Knock Tobacco Out of the Park campaign persuaded Major League Baseball to prohibit tobacco use before, during, and after games.

Courtesy of The Campaign for Tobacco-Free Kids.

their use. Even using it for a short time can cause bad breath and yellowish stains on your teeth. Almost three-quarters of people that use spit tobacco get mouth sores. The more often people use smokeless tobacco on a daily basis and over longer periods of time, the more serious the consequences can be. The gums may recede and can cause dental problems. The nicotine—like in smoked tobacco—causes increased heart rate, high blood pressure, and sometimes irregular heartbeats. These can all contribute to cardiovascular disease. Oral cancers are greatly increased in smokeless tobacco users. These include cancers of the tongue, lips, gums, and cheeks. In some cases cancer-causing aspects of smokeless tobacco can reach the esophagus, stomach, and even the bladder. There are not nearly as many treatment programs for smokeless tobacco users as there are for smokers, but the quitline (1-800-QUIT-NOW) helps both smokers and smokeless tobacco users (often in English or Spanish and other languages in some communities). Since the nicotine levels in smokeless tobacco users often reach higher levels than in smokers, the treatment is very likely to use medical nicotine replacement products.

In 2009, the U.S. Food and Drug Administration (FDA) was given authority to regulate tobacco, including the ability to ban certain tobacco additives (e.g., menthol), though it has yet to do so. The FDA also has the authority to stop the use of terms such as "light" and "low tar" and other marketing tactics.

In recent years, young people themselves have taken the lead on some countermarketing (anti-tobacco marketing) initiatives. Students have learned to increase their **media literacy** through efforts such as the Media Literacy Project, which, along with other organizations, helps them

- develop critical thinking skills;
- understand how media messages shape culture and society;
- identify target marketing strategies such as sports that traditionally have been associated with tobacco use;
- recognize what the media maker wants them to believe or do;
- name the techniques of persuasion used;
- recognize bias, spin, misinformation, and lies;
- discover the parts of the story that are not being told;
- evaluate media messages based on their own experiences, skills, beliefs, and values;
- create and distribute their own media messages; and
- advocate for a changed media system.

One of the most successful counter-tobacco advertising initiatives is TheTruth.com campaign. This campaign started in Florida and included young people in all aspects of the marketing plan. It does not demonize smokers; instead, it counters the tobacco industry's marketing campaigns. This type of social marketing, applying commercial marketing to noncommerical purposes, is used by many anti-tobacco campaigns. You can learn more about smoking cessation by visiting the student section of the Health Opportunities Through Physical Education website.

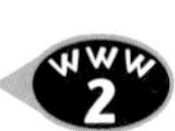

Smoking Cessation

It's hard to stop smoking or using smokeless tobacco. People who smoke get more out of it than just an addiction that causes diseases and disorders. Any habit that is repeated so frequently for such a long time is hard to change. Add to that the addictive nature of nicotine, and you have quite a challenge for behavior change. Of course, millions of people have been able to stop smoking. How did they do it? The answer varies.

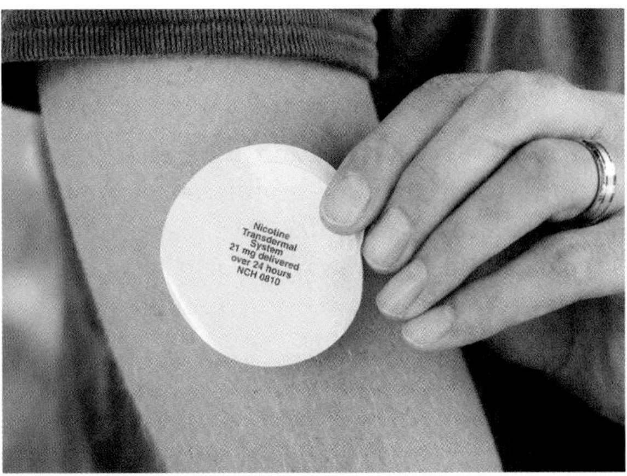

The most successful smoking cessation programs use counseling and social support, along with an alternative nicotine delivery option, such as nicotine patches.

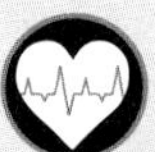

HEALTH TECHNOLOGY

A relatively new product has been introduced to the market—electronic cigarettes, or e-cigarettes. These products liquefy and vaporize nicotine into an aerosol mist. Users puff (sometimes called "vape") on the e-cigarette to get the nicotine that they crave. It looks like a cigarette and has the approximate feel of a cigarette, but the vapor is not smelly to the user or to those nearby. E-cigarettes have helped many people cut back on traditional cigarettes, but because there is not enough research about the possible harmful effects of e-cigarettes, there has been considerable debate among experts about what to do about these new nicotine delivery systems. Some experts want to ban or regulate e-cigarettes until more is known about the possible harmful effects. Others believe that e-cigarettes are valuable in harm reduction. This means they believe that e-cigarettes are safer than traditional cigarettes. Regardless of the possible levels of harm that may be found, there are no health or medical experts who recommend the use of e-cigarettes by people who do not currently use nicotine products.

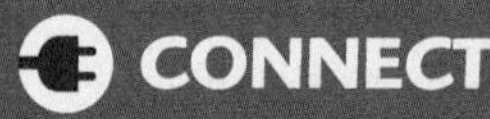

CONNECT

Would you consider trying an e-cigarette? Why or why not?

For one thing, all U.S. states have a quitline (1-800-QUIT-NOW) that enables you to talk with a trained counselor. The smoking cessation programs that are most successful use counseling and social support, along with an alternative nicotine delivery option, such as nicotine gum, patches, inhalers, tablets, or lozenges. Some smoking cessation aids are available over the counter, and others require a prescription. Smokers can also use various other tactics to stop smoking, such as substituting a lollipop for a cigarette or placing a rubber band on the wrist and snapping it each time they crave a cigarette.

There are many organizations such as the American Cancer Society, the American Heart Association, and the American Lung Association that offer tobacco cessation programs either in person or online. Your health care professional can also recommend effective programs to you. Programs offer many ways to help tobacco users to quit—counseling, support groups, quitlines, smartphone apps, nicotine replacement products, and other techniques. To be successful, most people need to be motivated to quit. They need to believe that they can succeed and they need to identify the triggers associated with tobacco use (e.g., smoking after a meal). Some tobacco cessations programs are designed especially for teens.

As with most behavior change strategies, no single program works for everyone. There are enough options, however, that one is bound to work for you. It may take several tries, but persistence pays off. Just as you can't become a great athlete or musician (or anything) without making lots of mistakes, you can't stop smoking without facing some setbacks. But each setback you overcome makes it more likely that you'll eventually succeed.

Quitting smoking is easy. I've done it a thousand times.

—Mark Twain, author and humorist

Comprehension Check

1. Are smoking rates in the U.S. higher now than they were 10 years ago? Why or why not?
2. Give two examples of policies that help reduce smoking.
3. Describe one method of smoking cessation.

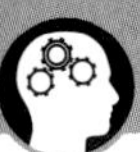

MAKING HEALTHY DECISIONS: Preventing Relapse

Nikko is a high school student who moved to the United States from Greece, where he spent his early years around an extended family of smokers and where smoking seemed to be allowed most everywhere. Now, his parents both still smoke, and Nikko has been smoking since he was 13, but he doesn't know as many smokers as he used to. Most of his friends don't smoke, and they even make comments to him about how gross it is. His best friend James won't let him smoke in his car or house, and the campus where Nikko goes to school just became a tobacco-free zone.

When Nikko told his parents that he wanted to quit smoking and that he wanted both of them to quit, they were not receptive: "Everyone in the family smokes, and Uncle Leo lived to be 92, so it can't be that bad. Besides, we've tried quitting, and it's no use." Nikko feels frustrated because he knows how unhealthy it is, but he has a hard time quitting when cigarettes and smoke are all around the house. He has quit three times but always ended up smoking again after a few weeks; the longest he's managed to quit was for three months last summer. He also wants James to come to the house sometimes to play video games, but James complains about the smoke and won't come over.

For Discussion

What are some strategies Nikko could use to help himself stop smoking? What options might help him avoid another relapse? What are some strategies Nikko might use to help his parents quit smoking? To help you organize your thoughts, refer to the Skills for Healthy Living feature.

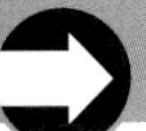

SKILLS FOR HEALTHY LIVING: Preventing Relapse

Relapse occurs when you stop implementing a healthy decision or return to an unhealthy habit. One example of relapse would be a smoker who quits for a month, then starts smoking again when facing a stressful situation. Once you stop a negative behavior, or begin a positive behavior, take the following steps to help prevent relapse.

- **Do a self-assessment.** Understand what might trigger your change in behavior.
- **Set goals.** You can use goals to maintain a behavior and to avoid relapse in the same way you can use them to start or stop a behavior in the first place. Use a series of short-term goals to keep you on track and motivated to stick with the behavior change.
- **Monitor your behavior.** Keep a journal or log that tracks your behavior. Doing so allows you to see patterns that might help you prevent a relapse such as recognizing that you automatically reach for a cigarette after a meal.
- **Tell other people what you're trying to accomplish.** When friends and family members know your goals, they can support you and help you stay accountable.
- **Don't let a small failure do you in.** If you have a setback, don't use it as an excuse. For example, if you try to quit smoking but take a puff of a friend's cigarette, don't use that as an excuse to give up on your efforts altogether. Acknowledge the mistake and get back on track right away.
- **Find a healthy distraction.** When you feel tempted to do something that could start a relapse, find a better activity. For example, instead of grabbing a cigarette, get a stick of gum or a piece of candy. Instead of drinking a can of soda, drink a glass of water to quench your thirst and fend off the urge.

What's in That Cigarette You're Smoking?

The main ingredient in cigarettes is tobacco—a leafy plant grown in warm climates. But that isn't the only thing. If you smoke, you're also ingesting more than four thousand chemicals, fifty-one of which are known to be carcinogenic (cancer causing). These chemicals also contribute to other serious health problems, such as emphysema, asthma, and heart disease. In fact, many of them are actually poisonous. See table 31.1 for a partial listing of chemicals found in cigarettes.

Three of the most widely known chemicals in cigarettes are nicotine, tar, and carbon monoxide. Nicotine is a strong poisonous drug that has been used in insecticides. In its pure form, just one drop on a person's tongue can be deadly. Tar is the oily material that remains after tobacco passes through a cigarette filter. When a smoker inhales, a lot of the tar sticks to and blackens his or her lungs. Carbon monoxide is a poisonous gas also found in car exhaust. When a smoker inhales carbon monoxide, it interferes with his or her respiratory and circulatory systems. It also gets into the smoker's bloodstream, where it reduces the amount of oxygen going to the person's heart. In addition, chemicals in cigarette smoke narrow the walls of the smoker's arteries, which means the person's heart must work harder and his or her blood pressure goes up.

"Choosing to smoke cigarettes is like choosing to stand in the middle of a toxic chemical plant, inhaling car exhaust and tar, while gradually suffocating to death," says anti-smoking advocate and public health official Madison Montgomery.

For Discussion

Do you think most smokers are fully aware of what is in their cigarettes? Do you think it would affect their smoking habit if they were fully aware? Why or why not? If you had the opportunity to educate the public about the chemicals in cigarettes, what would you tell them?

TABLE 31.1 Chemicals Found in Cigarettes

Chemical	Found in
Acetone	Nail polish remover
Ammonia	Cleaning products
Arsenic	Rat poison
Butane	Cigarette lighter fluid
Carbon monoxide	Car exhaust
Cyanide	Deadly poisons
DDT	Insecticides
Formaldehyde	Embalming fluids
Hydrogen cyanide	Gas chamber poison
Methoprene	Pesticides
Nicotine	Bug sprays
Sulfuric acid	Car batteries
Tar	Material similar to that used to make roads

Reviewing Concepts and Vocabulary

As directed by your teacher, answer items 1 through 5 by correctly completing each sentence with a word or phrase.

1. ____________ ____________ is the practice of showing a product in use by a TV or movie character to help promote the use of the product without direct advertising.
2. Two diseases that can be caused by smoking are ____________ ____________ and ____________ ____________.
3. The addictive component of tobacco is called ____________.
4. Cigarette smoke inhaled by a nonsmoker is called ____________ ____________.
5. Smokeless tobacco has been regulated in the sport of ____________.

For items 6 through 10, as directed by your teacher, match each term in column 1 with the appropriate phrase in column 2.

6. compliance check	a. when you discontinue implementing a healthy decision or return to a negative habit
7. 46,000	b. deaths each year by cigarette smoking
8. relapse	c. neurotransmitter released when the brain is exposed to nicotine
9. dopamine	d. enforcing laws related to age and cigarette sales
10. more than 400,000	e. deaths each year by secondhand smoke

For items 11 through 15, as directed by your teacher, respond to each statement or question.

11. What was the result of the Knock Tobacco Out of the Park campaign?
12. Why are laws related to purchasing tobacco products different for young people than for adults?
13. Why is quitting smoking so difficult for many people?
14. Name two types of institutions leading the way in banning smoking.
15. What is the federal agency that regulates tobacco in the United States?

Thinking Critically

Write a paragraph in response to the following question.

The legal age for purchasing alcohol in the U.S. is 21, whereas the legal age for purchasing tobacco products is 18 in most states. Tobacco kills more people than alcohol, and there is a movement to raise the legal age for purchasing tobacco products to 21 as they did in New York City. Opponents believe that if a person is old enough to vote, serve in the military, and sign a contract without a parent's or guardian's permission, then he or she should be able to make a decision—such as buying tobacco or alcohol. If you had the opportunity to vote on raising the age of tobacco purchase to 21, how would you vote? Explain your decision.

Take It Home

Share your response to the Thinking Critically question above with a parent or guardian. Ask for his or her opinion and compare it with your own. Does hearing this person's perspective change your thinking about the issue? Why or why not?

PhotoDisc

32

Alcohol

In This Chapter

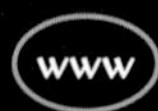

Student Web Resources

www.HOPEtextbook.org/student

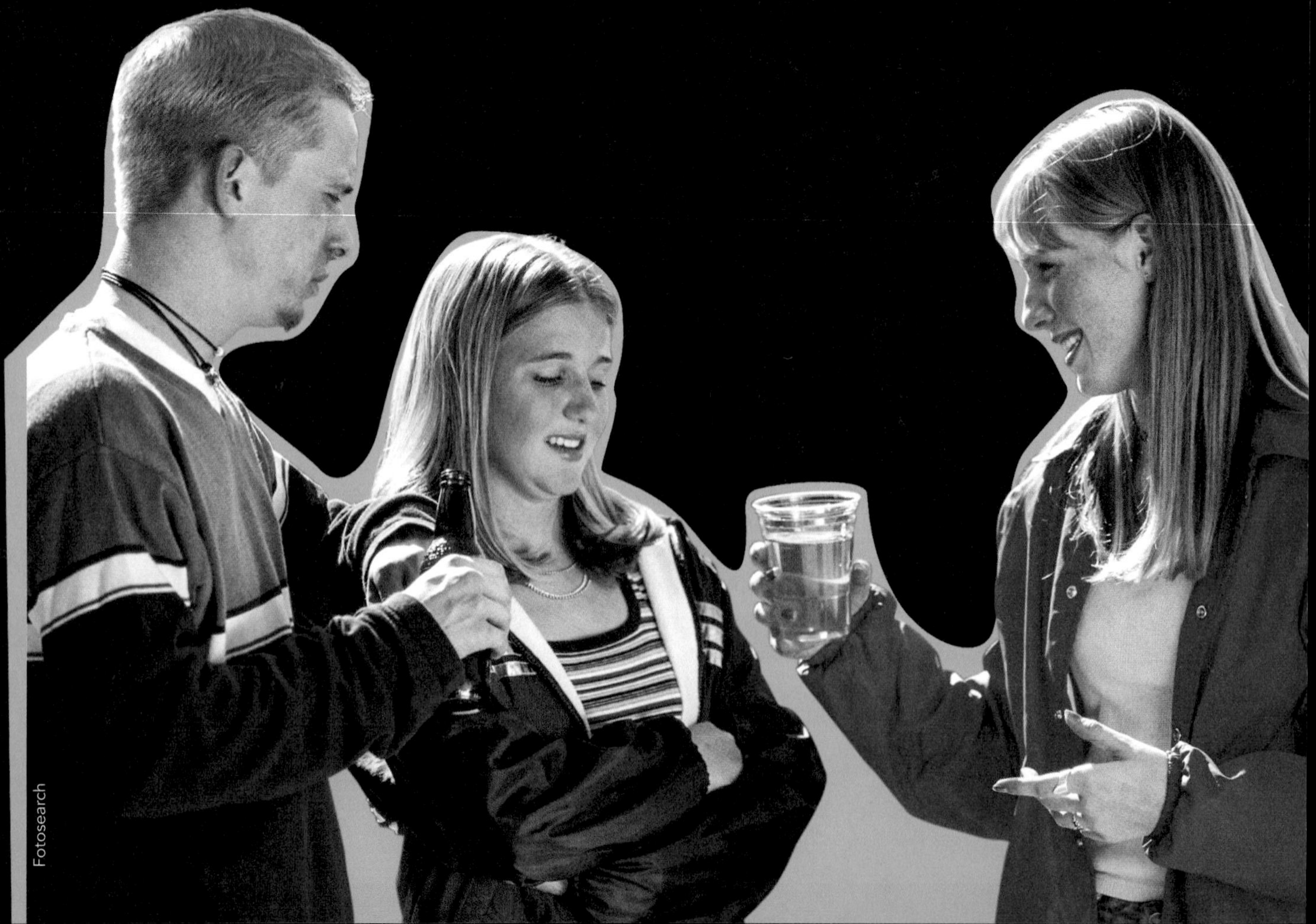

Fotosearch

Lesson 32.1

Alcohol Use, Misuse, and Health

Lesson Objectives

After reading this lesson, you should be able to

1. list two health problems associated with drinking alcohol,
2. explain the differences in how alcohol affects males and females, and
3. define *binge drinking*.

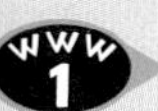

Lesson Vocabulary

acute alcohol poisoning, alcohol dehydrogenase, alcoholism, alcohol tolerance, binge drinking, ethyl alcohol (ethanol), heavy drinking, Prohibition

Alcohol has been part of human culture for thousands of years. Yet many societies still have a difficult time walking the tightrope between the positive and the negative aspects of its use. This lesson explains what alcohol is, discusses healthy and unhealthy levels of alcohol consumption, and addresses the short- and long-term health risks of alcohol consumption.

> "Always do sober what you said you'd do drunk."
>
> —Ernest Hemingway

History

Given the use of alcohol throughout history, many people feel an attraction to it despite the negative consequences associated with drinking it. Alcohol has been viewed as a medicine, a stress reducer, a social lubricant, an evil, a killer, and a destroyer of families. Behavior associated with alcohol consumption is also connected with many types of crime, and alcohol misuse has been referred to as sinful, criminal, immoral, and sick.

Despite the millions of adults who regularly use alcohol with no adverse effect, a sizable portion of drinkers have mild, severe, or even deadly effects. As a result, most countries in modern society have restricted alcohol access only to adults. In the United States, the current legal age for drinking or purchasing alcoholic beverages is 21. U.S. laws regulating the drinking age have changed several times. In recent history, for example, the legal age has been 18, 19, and 21. At one time, the legal age was even reduced from 21 to 18, but alcohol-related deaths then greatly increased, and the age was reset at 21.

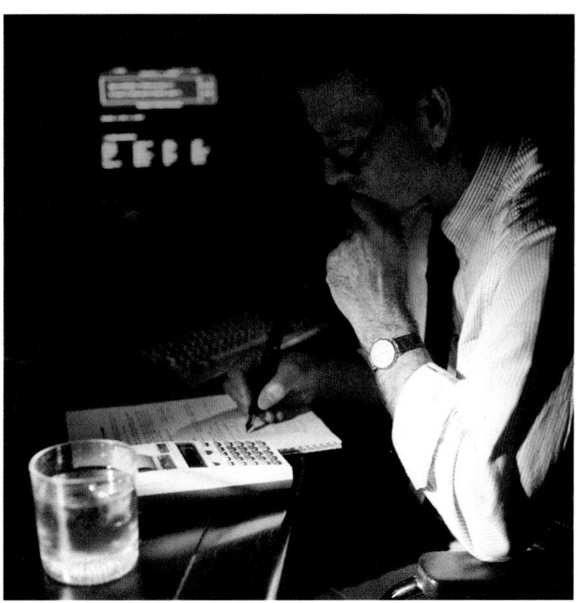

Some people view alcohol as a tool to reduce stress.
Photodisc

HEALTHY COMMUNICATION

Do you think 21 is an appropriate legal age for alcohol use? Do you think that teenagers can be responsible consumers of alcohol? Debate the issue with a classmate who sees it differently. Support your position with facts and be respectful of each other's opinions.

In your history classes, you've probably learned about **Prohibition**, which, through an amendment to the U.S. Constitution in 1920, made the sale and distribution of alcohol illegal. Many people ignored the laws, and criminal activity and corruption increased. In 1933, the amendment was repealed, and alcohol manufacturing and sales were once again legal. Several other countries, however, currently prohibit the sale and consumption of alcohol; in some other countries, the legal age for buying alcohol is 18.

Sound confusing? Well, it is. Why are there different legal ages for driving a car, buying tobacco, consuming alcohol, and getting married without a parent's or guardian's consent? The short answer is that the risks for these different behaviors are considered to be different. Of course, other cultural explanations go beyond the scope of this chapter. For our purpose here, it is enough to say that recent research reveals that drinking alcohol when you're young—when your brain is still developing—can hamper your ability to learn life skills. At least there is consistency in laws: A blood alcohol content (BAC) of 0.08 percent is the legal level of intoxication in all states (see lesson 2 for more information on BAC). Many of the health risks, policies, and laws associated with drinking alcohol (and a few possible benefits for adults) are summarized later in this chapter.

Alcohol and Alcohol Use

Ethyl alcohol (ethanol), the type of alcohol that people drink, is poisonous. Alcohol is also a depressant drug. Specifically, it depresses the parts of the brain that allow people to exercise good judgment. If consumed rapidly and in large amounts, it can also depress the part of the brain that controls breathing and heartbeat, which can result in coma or death. For example, people who drink a large amount of alcohol in a short time—as in a drinking contest or game—can suffer potentially fatal **acute alcohol poisoning**.

Fortunately, in most circumstances, the body automatically reacts to too much alcohol by causing the drinker to vomit or pass out. Vomiting protects the body by getting rid of some of the alcohol. However, if a person is somewhat conscious or passed out, he should not be induced to vomit because he could choke on his own vomit. It is never a good idea to leave someone alone who has passed out from drinking too much. Passing out, of course, stops a person from drinking more. However, if people drink too much too fast, they can bypass these safeguards of vomiting or passing out and the alcohol can kill them. A common misperception is that drinking coffee will speed up the sobering process. The body metabolizes alcohol at its own pace regardless of other drugs—like caffeine—that might be consumed.

Contrary to popular belief, being able to drink more than other people is not a good sign, because people who can drink a lot often do exactly that in the mistaken belief that alcohol can do them no harm. Furthermore, as people become more experienced drinkers, they develop an **alcohol tolerance**, which means that it takes more and more of the substance to feel the desired effects that they used to get by drinking less. This process can lead to a cycle of drinking more and more, thus increasing the likelihood of alcohol poisoning and many other health risks associated with **heavy drinking**.

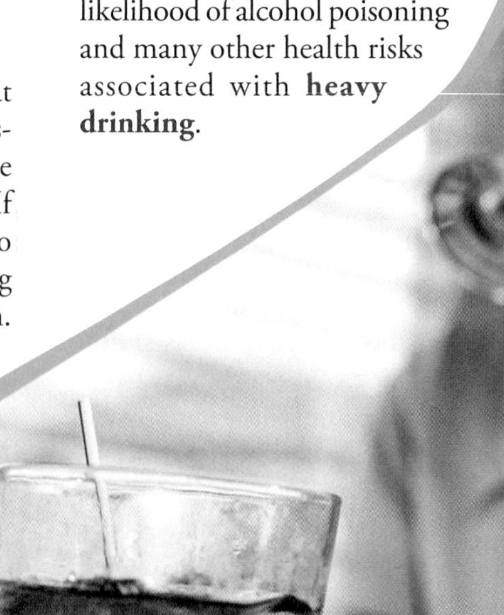

Alcohol tolerance means that it takes more and more of the substance for drinkers to feel the desired effects that they used to get by drinking less.

Photodisc

A beverage's alcohol content depends on its alcohol concentration, or percent alcohol. A standard drink of wine contains 5 ounces (148 milliliters), whereas a standard drink of hard liquor contains 1.5 ounces (44 milliliters). This means that the glass of wine and the shot of liquor, in their respective standard amounts, contain about the same amount of alcohol (see figure 32.1 for more examples).

Problematic drinking has several categories. **Binge drinking** involves consuming a lot of drinks on a single occasion, typically five or more drinks within two hours for males and four or more drinks within two hours for females. Heavy drinking refers to the average number of drinks a person has on a daily basis over a long time ranging from months to years. More specifically, heavy drinking refers to consuming two or more drinks per day for men and one or more per day for women. *Excessive drinking* is a more general term that can refer to binge drinking, heavy drinking, or both. **Alcoholism** is a disease in which a person is dependent on alcohol. Symptoms include strong cravings for alcohol, loss of control over how much alcohol is consumed, high tolerance for alcohol, and physical dependence on alcohol.

Differences in Alcohol Tolerance Between Males and Females

For several scientific reasons, males and females tolerate alcohol differently. The most obvious reason is that the average adult female is smaller than the average adult male. The smaller a person's body is (whether male or female), the less alcohol it takes to raise blood alcohol content. Of course, this is not the only reason, especially since many females are larger than many males.

The second reason is that the average female has a higher percent of body fat than the average male. Body fat contains little water, so most females have less body water than most males. Alcohol is not absorbed into body fat; therefore, BAC is increased in those with more body fat. Of course, there are many males who have more body fat than females.

There are also two more reasons. First, women have less **alcohol dehydrogenase** (an enzyme) than men, which allows more of what women drink to enter the bloodstream as pure alcohol. Finally, the level of the hormone estrogen varies with the female menstrual cycle (and in women who take birth control pills), and increased estrogen can result in a higher level of blood alcohol.

Immediate Health Risks of Alcohol Use

Excessive drinking has immediate effects that increase your risk of many harmful health conditions. These immediate effects, which result most often from binge drinking, include the following:

- Unintentional injuries increase, including traffic-related injuries, falls, drownings, burns, and firearm injuries.
- Violent acts increase, including intimate partner violence and maltreatment of children. In fact, alcohol use is associated

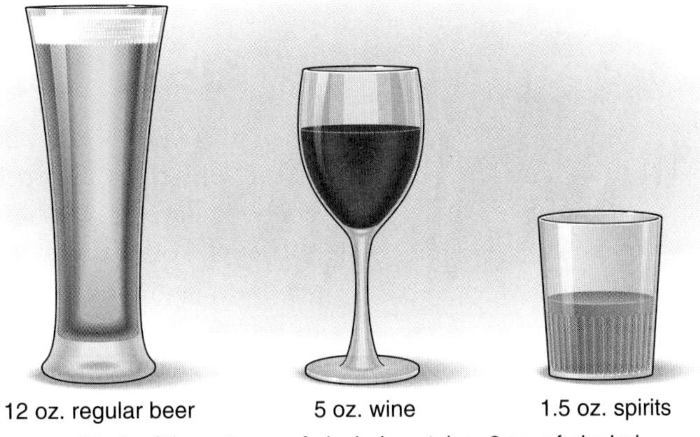
12 oz. regular beer
5 oz. wine
1.5 oz. spirits
Each of these types of alcohol contains .6 oz. of alcohol.

FIGURE 32.1 Examples of what constitutes a standard drink for different beverages.

with two out of three incidents of intimate partner violence.

- Risky sexual behavior increases, including unprotected sex, sex with multiple partners, and risk of sexual assault. These behaviors can also result in unintended pregnancy and sexually transmitted infection.
- Miscarriage and stillbirth increase among pregnant women, along with the risk of physical and mental birth defects in their children.
- The risk increases for acute alcohol poisoning—a medical emergency resulting from a high blood alcohol level that suppresses the central nervous system and can cause loss of consciousness, low blood pressure, low body temperature, coma, respiratory depression, and death.

Excessive alcohol use accounts for about 79,000 deaths each year in the United States, making it the third-leading cause of death related to lifestyle. In 2005 alone, for example, more than 1.6 million hospitalizations and 4 million emergency room visits resulted from alcohol-related conditions, according to the U.S. Centers for Disease Control and Prevention.

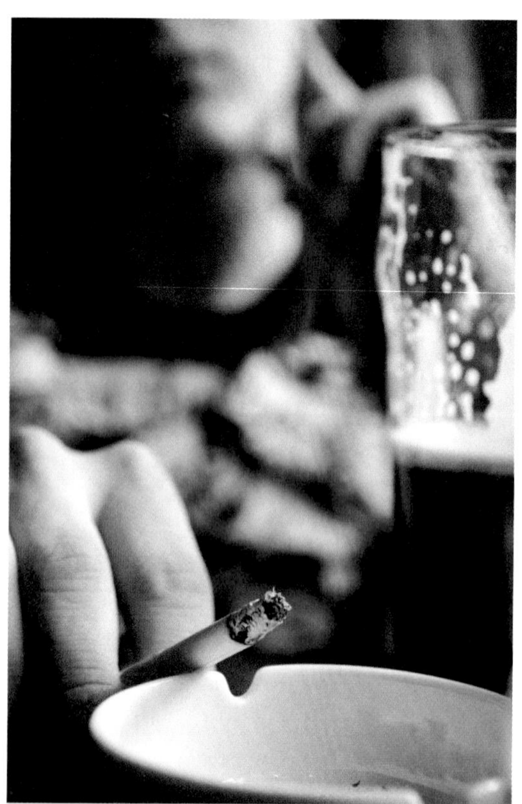

Smoking too many cigarettes in a short time span will not kill you, but binge drinking can.

Although a large percentage of people who smoke also drink, there are important differences between those who commonly drink and those who regularly smoke. For example, smoking too many cigarettes in a short time span will not kill you, but binge drinking can. Heavy smokers, unlike heavy drinkers, are not likely to have impaired judgment. Males are more likely than females to be drinkers, and whites are more likely than blacks and Latinos to be drinkers.

Tobacco and alcohol use are similar in that many of the diseases and disorders related to both of them occur later in life among regular, lifelong users. As a result, many young people are not concerned about what might happen to them in 20 or 30 years, because they haven't even been alive for that long. Unlike tobacco use, however, alcohol use also poses many health risks in the short term.

Long-Term Health Risks of Heavy Alcohol Use

Those who drink heavily over an extended period (months or years) can develop a range of chronic health problems (see table 32.1). In addition to increasing the risk of heart disease, cancer, and high blood pressure, heavy drinkers can experience disruptions in their social structure and livelihood. Common results of chronic drinking include family problems, broken relationships, job and career difficulties, and an increased risk of unintentional injury (e.g., in firearm and automobile crashes).

Alcohol and Calories

Since overweight and obesity are on the increase in the United States, people need to know that alcoholic beverages are high in calories and low in nutrients. For example, alcohol contains 7 calories per gram (a gram is the weight of an average paper clip), whereas carbohydrate and protein each contain only 4 calories per gram (fat contains the most, at 9 calories per gram). If a person drinks sweetened drinks (e.g., wine coolers) or mixes alcohol with sweetened soda, then the number of calories

TABLE 32.1 Health Problems Resulting From Long-Term Heavy Alcohol Use

Anemia—drinking lowers the number of oxygen-carrying red blood cells.	Gout—this painful condition occurs when uric acid builds up in the joints; it is made worse by alcohol use.
Cancer—alcohol can raise the level of carcinogens (cancer-causing agents) in the body.	High blood pressure—drinking more than three drinks within an hour can temporarily raise blood pressure; repeated binge drinking can result in long-term high blood pressure.
Cardiovascular disease—heavy drinking causes blood platelets to clump together, thus increasing the risk of blood clots.	Infectious disease—drinking suppresses the immune system, thus leaving you more susceptible to illness and infectious disease.
Cirrhosis—heavy drinking commonly damages the liver by scarring.	Nerve damage—alcohol-related nerve damage can result in numbness and a pins-and-needles sensation.
Dementia—heavy drinking causes the brain to shrink at a faster rate than normal, which can contribute to the development of dementia.	Seizures—heavy alcohol use can cause seizures even in people without a history of epilepsy.
Depression—drinking and depression go hand in hand, often creating a vicious cycle.	

is further increased. People who are trying to lose weight or maintain their current weight are often advised not to consume the "empty calories" that come from alcoholic beverages.

Alcohol Use and Pregnancy

According to the CDC, there is no known safe amount of alcohol consumption during pregnancy. This doesn't mean that drinking during pregnancy will definitely cause problems in a newborn. It does mean that drinking increases the chance of something going wrong—and the more the mother drinks, the greater the risk.

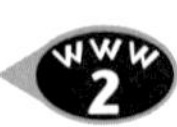

Potential problems include miscarriage, stillbirth, and increased risk of fetal alcohol spectrum disorders (FASD). Figure 32.2 lists problems that can be caused by drinking alcohol during pregnancy. Of course, many women don't immediately know that they're pregnant, and most women quit drinking once they do know. However, a woman who is a drinker and is not yet aware of being pregnant will

When a woman drinks alcohol during pregnancy, her baby may suffer the consequences.
Here are some of the major complications of drinking during pregnancy.

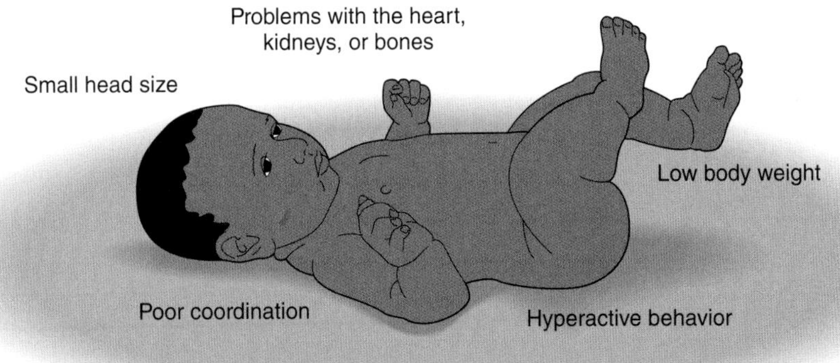

FIGURE 32.2 Problems related to drinking alcohol during pregnancy.

continue drinking, thus increasing health risks for the embryo. Therefore, a woman who is sexually active and not using reliable birth control should not drink alcohol.

Health Benefits of Drinking Among Adults

Some recent studies have shown that moderate drinkers (no more than two drinks per day if male, one if female) have less risk of developing heart disease than either people who don't drink at all or people who drink more than one or two drinks per day. However, although these studies show that alcohol consumption is not always bad for one's health, they are studies of adults—not young people. Recall that the younger a person starts drinking alcohol, the greater the risk of having alcohol-related health problems later in life. In addition, even if moderate drinking can improve some aspects of health, no medical or scientific organization recommends that you start drinking if you don't already drink. That's because of the many serious health risks associated with alcohol consumption. By way of emphasis, Utah, the U.S. state with the lowest alcohol consumption, also has the lowest rate of alcohol-related traffic deaths. Other factors may be involved, but the main reason is likely to be low alcohol consumption.

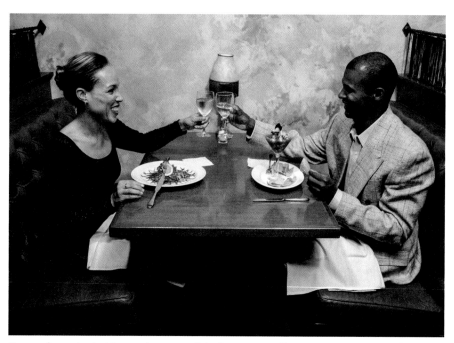

Even when alcohol is used responsibly, it can contribute excess empty calories to the diet.

Comprehension Check

1. What are two health problems associated with drinking alcohol?
2. How does alcohol affect males and females differently?
3. Explain the meaning of binge drinking.

SELF-ASSESSMENT: My Alcohol Knowledge

Answer *true* or *false* for the following questions. For a variation, compare your answers with those of a few friends or fellow students. See if you can all agree on the right answers.

1. Alcohol is a mood-altering stimulant.
   a. true
   b. false
2. Drinking coffee or taking a cold shower will sober a person up.
   a. true
   b. false
3. Alcohol's effects on the body vary according to the individual.
   a. true
   b. false
4. The most serious consequence of consuming alcohol is a hangover in the morning.
   a. true
   b. false
5. Blood alcohol charts that help you estimate your BAC based on your weight and the number of drinks that you had provide a safe and accurate means of determining how much alcohol is circulating in your bloodstream.
   a. true
   b. false
6. If an intoxicated person is semiconscious, you should encourage vomiting.
   a. true
   b. false
7. Women and men respond differently to alcohol.
   a. true
   b. false
8. Alcohol increases your sexual functioning.
   a. true
   b. false
9. If a person is passed out from drinking, he or she should be put in bed to "sleep it off."
   a. true
   b. false
10. The legal blood alcohol limit for driving for people under age 21 is 0.08 percent.
    a. true
    b. false

Here are the correct answers: 1 b, 2 b, 3 a, 4 b, 5 b, 6 b, 7 a, 8 b, 9 b, and 10 b. If you got nine or ten answers right, you're very knowledgeable about alcohol. If you got seven or eight right, you're above average in your knowledge. If you got six or fewer right, spend some time learning about alcohol to protect yourself and your family and friends.

Planning for Healthy Living

Use the Healthy Living Plan worksheet to help you avoid engaging in underage drinking or to stop drinking alcohol if you already do.

Lesson 32.2

Culture, Advertising, and the Law

Lesson Objectives

After reading this lesson, you should be able to

1. describe how alcohol is marketed and advertised to young people,
2. define *BAC* and *DUI* and explain the relationship between them, and
3. explain what an alcohol diversion program is.

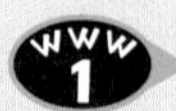

Lesson Vocabulary

addiction, alcopop, blood alcohol content (BAC), diversion program, DriveCam, driving under the influence (DUI), ignition interlock

In this lesson, you'll learn about alcohol advertising and how individual students and student groups have been and continue to be involved in alcohol issues. You'll also be introduced to programs that treat people who have alcohol problems, and you'll learn how modern technologies are used to help people with alcohol problems.

> "Water is the only drink for a wise man."
>
> —Henry David Thoreau

Alcohol and Popular Culture

For some reason, a culture has developed in the United States and other countries wherein many people believe that drinking is the best and perhaps only way to have fun. The fact is that most teens do not drink to excess, but the ones who do tend to be the most vocal. In addition, movies and TV shows often glorify drinking. It's a telling commentary that, according to Guinness World Records, the word *drunk* has more synonyms than any other word in the English language—more than 2,200! Clearly, then, the word is important in U.S. culture.

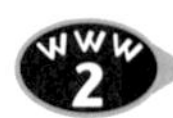

How many synonyms for *drunk* do you know? Since many of these terms strike many people as funny, they can suggest that being drunk has no negative consequences. As you've already learned, that is far from true. Even so, our slang has developed a bias toward a social, fun, and partying view of alcohol—much like alcohol advertising itself. What does it say about a culture when it spends so much time talking about drinking? American humorist Fran Lebowitz once said, "Great people talk about ideas, average people talk about things, and small people talk about wine." She made the statement in jest, but it does make one wonder about the overemphasis on alcohol in conversation, on television, in movies, and in advertising.

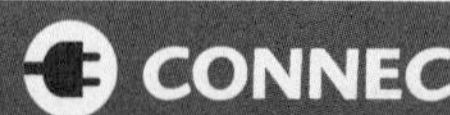

CONNECT

Do you think getting drunk is glamorized? Why or why not? What effect do you think social expectations have on your decision to drink alcohol or not? What other influences may play a role in your decision? Does advertising have much of an influence on you?

Advertising to Youth

For many years, alcohol advertising has been monitored by the Center on Alcohol Marketing and Youth (CAMY) at the Johns Hopkins Bloomberg School of Public Health. CAMY found that in 10 years, "youth exposure to alcohol advertising on U.S. television increased 71 percent . . . more than the exposure of either adults ages 21 and above or young adults ages 21 to 34." The center also noted that during the same time frame, alcohol advertising in magazines dropped dramatically. This is probably because young people have gravitated more to the Internet and less to magazines. Alcohol is also advertised on the radio through ads promoting **alcopops** (sweetened alcoholic beverages), distilled spirits, and wine. These ads are more likely to be heard by girls between the ages of 12 and 20 than by boys of the same age.

What about ads and public service announcements (PSAs) that deliver messages to counter underage alcohol use and alcohol abuse? It's true that messages such as "don't drink and drive" sometimes appear in alcohol advertising. But young people are 22 times more likely to see an ad promoting an alcohol product than one with a message like "drink responsibly." Furthermore, no definition of responsible drinking is given. As much as we don't like to admit it, advertising works—not just on others, but also on us—and alcohol advertising is all around us. It's not just in magazines, on the radio, on TV, on billboards, and in the in-store ads in grocery stores, convenience stores, and gas stations; it's also online and in product placement in movies.

The alcohol ads that have proven most effective at influencing young people use pitches aimed specifically at them. For example, they feature animals as lead characters and portray alcohol as providing instant gratification, thrills, and social status. In fact, according to most alcohol advertising, alcohol makes people more pleasing—to both themselves and others. Clearly, however, this is not true. In fact, people who binge-drink are more likely to damage property, get into arguments and fights, sexually assault someone, interrupt someone's sleep (as in a college dorm room), miss class, and do any number of other problematic things.

In addition to conventional advertising, alcohol is marketed to youth through products designed to appeal to young people. Consumer advocacy groups argue that companies use these products to intentionally—and illegally—target underage people and promote underage drinking. Of particular concern are sweet-flavored alcopop drinks such as hard lemon malt beverages and hard cola. These drinks often come in brightly colored packages that are attractive to young people. The combination of advertising and products designed to appeal to youth creates a powerful influence on underage drinking.

Alcohol Laws

Alcohol laws govern the sale, distribution, advertisement, and use of alcohol. Federal alcohol laws apply to everyone across the country; other alcohol laws vary by jurisdiction (city, county, or state). All of these laws govern where and when alcohol can be sold and when it can be consumed in public. For example, some states and local governments prohibit alcohol consumption in parks or on beaches. Others make it illegal for bars to sell alcohol after a given time (often 2 a.m.). Still others restrict or prohibit the sale of alcohol on Sundays. Open container laws make it illegal, as the name indicates, to have an open container of alcohol in certain areas, even if you're not actively drinking.

The consequences of breaking these laws vary by jurisdiction but can include fines, jail time, probation, suspension of driver's license, and the loss of a liquor license (e.g., in the case of stores and bars). In addition, schools and workplaces can enforce their own penalties for violation of their policies governing alcohol use.

Dangers of Caffeinated Alcoholic Beverages

When caffeine or another stimulant is mixed with alcohol, the combination can mask the depressant effects of alcohol, thus leading people to drink more. This is particularly dangerous because the stimulant does not reduce the underlying physiological effects of alcohol on the body. For a while, caffeinated alcoholic beverages (CABs) grew in popularity and were heavily marketed to teens and young adults. However, the risks associated with these drinks led the U.S. Food and Drug Administration to ban them. Teens and others who skirt this ban by combining energy drinks with alcohol put themselves at high risk of impaired judgment, alcohol poisoning, and other risks associated with excessive alcohol consumption.

Minimum Drinking Age Act

Despite the cultural influences and advertisements that promote drinking among teens, the National Minimum Drinking Age Act of 1984 makes it illegal to drink under the age of 21 anywhere in the United States (with the exception of parents being allowed to serve alcohol to their children in their own home). This law also makes it illegal to sell alcohol to minors or purchase alcohol for minors. In addition, laws in many states are getting stricter regarding adults who purchase alcohol for minors and for people who use fake identification cards to purchase alcohol. Punishment can include a large fine, probation, or jail time. If an adult purchases alcohol for a minor who is then seriously injured or dies due to an alcohol-related cause, the adult may receive a long jail sentence.

Alcohol and Driving

Laws also regulate the use of alcohol while driving for people of all ages. Currently, most states use a **blood alcohol content (BAC)** of 0.08 percent as the legal limit when driving for people ages 21 and over. For those under the age of 21, the BAC level is 0.02 percent in most places. It is not zero percent to allow for the use of some medications that contain alcohol. Blood alcohol content is the percentage of alcohol in the bloodstream. A BAC of 0.08 percent indicates that a person has 0.8 part alcohol per 1,000 parts of blood in the body. Because alcohol is absorbed directly through the walls of the stomach and small intestine, blood alcohol can be measured 30 to 70 minutes after a person has had a drink.

Table 32.2 summarizes the physiological and psychological effects of selected BAC levels. The table shows the BAC level at which each effect is usually first observed. Getting behind the wheel with a BAC above the legal limit is known as **driving under the influence (DUI)** or driving while intoxicated (DWI). Most deaths and injuries related to alcohol consumption result from vehicle crashes. According to the U.S. National Highway Traffic Safety Administration, more than 10,000 people died in alcohol-related crashes in 2009. Each year, one-third to one-half of these deaths occur in teens and young adults (under the age of 21).

Fortunately, recent years have brought decreases in both the total number of traffic deaths per mile driven and the number of alcohol-related crash deaths. Organizations such as Mothers Against Drunk Driving (MADD) have helped raise awareness and increase penalties for drinking and driving. In addition, roads and vehicles have become safer, and more people wear seat belts and use child safety seats. Despite these improvements, far too many alcohol-related traffic deaths still occur.

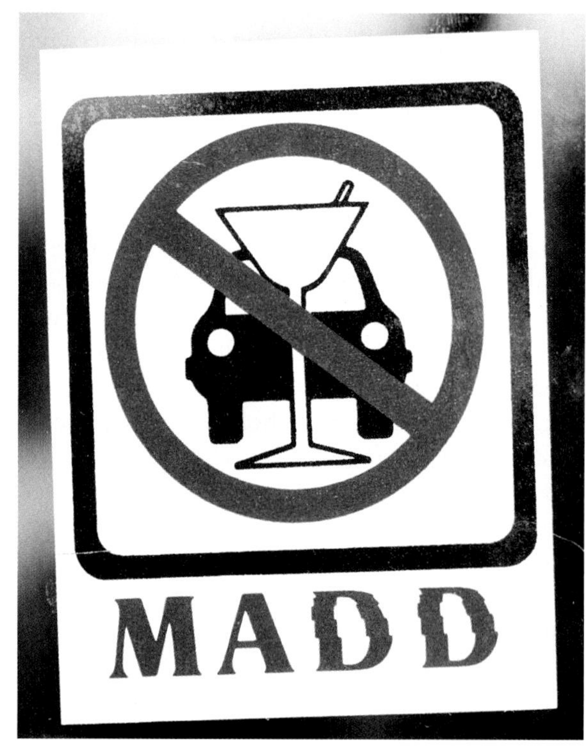

Mothers Against Drunk Driving is an organization that works to stop drunk driving.

Photodisc

School Policies and Youth Courts

Schools have their own policies governing students who consume alcohol before coming to school, during school, or at school events. These policies, and the associated punishments, vary from school to school and from school system to school system. Most schools maintain a student code of conduct that explains the behaviors expected of students.

TABLE 32.2 Psychological and Physical Effects of Selected Blood Alcohol Content (BAC) Levels

BAC	Typical effects	Predictable effects on driving
0.02	• Some loss of judgment • Relaxation • Slight body warmth • Altered mood	• Decline in visual functions (e.g., rapid tracking of a moving target) • Decline in ability to perform two tasks at the same time (divided attention)
0.05	• Exaggerated behavior • Possible loss of small muscle control (e.g., focusing the eyes) • Impaired judgment • Lowered alertness • Release of inhibition	• Reduced coordination • Reduced ability to track moving objects • Difficulty steering • Reduced response to emergency driving situations
0.08	• Poor muscle coordination (e.g., for balance, speech, vision, reaction time, hearing) • Impaired detection of danger • Impaired judgment, self-control, reasoning, and memory	• Reduced concentration • Short-term memory loss • Greatly reduced coordination • Reduced information-processing capability (e.g., signal detection, visual search) • Impaired perception
0.10	• Clear deterioration of reaction time and control • Slurred speech, poor coordination, and slowed thinking	• Reduced ability to maintain lane position and brake appropriately
0.15	• Far less muscle control than normal • Vomiting (unless this level is reached slowly or the person has developed a tolerance for alcohol) • Major loss of balance	• Substantial impairment in vehicle control, attention to driving task, and visual and auditory information processing

Reprinted, by permission, from Human Kinetics, 2009, *Health and wellness for life* (Champaign, IL: Human Kinetics), 398.

DIVERSE PERSPECTIVES: Alcoholism

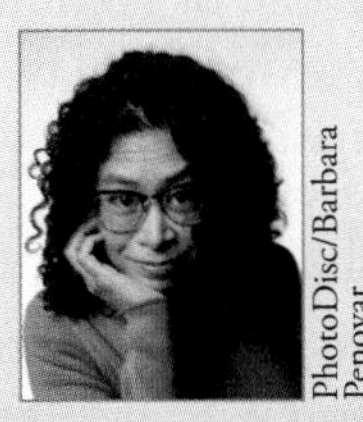

PhotoDisc/Barbara Penoyar

Hi. My name is Brenda, and I have always enjoyed alcohol. When I was single and in my early 20s, I would stay out late with my friends and would often drink until I passed out. Later on, after I was married and had a child of my own, I began to question my drinking habits. I noticed that I couldn't stop after just one glass of wine with dinner. I got to the point where I was having two drinks before my husband got home, then wine with dinner, and then I was sneaking into the kitchen after dinner for another round. One night, I drank so much that I passed out and cracked my head open. It was then that I realized I had to stop.

During the first year, learning how to live my life and get through big events like weddings and holidays without drinking was tough. I realized that life is hard, and getting and staying sober aren't easy. It was, and still is, a struggle. But my life is so much more interesting and adventurous now without drinking. I felt for years that I was anesthetized—numb. Today, I'm living in the moment. I feel my emotions, and I'm aware of everything with much more clarity. It's not boring—which is what you think life without alcohol must be when you're an alcoholic. I've learned the hard way that the opposite is actually true—it's exciting.

HEALTH TECHNOLOGY

Technological developments related to alcohol consumption include smartphone apps that can help people with various needs. Some, for example, help adult drinkers count their calories (people are often unaware of how many calories alcoholic beverages contain). Other apps can estimate an adult drinker's blood alcohol level based on height, weight, and what drinks he or she has consumed.

In addition, some auto insurance companies are offering driver cameras (one brand, for example, is called **DriveCam**) for use in cars driven by teenagers. These cameras monitor for erratic driving and send notifications to a parent's or guardian's computer. Some insurance companies even monitor the cameras themselves and raise the insurance rate if a teen driver often drives dangerously or erratically. Other companies leave it to parents and guardians to decide how to deal with bad driving.

Another form of technology that is growing in popularity is the **ignition interlock**, which tests the driver's BAC before allowing him or her to drive. This technology can be court-ordered for people who are found guilty of alcohol-related driving offenses. The device is installed in the vehicle at the offender's expense (usually about US$70 to US$100 per month, plus an installation fee of US$100 to US$200). Before the person can start the vehicle, he or she must breathe into the device, which determines the person's blood alcohol level. If it is above the legal limit, the car will not start. Some of the more sophisticated ignition locks include a camera to ensure that the proper person is blowing into the device. The intent, of course, is to keep people from driving under the influence of alcohol.

CONNECT

Do you think advanced technologies (e.g., apps or online calculators that estimate BAC) help prevent drinking and driving? Why or why not? Share your perspective with your peers. Identify the specific points where you agree and disagree.

Some schools also use student courts, in which students serve as judge, jury, prosecutor, and defense counsel under the supervision of adults. Students also decide on the punishment when a student is found guilty. For example, a student court might address a case in which a student is accused of bringing alcohol to school or providing it to other students. Student court systems are not, however, appropriate for dealing with very serious offenses such as an alcohol-related car crash or a fight that resulted in an injury. The most common forms of restitution ordered by student courts are community service, oral and written apologies, and written essays reflecting on one's behavior and discussing how one plans to change it. Student courts do not take the place of formal legal actions that may also be pursued against the offender.

Diversion Programs

In some U.S. jurisdictions, youth and sometimes other first-time offenders in alcohol-related cases have the option of attending classes (often led by a specially trained counselor) instead of receiving a large fine, being placed on probation, or spending time in jail. The offender has to pay for the classes, and young people may be required to attend the classes with a parent or guardian. In some programs targeting DUI offenses, an offender who successfully completes the course may be able to have the offense removed from his or her police record. If so, the person's car insurance costs may stay the same, whereas offenders who do not complete a **diversion program** usually face a substantial cost increase for their vehicle insurance.

Alcohol Dependence and Treatment

Some people who drink alcohol develop a physical dependence (**addiction**). They crave alcohol and don't feel right unless they drink it. What this means is that for some people, drinking gets out of control. They are alcoholics. Many programs are available to help people stop drinking. They include treatment centers, counseling, behavior modification, 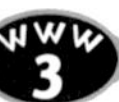 medication, an Alcoholics Anonymous (AA) group or other support group, and even technology (e.g., smartphone apps and text messages). Groups also exist to help family members and friends of problem drinkers; examples include Al-Anon and Alateen. These groups are self-help groups or support groups, in which people with similar problems work together to help each other. Group support offers help for people with alcohol addiction. People who have taken control of their own alcohol problems help others who are trying to quit. In AA, a person who helps another person is called a sponsor. Since the sponsor has experienced similar problems and challenges, he or she serves as a guide for the person who is trying to stop drinking. It is difficult to change addictive behavior. Whenever possible, problem drinkers should seek help from others and know their options. Your school counselor or school nurse can inform you about local groups that help people with alcohol problems as well as their family members and friends. Make no mistake about it, quitting drinking for an alcoholic is very difficult, but with the right treatment, people can and do overcome their addiction. Most alcohol treatment programs believe that alcoholics should completely refrain from drinking because if the person starts to drink even small amounts, the drinking is likely to escalate to out-of-control again.

Comprehension Check

1. Give one example of how alcohol is marketed and advertised to young people.
2. How are BAC and DUI related?
3. How does a diversion program work?

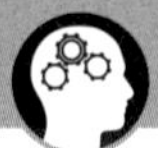

MAKING HEALTHY DECISIONS: Finding Social Support

Social support happens when people close to you, along with members of your community, support your positive health choices and encourage you to stick with them. You're more likely to stay on track when the people around you are supportive and encouraging.

Kerri has never had a drink of alcohol. Next week, she turns 21, and all of her friends are planning a big party for her at a local bar. Kerri is excited about celebrating her birthday with friends but doesn't want things to get out of control. She's curious about alcohol but also knows that she may be easily affected by it. Her mom struggled with alcoholism for years, and Kerri sees how hard it is for her to stay sober. Most of Kerri's friends have already turned 21, and many of them drink on a regular basis. One of the girls in the group drinks only once in a while because she doesn't want the extra calories in her diet. Kerri respects her friends' choice to drink but still isn't sure she wants to start down that road.

Ted is a popular guy at school, and as a student-athlete he attracts a lot of like-minded people. However, while almost all of his friends are physically active and eat well, they like to celebrate their victories on the field by drinking. Neither Ted nor any of his friends are of legal age to drink. Ted's older brother Matt is a pretty heavy drinker, and he has no problem supplying Ted and his buddies with alcohol when their parents are out of the house. At the last celebration, things got a little out of hand, and one of Ted's buddies passed out. Though this caused Ted a lot of anxiety and stress, his brother said it was no big deal, and his buddies blamed it on not eating enough while they were drinking. Ted is pretty worried about how much everyone is drinking now, but no one else seems to share his concern.

Kerri and Ted both need social support but for different reasons. Kerri needs to be supported in making a decision that might differ from the decision most of her friends make. Ted needs to be supported in his wish to keep his own and his buddies' behavior under control.

For Discussion

How might Kerri approach getting the support she needs? Who in her life might give her the best social support? Why? What should Ted do to build up his social support structure so that he can change his behavior and maybe help others as well? What are some long-term consequences for Kerri and Ted if they fail to get the social support they need in life? To guide your thinking about these questions, use the Skills for Healthy Living feature.

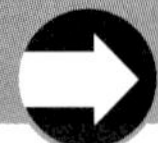

SKILLS FOR HEALTHY LIVING: Finding Social Support

The ability to find and use a strong social support system helps you engage in healthy behaviors and avoid unhealthy ones. Social support has been shown to increase positive behaviors (e.g., physical activity, healthy eating) and prevent negative behaviors (e.g., smoking, alcohol abuse). Use the following guidelines to help you find and make use of strong social support.

- **Assess your current level of social support.** A key first step is to become aware of your existing social support structure. Make a list of your closest friends and relatives and the groups you belong to. Rate each person or group on your list as either a positive or a negative influence on your health.
- **Set goals.** If you don't already have strong social support, set some goals to help you improve it. For example, do some research or clubs or other groups that include people who engage in the healthy behavior you're trying to adopt, then attend a meeting or gathering.
- **Find friends with similar interests and values.** People with common interests can help make positive lifestyle choices easier and more enjoyable. For example, if you want to quit drinking, spend more time with your nondrinking friends while

you're working to quit. If you want to become more active, find friends who enjoy the same physical activities that you do and make plans to do the activities together.

- **Start your own club or team.** If you can't find a club or group that supports your needs, consider creating your own. Chances are good that others share your interest and can provide you with new forms of social support.
- **Talk about your interests.** Letting others know what you like can help you attract like-minded friends. Speak up when you're given a chance to share about yourself. If you like working out or eating a healthy diet, share that information during class discussions or activities, or make it a clear part of your social media communications.
- **Encourage others to join you.** If you want to make a change and stick with it, create a group challenge related to the activity. For example, set a healthy goal and see who can reach it first. Friendly competition can go a long way toward giving you the social support you need.

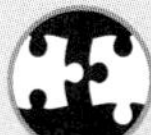

ACADEMIC CONNECTION: Mathematical Conversions

The metric system is most often used as the system of measurement in scientific research, including health and fitness research. To understand measures in the metric system or to compare data expressed using the metric system to data expressed using U.S. customary units (pounds, inches), you need to be able to calculate conversions. A conversion is a change or transformation. When converting measures, you will multiply the original value by a known factor to get the desired value. For example, if 1 kilogram is equivalent to 2.2 pounds, you would need to multiply the weight in kilograms by a factor of 2.2 to get the equivalent weight in pounds. Following are some commonly used factors for metric to U.S. customary units. If a research study suggested that a person who weighs 65 kilograms suffered a decrease in motor function after consuming 200 milliliters of wine, would you be able to convert that finding to pounds and ounces?

Multiply	By factor of	To find
Milliliters	.0353	fluid ounces
Kilograms	2.2046	pounds
Meters	3.2808	feet
Meters	39.37	inches

Are Americans Set Up to Become Alcoholics?

Different societies not only have different beliefs and rules about drinking, but they also show very different outcomes when people do drink (see table 32.3). For example, societies where daily drinking is the norm may have a higher rate of cirrhosis and other medical problems but fewer accidents, fights, homicides, or other violent alcohol-associated traumas. This may be because drinking itself is socially acceptable but drunkenness is not. Similarly, a culture that views drinking as a ritually significant act is not likely to develop many alcohol-related problems.

"One striking feature of drinking . . . is that it is essentially a social act," says Professor Kaufman, a social anthropologist specializing in the societal aspects of alcohol use. "The solitary drinker, so dominant an image in relation to alcohol in the United States, is virtually unknown in other countries. The same is true among tribal and peasant societies everywhere. In Italy, in contrast to America, drinking is institutionalized as part of family life and dietary and religious custom; alcohol (wine) is introduced early in life, within the context of the family, and as a traditional accompaniment to meals and a healthful way of enhancing the diet." Alcohol consumption is determined by many factors, such as social rules and expectations, customs and traditions, family history and beliefs, and religious beliefs.

"Such an approach to the socialization of alcohol use makes it less likely that drinking will be learned as a way of trying to solve personal problems or of coping with inadequacy and failure," says Randall Jessep, a social psychologist at a leading U.S. university.

For Discussion

What factors do you think contribute most to how a young person in America learns to use, abuse, or not use alcohol? Do you think our society promotes the responsible use of alcohol? Why or why not?

TABLE 32.3 Deaths From Alcohol Consumption per 100,000 People in Selected Countries

Rank	Country	Deaths per 100,000	Rank	Country	Deaths per 100,000
1	Turkey	0.0	6	Somalia	1.4
2	Italy	0.2	7	United States	1.6
3	Costa Rica	0.5	8	Kazakhstan	3.0
4	Kenya	0.7	9	Germany	3.8
5	United Kingdom	1.1	10	France	4.0

CHAPTER REVIEW

Reviewing Concepts and Vocabulary

As directed by your teacher, answer items 1 through 5 by correctly completing each sentence with a word or phrase.

1. Two natural physiological responses to drinking that protect people from acute alcohol poisoning are ____________ and ________ ________.
2. A device that lets others monitor your driving is called a(n) ____________.
3. When a person who drinks alcohol regularly over a long time no longer gets the same effect from drinking the same amount, she or he has developed a ________________.
4. Alcohol has a ________________ effect on the brain.
5. The English word with the most synonyms is __________.

For items 6 through 10, as directed by your teacher, match each term in column 1 with the appropriate phrase in column 2.

6. BAC	a. driving with too much alcohol in the blood
7. DUI	b. consuming a large amount of alcohol in a short time
8. binge drinking	c. a person with an addiction to alcohol
9. heavy drinking	d. the concentration of alcohol in the blood
10. alcoholic	e. consuming more than one drink (females) or two drinks (males) each day

For items 11 through 15, as directed by your teacher, respond to each statement or question.

11. Identify two things that make underage drinking unhealthy or dangerous.
12. What are two possible complications of drinking while pregnant?
13. How is drinking related to obesity in adults?
14. Name two treatments for alcohol dependence.
15. How is a diversion program for teen alcohol offenders different than going through the court system?

Thinking Critically

Write a paragraph in response to the following questions.

Alcohol use has some known health benefits among adults and is part of many social experiences. It also poses significant risks to individuals and society. Do you think society does a good job of balancing the benefits and risks of alcohol use? If you could change one thing about society's treatment of alcohol, what would it be? Why?

Take It Home

Have a discussion with your parents or guardians about their perspectives on drinking alcohol. What rules or expectations do they apply to themselves in regard to drinking? What expectations do they have for you, both now and as you approach the legal drinking age? Do their own experiences influence their thinking on this topic? Write a summary of what you learn; include your own response to their perspectives.

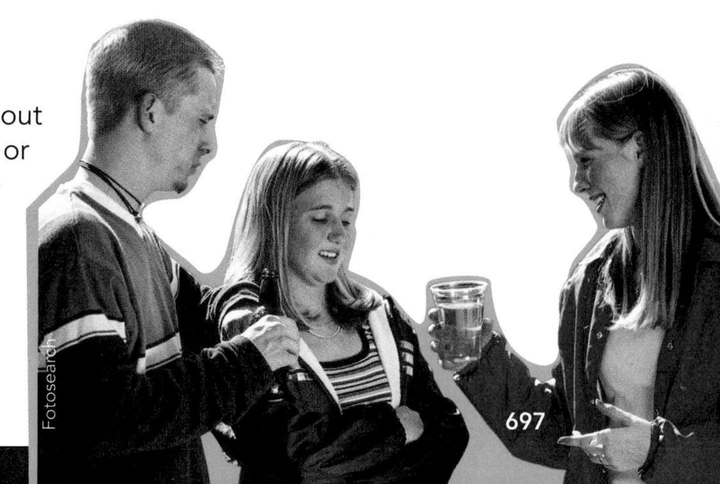

Fotosearch

33

Drugs and Medicine

In This Chapter

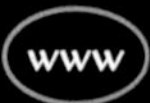

Student Web Resources

www.HOPEtextbook.org/student

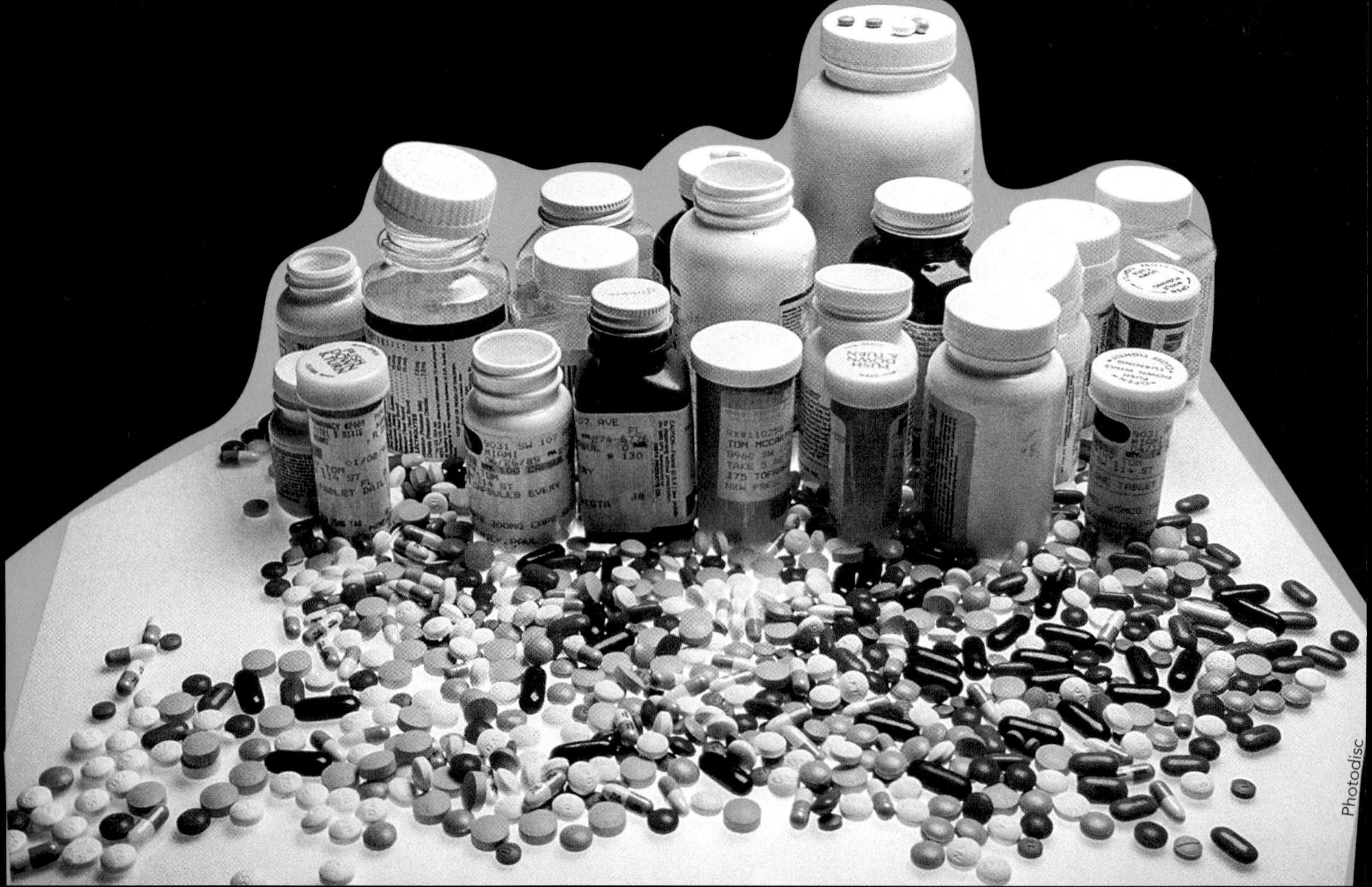

Photodisc

Lesson 33.1

Drug Classifications and Illicit Drugs

Lesson Objectives

After reading this lesson, you should be able to

1. explain what drug schedules are and what information they provide,
2. understand factors that contribute to illicit drug use, and
3. name examples of illicit drugs and identify the risks associated with each one.

Lesson Vocabulary

drug addiction, drug dependence, drug tolerance, illicit drug, licit drug, opiates, patent medicine, psychoactive drugs, withdrawal

In this chapter, you'll explore the roles that **licit** (legal) and **illicit** (illegal) **drugs** play in society. This first lesson focuses on the history of drug use in the United States and how drugs are classified based on their safety and effectiveness. It includes information about illegal drugs.

> "Let food be thy medicine and medicine be thy food."
>
> —Hippocrates

History

As with alcohol and tobacco, drug use and abuse have been around almost as long as people have existed. Aztec priests, for example, used drugs for various ceremonies, and Incas used coca plant extracts in their religious ceremonies to build group togetherness. You may have read about Native American tribes passing the "peace pipe" or calumet, which contained tobacco. However, even though some people had religious or spiritual experiences under the influence of certain drugs, they did not use these drugs recreationally, meaning just for fun, as many people do now in the United States.

In the early days of the United States, drugs were not regulated by law. As a result, companies and so-called snake oil salesmen freely and openly sold **opiates** and cocaine products as cure-alls. The product's claims were, of course, too good to be true. Like a gambler who talks only about winnings and never about losses, snake oil salesmen talked only about the supposed positive effects of their products—not the possible addictive properties. They also didn't mention side effects or the fact that flawed self-treatment could delay proven treatments of the diseases or disorders from which their customers suffered.

As shown in figure 33.1, even something as common as Coca-Cola was originally sold as both a beverage and a tonic for "nervous affections." In fact, the first part of the name (Coca) refers to the coca plant—the same one that produces cocaine. The second part (Cola) refers to the kola nut, an extract of which is still an ingredient in Coca-Cola today.

The reality is that, in those bygone days, there was no effective treatment for many conditions. Even today, modern medicine cannot cure all ailments. Nevertheless, in the late 1800s, it became

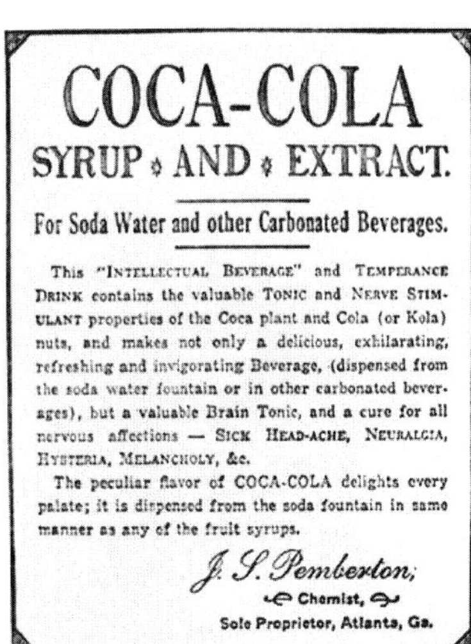

FIGURE 33.1 An early advertisement for Coca-Cola.

obvious that some of the **patent medicines** (i.e., nonprescription proprietary drugs) just described were worse than the conditions they were promoted as treating. As a result, the Pure Food and Drug Act was passed in the United States in 1906. The intent of this law was to protect the public from tainted or otherwise unsafe food and drug products. In 1930, these protections were expanded with the creation of the U.S. Food and Drug Administration (FDA).

Drug Classifications

To regulate drugs, the FDA, along with the U.S. Drug Enforcement Administration (DEA), assigns each drug to one of five categories or schedules (see table 33.1). The higher the schedule number, the less dangerous the drug is considered to be. For example, drugs included in schedule I are considered very dangerous and not suited for medical use. Schedule V drugs, on the other hand, have little potential for abuse but may be useful in treating certain medical conditions. Drug schedules are used to determine which drugs should require a prescription, which should be available over the counter, and which are illegal.

As with many other aspects of drug use and regulation, the schedule system is the subject of some controversy. For example, marijuana is listed in schedule I, which means that the DEA and FDA view it as having no medical value. Nevertheless, many states and the District of Columbia have enacted laws to make medical marijuana legal by prescription. Adding to the confusion, these differences pit state laws against federal laws.

Illicit Drugs

Illegal drugs are generally referred to as illicit drugs. These are the drugs that you are most likely to see depicted on TV shows and in movies—for example, heroin, cocaine, and methamphetamine (meth). In the United States, some laws governing illicit drugs

TABLE 33.1 Definitions of Controlled Substance Schedules

Schedule and definition	Examples
Schedule I Substances in this schedule have no currently accepted medical use in the United States, a lack of accepted safety for use under medical supervision, and a high potential for abuse.	Heroin, LSD, marijuana, Ecstasy
Schedule II Substances in this schedule have a high potential for abuse which may lead to severe psychological or physical dependence (addiction).	Oxycodone (OxyContin, Percocet), morphine, opium, codeine, amphetamines, methylphenidate (Ritalin)
Schedule III Substances in this schedule have a potential for abuse less than substances in schedules I or II. Abuse may lead to moderate or low physical dependence (addiction) or high psychological dependence.	Combination products containing less than 15 mg of hydrocodone per dosage unit (Vicodin) and products containing not more than 90 mg of codeine per dosage unit (Tylenol with Codeine)
Schedule IV Substances in this schedule have a low potential for abuse relative to substances in schedule III.	Alprazolam (Xanax), clorazepate (Tranxene), diazepam (Valium), lorazepam (Ativan), midazolam (Versed)
Schedule V Substances in this schedule have a low potential for abuse relative to substances listed in schedule IV and consist primarily of preparations containing limited quantities of certain narcotics.	Cough preparations containing not more than 200 mg of codeine per 100 ml or per 100 g (Robitussin AC, Phenergan with Codeine)

In the United States, drugs and other controlled substances are categorized into five schedules under the Controlled Substances Act (CSA).

From www.deadiversion.usdoj.gov/schedules/#define.

are federal (national), whereas others vary from state to state. These laws make it illegal not only to use certain drugs but also to give illegal drugs (or your own prescription drugs) to another person, to manufacture or grow illegal drugs, to sell or buy illegal drugs, or to possess illegal drugs.

Using or distributing illicit drugs not only poses potential legal and health problems; there is also a good chance that an illegal, or "street," drug does not contain what the buyer intends to obtain. Studies have found that street drugs are often "cut" with dangerous substances or replaced by other drugs. For example, cocaine has been found to be cut with substances such as flour, powdered milk, ground drywall, rat poison, and battery acid. As a result, if a user has an adverse reaction (bad experience) with the drug, emergency room staff will not know how to treat the person properly because they don't know what drug, or poison, the person has ingested.

Risks of Illicit Drugs

Illicit drug use poses many other dangers. For one thing, loss of inhibition can lead a person to take risks that he or she normally wouldn't take—for example, engaging in risky sexual behavior (which might result in pregnancy or a sexually transmitted infection), driving while impaired, getting in a car with someone who is impaired, taking other drugs, and sharing infected needles. Illicit drugs also carry other physical and emotional health risks; for some examples, see table 33.2. Teens who use illegal drugs have most likely obtained them from friends or siblings.

TABLE 33.2 Some Illicit Drugs and Their Risks

Drug	Short-term risks	Long-term risks
Cocaine	Euphoria; increased energy; chatty; anxiety; tremors; mentally alert to sights, sounds, and touch; irregular heartbeats	Headaches; irregular heartbeats; chest pains; heart attack; stomach pain; nausea; stroke; seizures
Ecstasy	Euphoria; increased energy; alertness and tactile sensitivity; anxiety; increased or irregular heartbeat; dehydration; chills; sweating; impaired cognition and motor function; reduced appetite; muscle cramping; teeth grinding; muscle breakdown; death	High risk for people with cardiovascular disease; dehydration leading to liver and kidney failure; disturbing emotional reactions, confusion, depression, sleep problems, anxiety, and heart palpitations; toxic to the brain; impairs memory; possibly brain damage
Heroin	Euphoria; warm flushing of skin; dry mouth; heavy feeling in extremities; clouded thinking; alternating wakeful and drowsy states; itching; nausea; depressed respiration	Addiction; physical dependence; collapsed veins and abscesses from injecting; infection of heart lining and valves; arthritis and other rheumatologic problems; HIV; hepatitis C
LSD	Elation; depression; arousal; paranoia; panic; impulsive behavior; rapid shifts in emotion; distortions in perception; increased body temperature, heart rate, and blood pressure; nausea; loss of appetite; sweating; dry mouth; jaw clenching; numbness; sleeplessness; dizziness; weakness; tremors	Frightening flashbacks; hallucinogens; addiction (low potential); tolerance
Methamphetamine	Enhanced mood; stimulant effect of increased heart rate, blood pressure, body temperature, energy, and activity; decreased appetite; dry mouth; increased sexuality; jaw clenching	Addiction; memory loss; weight loss; impaired cognition; insomnia; anxiety, irritability; confusion; paranoia; aggression; mood disturbances; hallucinations; violent behavior; liver, kidney, and lung damage; severe dental problems; cardiac and neurological damage; HIV; hepatitis

From drugabuse.gov.

Drug use can also result in **drug dependence**, which means a person needs a drug in order to function. A person with drug dependence typically exhibits signs and behavior changes such as withdrawing from school activities, being easily aggravated, and being physically sloppy and unclean (see figure 33.2). **Drug addiction**, on the other hand, is the compulsive use of a substance despite negative or dangerous effects. A person can be physically dependent on a substance without being addicted to it.

Addiction often includes **drug tolerance**—needing an increasingly high dose to attain the same effect. And, of course, once a person is addicted to a drug, he or she must also deal with emotional and physical **withdrawal** symptoms when quitting the drug (see figure 33.3).

Despite all of the possible dangers of using illicit drugs, millions of Americans do use them, including a significant proportion of teens (see figure 33.4). For some reason, people often believe they will experience only the positive aspects of drug use—that the negative aspects will happen only to other people. However, just as many people don't know they have an allergy until they use a certain substance or eat a certain food, there is no way to know how any

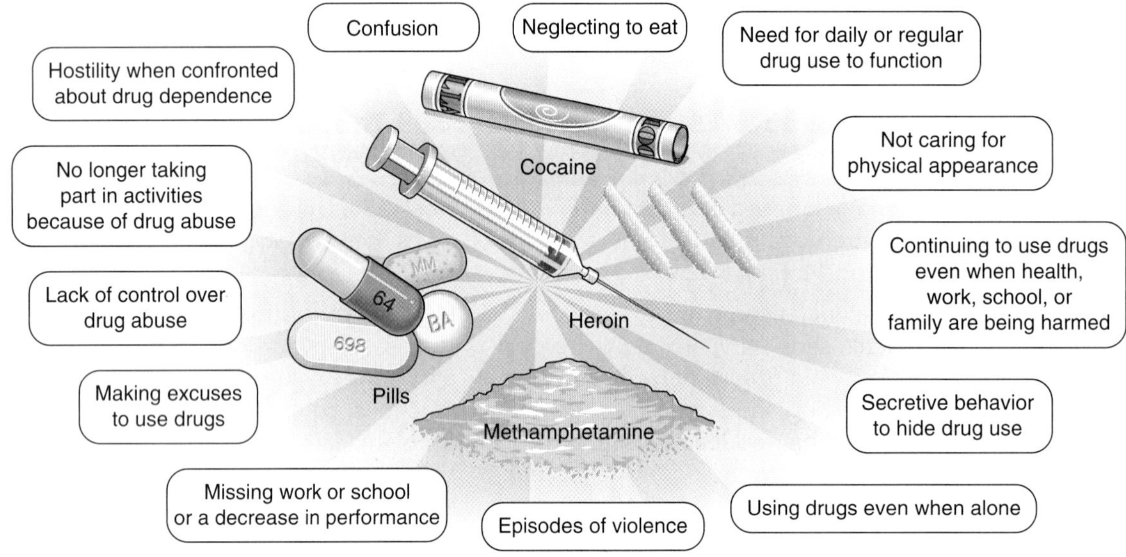

FIGURE 33.2 Symptoms and behaviors of drug dependence.

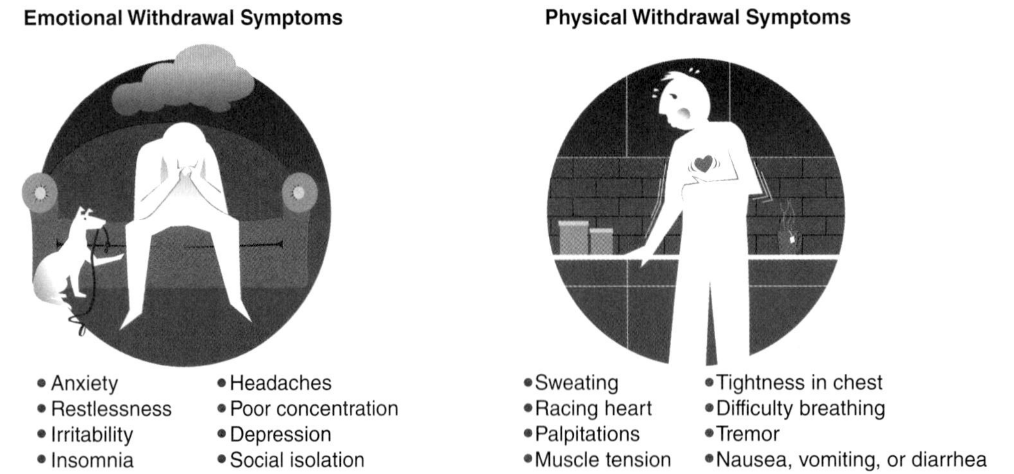

FIGURE 33.3 Emotional and physical symptoms of withdrawal.

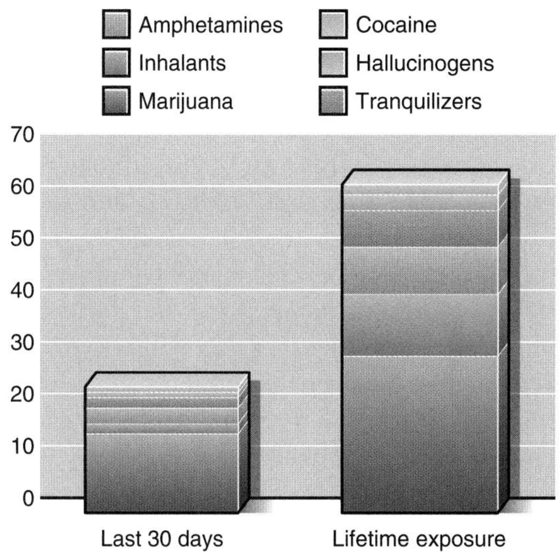

FIGURE 33.4 Percentage of teens reporting illicit drug use.

given person will respond to a specific drug, dosage, or mixture of drugs and alcohol until it happens. As you'll see in the next lesson, this is also true of prescription and over-the-counter drugs.

Marijuana

For marijuana, laws are changing so fast in many states that it is difficult to say what the legal status of marijuana is for adults. There are no states or organizations—even the National Organization for the Reform of Marijuana Laws (NORML)—that advocate for marijuana use by young people not suffering from disease. Of course, the marijuana laws are changing because there are disagreements, even among experts, about the medical value of marijuana. Some people believe that the possible harms from marijuana use are less than already legal drugs (e.g., tobacco and alcohol for adults). Numerous states have legalized marijuana for certain medical conditions like treating the symptoms of cancer and for the nausea that chemotherapy might cause. Some people believe the use of marijuana should be a personal choice for adults. Others argue that marijuana has not been subjected to the rigorous testing that is required by other drugs to be approved by the FDA. The American Medical Association is against the legalization of marijuana.

As you read earlier in this chapter, marijuana is still classified as a schedule I drug, meaning that the FDA and the DEA haven't taken it out of the category that is considered *not for medical use*. Colorado was the first state to legalize the recreational use of marijuana by adults. This law comes with provisions about taxation and who can be licensed to sell marijuana. Since this law started on January 1, 2014, it is hard to see what the advantages and disadvantages will be, both short term and long term. The inhalation of smoke on a regular basis and over a long period of time is not good for the lungs and the rest of the respiratory system. The chapter on tobacco pointed out the hazards of tobacco smoke. Less is known about the long-term effects of ingesting marijuana.

Suffice it to say that marijuana is not suitable for use by young people. Their bodies are still growing and developing and should not be exposed to any known or unknown harms that marijuana use can cause.

Drug Use to Enhance Performance

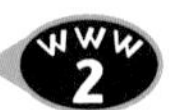

As discussed in this book's chapter on emotional health and wellness, muscle dysmorphia is a condition in which a person sees one's own body very differently from its actual appearance. As a result, the person may resort to using steroids or other substances to gain muscle mass. Bulking up in this way to look more muscular or gain a performance advantage is tempting to many athletes, but it is also dangerous, illegal, and unethical. Most people agree that taking performance-enhancing drugs violates the spirit of good sporting behavior—sort of like having a secret motor in a sailboat race. It's just not fair, and it's not right. The Olympics and most sport organizations have strict rules against the use of performance-enhancing drugs such as steroids.

HEALTHY COMMUNICATION

Do you think marijuana use is more or less dangerous than cigarette smoking? Write a summary (one paragraph to one page long) of your answer; support your position with facts.

Why Do People Use Illicit Drugs?

Drugs occurring in nature (e.g., in plants or animals) were probably originally consumed by accident a long time ago. Someone ate the bark of a tree; accidentally ingested mold in a food item; or picked up a frog, thus getting a certain substance on his or her hand, and later put the hand in his or her mouth—and as a result experienced an altered state of consciousness. Many people in various cultures viewed such experiences as supernatural, allowing them to talk to the gods (many ancient people believed in many gods).

We now know that most **psychoactive drugs** distort people's judgment. These are generally the drugs that people take for thrill seeking, consciousness raising (i.e., people believe they have special insights into the meaning of life), or mood elevation. People who take psychoactive drugs may think they are stronger, braver, or more intelligent, but to outside observers this is not so. Still, some people are attracted to the prospect of an altered state of consciousness, and drugs offer a relatively easy—but often unsafe—way to experience it.

Many factors are known to influence a person's likelihood of using illicit drugs. For example, there is a strong connection between drug use and mental illness, especially for people with depression, bipolar disorder, anxiety disorder, and schizophrenia.

Young people often feel invincible and believe that bad things happen to other people but not to them. These types of beliefs may contribute to risky behavior. In addition, young people may be tempted to take "dares" thinking that they will be perceived as weak if they don't do something dangerous for the benefit of impressing their friends. People are also more likely to use drugs if they have easy access to drugs, their parents use drugs, they have low self-esteem, they are in stressful economic or emotional circumstances, or they live in a culture with high acceptance of drug use. The main reason that teens in the United States try illegal drugs is to help them deal with the pressures of school. The second reason is related to low self-esteem or to enhance social acceptance, according to a study by Partnership for a Drug-Free America.

Some people think that the attraction of drugs is similar to the lure of magic potions described in fairy tales. People may believe that a substance can make them happier, more beautiful, stronger, more likable, thinner, or more lovable. Drugs are also sometimes used to provide a temporary sense of escape or for producing the sensations and feelings they bring. In other words, people often look for external solutions to their problems rather than working to solve problems internally. This book's stress management chapter discusses the fact that people can learn to alter their consciousness without drugs—for example, through mindfulness techniques or yoga. Although it may take longer to solve problems internally, the resulting solutions

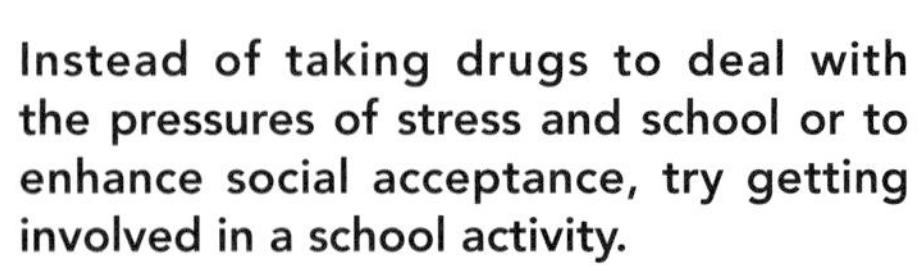

Instead of taking drugs to deal with the pressures of stress and school or to enhance social acceptance, try getting involved in a school activity.

Getty Images/DAJ

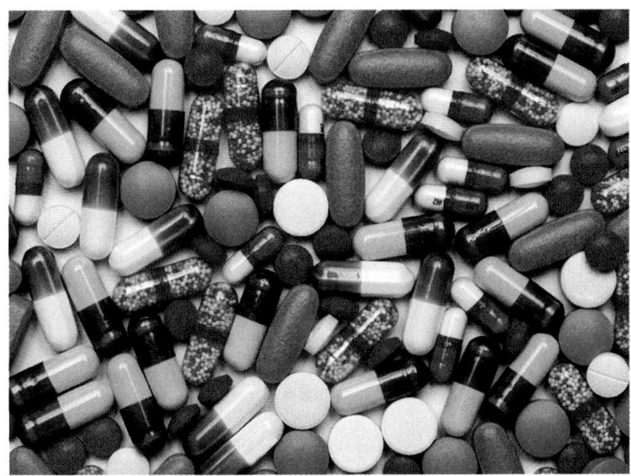

There are no magic potions to solve all of our problems.
Photodisc

are more likely to be more permanent, and they are certainly healthier.

You may have heard of famous artists who used drugs and even attributed some of their creativity to their drug use. But drugs do not teach people how to play a musical instrument, write a book, or be a good actor or dancer. Talented people practice their art over and over. Alcohol and drugs didn't make Amy Winehouse or Whitney Houston great singers or make Michael Jackson a great singer and dancer. In fact, drugs made it harder for them to perform and ultimately contributed to their deaths. Unfortunately, people who are dependent on drugs may deceive themselves into thinking that the drugs are essential to their performance. Add to this the addictive nature of drugs, and it's easy to explain why some people keep taking more and more drugs despite the risk of disease, injury, and death.

CONNECT

Do you think famous people (e.g., singers, actors) are more likely to use and abuse drugs than the rest of us? Why or why not? What aspects of society might contribute to drug use and abuse? Are these factors more prevalent among famous people? Discuss your perspective with your peers. Support your perspective with facts and respect each other's opinions.

Comprehension Check

1. Explain what the different levels of drug schedules represent.
2. Give two reasons why people use illegal drugs.
3. Aside from the toxic effect of illegal drugs, name another safety concern about street drugs.

✓ SELF-ASSESSMENT: My Drug Knowledge

Your knowledge about drugs and medicine can help you make informed decisions and stay safe. Use the following self-assessment to help you get a sense of your drug knowledge. Answer each question with the best choice.

1. Using cocaine can result in which of the following?
   a. anxiety and tremors
   b. irregular heartbeat
   c. high energy
   d. all of these
2. The Aztecs used drugs in religious ceremonies.
   a. true
   b. false
3. It is illegal in the U.S. to take a prescription drug prescribed for someone else.
   a. true
   b. false
4. A person is at greater risk of abusing drugs if a parent has abused drugs.
   a. true
   b. false
5. What is the number one reason why U.S. teens say they *begin* using alcohol or drugs?
   a. pressured by their peers
   b. influenced by the media
   c. the pressures and stress of school
   d. anxious, depressed, or stressed
6. The original Coca-Cola product contained extracts from which of the following?
   a. coca leaves
   b. the opium poppy
   c. malt and barley
   d. none of these
7. Which of the following best defines a psychoactive drug?
   a. a drug used to treat infections
   b. a drug that only comes from natural sources
   c. a drug that causes mood elevation
   d. a drug that has no active ingredient
   e. none of these
8. What does it mean when a person has developed a tolerance to a drug?
   a. she is addicted
   b. the drug makes her sick
   c. over time she requires more of the drug to produce the original effect
   d. her habit has been broken

9. Which of the following is not a common reason why people use illegal drugs?
   a. living in a culture where drug use is common
   b. curiosity
   c. social pressure
   d. its category on the DEA and FDA drug schedule
   e. none of these
10. More than half of sports governing organizations approve of performance enhancing drugs.
   a. true
   b. false

Here are the correct answers: 1 d, 2 a, 3 a, 4 a, 5 c, 6 a, 7 c, 8 c, 9 d, and 10 b. If you got nine or ten questions right, you're very knowledgeable about drug issues. If you got seven or eight right, you're above average in your knowledge. If you got six or fewer right, spend some time learning about drugs to help protect yourself and your family and friends.

✓ Planning for Healthy Living

Use the Healthy Living Plan worksheet to help you prevent drug use now and in your future or to help you stop or gain control over existing drug use.

Lesson 33.2

Prescription and Over-the-Counter Drugs

Lesson Objectives

After reading this lesson, you should be able to

1. identify the three types of prescription drugs that are most commonly abused,
2. explain the risks associated with misuse of over-the-counter drugs, and
3. explain what the acronym SAFER stands for.

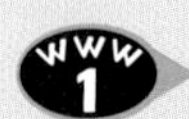

Lesson Vocabulary

depressants, over-the-counter (OTC) drug, prescription drug, stimulants

Drug abuse doesn't occur only with illicit drugs. In fact, the misuse and abuse of both prescription and over-the-counter medications is a growing concern in the United States. This lesson gives you information about prescription and over-the-counter medications, including guidelines for safe use and the risks associated with misuse.

> Always laugh when you can, it is cheap medicine.
>
> —George Gordon Byron

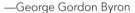

Prescription Drugs

The purpose of **prescription drugs** is to help people treat illnesses or symptoms, such as pain and discomfort. The differences between prescription drugs and over-the-counter drugs are summarized in table 33.3. Prescription drugs have helped millions of people suffering from a wide range of diseases and disorders, and they have saved millions of lives, but no drug is free of potentially harmful side effects. A prescription should always do more good than harm; if it doesn't, it should be discontinued or replaced by a different one.

Prescription drugs can also be abused, particularly when they are used for nonmedical purposes. According to the U.S. National Institute on Drug Abuse (NIDA), about 12 million Americans used prescription drugs for nonmedical (i.e., recreational) reasons in 2010. The most commonly misused and abused prescription drugs are called opiates (used for pain relief), central nervous system **depressants** (used to treat anxiety disorders and depression), and **stimulants** (used most often to treat ADHD).

Another issue is overdose from prescription drugs. It is estimated that 2 people die each day in the United States from a prescription drug overdose, and another 40 are admitted to emergency rooms

TABLE 33.3 Prescription Versus Over-the-Counter Drugs

Prescription	Over-the-counter
• Prescribed by a doctor • Bought at a pharmacy • Prescribed for and intended to be used by one person • Regulated by the U.S. Food and Drug Administration (FDA) through an application process requiring research data, analysis of the drug's behavior in the body, and information about how the drug is manufactured	• Doctor's prescription not needed • Bought off the shelf in stores • Regulated by the FDA through monographs (in effect, recipe books that cover acceptable ingredients, doses, formulations, and labeling and that are updated when ingredients change)

Drug Controversies

If you do even a little research, you'll find considerable disagreement about many drug-related issues in the United States—for example, current laws, drug classifications, punishment for drug offenders, whether FDA regulations are too strict or too lenient, whether certain drugs should be legalized, whether the "war on drugs" has been successful, and why there is so much demand for illegal drugs. One prime example is the ongoing debate over the legalization of marijuana; see the earlier section about marijuana. Despite these debates, there is widespread agreement that drugs can be harmful and that we need to be careful to ensure the health and safety of all people.

with life-threatening conditions. Both of these problems may be made worse by the increasing availability of prescription drugs. NIDA notes that enough painkillers were prescribed in the United States to medicate every American adult around the clock for a month and that prescriptions for opiates and stimulants have increased steadily since 1991.

Blame for prescription abuse can be assigned to many factors: consumers themselves, ineffective tracking systems, illegal sources, and improper prescribing, to name a few. Experts are beginning to pay more attention to the misuse and abuse of prescription drugs. More studies are being done, and more conferences held, to address the problem.

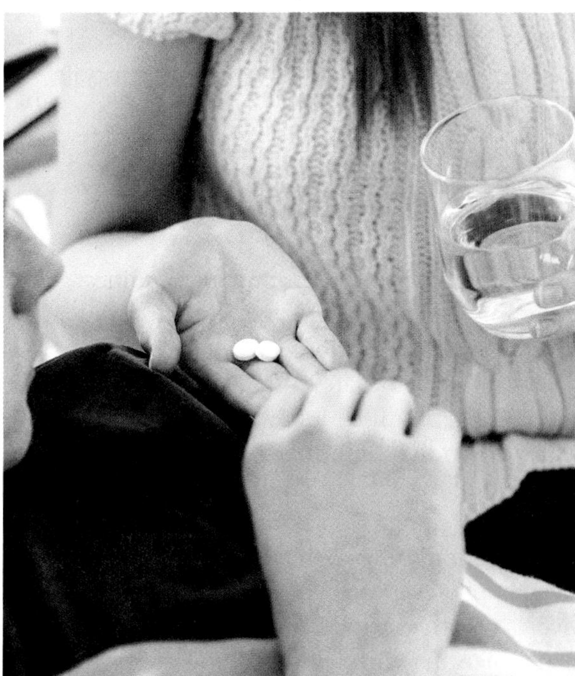

To help prevent problems with prescription drugs, always follow your doctor's instructions, and don't share your prescription or improvise on your dosage.

Although experts are far from solving the problem of prescription drug use, people can follow certain good practices to help prevent problems associated with prescription drugs. First, remember that prescription drugs are intended to help people who have medical problems. Prescription drugs should not make people feel worse or be used for recreational purposes. The sidebar titled Guidelines for Taking Prescription Medicines presents some of the most important practices you can follow to prevent problems with prescription medicines.

Over-the-Counter Drugs

Over-the-counter (OTC) drugs are available on the shelf in stores, rather than by prescription, because they are less likely to cause harm and less likely to need close monitoring (see table 33.3). OTC drugs can be helpful in treating minor disorders, aches, and pains. They are generally indicated for short-term use, but that doesn't mean they can't be harmful. Any drug can be harmful if not taken for the intended purpose, according to the instructions provided, and in the recommended dosage.

Abuse of over-the-counter drugs is most common among teens between the ages of 13 and 16. Young people may experiment with OTC medicines to which they have access in the medicine cabinet at home. This type of experimentation may seem less harmful than abusing prescription drugs or using illicit drugs, but it carries real risks. It also often leads to the use and abuse of more addictive drugs. Table 33.4 identifies some of the most commonly abused OTC drugs and their risks.

Guidelines for Taking Prescription Medicines

1. Make sure you understand why your medicine has been prescribed.
2. Make sure you get complete instructions about how and when to take the medication. If you don't understand the instructions, ask your doctor or pharmacist to explain them in simpler terms.
3. Know the common side effects of your medicine. Ask your doctor or pharmacist to explain them. If you don't understand the wording on the package insert, ask the doctor or pharmacist to give you a printout in language that is easier to understand.
4. Always tell your doctor and pharmacist about any other medications (prescription or otherwise) that you take so they can account for any possible drug interactions.
5. Don't improvise on your dosage—if you start to feel better, don't stop taking the medication without consulting your doctor or pharmacist.
6. Don't share your prescription with anyone else. Doing so is dangerous and against the law.
7. Make sure the medication is current. Don't save old medications after they have expired. Many communities have prescription drug take-back events where you can drop off unused or expired drugs and they will be disposed of properly.
8. If you have to take more than one medication, develop a system for keeping track of them.
9. Find out whether your medication requires you to avoid or limit certain foods or beverages. If so, there will often be a warning on the bottle or package insert. That's not always the case, so you should ask your doctor or pharmacist to be sure.
10. Alcohol reacts badly with many of the most commonly prescribed drugs. Not only is it illegal for minors to consume alcohol (except in states where it is legal to consume it in your own home under the supervision of a parent or guardian), but it is also dangerous when consumed with many prescription drugs.

Fads and Fantasies

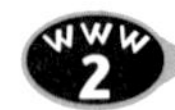

Drug use tends to go in social cycles, and the rise of social media (e.g., YouTube, Vimeo, Twitter, Facebook) enables fads to catch on faster and spread further than ever before. Fads range from drinking cough medicine to using newer, more exotic-sounding substances, such as bath salts, K2, and Spice. Some people even post online videos of drug use, such as taking "eyeball shots" of vodka, which does not get a person drunk but can permanently damage the eye. All of these practices can be very dangerous, but since people see them online or on TV shows, they tend to think of them as safe and even funny.

In fact, there seems to be no end to the various substances that some people will try to sell or convince others to use with the promise of happiness, bliss, enlightenment, or just plain fun. It would take several books to describe all of the fads and fantasies associated with the latest drug, but the usual pattern involves big promises, followed by experimentation, followed by disappointment (including adverse side effects), followed by the next fad that comes along.

Perhaps some people will always believe that a magic potion somewhere out there will make them live happily ever after. In reality, no substance can live up to this expectation in the long run, and experimenting with fad drugs often leads to use of even harder and more dangerous drugs—and to addiction.

As discussed in this book's stress management chapter, you can learn to safely alter your consciousness through practices such as mindfulness

TABLE 33.4 Commonly Misused Over-the-Counter (OTC) Drugs and Their Risks

Drug	Risks from heavy dosing or long-term use
Dextromethorphan This is the active ingredient in more than 100 cough and cold medicines (e.g., Robitussin, NyQuil). Ten percent of teens report abusing cough medicine to get high.	Impaired judgment, vomiting, loss of muscle movement, seizure, blurred vision, drowsiness, shallow breathing, fast heart rate, death (from large dose combined with alcohol or other drugs)
Pain relievers These medications (e.g., acetaminophen, ibuprofen) are sometimes taken in doses higher than recommended to try making them work faster.	Liver failure, stomach bleeding, kidney failure, cardiac risks
Caffeine medicines and energy drinks OTC caffeine pills (e.g., NoDoz), energy drinks (e.g., 5-hour Energy), and pain relievers with caffeine have all been abused for the buzz or jolt of energy they seem to impart.	Serious dehydration, gastric reflux, panic attacks, heart irregularities, accidental death (particularly in people with an underlying heart condition)
Diet pills In large doses, diet pills can create a mild buzz. Misuse of diet pills can also signal a serious eating disorder. Abuse of diet pills often starts with trying just a few in order to lose weight, but some OTC medicines and herbal preparations can be addictive.	Nervousness, tremor, digestive problems, hair loss, insomnia, anxiety, irritability, extreme paranoia, blurred vision, kidney problems, dehydration, rapid and irregular heartbeat, high blood pressure, stroke, heart failure, death
Laxatives and herbal diuretics (water pills) As with diet pills, some teens and young adults abuse these drugs in an attempt to lose weight. Examples include uva-ursi, goldenseal, dandelion root, and rose hip.	Serious dehydration; life-threatening loss of important minerals and salts that regulate the amount of water in the body, the acidity of the blood, and muscle function; physical dependence from long-term use of laxatives
Pseudoephedrine This substance is sought out to make the illegal drug methamphetamine. It has also been taken as a stimulant to cause an excitable, hyperactive feeling.	Heart palpitations, irregular heartbeat, heart attack, episodes of paranoid psychosis (when combined with other drugs, e.g., narcotics)
Herbal ecstasy This combination of inexpensive herbs is sold legally in pill form. It is swallowed, snorted, or smoked to produce euphoria, increased awareness, and enhanced sexual sensation.	Muscle spasm, increased blood pressure, seizure, heart attack, stroke, death

techniques. And as corny as it may sound, people *can* get high on life. The key is to focus on finding internal solutions to problems. People often ask the wrong questions. For example, if a person gets frequent headaches, she may ask herself, "What drug can I take to make the pain go away?" It's natural to want to relieve pain, but it's also necessary to get to the real cause of the problem. A good question to ask in this situation is "Why do I have so many headaches?" Depending on the cause, the person might find relief by exercising, practicing a stress management technique, or eliminating a certain food from the diet. Self-treating when you don't know the cause is unlikely to work.

Drug Treatment

Just as different drugs can affect different people in different ways, some treatments work for some people but not for others. As discussed in the chapters on tobacco and alcohol, it is difficult to overcome dependence or addiction. Drug addiction

CONSUMER CORNER: Selecting and Using Over-the-Counter Drugs

Over-the-counter drugs include a range of familiar medicines, such as aspirin, decongestants, antacids, NSAIDs (e.g., ibuprofen), sleep aids, and antihistamines. When purchasing OTC medications, you need to be a wise consumer. All OTC medications should be used only for their intended purpose, according to the directions provided, and in the recommended dosage. When buying and using OTC drugs, use the FDA's SAFER guidelines.

- **S**peak up (if the drug doesn't work or may be producing bad side effects).
- **A**sk questions (about what the drug can be expected to do).
- **F**ind the facts (ask your doctor or health care professional if he or she recommends this drug).
- **E**valuate your choices. (Is the OTC drug you want to buy the best way to treat your condition?)
- **R**ead the label (make sure this drug is appropriate for you and that it won't interact with any other drug you're taking).

Consumer Challenge

What are the main differences between prescription drugs and over-the-counter drugs? To help you research your answer, visit the student section of the Health Opportunities Through Physical Education website.

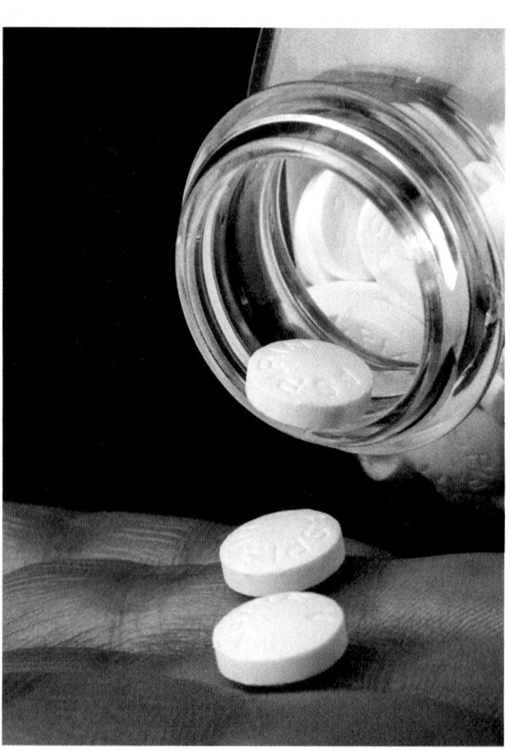

Use the SAFER guidelines when selecting and using OTC drugs.

Photodisc

is often recognized on the basis of the drug user developing a drug tolerance and thus craving more and more of the drug to get the same feeling. If the user is deprived of the drug, he or she goes through withdrawal, which (as discussed in this chapter's first lesson) can be emotional and physical. These are difficult problems to solve. Even if a person is not drug dependent or addicted, it can still be difficult to change or reverse a drug habit.

For people who are physically dependent or addicted, treatment can involve a range of responses, including counseling, medical intervention, behavior therapy, support groups (e.g., Narcotics Anonymous), and participation in a rehabilitation program. Some communities have drug courts in which minor drug offenders go through a program to help them stop using drugs instead of going to jail. Treatment can be complicated by dependence on more than one substance and by other medical problems. Despite these various challenges, hundreds of thousands of people in the United States have been able to return to a life free of drug dependence, misuse, and abuse. Of course, it is better to prevent drug problems than to have to treat them.

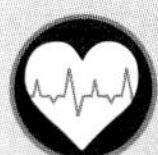

HEALTH TECHNOLOGY

Recovery from drug addiction is a challenging and continuing process. It is not uncommon for people to relapse during treatment or after active treatment ends. Could text messages help people who are recovering from drug dependence? Some researchers are experimenting with sending short messages to clients during and after their initial recovery. The messages are intended to encourage and motivate clients to continue their new, healthier behaviors.

Initial evaluations indicate that such text messaging may be helpful. In one study, Frederick Muench of the psychiatry department at Columbia University surveyed people in an addiction treatment program to find out what they wanted. He discovered that most of them wanted to receive text messages that, for example, recognized them for achieving milestones, such as a certain number of days clean. In addition, 96 percent wanted a friend to be notified (and 78 percent wanted a therapist to be notified) if they felt they were going to relapse. Overall, text messaging may help people who are recovering from drug addiction.

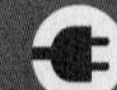

CONNECT

How might text messaging be a tool for helping people maintain positive behavior changes when recovering from drug or alcohol abuse? For promoting other healthy behaviors, such as exercise and healthy eating? Do you think you would ever subscribe to such a service? Why or why not?

Comprehension Check

1. What are two reasons why people misuse prescription drugs?
2. How can OTC drugs be harmful?
3. What government agency created the acronym SAFER to help people safely take OTC drugs and what does the S represent?

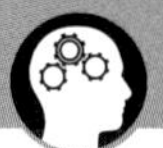

MAKING HEALTHY DECISIONS: Building Refusal Skills

Everyone says no to something at least once in a while, but sometimes it's more important than others. Being able to say no—that is, having strong refusal skills—helps you navigate risky or complicated situations with better results. Saying no may seem like a simple skill, but doing it effectively and comfortably requires confidence and practice. It's important to be able to say no without feeling guilty or self-conscious.

Emily was invited to her new friend Amelia's house after school. She liked Amelia and was excited to go, but when they got to the house she quickly realized that things weren't right. Amelia's parents weren't home, and her older brother was drinking beer and seemed to be on some sort of drug. When she asked Amelia about it, she said, "Yeah, my brother scores marijuana from a guy at work, and we light up out back when no one else is home." Emily immediately felt nervous because she doesn't agree with using drugs for recreation. Her stomach was in knots, and she felt really uncomfortable when she saw Amelia get a small package out of her brother's bag.

Charles was working hard to lose a few pounds and get in better shape. So far, he had lost 6 pounds (2.7 kilograms) in just under three weeks. Then a few of his buddies invited him over to watch the Super Bowl, and they were all bringing food with empty calories. He knew that they'd be eating a lot and that food would be a big part of the event. As part of his diet, however, Charles was eating only lean meats, fruits, vegetables, and whole grains, and he was drinking only water and tea. Last time the guys had watched a game together, they had all gotten sick on chicken wings, nachos, chili, and soda. Charles knew his friends would pressure him to join the party and tell him he could just take some diet pills the next day.

For Discussion

Both Emily and Charles need to use refusal skills. Emily is in a dangerous situation and is feeling uncomfortable. Charles isn't in danger, but he doesn't want to wreck his hard work or feel bad about his choices the next day. What strategies can Emily use to say no? What strategies can Charles use? What might some of the long-term consequences be if Emily can't develop effective refusal skills? What about Charles? To help you develop your answers, review the Skills for Healthy Living feature.

SKILLS FOR HEALTHY LIVING: Building Refusal Skills

Being able to say no is a key part of building refusal skills. Throughout your life, you'll be presented with opportunities and choices that may require you to say no in order to be true to your beliefs and values and maintain your health and safety. Use the following tips to help you say no when necessary.

- **Know what you believe and stick to it.** Having a strong and clear sense of your personal values goes a long way in helping you say no when you need to.
- **Be assertive.** When you say no, do it with conviction. You don't need to be mean or aggressive. Instead, stand tall, make eye contact with the person or people you're talking to, and simply say, "No, thank you" or "No, that is not something I am willing to do."
- **Don't apologize for saying no.** If you feel strongly about a choice you're making, don't apologize for it. Apologizing makes it easier for others to talk you out of your decision. Rather than saying, "I'm sorry, guys, but I don't want to do that," say, "I understand that you want to do this, but I don't want to, and I am saying no."
- **Offer alternatives.** If someone pressures you to do something you don't want to do, say no and also consider offering an alternative choice. If you don't want to smoke, suggest going for coffee instead.

If you don't want to be alone with someone else, suggest meeting in a public place like a park.

- **Support others when they say no.** If you offer your support when a friend or family member refuses something, that person will likely support you when you do so. You often get the same treatment from others that you give them.
- **Have a plan.** If you're going out with friends, know what your plan is and stick to it. Making spontaneous decisions may seem fun, but it often leads to situations where you feel pressured or uncomfortable. Having a plan for healthy living also makes it easier to say no to unhealthy food choices and to choose an active pursuit rather than a sedentary one.

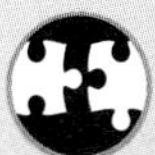

ACADEMIC CONNECTION: Understanding Risk (Probability)

In general terms, risk is the probability that an event will happen. Many things, like diseases, can't be predicted with certainty. The best you can do is estimate the likelihood that the disease will occur based on the information available to you. To understand how probabilities work, consider what happens when a coin is tossed. There are two possible outcomes: heads or tails. Given that reality, we say that the probability of the coin landing on heads is one in two, or 1/2, or 50%. The probability of the coin landing on tails is also one in two, or 1/2, or 50%. Similarly, when rolling a single die, there are six possible outcomes: 1, 2, 3, 4, 5, or 6. So, the probability of any one of those numbers occurring is one in six, or 1/6. When talking about a disease, such as in this chapter's Living Well News feature, risk is used to describe the chance that a person will develop the disease or have a recurrence of the disease. This risk, or probability, is based on research findings that look at the possible outcomes of a situation and determine the likelihood of each possible outcome based on all of the factors involved.

Is Aspirin a Miracle Drug?

"Taking a low dose of aspirin every day can prevent and possibly even treat cancer," BBC News reported in 2012. The painkiller is already taken by millions in order to cut the risk of heart attack and stroke (see table 33.5), but widely reported recent research suggests that it may play a role in fighting cancer as well.

In three research papers published simultaneously, doctors and researchers looked at cancer data recorded during dozens of trials that tested aspirin use for heart and circulatory health. They found that daily use of aspirin was linked to a drop in the short-term risk of developing cancer and could reduce both the risk of cancer spreading through the body and the risk of death due to cancer.

The reason for the potential beneficial effects is a particular chemical found in the drug that influences cell growth and development. Overall, a person's risk of cancer may drop 20 percent after 20 years of aspirin use. "The physiological reactions in the cells are similar to those seen from a dose of exercise," says medical researcher Patricia Rothchild of Oxford University.

It isn't all good news, however. Aspirin can cause painful stomach irritation, and there is a small but serious risk of bleeding associated with its use. Because of these risks, physician David Danielson says, "It is too soon to recommend that people should start taking daily aspirin simply for cancer prevention unless it has been specifically recommended to them by their doctor." There is certainly no reason for people under 18 to start on a daily low-dose aspirin.

However, Dr. Rothchild points out, "Studies suggest that 769 people would need to be treated with low-dose aspirin for one extra person to be harmed with major bleeding as a result, so it seems the known benefits might already outweigh the risks." For now, it appears the verdict is still out.

For Discussion

Based on the information in the table, who are the most likely people to use aspirin daily or every other day? Why do you think this is the case? Explain your answer.

TABLE 33.5 Aspirin Use By Adults Ages 18 to 65 in the United States

Characteristic	Aspirin use daily or every other day (%)	
Aspirin use by gender	Males	61.3%
	Females	47.4%
Aspirin use by age	18-44	4.6%
	45-65	27.0%
	Over 65	48.5%
Aspirin use by ethnicity	White non-Hispanic	22.3%
	Black non-Hispanic	15.1%
	Asian non-Hispanic	11.5%
	Hispanic	10.0%

Source: Agency for Health Care Research and Quality, Statistical Brief #179 (2007).

CHAPTER REVIEW

Reviewing Concepts and Vocabulary

As directed by your teacher, answer items 1 through 5 by correctly completing each sentence with a word or phrase.

1. The federal drug schedule for drugs considered to be the most dangerous is schedule ______.
2. The acronym SAFER can help you remember how to safely use what kind of drugs? ______________
3. A drug requiring a physician's approval is called a _______________ drug.
4. ____________ drugs are generally the ones that some people take for thrill seeking, consciousness raising, and mood elevation.
5. Methamphetamine is an example of a(n) ____________ drug.

For items 6 through 10, as directed by your teacher, match each term in column 1 with the appropriate phrase in column 2.

6. dependence	a. legal drug
7. drug addiction	b. physical and emotional condition that occurs when a drug is stopped
8. withdrawal	c. needing more of a drug because the body has adjusted to its effects
9. drug tolerance	d. needing a drug to prevent feeling sick
10. licit drug	e. compulsive use of a substance

For items 11 through 15, as directed by your teacher, respond to each statement or question.

11. Compare prescription and over-the-counter drugs.
12. Identify two guidelines for properly obtaining and using prescription drugs.
13. What does the acronym SAFER stand for, and what does it help you understand?
14. What are two ways to alter consciousness without using drugs?
15. What are some signs and behaviors associated with drug dependence?

Thinking Critically

Write a paragraph in response to the following questions.

Do you think that people who break the law while under the influence should be required to go to jail or to treatment? Explain your answers and use specific facts to support your positions.

Take It Home

Talk with your family members about safe use of over-the-counter medications. Take a written inventory of all OTC medications in your home and indicate where they are located. Make a list of tips or guidelines to help your family members be good consumers when buying, using, and storing medicines.

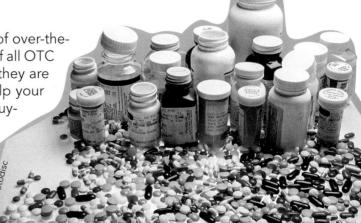

Photodisc

UNIT XII

Creating Healthy and Safe Communities

Healthy People 2020 Goals

- Reduce total injury rates in the population.
- Reduce rates of traumatic brain injury and traumatic spinal cord injury.
- Reduce rates of poisonings.
- Reduce rates of fatal and nonfatal unintentional injuries from fire, motor vehicle crashes, falls, suffocations, drowning, and sport and recreation accidents.
- Reduce the proportion of teens who report that they rode with a driver who was drinking alcohol.
- Decrease the rate of alcohol-impaired driving.
- Increase safety belt use.
- Increase bicycle helmet laws and motorcycle helmet use.
- Reduce homicides and firearm-related deaths and injuries.
- Reduce nonfatal physical assault injuries and physical assaults.
- Reduce fighting and bullying among teens.
- Reduce weapon carrying by adolescents on school property.
- Reduce child maltreatment.
- Reduce intimate partner and sexual violence.
- Reduce air toxic emissions to decrease the risk of adverse health effects.
- Reduce the amount of toxic pollutants.
- Increase recycling of municipal solid waste.
- Reduce indoor allergen levels.
- Increase the proportion of schools that engage in practices that promote a healthy and safe physical school environment.
- Reduce exposure to selected environmental chemicals in the population.
- Improve quality, utility, awareness, and use of information systems for environmental health.

Self-Assessment Features in This Unit

- My Injury Prevention and Emergency Preparedness
- How Green Are You?
- How Healthy Is My School Community?

Making Healthy Decisions and Skills for Healthy Living Features In This Unit

- Skill Building
- Overcoming Barriers
- Positive Attitudes

Special Features in This Unit

- Consumer Corner: Buying a First Aid Kit
- Advocacy in Action: Promoting Recycling
- Consumer Corner: Donating to Charities

Living Well News Features in This Unit

- Personal Watercraft Safety
- Can Earbuds Damage Hearing?
- Are We Failing at Community Health?

34

Safety and First Aid

In This Chapter

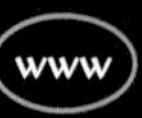

Student Web Resources

www.HOPEtextbook.org/student

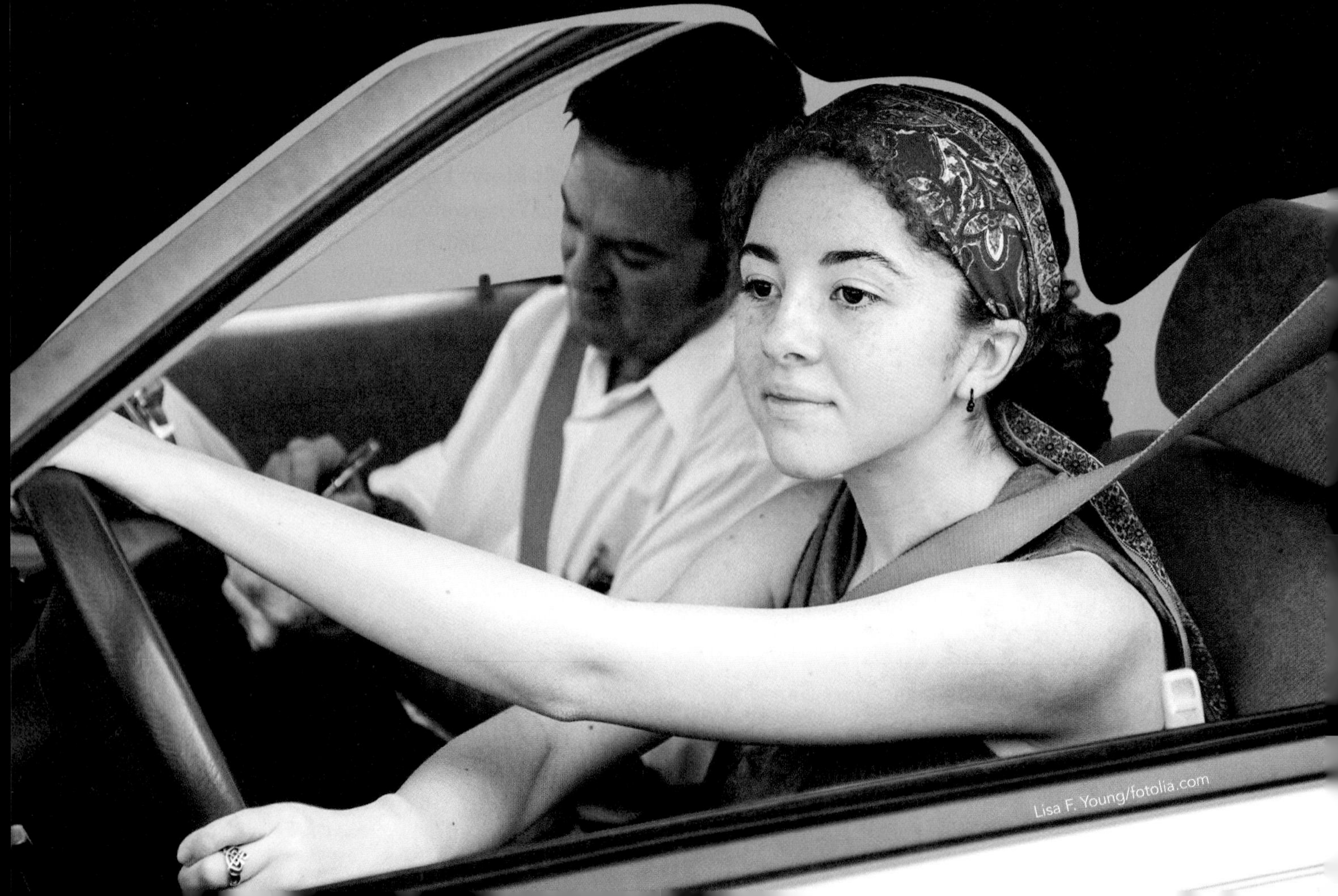

Lisa F. Young/fotolia.com

Lesson 34.1

Safety

Lesson Objectives

After reading this lesson, you should be able to

1. identify the major causes of unintentional injury in youth,
2. explain four ways to reduce the risk of being in an automobile crash, and
3. identify the major types of intentional injury and explain the steps you can take to avoid becoming a victim.

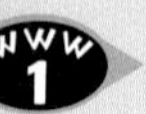

Lesson Vocabulary

assault, battery, distracted driving, homicide, inattention blindness, intentional injury, road rage, traumatic brain injury, unintentional injury

While your teenage years are a critical time for developing healthy habits and setting the stage for living a healthy adult life, accidents and violence pose the greatest immediate threats to your life as a teen. Accidents, or **unintentional injuries**, are caused by unplanned events, such as automobile crashes, poisonings, fires, and drownings. Unintentional injury is the leading cause of death among teenagers, and motor vehicle accidents alone account for 73 percent of all accidental deaths. The leading causes of unintentional death among teenagers can be seen in figure 34.1. **Intentional injury** includes violence, suicide, self-injury, and homicide. Homicides are the second leading cause of death among teens in the United States and the majority of these homicides involve a firearm. Understanding gun safety is an important aspect of overall safety.

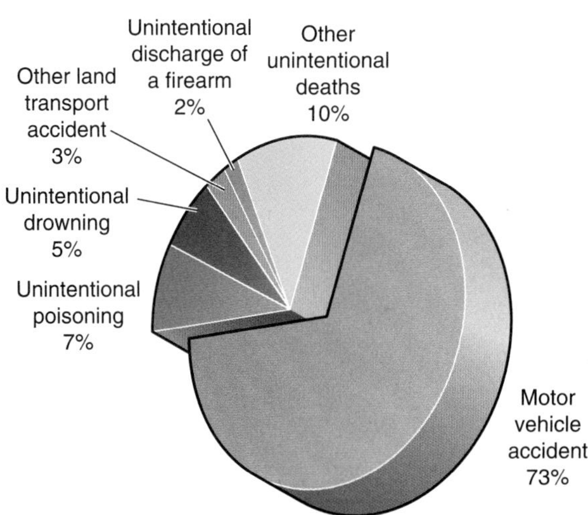

FIGURE 34.1 The leading causes of unintentional death among teenagers.

From USDHHS NCHS Data Brief, May 2010.

Staying Safe on the Road

Streets and highways can be dangerous places. The odds are that you will be in three or four traffic accidents in your lifetime, and about 30 percent of us willon be in a serious accident at some point. According to the National Highway Traffic Safety Administration, 20,000 people die from motor vehicle accidents each year. Motor vehicle accidents are the leading cause of death among teenagers. Fortunately, there are many safety precautions you can take to help you avoid accidents and limit your chances of being seriously hurt or killed if you are in an accident.

Seat Belts and Airbags

An average of eight teens between the ages of 16 and 19 die every day from motor vehicle injuries. In fact, one in every three teenage deaths results from an accident related to a motor vehicle. Teen drivers (age 16 to 19) are four times more likely than older drivers to crash, and teenage males are at the highest risk for accidents. To help keep yourself safe while driving or riding in a vehicle, always use your seat belt properly. Research shows that seat belt use reduces the severity of injuries by 60 percent and decreases the likelihood of death by 45 percent. American males aged 19 to 29 are the least likely to wear seat belts, and it is estimated that two-thirds of people killed by automobile accidents were not wearing a seat belt at the time.

Drivers are not the only ones who can be saved by regular seat belt use. When everyone in the car buckles up, one out of every six deaths is avoided. Passengers who are not wearing a seat belt can be thrown from the vehicle or thrown into other passengers, thus causing additional injuries or deaths. Airbags further reduce the risk of death and serious injury from automobile accidents. However, they can be dangerous to children due to a child's small size, and most states require that children ride in the backseat.

Distracted Driving

According to the U.S. National Highway Traffic Safety Administration, driving while distracted increases your risk of an accident by 20 percent to 30 percent. **Distracted driving** includes driving while talking on the phone, texting, eating, drinking, applying makeup, or engaging in other activities that take your attention away from the road.

The number one cause of distracted driving is cell phone use, even when hands-free devices are used. Cell phone conversations result in what is called **inattention blindness** because the conversation leads the driver's attention away from the visual environment, distracting both the brain and the eyes. In fact, it is estimated that the distraction effect from talking on a cell phone while driving lasts for up to two minutes after the phone conversation is over. Talking to a passenger in the car is less distracting because one's attention remains focused within the vehicle. Your passenger can also alert you to any dangers.

Texting while driving is even more distracting and more dangerous, since it takes your focus and attention completely off of the road and other drivers. Texting while driving dramatically increases your risk of an accident; some estimates show the risk to be 23 times greater. Most states have passed laws prohibiting the use of cell phones while driving, and the concern over distracted driving is so great that a U.S. government website has been developed specifically to address the issue (www.distraction.gov). Florida and some other states have a law prohibiting texting while driving as well.

HEALTHY COMMUNICATION

Have you ever engaged in texting while driving? Have you seen others engage in this behavior? What are some specific things you could do to keep yourself and your friends and family members from texting while driving? Share your perspectives and ideas with your classmates.

Safe Driving Checklist

- Always wear a seat belt when driving or riding in a vehicle.
- Pay attention to the actions of other drivers.
- Keep your eyes on the road.
- Never text or use a handheld device while driving.
- Pull over or exit the road to take a phone call.
- Follow all rules of the road.
- Stay calm and do not react to aggressive or impatient drivers.
- Never drive under the influence of alcohol or drugs.
- Avoid driving when drowsy or sleepy.
- Keep passengers from becoming rowdy or distracting.
- Limit the number of passengers in your car (some state laws set limits) especially for new drivers.

Driving Under the Influence

Alcohol plays a role in 25 percent of all fatal car crashes. Across all age groups, men are significantly more likely than women to engage in driving under the influence (DUI). And although young men between the ages of 21 and 34 make up only 11 percent of the adult U.S. population, they account for 32 percent of all instances of drinking and driving.

Alcohol has also been shown to be a factor in many car crashes involving people under the legal drinking age of 21. In fact, 25 percent of young men (aged 15 to 20) killed in crashes were under the influence of alcohol at the time of their death. Alcohol impairs both judgment and coordination, thus making it hard to control reactions, speed, steering, and braking (see figure 34.2). Impairment begins after only one or two drinks; thus mixing *any* amount of alcohol with driving is dangerous.

Road Rage

Many people become impatient while driving, and some engage in emotional outbursts known as **road rage**. These outbursts can involve extremely aggressive driving, in which the car itself is treated as a weapon; they can also involve the use of guns or other weapons. Road rage is thought to play a part in as many as two-thirds of all fatal car crashes and one-third of nonfatal crashes.

People who display road rage may be experiencing frustration in other parts of life. That frustration can spill over when traffic is heavy or when another driver does something they think is stupid or annoying. The truth is that people often see other vehicles on the road merely as things; we may fail to remember that there is a living, breathing, feeling person behind the wheel. Road rage is also more common among individuals who are involved in an argument or difficult conversation on a cell phone while driving. The emotions stirred up in the conversation can spill over into aggressive driving behaviors. Alcohol use also contributes to road rage. Some psychologists have also suggested that individuals prone to road rage may have witnessed road rage and aggressive driving by their parents when they were younger and are now repeating these behaviors.

Regardless of the root cause, road rage poses a danger to the angry driver, any passengers, and fellow motorists. One way to reduce the chance of being a victim of road rage is to practice defensive driving. This approach to driving involves paying

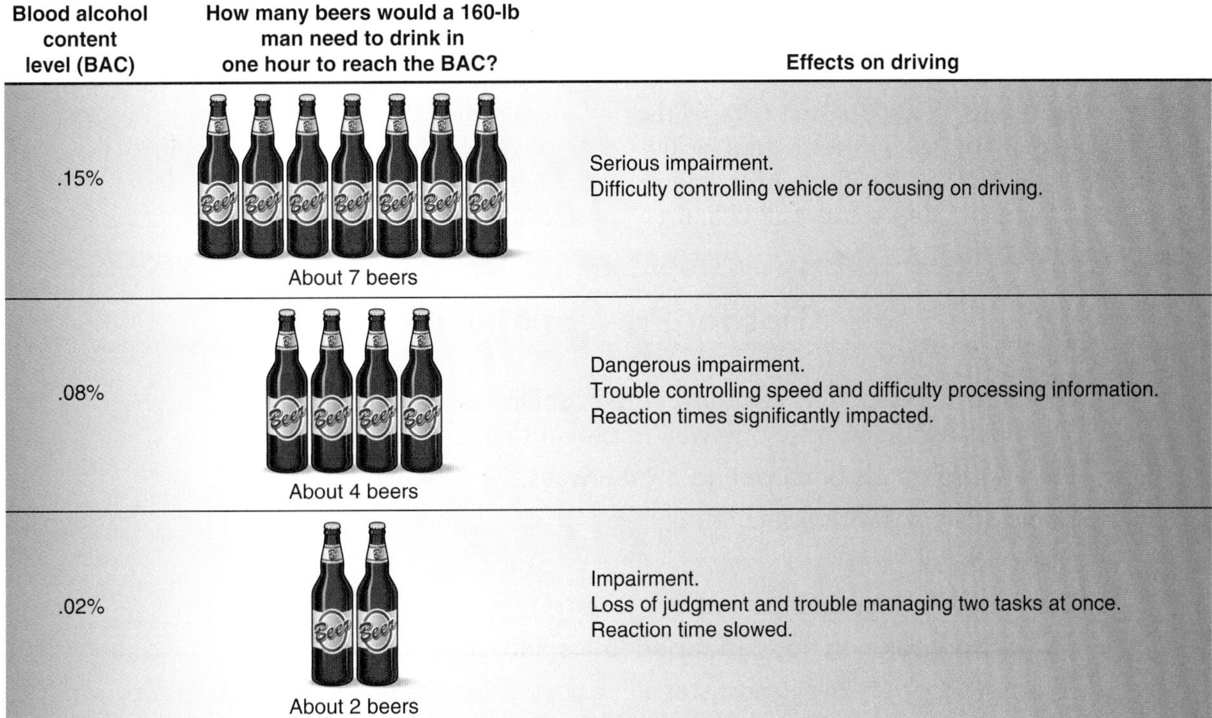

Blood alcohol content level (BAC)
How many beers would a 160-lb man need to drink in one hour to reach the BAC?
Effects on driving
.15%
About 7 beers
Serious impairment.
Difficulty controlling vehicle or focusing on driving.
.08%
About 4 beers
Dangerous impairment.
Trouble controlling speed and difficulty processing information.
Reaction times significantly impacted.
.02%
About 2 beers
Impairment.
Loss of judgment and trouble managing two tasks at once.
Reaction time slowed.

FIGURE 34.2 The effects of blood alcohol on driving ability.

close attention to other drivers but not expecting them to always do what you think they should. Other useful tactics include taking deep breaths to remain calm and talking with yourself rationally about how to respond if you're confronted by an enraged driver. Even if you feel the other driver is at fault, keeping your cool and letting the situation go could save your life.

Staying Safe at Home

Home accidents are among the leading causes of death among young children and injury among adults. People often feel secure at home and forget that real and serious risks are present. The most common categories of home injury include falling, fire, and poisoning; another home safety issue involves heavy computer use. Each is discussed here.

Falling

Falls are the second-leading cause of death from unintentional injury, following motor vehicle crashes. The risk of falling is increased by poor lighting, uneven surfaces, high-heeled shoes, objects on the ground, and even distracted walking. Tips for preventing falls are provided in the accompanying text box.

Fire

In 2010, there were 384,000 home fires in the United States, resulting in 2,640 deaths (not including firefighter deaths) and 13,350 injuries. Home fires account for about 85 percent of all U.S. fires. The number one cause of these fires is cooking, but smoking causes the most fire-related deaths.

The majority of deaths involving fire result not from burns but from smoke inhalation. Smoke from any type of fire contains a mixture of heated particles and gases. The particular type of smoke is influenced by what is burning, the fire's temperature, and the amount of available oxygen. However, any type of fire smoke is potentially deadly. Death from smoke inhalation can occur when oxygen is absent (simple asphyxia), when inhaled chemicals damage respiratory tissues and cause swelling or airway collapse (chemical irritation), or when chemicals interfere with oxygen use at a cellular level (chemical asphyxia). The leading cause of death related to smoke inhalation is carbon monoxide—an o dorless, colorless, tasteless gas that causes chemical asphyxia.

Poisoning

Poisoning occurs when any substance interferes with normal body function after it is swallowed, inhaled, injected, or absorbed. Every day, 87 people die from unintentional poisoning in the United States. Those most likely to suffer illness or death from accidental poisoning are children under the age of five. Each year, half a million children swallow poisonous material, including medication not intended for them as well as cleaning supplies.

Adults are most likely to suffer accidental poisoning when they take someone else's prescription drug or when they consume a combination of drugs (whether over-the-counter or prescription) without medical clearance. The leading cause of medication-

Tips for Preventing Falls

- Get regular exercise, which the Centers for Disease Control and Prevention (CDC) identifies as the number one way to prevent falls.
- Put nonslip treads or carpeting on stairways.
- Equip stairways with a secure rail.
- Clear floors of small objects.
- Firmly secure rugs and carpets.
- Equip bathtubs with nonskid rubber mats and grab bars.
- Keep outdoor walkways and steps in good repair. Regularly clear snow, ice, and debris. Be aware of pets that may be in the way.

HEALTH SCIENCE

Different types of fire require different types of fire extinguisher. For example, a grease fire and an electrical fire require the application of different types and concentrations of chemicals. Extinguishing agents are separated into five major types, and fire extinguishers are labeled to indicate which types of fire they will safely put out. Class A extinguishers are used for ordinary combustible materials, such as wood, clothing, and paper; class B extinguishers are for putting out fires involving flammable liquids, such as grease and gasoline; class C extinguishers are suitable for use on fires involving appliances and other electrical equipment; class D extinguishers cover flammable metals; and class K extinguishers are typically used in industrial kitchens with large amounts of flammable cooking oil.

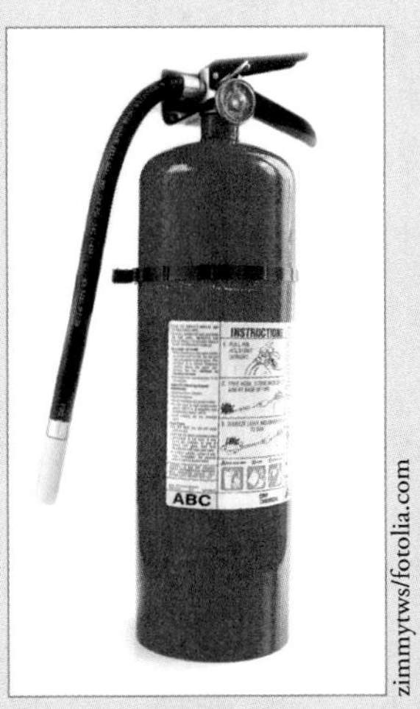

zimmytws/fotolia.com

Most homes benefit from a multipurpose class A/B/C fire extinguisher. Extinguishers can be heavy, and they require regular maintenance because of the chemicals and pressures involved.

related unintentional poisoning among adults is prescription painkiller medication. You should never take any medication prescribed for someone else. Medications are prescribed with specific consideration for the person's body weight, metabolic conditions, and other medications or supplements in use. Taking a medication not intended specifically for your needs is dangerous and potentially deadly. Keep all medications carefully labeled and stored out of the reach of both children and any adults for whom addiction or drug abuse is a problem.

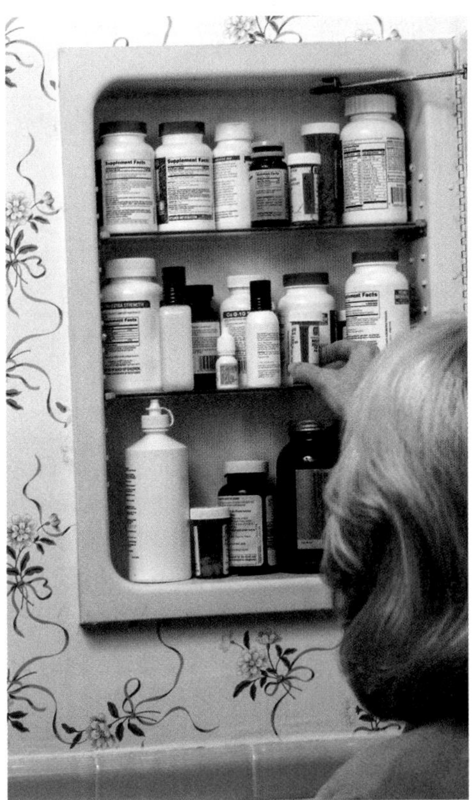

The leading cause of medication-related unintentional poisoning among adults is prescription painkiller medication. You should never take any medication prescribed for someone else.

Bill Crump/Brand X Pictures

Computer Use and Injury

Repetitive strain injury (RSI) occurs when too much stress is placed on a part of the body, resulting in inflammation (pain and swelling), at playmuscle strain, or tissue damage. This stress generally occurs from repeating the same movements over and over again. RSI is common in sport- and work-related settings, and is especially common among people who spend a lot of time using a computer keyboard.

Though most common in adults, RSI is becoming more prevalent among teens because they spend more time than ever playing video games and using computers, smartphones, and tablets for both schoolwork and social communication. Common signs and symptoms of RSI include tingling, numbness,

General Care for Poisoning

- Remove the person from the source of the poison.
- Check for consciousness, breathing, and signs of life.
- Care for any life-threatening conditions such as lack of breathing or pulse.
- If possible, ask questions of the victim to get more information (e.g., What substance was ingested? How much was ingested? When was it ingested?).
- Look for any nearby containers, and take them with you to the telephone.
- Call a poison control center—in the United States, the American Association of Poison Control Centers (1-800-222-1222)—or 911.
- Follow the directions provided to you by the poison control center or emergency services call taker.

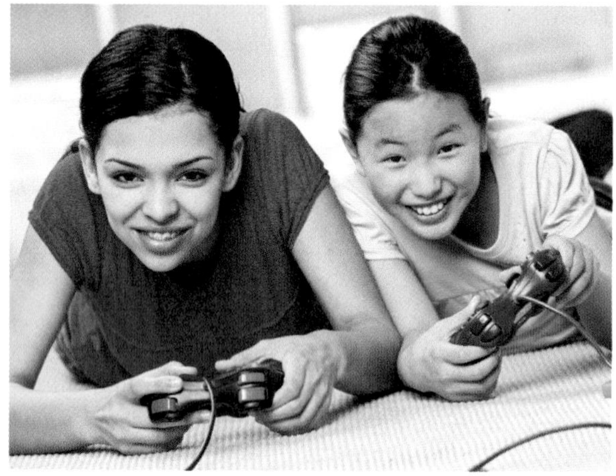

Take regular breaks when texting or playing video games.
AVAVA/fotolia.com

or pain in the affected area; stiffness or soreness in the neck or back; feelings of weakness or fatigue in the hands or arms; and popping or clicking sensations in the joints. To help prevent RSI, take regular breaks every 30 minutes or so when you are engaged in any repetitive task. If you experience symptoms, see a physician.

Staying Safe at Play

Recreational activity is an important and necessary part of living a healthy life. However, many recreational activities carry some risk of injury or even death. Therefore, whenever you're engaged in a recreational activity, consider your safety first. Guidelines vary by the activity, but it's always a good idea to carry a cell phone and a small first aid kit and to participate in the activity with at least one other person. Whether you're with others or alone, always inform someone else of your plans. If your plans take you outside, know the weather forecast and dress appropriately (the next lesson provides more information about weather-related risks).

Drowning

About ten people die from unintentional drowning each day in the United States, and half of drowning

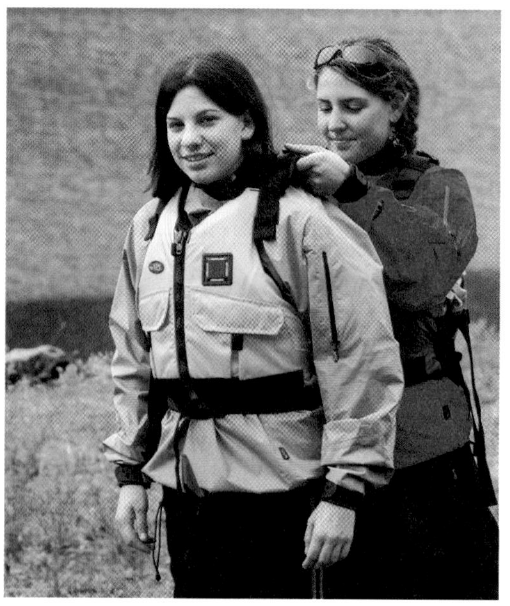

Making sure your life jacket fits properly is the first step before being on open water.
Human Kinetics/Mark Anderman/The Wild Studio

deaths occur in children under the age of 14. A majority of drowning deaths occur in swimming pools. Contributing factors include lack of swimming ability, absence of protective barriers (e.g., fences) around pools, and lack of supervision. The risk of drowning in open water settings is increased by alcohol use and failure to use a life jacket. Drowning can also occur in a bathtub, especially if a seizure disorder is involved. The most effective way to protect yourself from drowning is to learn basic swimming skills.

Bicycling and Skateboarding

Bicycle accidents account for nearly 2 percent of transportation-related deaths in the U.S. In 2010, 618 people died from bicycle-related accidents. The most effective way to reduce serious injury while bicycling is to wear a helmet, and many states require helmet use, especially among youth. Other good safety practices include wearing bright colors, avoiding night riding, and staying clear of road hazards and construction zones. You should also keep your bike in good repair, remain alert while riding, and follow all rules of the road.

Skateboarding remains a popular recreational activity, as well as a mode of transportation for some young people. When boarding, wear a helmet, knee and elbow pads, and wrist guards. Stay away from roads with heavy traffic, do not skate in areas with blind hills or turns, and practice stunt skateboarding only in designated skate parks.

High-Risk Recreational Activities

Not surprisingly, the risk of unintentional injury can be high when doing risky or thrill-seeking activities such as bungee jumping, ski or snowboard jumping, and parachuting. Young people often feel full of life and have a sense of being invincible and therefore may place themselves in risky situations more often than others do. Thus it's critical for you to recognize the risks in any activity you choose to do and protect yourself against unnecessary risk. Always maintain and use appropriate protective equipment and exercise reasonable judgment about your skills and abilities and the environment you're in.

Concussions

Traumatic brain injury (TBI) is a serious public health problem in the United States. A TBI is caused by a bump, blow, or jolt to the head and is a penetrating (or open) head injury that disrupts the normal function of the brain. Most traumatic brain injuries are concussions. The severity of these injuries may range from mild (limited interruption in cognitive function) to severe (causing a prolonged period of unconsciousness). Some contact sports such as football have come under increased scrutiny because of the relatively high risk of players getting concussions. Properly fitting protective equipment such as helmets can help reduce the risk of getting a concussion. Any bump, blow, or jolt to the head should be checked by a physician.

CONNECT

How do you think society views high-risk recreational activity, such as skydiving, bungee jumping, and base jumping? Do you think risk takers are viewed as more courageous or heroic than the average person? How might social norms about high-risk behavior influence your choices now or in the future? Under what circumstances might you be more likely to engage in a high-risk recreational activity? Discuss your answers with your peers.

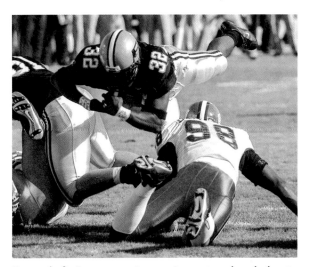

Properly fitting protective equipment such as helmets can help reduce the risk of getting a concussion.

Staying Safe at Work

Most Americans spend a significant amount of their time on the job and at the workplace. Injury risks in the workplace can include a wide range of things such as falling objects and debris, tripping hazards, lifting heavy or awkward items, performing repetitive tasks, and being exposed to hazardous chemicals, substances, and materials, to name a few. All workers in the U.S. have the right to a safe workplace; the rates of workplace injury, illness, and death have declined by 67 percent since 1970. These improvements are partly due to the passage of the Occupational Safety and Health Act of 1970. The law requires employers to provide their employees with working conditions that are free of known dangers and that follow all Occupational Health and Safety Administration (OSHA) standards. Employers must work to eliminate hazards as a first line of defense against illness and injury rather than simply relying on the use of masks, gloves, ear plugs, or other protective equipment.

Young workers (under the age of 18) are also protected under OSHA guidelines. In addition, the Fair Labor Standards Act (FLSA) sets limits on the number of hours youth under the age of 18 may work and on the occupations for such young workers. Following general health and safety guidelines, exercising caution in job tasks, following all job-specific rules and regulations, and reporting hazardous working environments are important steps for preventing worksite injury and illness. You can learn more about occupational health and safety by visiting the student section of the Health Opportunities Through Physical Education website. WWW 3

Intentional Injuries

Intentional injuries include any injury that has been purposely inflicted, either by oneself or another person. Examples are assaults, homicides, self-inflicted injuries, and suicides. Self-inflicted injuries and suicide are covered in the chapter on emotional health and wellness. Bullying and relationship vio-

Avoiding Risky Situations

- Keep doors and windows at your home locked. Never let a stranger into your home and never let a stranger know that you are or will be home alone.
- If you are meeting someone you do not know or who you met on the Internet, agree only to meet in a public place and take a friend with you.
- Don't hide keys to your home in obvious places, like under a doormat.
- Always be alert when walking, especially if you are alone. Avoid being distracted with electronic devices (e.g., phone, tablet). Take headphones off or keep the volume down so that you can hear what is happening around you. Walk confidently and briskly if you are feeling uneasy. Attackers often prey on people they think are confused, scared, or uncertain.
- Avoid dark and deserted places. If you must go to a dark or isolated area, make sure you have at least one other person with you. Also make sure someone else knows where you are going and when you expect to be back.
- Park your car in well-lit areas and always do a quick scan under the car and in the backseat before getting in the vehicle.
- When driving, keep car doors locked. If your car breaks down, stop and call the police, turn on the hazard lights, pop the hood, and remain in the locked vehicle. If someone stops to offer help, remain in your car until police arrive. If you do not have a phone, ask the person to call for you.
- Do not give rides to strangers or hitchhikers.
- If someone tries to rob you, give up your possessions and get away as quickly as possible.
- Call the police immediately if you witness a crime in progress.

lence are addressed in the chapter on family living and healthy relationships.

Assault, Battery, and Homicide

According to the CDC, almost one-third of U.S. high school students reported being in a physical fight in 2011, and almost 8 percent reported having been threatened with a weapon. **Assault** is an act of immediate harmful or offensive contact that creates fear for a person. **Battery** is harmfully or offensively touching another person. Both assault and battery should be reported to legal authorities.

Homicide refers to taking the life of another person. In 2010, 4,828 young people aged 10 to 24 were victims of homicide in the U.S. This is an average of 13 deaths each day. Over 80 percent of these homicides involved a firearm.

Gun Safety

In addition to being used in homicides, guns can be a cause of intentional and unintentional injury. Basic gun safety can help reduce the risks associated with firearms. Gun safety includes the following basic rules.

- Treat every gun as if it were loaded.
- Never treat a gun as a harmless toy or prop.
- Always store guns unloaded.
- Lock guns in a rack or safe and hide the keys or combination.
- Store ammunition away from guns and keep it locked.
- Don't keep guns in your home if someone in your family has a mental illness, severe depression, or potential for violence.

Recognizing and Preventing Violence

There is no way to guarantee that you will not be the victim of a violent act. However, there are general steps you can take to avoid risky situations and to help minimize the chances that you or others will become the victim of a violent crime. In addition, people who commit violent acts may display certain warning signs (see Warning Signs of Violent Behavior sidebar). If you see these signs in someone, it is important to tell a trusted adult. Individuals who commit acts of violence may suffer from mental illness (e.g., depression and suicidal tendencies) or may have issues with substance abuse, although most people with mental illness are not violent. Reporting observations and concerns will help save the lives of innocent victims.

Warning Signs of Violent Behavior

- Sudden lack of interest in school and regular activities
- Obsessions with violent games and movies
- Depression and mood swings
- Writing that shows despair and isolation or is extremely angry or violent
- Lack of anger management skills (i.e., losing one's temper often or is easily made angry)
- Talking about death or suicide
- Bringing weapons to school or work
- Violence toward animals

Comprehension Check

1. Identify two causes of unintentional injury in youth.
2. Explain one way to reduce the risk of being in an automobile crash.
3. Explain three specific actions to limit your risk of becoming a victim of violent crime.

SELF-ASSESSMENT: My Injury Prevention and Emergency Preparedness

Answer each question yes or no, then add up the total number of yes responses and evaluate your score according to the guide at the end of the assessment.

There is a fire extinguisher in my home, and I know where it is.	Yes	No
There are smoke detectors installed in my home.	Yes	No
There are first aid kits or first aid supplies in my home, and I know where they are.	Yes	No
I always wear a seat belt when I am in a motor vehicle.	Yes	No
There is a first aid kit in my car.	Yes	No
I always follow safety guidelines when riding my bike or skateboard.	Yes	No
I am confident in my ability to administer CPR to an adult.	Yes	No
I know what to do if a person chokes and becomes unconscious.	Yes	No
I know how to treat injuries such as sprains and strains.	Yes	No
I know what to do if someone shows signs of becoming suddenly ill.	Yes	No
I have successfully treated minor scrapes and bruises in the past.	Yes	No
I have practiced my first aid skills in a variety of situations.	Yes	No
I am confident in my ability to stay calm in an emergency situation.	Yes	No
I keep emergency numbers stored in my phone or another handy location.	Yes	No
I know how to use an AED for victims of sudden cardiac arrest.	Yes	No

My score for Injury Prevention and Emergency Preparedness = ____________ (total number of yes answers)

If you gave 13 to 15 yes responses, you're well prepared to both avoid and deal with a variety of emergency situations. If you gave 10 to 12 yes responses, you're somewhat prepared to avoid and deal with a variety of emergency situations. If you gave 9 or fewer yes responses, you may be putting yourself at risk and may not be ready to deal with an emergency situation.

Planning for Healthy Living

Use the Healthy Living Plan worksheet to improve your emergency readiness.

Lesson 34.2

First Aid and CPR

Lesson Objectives

After reading this lesson, you should be able to

1. describe the three basic emergency action steps for administering CPR,
2. explain basic first aid procedures for common emergency scenarios, and
3. identify the signs of sudden illness that might require medical attention.

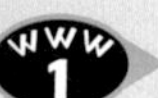

Lesson Vocabulary

closed fracture, closed wound, dislocation, heatstroke, Heimlich maneuver, hypothermia, open fracture, open wound, sprain, strain

We can find ourselves in the midst of an emergency at any time. You can help keep yourself and others safe in an emergency by learning basic steps for cardiopulmonary resuscitation (CPR) and first aid.

Emergency Action Steps

At some point, we will all face an emergency, and that emergency is more likely to involve a loved one than someone we don't know. As a result, emergencies are often particularly stressful and emotional. Remaining calm and thinking quickly can make the difference between saving and losing a life. Regardless of the type of emergency, you should always follow three basic steps: check, call, and care (the three Cs).

Check

Emergency scenes can be unsafe both for those involved in an accident and for those wanting to help. Always check the scene for safety. Use your senses—hearing, sight, and smell—to check for anything out of the ordinary that could signal danger, such as smoke, spilled chemicals, strange odors, screaming or crying sounds, downed electrical wires, and confused or disoriented people. If a scene is clearly dangerous, do not go near it. Instead, call 911 and wait for professionals to arrive.

If the scene does not appear dangerous, look for clues about what happened. Check for fallen items, such as a ladder or step stool, a spilled medicine bottle, tire tread marks, broken glass, or anything else that might indicate what happened. Check carefully to see how many people are hurt and if anyone else is available to help. Your observations will be important when you communicate with emergency personnel in the next step.

Call

Most of the time, calling for help is the most important thing you can do to help an ill or injured

Calling 911

When you call 911, an emergency call taker, or dispatcher, will answer the phone. Call takers are specifically trained to deal with crises over the phone. The caller will ask for your phone number and address or location and will want to know the nature of the emergency. When using a wireless phone to make a 911 call, it is especially important to be able to provide your location since it will not be automatically indicated to the dispatcher. If you are in an unfamiliar location, look for street signs or major landmarks, such as buildings with specific business names or logos.

The call taker will likely ask you a lot of questions in order to determine the most appropriate action to be taken. Remain calm and focus on answering the questions without panicking or becoming frustrated. Call takers may also provide you with basic CPR or first aid information to assist you until help arrives.

person. When calling, remain calm and observant. Answer the questions that the call taker asks. Be prepared to provide information about the location and describe the emergency and each victim's condition.

In situations where a victim's breathing might be impaired, you may need to provide care before placing a call to emergency services. If other people are around, you can instruct someone else to call 911 while you provide immediate care. Care-first situations include the unwitnessed collapse of a person younger than about 12 years and any instance of drowning. In these cases, try to provide oxygen as quickly as possible. See sidebar titled Learn Cardiopulmonary Resuscitation (CPR). If you are alone with the victim in these situations, attempt to provide care before you call.

Care

You may need to provide care in an emergency situation. Fundamental first aid guidelines for several common conditions are provided in the remainder of this chapter.

Helping a Conscious Choking Victim

The **Heimlich maneuver** is used to dislodge a piece of food or other object from a conscious person who is choking. The maneuver is safe for children over one year old and adults. A separate technique is used for infants. You can also perform the Heimlich maneuver on yourself. In any case, you may need to repeat the procedure several times before the object is dislodged. Each technique is described below.

When performing the Heimlich maneuver on a child over one year old or an adult, complete the following steps.

1. For a conscious person who is sitting or standing, position yourself behind the person and reach your arms around his or her waist (figure 34.3).

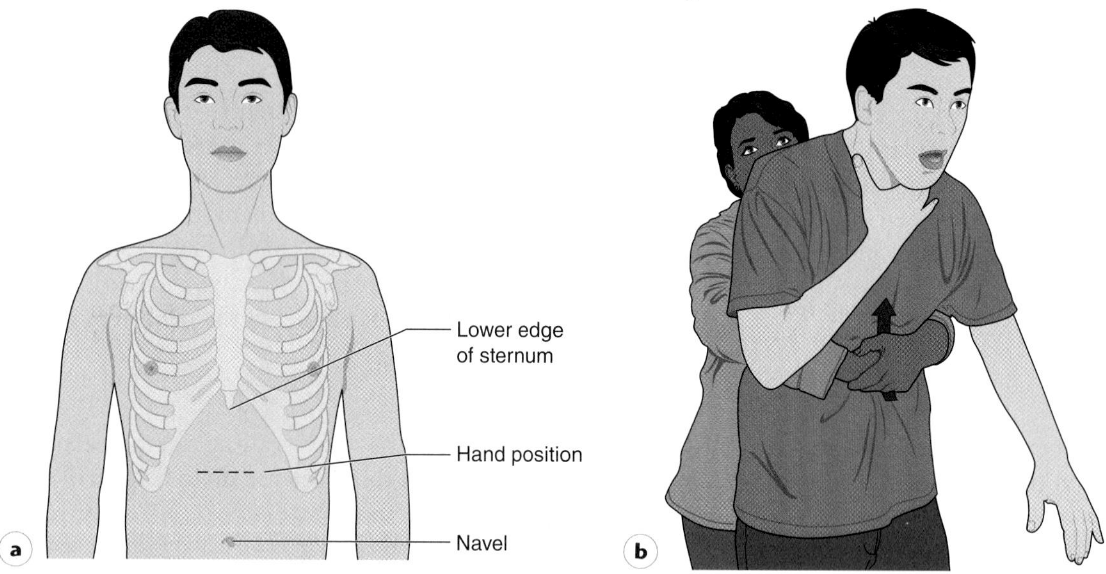

FIGURE 34.3 *(a)* Locating hand position, and *(b)* performing the Heimlich maneuver.

Basic Care Guidelines

- Do no harm.
- Monitor the person's breathing and consciousness.
- Keep the person from getting chilled or overheated.
- Help the person rest in the most comfortable position possible. If the person may have a spinal injury, do not move him or her unless there is immediate danger.
- Reassure the person and help him or her stay calm but alert.
- Give any specific care needed.

2. Place your fist, thumb side in, just above the person's navel and grab the fist tightly with your other hand.
3. Pull your fist abruptly upward and inward to increase airway pressure behind the obstructed object and force it from the windpipe.
4. If the person is conscious and lying on his or her back, straddle the person facing the head. Push your fist upward and inward in a maneuver similar to the one above.
5. If the person becomes unconscious, call 911 and begin CPR.

If you are alone and choking, you can perform the Heimlich maneuver on yourself with the following steps.

1. Make a fist. Place the thumb below your rib cage and above your navel.
2. Grasp your fist with your other hand. Press it into the area with a quick upward movement.
3. You can also lean over a table edge, chair, or railing. Quickly thrust your upper abdomen against the edge of the surface.

If an infant is choking (i.e., unable to cough or cry forcefully, demonstrating difficulty breathing and turning a bluish color), follow these steps.

1. Lay the infant facedown along your forearm. Use your thigh or lap for support. Hold the infant's chest in your hand and jaw with your fingers and firmly support the head. Point the infant's head downward, lower than the body.
2. Give up to five quick and forceful blows between the infant's shoulder blades using the palm of your free hand.

Follow these steps if the object does not come out of the airway after five blows.

1. Turn the infant faceup. Use your thigh or lap for support. Support the head.
2. Place two fingers on the middle of the infant's breastbone just below the nipples.
3. Give up to five quick thrusts down, compressing the chest 1/3 to 1/2 the depth of the chest.
4. Continue with five back blows followed by five chest thrusts until the object is dislodged or the infant loses alertness (i.e., becomes unconscious).
5. If the infant becomes unconscious, call 911 and begin CPR.

Basic First Aid

If you've ever cleaned a cut or scrape, then applied antibiotic ointment and covered the area with a bandage, you've performed first aid. Being skilled in first aid includes knowing how to recognize injuries and illnesses and how to manage or treat them. Using proper first aid procedures can prevent infection, slow bleeding, aid healing, and even save a life.

> "Take some time to learn first aid and CPR. It saves lives."
>
> —Bobby Sherman, actor and singer

Minor Burns

Burns are soft tissue injuries that can affect the skin and the layers of fat, muscle, and bone beneath the skin. Burns are classified by their source (heat, chemical, electricity, or radiation) and their depth. The deeper the burn, the more severe it is. First-degree burns affect only the top layer of skin and generally heal within a week without permanent scarring. Second-degree burns, or partial-thickness burns, affect several layers of skin and often include blistering. Healing is slower, and scarring may occur. Third-degree burns, or full-thickness burns, destroy all layers of the skin and some of the underlying tissue. Treatment will likely include skin grafting (surgery) and painful rehabilitation. All types of burn can be serious and can require medical care; even a first-degree burn can be considered critical if it affects a large area of the body or affects a particularly sensitive area.

Small thermal (heat) burns are common and can be treated by running cool water over the affected area, then covering it loosely with a sterile dressing to prevent infection. Chemical burns from a liquid source can be treated in the same manner. Chemical burns from dry powders should first be gently brushed off to remove the burning substance before applying running water. To reduce the risk of burns, follow safety practices around heat, chemicals, and electricity. Also follow all manufacturer

Learn Cardiopulmonary Resuscitation (CPR)

When a person's breathing and heart stop, time is critical. Brain damage can begin after 4 minutes without oxygen, and it becomes likely after 6 to 10 minutes. A person's chances of survival are directly affected by early recognition of symptoms, followed by early CPR and defibrillation (restoration of normal heart rhythm) and early access to advanced medical care. This sequence is known as the chain of survival, and it often depends on the initial steps taken by the person who is present when a cardiac event occurs.

Cardiopulmonary resuscitation (CPR) is a first aid procedure that is performed when the heart or breathing has stopped, and it saves many lives each year. The procedure uses chest compressions to keep blood flowing, preventing brain damage and death until expert medical help arrives. CPR training is strongly recommended, and many schools and several national organizations offer CPR classes and certification. According to the National Institutes of Health, "Even if you haven't had training you can do 'hands-only' CPR for a teen or an adult whose heart has stopped." Hands-only CPR is *not* recommended for use with children.

The American Heart Association recommends "two steps to staying alive": First, call 911 or direct someone else to call 911. Second, start chest compressions—push hard and fast at the center of the chest. The technique for chest compression is shown in the figure.

CPR techniques and procedures are often revised based on new research and findings. For this reason, a regular check of the National Institutes of Health website for the latest information is recommended.

Using an Automated External Defibrillator

If an automated external defibrillator (AED) is immediately available, use it as soon as you have determined that the individual in need is unresponsive and without a pulse. All AED devices will include written or verbal instructions as part of the device. Follow these general guidelines when using an AED.

1. Turn on the AED.
2. Wipe the person's bare chest dry and apply the pads. Place one pad on the person's upper right chest and the other pad on the person's lower left side of the chest.

guidelines and wear appropriate clothing and safety gear when dealing with chemicals or working in an environment where burns might occur.

Any major burn requires immediate medical attention. Call 911 immediately if you come across a person with large burns, suspected lung burns, or burns of the head, neck, hands, feet, or genitals. Immediate medical care is also required for any burn where the skin is clearly charred and underlying tissues look exposed or damaged, as well as any burn suffered by a person under age 5 or over age 60.

Wounds

Any injury to the body's soft tissue is commonly referred to as a wound. **Closed wounds** occur when the skin's surface is not broken but damage occurs below the surface. **Open wounds** involve damage to the skin's surface and typically include some bleeding. Most small closed wounds, such as bruises, do not require special care; they generally heal themselves. Larger bruises can be treated with light pressure, to control the internal bleeding. Ice should be applied for 20 minutes at a time, and you

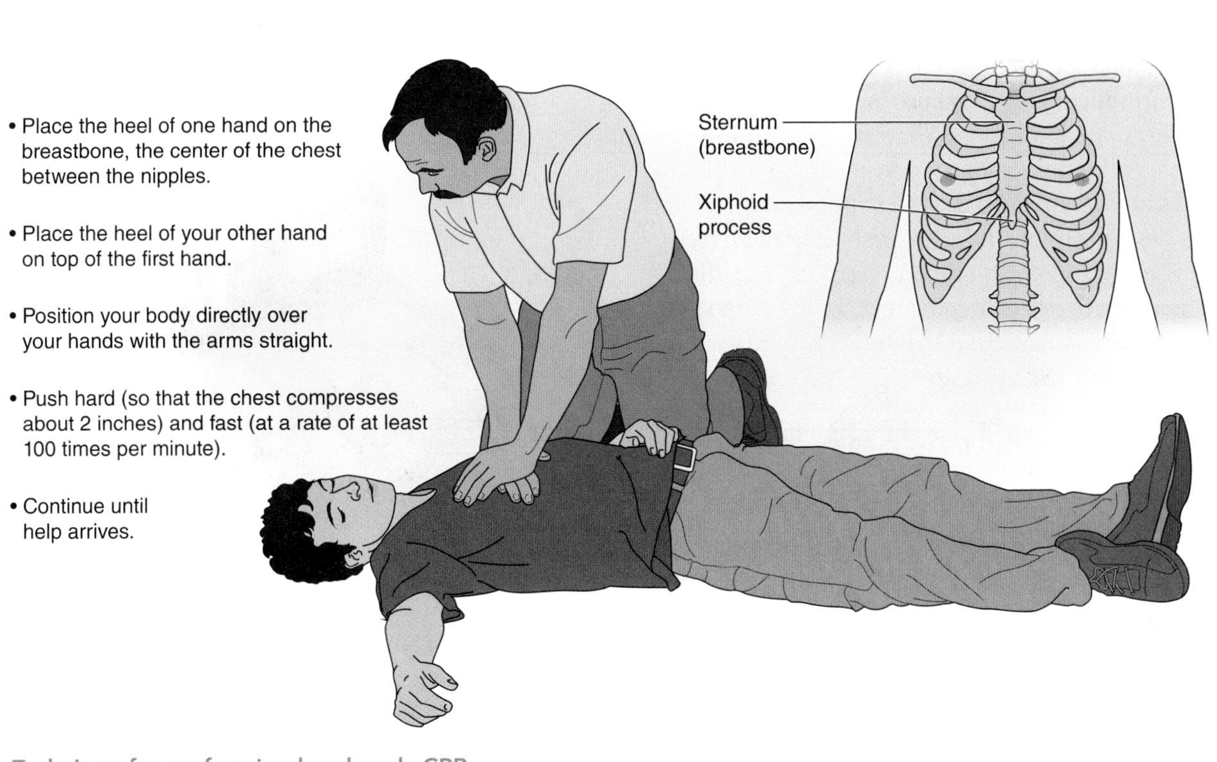

• Place the heel of one hand on the breastbone, the center of the chest between the nipples.
• Place the heel of your other hand on top of the first hand.
• Position your body directly over your hands with the arms straight.
• Push hard (so that the chest compresses about 2 inches) and fast (at a rate of at least 100 times per minute).
• Continue until help arrives.
Sternum (breastbone)
Xiphoid process

Technique for performing hands-only CPR.

3. Plug the connector into the AED.
4. Allow the AED to analyze the heart rhythm. Advise all bystanders to "stand clear" and do not touch the person.
5. Deliver a shock by pushing the button if indicated and prompted to do so by the AED. Be sure that no one is touching the AED and that there are no hazards present (e.g., water, wires) when delivering the shock.

should use a barrier such as a towel between the ice bag and the skin. A closed wound may be very serious if the individual cannot move the affected body part or is in obvious pain. Serious internal damage may also be indicated if an injured extremity is blue or extremely pale. In such cases, call 911 for assistance.

Open wounds include abrasions (scrapes), lacerations (cuts), avulsions (tearing), and punctures (holes). All open wounds require some sort of dressing, or covering, to control bleeding and prevent infection. For minor open wounds, apply direct pressure using a clean hand or sterile dressing (e.g., gauze) to control bleeding. Once the bleeding has stopped, wash the wound with warm water and soap. An open wound needs to be cleaned thoroughly. Any wound with dirt present should be rinsed in warm water for at least five minutes.

Finally, apply antibiotic ointment to the wound and cover it with a sterile bandage. Any major open wound that is bleeding profusely must be treated immediately with direct pressure to control the bleeding, and you should call 911. Never remove

CONSUMER CORNER: Buying a First Aid Kit

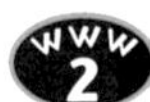

First aid kits are recommended for all homes and automobiles. You may also need one in other settings, such as a workshop, with camping or hiking supplies, or in a workout bag. Most first aid kits contain all of the basic supplies you need for treating minor injuries, including bandages, antiseptic and antibiotic ointment, and medical tape. Some kits are much larger and contain special items. When selecting or preparing a first aid kit, ask yourself the following questions.

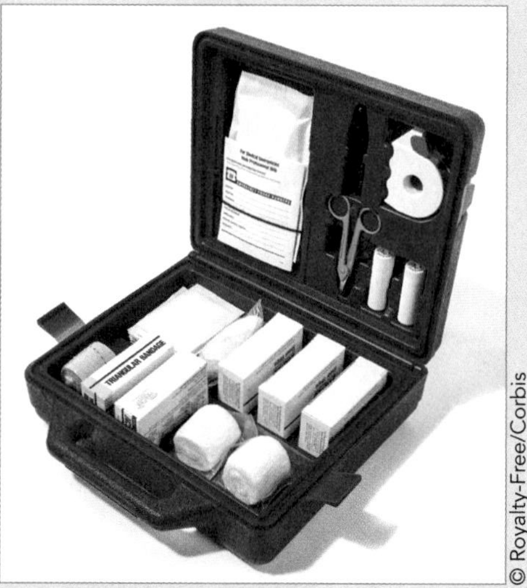

© Royalty-Free/Corbis

- **Where will I use the kit?** For home or automobile use, a basic kit is sufficient. If you'll be in a remote wilderness location or other high-risk situation (e.g., a workshop), you need a larger, more comprehensive kit.
- **What sort of container is best for my needs?** A home kit will do fine in a soft-sided bag. However, a kit for use outdoors is best kept in a hard-shelled container. The size of the container is also important. If you want the kit to be handy, make sure it fits in the space you have available.
- **How much do I want to spend?** If money is an issue, start with a basic kit. You can always add items to the kit over time.
- **What unique needs do I have?** If you have allergies, asthma, diabetes, or another condition that requires you to carry medication or supplies, buy a kit with enough room to add those items. If you live in a cold climate where you might be without power or get stranded in poor weather, choose a kit designed for outdoor use that includes emergency blankets and food. Consider any other particular needs you have.

Regardless of what kind of kit you buy or create, check it regularly to ensure that any medications and ointments are not outdated and that the supplies remain intact.

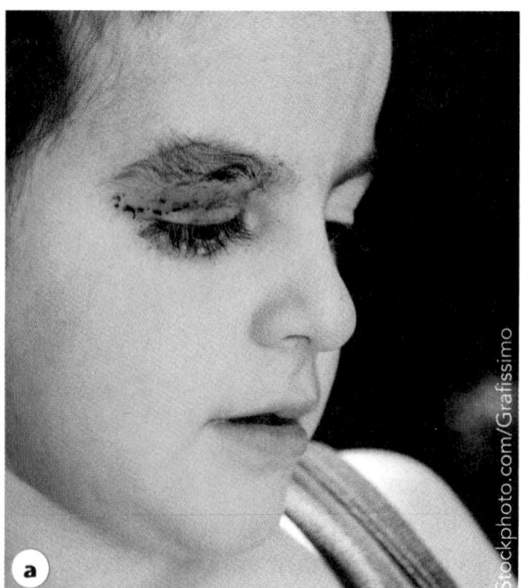

iStockphoto.com/Grafissimo

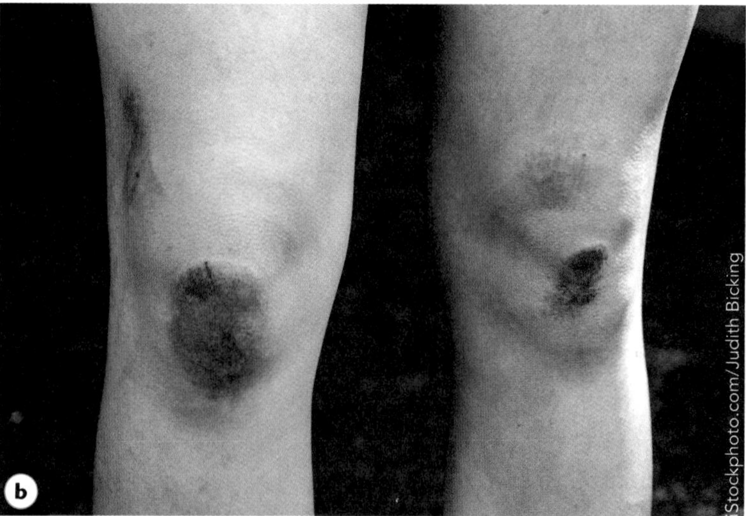

iStockphoto.com/Judith Bicking

Open wounds can include *(a)* lacerations (cuts) and *(b)* abrasions (scrapes).

blood-soaked dressings from a serious open wound; instead, continue to add clean dressings to absorb the blood. Removing bloody dressings can increase bleeding or bring germs into the site. Once the bleeding is under control, use a sterile bandage (wrap) to provide compression.

Muscle, Bone, and Joint Injuries

Injuries to muscles, bones, and joints happen often and to people of all ages. These injuries can happen at school, home, work, or play. They can be painful and often have long recovery periods that can make life difficult. Fortunately, they are rarely life threatening, but if left untreated they can cause serious problems, including disability. The general care appropriate for most muscle, bone, and joint injuries is to follow the RICE formula (see the accompanying text box). Serious bone or joint injuries such as a broken bone require immediate medical care.

Fractures

The term *fracture* refers to a break, chip, or crack in a bone. The most common kind is a **closed fracture**, which does not break through the skin. If the affected bone tears through the skin, the injury is an **open fracture**. Another type of bone injury is **dislocation**, in which the bone moves away from its normal position near a joint; as a result, motion at that joint is lost or severely impaired. All suspected fractures and dislocations must be treated by a physician.

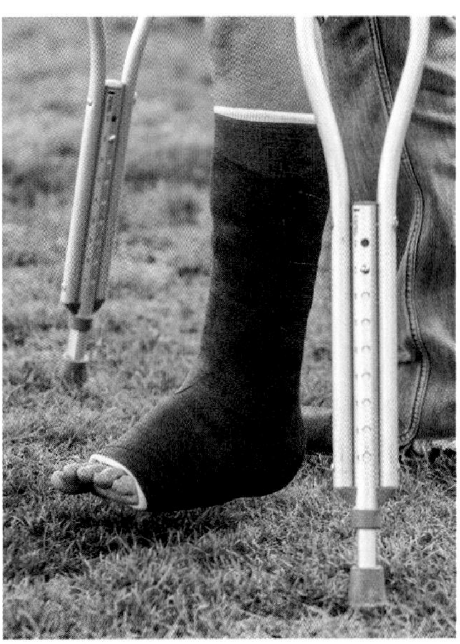

Broken bones require immobilization by a cast to allow them to heal.

Sprains and Strains

Sprains and **strains** are relatively common. A sprain involves the tearing of a ligament, whereas a strain involves the stretching or tearing of a muscle or tendon. Severe sprains and strains often cause extreme pain, swelling, bruising, unusual appearance in the injured area, and a temporary loss of functioning. Once the initial swelling has been treated with the RICE formula, severe strains and sprains may require immobilization by a cast, brace, or splint and surgery to repair the tissue may be needed.

The RICE Formula for Treating Injury

R is for rest. After first aid has been given for the injury, the body part should be immobilized for two to three days to prevent further injury.
I is for ice. A sprain or strain should be immersed in cold water or covered with ice in a towel or plastic bag. Ice the area for 20 minutes, starting immediately after the injury occurs, to reduce swelling and pain. Ice or cold should be applied several times a day for one to three days.
C is for compression. Use an elastic bandage to limit swelling. For a sprained ankle, keep the shoe laced and the sock on the foot until compression can be applied with a bandage (the shoe and sock compress the injured area in the meantime). The compression should not be too tight, and it should be taken off periodically so as not to restrict blood flow.
E is for elevation. Raise the body part above the heart to reduce swelling.
Note: Many people use the PRICE system where the P stands for protection.

Sudden Illness

It's usually easy to tell when an accident has occurred, but it can be more challenging to know what to do if someone becomes suddenly ill. Many chronic health conditions (e.g., diabetes, cardiovascular disease) can result in the onset of a sudden and serious situation, such as a stroke, diabetic reaction, or seizure. If a person demonstrates signs of a sudden and serious injury, call 911 and be prepared to describe the signs you're seeing. Don't be afraid to speak directly to the individual to help you determine what might be causing the signs. People with a chronic disease may understand what they are experiencing and may have medications available.

Weather-Related Emergencies

Weather conditions affect how our bodies function. Extremely hot and extremely cold conditions can quickly become life threatening. Even when weather conditions don't seem extreme, you can face weather-related risks depending on what you're wearing, what you're doing, and how well you're fed and hydrated.

Heat-Related Emergencies

Common heat-related emergencies include heat cramps, heat exhaustion, and **heatstroke**. Heat cramps (muscle spasms) can be an early sign of a more serious heat-related emergency. If a person experiences heat cramps, especially in the legs or abdomen, help him or her rest in a cool place and if possible provide cool water or a commercial sport drink.

In heat exhaustion, body temperature rises, and the person becomes nauseous, dizzy, exhausted, or weak and may have skin that is cool, moist, pale, or flushed. The most severe form of heat emergency is heatstroke, which is a serious medical emergency because body systems begin to shut down. Clear signs of heatstroke include changes in consciousness, along with rapid, shallow breathing and a weak pulse. For both heatstroke and heat exhaustion, seek medical assistance and have the person rest in a cool place and loosen any tight clothing. Apply loose, cool, wet clothing. Give water slowly, about 4 ounces (118 milliliters) every 15 minutes. Physical activity should be stopped for the remainder of the day, and 911 should be called if any changes occur in consciousness.

Cold-Related Emergencies

Two types of emergencies related to cold weather are frostbite and **hypothermia**. You can reduce your risk for both by wearing proper attire when engaged in outdoor activities in cold weather. Symptoms of frostbite include a lack of feeling in the affected area and skin that appears waxy, is cold to the touch, or is discolored. Avoid rubbing the frostbitten area and do not attempt to rewarm the area if there is any chance of refreezing. Call 911 or get the person to a hospital for proper care. Hypothermia results when the entire body cools below normal temperature; if untreated, it causes death. Hypothermia can be signaled by shivering, numbness, a glassy stare, indifference, or loss of consciousness. Keep the person warm and dry and seek immediate medical or emergency care.

Signs of Sudden Illness

- Changes in consciousness (e.g., severe dizziness, light-headedness, unconsciousness)
- Nausea or vomiting
- Difficulty speaking or slurred speech
- Numbness or weakness
- Changes in breathing or difficulty breathing
- Blurred vision or loss of vision
- Changes in skin color
- Profuse sweating

HEALTH TECHNOLOGY

Automated external defibrillators (AEDs) are portable, battery-operated devices that can deliver an electric shock to the heart. An AED is an essential tool for treating cardiac arrest and ventricular fibrillation, in which the heart contracts in an uncontrolled way and is therefore unable to deliver adequate blood to the body. The practice of delivering an electric shock to the heart dates back to 1899, when two French physiologists delivered an electric shock to a dog in ventricular defibrillation and successfully restored normal heart rhythm. With the AED, modern technology has made defibrillation possible in an affordable, self-contained device that is now found in many public places and buildings.

AEDs are simple and safe to use. Sticky pads with sensors (called electrodes) are attached to the chest of the person who is having a cardiac event, and the device itself provides step-by-step verbal and visual instructions. The electrodes can detect the person's heart rhythm and determine whether normal heart functioning has been restored by the delivery of the electric shock. Prompt use of an external defibrillator can save up to 60 percent of treated victims.

CONNECT

Do you know how to use an external defibrillator? What types of facility might benefit from having a defibrillator on site? What circumstances might make it important for a family to consider purchasing a defibrillator? To research your responses, visit the website of the American Heart Association (www.heart.org).

Emergency Preparedness

Everything discussed in this chapter should be taken into consideration when creating an emergency preparedness plan. An emergency preparedness plan involves taking actions to keep yourself and your loved ones safe before an emergency occurs so that you can remain safe during the emergency. You may need to activate your emergency preparedness plan in the event of natural disasters, pandemic emergencies (rapidly spreading disease), technological emergencies (e.g., a blackout or nuclear power plant disaster), or terrorist attacks. Each type of emergency requires specific consideration, but all emergencies share some common considerations. First, consider your physical safety. Many emergencies will require either sheltering in place or evacuating. Determine the safest place to be in each type of emergency you may face and make sure every member of the family knows the plan. Develop a family communication plan so that you know how you will get and stay in contact during an emergency. It is also important to make an emergency supply kit that will prepare you for any type of disaster. Nonperishable food, water, sanitation needs, light sources, blankets, first aid supplies, and other items unique to your circumstances need to be part of your disaster kit. You should also learn about the emergency alert systems in place at your school, workplace, and community. Getting early warning about dangers is one of the most effective tools for staying safe in all types of situations. It is also important to be familiar with local emergency plans. Many communities have designated shelter facilities where aid, medical help, and food are available during emergencies. You can learn more about emergency preparedness in the student section of the Health Opportunities Through Physical Education website.

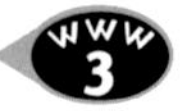

Comprehension Check

1. What are the three emergency action steps that should be followed for administering CPR?
2. What are the basic first aid procedures for common emergency scenarios such as treating an open wound?
3. How do you know if a person has a sudden illness that might need medical attention?

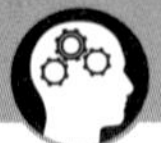

MAKING HEALTHY DECISIONS: Skill Building

David is a high school sophomore who was in a serious car crash during middle school. His dad had often been impatient on the road and had driven aggressively. David suffered only minor injuries in the crash, but his dad was more severely injured (abrasions and broken bones). At the scene, David felt helpless and didn't know what to do to help himself or his dad. Ever since that night, David has been studying first aid almost obsessively. He never wants to feel unprepared again. When his school has emergency preparedness days, David is very particular and criticizes others who are learning and practicing their skills. He obsesses over the details of the scenario and argues with others about the right thing to do.

Jennifer, also a sophomore, doesn't understand David's obsession with being prepared for emergencies. She figures nothing will really happen to her, and if it does she can just look up the answers online or rely on someone nearby to help. On emergency preparedness days at school, Jennifer goofs off, and she thinks that learning CPR and first aid is a waste of time.

For Discussion

Neither David nor Jennifer is building skills in the right way. What would you tell David about his approach to skill building? How might you encourage Jennifer to take her skill building seriously? Which of the two do you most resemble when it comes to developing your CPR and first aid skills? See the Skills for Healthy Living feature to help you address these questions.

SKILLS FOR HEALTHY LIVING: Skill Building

Emergency situations can be stressful and cause a sense of panic and fear. In order to help yourself and others during an emergency, keep your CPR and first aid skills fresh.

- **Get good training.** High-quality CPR and first aid instruction is readily available in most communities. Seek out training opportunities, for example, at your local Red Cross chapter, community center, fire or police station, safety council, or school. Some communities offer free training for community members at CPR events.
- **Revisit your training as often as needed.** Most CPR cards are good for 12 months, and most first aid cards for 3 years, but research shows that much of what is learned is forgotten within 3 months. Don't be shy about attending training more often than required or reviewing resource materials regularly.
- **Practice responding to emergency situations before they occur.** As with sport, music, and other skills, the more you practice your CPR and first aid skills, the more likely you are to use them effectively during a real emergency. To prepare yourself to respond in a variety of situations, think about realistic emergency scenarios and rehearse your responses in your mind. Don't, however, try to imagine every possible scenario; focus on general situations and the skills they might require.
- **Don't wait for an emergency to occur to learn how to respond.** Learn a variety of first aid and CPR skills, even if they don't seem to apply to you or your current life. For example, a person may not think to learn how to provide CPR for an infant if he or she doesn't have children, and someone living in a tropical climate might not think to learn how to treat cold-related emergencies. However, emergencies occur in all sorts of unexpected situations, and being prepared before the fact is the only way to ensure that you can be effective in helping.
- **Communicate about emergency plans with others.** Talking about emergency plans and skills can help you remember what you need to do in a given situation

and can enable a sense of calm when an emergency occurs. For example, you can help reduce the risks associated with emergencies by reviewing fire exits, locations of fire extinguishers, and basic fire safety with family members and reminding teammates to dress properly to prevent heat- or cold-related injuries.

- **Remain focused and calm.** The better your skills—and the more regularly you practice them—the more likely you are to remain calm and focused during an emergency. When facing an emergency, take deep breaths, focus on the situation, and think one step at a time. If you have trouble remembering all of the specifics, calmly think through the situation and do the best you can.

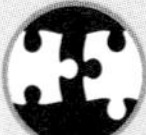

ACADEMIC CONNECTION: Causation and Correlation

One of the most common causes of confusion when reading scientific and health-related studies is the difference between causation and correlation. Causation means that one thing results in a specific change in another. The first is the reason why the second happens. For example, we now have enough evidence to know that smoking (the first thing) causes lung cancer (the second thing). Correlation means that two things are related to one another. For example, smoking is correlated to alcoholism, but smoking does not cause alcoholism. If one thing causes another, then the two things are also most certainly correlated. But just because two things occur together does not mean that one caused the other, even if it seems to make sense. For example, as stated in this chapter, mental illness is correlated (related) to incidences of violence. This means that these two factors have been shown to occur together more often than chance alone would predict. However, just because this correlation exists, it doesn't mean that mental illness directly causes violent acts. As a consumer of health information, you need to distinguish correlation from causation in order to accurately interpret and apply the information you learn.

Personal Watercraft Safety

In 2008, Michigan passed a law setting the minimum age for operating a personal watercraft at 14. Personal watercraft are vehicles that are propelled by machinery and are designed to be operated by a person sitting, standing, or kneeling on the vessel. Like many states, Michigan had previously allowed children as young as 12 to operate personal watercraft if they had a boater safety certificate and a parent on board. The new law bans anyone under 14 from operating a personal watercraft under any circumstances and allows only those over age 16 to do so without a supervisor on board. Supporters of the law believe that young teens do not have the maturity to maneuver what is essentially a motorcycle on water, and they support their position by citing accident statistics—personal watercraft make up only about 10 percent of water traffic but are involved in 30 percent of water traffic accidents.

Opponents of the law note that personal watercraft are no more dangerous than other forms of boating and that evidence is lacking against younger operators. U.S. Coast Guard data show fatal drownings while using a personal watercraft are quite low when compared with those associated with paddle boats, open motorboats, and cabin motorboats. This difference results primarily from the fact that most states require personal watercraft operators and passengers to wear life jackets. Studies show that only 9 percent of people who drown while using a personal watercraft are wearing a life jacket.

More generally, the most common injury sustained by personal watercraft users is blunt force trauma (trauma caused by injury, impact, or attack). Overall, the top five causes of boating accidents are operator inattention, operator inexperience, excessive speed, improper lookout, and alcohol (see table 34.1 for details). Of these factors, alcohol is the leading secondary factor in fatal personal watercraft accidents. It contributes to excessive speed, improper lookout, and operator inattention.

For Discussion

Have you ever been in a risky situation involving swimming or a personal watercraft? If so, what happened, and what did you do to minimize your risk? If you haven't been in this situation, what steps could you take to minimize the chances that you will experience such an incident?

TABLE 34.1 Top Five Contributing Factors in Personal Watercraft Accidents

Contributing factor	Accidents	Deaths	Injuries requiring medical attention
Operator inattention	624	58	426
Operator inexperience	553	49	321
Excessive speed	407	53	297
Improper lookout	398	37	305
Alcohol use	365	94	248

Source: United States Coast Guard Boating Safety Division, *2012 Boating Statistics.*

CHAPTER REVIEW

Reviewing Concepts and Vocabulary

As directed by your teacher, answer items 1 through 5 by correctly completing each sentence with a word or phrase.

1. Prescription ______________________ are the leading cause of death from unintentional poisonings among adults.
2. ________________ is the harmful or offensive contact of another person.
3. When performing adult CPR, give _______ compressions per minute.
4. Wearing a ____________ helps reduce the risk of injury while bicycling or skateboarding.
5. The term ________________ refers to a break, chip, or crack in a bone.

For items 6 through 10, as directed by your teacher, match each term in column 1 with the appropriate phrase in column 2.

6. alcohol	a. number of teens (aged 16 to 19) who die each day in a motor vehicle crash
7. distracted driving	b. least likely to wear a seat belt
8. males aged 19 to 29	c. four times more likely to crash
9. eight	d. plays a role in 25 percent of all fatal car crashes
10. teens aged 16 to 19	e. increases accident risk by 20 to 30 percent

For items 11 through 15, as directed by your teacher, respond to each statement or question.

11. Describe the three emergency action steps.
12. What does the acronym RICE stand for?
13. What is the difference between a sprain and a strain?
14. Provide two examples of intentional injuries.
15. What are three warning signs that a person might become violent against others?

Thinking Critically

Write a paragraph in response to the following questions.

You're walking home from work one day when you notice an older gentleman lying on the sidewalk. He is moaning, and his dog is standing near him on a leash. It's a sunny day, and you don't see any notable objects or blood on the sidewalk. What are some possible reasons that the man is on the ground? What are your next steps?

Take It Home

With the help of a parent or guardian, develop an emergency preparedness plan for your family. Identify potential emergencies. Address the following in your plan.

1. Determine your evacuation and communication plans.
2. Create an emergency supply kit.
3. Determine the local evacuation and emergency plans and services.

Then, write down your emergency plan and share it with family members.

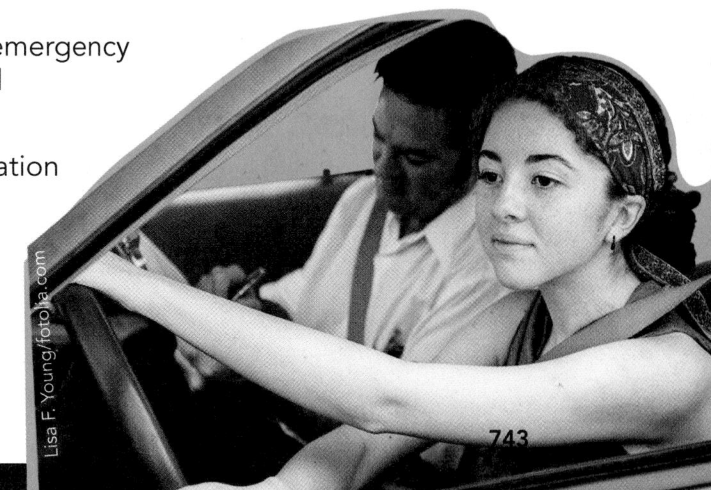
Lisa F. Young/fotolia.com

35

A Healthy Environment

In This Chapter

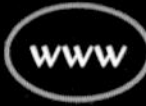

www **Student Web Resources**

www.HOPEtextbook.org/student

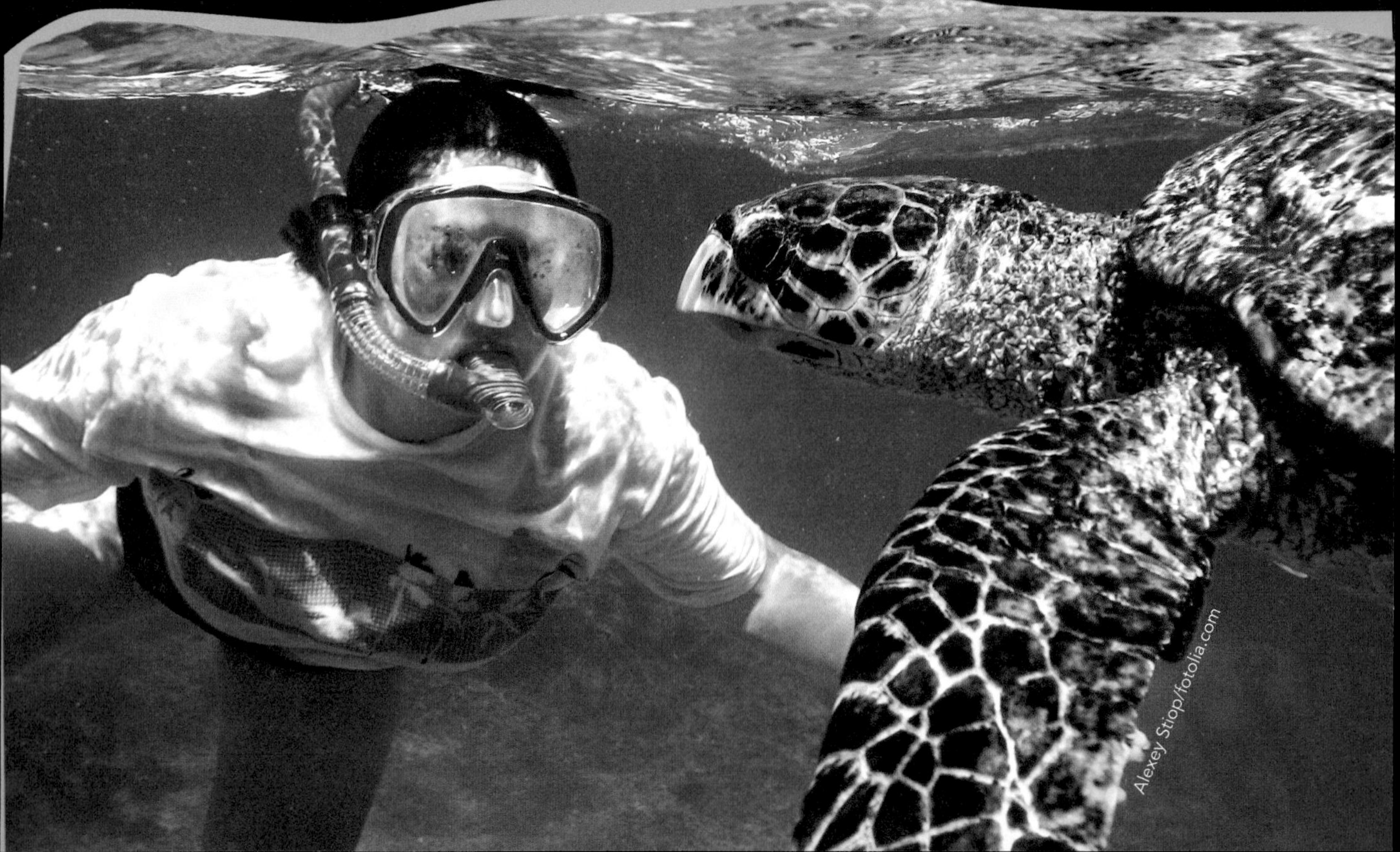

Alexey Stiop/fotolia.com

Lesson 35.1

Our Changing Environment

Lesson Objectives

After reading this lesson, you should be able to

1. list Barry Commoner's laws of ecology,
2. explain the importance of the four Rs, and
3. explain what is meant by the term *climate change*.

WWW 1 **Lesson Vocabulary**

biodegradable, climate change, ecology, global warming, sanitary landfill

Four basic laws of ecology have been formulated to help us better understand how our choices affect the environment. These laws, developed by American biologist Dr. Barry Commoner and others, are described in this lesson.

Human Impact on the Environment

The study of the interaction between people and the environment is known as **ecology**. Of course, humans have interacted with the environment as long as they have existed. However, as the human population has grown and technologies have evolved, our environmental impact has increased, and ecology has become an increasingly important area of study. The earth is home to seven billion people, all of whom eat, travel, go to the bathroom, and use various products. We throw things away and use energy in various forms and for various reasons. In addition, we have developed farming practices and advanced industry in ways that are not always friendly to the environment. Over time, we've discovered that we have to be careful about how much we consume, how we dispose of our waste, and how we affect the environment through our farming, industry, and technology.

Four Laws of Ecology

Barry Commoner (1917–2012) was an American biologist who once ran for U.S. president and who formulated four laws of ecology. These laws help us better understand how our choices affect the environment.

1. Everything is connected to everything else (what affects one organism affects us all). The earth is very complex, and all living things are in some way dependent on, or affected by, other living things. For example, honeybees pollinate many of the plants that humans rely on for food. In fact, one in every three bites of human food depends on the work of honeybees. However, when we humans use pesticides to control other insects, they can also hurt honeybees, thus dramatically affecting our own food supply.

2. Everything must go somewhere (when we throw something away, we have to realize there is no "away"). Our globe is a closed system. When we burn firewood, the fire produces smoke, which can fall back to earth as sediment when the embers cool or can be absorbed by plants, bacteria, and algae, in which it is broken down and used for energy or other processes. Unused gases from the smoke can also linger in the atmosphere and form pollution. In other words, the wood, like everything we use, never simply disappears.

3. Nature knows best (humans learn from nature and depend on nature to live; it is difficult to improve on nature and natural laws). In essence, this law suggests that the whole is greater than the sum of its parts. The earth is always changing, and the delicate balance of each part of nature plays a role in that change. For example, new forests are formed over thousands of years when seeds from briars, shrubs, vines, and trees are blown or carried by animals or water into a new area. Eventually, the seeds take root, and trees and shrubs start to grow and eventually dominate the grasses and herbs. Over time, the animal life also changes,

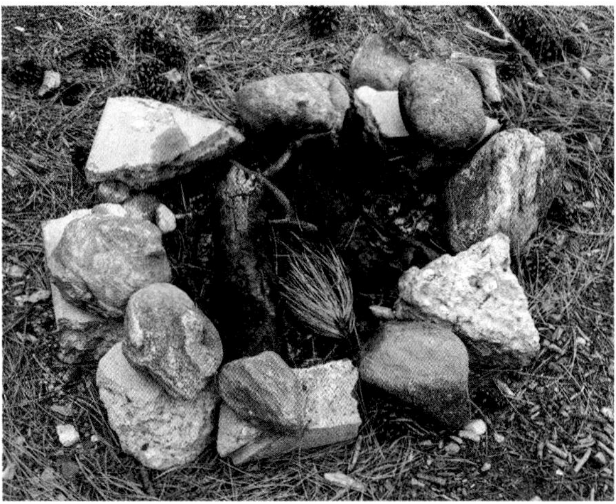

A fire ring represents the second law of ecology that says everything must go somewhere.

as field mice and rabbits who thrived on grasses make way for the animals of the forest, such as deer, squirrels, and owls. If humans clear a field and then plant a forest, our quick actions can devastate the naturally occurring habitats of animals and plants, displacing animals and upsetting the area's natural food supply.

4. There is no such thing as a free lunch (everything has a cost, which can come, for example, in the form of pollution-related health problems or the money we pay to light and heat our homes, businesses, and schools). Every action we take carries consequences—sometimes positive, sometimes negative. For example, if we overfish a particular body of water, we might increase the number of fish available for sale as food, which might reduce the cost to the consumer in the short term. However, we would also reduce the number of fish alive to reproduce and sustain the species, perhaps ultimately leaving it endangered or extinct.

> "I believe that you shouldn't have to leave your neighborhood to live in a better one."
>
> —Majora Carter, activist

The Four Rs

The four Rs refer to actions we can take to support a healthy environment (see figure 35.1):

- Refuse
- Reduce
- Reuse
- Recycle

Originally there were only three Rs, but many people saw an important distinction between reducing the use of something (e.g., a plastic bag), which means you'll continue to use it, and simply refusing to use it at all. Some people suggest that in order to really reduce, we have to refuse at least some of the time.

Whether you prefer four Rs or three Rs, the message should be clear: Don't use things that you don't need. Do avoid single-use items. Most plastic bags, for example, are used only once, usually for a short time, and then thrown away. Reuse means using the bag again—for example, on your next shopping trip, to carry a wet bathing suit, or to store things in. Recycling, in turn, means making sure that the plastic bag gets to a recycling center where it can be turned into another product. Not only are most plastic bags not taken to recycling centers, but even when they are, they are difficult to convert into new products, since that involves a costly and difficult process. WWW 2

A cloth bag, on the other hand, addresses all four Rs. If you have a cloth bag (the key is to remember

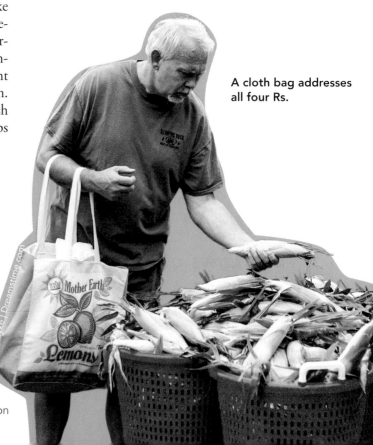

A cloth bag addresses all four Rs.

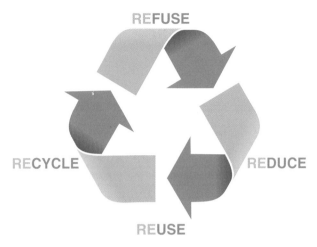

FIGURE 35.1 The four Rs.

to take it with you when you shop!), you can *refuse* to use a plastic or paper bag. Thus you have *reduced* the need for plastic bags, and you can also *reuse* your cloth bag over and over. When it finally does get torn or worn out, you can *recycle* it or, depending on the type of cloth, perhaps even compost it.

The four Rs are listed in the order of their importance. If you refuse a product, you don't need to worry about the next three Rs. If you reduce the amount of the product, you have fewer products to reuse. And if you reuse a product, you don't need to recycle it, at least not yet.

CONNECT

How do your peers affect your adoption of the four Rs? Do you experience peer pressure related to these practices? What could you do to encourage yourself and your friends to adopt the four Rs? Do you belong to any groups or organizations that help protect the environment?

Conspicuous Consumption

On average, each person in the United States generates 4.6 pounds (2.1 kilograms) of waste material every day—up from 2.7 pounds (1.2 kilograms) in 1960. As a result, some people refer to the nation as a "throwaway society" in which products either don't last very long or get discarded quickly in favor of a newer model. This way of life is becoming more and more problematic, in part because much of the stuff we throw away neither gets recycled nor goes to a sanitary landfill. So where does it go?

Captain Charles Moore has an answer. He has spent many years studying the items that end up in ocean waters. In his book *Plastic Ocean,* he describes the largest garbage dump in the world—an area twice the size of Texas in the Pacific Ocean that is strewn with plastic debris. Dubbed the Great Pacific Garbage Patch, this massive area serves as a stark warning about human consumption. Recycling efforts have not kept pace with our production of trash.

Captain Moore believes that plastic producers should be held responsible for making products that can be more easily recycled, that last longer, and that are not toxic to animals (including people). Of course, it is also everyone's responsibility to do a better job of recycling and making sure that our discarded products are disposed of appropriately. With this need in mind, it's always good to remind yourself of the four Rs as you go through your daily life: refuse products you don't need, reduce the number and amount of products you use, reuse any product that you can, and, if you can't do any of the first three Rs, recycle the product.

Sanitary Landfills

Plastics of all sorts have also become problematic for the environment beyond the Great Pacific Garbage Patch. Most plastics are petroleum based, which means they require fossil fuels to be manufactured. Fossil fuels contribute to air, land, and water pollution. Plastics also disturb or endanger animals that accidentally eat them or get entangled in them. And they are not **biodegradable**—that is, they do not break down or decompose. As a result, they take up space in **sanitary landfills**—sites where waste (the stuff we throw away) is taken to keep it separated from the rest of the environment.

Despite these issues, plastics keep increasing in availability. In fact, a large number of the goods we buy are either made of plastic or packaged in plastic. The more things we throw away (not just plastics), the more trips have to be made to the landfill, and the more energy is consumed in doing so.

In sanitary landfills, each day's waste is covered by dirt to prevent attracting birds or rodents. Sanitary landfills are located in places that minimize the

 ADVOCACY IN ACTION: Promoting Recycling

Not surprisingly, people are more likely to recycle when appropriate recycling bins are readily available. Evaluate your school to determine whether an *effective* recycling program is in place.

If your school doesn't provide recycling bins or lacks some needed options (e.g., paper, plastic, refuse, glass), determine what bins the school should add and what company or community organization will recycle the materials. You can even create a map showing where recycling bins should be located. Then write a one-page letter to the school board advocating for the purchase and appropriate placement of the needed recycling bins. Include information about the four Rs and explain why recycling is important for both environmental and personal health.

If your school already has adequate recycling bins, create posters to place above the bins that explain their importance and encourage students, teachers, and staff members to use them regularly.

likelihood of contaminating water sources and they have liners to prevent contaminants from leaching into water systems. When full, they can be turned into parks or recreation areas. In some landfills, the methane gas that is given off by the biological action of the buried materials can help to produce electrical power (see Health Science sidebar in this chapter). Poorly managed sanitary landfills can contaminate bodies of water and wells. Even in well-managed landfills, there is a concern about how effective they will contain contaminants 50 or more years into the future.

Climate Change

The term **climate change** is often used interchangeably with the term **global warming**, but, according to the U.S. Environmental Protection Agency (EPA), "Global warming is causing climate patterns to change. However, global warming itself represents only one aspect of climate change. *Climate change* refers to any significant change in the measures of climate lasting for an extended period of time." Some of these changes are shown in figure 35.2.

Climate change can result from

- natural factors such as changes in the sun's intensity;
- natural processes within the climate system, such as changes in ocean circulation; and
- human activities that change the atmosphere's composition (e.g., through the burning of fossil fuels) or the land surface (e.g., deforestation, reforestation, urbanization, desertification).

Global warming refers to an average increase in the temperature of the atmosphere near the earth's surface and in the troposphere (i.e., the layer of the atmosphere from the earth's surface to about six miles above the earth), which can contribute to changes in global climate patterns. The warming can result from a variety of causes, both natural and human induced. In common usage, the term often refers to the warming that can occur as a result of greenhouse gas emissions related to human activity.

Most climate scientists have concluded that climate change is placing great stress on the environment and that we must make major environmental changes. We can't depend on fossil fuels forever. Experts agree that we need to diversify our energy usage by increasing our use of renewable energy sources, such as wind, solar power, and biomass (animal waste and mostly plant material). We can also make houses and businesses more energy efficient. If we work together to create a more energy efficient society, we will be able to affect climate change for the better.

HEALTHY COMMUNICATION

Is your community a leader in addressing climate change? Should individuals be primarily responsible for changing their behaviors, or should society enact laws and regulations that require changes in how cars, houses, businesses, and manufacturing operations are powered? Debate your position with your peers. Support your position with facts and be respectful of others' opinions.

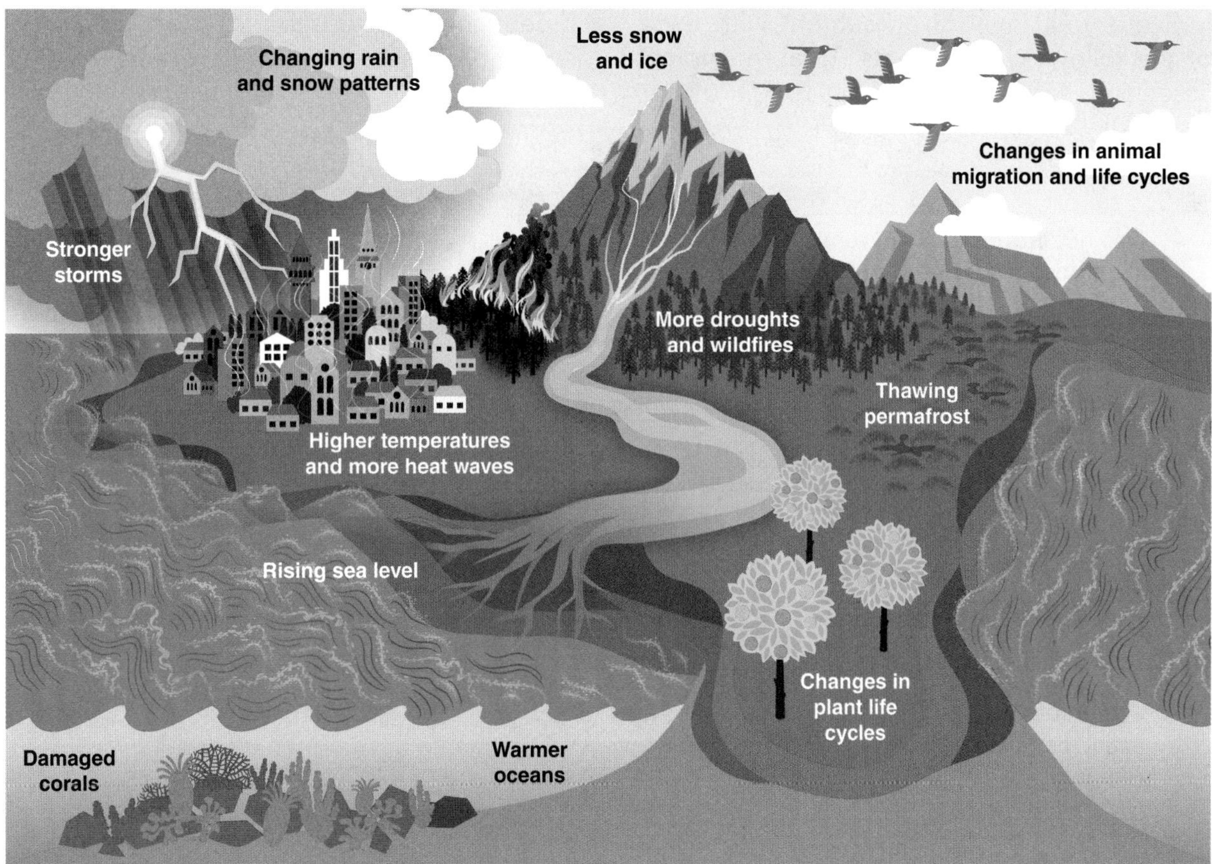

FIGURE 35.2 Effects of climate change.

HEALTH SCIENCE

Landfills are large sources of U.S. methane gas emissions—a major contributor to the erosion of the ozone layer that helps protect us from the sun's ultraviolet radiation. Landfill methane is produced when organic materials (e.g., yard, household, and food wastes) are decomposed by bacteria under anaerobic conditions (i.e., in the absence of oxygen). Methane production varies greatly from landfill to landfill, depending on site-specific characteristics such as moisture content, landfill design, operating practices, and climate.

Methane generated by a landfill is emitted when it migrates through the landfill cover. During this process, the soil oxidizes approximately 10 percent of the generated methane, and the remaining 90 percent is emitted. Landfill methane can be captured and used as fuel to generate electricity through the development of well fields and collection systems at the landfill. Collected methane can be used for on-site power generation or piped to a nearby generating station.

Comprehension Check

1. Which of Barry Commoner's laws of ecology best relates to sanitary landfills?
2. Explain why the order of the four Rs is important.
3. What is the difference between global warming and climate change?

SELF-ASSESSMENT: How Green Are You?

Indicate your level of agreement with each of the following statements. Total the points associated with your responses to figure your green score, then use the scale provided at the end of the assessment to interpret your score.

	Always	Sometimes	Never
1. I do not leave the water running when I am washing dishes or brushing my teeth (I turn it off and on as needed).	3	2	1
2. I use a cloth bag when I buy items at the store.	3	2	1
3. I walk, ride a bike, or use public transportation.	3	2	1
4. I participate in recycling programs.	3	2	1
5. I eat food from my own garden, a community or school garden, or a farmer's market.	3	2	1
6. I help conserve energy by keeping the thermostat at 68°F (20°C) or below in the winter and 78°F (26°C) or above in the summer.	3	2	1
7. I volunteer for projects, organizations, or school activities that help protect or clean up the environment.	3	2	1
8. I refuse to buy products that I don't really need.	3	2	1

Add up your points. My green score is ____________.

A score of 19 to 24 suggests that you have habits and behaviors that help protect the environment and your health.

A score of 16 to 18 suggests that you have some green habits and behaviors but also have room for improvement. Try to change at least one behavior to make your lifestyle more green.

A score of 15 or lower suggests that you have habits and behaviors that are not very green. It's time to make some changes. Try to change at least two behaviors to make your lifestyle more green.

Planning for Healthy Living

Use the Healthy Living Plan worksheet to help you change your environmental health habits.

Lesson 35.2

Green Schools and Communities

Lesson Objectives

After reading this lesson, you should be able to

1. explain two steps that individuals can take to reduce water pollution,
2. list at least two air pollutants and identify two actions that individuals can take to reduce their contribution to air pollution, and
3. define the term *conservation* and identify two types of conservation.

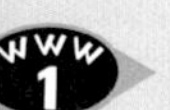

Lesson Vocabulary

built environment, complete streets, conservation, farm-to-school, green school, LEED certified

Water, air, soil, and noise pollution affect the health of both people and the environment. For example, more than a billion people in the world lack access to safe drinking water, and five thousand people die each day from drinking unsafe water. In the United States, almost half of all lakes, rivers, and streams are too polluted for safe fishing or swimming. Similarly, individuals who live in areas with heavy air pollution are 20 percent more likely to die from lung cancer than those who live in environments with clean air. And though the United States contains only 5 percent of the world's population, it consumes 25 percent of the world's resources.

As a result, improving our use and conservation of resources can improve both individual and environmental health. This lesson focuses on air pollution, water pollution, and conservation. In addition, the Living Well News feature addresses the effect of noise pollution on personal health.

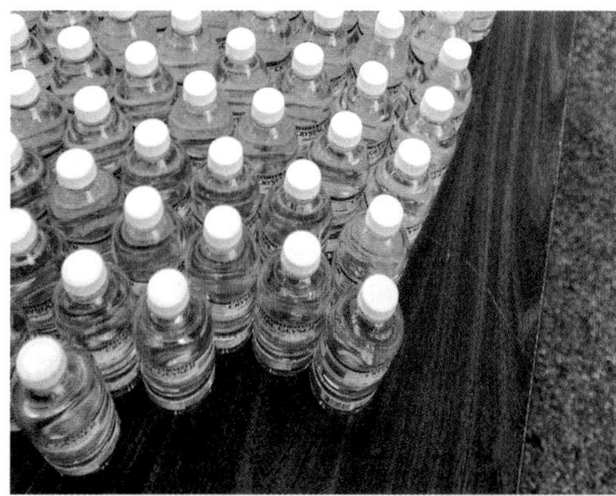

Some people drink from water bottles because they think public drinking water is unsafe. This is untrue for the majority of public water systems, and water bottles contribute to the problem of plastic waste.

Water Pollution

Water is one of our most important resources; in fact, we literally can't live without it. Therefore, we must conserve our clean water supply and keep it clean and free of chemicals and other pollutants.

Water pollution is not new. With the advent of the Industrial Revolution, factories began releasing large amounts of pollutants directly into rivers and streams. People were also dumping raw sewage into rivers and lakes, and over the years more and more chemicals were handled in the same way. In 1969, chemical pollution caused a fire on the Cuyahoga River that drew national attention, and the burning river became a symbol of how industrial water pollution was destroying America's natural resources. In response, the public demanded better pollution controls, and science supported the demand to clean up water supplies in the interest of public health.

As you may recall, microorganisms can cause illness and many of these microorganisms can live in water. That's why we have to treat water in order to make it safe. Fortunately, the overwhelming majority of public water systems in the United States provide safe drinking water. This is due in part to the work of the U.S. Environmental Protection Agency (EPA), which helps regulate the quality of water, air, and soil.

The general safety of public drinking water in the United States makes it unnecessary to drink bottled water. In fact, drinking water from plastic bottles contributes to the problem of plastic waste. Not only do most plastic bottles not get recycled, but also the bottling and transporting of water uses a lot of energy. In addition, certain types of plastic bottles may leach toxins into the liquid in the bottles.

Since water is all around us in streams, rivers, wells, lakes, and oceans, we need to actively protect it from contamination. Contaminated water can contribute not only to infections but also to some types of cancer, kidney damage, skin irritations, nervous system problems, and fertility problems. We can all do our part to help keep water safe (see table 35.1).

Air Pollution

Like water pollution, air pollution poses many risks to human health, including lung and heart disease. Also like water pollution, air pollution is not new. The main cause of air pollution is the burning of fuel that releases chemicals into the air—for example, at power plants and other industrial operations, as well as in the combustion engines that power cars, trucks, and airplanes.

The United States, like many countries, has enacted laws to protect the quality of the air we breathe, most notably the Clean Air Act Extension of 1970. This comprehensive federal law (since updated) regulates air emissions from stationary and mobile sources. Among other things, it authorizes the EPA to establish the National Ambient Air Quality Standards to protect the public's health and welfare and specifically to regulate the emission of air pollutants.

Throughout history, people have debated what pollutant levels are safe and to what extent governments should control businesses' and individual's activities related to air pollution. It is not always easy to decide, for example, where to draw the line and when there is a conflict between earning a living and protecting the environment. For example, some people think the EPA's rules are too strict and that they make it too difficult or expensive to do business. Others see the rules as too lenient and think they should regulate even more substances to protect people from harm. Scientific research can help people decide which substances should be regulated and to what extent. Table 35.2 summarizes four of the main air pollutants, their origins, and the health problems associated with them. In 2013, the World Health Organization added air pollution to its list of known carcinogens (i.e., something that causes cancer).

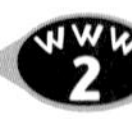

The EPA offers many suggestions for reducing air pollution (see the student section of the Health Opportunities Through Physical Education website). Examples include deciding not to buy things you don't need, recycling as many things as you can, turning off (or better yet, unplugging) appliances and lights you aren't using, and choosing rechargeable batteries to power devices that you use frequently.

TABLE 35.1 How to Keep the Water Supply Safe

Action item	Notes
Don't put anything except water down storm drains.	Contaminants (e.g., motor oil, detergent, fertilizer, pesticide) get carried by storm water to local waterways and cause unnecessary harm.
Whenever possible, avoid using pesticides and chemical fertilizers.	They pose a serious threat to your health and safety and pollute both ground and surface water, which can harm fish, other animals, and humans.
Choose nontoxic household products whenever possible.	Dangerous fumes from toxic products can contaminate the air, and toxins can enter the water supply. The best way to avoid polluting is to use products that are not dangerous to the environment in the first place.
Don't flush unwanted or out-of-date medicine down the toilet or put it down the drain.	Find out if your county or city has a program for collecting unwanted pharmaceuticals. If not, remove all labels and wrap the product up before putting it in the garbage. If possible, pour water or vinegar into the bottle to destroy pills and make them inaccessible to children.

TABLE 35.2 Selected Major Air Pollutants

Pollutant	Source(s)	Human health effects
Particles (often referred to as particulate matter or PM)	• Internal combustion engines (e.g., cars, trucks) • Industry (e.g., factories) • Burning wood and coal • Cigarette smoke • Bush and forest fires	Long-term exposure is linked to health problems, such as lung disease (including cancer), heart disease, and asthma attacks.
Ozone (O_3)	Ozone is formed by complex chemical reactions involving oxides of nitrogen and some hydrocarbons. It is the main ingredient of smog in summer and early autumn.	Ozone affects the lining of the lungs and respiratory tract and causes eye irritation. It also damages plants, buildings, and other materials.
Carbon monoxide (CO)	• Motor vehicle exhaust • Burning of various materials (e.g., coal, oil, wood) • Industrial processes (e.g., waste incineration)	Inhaled carbon monoxide enters the bloodstream and disrupts the supply of oxygen to the body's tissues. Health effects depend on the extent of exposure. Depending on which organizational guidelines you choose, the permissible exposure amount ranges from 25 parts per million to 50 parts per million.
Carbon dioxide (CO_2)	Burning of fossil fuels in, for example, coal and natural gas energy plants, motor vehicles, and airplanes	Carbon dioxide is the main greenhouse gas that contributes to global warming, which in turn contributes to increases in asthma, respiratory disease, heart and lung disease, and cancer. It also contributes indirectly to increases in malaria, Lyme disease, encephalitis, hantavirus, cholera, cryptosporidiosis, and salmonella.

Adapted, by permission, from EPA Victoria. Available: www.epa.vic.gov.au/air/aq4kids/main_pollutants.asp.

You can also help prevent pollution when you travel by using public transportation, walking, or riding a bike whenever possible. If you do drive, plan thoughtfully so that you can get several things done in one trip instead of going back and forth to the same area. You can also keep your tires properly inflated and aligned to improve gas mileage. Avoid spilling gas (don't "top off" the tank; do replace the gas cap tightly) and have your car tuned up regularly for better gas mileage and to reduce emissions. You can also carpool or ride the bus to school.

If you have a respiratory condition (e.g., asthma) or want to prevent a respiratory problem, check the daily air quality forecast online. If you have a smartphone, try one of the free apps available to keep you updated about the air quality where you live.

Conservation

Conservation involves the preservation, protection, and restoration of natural ecosystems (see table 35.3). It is closely related to sustainability, which involves using a resource in such a way that it is not permanently damaged or depleted. Water and energy conservation are two types of conservation that you can practice every day.

For example, if we let a faucet run, we not only waste water but also add to the water that must be treated (it goes down the drain just like the water we actually use). Fortunately, there are lots of actions we can take to conserve water on a daily basis; for some examples, see figure 35.3. Similarly, if you walk, bike, or take public transportation, you help

TABLE 35.3 Types of Conservation

Type	Significance
Water	Only 1% of the earth's water is freshwater. Therefore, gathering, cleaning, storing, and distributing freshwater is critical to human survival and global health.
Soil	Topsoil holds most of the nutrients needed to support plant life. It is eroded, however, by deforestation, poor farming practices, and other human actions.
Wetland	Wetlands provide valuable flood protection, as well as habitat for plants and wildlife. The U.S. Environmental Protection Agency estimates that one-third of the nation's threatened and endangered species depend strictly on wetlands, making wetland conservation necessary if we are to prevent further environmental losses.
Prairie	Prairies are some of the most endangered ecosystems in the world, and they have experienced losses of more than 90% in some states (e.g., Iowa, Illinois). Like wetlands, prairies provide valuable habitat for plants and wildlife. They can also play a role in conserving other natural resources, such as soil.
Energy	The rising cost of fossil fuels and growing environmental concerns have made energy conservation a priority for many governments and individuals. The goal of energy conservation is to properly balance the need for energy with the environmental impact of fulfilling that need.

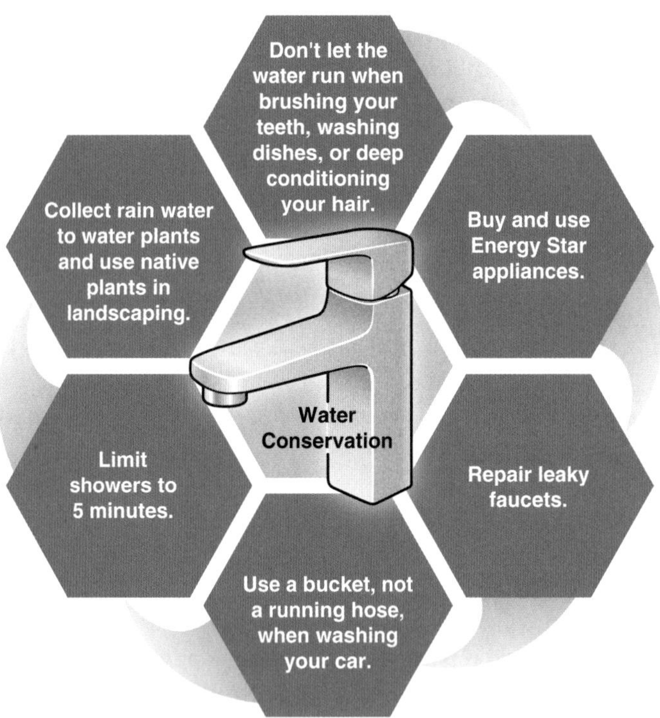

FIGURE 35.3 Ways to conserve water.

conserve energy (and you're reducing the air pollution emitted by car engines). Other daily choices you can make to conserve energy are shown in figure 35.4. Conserving water, energy, and other resources is an excellent way to reduce pollution that can adversely affect health.

Complete Streets

Conserving energy doesn't just mean reducing energy use or advocating for renewable fuel sources. It can also be incorporated into building and urban design (see the Health Technology feature for more information). For example, many organizations

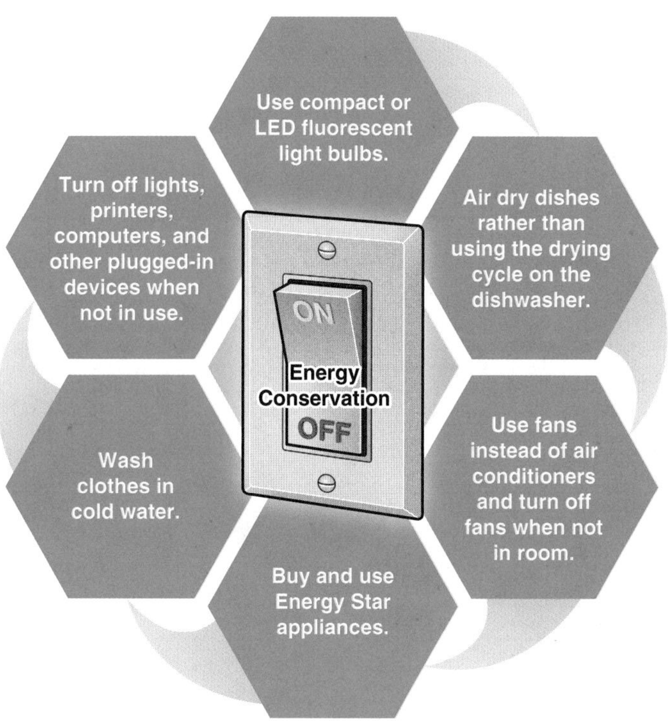

FIGURE 35.4 Ways to conserve energy.

in the United States and around the world now advocate for **complete streets**—that is, streets designed and operated to enable safe access for all users, including pedestrians, bicyclists, motorists, and transit riders of all ages and abilities. Complete streets make it easy to cross the street, walk to shops, and bicycle to work. They allow buses to run on time and make it safe for people to walk to and from train stations. This initiative is an example of how energy conservation can be integrated even into a modern endeavor such as urban (city) design. The value of complete streets is summarized in figure 35.5.

Green Schools

The movement for creating **green schools** is growing. The Green Schools Initiative advocates for schools to address what it calls the four pillars (see figure 35.6). The first pillar involves striving to be free of toxic substances, which means re-evaluating the chemicals used in cleaning supplies, in chemistry classes, and as pesticides. Pillar two involves using resources in a sustainable way—for example, using recycled paper whenever possible and recycling as many materials as possible. Pillar three calls for each school to have or be involved with healthy, green spaces. This might mean growing food in a school garden or having a local farm deliver fresh food to the school cafeteria. This is called **farm-to-school**, where farms deliver fresh foods directly to the schools. The fourth pillar involves teaching students about the environment and encouraging them to get involved in organizations and in the community to help maintain or improve the environment. An overarching theme of green schools is they observe the precautionary principle, which can best be summarized by the phrase *better safe than sorry*. If you are not sure if an action or behavior is safe or not, you should not do it. At the very least, do more research before you act.

School Gardens

School gardens are becoming increasingly popular, and they can meet many needs. Food grown in a school garden can be served in the cafeteria, thus providing fresher food that doesn't have to be transported, which saves energy. Gardens also help students and teachers learn about nature and where food comes from. In addition, gardening is a good form of exercise and a good way to socialize and build community. Many organizations support school gardens and provide resources that can

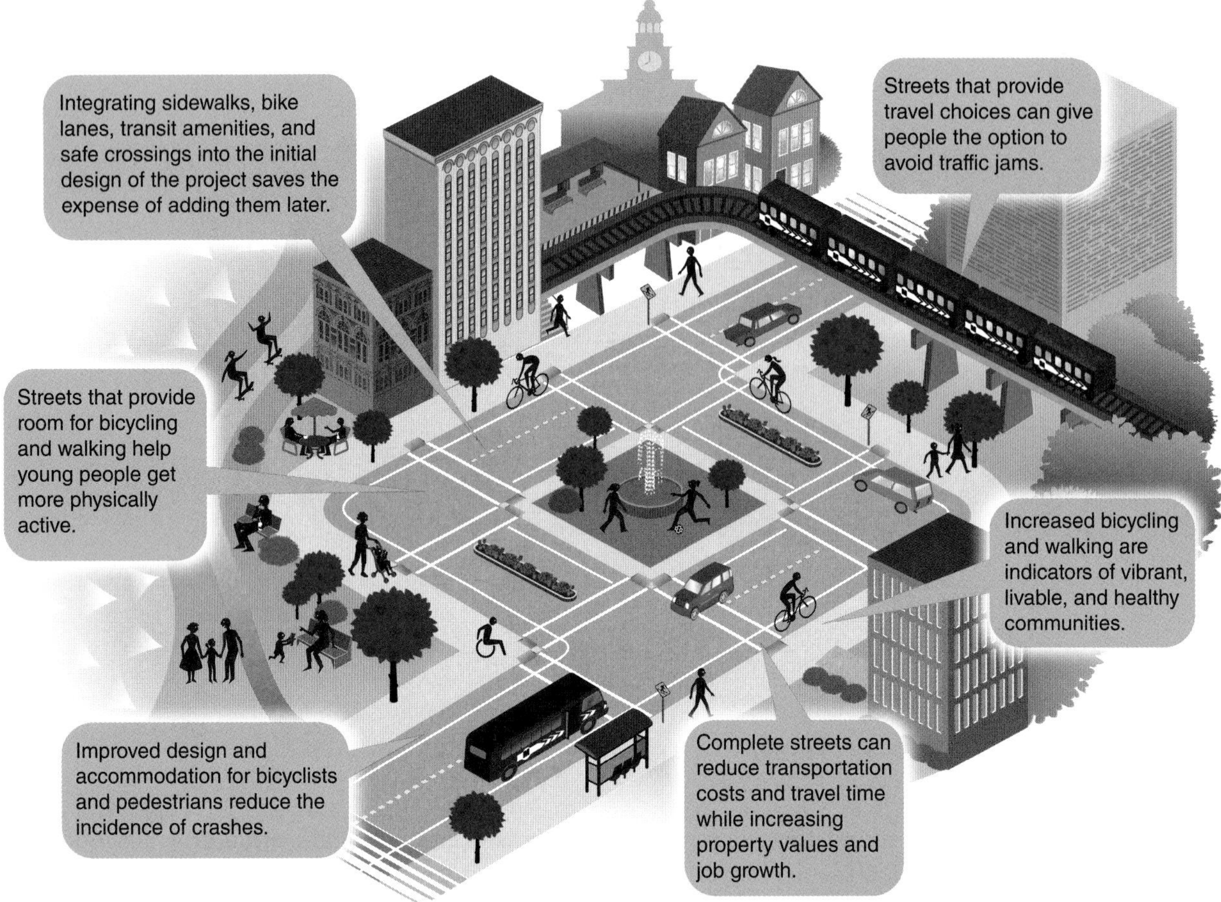

Integrating sidewalks, bike lanes, transit amenities, and safe crossings into the initial design of the project saves the expense of adding them later.
Streets that provide travel choices can give people the option to avoid traffic jams.
Streets that provide room for bicycling and walking help young people get more physically active.
Increased bicycling and walking are indicators of vibrant, livable, and healthy communities.
Improved design and accommodation for bicyclists and pedestrians reduce the incidence of crashes.
Complete streets can reduce transportation costs and travel time while increasing property values and job growth.

FIGURE 35.5 Streets are not complete until they are safe and convenient for travel by foot and bicycle, as well as for transit users, people with disabilities, and people in automobiles.

Facts are adapted from The National Complete Streets Coalition *Benefits fact sheet, and the Bicycle Coalition of Maine*, April 2009. www.bikewalklee.org/BWL_PDFs/BWL_facts/051109completeStreets.pdf.

help you start, operate, and maintain a garden at your school. To find them, just do a web search for information about school gardens.

Other Ways to Help Solve Environmental Health Problems

Numerous groups and organizations are dedicated to protecting the environment and improving human health, and many of them are led by young people. These organizations take a variety of focuses—for example, policy change, community cleanup, and community togetherness.

Some schools follow their own environmental checklists through cooperation among students, teachers, and staff. One example is the Georgia School Environmental Checklist, which includes questions such as the following: Are cleaning products and science and art supplies free of toxic substances? Does the school control pests and unwanted weeds without the use of pesticides?

In addition, groups such as Youth Service America and Do Something organize youth service and youth involvement projects, some of which provide opportunities for which groups can receive funding. Not all the projects are related to the environment, but many are. As the saying goes, "if you're not part of the solution, you're part of the problem."

HEALTH TECHNOLOGY

The environment created by people is referred to as the **built environment**, and it can include elements such as green (environmentally friendly) buildings; bicycle lanes and bike racks; complete streets; sidewalk cafes; playgrounds; water parks, fitness parks, and traditional parks; fountains and public art; and community and school gardens. When people—planners, architects, politicians, public health professionals, and everyday citizens—work together thoughtfully on the built environment, they can create healthier communities.

For example, designers can use new computer technology to test their designs and see which type of home is most energy efficient or which type of street is safest. If, for example, a building meets the standards required to become **LEED certified**, it will use less energy and water. If a building has solar panels, the occupants can use their personal computers to track, in real time, how much solar energy is being produced. They can also view an estimate of the money they're saving and the carbon they're preventing from being released into the atmosphere. They can even use a smartphone to monitor how much solar energy they are producing in the building where they work or live.

CONNECT

How important do you think it is for new buildings to be built to green standards? If you were renting an apartment or buying a home, how important would it be to you that it meet green standards? Explain your perspective.

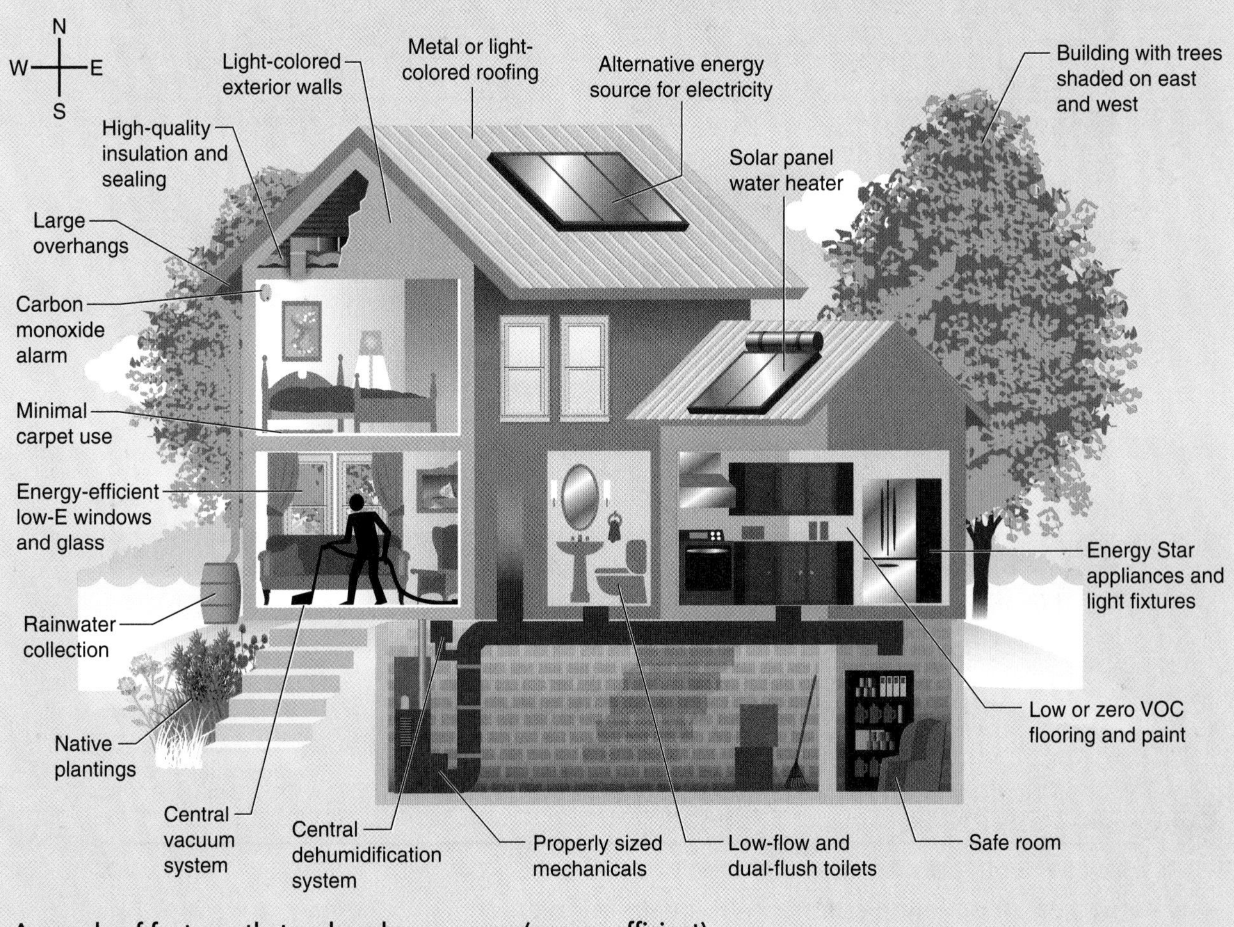

A sample of features that make a house green (energy efficient).

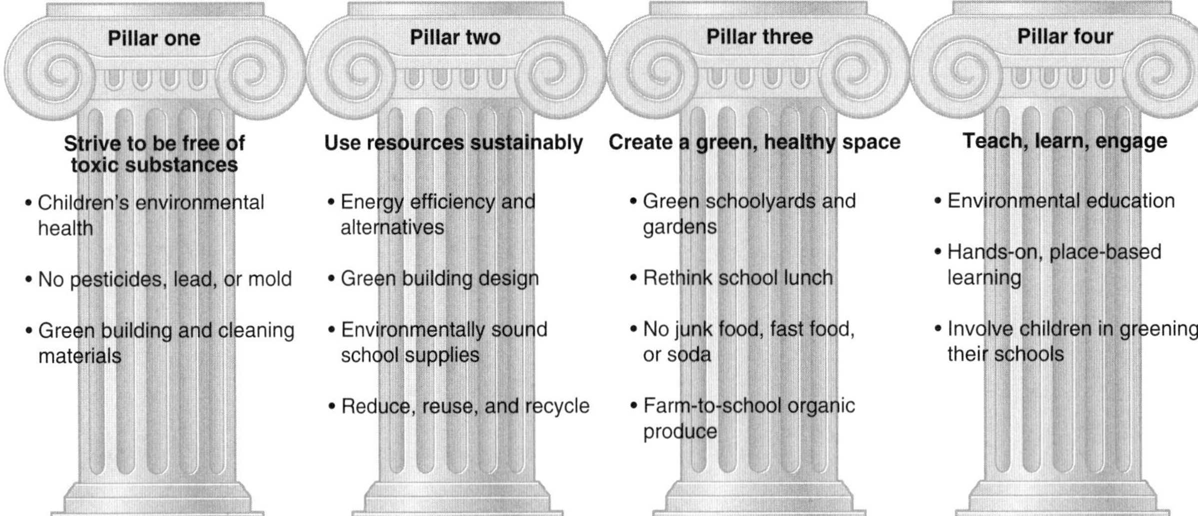

Pillar one
Strive to be free of toxic substances
• Children's environmental health
• No pesticides, lead, or mold
• Green building and cleaning materials
Pillar two
Use resources sustainably
• Energy efficiency and alternatives
• Green building design
• Environmentally sound school supplies
• Reduce, reuse, and recycle
Pillar three
Create a green, healthy space
• Green schoolyards and gardens
• Rethink school lunch
• No junk food, fast food, or soda
• Farm-to-school organic produce
Pillar four
Teach, learn, engage
• Environmental education
• Hands-on, place-based learning
• Involve children in greening their schools

FIGURE 35.6 The four pillars of a green school.

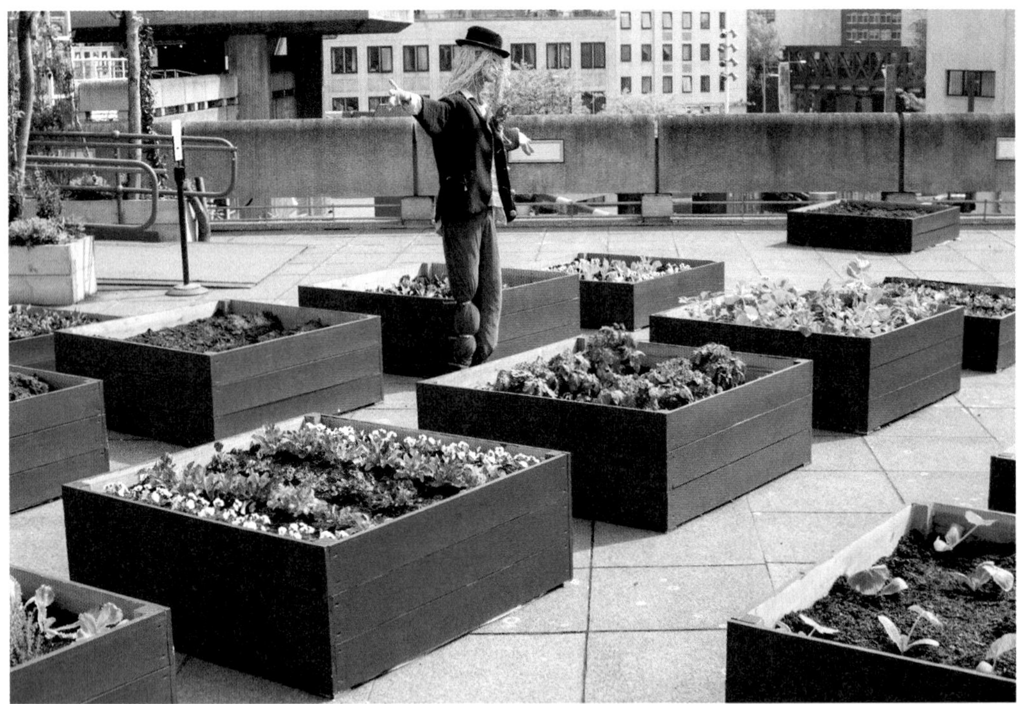

Rooftops make school gardens possible in urban areas.

nickos - Fotolia

Comprehension Check

1. How can you reduce water pollution?
2. How can air pollution contribute to health problems?
3. What is the relationship between conservation and reducing the amount of things you buy?

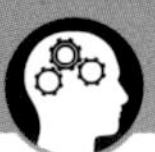

MAKING HEALTHY DECISIONS: Overcoming Barriers

Jerry wanted to eat a healthier diet but found it easier to eat at the convenience store beside his workplace. Their hot dogs and nachos were regularly on special, he could get plenty to eat for very little money, and there were no other convenient places within walking distance (he didn't have a car). As for dinner, he was often too tired to care.

One of Jerry's co-workers with a car usually drove to a sandwich shop a few miles away for lunch, but Jerry didn't feel comfortable asking for a ride. Besides, their lunch hours didn't always line up. In addition, Jerry sometimes had only a couple of dollars and wouldn't be able to buy a sandwich anyway. True, his parents usually kept carrots and apples in the house, but he always seemed to forget about them. When his friend Samson asked why he didn't just bring a healthy lunch to work, he said, "A guy can't live on carrots and apples anyway, so I'd still be buying this other stuff, so it really doesn't matter."

For Discussion

What barriers does Jerry have to overcome in order to change his eating habits? What is one strategy Jerry might use to overcome his barriers? What are three specific action steps Jerry could take? In answering these questions, consider the guidelines presented in the Skills for Healthy Living feature.

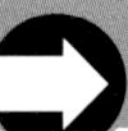

SKILLS FOR HEALTHY LIVING: Overcoming Barriers

People can face many barriers when trying to make healthy behavior changes. Some barriers involve the environment (e.g., access to food choices, exercise facilities, health care, and support groups), some involve personal characteristics (e.g., existing health conditions), and some are psychological (e.g., low self-confidence, lack of time management skills). Overcoming such barriers is a necessary skill for successfully adopting any healthy behavior—or quitting any unhealthy behavior. Here are some helpful strategies.

- **Identify and evaluate your barriers.** The first step in overcoming a barrier to behavior change is recognizing the barrier in the first place.
- **Set goals.** Set both short- and long-term goals to give you direction and purpose.
- **Take small steps.** Use small, manageable action steps that help you progress toward your goals.
- **Develop a new way of thinking.** Avoid negative self-talk. Do use positive self-talk to improve your self-perceptions and self-confidence. Focus on things you can do and use phrases like "I can" and "I will" in place of "I can't" or "I won't."
- **Get active.** Join a community or school group that provides social support.
- **Don't quit.** If a barrier seems too big to overcome and you begin to feel discouraged, don't quit. Stick to your action steps.

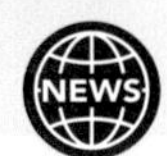

LIVING WELL NEWS, ISSUE 35

Can Earbuds Damage Hearing?

A stunning number of teens—nearly one in five—have lost some of their hearing, and the problem has increased substantially in recent years, according to a new study based on data from the U.S. Centers for Disease Control and Prevention. The researchers compared hearing loss in about three thousand teenagers tested between 1988 and 1994 with hearing loss in nearly two thousand students tested in 2005 and 2006. They found that hearing loss was more common in the more recently tested group (20 percent versus 15 percent).

In most cases, the loss was mild, affecting only the ability to hear sounds at 16 to 24 decibels (e.g., a whisper or dripping water; see table 35.4 for decibel levels for various sounds). However, that loss can have an effect in daily life. Students with slight hearing loss "will hear all of the vowel sounds clearly, but might miss some of the consonant sounds," such as *t*, *k*, and *s*, says Dr. Gary Curhan. "Although speech will be detectable, it might not be fully intelligible."

Although the researchers didn't single out ear phones or earbuds or any other listening device for blame, they did find a significant increase in high-frequency hearing loss, which they said may indicate that noise caused the problems. And they cited a 2010 Australian study that linked the use of personal listening devices with a 70 percent increase in the risk of hearing loss among children. In fact, some young people turn their digital players up to 85 decibels (about as loud as a hair dryer or vacuum cleaner)—a level that approaches U.S. workplace exposure limits (see table 35.5). Habitual listening at such a level can turn microscopic hair cells in the inner ear into scar tissue.

TABLE 35.4 Environmental Noise

Sound	Decibel level
Threshold of hearing	0
Whisper-quiet library at 6 ft. (about 2 m)	30
Normal conversation at 3 ft. (about 1 m)	60–65
City traffic (inside car)	85
Train whistle at 500 ft. (about 150 m), truck traffic	90
Subway train at 200 ft. (about 60 m)	95
Sustained exposure at this level may result in hearing loss.	*90–95*
Hand drill	98
Snowmobile, motorcycle	100
Sandblasting, loud rock concert	115
Pain begins.	*125*
Even short-term exposure can cause permanent damage (this is the loudest recommended exposure when hearing protection is used).	*140*
Jet engine at 100 ft. (30 m)	140
12-gauge shotgun blast	165
Death of hearing tissue	180
Loudest sound possible	194

Reprinted, by permission, from Galen Carol Audio. Available: www.gcaudio.com/resources/howtos/loudness.html.

TABLE 35.5 Noise Safety Levels

OSHA* daily permissible noise level exposure	
Hours	**Sound level (decibels)**
8	90
4	95
2	100
0.5	110
0.25 or less	115

*U.S. Occupational Safety and Health Administration.

Reprinted, by permission, from Galen Carol Audio. Available: www.gcaudio.com/resources/howtos/loudness.html.

For Discussion

Do you think earbuds have affected your hearing or the hearing of someone you know? Will the information presented in this article change how you listen to your personal entertainment? Why or why not?

Reviewing Concepts and Vocabulary

As directed by your teacher, answer items 1 through 5 by correctly completing each sentence with a word or phrase.

1. The four Rs stand for ____________, reduce, reuse, and recycle.
2. The precautionary principle is the saying "better _____ than sorry."
3. The U.S. governmental unit charged with looking out for the environment is the Environmental ______________ Agency.
4. One of Barry Commoner's laws of ecology is that ____________ knows best.
5. One disease or disorder that can be caused by air pollution is ______________.

For items 6 through 10, as directed by your teacher, match each term in column 1 with the appropriate phrase in column 2.

6. climate change	a. made by humans
7. complete street	b. buying products that you don't really need
8. conspicuous consumption	c. can be broken down by microorganisms
9. biodegradable	d. accommodates all types of transportation for people of all ages and abilities
10. built environment	e. long-term change in temperature, precipitation, or wind

For items 11 through 15, as directed by your teacher, respond to each statement or question.

11. Explain one of the four laws of ecology.
12. What is a sanitary landfill?
13. Which international organization formally recognized the connection between air pollution and cancer?
14. What is one of the four pillars of a green school?
15. Identify one major air pollutant and one of its main sources.

Thinking Critically

Write a paragraph in response to the following question.

What type of conservation (from table 35.3) do you think is most important for the world today? Support your opinion with fact and reason.

Take It Home

Save all of the plastic items that your family uses in a one-week period. Include wrappers, bottles, caps, lids, straws, and everything else you use that is plastic. At the end of the week, take a picture of your plastic and compare it with a picture from a friend who has a family of similar size. After you photographed the plastic, did you recycle all of it that could be recycled?

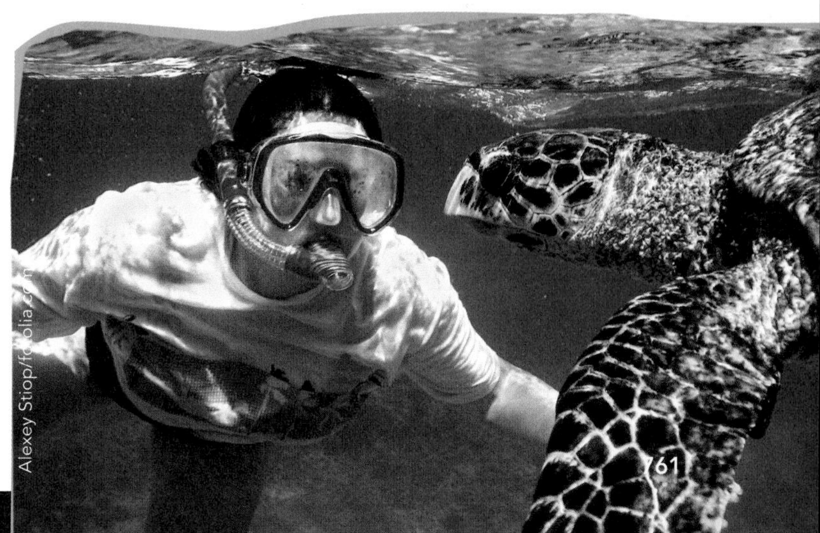
Alexey Stiop/fotolia.com

36

Community and Public Health

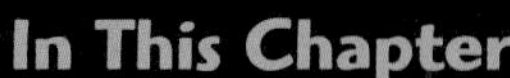

In This Chapter

www Student Web Resources
www.HOPEtextbook.org/student

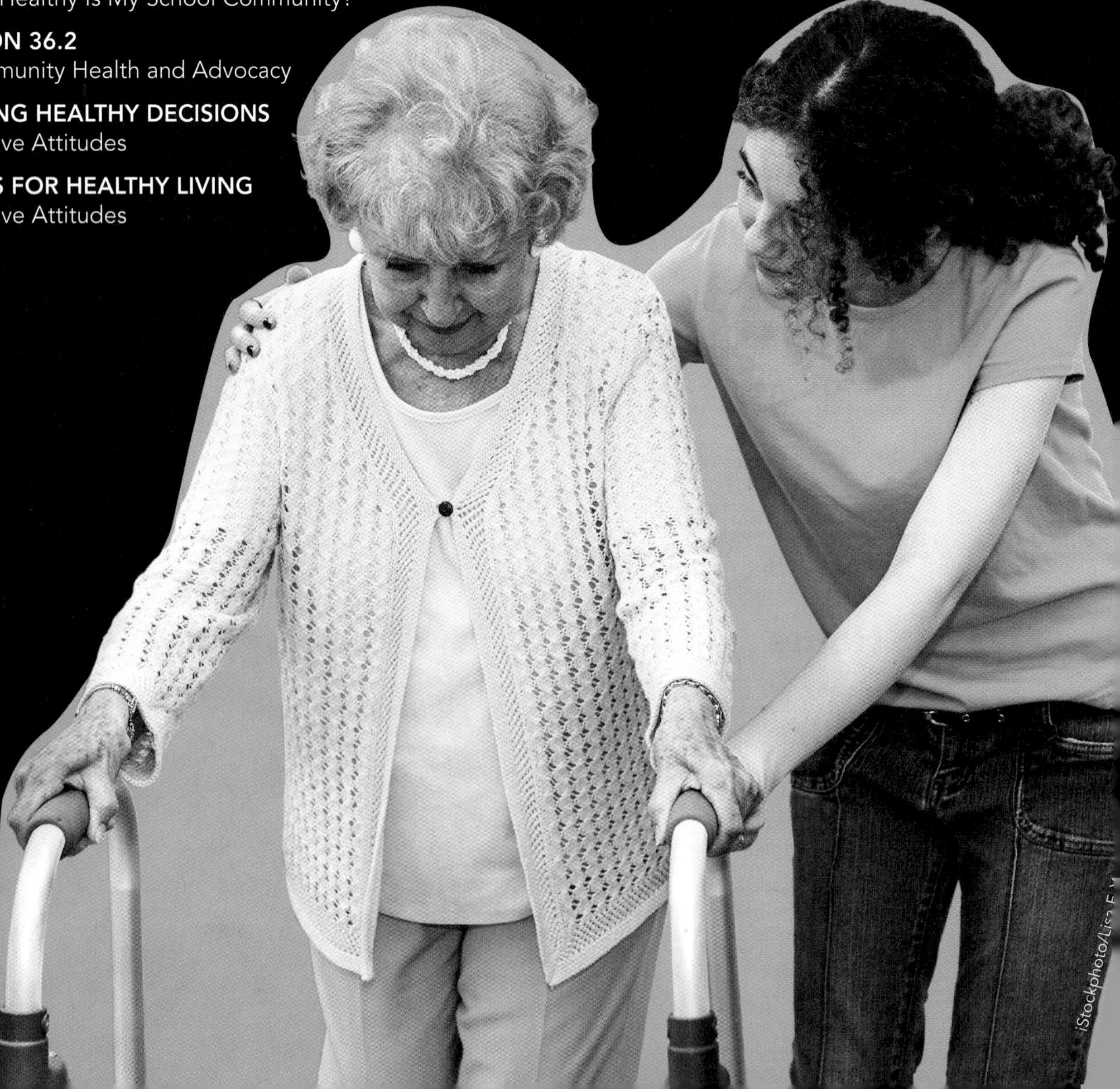

iStockphoto/Lisa F.

Lesson 36.1

Public Health

Lesson Objectives

After reading this lesson, you should be able to

1. define *public health* and identify types of public health providers;
2. understand the difference between primary, secondary, and tertiary prevention efforts; and
3. explain the difference between the prevalence and the incidence of a disease.

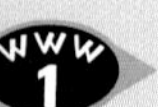

Lesson Vocabulary

developing nations, epidemiologist, health disparities, incidence, prevalence, primary prevention, public health, secondary prevention, tertiary prevention

Have you ever wondered who inspects restaurants for cleanliness? Who writes the public service announcements you see on television? Who tracks illness and outbreaks in communities? Or who decides which vaccinations are required for attending school? These issues and many others are part of the general activity of **public health**—the art and science of protecting and improving the health of individuals and groups of people.

Public health officials carry out educational campaigns, such as public service announcements, and deliver a range of programming designed to inform the public about health issues. They also seek to affect the health behaviors of large groups of people. Other aspects of the public health system are research and policy making. Overall, public health efforts are made by local and state health departments, federal agencies, private organizations, and international agencies. See figure 36.1 for the 10 essential public health services.

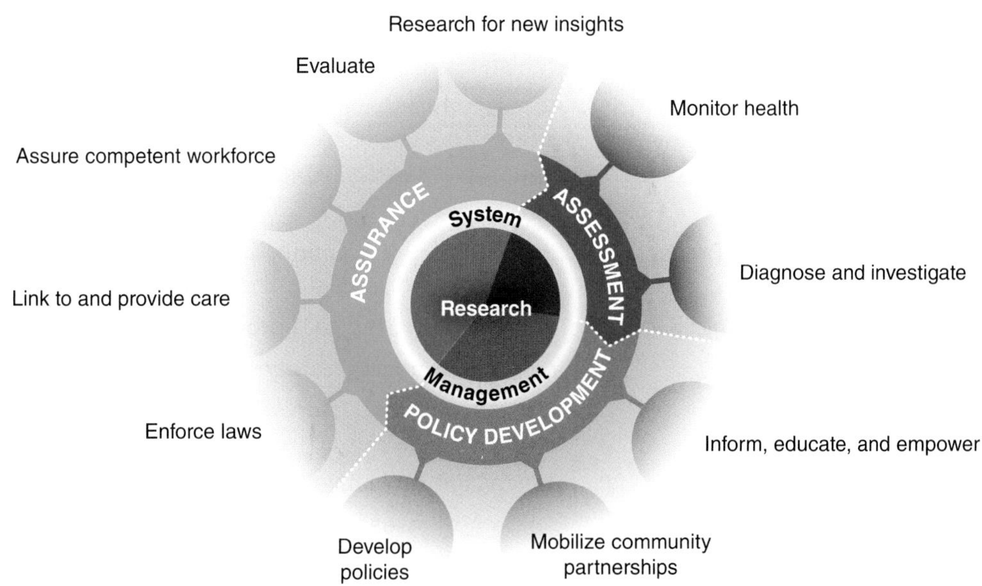

FIGURE 36.1 The public health wheel illustrates the relationship among core functions, specific responsibilities, and the 10 essential public health services.

Local and State Health Departments

In most U.S. states, public health services are provided by county, city, and state health departments. Many public health department services are provided free of charge to the consumer, whereas others are priced on the basis of the individual's socioeconomic status. One major charge for all health departments is to help limit the effect of **health disparities**. These disparities are defined by the Centers for Disease Control and Prevention (CDC) as the preventable differences in the burden of disease, injury, violence, or opportunity for optimal health that people in socially disadvantaged populations experience. These populations may be characterized by certain race or ethnicity identifications, gender, education, income, disability, geographic location, or sexual orientation. Providing essential services to people disadvantaged by these disparities ensures the health and productivity of the nation.

Federal Agencies

The federal agency with the widest reach and biggest effect on public health in the United States is the Department of Health and Human Services (HHS). This agency includes many operating divisions, such as CDC and the National Institutes of Health (see table 36.1 for a complete listing). HHS establishes most U.S. health and safety standards, compiles and analyzes health information, supports state and county health departments, and supports research and education efforts. The websites maintained by the HHS operating divisions are excellent sources of public health information.

Other U.S. agencies involved in public health include the Occupational Safety and Health Administration (often referred to by its acronym OSHA), which regulates worksite health and safety; the Department of Agriculture, which is responsible for the inspection of meat and agricultural products; and the Environmental Protection Agency, which oversees areas related to environmental health.

TABLE 36.1 Divisions of the U.S. Department of Health and Human Services (HHS)

Division	Responsibilities
Administration for Children and Families	Programs that improve the lives of children from low-income families, as well as individuals with disabilities
Administration for Community Living	Promotes the economic and social well-being of families, children, individuals, and communities through a range of educational and supportive programs in partnership with states, tribes, and community organizations
Agency for Healthcare Research and Quality	Access to health care and improved quality of health care
Agency for Toxic Substances and Disease Registry	Monitoring and investigation of risks to human health from toxins
Centers for Disease Control and Prevention	Research, data collection, and information distribution on almost all diseases and disorders
Centers for Medicare and Medicaid Services	Medicare and Medicaid programs
Food and Drug Administration	Food and medicine safety
Health Resources and Services Administration	Assistance for underserved groups such as homeless people
Indian Health Services	Health care for Native American populations
National Institutes of Health	Biomedical research
Substance Abuse and Mental Health Services Administration	Prevention and treatment of substance abuse and mental illness

Nongovernmental Organizations

Many private organizations are also invested in public health. They include charitable and religious organizations and private for-profit organizations. Well-known examples are the American Heart Association, the American Cancer Society, and the American Diabetes Association. Smaller organizations—such as community centers, churches, and local nonprofit agencies—are also involved in public health efforts. For example, they operate food banks and shelters for people who have low income or are homeless. Hospitals also serve public health needs by providing free clinics, screenings, and vaccination services.

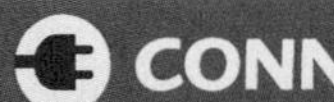

CONNECT

Is there a food bank in your community? Is there a homeless shelter? What are two ways that a food bank or homeless shelter can help the community it serves? What is one thing you could do to support a food bank or shelter this year?

Public Health and Prevention

Public health efforts fall into three categories based on the type of prevention they seek: primary, secondary, and tertiary (see figure 36.2). **Primary prevention** includes actions and services that reduce risk and avoid health problems—for example, efforts to keep underage people from drinking. **Secondary prevention** involves recognizing risks for (or beginnings of) problems and intervening before serious illness or effects arise. One example is an educational program aimed at college students who engage in social drinking; the goal is to help young people understand the risks of drinking and avoid becoming alcoholics.

CONSUMER CORNER: Donating to Charities

One great way to support a community and develop an altruistic (giving) attitude is to make a financial donation to a charity that supports a cause you find meaningful. Unfortunately, we live in a world where some people take advantage of others' generous hearts by organizing scams and committing fraud. Use the following guidelines to help you determine whether a charity is legitimate and worthy of your donation. Be suspicious of any charity that

- fails to provide detailed information about its identity, mission, costs, and planned use of your donation;
- refuses to provide proof that a contribution is tax deductible;
- uses a name closely resembling the name of a better-known, reputable organization (this could be a sign that someone is trying to trick you);
- thanks you for a pledge you don't recall making, then asks you to consider giving more;
- uses high-pressure tactics, such as trying to get you to donate immediately;
- asks for donations in cash or asks you to wire money (all reputable charities accept multiple forms of payment, such as check, credit card, and direct pay options);
- offers to come collect the donation immediately; or
- guarantees sweepstakes winnings in exchange for a contribution (by law, you never have to give a donation to be eligible to win a sweepstakes).

Consumer Challenge

Identify three charities of your choosing and visit their websites. Look for information about mission, costs, planned uses of the donations, tax status, and donation methods. Evaluate the charities using the information you gather and determine your willingness to contribute to each cause based on what you learn.

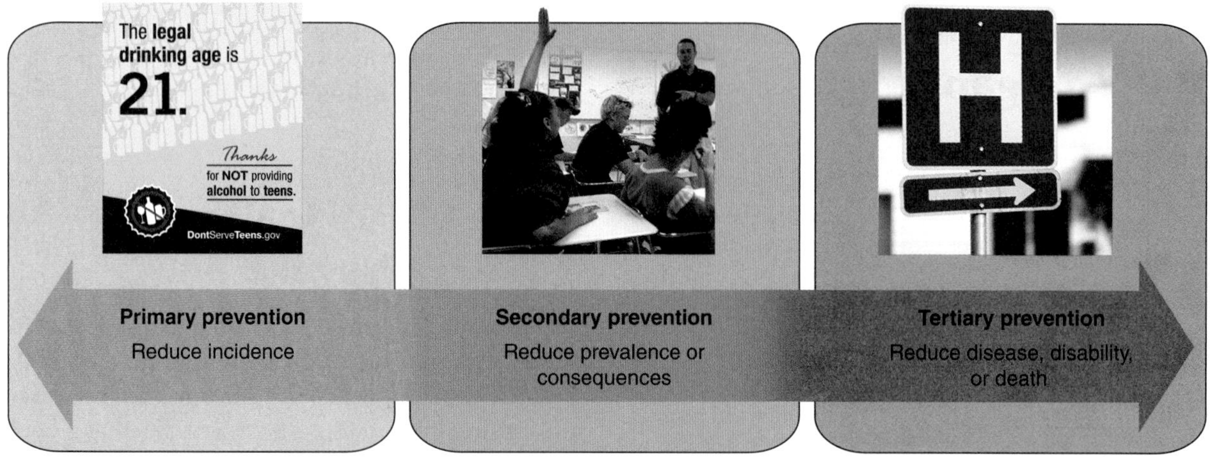

FIGURE 36.2 Levels of prevention in public health.

Finally, **tertiary prevention** is best thought of as the prevention of death. It involves treatment and rehabilitation of a person who is already sick, such as a person being treated for liver damage due to a lifetime of alcohol abuse. As you might expect, public health efforts are most effective at the primary and secondary levels of prevention.

One major public health goal is to reduce both the incidence and the prevalence of disease and disability. **Incidence** refers to the number of new cases that occur in a year. **Prevalence** refers to the number of existing cases. Both the incidence and the prevalence of diseases, disabilities, and related health behaviors are tracked and studied by public health workers called **epidemiologists**. Tracking the incidence rate of a communicable disease, for example, can help public health officials determine whether there is an epidemic—a widespread occurrence of an infectious disease in a community at a particular time.

Following the prevalence of a disease over time can also help officials determine how effective public health interventions are. For example, studying how positive health behaviors (e.g., healthy eating and regular physical activity) affect disease rates and quality of life can help us better understand and promote the benefits associated with these behaviors. You can learn more about the study of epidemiology by visiting the student section of the Health Opportunities Through Physical Education website.

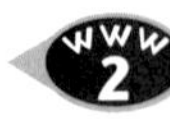

Global Public Health Organizations and Issues

Public health is a concern not only in the United States; all developed countries maintain public health services. In addition, global organizations provide public health guidance, programming, and support. Examples include the World Health Organization, the United Nations Children's Fund (UNICEF), and the Peace Corps. While prosperous countries such as the United States must address issues such as excessive food consumption and lack

Healthy People 2020

This book's chapter on the introduction to health and wellness discusses the *Healthy People 2020* report, which plays a significant role in guiding public health efforts in the United States. The goals established by the report help public health departments and private agencies prioritize their efforts. For example, one public health goal established in *Healthy People 2020* is to reduce by 10 percent the number of schools that have a serious violent incident. This goal encourages schools and local health departments to work together to create anti-bullying and anti-violence education, policies, and programs. A web link to the *Healthy People 2020* report is included in the student section of the Health Opportunities Through Physical Education website, and relevant *Healthy People 2020* goals are listed at the start of each unit in this book.

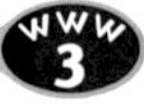

HEALTH SCIENCE

Malaria was eliminated in the United States by a concerted effort made from 1947 to 1951, yet somewhere in the world a child dies from malaria every 30 seconds. In Africa, one in every five childhood deaths is attributed to malaria. Poorer individuals are at highest risk because their homes and dwellings provide little protection from infected mosquitoes. They can't afford preventive medication or, if symptoms arise, medical care. The elimination of malaria in the United States was aided by spraying homes with mosquito-killing insecticides, spraying insecticides over large land areas, and removing mosquito nesting sites. In addition, U.S. residents have access to medicine that helps prevent and treat malaria.

The advances in chemical and medical science that contributed to effective insecticides and medications are certainly not new, yet malaria remains a global threat. This disparity illustrates the fact that even when science can solve a particular health problem, challenges may still exist in distributing the solution to those most in need. In addition, many developing countries have little in the way of organized public health services, and citizens often have no education or awareness of options that might exist. Therefore, humanitarians and scientists must often work together to make the greatest gains in global public health.

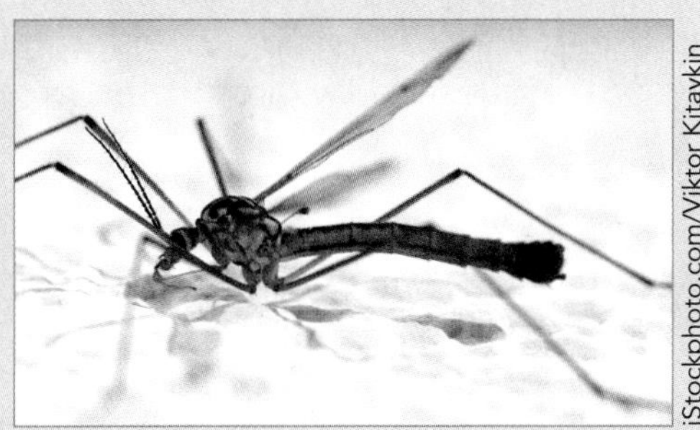
iStockphoto.com/Viktor Kitaykin

of exercise, much of the world faces very different public health issues, and the biggest challenge in global public health is poverty.

Countries with a poor economy and low standards of living are sometimes referred to as **developing nations**, and these are the places where the majority of the world's people live. These countries often face particularly intense public health problems, including malnutrition and widespread disease (e.g., malaria, AIDS). As a result, major global health initiatives are focused on bringing vaccinations, antibiotics, safe water, and sustainable farming techniques to developing countries.

Another key effort focuses on creating educational opportunities for more children around the world. Access to education is considered a primary way to end the cycle of poverty and improve global public health. It opens doors for employment, which can bring individual freedom as well as opportunities for acquiring healthier food, safer living conditions, and higher-quality health care.

HEALTHY COMMUNICATION

If you had US$1,000 to donate to a group addressing a serious health problem, what would it be? Why? Would you choose to support a cause in the United States or donate to a group addressing a global health issue? Why? Share your response with a group of classmates or peers.

> "Of all the forms of inequality, injustice in health care is the most shocking and inhumane."
>
> —Martin Luther King, Jr.

Comprehension Check

1. What types of organization serve the public health in the United States? Provide three specific examples.
2. What are the three levels of prevention addressed by public health services? Which are the most effective in improving public health?
3. What is the difference between the prevalence and the incidence of a disease?

SELF-ASSESSMENT: How Healthy Is My School Community?

Your school is an important community to which you belong. This assessment asks you to think about aspects of a healthy school community and consider your connection to your school. Answer each question by circling the proper response, then add up the total number of points as directed in the assessment. You may need to ask a teacher or school staff member for help in answering some of the questions in parts 1 and 2.

	Yes (2 points)	No (0 points)
Part 1: Health and safety		
My school . . .		
has a no tolerance policy for harassment or bullying.	2	0
has emergency plans, like evacuation routes, in place.	2	0
has active supervision in place to ensure safety and reduce violence.	2	0
is a safe physical environment.	2	0
does not allow smoking on campus.	2	0
is kept clean and bright.	2	0
provides help to those who want to quit smoking.	2	0
has at least one full-time nurse on campus.	2	0
provides counseling and mental health services.	2	0
Part 2: Nutrition and physical activity services		
My school . . .		
requires students to take physical education.	2	0
provides physical activities after school.	2	0
requires students to take health education.	2	0
promotes healthy food and beverage choices.	2	0
provides healthy and low-fat food.	2	0
has a clean and pleasant cafeteria.	2	0
Total points from parts 1 and 2: ________________ *The higher the score, the healthier and safer the school community.*		
Part 3: My school engagement		
As a member of my school, I . . .		
am involved in at least one club or organization at school.	2	0
feel comfortable at my school.	2	0
feel connected to my school and have school pride.	2	0
feel safe from violence or bullying.	2	0
know how to get help if I feel stressed, am depressed, or have anxiety.	2	0
am physically active almost every day.	2	0
make healthy food choices most of the time.	2	0
Total points from part 3: ________________ *The higher the score, the more your school community is helping you be a healthier person.*		

Planning for Healthy Living

Use the Healthy Living Plan worksheet to address an aspect of community or public health—for example, getting more involved in your neighborhood or advocating for ways to meet a specific community health need.

Lesson 36.2

Community Health and Advocacy

Lesson Objectives

After reading this lesson, you should be able to

1. explain the various meanings of *community* and identify ways in which communities affect personal health,
2. understand the steps for developing healthy communities, and
3. define *advocacy* and explain the keys to being an effective advocate.

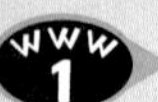

Lesson Vocabulary

advocacy, community, community health, stakeholder

One part of public health is **community health**, which is concerned with issues affecting the health of a specific community of people, usually defined by a specific geographic area. Community health efforts take into account the unique features of the community and its environment; they also use input from community members when generating programs and services. Community health efforts address public health issues identified as most important at the local level—for example, sanitation, safe water, public safety, and laws and policies that promote good health. They may also include services and programs targeting groups of people at risk for particular health problems. This lesson will help you understand the types of community around you and how to advocate for positive change related to health issues in those communities.

Communities

What communities do you belong to? Are you part of a neighborhood or school? Are you a member of a club or team? Do you have a religious or cultural community? All of us belong to multiple communities. A **community** is any group of people who share common characteristics or interests. Examples include your city or town, your neighborhood, your school, your family, and your cultural groups. Each of these communities can affect your health.

Your Neighborhood and Your Town or City

Where you live can dramatically influence your health. Each city, town, and state has its own characteristics, people, laws, opportunities, and basic health services (e.g., emergency medical services and access to community health centers). Some communities also have laws that affect health, such as bans on smoking in public areas. Others promote healthy living in their design itself—for example, by including lots of parks, bicycle lanes, and sidewalks to facilitate active living. Local crime patterns can also affect both individual health behaviors and the overall community's health. With this reality in mind, some neighborhoods organize watch programs so that children can safely play outside and travel to and from school. Some schools make their gyms, playgrounds, and tracks accessible to the public when they aren't being used for school activities. Some schools also have afterschool programs that have physical activity components.

Your School

Your school is a strong community that influences your health in many ways—for example, breakfast and lunch choices, mental health counseling, nursing services, and vaccination clinics. Your school environment, if clean and well lit, can also enhance your mental health. In contrast, schools that are dirty, moldy, dark, run-down, or unsafe increase the risk of injury and illness. Schools can also implement policies to protect health, as in anti-bullying and anti-smoking programs. In addition, schools can provide opportunities to engage in health-enhancing behaviors, such as physical activity, through physical education and afterschool programs.

The bottom line is that all schools should establish services, environments, policies, and programs that promote the health and well-being of their students, faculty, and staff. One strategy is provided by the CDC in its coordinated school health model (see figure 36.3). You can learn about other tools used to promote healthy schools in the student section of the Health Opportunities Through Physical Education website.

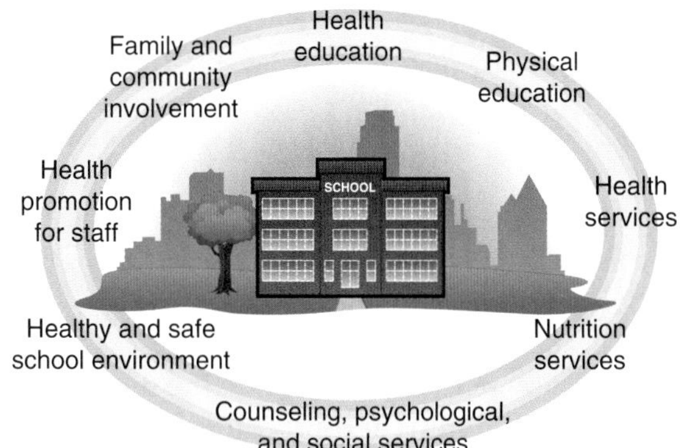

FIGURE 36.3 The coordinated school health model.

Your Cultural Community

The word *culture* can refer to many things. For example, you may belong to an ethnic cultural group with a strong tradition of gathering, supporting each other, and celebrating life together. You may also have a culture defined by your religion, your politics, or your sexual orientation. Regardless of its basis, a cultural community can provide you with strong social support and increase your sense of belonging through its rituals and traditions. In fact, a cultural community can influence many aspects of your life, such as your diet, your attitude toward exercise, and the choices you make about smoking and drinking.

Developing Healthy Communities

Healthy communities don't just happen. People in a community must work together to make it healthy. To do so, they must feel a sense of belonging and care about the outcome of community health efforts. When people feel interested or concerned—particularly when they are affected by the outcome of an action—they are referred to as **stakeholders**. An invested group of stakeholders and advocates is crucial to the success of any community project. Do you care about the health of your community? Are you involved in it? To make a difference in your community's health, you must do three things: get informed, get involved, and become an advocate.

Getting Informed

If you want to make a positive difference, you must understand the issues that people in your community care about. You can learn about local issues in various ways, such as reading local newspapers or blogs, listening to news radio shows, watching informative shows on local and public television stations, and attending community meetings. Social media outlets also provide forums where people express their concerns about their communities. Using social media to follow public leaders or local organizations can give you a sense of important issues and the types of actions the community tends to support. Other strategies include interviewing local officials and leaders and surveying peers and community members about key topics.

Getting Involved

Once you're aware of the issues facing your community, you should get involved with one

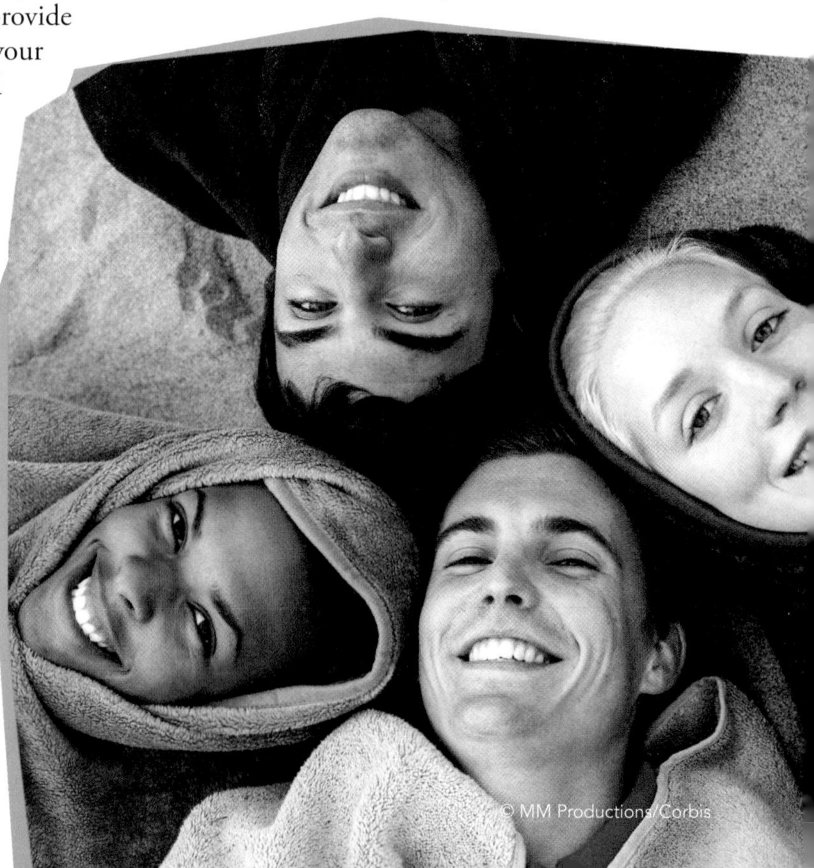

or more causes that you care about. You can get involved by joining an organization, voicing your opinion at community and civic meetings, or taking on a leadership role in a school organization. Another great way to engage with your community is to volunteer your time and energy. Select a cause that you're passionate about and ask around about ways to help.

For example, if you care about literacy, you might choose to volunteer your time tutoring children. If you're passionate about the environment, you might participate in local cleanup days or even organize your own cleanup club. You can also choose volunteer opportunities that allow you to help someone while also building your own skills and exploring an area of interest. Examples include volunteering in a hospital, senior center, youth club, or afterschool program. Whatever you choose to do, volunteering can be rewarding for both you and your community.

Becoming an Advocate

Advocacy is a critical skill. It involves speaking, writing, or organizing in support of an individual or cause. To be an effective health advocate, you must first know and believe in the positive and health-enhancing nature of what you're advocating. A good health advocacy effort educates other people about the particular behavior or issue, provides strategies and solutions to influence others' health behaviors, and provides support to encourage the necessary behavior changes or other actions. Advocacy can be focused at the individual level (benefitting a friend or peer), the classroom level (supporting policies and practices that promote healthy behavior), the school level (involving the entire school community in policies, actions, or improvements), or the societal level (writing to government representatives or taking other actions to influence change on a larger scale).

Becoming an advocate takes courage, and it is rarely done without facing some opposition. People are passionate about issues they care about, and their opinions often differ from yours. When advocating on any issue or cause, you need to respect the views of others while working calmly and rationally to share your own perspectives and ideas.

How to Advocate Effectively

Step 1: Understand and define the issue. Learn what issues matter to the community you're involved in. Ask a lot of questions, conduct a survey, read, and listen. Clearly define the issue you're working on and seek to understand it from as many perspectives as you can. Share your knowledge with others.

Step 2: Create solutions. Identify realistic solutions to the problem. Start by brainstorming as many solutions as you can. Be specific and offer concrete suggestions for how the community might improve. Check community resources and policies to ensure that your solutions can be supported and the actions you take do not violate any existing laws or regulations.

Step 3: Gather support. Your strategy for gathering support will vary depending on the issue you're addressing and the goal you're working toward. In some cases, you might need to gather the support of community leaders and officials by writing thoughtful letters or circulating a petition. In other instances, you might need to gather the support of peers to implement a change. Examples of strategies for gathering support are social media, web pages, flyers, and public speaking (e.g., at club or organizational meetings). If you're trying to influence a group of people with whom you do not usually interact, approach their leaders and influential members of the group. In all cases, be thoughtful about whom you want to reach with your message, then use appropriate means to gather their support.

Step 4: Implement your plan. Take action, be persistent, and expect to face challenges along the way. Stay positive in your message and be respectful of others.

HEALTH TECHNOLOGY

Social media has emerged as a major force for change in community health and advocacy because it makes it easier than ever before to communicate with large numbers of people in a community or even across the globe. The most common social media outlets for advocating community change are the electronic newsletters of agencies and nonprofit organizations, Facebook, Twitter, YouTube, and blogs.

Social media also allows people to stay updated on issues in a community and to follow community leaders. For example, more than 80 percent of government officials, including members of the U.S. Congress, use Twitter at least once a week, allowing constituents to follow their actions and decisions. During the 2008 U.S. presidential election, social media was used strategically for the first time to motivate a large youth vote that significantly affected the results. When used appropriately, social media can also help bring about positive community changes that promote good health and wellness.

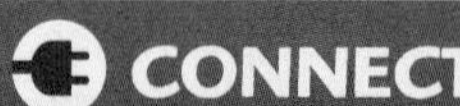

CONNECT

Using your favorite forms of social media, find a way to connect to a public health service or official. Share your chosen connection with your classmates. Consider making a directory of social media sites that students can use to become informed and stay updated about important health issues in your community.

Accessing Community and Public Health Resources

Most communities provide a range of health resources for members of the public. Knowing the community resources available to you and others when in need is an important part of being a healthy citizen. If you're in need of a resource, or aren't sure of what's available, begin by asking a trusted adult. Adults often know of resources because they've used them; they may also have advice about where to look. Another good source is your local phonebook. Check the government listings under titles such as "Community Health Services" and "Human Health and Safety."

You can also conduct a web search to find a good list of resources. Begin your web search with established organizations, such as those mentioned in table 36.1 or elsewhere in this chapter. Also consider looking at the website of your local city or county government or health department and the local chapters of aid organizations such as the American Red Cross. Once you've located a few resources, make calls or inquiries to see which organization provides the services you need. If a particular group doesn't meet your need, ask someone there for a reference to other resources that might be of help to you.

Comprehension Check

1. How does your neighborhood, city, or another community influence your health?
2. How can becoming informed and involved in a community help you to make the community healthier?
3. What are the four steps involved in effective advocacy?

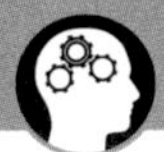

MAKING HEALTHY DECISIONS: Positive Attitudes

Malcolm is one of only a dozen African Americans in his high school; most of his school community consists of Latinos and Asian Americans. His school is in an area of the city that has a long history of serving immigrants and their families, and many of the students come from lower socioeconomic conditions. Malcolm's immediate family is small, including just his parents and himself, and they are financially comfortable. He also has a large extended family, but all of them live in a different state.

Malcolm is a good student and wants to go to college to study business. Some of the kids at school harass him for being too studious and others just ignore him altogether. Lately, Malcolm has been feeling isolated and discouraged about life. Going to school is becoming more stressful, and he recently started smoking cigarettes to help him cope and try to fit in better at school. His grades have slipped a little, and he's starting to question his own ambition. Everything seems less interesting, and his attitude is increasingly negative.

For Discussion

Do you understand Malcolm's attitude toward his situation? What things would you advise him to do to improve his attitude? How has his community affected his attitude and health behaviors? What community resources might be available to help Malcolm improve his situation? In answering these questions, refer to the Skills for Healthy Living feature for guidance.

SKILLS FOR HEALTHY LIVING: Positive Attitudes

Maintaining positive attitudes is an important part of having good mental and physical health. For some people, positive attitudes seem to come easily; for others, it requires conscious effort and practice. Everyone, however, can develop and maintain a positive mental outlook and a positive attitude. Here are some suggestions to help you build and maintain a positive attitude.

- **Use positive language.** Avoid using negative words and phrases, such as "I can't," "never," "I don't," "always," and "I won't." Instead, practice framing your sentences with positive phrases, such as "I choose," "I can," "I will," or, when referring to something you feel less confident about, "I might."
- **Surround yourself with positive friends.** You and your friends influence each other. When someone in a group is negative, others in the group also tend to act and feel negative more often. Similarly, when members of a group are positive and hopeful, others in the group will more often be hopeful and positive as well.
- **Smile.** Though it may sound funny, it's been proven that smiling or laughing intentionally for 30 seconds can help you feel happier. Try smiling at strangers in public or when you are alone. Do things that make you laugh. When you feel happy, you tend to be more optimistic and positive in your attitudes.
- **Pay attention to your emotions.** When you do feel angry, frustrated, hopeless, or negative, attend to how you feel and what caused your feelings. Don't avoid these feelings. Instead, acknowledge that you have them, explore why you have them, and address them with positive thoughts and actions. You can't always control what happens to you or around you, but you can control how you react to it.
- **Limit your screen time.** Unrealistic media images and messages can lead people to feel inadequate and unattractive. Pay attention to what you watch and how it makes you feel. Avoid shows, magazines, and other media sources that leave you feeling bad about yourself.

- **Keep a gratitude journal.** Write down three things each day that you feel thankful for. Do this every day for a week and see how it affects your attitude.
- **Keep a success journal.** Write down three things each day that you achieved or did well. Periodically, read through your successes and remind yourself how capable you are.
- **Share your feelings.** Share how you're feeling with someone you trust to be supportive. Keeping negative emotions tied up inside can hurt your physical and emotional health, and it can get worse over time. Share how you feel and talk about ways in which you might handle a challenging situation and improve your attitude toward it.
- **Take time to play.** Do things you love. Play a sport or make music. Draw, write, or cook. Spend time following your passions and doing things you love.
- **Give to others.** Do things to help others and serve your community. Helping others in need can remind you of what's most important and help you feel proud of who you are.

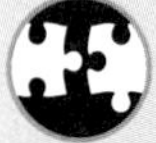

ACADEMIC CONNECTION: Making Sense of Concentrations

Mercury, often found in fish, is considered toxic to humans at concentration levels of one part per million. Just how much is that? Concentrations are mathematical measures often used in health science to help researchers and consumers understand how much of a substance is present in a particular liquid or solid. For example, visualize an object 1 inch (2.5 cm) long in a space that is 16 miles (26 km) long. That's the equivalent of one part per million. Another example is to think of a 55-gallon (208 L) barrel of water. It would take only four drops of mercury in the barrel to reach a concentration of one part per million. A single minute over the course of two years is also equivalent to one part per million.

Concentrations can be expressed in other ways. One is milligrams per liter (mg/L). Another is milligrams per deciliter (mg/dL). Concentrations such as mg/dL are used in laboratory reports that show how much of a particular element is found in the blood. For example, a healthy total blood cholesterol reading is considered to be less than 200 mg/dL (milligrams per deciliter). Since a deciliter is equal to 1/10 of a liter, this is equivalent to 2,000 mg of cholesterol per liter of blood, or 2,000 parts per million.

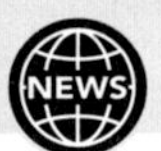

Are We Failing at Community Health?

More than 20 million Americans sought care at community health centers in 2011. These centers provide much-needed services, such as prenatal care, diabetes prevention and care, and childhood immunization. Unfortunately, a recent analysis of federal data by Kaiser Health News (a nonprofit, nonpartisan health policy research and communication group) found that many community health centers are failing Americans in diabetes care, childhood immunization, and cervical cancer screening for women, among other areas (see table 36.2).

"We feel good about quality overall, but there is clearly room to improve," says Mary Wakefield, who oversees community health centers for the U.S. Health Resources and Services Administration. She points out that some community health centers do perform better than private health service facilities in certain areas. For instance, 75 percent of centers performed significantly better in helping individuals with high blood pressure manage their condition, and more than 40 percent do significantly better than the national average in making sure women get timely prenatal care.

Elizabeth Rayes, 38, of Warner Robins, Georgia, credits a nurse at her local community health center for counseling her on how to control her diabetes even though she can't afford a blood glucose meter to test herself. "They do a great job," she says.

Compared with the clientele at a typical doctor's office, community center patients are nearly six times as likely to be poor, more than twice as likely to be uninsured, and nearly three times as likely to be on Medicaid, the combined state and federal health insurance program for people who are poor. "Given the complex nature of diseases and the many factors that contribute to them, it might be unreasonable to expect centers that serve the poor to perform above the average when compared to the well-staffed and financially sound medical centers and hospitals," says Dr. Jonathon Starkovich, who runs a community center outside of Athens, Georgia.

For Discussion

What do community health centers do, and who do they serve? What did this article teach you about how income level can affect the quality of health care that a person receives?

TABLE 36.2 Sampling of Community Health Centers: Performance on Key Measures

Center	State	Diabetes control*	Hypertension control**	Childhood immunization***
Yakima Valley Farm Workers Clinic	Washington	64	77	80
Shackelford County Community Resource Center	Texas	60	Not available	58
Family Health of Darke County	Ohio	83	96	70
Camillus Health Concern, Inc.	Florida	49	Not available	100
National average (all health service providers)	—	88	68	67

*Diabetes control: Percentage of adults, aged 18 to 75, with diabetes whose blood sugar is under control.

**Hypertension control: Percentage of adults, aged 18 to 85, with hypertension whose blood pressure is under control.

***Childhood immunization: Percentage of children who receive all seven federally recommended vaccines by age two.

Source: 2010 Health Center Data, Department of Health and Human Services.

Reviewing Concepts and Vocabulary

As directed by your teacher, answer items 1 through 5 by correctly completing each sentence with a word or phrase.

1. ________________________ involves taking action in support of an individual or cause.
2. In order to help develop a healthy community, you need to get informed, get ________________, and become an advocate.
3. _________ _________ is the art and science of protecting and improving the health of individuals and the nation.
4. ____________ ____________ refer to differences in health status between people that are related to social or demographic factors.
5. Countries with a poor economy and low standards of living are sometimes referred to as _____________ nations.

For items 6 through 10, as directed by your teacher, match each term in column 1 with the appropriate phrase in column 2.

6. primary prevention	a. intervening before serious illness or effects occur
7. secondary prevention	b. the number of new cases of disease in a year
8. tertiary prevention	c. prevention of death
9. incidence	d. the number of existing cases of disease
10. prevalence	e. actions and services designed to reduce risk and avoid health problems

For items 11 through 15, as directed by your teacher, respond to each statement or question.

11. Name two divisions of the U.S. Department of Health and Human Services.
12. Which government agency oversees worksite health conditions?
13. Explain the difference between the incidence and the prevalence of a disease.
14. List the four steps of effective advocacy.
15. What are two things a person can do to develop a more positive attitude?

Thinking Critically

Write a paragraph in response to the following prompt.

Think about all the services and policies at your school that are designed to positively affect your health. Write down as many as you can think of. For each service or policy on the list, identify what purpose it has and what health behavior or disease it is meant to affect.

Take It Home

Make a list of the communities to which you and your family belong. How do you think your family's health is positively or negatively influenced by each community? Write down as many influences as you can for each community and share your list with a family member.

Glossary

1-repetition maximum (1RM)—Test of muscle strength in which you determine how much weight you can lift (or how much resistance you can overcome) in one repetition.

absolute strength—Strength measured by how much weight or resistance you can overcome regardless of your body size.

abstract thinking—Ability to consider ideas that are not visible, immediate, or concrete.

acceleration—Increase in velocity.

accelerometer—Device that measures movement; frequently used to measure steps, intensity of movement, and duration of physical activity.

accountability—Following through with the commitments you make to yourself and others.

acquired immune deficiency syndrome (AIDS)—Infectious disease caused by the human immunodeficiency virus (HIV).

acronym—Specific kind of mnemonic in which the first letters of each word in a phrase are combined to form an easy-to-remember word (for example, SMART—specific, measurable, attainable, realistic, and timely).

action steps—Things you can do immediately to begin progressing toward your goal.

active stretch—Stretch caused by contraction of your own antagonist muscles.

activities of daily living—Tasks one does on a regular basis, such as bathing, eating, dressing, and grooming.

activity neurosis—Condition in which a person feels overly concerned about getting enough exercise and upset if he or she misses a regular workout.

acute alcohol poisoning—Potentially fatal overdose of alcohol or a medical emergency resulting from binge drinking.

addiction—Physical dependency on a chemical substance such as alcohol, nicotine, or heroin.

adolescents—People transitioning through puberty.

adventure education—Physical education approach focused on challenging recreational activities, such as rock climbing, orienteering, and rafting.

advocacy—Taking action in support of an individual or cause.

aerobic—Term often used to describe moderate to vigorous physical activity that can be sustained for a long time because the body can supply adequate oxygen to continue activity; means "with oxygen."

aerobic activity—Activity that is steady enough to allow your heart to supply all the oxygen your muscles need.

aerobic capacity—The ability of the cardiorespiratory system to provide and use oxygen during very hard exertion over a specific amount of time. The maximal oxygen uptake test measures aerobic capacity.

aerodynamics—Study of motion in the air.

agility—Ability to change your body position quickly and control your body's movements.

air quality index—Scale used to rate pollution levels ranging from good air quality to very unhealthful.

alcohol dehydrogenase—The *de–* prefix means "to remove." When a word ends in *–ase* it means that it is an enzyme. The *hydrogen* means just that, hydrogen. Dehydrogenase is an enzyme that removes hydrogen atoms. Alcohol dehydrogenase is an enzyme that removes hydrogen atoms from the alcohol molecule; it breaks down the majority of the alcohol that enters the human body.

alcoholism—Disease in which a person is dependent on alcohol.

alcohol tolerance—After continued drinking of alcohol over a long time, the consumption of a the same amount of alcohol creates less effect.

alcopop—Flavored alcoholic beverage to which various fruit juices or other flavorings have been added, such as wine coolers and some malt beverages.

alveoli—Small air sacs in the lungs that exchange gases with the blood through capillary beds.

Americans with Disabilities Act—Ensures the civil rights of all Americans who have mental or physical disabilities.

anabolic steroid—Synthetic drug that resembles the male hormone testosterone but that has health risks. It produces lean body mass, weight gain, and bone maturation.

anaerobic activity—Activity so intense that your body cannot supply adequate oxygen to sustain it for a long time.

anaerobic capacity—The ability of the body to perform all-out exercise using the body's high energy fuel sources (ATP-PC and glycolytic systems); commonly measured using the Wingate Test.

androstenedione—Substance considered to be a steroid precursor because it is converted into anabolic steroids such as testosterone (male hormone) after it enters the body; also called andro.

anorexia athletica—Eating disorder with symptoms similar to anorexia nervosa; most common among athletes involved in sports in which low body weight is desirable (such as gymnastics and wrestling).

anorexia nervosa—Eating disorder characterized by starvation, weight loss, and intense feelings of being fat or overweight.

antagonist—Muscle or muscle group having the opposite function of another muscle or muscle group.

antibiotic—Prescription drug that kills or inhibits bacteria that cause disease.

anxiety disorder—When feelings of anxiety occur regularly or interfere with a person's ability to function normally.

appetite—Psychological need for food.

arteriosclerosis—Hardening of the arteries.

artery—Vessel that carries blood from your heart to another part of your body.

asanas—Postures or positions in yoga.

assault—An act of immediate harmful or offensive contact that creates fear for a person.

assertive behavior—Behavior that involves making a firm verbal statement letting another person know how you feel.

assertiveness—Act of being honest and direct in communication.

atherosclerosis—Clogging of the arteries.

athlete's foot—Fungal infection of the feet that results from a warm, moist environment.

attention-deficit/hyperactivity disorder (ADHD)—Most common mental disorder diagnosed in children and young adults. Factors include hyperactivity, inattention, and problems with impulse control.

attitude—Your feelings about something.

autonomy—Self-direction; ability to make decisions for yourself.

bacteria—Simple single-cell organisms that are commonly found in air, soil, and food and on the bodies of plants and animals and that can produce toxins and cause illness.

balance—Ability to maintain an upright posture while standing still or moving.

ballistic stretch—Series of gentle bouncing or bobbing motions that are not held for a long time.

basal metabolism—Amount of energy your body uses just to keep you living.

battery—Harmfully or offensively touching another person.

binge drinking—When men consume 5 or more drinks and when women consume 4 or more drinks in about a 2-hour span.

biodegradable—Capable of breaking down (decomposing) by bacteria or other micro-organisms.

biofeedback—Technique, often using special equipment, that enables a person to gain some element of voluntary control over what people often believe are involuntary body functions.

biomechanical principles—Basic laws of physics that are used to help people perform physical tasks efficiently and effectively.

biomechanics—Branch of kinesiology that uses principles of physics to help us understand the human body in motion.

blended family—Formed when a parent remarries.

blood alcohol content (BAC)—Percentage of alcohol in the bloodstream. A BAC of 0.08 percent is the legal level of intoxication in all states.

blood pressure—Force of blood against your artery walls.

body composition—The proportional amounts of body tissues, including muscle, bone, body fat, and other tissues that make up your body.

body dysmorphia—Condition in which a person is obsessed with building muscle.

body fat level—Percentage of body weight that is made up of fat.

body image—Thoughts, feelings, and actions in response to your body shape, size, or appearance.

body mass index (BMI)—Measure of body weight in relation to body height that is associated with certain health risks.

bodybuilding—A competitive sport in which participants are judged primarily on the appearance of their muscles rather than how much they can lift.

built environment—Any human-made structure or system such as buildings, parks, roads, or bicycle paths.

bulimia—Eating disorder characterized by overeating and purging (vomiting, engaging in excessive exercise, using laxatives) in order to rid the body of unwanted calories.

bullying—The act of repeatedly doing or saying something to intimidate or dominate another person.

calisthenics—Exercises done using all or part of the body weight as resistance.

calorie—Unit of energy or heat that describes the amount of energy in a food (the true term is *kilocalorie*).

calorie expenditure—Calories (energy) used in physical activity.

calorie intake—Calories (energy) ingested.

cancer—Uncontrolled growth of abnormal cells in the body.

carbohydrate—One of the six major classes of nutrients composed of sugar, starch, and fiber.

cardiac muscle—Heart muscle.

cardiorespiratory endurance—Ability to exercise your entire body for a long time without stopping.

cardiovascular disease (CVD)—A physical illness that affects the heart, blood vessels, or blood. Examples include heart attack and stroke. It's the leading cause of death in the United States.

cardiovascular system—Body system that includes your heart, blood vessels, and blood; provides oxygen and nutrients to the body.

casual friendship—A friendship between individuals who share some commonalities (e.g., classmates or co-workers) that is not characterized by the formation of a deep bond.

center of gravity—The location of the center or midpoint of the total body weight.

cholesterol—Waxy, fatlike substance found in meat, dairy products, and egg yolk; a high amount in the blood is implicated in various types of heart disease.

chronic disease—Disease that lasts a lifetime.

chronological age—Number of years a person has been alive.

circuit training—Performance of different exercises one after another, separated only by brief breaks, with the goal of keeping your heart rate in your target zone and building various components of health-related fitness.

climate change—Any significant change in measures of climate (such as temperature, precipitation, or wind) lasting for decades or longer.

close friendship—A friendship with emotional ties and the sharing of intimate personal information. Close friends provide support and guidance.

closed fracture—Break in a bone where the damage has occurred below the surface and has not punctured through the skin.

closed wound—When the skin's surface is not broken and damage and has occurred below the surface.

cognitive development—Acquisition and development of skills such as language use, problem solving, and reasoning.

cognitive skills—Abilities that help you gain knowledge from information; examples include being able to concentrate and focusing your attention.

cognitive theory—Theory that addresses a person's ability to use information to make reasonable decisions and create reasonable solutions to problems.

community—Any group of people who share common characteristics or interests.

community health—Concerned with issues affecting the health and wellness of a specific community of people.

compendium—List of physical activity that tells you the intensity of various activities.

complete streets—Streets that provide for safe, convenient, efficient, and accessible use by all users: motor vehicles, pedestrians of all ages and abilities, people with disabilities, bicyclists, and people who use public transportation.

complex skill—Task that involves complicated movement sequences (for example, serving a tennis ball, hip-hop dancing) or integrating several movements at the same time (for example, stroking, kicking, and breathing in swimming).

compulsive behavior—Unreasonable behavior done in an attempt to prevent a feared outcome.

con artist—Person who practices fraud.

concentric—A shortening isotonic muscle contraction.

conservation—Involves the preservation, protection, and restoration of natural ecosystems.

controllable risk factor—Risk factor that you can act on to change.

cool-down—Activity performed after a workout to help you recover.

cooperative game—Game in which teams work together rather than compete.

coordination—Ability to use your senses together with your body parts or to use two or more body parts together.

coronary artery disease (CAD)—Specific kind of cardiovascular disease in which the arteries in the heart become clogged.

coronary circulation—Process of providing the heart tissue with necessary blood and nutrients.

coronary heart disease—When the arteries that send blood to the heart become clogged or hardened.

countermarketing—Methods to reduce demand for a product (like tobacco) by revealing the products' unhealthy aspects or bad effects on society.

CRAC—Contract-relax-antagonist-contract; a type of PNF stretch that first requires the muscle or muscles to contract and then relax before being stretched by the contraction of the opposing muscle or muscles.

creatine—Natural substance manufactured in the body by meat-eating animals including humans and needed in order for the body to perform anaerobic exercise, including many types of progressive resistance exercise.

criterion-referenced health standards—Fitness ratings used to determine how much fitness is needed to prevent health problems and to achieve wellness.

culturally and linguistically appropriate services (CLAS)—Standards primarily directed at health care organizations, but they are recommended to be used by any health care provider to ensure that a patient understands the treatment within the bounds of their cultural practices.

culture—A set of rules governing behavior in a society. It is influenced by morals, values, and religious beliefs.

cyberbullying—Bullying that takes place through electronic technology, such as cell phones, computers, tablets, and social media sites.

cystic fibrosis—Genetic disorder caused by inheriting a particular defective gene from each parent.

dance education—An approach to physical education (or a separate program) that focuses on teaching various forms of dance, both in and out of school.

date rape—Forced sex that occurs between two people who already know each other.

dating violence—Various kinds of physical, emotional, and sexual abuse that take place in a dating relationship.

deceleration—Decrease in velocity.

dementia—Loss of brain function over time; affects memory, judgment, behavior, thinking, and language.

depressants—Prescription drugs used to treat anxiety disorders and depression.

depression—Mood disorder characterized by extreme sadness and hopelessness that interferes with normal functioning.

determinant—Factor affecting fitness, health, and wellness.

developing nations—Countries with poor economies and low standards of living.

developmental milestones—Major physical and behavioral signs one expects to see in a normally developing infant or child during a particular period or at a particular age.

diabetes—Disease in which a person's body is unable to regulate sugar levels, leading to an excessively high blood sugar level.

diastolic blood pressure—Pressure in your arteries just before the next beat of your heart.

dietitian—Expert in nutrition who helps people apply principles of nutrition in daily life; has a college degree and certification by a reputable national organization.

disability—Restriction or impairment that makes a person unable to perform activities or actions in a way that they would normally be performed.

dislocation—When the bone moves away from its normal position near a joint and motion at the joint is lost or severely impaired.

distracted driving—Driving while talking on the phone or texting or while eating, drinking, applying makeup, or engaging in similar activities.

distress—Bad or unhealthy stress that contributes to anxiety and a feeling of being overwhelmed.

diversion program—Program that substitutes classes or training instead of fines or punishments, usually for minor or first-time offenses.

divorce—Legal termination of marriage.

double progressive system—The most-used method of applying the principle of progression for improving muscle fitness—first by increasing repetitions (reps) and second by increasing resistance or weight.

DriveCam—Cameras typically installed in a teenager's car to monitor for erratic driving and send notifications to a parent's or guardian's computer.

driving under the influence (DUI)—Driving while under the influence of alcohol or drugs.

drug addiction—Compulsive use of a substance despite negative or dangerous effects.

drug dependence—When a person needs a drug in order to function.

drug tolerance—Condition that occurs when a person who is a regular and excessive user of an addictive drug needs more of that drug to get the same effect that they used to get with a smaller amount of that same drug.

dynamic movement exercises—Exercises such as jumping, skipping, and calisthenics that are often used in a warm-up for activities requiring strength, power, and speed. They move the joints beyond normal resting ROM and cause the muscles and tendons to stretch. The stretch caused by dynamic movement exercise is followed by a contraction of the stretched muscle.

dynamic stretch—Slow movement exercises designed to lengthen the muscles.

dynamic warm-up—Dynamic movement exercises that increase body temperature and get muscles ready for more vigorous exercise; can serve as all or part of the general warm-up.

dynamometer—Device that measures the amount of force produced by a muscle or group of muscles.

eating disorder—Condition that involves dangerous eating habits and often excessive activity to expend calories for fat loss.

eccentric—A lengthening isotonic muscle contraction.

ecology—Study of living organisms and how they interact with the environment.

electrolytes—Minerals in your blood and body fluids that are important for normal body functioning and prevention of water loss during exercise.

electronic medical records (EMR)—Medical records that are stored electronically or digitally to make the exchanging of medical records faster. An EMR system may be part of a stand-alone health information system that allows the secure storage, retrieval, and modification of medical records. The records might include X rays and other diagnostic tests, medical histories, and any other information that may enable the health care provider to help the patient.

emotional wellness—How you feel and how you react to situations as a result of how you feel.

empty calories—Non-nutritional calories in foods that come from solid fat or added sugar.

empty nest—In child-rearing families when the last child leaves home and parents find themselves at home alone.

enabler—People who make it easier (enable you) to engage in a certain habit. Negative enablers make it easier to engage in a destructive habit or make it harder to stay on track with your positive behavior changes.

energy balance—Balance between calorie intake and calorie expenditure.

epidemiologist—Public health worker who tracks, monitors, and studies the incidence and prevalence of diseases and disabilities.

ergogenic aid—Anything done to help you generate work or to increase your ability to do work, including performing vigorous exercise.

ergolytic—Term referring to substances that negatively affect performance (*ergo* meaning work, and *lytic* meaning destruction).

essential amino acid—One of the nine amino acids that must be eaten in the diet for normal protein metabolism to occur.

essential body fat—The minimum amount of body fat that a person needs to maintain health.

ethyl alcohol (ethanol)—Name of the alcohol in beer and liquor.

etiquette—Typical or expected behavior of a social group.

eustress—Good or healthy stress that motivates a person or provides fulfillment.

exercise—Form of physical activity specifically designed to improve your fitness.

exercise anatomy—Study of how muscles work together with bones, ligaments, and tendons to produce human movement.

exercise physiology—Branch of kinesiology focused on how physical activity affects body systems.

exercise psychology—Study of human behavior in all types of physical activity, including exercise for fitness and sport.

exercise sociology—Study of social relationships and interactions in physical activity, including sport.

extended family—Grandparents, aunts, and uncles.

extension—A movement that increases the angle between the bones at a joint.

extrinsic motivation—Reason for doing something that comes from an outside source (for example, prizes, approval, or acceptance).

family role—The role that a person plays in a family including financial duties, household chores, and child rearing. Roles vary from family to family.

farm-to-school—Program that connects schools and local farms with the intention of serving healthy meals at school, improving student nutrition, providing education about growing food and the connections between health and nutrition, and supporting local farmers.

fast-twitch muscle fiber—Fiber that contracts quickly, is white because it receives less blood flow delivering oxygen, and generates more force than slow-twitch muscle fiber when it contracts (thus, muscles with many fast-twitch fibers are important for strength activities).

feedback—Information you receive about your performance, including suggestions for making changes in order to perform better.

fibrin—Substance involved in blood clotting.

fight-or-flight response—Body's response to stress, which includes an increase in heart rate and blood pressure and elevation of blood sugar level. This prepares the body to either fight or flee from a perceived threat.

fitness education—Classes or units in physical education focused on learning fitness and activity concepts and self-management skills that can help you be active throughout your life.

fitness profile—Brief summary of your fitness self-assessment results.

fitness target zone—Optimal range of physical activity for promoting fitness and achieving health and wellness.

FITT formula—Prescription or recipe (based on the ingredients of frequency, intensity, time, and type) for appropriate physical activity.

flexibility—Ability to use your joints fully through a wide range of motion without injury.

flexion—A movement that reduces the angle between the bones at a joint.

force—In physical activity, it is energy exerted by the muscles to cause movement or resist movement; other uses include military force (ships and troops), violent force (a physical attack), or resistance force (stopping a moving body or object).

fraud—Intentional use of deception to get you to buy products or services known to be ineffective or harmful.

frequency—How often a task is performed; in the FITT formula, it refers to how often physical activity is performed.

functional fitness—Capacity to function effectively when performing normal daily tasks.

fungi—Single-cell or multi-cell plantlike organisms that thrive in warm, humid environments and can infect the skin or other body systems.

gender—The social and cultural roles of people (masculine or feminine).

gene—Basic unit capable of transmitting characteristics from one generation to the next.

generalized anxiety disorder—Class of mental illness that includes intense feelings of worry, fear, or severe uneasiness that do not stem from a specific source or cause.

global health—Health of everyone on our planet.

global warming—Average increase in the temperature of the atmosphere near and above the earth's surface, which can contribute to changes in global climate patterns.

goal setting—Process of establishing objectives to accomplish; the objectives for lifetime fitness are to achieve good fitness, health, and wellness and to adopt a healthy lifestyle.

graded exercise test—Test used to detect potential heart problems by having you exercise on a treadmill while your heart is monitored by an electrocardiogram.

green school—Four main areas, or pillars: strive to be free of toxic or poisonous materials, use sustainable products like recycled paper and promote the 4Rs, promote green spaces around the school, and teach the students about the environment as part of a planned curriculum.

group cohesiveness—Sticking together in working toward a common goal.

growth spurts—Rapid period of growth when the bones get longer and may ache or cause pain.

habituate—To get used to something because of repeated exposure to it.

harassment—Includes name calling, teasing, or bullying.

health—Freedom from disease and a state of optimal physical, mental, social, intellectual, and spiritual well-being (wellness).

health and medical science—Area of study that focuses on preventing and treating illness and promoting wellness.

health behavior—Behavior taken by a person to maintain or gain good health.

health behavior contract—Agreement you make with yourself to change a specific health behavior.

health claim—Regulated statement about a food product that relates directly to a health condition or disease such as "heart healthy" or "helps prevent osteoporosis."

health disparities—Differences in health status between people that are related to social or demographic factors such as race, gender, income, or geographic region.

health literacy—Degree to which individuals have the capacity to obtain, process, and understand basic health information and services needed to make appropriate health decisions.

health psychology—Study of human health behaviors.

health-related physical fitness—Parts of physical fitness that help a person stay healthy; includes cardiorespiratory endurance, flexibility, muscular endurance, strength, power, and body composition.

healthy lifestyle—Way of living and making healthy choices such as eating well and doing regular physical activity that help you prevent illness and enhance your wellness.

Healthy People 2020—Document that identifies health goals to be accomplished by the year 2020.

heart attack—Condition in which the blood supply within the heart is severely reduced or cut off, which can cause an area of the heart muscle to die.

heart rate reserve (HRR)—Difference between the number of times that your heart beats per minute at rest and during maximal exercise.

heat index—Scale that rates the safety of the environment for exercise based on temperature and humidity.

heatstroke—Condition caused by excessive exposure to heat and resulting in a high body temperature and dry skin.

heavy drinking—Consuming two or more drinks per day for men and one or more per day for women over a long period ranging from months to years.

Heimlich maneuver—Used to dislodge a piece of food or other object from a conscious person who is choking.

high-density lipoprotein (HDL)—Lipoprotein often referred to as good cholesterol because it carries excess cholesterol out of your bloodstream and into your liver for elimination from your body.

homicide—Taking the life of another person.

hormones—Also called chemical messengers; they communicate information from one cell to another and coordinate functions throughout the body.

human growth hormone (HGH)—Illegal drug that is exceptionally dangerous, especially for teens; causes premature closure of bones and can have deforming and even life-threatening effects.

human immunodeficiency virus (HIV)—Virus in bodily fluids of infected people and can be transmitted to others through sexual contact and in blood.

humidity—Relative amount of moisture in the air.

hunger—Physiological drive to eat.

hydrodynamics—Study of motion in fluids.

hyperkinetic condition—Health problem caused by doing too much physical activity.

hypermobility—Unusually large range of motion in the joints; sometimes referred to as double-jointedness.

hypertension—Condition in which blood pressure is consistently higher than normal.

hyperthermia—Exceptionally high body temperature often associated with exposure to hot or humid environments.

hypertrophy—Increase in muscle fiber size.

hypokinetic condition—Health problem caused partly by lack of physical activity.

hypothermia—Abnormally low body temperature often associated with exposure to cold and windy environments.

ignition interlock—Device installed in a motor vehicle that is designed to keep people from driving if they have been drinking. The driver has to blow into a monitor that determines if the driver has been drinking. If so, the vehicle will not start.

illicit drug—Drug that is illegal to use, such as heroin or alcohol, which is illegal for people under age 21.

immune system—Body system that protects against infections.

implement—Device or tool used to perform a task.

impulse control—Ability to resist making rapid decisions without fully considering the consequences.

inattention blindness—When a distraction disrupts the driver's attention to the visual environment, distracting both the brain and the eyes.

incidence—Refers to the number of new cases of a disease that occur in a year.

influenza—Common viral infection that attacks the upper respiratory system.

insoluble fiber—Fiber that cannot be broken down by the digestive system.

intensity—Magnitude or vigorousness of a task; in the FITT formula, it refers to how hard you perform a physical activity.

intentional injury—Includes violence, suicide, self-injury, and homicide.

intermediate muscle fiber—Fiber with characteristics of both slow- and fast-twitch fibers.

interval training—Type of training that uses bouts of high-intensity exercise followed by rest periods.

intrinsic motivation—Reason for doing something that comes from within (for example, enjoyment, desire to be more fit).

isokinetic exercise—Type of isotonic exercise in which movement velocity is kept constant through the full range of motion.

isometric contraction—Contraction in which muscles exert force but do not cause movement at a joint.

isometric exercise—Exercise involving isometric contractions in which body parts do not move.

isotonic contraction—Muscle contraction that pulls on bone and produces movement of a body part.

isotonic exercise—Exercise involving isotonic contractions in which body parts move.

jai alai—Sport played on a large enclosed court similar to handball but using a wicker basket glove and a pelota (ball).

kidney dialysis—Process of filtering the blood through a machine when the kidneys are damaged.

kinesiology—Study of human movement.

kyphosis—Posture problem characterized by rounded back and shoulders.

laws of motion—Rules of physics that help us understand human movements.

leadership—Ability to motivate and help people in a group work toward a common goal.

lean body tissue—All tissue in the body other than fat.

LEED certified—Stands for leadership in energy and environmental design. To be LEED-certified buildings, homes or neighborhoods must meet certain standards for energy efficiency, green building materials, and indoor environmental quality.

leisure time—Time free from work and other commitments; also called discretionary time.

licit drug—Drug that is legal to use, such as prescribed drugs or over-the-counter drugs.

lifestyle physical activity—Activity done as part of daily life (such as walking to school or doing yardwork).

lifetime sport—Sport in which you're likely to participate throughout your life.

ligament—Tough tissue that holds bones together.

lipoprotein—Protein that carries lipids and cholesterol through your bloodstream.

localized infections—Infection that affects only one body part or organ.

locomotion—Movement of the body from place to place.

long-term goal—Goal that takes months or even years to accomplish.

lordosis—Posture problem characterized by too much arch in the lower back; also called swayback.

low-density lipoprotein (LDL)—Type of lipoprotein often referred to as bad cholesterol because it carries cholesterol that is most likely to stay in your body and contribute to atherosclerosis.

lower body fat—Fat located in and around the hips and thighs that does not pose significant health risks and may have some protective benefits.

macronutrients—Nutrients needed in large quantities.

manic-depressive disorder—Episodes of depression that alternate with periods of extreme excitability and restlessness (also called bipolar disorder).

manipulation—Indirect pressure to get someone to do something inappropriate or harassing.

maturation—Process of becoming fully grown and developed.

maximal heart rate—Number of times your heart beats per minute during very vigorous activity; the highest your heart rate can go.

maximal oxygen uptake—Lab measure considered to be the best for assessing fitness of the cardiovascular and respiratory systems; see also *aerobic capacity*.

media literacy—Having the skills to analyze, evaluate, and create messages in a variety of media, including knowing how to figure out if you are being manipulated.

medical history—Record of person's current state of health, which includes a list of past diseases, injuries, treatments, medications, and other health and medical information.

medical home—Having a personal physician who provides comprehensive, culturally appropriate care. Your physician also helps to coordinate care with other providers.

medical scientist—Expert who conducts research in hopes of improving overall human health.

mental disorder—Illness that affects the mind and reduces a person's ability to function.

metabolic equivalent (MET)—Measure that refers to metabolism (the use of energy to sustain life), with 1 MET representing the energy you expend while resting; multiples are used to describe the intensity of all types of physical activity.

metabolic syndrome—Condition in which a person has high body fat, large girth, and other health risks, such as high blood pressure, high blood fat, and high blood sugar.

micronutrients—Nutrients needed in smaller quantities (also called non-energy-yielding nutrients).

microtrauma—Invisible injury, caused by repeated use or misuse of a body part, that may not result in immediate pain, soreness, or symptoms.

mindfulness—Purposefully paying attention to what you are doing by being present in the moment.

mineral—Essential nutrients that help regulate the activities of cells.

mnemonic—A term that is useful in remembering specific information, such as an acronym (for example, SMART).

moderate physical activity—Activity that requires energy expenditure four to seven times greater than that required by being sedentary (that is, 4 to 7 METs).

motor learning—Process of acquiring a motor skill; also an area of study within kinesiology that relates to acquiring motor skills.

motor skill—The learned ability to use the muscles and nerves together to perform a physical task (for example, throwing, running).

motor unit—A group of nerves and muscle fibers working together to cause movement. The nerves cause the muscle fibers to contract.

muscle bound—Having tight, bulky muscles that inhibit free movement.

muscle dysmorphia—Disorder typically seen in males that involves an intense desire to become more muscular accompanied by excessive exercise, extreme dietary practices, or steroid abuse.

muscle-tendon unit—Skeletal muscles and the tendons that attach them to bones.

muscular endurance—Ability to use your muscles many times without tiring.

negative energy balance—State that the body is in when energy output is greater than energy input.

nephrons—Filtering units of the kidney that remove toxins from the bloodstream.

neurotransmitter—Chemical substance that is produced by a nerve cell that allows nerve cells to complete a circuit to send messages from nerve cells to nerve cells.

nuclear family—A father and mother with children, sometimes referred to as a traditional family.

nutrient claim—Regulated statement about a food product that relates to the nutrition content of the food, such as "low fat" or "fat free."

nutrient-dense food—Foods that contain a lot of vitamins and minerals and fewer calories.

nutrition science—Study of the processes by which a plant or animal uses food to grow and sustain life.

nutritionist—Ungoverned term that anyone can use to claim that they have nutrition information.

obesity—Condition of being especially overweight or high in body fat.

object—An item used in sport and physical activity (for example, a ball or hockey puck).

obsession—Unwanted thought or image that takes control of the mind.

online dating—The process of searching for a romantic partner on the Internet. It is also called Internet dating.

open fracture—Break in a bone where the bone has pushed through the skin's surface.

open wound—Involves damage to the skin's surface and typically involves some bleeding.

opiates—Natural or synthetic drug that has a depressant or calming effect on the central nervous system (originally opiates were only drugs that came from the opium poppy).

optimal challenge—Activity that is neither too hard nor too easy; activity that isn't too distressful compared to the competitive situation.

osteoporosis—Condition in which bone structure deteriorates and bones become weak.

outdoor education—An approach to physical education that occurs in an outdoor classroom.

over-exercising—Doing so much exercise that you increase your risk of injury or soreness.

over-the-counter (OTC) drug—Drug that can be bought without a doctor's prescription.

overuse injury—Injury resulting from repeated movement that causes wear and tear in your body.

overweight—Condition of weighing more than the healthy range.

passive exercise—Use of a machine or device that moves your body for you. Programs using passive exercise are ineffective.

passive stretch—Stretch requiring an assist from an external source (gravity, a partner, or some other source).

patent medicine—Drug that is intended to prevent or alleviate the symptoms of a disease or disorder that is produced and owned by a company.

pathogen—Dangerous microorganism that causes a disease is known as a pathogen.

patient education—Planned learning experience that may use a variety of methods such as teaching, counseling, and behavior modification techniques to help patients deal more effectively with any disease, disorder, or health condition.

peak bone mass—Highest bone density achieved during life; typically occurs in late adolescence or early adulthood.

pedometer—Small battery-powered device that can be worn on your belt to count your steps.

peer pressure—The pressure an individual can feel from peers. It can be positive where peers serve as role models encouraging us to try new things and be better in some way, or it can be negative by encouraging us to make poor decisions and behave badly, thus ultimately leading to negative consequences.

pelota—Ball used in jai alai.

periodization—Way of scheduling muscle fitness exercise in which you perform a given plan for a while, then alter it to perform different exercises or change the way you do your exercises.

personal health—Choices and actions you take as an individual (related to health and wellness) that affect your health. Some of these include regularly brushing and flossing your teeth, washing your hands before meals and after using the bathroom, and getting enough sleep.

personal lifestyle plan—Written schedule of activities designed to improve fitness, health, and wellness.

personal needs profile—Chart listing self-assessment scores and corresponding ratings.

personal program—Written individualized plan designed to change behavior (the way you live) to improve fitness, health, and wellness.

personality—Unique mixture of qualities and traits that distinguish you from others.

phenotype—Visible characteristics of an organism resulting from the interaction between its genetic makeup and the environment.

phobias—Intense fears and anxieties that relate to a specific situation or object.

physical activity—Movement using the large muscles; includes sport, dance, recreational activity, and activities of daily living.

Physical Activity Pyramid—Diagram or model that describes the various types of physical activity that produce good fitness, health, and wellness.

Physical Activity Readiness Questionnaire (PAR-Q)—Seven-question assessment of medical and physical readiness that should be taken before beginning a regular physical activity program for health and wellness.

physical development—Changes in weight, height, motor skills, and sensory perceptions as a person develops.

physical fitness—Capacity of your body systems to work together efficiently to allow you to be healthy and effectively perform activities of daily living.

physical literacy—Being physically educated; a physically literate person does regular activity, is fit, has skills, values activity, and knows the implications and benefits of physical activity.

physiological age—How well the body systems are aging relative to what is expected at a particular age.

Pilates—Form of training, quite popular in recent years, designed to build core muscle fitness; named for Joseph Pilates, who described core exercises and developed special exercise machines for building core muscles.

platonic friendship—A relationship, often with a member of the opposite sex, in which there is no romantic involvement.

plyometrics—Type of training designed to increase athletic performance using jumping, hopping, and other exercises to cause lengthening of a muscle followed by a shortening contraction.

PNF stretching—Flexibility exercise using proprioceptive neuromuscular facilitation; a variation of static stretching that involves contracting a muscle before stretching it.

positive energy balance—State that the body is in when energy intake is greater than energy output.

post-traumatic stress disorder—A person who has experienced or witnessed a traumatic event, such as a war or terrorist attack, experiences intense flashbacks or nightmares that produce high anxiety and may interfere with sleep, concentration, and relationships.

power—Capacity to use strength quickly; involves both strength and speed.

powerlifting—Competitive sport using free weights and involving only three exercises: bench press, squat, and deadlift.

prescription drug—Drug prescribed by a doctor to help treat illnesses or symptoms, such as pain and discomfort.

prevalence—Refers to the number of existing cases of disease and disability.

primary prevention—Actions and services designed to reduce risk and avoid health problems.

principle of overload—The most basic law of physical activity, which states that the only way to produce fitness and health benefits through physical activity is to require your body to do more than it normally does.

principle of progression—Principle stating that the amount and intensity of your exercise should be increased gradually.

principle of rest and recovery—Principle stating that you need to give your muscles time to rest and recover after a workout.

principle of specificity—Principle stating that the type of exercise you perform determines the type of benefit you receive.

priority healthy lifestyle choice—One of the key lifestyle choices (regular physical activity, sound nutrition, and stress management) that help you prevent disease, get and stay fit, and enjoy a good quality of life.

process goal—Goal relating to what you do rather than the product resulting from what you do.

product goal—Goal relating to what you get as a result of what you do.

product placement—Form of advertising where products are placed where they are not generally associated with advertising, such as movies, TV shows, music videos, or news programs.

progressive resistance exercise (PRE)—Exercise that increases resistance (overload) until you have the amount of muscle fitness you want; also called progressive resistance training (PRT).

Prohibition—The 18th amendment (1920), which made the sale and distribution of alcohol illegal until it was repealed by the 21st Amendment in 1933.

protein—Provides the body with energy and builds, repairs, and maintains body cells. Protein is easily found in animal products.

protozoan—Large single-cell organism that can move through the body in search of food. It attacks the body by releasing enzymes or toxins that can destroy or damage cells.

psychoactive drugs—Drugs that change a person's perceptions or mood.

psychotherapy—Method of treating mental disorders that involve talking about your condition and related issues with a mental health provider.

ptosis—Posture problem characterized by protruding abdomen.

puberty—Time when the pituitary gland triggers production of testosterone in boys and estrogen and progesterone in girls. Puberty typically begins between ages 9 and 12 for girls and between ages 11 and 14 for boys and includes such body changes as hair growth around the genitals, menstruation in girls, and sperm production in boys.

public health—Practice of preventing disease and protecting, improving, and promoting good health within groups of people using research, policies, and health communications. Public health is sometimes referred to as population health because it focuses on groups of people in a community, state, or country.

public health scientist—Expert who studies disease prevention and wellness promotion in communities.

pulmonary circulation—Process of moving blood from the heart to the lungs and back to the heart again.

quack—Person who practices quackery.

quackery—Method of advertising or selling that uses false claims to lure people into buying products that are worthless or even harmful.

range of motion (ROM)—The amount of movement in a specific joint that is considered to be healthy (neither too much nor too little).

range-of-motion (ROM) exercise—Exercise that requires a joint to move through a full range of motion by using either your own muscles or the assistance of a partner or therapist.

reaction time—Amount of time it takes to move once you recognize the need to act.

reasoning skills—Ability to solve problems and make decisions. Changes allow you to think more critically and evaluate ideas more carefully.

recreation—Something you do during your free time.

reframing—Method of viewing a situation or event differently, such as instead of complaining about having to wait in a long line, view it as a time to listen to music or audiobooks or a time to tweet, text, e-mail, or phone a friend.

refusal skills—Techniques for saying no and sticking with it.

registered dietitian (RD)—Formally educated and licensed nutrition practitioner.

relative strength—Strength adjusted for your body size.

reps—Short for *repetitions* (the number of consecutive times you do an exercise).

respiratory system—Body system made up of your lungs and the passages that bring air, including oxygen, from outside of your body into your lungs.

resting metabolic rate—Calories used each day to maintain normal physiological function.

rhabdomyolysis—Condition in which muscle fibers break down and the bloodstream absorbs muscle fiber elements.

RICE—Formula in which each letter represents a step in the treatment of a minor injury: R = rest; I = ice; C = compression; E = elevation.

risk factor—Any action or condition that increases your chances of developing a disease or health condition.

road rage—Emotional outbursts that occur while driving.

role model—A person who imparts values and information to others.

rule—Guideline or requirement for conduct or action.

sanitary landfill—Site where waste is isolated from the rest of the environment. It is daily covered in layers of dirt to reduce attracting birds and rodents. When sanitary landfills are full, the land can be reclaimed as a park or recreation area and sometimes the methane gas that the landfill produces can be used to produce electricity.

satiety—Comfortable state between meals without feeling hungry or full.

saturated fat—Fat that is more dangerous to health and comes mostly from animal sources.

secondary prevention—Recognizing risks or the beginning of problems and intervening before serious illnesses or effects take over.

secondary sex characteristics—Physical changes that occur during puberty; the start of ovulation in girls and sperm production in boys.

secondhand smoke—Tobacco smoke that is inhaled involuntarily or passively by someone who is not smoking. Also referred to as sidestream smoke or environmental tobacco smoke.

sedentary—Not engaging in regular physical activity from any of the steps of the Physical Activity Pyramid.

self-assessment—Test that helps you figure out your current health status and set goals for good health.

self-care—A person's decisions and behaviors in coping with a health problem, or improving health, or preventing certain health problems. Self-care is in addition to medical care, not instead of medical care.

self-esteem—How a person perceives oneself.

self-management skill—Skill that helps you adopt a healthy lifestyle now and throughout your life.

self-regulation skills—Self-management skills.

self-reward system—System for gradually building skills and finding success and, ultimately, intrinsic motivation; involves rewarding yourself rather than expecting others to reward you for your efforts.

separation—A test period for married couples to separate that is not legally recognized.

set—One group of repetitions.

sex—Refers to the biological factors (male or female) that influence your fitness, health, and wellness.

sexual coercion—The use of force, manipulation, or intimidation to get someone to participate in unwanted sexual activity.

short-term goal—Goal that can be reached in a short time, such as a few days or weeks.

side stitch—Pain in the side of the lower abdomen that people often experience during sport activity, especially running.

skeletal muscle—Muscle attached to bones that makes movement possible.

skill—Ability to perform a specific task effectively that results from knowledge and practice.

skill-related physical fitness—Parts of fitness that help a person perform well in sports and activities requiring certain skills; the parts include agility, balance, coordination, reaction time, and speed.

skills for healthy living—Skills that can help you accomplish a desired goal or keep doing a good thing that you already do.

skinfold—Fold of fat and skin used to estimate total body fat level.

sleep apnea—Disorder that results in poor sleep or inability to sleep, characterized by pauses in breathing or shallow breathing during sleep.

slow-twitch muscle fiber—Muscle fiber that contracts at a slow rate, is usually red because it has a lot of blood vessels delivering oxygen, and generates less force than fast-twitch muscle fiber but is able to resist fatigue.

SMART goal—Goal that is specific, measurable, attainable, realistic, and timely.

smokeless tobacco—Tobacco that is not smoked, such as chewing tobacco and snuff.

smooth muscle—Involuntarily controlled tissue found in the walls of hollow organs.

social marketing—Applying commercial marketing concepts and techniques to noncommercial purposes.

socioemotional development—Emotional and social development; markers of growth are self-esteem, empathy, and friendship.

soluble fiber—Fiber that can be partially broken down by the digestive system.

spa—Facility offering saunas, whirlpool baths, and other services such as massage and hair or skin care.

speed—Ability to perform a movement or cover a distance in a short time.

spirituality—Person's sense of purpose and meaning in life, beyond material values.

sport—Physical activity that is competitive (has winners and losers) and has well-established rules.

sport education—Approach that seeks to make physical education both fun and interesting by dividing the year into seasons similar to those found in the sport world.

sport pedagogy—Art and science of teaching physical activity; includes applying motor learning principles to help people learn motor skills and studying the best ways to teach and learn the principles of physical activity derived from the sciences.

sportsmanship—Having respect for people on opposing teams; being a good winner and not being a poor loser.

sprain—Injury to a ligament.

stages of health behavior change—Precontemplation, contemplation, preparation, action, and maintenance.

stakeholder—Someone who has an interest or concern in something.

stance—Way of standing.

state of being—Overall condition of a person.

static stretch—Stretch performed slowly as far as you can without pain, until you feel a sense of pulling or tension.

stimulants—Prescription drugs most often used to treat ADHD.

storage fat—Additional body fat. Up to a certain point, it does not appear to be harmful for health.

strain—Injury to a tendon or muscle.

strategy—Master plan for achieving a goal or set of goals.

strength—Maximal amount of force your muscles can produce.

stressor—Anything that causes wear and tear on the body, whether physically or mentally.

stretching warm-up—A way of preparing for physical activity using flexibility exercises performed after several minutes of general exercise.

stroke—Condition in which the supply of oxygen to the brain is severely reduced or cut off resulting in damage to the brain.

structure/function claim—Statement found on a food or supplement, such as vitamins, that relates to a function or specific structure in the body such as "improves eyesight" or "builds strong bones." These claims are not regulated by the FDA.

sudden infant death syndrome (SIDS)—Sudden and unexpected death of an apparently healthy infant.

suicide—Ending one's own life.

support group—People with common diagnoses and conditions who provide informational, emotional, and moral support for one another.

systemic circulation—Process of delivering blood to all areas of the body aside from the heart and lungs.

systemic infections—Infections that affect the entire body, not just a single organ or body part.

systolic blood pressure—Pressure in your arteries immediately after your heart beats.

tactic—Specific method for carrying out a strategy.

tai chi—Ancient form of exercise that originated in China and whose basic movements have been shown to increase flexibility and reduce symptoms of arthritis in some people.

target ceiling—Your upper recommended limit of activity for optimally promoting fitness and achieving health and wellness.

teamwork—Cooperative effort of all team members to strive for a common goal in the most effective way.

telemedicine—Medical information exchanged electronically from one site to another to improve a person's health status.

tendon—Tissue that connects muscle to bone.

tertiary prevention—Treatment and rehabilitation after a person is sick to avoid further illness or death.

threshold of training—Minimum amount of overload you need in order to build physical fitness.

time—Length of a task; in the FITT formula (first *T*), it refers to the optimal length of an activity session designed to improve fitness and promote health and wellness.

toxic food environment—A place where high-calorie, high-fat food is abundant and inexpensive.

tracking—Using vision to follow the path of an object (for example, watching the path of a thrown ball).

traditional family—A father and mother with children, sometimes referred to as a nuclear family.

traumatic brain injury—Caused by a bump, blow, or jolt to the head and is a penetrating head injury that disrupts the normal function of the brain. Most traumatic brain injuries (TBIs) are concussions.

type—The specific kind of task; in the FITT formula (second *T*), it refers to the specific kind of physical activity that is performed.

uncontrollable risk factor—Risk factor that you cannot change.

underweight—Condition of weighing less than the healthy range.

unintentional injury—Injury caused by unplanned events such as automobile crashes, poisonings, fires, and drowning.

unsaturated fat—Fats that is less dangerous to health and comes mostly from plant sources.

upper body fat—Fat located in and around the abdominal organs that is associated with high blood cholesterol and heart disease risk.

vein—Vessel that carries blood filled with waste products from your muscle cells back to your heart.

velocity—Speed of movement.

vigorous aerobics—Aerobic activities intense enough to elevate your heart rate above your threshold of training and into your target zone for cardiorespiratory endurance.

vigorous recreation—Activity done during your free time that is fun and typically noncompetitive but intense enough to elevate your heart rate above your threshold of training and into your target zone for cardiorespiratory endurance.

vigorous sport—Sport activity that elevates your heart rate above your threshold of training and into your target zone for cardiorespiratory endurance.

viruses—Smallest of all pathogens; they take enter a cell and take over normal functioning.

vitamins—Organic compounds essential for normal growth, functioning, and maintenance of the body.

warm-up—A series of activities that prepares the body for more vigorous exercise.

web extension—Ending of a web address, such as .gov, .org, and .com.

weight cycling—Repeated bouts of gaining and losing weight.

weightlifting—Olympic sport involving free weights in which athletes try to lift a maximum load; includes two lifts—the snatch and the clean and jerk.

wellness—Positive component of health that involves having a good quality of life and a good sense of well-being as exhibited by a positive outlook.

wind-chill factor—Index used to determine when dangerously low temperatures and unsafe wind conditions exist.

withdrawal—Physical sickness that a person with a physical dependence (addiction) develops when he or she can't or isn't able to take the drug to which he or she is addicted.

workout—The part of the physical activity program during which a person does activities to improve fitness.

World Health Organization (WHO)—Organization that focuses on public health. They issued a statement proclaiming that good health is not merely the absence of disease or illness; rather, it is a more complete state of being that includes wellness.

yoga—Activity that originated in India and that in its traditional forms includes meditation as well as the exercises and breathing techniques common to modern forms; involves poses called asanas that are similar to many flexibility exercises and can offer improved flexibility and other health benefits.

Index